Ocular Manifestations of Systemic Diseases

Alexandr Stepanov · Jan Studnicka
Editors

Ocular Manifestations of Systemic Diseases

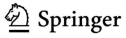

Editors
Alexandr Stepanov ⓘD
Department of Ophthalmology
Klaudian's Hospital in Mlada Boleslav
Mlada Boleslav, Czech Republic

Department of Ophthalmology
University Hospital in Hradec Kralove
Hradec Kralove, Czech Republic

Third Faculty of Medicine in Prague
Charles University
Prague, Czech Republic

Jan Studnicka ⓘD
Department of Ophthalmology
University Hospital in Hradec Kralove
Hradec Kralove, Czech Republic

Eye Centre VISUS, spol. s.r.o.
Nachod, Czech Republic

ISBN 978-3-031-58591-3   ISBN 978-3-031-58592-0 (eBook)
https://doi.org/10.1007/978-3-031-58592-0

Translation from the Czech language edition: "Oční Projevy Systémových Onemocnění" by Alexandr Stepanov and Jan Studnicka, © Grada Publishing 2021. Published by Grada Publishing. All Rights Reserved.

Originally published with the title: Oční Projevy Systémových Onemocnění

© The Editor(s) (if applicable) and The Author(s), under exclusive license to Springer Nature Switzerland AG 2024

This work is subject to copyright. All rights are solely and exclusively licensed by the Publisher, whether the whole or part of the material is concerned, specifically the rights of reprinting, reuse of illustrations, recitation, broadcasting, reproduction on microfilms or in any other physical way, and transmission or information storage and retrieval, electronic adaptation, computer software, or by similar or dissimilar methodology now known or hereafter developed.
The use of general descriptive names, registered names, trademarks, service marks, etc. in this publication does not imply, even in the absence of a specific statement, that such names are exempt from the relevant protective laws and regulations and therefore free for general use.
The publisher, the authors and the editors are safe to assume that the advice and information in this book are believed to be true and accurate at the date of publication. Neither the publisher nor the authors or the editors give a warranty, expressed or implied, with respect to the material contained herein or for any errors or omissions that may have been made. The publisher remains neutral with regard to jurisdictional claims in published maps and institutional affiliations.

This Springer imprint is published by the registered company Springer Nature Switzerland AG
The registered company address is: Gewerbestrasse 11, 6330 Cham, Switzerland

If disposing of this product, please recycle the paper.

Preface

We present to you *Ocular Manifestations of Systemic Diseases*, a book which introduces ocular complications of diseases primarily affecting other organs and tissues of the human body. This textbook is intended primarily for ophthalmologists, but also for medical students and specialists in other disciplines, including general practitioners.

Renowned experts from the ranks of ophthalmologists and specialists in various fields of medicine have participated in its preparation. The book is divided into twelve chapters, in which individual diseases are described, followed by a discussion by ophthalmologists who present an overview of the ocular complications of these diseases.

The textbook summarises the most common ocular manifestations of systemic diseases, specifically vascular, endocrine, autoimmune, rheumatological, pulmonary, gastrointestinal, hematological, infectious, cutaneous, neurological, sexually transmitted, and cancer. Successful treatment of these conditions requires early and usually long-term cooperation between the specialist and the ophthalmologist. The diseases can be manifested in all parts of the eye, depending on the overall way they spread throughout the body, whether through the blood, the lymphatic and nervous systems, or by affecting the avascular parts of the eye. Some diseases can already be demonstrated by ophthalmological examination before the onset of general symptoms. As the eye is the only organ whose structures, tissues, blood vessels, and inner wall can easily be examined, it can be described as a "window to the whole human body". Changes in the blood vessels on the fundus can be noted and inferences can be made about the condition of arteries and veins in other organs, especially in the brain. In some cases, these manifestations are an initial indicator of a serious disease which, without early diagnosis, could be severe or even fatal.

The book contains a rich pictorial documentation and a set of graphic diagrams. Thanks to these, ophthalmologists and specialists in various disciplines can quickly orient themselves to the most common symptoms, clinical pictures, differential diagnoses, and treatment of general human diseases and their ocular complications.

We wish to express our gratitude to the entire team of authors of this book for their excellent collaboration. Finally, we also wish to thank our families, without whose tremendous support this book would not have been possible.

Mlada Boleslav, Czech Republic
Hradec Kralove, Czech Republic

Alexandr Stepanov
Jan Studnicka

Contents

Cardiovascular Diseases 1
Jan Studnicka, Leos Pleva, Alexandr Stepanov, Pavel Poczos,
and Tomas Cesak

Blood Diseases 23
Alexandr Stepanov, Jakub Radocha, and Veronika Matuskova

Lung Diseases 79
Marketa Stredova, Vladimir Koblizek, Alexandr Stepanov,
Larisa Solichova, Vladimir Bartos, Vit Havel, Eva Kocova,
and Helena Hornychova

Gastrointestinal Diseases 127
Alexandr Stepanov, Marcela Kopacova, Ilja Tacheci, Marie Burova,
and Petr Hulek

Metabolic and Endocrine Diseases 153
Jan Studnicka, Marta Karhanova, Filip Gabalec, Alexandr Stepanov,
Vladimir Blaha, Martina Lasticova, Jana Kalitova, and Jan Schovanek

Rheumatic Diseases 207
Jan Nemcansky, Petr Bradna, and Veronika Kolarcikova

Skin Diseases 267
Marketa Stredova, Miloslav Salavec, and Andrea Bartlova

Sexually Transmitted Diseases 293
Jan Nemcansky, Miloslav Salavec, Sabina Nemcanska,
Dominika Linzerova, and Pavel Bostik

Cancer Diseases 341
Veronika Matuskova, Jiri Petera, Ondrej Kubecek,
and Ahmed Youbi Zakaria

Neurological Disorders 375
Zdenek Kasl, Pavel Poczos, Roman Herzig, Nada Jiraskova,
Martin Matuska, and Tomas Cesak

Neurosurgical Diseases 447
Pavel Poczos, Zdenek Kasl, Martin Matuska, Nada Jiraskova,
and Tomas Cesak

Infectious Diseases 499
Alexandr Stepanov, Michal Holub, Milan Zlamal, Ondrej Beran,
Zofia Bartovska, and Michal Ptacek

Cardiovascular Diseases

Jan Studnicka, Leos Pleva, Alexandr Stepanov⑩, Pavel Poczos, and Tomas Cesak

1 Arterial Hypertension

Arterial hypertension is a serious, often inadequately treated, health problem, especially in developed countries. Along with smoking, diabetes mellitus (DM), dyslipidaemia and obesity, it is one of the most serious risk factors for cardiovascular disease (CVD), especially stroke, coronary artery disease (CAD) and other clinical manifestations of atherosclerosis.

J. Studnicka · A. Stepanov
Department of Ophthalmology, University Hospital and Faculty of Medicine of Charles University in Hradec Kralove, Sokolska 581, 500 05 Hradec Kralove, Czech Republic
e-mail: jan.studnicka@ocni-visus.cz

J. Studnicka
Eye Centre VISUS, spol. s r.o., Nemcove 738, 547 01 Nachod, Czech Republic

P. Poczos · T. Cesak
Department of Neurosurgery, University Hospital and Faculty of Medicine of Charles University in Hradec Kralove, Sokolska 581, 500 05 Hradec Kralove, Czech Republic
e-mail: pavel.poczos@fnhk.cz

T. Cesak
e-mail: tomas.cesak@fnhk.cz

A. Stepanov (✉)
Ophthalmology Department, Klaudian's Hospital, Vaclava Klementa 147, 293 01 Mlada Boleslav, Czech Republic
e-mail: stepanov.doctor@gmail.com

Third Faculty of Medicine in Prague, Charles University, Ruska 2411, 100 00 Prague, Czech Republic

L. Pleva
Department of Clinic Subjects, Faculty of Medicine, Medical Research Center, University of Ostrava, Syllabova 19, 703 00 Ostrava, Czech Republic
e-mail: leos.pleva@volny.cz

© The Author(s), under exclusive license to Springer Nature Switzerland AG 2024
A. Stepanov and J. Studnicka (eds.), *Ocular Manifestations of Systemic Diseases*,
https://doi.org/10.1007/978-3-031-58592-0_1

Globally, an estimated 26% of the world's population (972 million people) has hypertension, and the prevalence is expected to increase to 29% by 2025, driven largely by increases in economically developing nations [41]. However, less than 50% of hypertensives are adequately treated [66].

Diagnosis and classification

Arterial hypertension is defined as a recurrent increase in blood pressure (BP) $\geq$ 140/90 mmHg measured on at least two different visits. The current classification according to BP level includes mild, moderate and severe hypertension [66].

In terms of aetiopathogenesis, a distinction is made between essential hypertension, without a clear causative factor (in 90% of cases), and secondary hypertension (the remaining 10%), arising from another disease (Table 1.1).

Secondary hypertension is more common at younger ages and should be kept in mind in patients with severe or resistant hypertension. Adequate diagnosis is important to allow subsequent targeted therapy of the causative disease. The most common causes of secondary hypertension are primary hyperaldosteronism and renal diseases.

Methodology of blood pressure measurement

Adequate measurement of pressure is the basis for the diagnosis and treatment of hypertension. Measurement is performed in the office (clinical BP) with the patient sitting for 5–10 min on the arm at heart level with the forearm resting loosely. During the first examination, BP is measured on both arms; later it is always measured on the same arm. The measurement is repeated 3 times and the average of the 2nd and 3rd readings is assessed.

Table 1.1 Secondary arterial hypertension

Endocrine	Primary hyperaldosteronism (*most common*) Cushing's syndrome, pheochromocytoma, primary hyperparathyroidism, acromegaly, thyreopathies
Nephrogenic	Polycystic kidney disease, glomerulonephritis, diabetic nephropathy, tubulointestinal nephritis
Renovascular hypertension	
Sleep apnoea syndrome	
Hypertension induced by drugs and addictive substances	Immunosuppressants, corticosteroids, non-steroidal anti-inflammatory drugs, hormonal contraceptives, sympathomimetics, cocaine, etc.
Coarctation of the aorta	
Neurogenic causes	

Cardiovascular Diseases

Table 1.2 Assessment of hypertension according to ambulatory BP monitoring

	Systolic BP (mm Hg)	Diastolic BP (mm Hg)
24-h average	≥ 130	≥ 80
Daily average	≥ 135	≥ 85
Night average	≥ 120	≥ 70

BP blood pressure

24-h ambulatory blood pressure monitoring

This is performed in newly diagnosed hypertension, when a discrepancy between ambulatory and home measurements is suspected (white coat syndrome), with significant variability of measured values during the day, to exclude episodes of post-medication hypotension or in resistant hypertension. The 24-h mean and the mean values of BP during day and night hours are assessed (Table 1.2).

Basic examination procedures and determination of overall cardiovascular risk

The diagnosis of hypertension is established based on the results of repeated BP measurements. Table 1.3 lists the basic investigations that are performed in all patients, with additional investigations appropriate in selected groups or to exclude secondary hypertension [49].

Table 1.3 Examination of the arterial hypertension

Basic examination
- Medical history (family, pharmacological)
- Physical examination (+ palpation and auscultation of peripheral arteries)
- BP, sitting or standing; on first examination on both arms
- Serum Na, K, Cl, glucose, uric acid
- Lipid spectrum (total cholesterol, LDL-, HDL-cholesterol, TAG)
- Urine chemistry + sediment
- Estimation of glomerular filtration rate
- Albuminuria
- Blood count
- ECG

Extended examinations, suitable for certain groups
- 24h ambulatory BP monitoring
- Ankle-brachial systolic BP ratio (ankle-brachial index)
- Echocardiography
- Doppler US of the carotid arteries
- Aortic pulse wave velocity
- Renal ultrasound
- Ocular background
- HbA1c, eventually glycaemic curve (at fasting glycaemia 5.6–6.9 mmol/l)

To exclude secondary hypertension
- Plasma renin activity (aldosterone/renin ratio)
- Doppler US of renal arteries
- Exclusion of sleep apnoea syndrome

An important part of the examination is the determination of the overall cardiovascular (CV) risk, as the aim of our treatment is obviously to positively influence the prognosis of patients [9]. This prognosis depends not only on the level of BP, but also on the presence of other risk factors for atherosclerosis, subclinical or manifest organ involvement and associated diseases.

In hypertensives without associated diseases and signs of organ damage (i.e. as part of primary prevention), CV risk is assessed according to SCORE tables, where the 10-year risk of a fatal CV event depends on sex, age, smoking, systolic BP and total cholesterol [48] (Piepoli et al. 2016).

Therapy

Treatment of hypertension reduces the incidence of CV events, especially stroke and heart failure and, to a lesser extent, coronary artery disease, renal failure, and atrial fibrillation.

The primary goal of antihypertensive treatment is to reduce BP < 140/90 mmHg in all patients. If treatment is well tolerated, further reduction to ≤ 130/80 mmHg should be sought. In patients < 65 years of age, achieving systolic BP values in the range of 120–129 mmHg is considered optimal; further reductions < 120 mmHg is no longer beneficial [66].

Overview of pharmacotherapy

The basis of treatment is the group of antihypertensive drugs for which there are data from clinical trials confirming their beneficial effect on CV mortality. These include angiotensin-I converting enzyme inhibitors (i-ACE), angiotensin II AT_1-receptor blockers (ARBs; sartans), long-acting calcium blockers, diuretics, and beta-blockers. Treatment with a fixed double combination of antihypertensive drugs is preferred.

Secondary hypertension

We refer to hypertension in which a specific underlying cause can be identified as secondary (Table 1.1). It occurs more frequently at younger ages and should be kept in mind in patients with severe, resistant hypertension or hypertension with specific accompanying symptoms.

Adequate diagnosis and subsequent targeted treatment are particularly important in young patients.

When to consider secondary hypertension?

- Hypertension with hypokalaemia—primary hyperaldosteronism
- Hypertension and decreased renal function or proteinuria—nephrogenic hypertension
- Recurrent, sudden onset pulmonary oedema, significant deterioration of renal function after i-ACE/sartan—renovascular hypertension
- Seizures, cephalea, palpitations, sweating and pallor—pheochromocytoma.

Cardiovascular Diseases

2 Ocular Manifestations of Arterial Hypertension

Hypertonic retinopathy is the most common manifestation of arterial hypertension, which is closely related to acute or chronic elevation of BP. It was first described in 1859 by Dr. Liebreich [39]. Data from worldwide studies show that retinal microvascular signs are present in 2–15% of adults aged ≥ 40 years [18]. Early recognition of hypertonic retinopathy is an important step in the risk assessment of patients with hypertension. Prolonged and inadequately compensated systemic hypertension results in disruption of the inner and subsequently the outer blood-retina barrier, leading to both focal and generalised retinal arteriolar changes [34].

Two processes play a role in the *aetiopathogenesis* of hypertonic retinopathy. Firstly, there is the acute effect of systemic arterial hypertension (vasoconstrictive phase), which results in vasospasm of retinal vessels. Arterioles respond to increased luminal pressure by vasoconstriction to reduce blood flow, but gradually endothelial damage, smooth muscle degeneration and fibrinous necrosis of endothelial cells occurs [18]. Secondly, there are the chronic effects of hypertension (sclerotic phase), manifested by thickening of the inner layer of the vascular wall, hyperplasia of the middle layer and hyaline degeneration [42]. The vascular changes include diffuse or local narrowing of retinal arterioles, intensification of arterial reflex, and compression of the vein by adjacent arteries [30, 31].

Retinal changes are a consequence of a breakdown of the blood-retina barrier and leakage of blood and plasma. They are manifested by necrosis of vascular smooth muscle and endothelial cells, exudation of blood and lipids and ischaemia of the retinal nerve fibre layer [32, 42].

With very high BP (malignant hypertension), swelling of the optic disc can occur, which is often a picture of hypertensive encephalopathy associated with increased intracranial pressure. These changes may not be progressive. For example, a patient with an acute increase in BP may present retinal changes without evidence of a sclerotic phase on the vessels.

Other complications of arterial hypertension are retinal vein and artery occlusion and retinal arterial macroaneurysms.

Risk factors

- Duration of arterial hypertension
- Age
- Systolic blood pressure level.

Clinical presentation

Clinical signs are the result of developing *macular oedema* and the presence of subretinal fluid. When the macula is affected, visual acuity and contrast sensitivity gradually decrease and the patient reports metamorphopsia. In the case of the development of optic disc oedema, positive scotomas on the perimeter are found. The treachery of hypertonic retinopathy lies in the absence of general symptoms. In the case of malignant hypertension, headaches, scotomas and photopsies may occur.

Objective findings

The modern classification by Wong and Mitchell includes *three stages* of hypertonic retinopathy [67]. In its mild degree, mainly vascular changes are found. There is an arteriovenous crossing change and generalised or focal spasm of arterioles. Furthermore, the *"copper wire"* phenomenon is observed, characterised by widening or accentuation of the arterial reflex, with the gradual development of the *"silver wire"* phenomenon when the blood column cannot be identified [30].

The moderate stage is characterised by retinal haemorrhages (dot, blot or flame shaped) (Fig. 1.1), the appearance of soft exudates resulting from nerve fibre ischaemia—*"cotton wool spots"* (Fig. 1.1) and the finding of microaneurysms of small vessels [34].

Another finding is the appearance of hard exudates, deposited typically in a *star shape*. The hard exudates represent lipid deposition due to a breakdown of the inner blood-retina barrier in the Henle's fibre layer (Fig. 1.2).

In severe hypertonic retinopathy (malignant hypertension), optic disc oedema occurs due to ischaemic axonal oedema (Figs. 1.1 and 1.2).

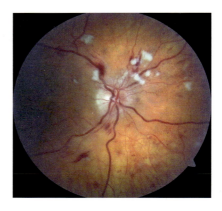

Fig. 1.1 Cotton wool spots and multiple intraretinal haemorrhages

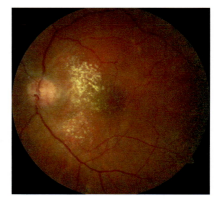

Fig. 1.2 Hypertonic neuroretinopathy. Oedema of the optic nerve and macula with multiple hard exudates

Cardiovascular Diseases

The traditional Keith-Wagener-Barker classification of hypertonic retinopathy divides the changes into four stages [27].

Stage 1: hypertensive angiopathy involves narrowing of the retinal arterioles and their increased tortuosity.

Stage 2: hypertensive angiosclerosis includes, in addition to the changes of the first stage, the arteriovenous crossing alteration.

Stage 3: hypertensive retinopathy adds retinal lesions (retinal haemorrhages and cotton wool spots) to the changes of the first and second stages.

Stage 4: hypertensive neuroretinopathy includes, in addition to the above changes, optic disc oedema, sometimes with formation of a star-shaped figure of hard exudates in the macula.

In the case of BP compensation, most of the retinal changes gradually recede, but the vascular changes persist. Prolonged macular oedema can lead to irreversible changes in photoreceptors and retinal pigment epithelial cells with a permanent decrease in visual acuity [8]. Chronic optic disc oedema leads to its atrophy, which also results in a permanent decrease in vision [34].

Complications

At the most advanced stage of hypertensive retinopathy, the development of exudative retinal detachment and ischaemic choroidopathy can be observed. The choroidal capillaries undergo fibrinoid necrosis in acute hypertension, which is manifested by the presence of Elschnig's spots (round, deep, grey-yellow spots at the level of the retinal pigment epithelium) and Siegrist´s streaks (linear hyperpigmented lines along the choroidal arteries) [34].

Diagnosis

The diagnosis of hypertonic retinopathy relies on biomicroscopy, digital fundus photography, and OCT examination to demonstrate and monitor the development of macular oedema and optic disc oedema (Fig. 1.3).

In severe cases, fluorescein angiography (FAG) is an indispensable diagnostic method to detect retinal ischaemia. The Amsler grid examination is considered as a complementary examination to detect macular involvement early.

Differential diagnosis

- Diabetic retinopathy
- Anemia
- High altitude retinopathy
- Ocular ischaemic syndrome
- Radiation retinopathy
- Central retinal vein occlusion.

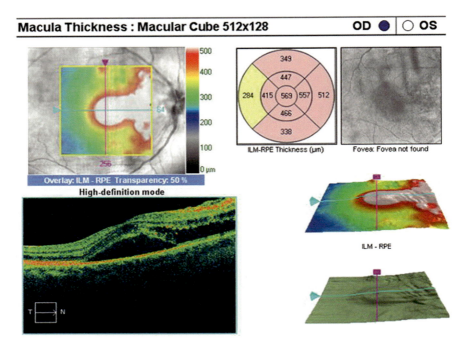

Fig. 1.3 OCT of the macula. Finding of free fluid between the neuroretina and retinal pigment epithelium (RPE), oedema of the neuroretina that continues toward the optic disc

Therapy

In the treatment of hypertonic retinopathy, early compensation of arterial hypertension and the cooperation of the patient and the general practitioner are essential. In the case of malignant hypertension with chronic macular oedema, the effectiveness of intravitreal injection of vascular endothelial growth factor (VEGF) inhibitors has been demonstrated [1].

Prognosis

Patients with severe hypertonic retinopathy and arteriosclerotic changes have an increased risk of coronary disease, peripheral vascular disease, and stroke. As arteriosclerotic changes in the retina do not recede, these patients remain at increased risk of retinal artery occlusions, retinal vein occlusions and retinal macroaneurysms.

Cardiovascular Diseases

3 Carotid-Cavernous Fistula

Carotid-cavernous fistula (CCF) is an abnormal communication between an artery and a vein within the cavernous sinus. According to the etiological aspect, two types of fistulas are distinguished: *posttraumatic* and *spontaneous.* Posttraumatic fistulas occur in approximately 0.2% of craniocerebral injuries [6]. Spontaneous CCFs are classified according to Barrow into four groups: direct fistulas (Barrow type A) and indirect (dural) fistulas (Barrow types B, C and D) [12]. *A direct fistula* represents a direct pathological communication between the internal carotid artery (ACI) and the cavernous sinus. It is usually a high-flow fistula, accompanied by significant clinical signs, most often caused by rupture of the ACI bulge in the cavernous sinus, often in association with systemic connective tissue defects, e.g., in Ehlers-Danlos syndrome [22]. It can also be iatrogenic following an endovascular procedures or neurosurgical interventions in the cavernous sinus [45]. *Indirect* or *dural fistulas,* usually low-flow ones, involve the communication between the cavernous sinus and the cavernous arterial meningeal branch. The arterial component of the fistula in Barrow type B is the meningeal branch of the ACI, in type C the meningeal branch of the external carotid artery (ACE) and, in type D, both the ACI and ACE meningeal branches are involved. Spontaneous fistulas are more common in type D [12].

Risk factors

- Arterial hypertension
- ACI dissection
- Fibromuscular dysplasia, Ehlers-Danlos syndrome type IV
- Female sex (postmenopausal period)
- Primary thrombosis of the cavernous sinus (more likely in dural fistulas).

Clinical presentation

Subjective complaints include retro-orbital pain, diplopia, tearing, foreign body sensation in the eye and blurred vision, which in more severe cases can lead to loss of vision. A ventrally draining fistula causes more ocular symptoms. Just like subjective complaints, they are usually homolateral to the side of the fistula. Patients with a venous drainage fistula that courses dorsally may suffer from confusion, expressive aphasia, oculomotor nerve disorder, etc. The fistula will cause more pronounced symptoms if it is a direct fistula (i.e., the flow is greater) and if the retrograde filling of the veins is more pronounced anteriorly—towards the orbital region. The classic clinical triad is *pulsatile exophthalmos, orbital bruit*, and *chemosis.* The bruit is audible over the carotid artery in the neck, sometimes temporally or over the eye. Exceptionally, there are also manifestations of ischemia in a case of a large opening in the ACI, which may lead to "steal syndrome" [28]. When *traumatic* carotid-cavernous fistulas occur, symptoms may appear with a delay. They arise based on venous hypertension, most often in the orbit on the same side [38].

Diagnosis

Both CT angiography (CTA) and MR angiography (MRA) are highly sensitive imaging methods to detect direct and dural fistulas. The gold standard is angiography, which is not only a diagnostic method but also a therapeutic one, as it allows endovascular treatment of the fistula in one session.

Differential diagnosis

- Tumours with compression of the cavernous sinus
- Endocrine orbitopathy
- Thrombosis of the cavernous sinus
- Retrobulbar intraorbital expansion.

Therapy

The aim of treatment is to eliminate, or at least alleviate, clinical symptoms, with vision preservation. Methods aimed at disrupting arteriovenous communication in the cavernous sinus are currently performed exclusively by interventional neuroradiologists using endovascular techniques. They consist of placing embolic agents (glue, spirals) or stents into the fistula site, either by transvenous, transarterial or combined methods [37]. The surgical solution of trapping the internal carotid artery (ACI trapping) is reserved only for very exceptional situations of unusual anatomical conditions that prevent endovascular treatment. Rapid visual loss presents an indication for urgent treatment.

4 Ocular Manifestations of Carotid-Cavernous Fistula

CCF is the result of an abnormal vascular connection between the internal or external carotid artery and the venous channels of the cavernous sinus. After the fistula is formed, arterial and venous blood mixes and under high pressure it penetrates mostly through the v. ophthalmica superior into the orbit. The vein dilates under the influence of high pressure, gradually changing the vascular wall and transmitting arterial pulsation to the contents of the orbit. At the same time, the outflow of venous blood from the orbit is impaired, resulting in proptosis, eyelid edema, and conjunctival hyperemia and chemosis. After the formation of a fistula within the cavernous sinus, the pressure in the supracavernous carotid segment decreases with a subsequent decrease pressure in the ophthalmic artery. The result is chronic hypoxia of the ocular and orbital structures [46]. Direct CCFs have an acute manifestation of clinical symptoms, whereas indirect CCFs are associated with a more gradual onset and chronic course. The earliest clinical signs usually include orbital manifestations due to venous congestion and venous drainage pathological communication.

Cardiovascular Diseases

Objective findings

Anterior eye segment

Ocular symptoms seen in *direct CCF* include pulsating proptosis, eyelid oedema, ptosis, chemotic conjunctiva, tortuous perilimbal corkscrew veins (caput medusae sign), secondary elevation of intraocular pressure, and disorders of pupillary reaction. Anterior segment ischemia is characterized by corneal oedema, flare, iris atrophy, rubeosis and cataract.

Paresis of cranial nerves III, IV and/or VI can occur and change over time. Ophthalmoplegia and Horner's syndrome with VI cranial nerve palsy due to compression in the cavernous sinus can also be observed. CCF can also present as isolated *n. oculomotorius* palsy without orbital congestive symptoms.

Posterior eye segment

Ocular findings include optic disc oedema, dilated retinal veins, hypoxic retinopathy, ischaemic optic neuropathy, and occasionally central retinal vein occlusion [25, 46].

Patients complain of diplopia, redness of the eyes, orbital pain, pain behind the eye, swelling, head murmur, or a decrease of visual acuity. They may also have pulsatile tinnitus due to turbulent flow through the venous system. Symptoms are typically on the side of the fistula but may occur bilaterally depending on the severity and duration of venous congestion [35, 65].

Unlike direct high-flow CCFs, *indirect CCFs* with slower blood flow can be asymptomatic at the onset. The most common manifestation is the finding of dilated episcleral blood vessels. In advanced indirect CCFs, venous congestion and retrograde drainage into the orbital veins increase arterial flow to the *sinus cavernosus*. The symptoms are then similar to those of direct CCF.

Diagnosis

A complete anamnesis and detailed clinical examination with appropriate complementary methods will facilitate early diagnosis and initiation of treatment of CCF. Ultrasound examination will reveal dilatation of *the v. ophthalmica superior*, arterial flow within the *v. ophthalmica superior* or enlargement of the extrabulbar muscles. CT angiography and MR angiography are essential to demonstrate an existing fistula. Additional methods include exophthalmometry, auscultation of the periocular region, slit-lamp biomicroscopy and ophthalmoscopy [25, 46].

Differential diagnosis

- Sinus cavernous thrombosis
- Superior orbital fissure syndrome
- Graves orbitopathy
- Orbital apex syndrome.

Therapy

Patients with asymptomatic, incidentally discovered indirect CCFs can often be followed up without the need for invasive intervention. Patients with mild ocular symptoms are treated with topical medications and monitored for preservation of visual acuity, intraocular pressure, or changes in the eye fundus. In some cases, indirect CCFs may also heal spontaneously. Direct CCFs are rarely asymptomatic and are treated as early as possible. Embolisation of the fistula using an endovascular technique is performed by an interventional neuroradiologist [40].

5   Cardiac Myxoma and Its Ocular Manifestations

Primary cardiac tumours are very rare, mostly benign, and myxoma is their most common representative. It is a polypoid mass of gel-like consistency (several cm in size), which most often occurs in the left atrium (80%) and is usually sessile on the interatrial septum [17].

Clinical presentation

About 1/3 of patients with cardiac myxomas are asymptomatic; the remaining may present with non-specific influenza-like symptoms (subfebrile, weight loss, fatigue, myalgia) or cardiac symptoms (palpitations, weakness, dyspnoea, syncope) [51]. Cardiac myxoma also may be the cause of embolisation of tumour masses or thrombi into the arterial circulation (transient ischaemic attack/stroke, limb ischemia, myocardial infarction). Large myxoma may cause valve orifice obstruction or regurgitation when interfering with the valve tips [17].

The demonstration of myxoma is usually echocardiographic and treatment consists of surgical extirpation [58].

The most common ocular complications of cardiac myxoma are *thromboembolic events* in the retinal and choroidal vessels. Myxoma can cause embolism due to its susceptibility to crush, primarily affecting the midcerebral or supraclinoid internal carotid artery [2, 5]. Fragments from myxoma in the left atrium can travel to systemic vessels such as the retinal artery [14], whereas those from the right atrium do not [26]. In addition, all patients have other embolic symptoms, such as cerebral infarction, red spots, and pain in the extremities. Other ocular manifestations include homonymous hemianopia, diplopia, rotational and horizontal nystagmus [59].

Several cases of patients with retinal artery occlusion caused by left atrial myxoma have been reported in the literature since 1990. Schmidt et al. described a case of a 29-year-old patient with isolated central retinal artery occlusion, secondary to a previously undiagnosed left atrial myxoma [59]. Rafuse et al. presented a 45-year-old woman with sudden onset right-sided hemiparesis, central retinal artery occlusion, and aphasia [54]. Examination of the ocular posterior segment showed a pale ischaemic neuroretinal mass with no evidence of retinal or choroidal circulation. The echocardiography examination showed a mobile, multilobulated mass attached

Cardiovascular Diseases

to the septal wall of the left atrium. Pathological examination of the resected tumour confirmed the diagnosis of endocardial myxoma [54].

Diagnosis of ocular manifestations of cardiac myxoma is based on examination of the posterior segment of the eye with regular fundus photography.

Therapy includes administration of vasodilator infusions and management of any complications of thromboembolic events (e.g. macular oedema, neovascular glaucoma, tractional retinal detachment, etc.).

6 Atrial Fibrillation

Atrial fibrillation (AF) is the most common clinically significant arrhythmia. It is a supraventricular tachyarrhythmia with uncoordinated electrical activation of the atria, leading to their ineffective mechanical contraction. It is present in 2–4% of adults, more commonly in men, and its incidence increases with age (85% of patients with AF are over 65 years of age) [29]. The main risk factors are heart failure, valvular heart disease, coronary artery disease, hypertension, diabetes mellitus, chronic kidney disease, hyperthyroidism, obesity, chronic obstructive pulmonary disease, and others. The presence of atrial fibrillation is associated with increased mortality (1.5–3.5 fold), incidence of cardioembolic ischaemic stroke, heart failure, vascular dementia, and the need for hospitalisation [23].

Clinical presentation

Manifestations of AF include palpitations, fatigue, decreased exercise tolerance, shortness of breath, chest tightness, dizziness and more; but up to 50% of patients may be clinically mute.

Diagnosis

It is based on the ECG recording: irregular atrial activation (missing P waves, irregular f waves) and irregular R-R intervals. The classification of atrial fibrillation includes first diagnosed, paroxysmal, persistent, and permanent AF [23].

Therapy

Treatment of patients with atrial fibrillation is based on:

- Anticoagulation—prevention of ischaemic stroke
- Affecting symptoms—restoring and maintaining sinus rhythm ("rhythm control") or controlling heart rate ("rate control")
- Treatment of associated diseases (heart failure, hypertension, etc.)

Anticoagulation

Ineffective mechanical contraction of the left atrium in AF is associated with the risk of thrombus formation (most often in the left atrial appendage) and the risk of

Table 1.4 CHA_2DS_2-VASc score

Risk factor		Points
C	Congestive heart failure	1
H	Hypertension	1
A	Age $\geq$ 75 years[a]	2
D	Diabetes mellitus	1
S	Previous stroke/TIA	2
V	Vascular disease[b]	1
A	Age 65–74 years	1
S	Gender (females)	1
Maximum score		9

Note
[a] significant risk factor, therefore 2 points
[b] ischaemic heart disease, previous myocardial infarction, lower limb ischaemia

systemic thromboembolism, especially ischaemic stroke. The risk of cardioembolic stroke is increased fivefold in AF, but also depends on the presence of other risk factors. We assess the presence and influence of these risk factors according to the CHA_2DS_2-VASc score (Table 1.4), which allows us to determine the overall risk of ischaemic stroke (systemic thromboembolism).

Patients with atrial fibrillation and a CHA_2DS_2-VASc score of 0 (in men) or 1 (in women) have a low thromboembolic risk and do not require anticoagulation therapy. Conversely, in patients with a CHA_2DS_2-VASc $\geq$ 2 (men) or $\geq$ 3 (women), this risk is high and anticoagulation therapy is necessary. However, even in patients with CHA_2DS_2-VASc $=$ 1 (men) or 2 (women), anticoagulation should be considered [23].

Currently, anticoagulation therapy is based on the administration of non-vitamin K oral anticoagulants (NOACs; dabigatran, xabans), which, unlike warfarin, do not require dose titration according to INR. Their efficacy in preventing ischaemic stroke is at least comparable to warfarin, whereas the risk of intracranial haemorrhage is lower [60]. Contraindications to anticoagulation therapy include active major bleeding or recent intracranial haemorrhage, severe anaemia, or thrombocytopenia. The HAS-BLED score is used to assess the risk of bleeding complications with anticoagulation therapy [23].

Influence of symptoms

Rhythm control

It consists of restoring and maintaining sinus rhythm by cardioversion, antiarrhythmic therapy or catheter radiofrequency ablation. Cardioversion (electrical or pharmacological) can be performed in patients with a duration of atrial fibrillation < 12–48 h without prior anticoagulation. Patients with AF duration $\geq$ 48 h or unknown duration

Cardiovascular Diseases

require at least 3 weeks of effective anticoagulation before cardioversion or exclusion of left atrial appendage thrombus by transoesophageal echocardiography (risk of cardioembolism during cardioversion).

Electrical cardioversion is performed under short-term anaesthesia with a synchronous biphasic discharge; for pharmacological cardioversion and subsequent antiarrhythmic therapy we use propafenone or sotalol (in patients without structural heart disease) or amiodarone (reduced left ventricular systolic function, status post myocardial infarction, etc.), especially in view of their possible proarrhythmogenic side effects.

After cardioversion, we continue anticoagulation therapy in low-risk patients for at least 4 weeks until mechanical atrial contractility is restored. In patients at high risk of thromboembolism with CHA2DS2-VASc ≥ 2 (men) or ≥ 3 (women), anticoagulation therapy is permanent because of the possibility of recurrence of clinically silent paroxysms of atrial fibrillation.

Catheter ablation is a more effective method to restore and maintain sinus rhythm than antiarrhythmic drugs.

Rate control

Controlling the heart rate in atrial fibrillation alone can lead to relief. This option is chosen in low-symptom patients and in cases where efforts to maintain sinus rhythm with antiarrhythmic therapy repeatedly fail or are not feasible. Among the drugs we use are beta-blockers, verapamil, digoxin or amiodarone. Long-term anticoagulation therapy according to the CHA2DS2-VASc score is essential.

7 Patent Foramen Ovale

The foramen ovale is a slit-like opening in the atrial septum that is part of the foetal circulation. If it does not grow postnatally and incomplete closure of the foramen ovale persists, we speak of a foramen ovale patens (PFO). Its occurrence in the population is relatively frequent (25–30%). A patent foramen ovale does not cause a haemodynamically significant shunt, but it may be a pathway that, under certain conditions (increased pressure in the right-sided cardiac compartments, e.g. during the Valsalva manoeuvre), allows paradoxical embolisation of venous thrombi (most often in deep venous thrombosis of the lower limbs) into the arterial circulation.

Clinical presentation

Ischaemic stroke is one of the most important clinical manifestations associated with patent foramen ovale. The presence of patent foramen ovale is associated with cryptogenic strokes, especially in patients younger than 55 years of age, or with embolic occlusion of the central retinal artery [53].

Diagnosis

The diagnosis of PFO is based on the detection of a right shunt during the Valsalva manoeuvre by transcranial Doppler or transoesophageal echocardiography. Transoesophageal echocardiography allows the morphology of the PFO to be assessed and its significance to be quantified. A significant shunt is considered as being the penetration of > 20 microbubbles of echocontrast during the Valsalva manoeuvre through the PFO into the left atrium [53].

Therapy

In younger patients with cryptogenic ischaemic stroke and the presence of a PFO with significant shunt, closure can be performed by implantation of an Amplatz occluder. This is subject to the exclusion of other known causes of ischaemic stroke (stenosis or atherothrombotic plaques in the carotid watersheds, atrial fibrillation, etc.).

8 Ocular Manifestations of Atrial Fibrillation and Patent Foramen Ovale

In the field of FS, the conditions are very favourable for the formation of intracardiac thrombus (especially in the left atrial appendage), which can cause macro- and microembolism [3]. Macroembolic complications often manifest as transient ischaemic attacks and stroke. Complications that result from microembolic events are much more difficult to diagnose. Occlusion of the posterior ciliary arteries causes optic nerve ischaemia and the development of anterior ischemic optic neuropathy (AION). In this case, there is a sudden deterioration of visual acuity, with typical changes in the eye fundus, including optic disc oedema and peripapillary haemorrhage. Other ophthalmological complications of FS include retinal vessel occlusions [29] and a greater susceptibility to glaucoma, especially normotensive glaucoma [24, 50]. The prevalence of FS in patients with retinal thromboembolic events ranges from 1.16 to 15.2% [7, 52].

The prevalence of ocular blood supply disorders in patients with PFO is as high as 23% [61]. In the elderly with PFO, the most common cause of retinal artery occlusion is embolus due to atheromatous plaque in the carotid artery [33, 57, 64]. Phlebothrombosis may be another potential source of paradoxical embolism. Nakagawa et al. presented a case of bilateral CRAO in a patient with PFO and deep vein thrombosis [44]. The most common causes of retinal and choroidal thromboembolism in younger patients in addition to PFO include concomitant cardiac disorders (valvular heart disease [4], left atrial myxoma [36], and hypercoagulable states) [16]. Clifford et al. described CRAO and ischaemic optic neuropathy in a young patient with PFO [10]. If calcified emboli are found in the eye fundus, a thorough cardiological examination including echocardiography is recommended.

Cardiovascular Diseases 17

Diagnosis of ocular complications of FS and PFO includes examination of the posterior ocular segment and FAG.

Therapy includes administration of vasodilator infusions and management of other potential neovascular complications (e.g. neovascular glaucoma, tractional retinal detachment, etc.).

9 Infective Endocarditis

It is an inflammatory disease caused by various types of microorganisms affecting mainly the endocardium of the heart valves. The predisposing factor allowing the attachment of circulating pathogens is damage to the endocardial lining (valvular heart disease) or the presence of foreign material (valve replacements, pacing leads, etc.). At these sites or areas of turbulent flow, microtubules can form, which provide a favourable environment for the attachment and further multiplication of microorganisms, growing typical vegetations.

Clinical presentation

The manifestations of infective endocarditis (IE) are varied, ranging from rapidly progressive sepsis to slow-onset disease with non-specific symptoms (subfebrile, sweating, weakness, malnutrition, etc.). The most common symptoms are febrile and heart murmur (80–90% of patients) or septic embolisation (brain, spleen, kidneys). Findings of immunocomplex deposits (glomerulonephritis, Osler's nodosities or Roth's spots—retinal haemorrhages with central blanching) are now less common [19].

Diagnosis

Laboratory tests show signs of inflammation (leucocytosis, elevation of CRP, procalcitonin) and repeated positive haemocultures. Typical pathogens are Streptococcus viridans and bovis, Staphylococcus aureus or Enterococcus. In addition, there are more difficult-to-cultivate microorganisms of the HACEK group (Haemophlius, Actinobacillus, Cardiobacterium, Eikenella and Kingella) or Coxiella burnetii.

Echocardiographic findings include evidence of vegetations (mobile tuft-like formations overlying the heart valves) or paravalvular abscess or fistula [20]. New valvular regurgitation is also detected. Table 1.5 lists the modified Duke criteria for the diagnosis of infective endocarditis [19].

Therapy

Untreated IE is 100% fatal. The mainstay is long-term antibiotic therapy (intravenous, 4–6 weeks) according to ATB sensitivity. Most used are penicillins, cephalosporins or vancomycin, often in combination with aminoglycosides.

Table 1.5 Duke's modified criteria for the diagnosis of infective endocarditis [47]

Major criteria	Typical microorganisms from 2 different haemocultures (*Streptococcus viridans, S. bovis, Staphylococcus aureus*, Enterococcus, HACEK group)
	Other microorganisms consistent with dg. IE from repeatedly positive haemocultures (at least 2 samples > 12 h)
	Any positive haemoculture or antibody titre to *Coxiella burnetii*
	Echocardiographic evidence of IE (vegetations, abscess, fistula)
	New valvular regurgitation
Minor criteria	Predisposing cardiac defect or intravenous toxicity
	Febrile illness > 38 °C
	Vascular embolization (septic emboli, mycotic aneurysms, intracranial haemorrhage, Janaway lesions)
	Immunological manifestations (glomerulonephritis, Osler's nodosities, Roth spots)
	Positive haemocultures not meeting the major criteria
Assessment	
Confirmed IE	Meets 2 major criteria 1 major + 3 minor criteria 5 minor criteria
Possible IE	1 major + 1 minor criterion 3 major criteria

In the case of failure of ATB therapy, progression of heart failure (due to acute valvular regurgitation) or risk of systemic embolisation (large vegetations), surgical treatment is indicated, which consists of replacement of the infected valve.

10   Ocular Manifestations of Infective Endocarditis

Ocular manifestations of IE are nonspecific, caused by septic and, in rare cases, aseptic embolism. On average, 5% of patients with infective endocarditis have ocular symptoms, with Roth's spots being the most common manifestation [21]. Other findings are described in case reports and include focal retinitis, embolic retinopathy, subretinal abscesses, choroidal septic metastases, choroiditis, endophthalmitis, papillitis and optic neuritis [32].

Objective findings

Anterior eye segment

Iris abscess is a rare and the only manifestation of IE [55]. An iris abscess in a patient with bacterial endocarditis can be considered a septic embolus. This is an important clinical finding, because recurrent embolism in bacterial endocarditis may require surgical intervention, specifically valve replacement [11]. Other causes of iris abscesses as manifestations of endophthalmitis are as follows: secondary to septicaemia [62], after cataract extraction [56], and of unknown aetiology [15].

Posterior eye segment

Roth spots

The most common localisation of Roth spots in infective endocarditis is the peripapillary zone. The finding includes a typical picture of erythrocytes surrounding inflammatory cells in the area in response to septic embolism from valvular vegetations [32].

Retinal arterial occlusions

Retinal arterial occlusion occurs as a complication of septic or aseptic embolism. Clinical manifestations depend on the localisation of the occlusion.

Retinal and vitreous infiltration

Septic embolism can lead to the development of posterior uveitis (retinitis, chorioretinitis, choroiditis and vitreous infiltration). In most cases, posterior uveitis is misdiagnosed and is complicated by endophthalmitis.

Endophthalmitis

Endogenous bacterial endophthalmitis is a rare pathology that affects individuals of any age and accounts for 2–15% of all cases of endophthalmitis. The right eye is generally more affected than the left eye, which is probably due to direct blood flow from the heart [13]. Endocarditis is the second-most common cause of endogenous endophthalmitis after meningitis.

Choroidal neovascularisation

Choroidal neovascularisation (CNV) secondary to choroidal septic metastases is very rare. The occurrence of choroidal scarring tends to be variably delayed (10 months–5 years) [43].

Diagnosis

Haemoculture is positive in more than 90% of cases of infective endocarditis when endophthalmitis develops. The most common aetiological agent is Streptococcus (45.7%), and the heart valve is affected in 27.2% of cases.

Therapy

Systemic antibiotic treatment of intraocular inflammation in IE may be sufficient if the vitreous is not excessively affected. In advanced cases of endophthalmitis, antibiotic intravitreal injections and pars plana vitrectomy are necessary [63]. In the case of secondary CNV formation, intravitreal injections of anti-VEGF agents are the treatment of choice.

References

1. Abdelrahman GS. Intravitreal bevacizumab in persistent retinopathy secondary to malignant hypertension. Saudi J Ophthalmol. 2013;27:25–9.
2. Al-Mateen M, Hood M, Trippel D, et al. Cerebral embolism from atrial myxoma in pediatric patients. Pediatrics. 2003;112:e162–7.
3. Al-Saady NM, Obel OA, Camm AJ. Left atrial appendage: structure, function, and role in thromboembolism. Heart. 1999;82:547–54.
4. Barnett HJM. Embolization in mitral valve prolapse. Annu Rev Med. 1982;33:489–507.
5. Bayir H, Morelli PJ, Smith TH, et al. A left atrial myxoma presenting as a cerebrovascular accident. Pediatr Neurol. 1999;21:569–72.
6. Chang CM, Cheng CS. Late intracranial haemorrhage and subsequent carotid-cavernous sinus fistula after fracture of the facial bones. Br J Oral Maxillofac Surg. 2013;51:e296.
7. Chang Y-S, Chu C-C, Weng S-F, et al. The risk of acute coronary syndrome after retinal artery occlusion: a population-based cohort study. Br J Ophthalmol. 2015;99:227–31.
8. Chatterjee S, Chattopadhya S, Hope-Ross M, et al. Hypertensive and the eye: changing perspective. J Hum Hypertens. 2002;16(10):667–75.
9. Chobanian AV. Control of hypertension—An important national priority. N Engl J Med. 2001;345:534–5.
10. Clifford L, Sievers R, Salmon A, et al. Central retinal artery occlusion: association with patent foramen ovale. Eye. 2006;20:736–8.
11. Cunha B, Gill V, Lazar J. Acute infective endocarditis. Diagnostic and therapeutic approach. Infect Dis Clin North Am. 1996;10:811–31.
12. Ellis JA, Goldstein H, Connolly ES, et al. Carotid-cavernous fistulas. Neurosurg Focus. 2012;32(5):E9.
13. Forster RK. Endophthalmitis. In: Tasman W, Jaeger EA, editors. Duane's clinical ophthalmology. Philadelphia: JB Lippincott. 1998. Chapter 24.
14. Galvez-Ruiz A, Galindo-Ferreiro A, Lehner AJ, et al. Clinical presentation of multiple cerebral emboli and central retinal artery occlusion (CRAO) as signs of cardiac myxoma. Saudi J Ophthalmol. 2018;32(2):151–5.
15. Gass JD. Iris abscess simulating malignant melanoma. Arch Ophthalmol. 1973;90:300–2.
16. Greven CM, Slusher MM, Weaver RG. Retinal arterial occlusions in young adults. Am J Ophthalmol. 1995;120:776–83.
17. Griborio-Guzman AG, Aseyev OI, Shah H, Sadreddini M. Cardiac myxomas: clinical presentation, diagnosis and management. Heart. 2022 May 12;108(11):827–833.
18. Grosso A, Veglio F, Porta M, et al. Hypertensive retinopathy revisited: some answers, more questions. Br J Ophthalmol. 2005;89:1646–54.
19. Habib G, Lancellotti P, Antunes MJ, et al. 2015 ESC guidelines for the management of infective endocarditis: the task force for the management of infective endocarditis of the European Society of Cardiology (ESC). Endorsed by: European Association for Cardio-Thoracic Surgery (EACTS), the European Association of Nuclear Medicine (EANM). Eur Heart J. 2015;36(44):3075–128.
20. Habib G, Badano L, Tribouilloy C, Vilacosta I, Zamorano JL, Galderisi M, Voigt JU, Sicari R, Cosyns B, Fox K, Aakhus S; European Association of Echocardiography. Recommendations for the practice of echocardiography in infective endocarditis. Eur J Echocardiogr. 2010 Mar;11(2):202–19.
21. Hasbun R, Vikram HR, Barakat LA, et al. Complicated left-sided native valve endocarditis in adults: risk classification for mortality. JAMA. 2003;289:1933–40.
22. Helmke K, Krüger O, Laas R. The direct carotid cavernous fistula: a clinical, pathoanatomical, and physical study. Acta Neurochir. 1994;127(1–2):1–5.
23. Hindricks G, Potpara T, Dagres N, et al. Guidelines for the diagnosis and management of atrial fibrillation developed in collaboration with the European Association for Cardio-Thoracic Surgery (EACTS): the task force for the diagnosis and management of atrial fibrillation of

the European Society of Cardiology (ESC) Developed with the special contribution of the European Heart Rhythm Association (EHRA) of the ESC. Eur Heart J. 2021;42(5):373–498.

24. Ju-Chuan Y, Hsiu-Li L, Chia-An H, et al. Atrial fibrillation and coronary artery disease as risk factors of retinal artery occlusion: a nationwide population-based study. Biomed Res Int. 2015;2015:374616.

25. Kanski JJ. Clinical ophthalmology. A systemic approach. 4th ed. Reed Educational and Profesional Publishing Ltd.; 1999.

26. Keenan DJ, Morton P, O'kane HO. Right atrial myxoma and pulmonary embolism. Rational basis for investigation and treatment. Br Heart J. 1982;48:510.

27. Keith NM, Wagener HP, Barker NW. Some different types of essential hypertension: their course and prognosis. Am J Med Sci. 1974;268(6):336–45.

28. Keizer R. Carotid-cavernous and orbital arteriovenous fistulas: ocular features, diagnostic and hemodynamic considerations in relation to visual impairment and morbidity. Orbit. 2003;22(2):121–42.

29. Kewcharoen J, Tom ES, Wiboonchutikula C, et al. Prevalence of atrial fibrillation in patients with retinal vessel occlusion and its association: a systematic review and meta-analysis. Curr Eye Res. 2019;44(12):1337–44.

30. Klein R, Klein BEK, Moss SE, et al. Hypertension and retinopathy, arteriolar narrowing and arteriovenous nicking in a population. Arch Ophthalmol. 1994;112:92–8.

31. Klein R, Klein BEK, Moss SE. The relation of systemic hypertension to changes in the retinal vasculature. The beaver dam eye study. Trans Am Ophthalmol. 1997;95:329–50.

32. Klig JE. Ophthalmologic complications of systemic disease. Emerg Med Clin N Am. 2008;26:217–31.

33. Kollarits CR, Lubow M, Hissong SL. Retinal strokes. I. Incidence of carotid atheromata. JAMA. 1972;222:1273–5.

34. Kumudini S, Vikas K, Priyadarshini M, et al. Hypertensive retinopathy. Clin Queries Nephrol. 2013;2:136–9.

35. Lerut B, De Vuyst C, Ghekiere J, et al. Post-traumatic pulsatile tinnitus: the hallmark of a direct carotico-cavernous fistula. J Laryngol Otol. 2007;121:1103–7.

36. Lewis JM. Multiple retinal occlusions from a left atrial myxoma. Am J Ophthalmol. 1994;117:674–5.

37. Lewis AI, Tomsick TA, Tew JM. Management of 100 consecutive direct carotid-cavernous fistulas. Neurosurgery. 1995;36(2):239–45.

38. Liang W, Xiaofeng Y, Weiguo L, et al. Traumatic carotid cavernous fistula accompanying basilar skull fracture: a study on the incidence of traumatic carotid cavernous fistula in the patients with basilar skull fracture and the prognostic analysis about traumatic carotid cavernous fistula. J Trauma Injury Infect Critical Care. 2007;63(5):1014–20.

39. Liebreich R. Ophthalmoscopic findings in bright's disease. Albrecht von Graefes Arch Ophthalmol. 1859;5:265–8.

40. Luo CB, Teng MMH, Chang FC, et al. Bilateral traumatic carotid-cavernous fistulae: 35. Strategies for endovascular treatment. Acta Neurochir. 2007;149(7):675–80.

41. Mills KT, Stefanescu A, He J. The global epidemiology of hypertension. Nat Rev Nephrol. 2020;16(4):223–37.

42. Modi P, Arsiwalla T. Hypertensive retinopathy. StatPearls [Internet]. Treasure Island (FL): StatPearls Publishing; 2020.

43. Munier F, Othenin-Girard P. Subretinal neovascularization secondary to choroidal septic metastasis from acute bacterial endocarditis. Retina. 1992;12:108–12.

44. Nakagawa T, Hirata A, Inoue N, et al. A case of bilateral central retinal artery obstruction with patent foramen ovale. Acta Ophthalmol Scand. 2004;82:111–2.

45. Ono K, Oishi H, Tanoue S, et al. Direct carotid-cavernous fistulas occurring during neurointerventional procedures. Interv Neuroradiol. 2016;22(1):91–6.

46. Otradovec J. Klinická neurooftalmologie. Praha: Grada Publishing a.s.; 2003.

47. Otto CM, Nishimura RA, Bonow RO, et al. 2020 ACC/AHA guideline for the management of patients with valvular heart disease: a report of the American College of Cardiology/American Heart Association Joint Committee on clinical practice guidelines. J Am Coll Cardiol. 2021;77(4):e25–197.
48. Perk J, De Backer G, Gohlke H, et al. European Association for Cardiovascular Prevention & Rehabilitation (EACPR). European guidelines on cardiovascular disease prevention in clinical practice (version 2012): the fifth joint task force of the European society of cardiology and other societies on cardiovascular disease prevention in clinical practice (constituted by representatives of nine societies and by invited experts). Int J Behav Med. 2012;19(4):403–88.
49. Perrone-Filardi P, Coca A, Galderisi M, et al. Noninvasive cardiovascular imaging for evaluating subclinical target organ damage in hypertensive patients: a consensus article from the European Association of Cardiovascular Imaging, the European Society of Cardiology Council on Hypertension and the European Society of Hypertension. J Hypertens. 2017;35(9):1727–41.
50. Phan K, Mitchell P, Liew G, et al. Relationship between macular and retinal diseases with prevalent atrial fibrillation—an analysis of the Australian Heart Eye Study. Intl J Cardiol. 2015;178:96–8.
51. Pinede L, Duhaut P, Loire R. Clinical presentation of left atrial cardiac myxoma: a series of 112 consecutive cases. Medicine (Baltimore). 2001;80:159–72.
52. Ponto KA, Elbaz H, Peto T, et al. Prevalence and risk factors of retinal vein occlusion: the Gutenberg Health Study. J Thromb Haemost JTH. 2015;13:1254–63.
53. Pristipino C, Sievert H, D'Ascenzo F. European position paper on the management of patients with patent foramen ovale. General approach and left circulation thromboembolism. EuroIntervention. 2018. pii:EIJ-D-18-00622.
54. Rafuse PE, Nicolle DA, Hutnik CM, et al. Left atrial myxoma causing ophthalmic artery occlusion. Eye. 1997;11(1):25–9.
55. Ramonas KM, Freilich BD. Iris abscess as an unusual presentation of endogenous endophthalmitis in a patient with bacterial endocarditis. Am J Ophthalmol. 2003;135(2):228–9.
56. Romem M, Glasul Z. Late iris abscess after cataract extraction. Am J Ophthalmol. 1977;84(1):120–1.
57. Sabanis N, Zagkotsis G, Krikos VD, et al. Central retinal artery occlusion secondary to patent foramen ovale: the unexpected journey of a paradoxical embolus. Cureus. 2020;12(7):e9496.
58. Samanidis G, Khoury M, Balanika M, et al. Current challenges in the diagnosis and treatment of cardiac myxoma. Kardiol Pol. 2020;78(4):269–77.
59. Schmidt D, Hetzel A, Geibel-Zehender A. Retinal arterial occlusion due to embolism of suspected cardiac tumors—report on two patients and review of the topic. Eur J Med Res. 2005;10(7):296–304.
60. Steffel J, Verhamme P, Potpara TS, Albaladejo P, Antz M, Desteghe L, Georg Haeusler K, Oldgren J, Reinecke H, Roldan-Schilling V, Rowell N, Sinnaeve P, Collins R, Camm AJ, Heidbüchel H; ESC Scientific Document Group. The 2018 European Heart Rhythm Association Practical Guide on the use of non-vitamin K antagonist oral anticoagulants in patients with atrial fibrillation: executive summary. Europace. 2018 Aug 1;20(8):1231–1242.
61. Steuber C, Panzner B, Steuber T, et al. Open foramen ovale in patients with arterial vascular occlusions of the retina and optic nerve. Ophthalmologe. 1997;94:871–6.
62. Stokes DW, O'Day DM. Iris nodule and intralenticular abscess associated with Propionibacterium acnes endophthalmitis. Arch Ophthalmol. 1992;110(7):921–2.
63. Wathek C, Kharrat O, Maalej A, et al. Ophthalmic artery occlusion as a complication of infectious endocarditis. J Fr Ophthalmol. 2014;37(10):e161–3.
64. Wieder MS, Blace N, Szlechter MM, et al. Central retinal artery occlusion associated with patent foramen ovale:a case report and literature review. Arq Bras Oftalmol. 2021;84(5):494–8.
65. Williams ZR. Carotid-cavernous fistulae. Int Ophthalmol Clin. 2018;58(2):271–94.
66. Williams B, Mancia G, Spiering W, et al. 2018 ESC/ESH guidelines for the management of arterial hypertension. Eur Heart J. 2018;39:3021–104.
67. Wong TY, Mitchell P. Hypertensive retinopathy. N Engl J Med. 2004;351(22):2310–7.

Blood Diseases

Alexandr Stepanov, Jakub Radocha, and Veronika Matuskova

1 Anaemia

Anaemia is one of the most common diseases in the general population today. It is generally defined as a disease resulting from a decrease in haemoglobin concentration below 135 g/L in men and below 120 g/L in women.

Classification

Anaemias can be classified according to morphological or pathophysiological criteria, which may complement each other in the diagnosis [55].

The morphological classification is based on the morphology of red blood cells, namely their measurable parameters, especially:

- Mean Corpuscular Volume (MCV)

A. Stepanov (✉)
Department of Ophthalmology, Klaudian's Hospital, Vaclava Klementa 147, 293 01 Mlada Boleslav, Czech Republic
e-mail: stepanov.doctor@gmail.com

J. Radocha
4th Department of Internal Medicine - Hematology, University Hospital and Faculty of Medicine of Charles University in Hradec Králové, Sokolska 581, 500 05 Hradec Králové, Czech Republic
e-mail: jakub.radocha@fnhk.cz

V. Matuskova
Department of Ophthalmology, University Hospital Brno, Jihlavská 340/20, 625 00 Brno, Czech Republic
e-mail: v.matuskova@email.cz

A. Stepanov
Third Faculty of Medicine in Prague, Charles University, Ruska 2411, 100 00 Prague, Czech Republic

Department of Ophthalmology, University Hospital and Faculty of Medicine of Charles University in Hradec Kralove, Sokolska 581, 500 05 Hradec Kralove, Czech Republic

© The Author(s), under exclusive license to Springer Nature Switzerland AG 2024
A. Stepanov and J. Studnicka (eds.), *Ocular Manifestations of Systemic Diseases*,
https://doi.org/10.1007/978-3-031-58592-0_2

- Mean Corpuscular Haemoglobin (MCH)
- Mean Cell Haemoglobin Concentration (MCHC)
- Red cell distribution width (RDW).

According to MCV values, anaemias are divided into normo-, micro- and macrocytic. According to the MCHC values, they are divided into normo-, hypo- and hyperchromic anaemias, and according to the RDW values, into anaemias with a homogeneous distribution of erythrocytes (i.e. all red blood cells are similar in size) and anaemias with pathological anisocytosis (i.e. red blood cells show atypical variability in size) (Table 1).

The pathophysiological classification divides anaemic conditions into 4 groups, which are:

- Anaemia from impaired haematopoiesis
- Anaemia from increased erythrocyte destruction (haemolytic)
- Anaemia from blood loss (post-haemorrhagic)
- Anaemia of combined aetiology.

Both classifications of anaemias are an essential basis for the diagnostic and therapeutic process.

Clinical presentation

Clinical symptoms can be divided into nonspecific and specific. Nonspecific subjective manifestations of anaemia include fatigue, malaise, weakness, dizziness, tinnitus, impaired concentration, appetite loss, weight loss, shortness of breath on exertion, chest pain, palpitations. The objective findings are dominated by pallor of the skin and mucous membranes, including the conjunctivae, tachycardia, and tachypnoea may be present. However, there are also clinical signs specific to a certain type of anaemia, which are an integral part of the clinical presentation. For example, brittle, striated to spoon-shaped nails, angular cheilitis or glossitis are specific manifestations of iron deficiency anaemia. Jaundice accompanies haemolytic anaemia. All these manifestations should always be evaluated in relation to the general state of health.

Table 1 Classification of CLL

Stage according to Rai	
0	Lymphocytosis
I	Lymphocytosis + lymphadenopathy
II	Lymphocytosis + spleno- or hepatomegaly
III	Lymphocytosis + anaemia (haemoglobin < 110 g/L)
Stage according to Binet	
A	< 3 affected groups of lymphatic nodes
B	≥ 3 affected groups of lymphatic nodes
C	Anaemia—haemoglobin < 100 g/L or thrombocytopenia < 100×10^9/L

Blood Diseases

Diagnosis

The basic examination in the diagnosis of anaemias remains the blood count, always performed initially with a manual differential leukocyte count and determination of the reticulocyte count (immature forms of erythrocytes). Other laboratory tests (serum iron, ferritin, transferrin, soluble transferrin receptor, erythropoietin, vitamin B_{12}, folic acid, etc.) are also part of the diagnostic work-up. Only after evaluation of the patient´s anamnesis, physical examination and basic laboratory tests can specialised haematological investigations be carried out—such as bone marrow aspirate biopsy, which are indicated and performed by a haematologist.

1.1 Iron Deficiency Anaemia

Iron deficiency anaemia is the most common type of anaemia. It affects about 30% of the global human population. It is a typical microcytic and hypochromic anaemia, which is caused by iron deficiency in the human body, mainly resulting from long-term and gradual blood loss. Women with heavy menstrual bleeding are most frequently affected. Another common cause of iron deficiency anaemia is prolonged occult blood loss to the digestive tract accompanying various diseases (colorectal cancer, colonic adenomas, oesophageal varices, gastric and duodenal ulcer disease). Iron deficiency can also occur when iron is not absorbed sufficiently after resection procedures on the digestive tract (iron from food is absorbed in the duodenum and proximal jejunum). Increased iron requirements exist during growth and pregnancy.

When iron deficiency anaemia is suspected, serum iron concentration, iron binding capacity and ferritin level are investigated. In iron deficiency, the body's iron stores are first depleted, as indicated by a reduced serum ferritin value that falls below normal levels. Thus, an important sign of iron deficiency anaemia is a reduction in the level of storage iron, which distinguishes this anaemia from other types of microcytic anaemias. In the differential diagnosis, we mainly consider anaemia of inflammation (formerly anaemia of chronic disease, reduced iron levels, normal binding capacity, normal or high ferritin levels), thalassaemia (normal or higher iron metabolism parameters, positive family anamnesis) and rare congenital sideroblastic anaemia (age, elevated iron metabolism parameters).

The most important clinical symptom of iron deficiency anaemia is chronic fatigue. Pallor of the skin and mucous membranes (nail beds, soft palate, conjunctivae) and koilonychia (brittle, longitudinally striated to spoon-shaped nails) are often seen. Iron deficiency anaemia is also one of the three main symptoms of Plummer-Vinson syndrome or sideropenic dysphagia. The classic triad of symptoms consists of iron deficiency anaemia, dysphagia, and upper oesophageal strictures. One of the unusual symptoms is what is called pika (i.e. pathological eating of inedible substances, e.g. ice, clay, hair, plaster, etc.). The basic treatment for iron deficiency anaemia is to eliminate the causes of blood loss and to supplement iron, usually in oral form. Only rarely can iron be administered intravenously. The rate of disappearance of the symptoms of iron deficiency anaemia and the correction of the blood count depends on the cause of the anaemia and on the possibility of correcting the underlying cause.

1.2 Megaloblastic Anaemias

Megaloblastic anaemias are macrocytic anaemias characterised by the presence of large erythrocytes—macrocytes in the blood count and megaloblastic bone marrow remodelling with ineffective haematopoiesis. The cause of megaloblastic anaemias is most often cobalamin (vitamin B_{12}) deficiency, most often because of malabsorption (intrinsic factor deficiency, terminal ileum disease, etc.), less often because of insufficient dietary vitamin B_{12} (such as in vegans). The second more common cause of this anaemia is folic acid deficiency, common, for example, in alcoholics. Other causes of megaloblastic anaemia are rare.

The most frequently occurring megaloblastic anaemia is pernicious anaemia (M. Addison-Biermer). This is an autoimmune disease in which the main pathogenetic factor is the production of autoantibodies directed against parietal cells of the gastric mucosa, leading to its atrophy, achlorhydria and reduced production of the intrinsic factor, which fundamentally impairs the absorption of vitamin B_{12} from the digestive tract.

Macrocytosis (MCV > 100 fl) is found in the blood count. At the same time, the MCH value is elevated (often MCH > 40 pg). The anaemia is usually very severe due to its slow progression. Leukopenia and thrombocytopenia are also present. There is a reduced concentration of cobalamin or folic acid in the blood. In the differential diagnosis, it is necessary to consider myelodysplastic syndrome. It is also necessary to distinguish macrocytic anaemias in liver diseases, hypothyroidism and a number of other causes.

The development of subjective difficulties in pernicious anaemia is usually gradual and subtle. As a result of gradual adaptation, patients often come at an advanced or fully developed stage of the disease. In addition to the usual manifestations of anaemic syndrome, there is also inappetence, weight loss, dysphagia, diarrhoea, and sometimes sensory disturbances—impaired sense of smell, taste and vision. In the advanced stage of the disease, several (additional) neurological symptoms are present, which may mimic other neurological diseases. Vitiligo may also be present.

In the case of cobalamin deficiency, substitution is always necessary. Therapy is usually lifelong, consisting of parenteral administration of vitamin B_{12}. If the cause of the disease is folic acid deficiency, it is given long term in oral daily doses of 10–20 mg.

Blood Diseases 27

1.3 Anaemia of Inflammation

Anaemia of inflammation (recently called anaemia associated with chronic diseases), is a heterogeneous group of anaemias accompanying various chronic diseases. These are mainly protracted infectious, inflammatory, autoimmune, tumour, and sometimes post-traumatic conditions, in which anaemia is caused by increased production of certain cytokines (TNFα, IL-1, IFNβ, etc.) that induce a disturbance of iron homeostasis in the body. The organism does not suffer from true iron deficiency. Iron turnover is increased, iron stores are normal or increased in most cases, but erythropoiesis is insufficiently saturated. The survival of erythrocytes tends to be shortened. It is the second most common type of anaemia after iron deficiency anaemia. Reduced iron and transferrin levels, including reduced iron saturation, are demonstrated in the laboratory. However, in contrast to iron deficiency anaemia, ferritin levels are elevated. Anaemia is usually only mild, with a tendency to microcytosis. Anaemia of inflammation should be distinguished from iron deficiency anaemia, in which there is a reduced serum ferritin concentration, reduced transferrin saturation, increased circulating transferrin receptors, reduced bone marrow iron storage and evidence of sideroblasts.

The clinical manifestations of anaemia of inflammation are usually masked by symptoms of the causative diseases. It presents with only mild symptoms of anaemia, usually with haemoglobin concentrations greater than 90 g/L. Treatment is primarily applied to cure the underlying disease when possible. Other therapeutic options are limited and iron administration is not indicated.

1.4 Haemolytic Anaemias

Apart from the fact that they cause jaundice, haemolytic anaemias are a relatively marginal topic in ophthalmology. Haemolytic anaemia is concerned when the shortened survival of erythrocytes (the norm is 120 days) is the cause of a decrease in haemoglobin concentration values and the bone marrow is not sufficient to compensate for these losses by increased production. Haemolytic anaemias can be divided according to cause into corpuscular anaemias (if the cause of haemolysis is in the blood cell—membrane, metabolism or structure) and extracorpuscular anaemias, which are due to haemolytic mechanisms existing outside the cell. Sickle cell anaemia is an exception, with numerous manifestations in the eye. This disease is an autosomal dominantly inherited disorder of the synthesis of the globin chain, which produces haemoglobin S. In addition to haemolysis, pain of various localisations caused by occlusion of blood vessels due to microthrombolysis is also a common manifestation.

Haemolytic anaemia should be distinguished from other macrocytic anaemias, i.e. cobalamin and folate deficiency anaemias, and from myelodysplastic syndrome. Severe microangiopathic haemolytic anaemia, which is accompanied by severe thrombocytopenia and is accompanied by impending renal and central nervous system failure, should be excluded. The condition requires urgent treatment with plasmapheresis in a specialised unit.

2 Ocular Manifestations of Anaemia

A classic example of fundus manifestations in anaemias is the finding in sickle cell anaemia. Abnormalities in the fundus of the eye in sickle cell anaemia were first described in 1930 by Cook, who noted a fresh haemorrhage in the retina of a patient who died of subarachnoid haemorrhage [15]. However, ocular manifestations can occur in various structures of the eye, including the orbit, conjunctiva, iris, uveal tissue, and fundus. Visual loss in sickle retinopathy occurs in up to 10% of patients [3].

Risk factors

The presence of an abnormal allele of the haemoglobin beta gene.

Clinical signs include a gradual decrease in central visual acuity (due to perifoveolar capillary occlusion, with subsequent macular ischemia and neuroretinal atrophy), metamorphopsia, decrease in contrast sensitivity, and positive scotoma in the visual field in the case of retinal detachment. In the case of the development of orbital compression syndrome, periocular oedema and proptosis of the eye may be noted.

Objective findings

Orbit

Patients with sickle cell anaemia are predisposed to retroseptal cellulitis and to the development of orbital compression syndrome [45]. Orbital changes are usually confirmed by magnetic resonance imaging with contrast. Orbital compression syndrome is characterised by facial pain, fever, eyelid oedema, and proptosis.

Anterior eye segment

Conjunctiva

One of the first described findings in sickle cell anaemia was transient dilatation of the conjunctival vessels. Paton described these line-shaped capillary segments of a dark red colour in the lower part of the bulbar conjunctiva, which is covered by the eyelid, as a pathognomonic finding of sickle cell anaemia and called them the "conjunctival sign" [45]. Risk factors for these vascular changes are decreased haemoglobin levels and increased haematocrit. The pathogenesis of this finding is still controversial, although the most likely underlying mechanism is vaso-occlusion. A similar segmentation of the blood column has been described on the optic nerve papilla in patients with sickle cell anaemia and is referred to as the "disc sign". However, these changes are usually not severe enough to affect the patient's vision.

Fig. 1 Intraretinal haemorrhage "salmon spot" in the periphery of the retina in a patient with sickle cell anaemia

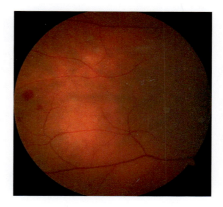

Iris

Sectorial iris atrophy with subsequent pupil irregularity may result from iris ischemia.

Posterior eye segment

The most common ocular complication of sickle cell anaemia is the development of retinopathy, which is divided into non-proliferative and proliferative [3].

Objective findings in non-proliferative retinopathy

Pathological changes in the fundus are the result of retinal vessel occlusions and neuroretinal ischemia. The first manifestation is the formation of *"salmon spots"* in the periphery of the retina, which represent intraretinal haemorrhages from superficial vessels (Fig. 1).

These lesions are round or oval and may be prominent into the vitreous. Although they are distinctly red in colour initially, they then acquire a salmon hue because of erythrocyte haemolysis. Gradually the haemorrhage is absorbed and only a deposit of hemosiderin remains in place of the original deposit. Another finding is the migration and proliferation of RPE cells at the site of subretinal haemorrhages, leading to the formation of dark *"sunspots"*. The term *"macular depression"* was first described by Goldbaum and represents thinning of the inner retinal layers due to macular ischemia [28]. Angioid streaks are present in approximately 1–2% of patients with sickle cell anaemia and result from choroidal ischemia and ruptures of Bruch's membrane. Nonspecific vascular changes such as arteriosclerosis and tortuosity are common findings.

Objective findings in proliferative retinopathy

Chronic ischemia leads to increased production of vascular endothelial growth factor (VEGF) with subsequent growth of newly formed blood vessels, complicated by vitreous haemorrhage and tractional retinal detachment. The current classification of proliferative retinopathy includes 5 stages of the disease. The first stage is characterised by the finding of peripheral retinal ischemia. Peripheral arteriovenous anastomoses belong to the second degree of the disease. Grade 3 is characterised by the appearance of newly formed vessels. Vitreous haemorrhage is a sign of Stage 4. Patients with Grade 5 have tractional or rhegmatogenous retinal detachment.

Other ocular findings have been described, including the development of epiretinal membrane, angioid streaks, macular holes, ischemic optic neuropathy, and central and branch retinal artery occlusion [4].

Diagnosis

It includes examination of the anterior segment of the eye using biomicroscopy, documentation of the findings on the posterior segment using digital fundus photography. Other methods used in patients with complications of sickle cell anaemia include optical coherence tomography (OCT) to demonstrate a decrease in central retinal thickness due to neuroretinal atrophy, fluorescence angiography (FAG) to detect zones of retinal ischemia, and fluorescein leakage from newly formed vessels.

Differential diagnosis

- Diabetic retinopathy
- Hypertonic retinopathy
- Sarcoidosis
- Eales disease
- Retinopathy of prematurity
- Familial exudative vitreoretinopathy
- Chronic myeloid leukaemia
- Ocular ischemic syndrome
- Hyperviscosity syndrome
- Vascular occlusive disease of the retina.

Therapy

The treatment focuses primarily on preventing the progression of proliferative retinopathy. In patients with severe retinal ischemia and with signs of neovascularisation, it is necessary to initiate early panretinal laser photocoagulation with possible intravitreal administration of VEGF inhibitors. Pars plana vitrectomy remains the method of first choice in patients with long-standing vitreous haemorrhage and retinal detachment.

3 Leukaemia

Leukaemias are a very heterogeneous group of diseases. The original meaning of the word leukaemia is loosely translated as "white blood". At the time the term was coined, it was not obvious to researchers at the time that not all leukaemias were the

Blood Diseases 31

same. Thus, although the nomenclature of the various clinical entities has persisted, the increasing knowledge of the biology of each disease has classified leukaemias into four basic subgroups which, apart from leucocytosis, i.e. white blood, have nothing in common.

3.1 Acute Myeloid Leukaemia

Acute myeloid leukaemia is the more common type of adult leukaemia [38]. It is rare in children. The average age at diagnosis is 66 years and the incidence increases with increasing age. It is a clonal hematopoietic disease with a complex pathogenesis. The aetiology is largely unknown, but it is a group of leukaemias linked both to previous anticancer therapy for another malignancy and to the possible transformation of another haematological disease into AML (e.g. myeloproliferative disorders or myelodysplastic syndrome). The incidence is 4 cases/100,000/year.

Clinical presentation

The clinical presentation of AML is mainly based on the suppression of healthy hematopoietic tissue. Subjective symptoms are nonspecific and include symptoms of anaemic syndrome, i.e. fatigue, malaise, dyspnoea, etc. Objectively, the patient tends to be pale. As a result of a decrease in platelet production, bleeding occurs, mainly cutaneous and mucous membrane bleeding, and the objective correlate is most often petechiae. Leukaemia is usually accompanied by leucocytosis. More severe bleeding due to a coagulation disorder may also occur in the presence of consumptive coagulopathy and/or fibrinolysis. With extreme leukocyte counts (above 50×10^9/L in the case of AML), manifestations of hyperviscosity from leukostasis may occur.

Diagnosis and classification

The basic examination for suspected AML is a blood count with a differential leukocyte count. Leukocytosis usually predominates, but the leukocyte count may be normal or lower. Thrombocytopenia and normocytic normochromic anaemia are typically present. The differential count is usually dominated by blast cells with suppression of other white blood cells.

Therapy and prognosis

The therapy relies on the administration of combination chemotherapy. The treatment philosophy is to administer induction chemotherapy to induce disease remission, which is then followed by consolidation therapy. Consolidation therapy then relies on the administration of chemotherapy or stem cell transplantation, which is the method used in most AML patients who meet the age limit for transplantation and do not have significant comorbidities. Therapy for patients who are unable to undergo intensive treatment is usually only palliative (cytoreduction, blood transfusion).

3.2 Acute Lymphoblastic Leukaemia

Acute lymphoblastic leukaemia (ALL) is a disease with a multifocal incidence in the population. It is the most common childhood leukaemia and the next peak comes after the age of 50 years. The incidence of the disease is 1.5 cases/100,000/year [66].

Clinical presentation

It is like that of AML (see Sect. 3.1); leukostasis in ALL occurs only at significantly higher leukocyte counts than in AML (the cells are usually smaller). The central nervous system is also significantly more often affected with leptomeningeal spread of the disease.

Diagnosis and classification

The diagnostic approach is the same as in AML.

Therapy and prognosis

The therapy is based on combination chemotherapy. Allogeneic stem cell transplantation is often a necessary part of the treatment.

3.3 Chronic Myeloid Leukaemia

Chronic myeloid leukaemia (CML) is a rare disease, with an incidence of approximately 1.5 cases/100,000/year. The median age at diagnosis is 56 years. CML is now classified as a myeloproliferative disease (together with polycythaemia vera, essential thrombocythemia and primary myelofibrosis). The presence of the fusion gene t(9;22), the Philadelphia chromosome, is essential for the development of the disease [32].

Clinical presentation

Extreme leukocytosis predominates, which is usually not symptomatic and may be found incidentally. Hepatomegaly and especially splenomegaly are usually present, which may also cause leading clinical symptoms (abdominal pain, discomfort, abdominal volume increase, ...).

Diagnosis and classification

Diagnosis is based on the blood count with a differential count. Usually a pronounced leukocytosis predominates, there is no pronounced anaemia or thrombocytopenia. In the differential count, virtually all elements of the white series are present in abundance. The diagnosis is definitively confirmed by the presence of the t(9;22) translocation by cytogenetic and molecular genetic testing.

Blood Diseases

Therapy and prognosis

The cornerstone of treatment are tyrosine kinase inhibitors (imatinib, dasatinib, nilotinib and others) that specifically prevents the activity of the kinase produced by t(9;22).

3.4 *Chronic Lymphocytic Leukaemia*

Chronic lymphocytic leukaemia (CLL) is a mature lymphoproliferation, unlike the above diseases. While the other leukaemias are progenitor cell diseases, CLL arises from mature B lymphocytes (there is no T lymphocytic chronic leukaemia). It is the most common leukaemia in the western population, with an incidence and median incidence in the decade.

Clinical presentation

CLL has a heterogeneous clinical presentation. It ranges from completely indolent forms that do not require therapy to very aggressive disease with a rapid course. Often the disease is found accidentally, e.g. during preoperative examination. If symptoms do occur, they are most often nodal enlargement in any location (which may be associated with compression of surrounding organs in large-scale disease), splenomegaly (abdominal pain and pressure) and symptoms caused by thrombocytopenia and anaemia in aggressive or advanced disease [21].

Diagnosis and classification

Diagnosis is based on blood counts, which are usually dominated by isolated leukocytosis, which can be extreme and is usually asymptomatic. The differential leukocyte count is dominated by mature lymphocytes. The diagnosis is confirmed by flowcytometric examination of peripheral blood, which is sufficient to diagnose CLL.

Therapy and prognosis

Therapy of early stages of CLL consists only of observation of patients (watch and wait strategy). Indications for treatment are advanced stages (III and IV), presence of significant lymphadenopathy (bulky disease), presence of B symptoms or rapid doubling time of leukocyte count. Treatment relies on the administration of combination chemoimmunotherapy, usually an anti-CD20 monoclonal antibody (most commonly rituximab) together with fludarabine and cyclophosphamide. Newer molecules in CLL therapy are more targeted molecules, which include Bruton's kinase inhibitors (ibrutinib), PI3K kinase inhibitors (idelalisib) and BCL-2 inhibitors (venetoclax).

4 Ocular Manifestations of Leukaemia

Currently, the incidence of ocular complications of leukaemia ranges from 9 to 90%, with primary leukemic infiltration occurring in 3% of patients, leukaemia-related findings in 39% and unrelated abnormalities in 20% [51, 57]. The ocular manifestations of leukaemia can be divided into primary (leukemic infiltrates), secondary (especially in anaemia, thrombocytopenia and blood hyperviscosity) related to the treatment of the underlying disease and manifestations of opportunistic infections [51, 57]. In leukemic patients, it may be difficult to distinguish between inflammatory and leukemic infiltration of ocular tissues. Classic signs of inflammation are often absent, due to immunosuppression of the patient.

Risk factors

- Previous cancer treatment
- Exposure to ionising radiation
- Some genetic diseases, such as Down syndrome, are associated with an increased risk of developing acute leukaemia
- Family anamnesis of acute leukaemia.

Clinical signs include a gradual decline in central visual acuity, contrast sensitivity and positive scotoma in the visual field associated with macular or optic nerve involvement. In the case of orbital infiltration, painful rapidly developing protrusion of the eyeball, eyelid oedema and conjunctival chemosis may be noted. Secondary complications of leukaemia are related to the growth of newly formed blood vessels and are manifested by vitreous haemorrhage, secondary glaucoma, etc.

Objective findings

Anterior eye segment

Infiltration of iris tissue causes diffuse thickening associated with crypt disappearance or nodular thickening of the iris with nodule formation at the pupil margin [61]. In more extensive infiltration of iris tissue, leukemic cells penetrate the anterior chamber to form a pseudohypopyon. Infiltration of the ventricular angle may manifest as an increase in intraocular pressure with the development of secondary glaucoma. In addition, orbital infiltration can be caused by all types of leukaemia, however, orbital involvement is more common in acute leukaemia than in chronic leukaemia and occurs more frequently in the lymphoid type than in the myeloid type. Avascular tissues of the lens are not primarily affected.

Posterior eye segment

Objective findings on the ocular fundus in *acute leukaemias* include dilatation and tortuosity of the veins, flame or patchy intraretinal haemorrhages with a typical pale centre, consisting of aggregates of leukocytes or platelets (Roth spots) (Fig. 2) [20, 61].

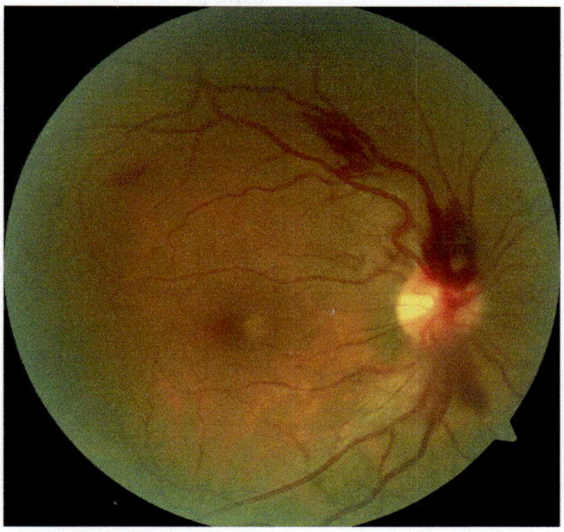

Blood Diseases

Fig. 2 Leukemic retinopathy. Numerous plaque haemorrhages, Roth spots, soft exudates, and preretinal haemorrhages

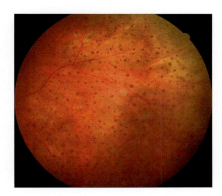

Fig. 3 RPE cell migration and hypertrophy in a patient with myeloid leukaemia. *Note* used with permission of Veronika Löfflerova, MD

The incidence of haemorrhages has been shown to correlate with the degree of thrombocytopenia. Other findings include soft exudates, hypertrophy, atrophy, or migration of RPE cells (Fig. 3) with subsequent photoreceptor atrophy and, in some cases, neuroretinal ablation.

In some cases, leukemic infiltration of the optic nerve, neuroretina, choroid, and vitreous can be noted (Fig. 4).

The intraocular complications of *CML* are in most cases mild, until the disease becomes acute leukaemia. The typical findings, unlike other leukaemias, are zones of capillary nonperfusion, microaneurysms in the midperiphery as a manifestation of chronic leukocytosis and a consequence of vascular wall disorders [51]. In severe cases, there is growth of newly formed vessels (Fig. 5A, B).

Optic disc oedema occurs as a complication of treatment of chronic myeloid leukaemia with imatinib, or as a manifestation of iatrogenic infection after bone marrow transplantation. Manifestations of choroidal infiltration, which is most affected, are best detected by ultrasonography as diffuse thickening.

Fig. 4 Acute myeloid leukaemia, leukemic infiltration of neuroretina

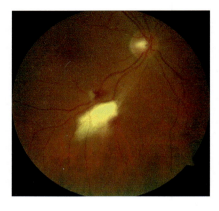

Fig. 5 Chronic myeloid leukaemia: **A** growth of neoplastic vessels along vascular arcades, finding of microaneurysms; **B** development of massive subhyaloid haemorrhage from neoplastic vessels

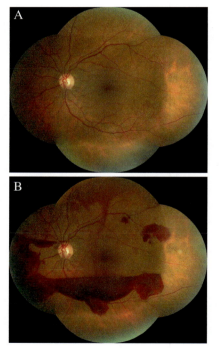

Ocular complications of immunosuppression

Ocular complications of long-term immunosuppression, whole-body irradiation, aggressive chemotherapeutic treatment and, last but not least, recurrent malignancy are mainly seen in the anterior segment and include manifestations such as dry eye syndrome, pseudomembranous conjunctivitis, bacterial and viral conjunctivitis, sterile or infectious corneal ulcer and cataract development. In the posterior segment

Blood Diseases

of the eye, manifestations of immunosuppression and haematological disproportions are less frequent but very severe and sight threatening [51]. These are mainly opportunistic infections of the eye, most commonly cytomegalovirus chorioretinitis. Patients with acute leukaemia undergoing intensive chemotherapy are also the most at-risk group for developing invasive mycotic infections caused by both yeasts and filamentous fungi.

Diagnosis

It includes examination of the anterior eye segment using biomicroscopy, and the posterior segment using digital fundus photography. Other methods used in patients with complications of leukaemia include FAG to identify zones of retinal ischemia and, in advanced cases, to visualise microaneurysms and newly formed vessels.

Differential diagnosis

- Diabetic retinopathy
- Hypertonic retinopathy
- Sarcoidosis
- Retinopathy in polycythemia vera
- Ocular ischemic syndrome
- Hyperviscosity syndrome
- Vascular occlusive disease of the retina.

Therapy

The basis of treatment is to compensate for the underlying disease. In patients with severe retinal ischemia and with signs of neovascularisation, it is necessary to initiate early panretinal laser photocoagulation with possible intravitreal administration of VEGF inhibitors. In the case of neovascularisation—treatment is aimed at possible complications (neovascular glaucoma, vitreous haemorrhage, etc.).

5 Multiple Myeloma

Monoclonal gammopathies are a highly heterogeneous group of clonal haematopoietic diseases of the bone marrow originating from plasma cells. The primary function of these cells under normal circumstances is the production of antibodies. In the case of clonal evolution, the cells produce monoclonal immunoglobulin (MIG), a paraprotein. It is the presence of paraprotein in the patient's serum or urine that is the basic characteristic of this group of diseases. Multiple myeloma (MM), the second most common haematological malignancy, is a highly genetically heterogeneous and unstable disease, whose clinical spectrum ranges from indolent slow-growing solitary tumours (solitary bone plasmacytoma and solitary extramedullary plasmacytoma) to highly genetically unstable plasma cell leukaemia with a very rapid malignant course and a poor prognosis for patients. The median age of onset is in the 6th decade, specifically 67 years, but patients younger than 50 years are no exception. Conversely, the incidence of the disease under the age of 40 is very rare. There is a slight male to female preponderance, with a ratio of 1.1:1.

Clinical presentation

In addition to the general symptoms of malignant disease (loss of appetite, weight loss, …), anaemia and bone disease, sometimes isolated renal failure and hypercalcaemia are the usual initial presentations. Thus, the first manifestation of the disease is very often back pain, most often in the lower back, which may initially make differential diagnosis difficult. Some patients with high MIG concentrations may have initial manifestations of hyperviscosity syndrome (vertigo, tinnitus, visual disturbances, cardiac decompensation, respiratory insufficiency, manifestations of cerebral and myocardial ischemia, etc.). In the protracted course of the disease, additional organ involvement is usually added and the disease reaches a refractory incurable phase after years of duration.

Diagnosis and classification

The diagnosis of multiple myeloma is based on the detection of MIG or free light chains in serum, bone marrow examination and exclusion/confirmation of organ involvement. Thus, the standard is a blood count, which is dominated by normocytic normochromic anaemia. Other blood series tend to be normal, including differential count. Serum biochemical examination may reveal hypercalcaemia and signs of renal failure. Complementary imaging is necessary. The gold standard today is a low-dose CT scan of the entire skeleton, or a PET/CT scan. The diagnostic classification used today follows the International Myeloma Working Group (IMWG) definition (Table 2).

In the absence of organ manifestations, we speak of the asymptomatic or smouldering multiple myeloma. If organ involvement is present, we speak of symptomatic multiple myeloma and treatment is indicated. Interesting and new is the introduction

Table 2 Diagnostic criteria for MM according to IMWG 2014

MGUS	Smoldering myeloma	Active myeloma
Risk of progression 1% per year	Risk of progression 10% per year	
Asymptomatic MIG < 30 g/L Plasma cells < 10% No CRAB criteria	Asymptomatic MIG ≥ 30 g/L and/or Plasma cells 10–60% No CRAB criteria No markers of malignancy	May or may not have symptoms MIG in serum or urine and/or ≥ 10% plasma cells in the KD Presence of CRAB criteria or presence of malignancy markers: • > 60% plasma cells • FLCr > 100 • 2 or more focal lesions on MRI ≥ 5 mm (in KD)

Blood Diseases 39

of the biomarkers of malignancy, where we indicate for therapy already myeloma, apparently asymptomatic, with a rapid risk of progression to symptomatic disease.

Therapy and prognosis

MM is a disease with a very low chance of recovery. Currently, treatment is indicated for symptomatic multiple myeloma, while asymptomatic myelomas are indicated for a "watch and wait" strategy.

Until the 1960s, treatment of multiple myeloma was only symptomatic. Since the 1960s, melphalan has been used together with corticosteroids as the basis of MM therapy, which has revolutionised the prognosis of patients. Autologous stem cell transplantation was introduced in the second half of the 1990s. In the late 1990s and the beginning of the new millennium, several drugs emerged that have by now almost completely replaced conventional therapy. The main groups of these drugs include IMIDs (thalidomide, lenalidomide and pomalidomide), proteasome inhibitors (bortezomib, carfilzomib and ixazomib) and, in recent years, monoclonal antibodies (daratumumab, isatuximab).

Supportive therapy plays a crucial role in the treatment of multiple myeloma. With an emphasis on bone involvement and the risk of skeletal fractures, treatment with bisphosphonates, primarily zoledronate, is indicated. Pain management and haemodialysis therapy are also essential complements in the complex therapy of myeloma, as are rehabilitation and orthopaedic treatment, including the possibility of vertrebroplasty or vertebral body kyphoplasty. A complementary but important method for patients with hyperviscosity syndrome is exchange plasmapheresis.

The prognosis of the disease today is quite favourable, due to its variable course it can be counted from a few months to several decades. Median overall survival in patients who can undergo autologous transplantation is over 10 years, in non-transplantable patients 4–5 years. The disease is curative in about 10–20% of cases.

6 Ocular Manifestations of Multiple Myeloma

The ocular manifestations of MM are both rare and variable. Most of them can be classified as primarily ocular, orbital or neuro-ophthalmological [37]. Two pathophysiologic processes that lead to most ocular symptoms include infiltration of tissue by plasma cells and disturbances in haematological balance. Common ocular findings include deposition of immunocomplex or copper crystals in the cornea, ciliary body cysts, and retinopathy based on hyperviscosity of the blood [54]. These findings tend to be asymptomatic and, in some cases, such as ciliary body cysts, can only be found at autopsy. Orbital involvement is rare, but when it occurs it is often the first manifestation of multiple myeloma.

Risk factors

- Age, MM complications are most common in people over 60 years of age
- Comorbidity with monoclonal gammopathy of undetermined significance

- Male gender.

Clinical symptoms are a manifestation of macular involvement and the main sign is a decrease in central visual acuity.

Objective findings

Anterior eye segment

Already in 1958, Burki et al. first described the deposition of *immunoglobulin crystals* in the cornea of MM patients [10]. Deposition of *copper* in the central cornea in the Descemet's membrane layer and in the anterior lens capsule is a manifestation of hypercupraemia in a patient with MM [42]. Orbital involvement in MM is rare and proptosis is the most common manifestation of orbital infiltration.

Another finding is *ciliary body cysts*, which occur in 33–50% of MM patients [37]. As they can only be found at autopsy, they are of minimal diagnostic significance. Other possible rare manifestations include periocular xanthogranuloma, paraproteinaemia-induced myositis or proptosis, and opportunistic infections of ocular structures.

Neuro-ophthalmic manifestations were the most common form of ocular findings with resultant dysfunction of cranial nerves II, III or VI. The length of the VI nerve is probably the reason for its vulnerability. It should be noted that nerves tend to be affected by several mechanisms, including compression, meningeal metastases, and haematological effects of myeloma or direct infiltration of the nerve itself.

Posterior eye segment

The classic manifestation of MM on the fundus is the complication of *hyperviscosity syndrome*, which results from overproduction of monoclonal immunoglobulin in the bone marrow, an increase in plasma viscosity with subsequent microcirculation disorder. Dilated and tortuous veins, intraretinal haemorrhages, microaneurysms, or soft exudates may be noted on the fundus (Fig. 6).

These changes are similar to those seen more commonly in patients with diabetic and hypertensive retinopathy. Therefore, if these fundus findings (especially soft

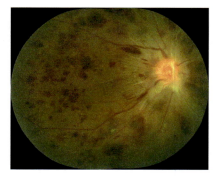

Fig. 6 Hyperviscous syndrome in multiple myeloma. Numerous intraretinal haemorrhages, soft exudates, fibroproliferation on the optic nerve papilla with subsequent contraction

exudates) are observed in the absence of diabetes or arterial hypertension, a comprehensive medical evaluation should be initiated to rule out other systemic diseases such as MM.

Diagnosis

Biomicroscopy of the anterior segment of the eye, examination of the posterior segment using digital fundus photography. Additional investigative methods include FAG with findings of progressive hyperfluorescence from microaneurysms (along the vascular wall in the case of vasculitis) and signs of hypoperfusion in zones of ischemic retina.

Differential diagnosis

- Retinal vasculitis
- Diabetic retinopathy
- Vascular occlusive disease of the retina.

Therapy

Localised ocular complications of MM are treated with radiotherapy. Surgery can be performed for residual ocular functional abnormalities. Melphalan was the first effective treatment for MM. Newer treatments include combining melphalan with steroids and autologous stem cells, angiogenesis inhibitors (thalidomide), proteasome inhibitors, and immunotherapy.

7 Lymphomas

Lymphomas account for about 4% of all cancers. The incidence is high at 35 cases/ 100,000/year and increases with age, with the median age at diagnosis for most lymphomas being 50 + years. Lymphomas are broadly divided into B- and T-cell lymphomas. Hodgkin's lymphoma is a separate entity. B lymphomas account for approximately 80% of all non-Hodgkin lymphomas. The aetiology of the disease is unknown. The pathogenesis of lymphomas is complex, genetic changes are very common, some are pathognomonic for certain types of lymphomas. Oncogenic viruses are also known to be involved in the pathogenesis of lymphomas (EBV: Epstein-Barr virus, HTLV-1: T lymphotropic virus and HHV-8: human herpesvirus 8).

Clinical presentation

Clinically, the most common manifestation of lymphomas is the development of lymphadenopathy. Enlarged nodes can appear in any location, the patient most often notices nodes in the neck, axillae and groin. The nodules are painless, firm and variable in size, with growth occurring over days to weeks in aggressive lymphomas and months in indolent lymphomas. In the thoracic cavity, the most alarming condition is the superior vena cava syndrome, which occurs when the *v. cava superior* is obstructed externally by a tumour mass. Clinically, it is manifested by stasis of blood in the upper half of the body. Swelling of the face and eyelids, facial plethora, headaches may predominate. There is a pronounced swelling of the neck and the expansion of venous plexi on the upper half of the chest can be observed. The condition requires urgent therapy. Frequent systemic manifestations of lymphomas are the B symptoms. This group includes night sweats, weight loss (over 10% in 6 months), fever and less frequently itchy skin. Lymphomas can manifest both as leptomeningeal spread and localised involvement of brain structures (less commonly, the spinal cord).

Diagnosis and classification

The diagnosis of lymphoma is exclusively histological. It is necessary to take sufficient tissue, ideally the entire affected lymph node. The histopathological classification is then based on a very rich immunohistochemical examination of the tissue, with the classification of the lymphoma into each category. The classification of lymphomas is based on the WHO classification. The Ann Arbor system is used for staging, which classifies lymphomas into 4 stages I-IV (see Fig. 7). This system is based on the extent of the affected nodal areas, with the main discriminant being the diaphragm, i.e. the extent below/above the diaphragm (Stage I or II) or both (Stage III). Lymphomas with extranodal involvement present are referred to as Stage IV (Fig. 7).

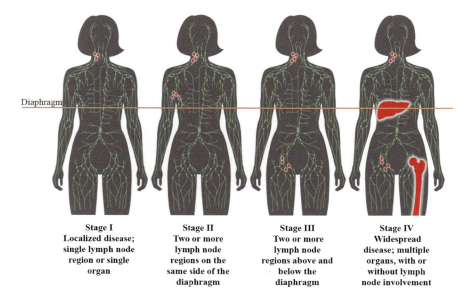

Fig. 7 Staging of lymphomas according to Ann-Arbor (With permission of Grada Publishing a.s.)

Blood Diseases

Therapy

The mainstay of lymphoma treatment is combined chemoimmunotherapy, sometimes radiotherapy. The mainstay of treatment for non-Hodgkin lymphomas is the use of the CHOP regimen, which is a combination of cyclophosphamide, doxorubicin, vincristine, and prednisone. This combination has been the gold standard therapy for most lymphomas for many years. Today, in addition, a monoclonal anti-CD20 antibody (rituximab) is also a standard part of therapy and is universally used in the treatment of virtually all B lymphomas.

The most common types of lymphomas

Hodgkin's lymphoma (HL)

HL is a specific type of lymphoma, not only because of its unique histological picture, but also in terms of treatment and prognosis. It is classified as a rather aggressive lymphoma. Clinically, nodal involvement predominates, extranodal manifestations are rare. The prognosis is usually excellent, relapses are rare (up to 10% of patients) and most patients are permanently cured.

Diffuse large B-cell lymphoma (DLBCL)

It is the most common type of B-cell lymphoma (about 40% of all cases). DLBCL is an aggressive lymphoma with rapid growth. Clinically, extensive nodal involvement usually dominates and extranodal manifestations are very common (over 40% of cases), including CNS involvement. In the CNS, it is the most common type of lymphoma.

Follicular lymphoma (FL)

A typical representative of indolent lymphomas is FL. It is the second-most common subtype of NHL (about 35% of all NHL). It is characterised by the expression of the BCL-2 gene causing apoptosis blockage. The development of symptoms is usually gradual and the growth of nodules is slow.

Burkitt's lymphoma (BL)

Burkitt's lymphoma is a typical representative of highly aggressive lymphomas with rapid development of symptoms, which are usually due to dramatic growth of nodules. Extranodal involvement, including the CNS, is common, but the abdominal cavity is most affected.

Peripheral T-cell lymphoma (PTCL)

T lymphomas represent a minority of lymphomas in the European population (10–15% of all NHLs). PTCL account for about 90% of all T-NHL. Their incidence is much higher in Asia, where they predominate over B lymphomas. It is an aggressive lymphoma with rapid nodal growth, extranodal involvement is possible, CNS involvement is rare.

8 Ocular Manifestations of Lymphomas

Intraocular lymphomas belong to the group of primary CNS lymphomas—primary central nervous system lymphoma—PCNSL. According to the Revised European-American Lymphoma Classification (REAL, [62]), intraocular lymphomas are divided into:

- Benign reactive lymphoid hyperplasia (BRLH)
- Non-Hodgkin B lymphoma
- Plasmocytoma
- Hodgkin's lymphoma
- T-cell lymphoma.

Benign reactive lymphoid hyperplasia (BRLH) is an idiopathic infiltration of the uveal tract with lymphocytes and plasma cells. It is sometimes classified as a well-differentiated small cell lymphoma. The aetiology is not entirely clear, but it is thought to be a benign immunological process with minimal risk of progression to malignant lymphoma. Rarely, it may be associated with Waldenström's macroglobulinaemia. BRLH can sometimes have a multisystem manifestation that is called the Castleman syndrome.

Most of all intraocular lymphomas are extranodal non-Hodgkin lymphomas from large cells within the B lymphocyte lineage (DLBLC lymphoma). Two forms are described: vitreoretinal and uveal.

Vitreoretinal lymphoma has the worst prognosis quod vitam of all primary intraocular tumours. It affects the retina, vitreous and optic nerve. It is closely associated with CNS involvement, i.e. involvement of the brain and brain envelope. Its incidence is 0.46/100,000. In 20% of patients with CNS lymphoma, ocular involvement is present. 80% of patients with intraocular lymphoma develop CNS involvement within 3 years. Vitreoretinal lymphoma affects patients around 60 years of age, more often immunosuppressed persons. There has been a substantial increase in the incidence of primary CNS lymphomas in recent years. This phenomenon is probably related not only to the higher number of immunosuppressed persons, but also to better diagnostic methods (Figs. 8 and 9).

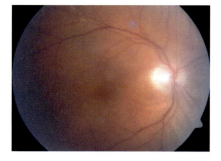

Fig. 8 Vitreoretinal lymphoma (without choroidal involvement)

Fig. 9 Vitreoretinal lymphoma (with choroidal involvement)

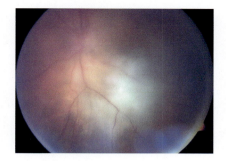

Fig. 10 Uveal lymphoma

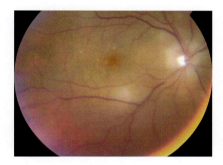

Uveal lymphoma is classified as an extranodal B-cell lymphoma from the marginal zone (low grade). It may be primary or secondary in systemic involvement of non-Hodgkin lymphoma. It is commonly associated with visceral (liver, spleen, GIT and lung) or nodal lymphoma. It typically affects patients around 60 years of age, without immunosuppression. The disease tends to be unilateral and may be associated with epibulbar involvement. It causes a slow decline in visual acuity and 20% of patients may be asymptomatic (Fig. 10).

Plasmacytoma is composed of plasma cells. It can be benign or malignant in nature and typically affects the uveal tract. It is present in the context of multiple myeloma or, less commonly, in isolation as a solitary extramedullary plasmacytoma [17, 62].

The term primary intraocular lymphoma (PIOL) is defined for lymphoma in which the intraocular structures are primarily affected, most commonly vitreoretinal lymphoma [27].

Risk factors

- Higher age
- Long-term immunosuppressive therapy
- Previous systemic involvement with non-Hodgkin B lymphoma
- Previous infection with Epstein-Barr virus.

Clinical signs

Clinical signs include a decrease in central visual acuity, unilateral "floaters" or photophobia.

Objective findings

BRLH is usually unilateral. The eye may show iris infiltration as a circumscribed mass or diffuse amelanotic thickening of the iris stroma. In choroidal involvement, the fundus shows one or more circumscribed yellow-orange foci, flat or prominent, isolated or confluent; sometimes diffuse choroidal thickening may occur. In some cases, several small yellowish foci resembling birdshot chorioretinopathy may be present. There is no evidence of inflammatory infiltration in the vitreous, but sometimes exudative retinal detachment may develop. Salmon-like masses can sometimes be seen on the conjunctiva [18].

Vitreoretinal lymphoma manifests as mild anterior uveitis in the anterior segment, with precipitates on the endothelium (Fig. 11), and rarely pseudohypopyon (Fig. 12).

The typical feature of lymphoma is vitritis with relatively good visual acuity. Abundant cells forming clusters without fibrin are seen in the vitreous [13]. The tumour cells are larger than the inflammatory cells and do not aggregate with other reactive inflammatory elements, leading to deposition of cells along the collagen fibrils. This leads to the image of the "aurora borealis" [46]. It is typical for lymphoma

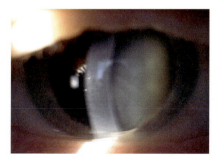

Fig. 11 Mild anterior uveitis in a patient with PIOL

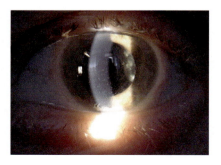

Fig. 12 Pseudohypopyon

Fig. 13 Vitritis without cystoid macular oedema

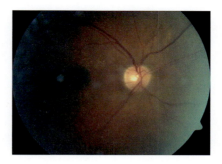

Fig. 14 Leopard spots on the fundus of a patient after IVT treatment with MTX

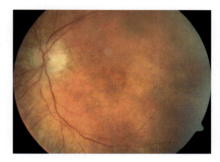

that vitritis is not associated with the presence of cystoid macular oedema (vitritis without CME—always susp. intraocular lymphoma!) (Fig. 13).

Multifocal, yellowish, confluent infiltrates are present on the fundus. They are located beneath the retinal pigment epithelium (RPE) and gradually increase in extent; sometimes the lymphoma may present as diffuse retinal or subretinal infiltration. Changes in the RPE lead to typical "leopard-spot" pigmentation overlying underlying yellow-whitish infiltrates (Fig. 14).

In the periphery, the foci may merge and form a whitish rim along the equator. Whitish streaks along the vessels mimic vasculitis (Fig. 8) or angiopathy of the frostbitten vessel type (angiocentric lymphoma). In some cases, optic nerve oedema is visible [5, 16]. Intraocular lymphoma is characterised by a good but short-term (2–3 weeks) response to systemic steroid administration (usually given as part of a misdiagnosis of uveitis).

Uveal lymphoma manifests in the same way as BHRL, but the lesion progresses rapidly and is usually more extensive. The lesion is more often unilateral with a solitary mass in the choroid. Very often the iris is also affected—pseudohypopyon may be present. Uveal lymphoma is usually associated with epibulbar involvement, so it is always necessary to thoroughly examine the conjunctiva including the eyelid.

Plasmacytoma is manifested by a yellow-pink circumscribed lesion of the choroid, often with collateral detachment [60, 65].

Fig. 15 Massive conjunctival infiltration in a patient with lymphoma

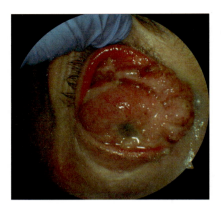

Complications

In the case of concomitant CNS involvement, neurological symptoms are usually present—headache, nausea, convulsions, motor or sensory deficits or cranial nerve palsy. In the case of frontal lobe infiltration, behavioural disturbances and cognitive alterations may occur [30].

Diagnosis

Diagnosis of lymphomas is based on the findings of fundus biomicroscopy. The uveal form of lymphoma may be associated with epibulbar involvement (salmon-like masses), both anterior and posterior (Fig. 15).

When lymphoma is suspected, the conjunctiva should be carefully examined. Digital fundus photography is used to monitor the evolution of the disease. On fluorescence angiography, hypofluorescent precincts, typically of a "leopard spot" character, are evident in the early arterial phase, while mild hyperfluorescence of the lesions is seen in the late phase (Fig. 16).

Fig. 16 Finding on FAG in the late stage

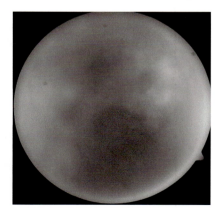

Blood Diseases

On indocyanine angiography, small hypofluorescent lesions may be visible in the arterial phase, becoming less distinct as the disease progresses. Ultrasound is important in excluding epibulbar involvement in the posterior parts of the eye. Furthermore, on ultrasound examination, diffuse choroidal thickening of lower or intermediate reflectivity is found [13, 23]. OCT is only an auxiliary method. It finds hyperreflective small nodules in the subretinal space, sometimes hyperreflective lesions can be seen in the inner layer of the retina, less commonly undulations of the RPE or deposition under the RPE are present (Fig. 17).

The key diagnostic method is tissue sampling for lymphoma [6]. Based on positive findings, systemic therapy is indicated by the haemato-oncologist. If present, a biopsy of the epibulbar mass (usually histologically the same as the tissue in the eye) may be performed. In most cases, a diagnostic and therapeutic pars plana vitrectomy (PPV) should be performed. Initially, the vitreous is harvested using a "dry vitrectomy"—harvesting the vitreous with saline infusion turned off while the number of vitrectomy incisions is reduced (approximately 500) and suction is increased to prevent damage to individual lymphoma cells. The vitreous fluid is either directly aspirated by assisted suction into a sterile syringe (Fig. 18) or withdrawn into the syringe by subsequent suction from the vitrectomy tubing (Fig. 19).

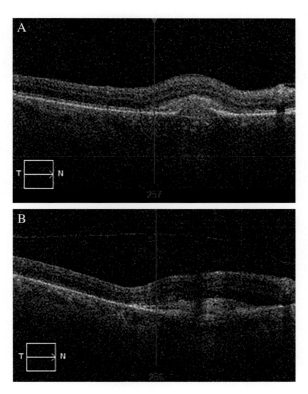

Fig. 17 A Finding on OCT. B Progression within 4 months (2.17B)

Fig. 18 Diagnostic and therapeutic PPV—collection of vitreous by assistance into the syringe

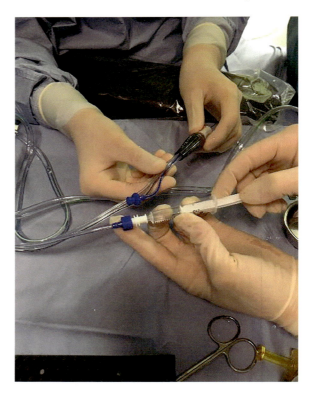

The samples are placed in a sterile tube. The main perioperative risks include hypotony at the start of surgery and the associated risk of choroidal ablation. After opening the infusion, further collection of diluted vitreous is performed. There is only minimal benefit in performing a sample collection on the eye after the PPV has taken place. Retinal biopsy during PPV is sometimes described in the literature. In the USA, fine needle aspiration biopsy (FNAB) of the vitreous is performed [43].

Sample processing is carried out in a specialised laboratory, usually only in the morning, and samples must be transported to the laboratory immediately from the operating theatre. Undiluted vitreous is processed by flow cytometry using fluorochrome-conjugated antibodies. After the sample is labelled with these antibodies, excitation with an argon laser is performed and the radiation emission is then measured. Through this process, individual CD antigens are identified (immunophenotyping). Primary intraocular lymphoma is usually composed of B lymphocytes, so if B lymphocytes (and not T lymphocytes) predominate in the sample, a diagnosis of lymphoma can be assumed. Monoclonality is also typical for lymphoma. Flow cytometry allows the processing of samples with a small volume and a small number of cells such as vitreous. Thinned vitreous is processed cytologically, usually in a pathology laboratory. It is first processed using cytospin (Fig. 20).

Fig. 19 Diagnostic and therapeutic PPV—vitreous extraction from vitrectomy tubes

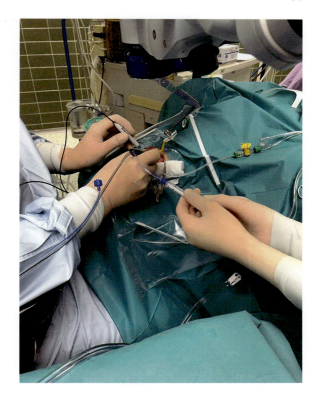

According to laboratory practice, 2 stains are used—common stains include May-Grünwald-Giemsa (MGG) and Papanicolaou stains (Fig. 21).

The specimen is evaluated by a pathologist under a microscope. Among the major problems in the laboratory diagnosis of intraocular lymphomas is the small amount of sample collected [48]. According to the literature, up to 30% of samples collected by PPV can be false negative, whereas only 10% false negative results have been described for FNAB [13]. Another laboratory method that could refine the diagnosis of intraocular lymphomas is the detection of interleukins in vitreous samples. While interleukin 6 (IL-6) is produced in large quantities by inflammatory cells in uveitis, interleukin 10 is produced by malignant B lymphocytes. The ratio of the two interleukins (IL-10: IL-6) is important. A ratio greater than 1 is typical for primary intraocular lymphoma [11, 14, 71].

In all patients with suspected PIOL, lumbar puncture is indicated to assess CNS involvement. In the case of CNS involvement by lymphoma, isodense or hyperdense lesions on brain CT are found, solitary or multiple periventricular homogeneous lesions on brain MRI. They are hypodense on T1-weighted images and hyperdense on T2-weighted images. Another option to identify CNS lymphoma lesions is to perform PET MRI [47].

Fig. 20 Cytospin to process vitreous sample

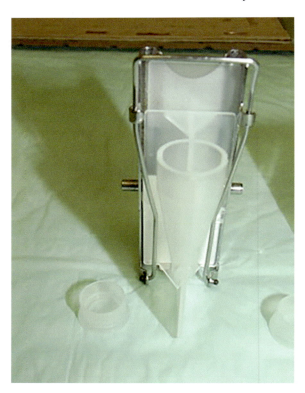

Fig. 21 Staining of the smear on the vitreous with MGG

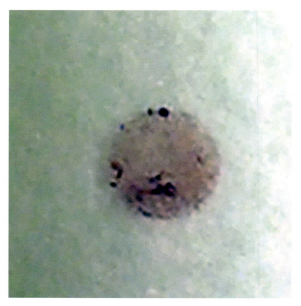

Blood Diseases

Differential diagnosis

- Pars planitis—intraocular lymphoma is characterised by a good but short-lived (2–3 weeks) response to systemic steroid administration and absence of macular oedema
- Chronic idiopathic uveitis (usually associated with macular oedema)
- Infectious chorioretinitis or retinitis (CMV retinitis, acute retinal necrosis)
- Leukemic infiltration
- Vitreous amyloidosis
- Amelanotic nevus
- Amelanotic melanoma (uveal lymphoma)
- Birdshot choroiditis (benign reactive lymphoid hyperplasia)
- Sarcoidosis (benign reactive lymphoid hyperplasia) [62].

Therapy

The treatment that affects survival is systemic administration of methotrexate, 5 or 7 cycles until remission is induced. Treatment is administered by a haemato-oncologist based on the detection of lymphoma cells in the vitreous (mainly by flow cytometry). Methotrexate belongs to the class of cytostatics—antimetabolites. It is an analogue of folic acid, which is necessary for DNA synthesis. Methotrexate, as its analogue, inhibits the enzyme dihydrofolate reductase and thus prevents DNA synthesis. The most serious adverse effects of systemic administration include hepatic toxicity (liver cirrhosis and fibrosis) and myelotoxicity (development of marrow attenuation). Another treatment option for methotrexate is its administration into the vitreous humour in patients without systemic or CNS involvement. A dose of 0.4 mg MTX/0.1 mL is administered repeatedly, usually one week apart. The most common adverse effects include corneal epitheliopathy, which typically occurs after the third application ([60, 66]).

A new development in the intravitreal treatment of PIOL is the administration of rituximab, an anti-CD20 monoclonal antibody, which is administered in CD 20-positive primary vitreoretinal lymphomas. A dose of 1 mg/0.1 mL is applied. Rituximab is less toxic than methotrexate and may be an alternative in case of severe side effects of methotrexate. Intravitreal treatment does not affect survival. Lenalidomide is another potential antiproliferative and immunomodulatory agent that has a therapeutic effect against some subtypes of (non-GC) lymphomas, including primary vitreoretinal lymphoma [26]. Another treatment alternative is external beam radiotherapy—high-dose (35–40 Gy) low fractionation (less than 5 doses per week). The main side effects include neurotoxicity, sometimes leading to severe depression [8, 47].

For the successful diagnosis and treatment of patients with vitreoretinal lymphoma, the cooperation of pathologist, haematologist-oncologist and ophthalmologist (uveal, oncological and vitreoretinal team) is necessary.

9 Blood Clotting Disorders

Disorders of blood coagulation represent a separate subfield of haematology. In a broad view, this category includes diseases of the vascular wall, diseases of primary haemostasis (platelets) and disorders of plasma coagulation. Diseases of the vascular wall fall more into the field of rheumatology (vasculitis) and will not be discussed further in this text. Although the diseases are very heterogeneous in nature, the clinical consequences are essentially the same for all groups, namely bleeding or thrombus development. Similarly, for the detection of the various diseases, the basic methods of investigation are practically universally applicable to all situations.

Platelet function tests—primary haemostasis

For primary haemostasis, a platelet count, i.e. a blood count, usually accompanied by a differential white blood cell count, is essential. A common laboratory phenomenon is a false thrombocytopenia, which is caused by precipitation of platelets in the preanalytical phase. This is not a disease and an experienced laboratory will always detect this error.

Platelet function can be investigated using several methods. The aggregometry method can be used. The test is performed after the addition of strong inducers of platelet aggregation (collagen, ADP) with measurement of the time of aggregation. A more modern test is the PFA-100 test, which is a test to measure the rate of clot formation during rapid blood flow. The bleeding time test (from a skin incision) is no longer practically performed.

Coagulation tests

These tests are among the basic screening tests for haemostasis and can be used to diagnose virtually all disorders. An overview of the principle of each test is given in Fig. 22 and the differential diagnosis of individual disorders in Table 3.

APTT (activated partial thromboplastin time)

The test mainly measures the intrinsic pathway of blood clotting and the common pathway of coagulation. It is performed by adding phospholipids (partial thromboplastin) to the patient's non-clotting plasma. The time to coagulum formation is then measured and this is then usually compared with the time of normal standardised plasma. The result is given in seconds and as the ratio of the patient's APTT to the control. The APTT can be used to monitor therapy with unfractionated heparin, but not low molecular weight heparin.

PT (prothrombin time)

The test mainly measures the external pathway of blood clotting and the common pathway of coagulation. It is performed by adding tissue factor (thromboplastin) and calcium to the patient's non-clotting plasma. The time to coagulum formation is then measured and this is then usually compared with that of normal standardised plasma. The result is given in seconds and as the ratio of the patient's PT to the

Blood Diseases

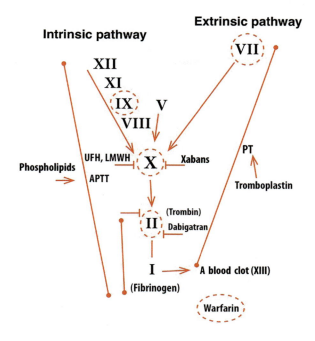

Fig. 22 Coagulation cascade, tests and treatment options

Table 3 Differential diagnosis of blood clotting diseases

Test				Clinical situation
PT	APTT	TT	Platelet count	Disorder
Prolonged	Normal	Normal	Normal	Deficit of factor VII
Normal	Prolonged	Normal	Normal	With thrombosis: circulating anticoagulants. With bleeding: von Willebrand's disease, haemophilia A, B, deficiency of other intrinsic pathway factors
Prolonged	Prolonged	Normal	Normal	Deficit of vitamin K, warfarin
Prolonged	Prolonged	Prolonged	Normal	Heparin, fibrinogen deficiency, liver disease, disseminated intravascular coagulation (DIC)
Normal	Normal	Normal	Reduced	Thrombocytopenia of various aetiology
Prolonged	Prolonged	Normal	Reduced	Liver disease (with cirrhosis)
Prolonged	Prolonged	Prolonged	Reduced	Acute liver disease, DIC

control. INR (international normalised ratio or Quick test) should be reserved for monitoring warfarin therapy only. The principle of the test is the same, but the result is amplified by a "normalisation" constant, so that the results are reproducible across laboratories.

Thrombin time (TT)

It measures the clotting time of plasma after the addition of thrombin and is therefore able to measure the conversion of fibrinogen to fibrin. The test is sensitive to the presence of heparin in the blood sample in addition to hypofibrinogenaemia. The result is again reported in seconds and as a ratio.

Fibrinogen level

This is a quantitative determination of the absolute concentration of fibrinogen. The result is usually given in grams/litre.

Mixed tests

The above tests can be performed as mixed tests. That is, a mixture of the patient's plasma enriched (usually in a 1:1 ratio) with plasma containing normal concentrations of clotting factors is tested. The aim is to detect an existing deficiency in a given pathway or, conversely, to highlight the presence of a clotting inhibitor (e.g. antiphospholipid antibody). The tests are carried out in the same way as the previous ones.

Examination of the concentration of individual factors

Almost every blood clotting factor can be tested. It is usually given as a percentage of normal values. Examination should be indicated by a specialist to verify the disease, after screening tests have been performed. Investigations are time-consuming and their results usually cannot be used (and are not usually needed) in routine clinical decision making.

9.1 Bleeding Disorders

As the name suggests, clinically, bleeding disorders are manifested by different types of bleeding [69]. Bleeding from platelet causes (primary haemostasis) is usually mucosal in nature. Most often, bleeding occurs in the skin and mucous membranes (oral cavity, but also other e.g. digestive tract). Usually, only superficial punctate haemorrhages form, which we call petechiae. Bleeding into deep structures and the CNS is relatively rare. In contrast, bleeding due to plasma coagulation disorders is usually more extensive; joint and intramuscular bleeding is common, and GIT bleeding is also common. The formation of large hematomas and suffusions on the skin is frequent.

Blood Diseases

9.1.1 Haemophilia A and B

Haemophilia is the prototype of haemorrhagic haematological disease. It is a genetic deficiency of Factor VIII (A) or IX (B). The diseases are linked to the X chromosome, so all men are sick and have healthy sons, and all women carry the gene for haemophilia. They themselves may have reduced levels of the factor, but do not usually suffer clinically significant bleeding. Haemophilia A occurs in 1/5000 male births and haemophilia B in 1/25,000. Up to one-third of haemophiliacs have a de novo mutation with a negative family anamnesis. Clinically, they have a similar phenotype. Bleeding is usually articular with a target joint (i.e. repeated bleeding into the same joint). Bleeding into deep muscle structures is also typically present. Although a haemophilic can bleed anywhere, other sites of bleeding are fortunately rare. Haemophilia is classified according to the factor concentration as severe (below 1%), moderate (1–5%) and mild (above 5%). Severe haemophiliacs usually suffer from spontaneous bleeding, while mild haemophiliacs bleed only during trauma and surgery. Diagnosis is based on prolongation of the APTT in screening tests and verification by determination of the concentration of the relevant factor. The mainstay of haemophilia treatment is the administration of concentrates of individual factors. Factors derived from human plasma or recombinant factors may be used. The dosage depends on the nature of the bleeding or the procedure and, as a guide, a 2% increase in Factor VIII activity can be expected with 1 IU/kg and a 1% increase for Factor IX. The current strategy for the treatment of severe haemophiliacs is to administer the factor prophylactically on a regular basis with the aim of achieving sustained factor activity above 1% (prophylactic therapy).

9.1.2 Von Willebrand's Disease

It is a congenital bleeding disorder caused by a decrease in the concentration of von Willebrand Factor (vWF) or its functional deficiency. It is the most common congenital coagulopathy (1 in 1000 births). Von Willebrand Factor is a large molecule produced by the endothelium in the form of large multimers that are cleaved by the metalloproteinase ADAMTS.13 The primary function of vWF is platelet adhesion to the injured vessel. Thus, deficiency effectively leads to a failure of primary haemostasis (platelet adhesion), which corresponds to the clinical presentation of the disease. Bleeding is therefore typically cutaneous and mucosal, and there is a risk of increased bleeding during surgery. The clinical presentation is variable. Diagnosis is quite difficult, because the disease has several functional subtypes and vWF concentrations are highly variable. Screening tests may be normal, and the diagnosis is confirmed by determination of vWF activity (vWF-RiCo test). Treatment is both replacement (vWF concentrates, usually together with f VIII) and desmopressin (DDAVD, a vasopressin analogue), which causes release of vWF from the endothelium, has also been used successfully.

9.1.3 Acquired Coagulopathies

Acquired coagulopathies may originate from a defect in the synthesis of individual factors, their significant consumption or drug induced. Impaired synthesis tends to be present in liver disease and in vitamin K deficiency, on which the synthesis of Factors II, VII, IX and X is dependent. A representative of acquired consumption coagulopathy is disseminated intravascular coagulation, the essential feature of which is a decrease in fibrinogen. Drug-induced coagulation disorders are the most common coagulation disorder encountered in clinical practice.

9.1.4 Immune Thrombocytopenia

Immune Thrombocytopenia (ITP) is probably the most common cause of thrombocytopenia. It is an acquired autoimmune reaction against platelets, with their subsequent destruction. The targets for antibody production on platelets are different. The most common is the primary form with no apparent cause. Secondary forms are usually seen in lymphoproliferative or autoimmune diseases (systemic lupus, rheumatoid arthritis) and post-infectious forms are also common (especially in younger patients). Clinically, petechial mucosal haemorrhage predominates, which fortunately is usually not severe. The blood count then shows isolated, usually severe thrombocytopenia with other laboratory findings quite normal. There is no confirmatory test; antiplatelet antibodies are usually not tested, and the diagnosis is made after excluding other causes. Corticosteroids are the drug of choice, followed by thrombopoietin receptor agonists (romiplostim, eltrombopag) rituximab in the second line; splenectomy and intravenous immunoglobulins can be used in acute situations.

9.1.5 Thrombotic Thrombocytopenic Purpura

This disease is a rare autoimmune or congenital disorder of the enzyme ADAMTS13. Although the disease is rare, due to the highly variable clinical manifestations in the central nervous system, we mention it here. Low ADAMTS13 activity results in the formation of vWF multimers and subsequent platelet aggregation in the microvasculature. Mechanical destruction of erythrocytes and development of haemolytic anaemia then occurs on the microtubules. Clinically, the disease presents with variable neurological symptomatology including convulsions, diplopia, visual disturbances, hearing loss, tinnitus, vertigo and many others. Jaundice, fever, renal insufficiency and of course bleeding due to thrombocytopenia are present. Diagnostically, anaemia and thrombocytopenia are present in the blood count and the schistocytes (erythrocyte fragments) are present. Hyperbilirubinaemia (unconjugated) and elevation of creatinine and urea are present. Untreated, the disease is fatal in virtually 100% of cases. The treatment of choice is exchange plasmapheresis (ADAMTS13 supplementation), which in turn leads to correction of the condition in virtually all patients. Early recognition of the disease is therefore crucial for successful therapy.

Blood Diseases 59

9.2 Thrombophilia

Thrombophilia represents a heterogeneous group of diseases or situations that result in the formation of a thrombus (venous or arterial). Thrombosis always arises when haemostasis is deflected towards its thrombogenic potential by the action of multiple factors [32]. Thus, usually not only one mechanism is pathogenetically involved, but the accumulation of multiple factors is responsible for the outcome. Clinically, it is of course essential to distinguish between arterial and venous thrombosis, which have their own pathogenetic specificities. While blood clotting factors are usually responsible for venous thrombi, arterial thrombi are usually platelet thrombi. Clinically, venous thrombosis is usually dominated by swelling in the outflow area of the vein (i.e. most often in the lower extremities) accompanied by pain. Venous thrombi in the CNS are usually accompanied by headache and variable, often very severe neurological symptomatology. Arterial thrombi obviously lead to ischemia of the supplied tissue, and a detailed list of symptoms is more a subject for cardioangiology (ischemic heart and lower extremity disease) and neurology (ischemic stroke). Each condition is usually divided into congenital and acquired.

9.2.1 Congenital Thrombophilia

Congenital thrombophilia conditions is relatively common in the population. The most common is the Factor V (Leiden) mutation, which causes resistance to activated protein C. It occurs in 3–15% of the Caucasian population. It is a moderate risk factor in the heterozygous form and a significant factor in the homozygous form (rare). Thrombosis usually occurs in combination with other factors. A mutation for Factor II (prothrombin mutation G20210A) increases prothrombin levels and slightly increases the risk of thrombosis in heterozygotes. Antithrombin deficiency is a rare disease, but with significant thrombophilia. In this disease, thrombosis occur as early as infancy, usually involving high thrombosis of the lower extremities. Protein C and S deficiencies are rarer.

9.2.2 Acquired Thrombophilia

The group includes a plethora of diseases and situations that are very common. They can be summarised into several basic groups, which in many ways replicate the classical Wirchov triad. These include mainly blood stasis (immobilisation after surgery, plaster fixation, trauma, mechanical venostasis e.g. by tumour, long flights), increased blood viscosity (dehydration, long flights, polycythaemia, paraproteinaemia), endothelial disorders (antiphospholipid syndrome, atherosclerosis, myeloproliferative diseases). Other important factors include age as an independent risk factor, the presence of malignancy (most commonly lung, prostate and pancreatic cancers) and, last but not least, smoking. In women, the use of hormonal contraceptives is a moderate risk factor, followed by pregnancy. Deep vein thrombosis is the most common manifestation of thrombophilia. It is manifested by swelling of the affected limb (most often the lower limb), pain and sometimes redness. Any vein can be affected and infarction of the affected organ occurs. This situation is particularly critical in the cerebral plexus and other veins of the central nervous system. The manifestations of arterial thrombosis are most often localised to organs with a dense terminal capillary network. Thus, again, it is mainly the central nervous system (ictus), the heart (myocardial infarction) or the lower limbs. Frequent manifestations of thromboembolism include repeated abortions in women.

Diagnosis

The key is a medical anamnesis with identification of risk factors. D-dimer testing is useful to identify the presence of thrombosis in the body. The test has a high negative predictive value (if negative, thrombosis is unlikely). Ultrasound with Doppler is a reliable imaging test. Investigation of inherited thrombophilic conditions is not routinely undertaken.

Treatment

Treatment of thrombosis relies on the use of anticoagulant therapy, usually at least 3–6 months after the event. Some conditions are then indicated for long-term or even permanent anticoagulation treatment.

Warfarin

Warfarin, which inhibits the synthesis of vitamin K-dependent factors in the liver, is still the most widely used anticoagulant. The main drawback of the drug is its long half-life and multiple drug interactions that increase both the risk of bleeding and the risk of ineffectiveness. Monitoring of the effect of warfarin is performed using the INR test. In the event of significant bleeding, the effect can be reversed using antidotes, which include administration of vitamin K, plasma or administration of prothrombin complex factors. For elective procedures, early discontinuation and transfer to another type of anticoagulation, e.g. low molecular weight heparin, is possible.

Heparin (UFH) and low molecular weight heparins (LMWH)

Heparins are used very frequently in the treatment and prevention of thrombotic complications. UFH is rarely used, due to its short half-life, unpredictable biological effect and the need for frequent monitoring with APTT. LMWH are probably the most used group of anticoagulants in the hospital setting. They have the advantage of a longer half-life and therefore only need to be administered 1–2 times a day. They are administered subcutaneously (rarely intravenously). In most patients, the pharmacokinetics are predictable and so monitoring is not necessary. Groups at risk include patients with renal insufficiency (renally excreted), obese patients (change in volume of distribution) and pregnant women. In these groups of patients, LMWH

Blood Diseases

can then be monitored using the antiXa test (3 h after the dose). The effect of LMWH and UFH can be abolished with protamine sulphate.

Dabigatran

Dabigatran is one of the new oral anticoagulants. Its target is Factor II (thrombin), of which it is a direct inhibitor. The drug has the advantage of oral administration and predictable pharmacokinetics. Indications are mainly atrial fibrillation, but also prevention of thromboembolic disease and treatment of venous thrombosis and pulmonary embolism. It is not necessary to monitor the effect of the drug. The presence of the drug is indicated by an extreme prolongation of the thrombin time, whereas a normal TT virtually excludes an effective drug concentration. Due to the short half-life, discontinuation of one dose of the drug before elective surgery is usually sufficient in most patients, without the need for conversion to other anticoagulants. The effect of the drug can be abolished with the specific antidote idarucizumab (a fragment of a monoclonal antibody against dabigatran). The drug is contraindicated in renal insufficiency.

Xabans

This group of drugs represents direct oral Factor X inhibitors. The most used representatives include rivaroxaban, apixaban and edoxaban. The indications are similar to dabigatran. It is not necessary to monitor the effect of the drugs. Due to the short half-life, discontinuation of one dose of the drug before elective surgery is usually sufficient in most patients, without the need to switch to other anticoagulants. The drugs are contraindicated in renal insufficiency. A specific antidote is called andexanet.

10   Ocular Manifestations of Blood Clotting Disorders

10.1   Haemophilia A and B

Although ocular and periocular haemorrhages may occur, especially after trauma or surgery, the ocular manifestations of haemophilia are primarily neuro-ophthalmological in nature due to CNS haemorrhage. Recurrent intraretinal haemorrhage and vitreous haemorrhage are associated with Factor VIII and Factor IX deficiency.

Clinical signs include a sudden decrease in central visual acuity (due to vascular occlusions, macular haemorrhages, and even choroidal detachment) and a positive scotoma in the visual field in cases of CNS haemorrhage or optic disc oedema.

Objective findings

Ocular findings associated with haemophilia can be broadly divided into spontaneous, post-traumatic, post-surgical and comorbid.

Spontaneous

Bleeding is common in haemophilia and causes 25% of ocular complications [52]. Although relatively harmless for normal patients, subconjunctival haemorrhage in haemophiliacs can be much more severe, with a risk of developing periocular and retrobulbar haemorrhage within 24 h. Optic disc oedema and a significant decrease in visual acuity may result.

Post-traumatic

Most post-traumatic complications of haemophilia manifest in the anterior segment of the eye, with typical findings of hyphema and secondary elevation of intraocular pressure. A common finding is that recurrent anterior chamber haemorrhage in children may reveal a previously undetermined diagnosis of haemophilia. Other complications include the development of subconjunctival suffusion, periocular hematoma, vitreous haemorrhage, choroidal effusion and, in severe cases, the development of retrobulbar haemorrhage with subsequent protrusion of the globe and risk of vision loss.

Diagnosis

It includes examination of the anterior segment of the eye using biomicroscopy, documentation of the findings on the posterior segment using digital fundus photography.

Therapy

It involves flushing out bleeding from the anterior chamber of the eye for reduce intraocular pressure. In the case of development of vitreous haemorrhage, pars plana vitrectomy is the method of choice.

10.2 Thrombotic Thrombocytopenic Purpura

The prevalence of ocular manifestations of thrombotic thrombocytopenic purpura (TTP) is estimated at 14–20% of cases [7]. Microthrombus formation and haemolysis in TTP can occur in any organ, including the retina and choroid. Secondary involvement of the cranial nerves due to thrombotic ischemia is common. Because of concomitant renal failure, TTP may be accompanied by malignant hypertension, with subsequent development of optic disc oedema.

Clinical signs include acute loss of vision due to retinal pathology, diplopia in the case of optic nerve involvement, and positive scotoma in the visual field when optic disc oedema develops.

Objective finding

Ocular complications of TTP include retinal haemorrhages, arterial or venous occlusions, and serous retinal detachment (Fig. 23) [41].

Fig. 23 Retinopathy in a patient with TTP, multiple retinal haemorrhages and soft exudates

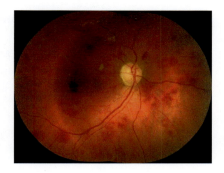

If the cranial nerves are affected, anisocoria or strabismus may be present. Papilledema caused by increased intracranial pressure, hypertensive choroidopathy, retinopathy, and optic neuropathy have also been described.

Diagnosis

It includes examination of the anterior segment of the eye using biomicroscopy, documentation of the findings on the posterior segment using digital fundus photography. The diagnosis of TTP is made based on the presence of microangiopathic haemolytic anaemia in association with thrombocytopenic purpura (two main criteria).

10.3 Leiden Mutations, Hyperhomocysteinaemia

Given the high prevalence of *Factor V Leiden* mutations in the general population and the small number of people with the mutation who develop venous occlusions, Factor V Leiden carriers develop thromboembolic events only in association with other risk factors, such as smoking, atherosclerosis and other genetic defects [9, 72].

Hyperhomocysteinaemia is a risk factor for the development of thrombophilia and is usually caused by genetic enzymatic defects in homocysteine metabolism or nutritional deficiencies in vitamin cofactors. Ocular manifestations of congenital homocysteinaemia include lens dislocation and retinal vessel occlusions. Overall, mild hyperhomocysteinaemia occurs in 5–7% of the general population but is present in a high percentage of bilateral CRVOs (55%) and ischemic CRVOs (30%). An association between hyperhomocysteinaemia and non-arteritic anterior ischemic neuropathy and a neovascular form of AMD has also been described.

11 Waldenström's Macroglobulinaemia

Waldenström macroglobulinaemia (WM) is a clonal disease, exclusively associated with the presence of IgM paraprotein and infiltration of the marrow by lymphoplasmacytic cells or a similar lymphocyte population. Thus, it can be stated that it is a lymphoplasmacytic lymphoma producing IgM paraprotein. WM is a rare B lymphoproliferative disease with an incidence of 3–3.8/1 million inhabitants. The median age at diagnosis is 63–75 years. As with other diseases, the aetiology of the disease is unknown.

Clinical presentation

WM patients may develop symptoms related to infiltration of hematopoietic or other tissues (e.g. anaemia, lymphadenopathy, hepatosplenomegaly) and/or symptoms related to IgM monoclonal protein in the blood (e.g. hyperviscosity, peripheral neuropathy). Most patients with WM have nonspecific constitutional symptoms, but up to one-quarter of patients may be asymptomatic at the time of diagnosis. The most common symptoms include weakness, fatigue, weight loss, and chronic bloody discharge from the nose or gums. Recurrent infections may also occur because of a relative decline in other immunoglobulins.

Hyperviscosity syndrome

Symptoms associated with hyperviscosity occur in up to 30% of patients and cause neurological problems, such as blurred vision or loss of vision, headache, vertigo, nystagmus, dizziness, tinnitus, sudden deafness, diplopia or ataxia.

Neuropathy

Approximately 20% of patients may have symptoms of neuropathy at the time of diagnosis. The most common neurological abnormality is a distal, symmetrical and slowly progressive sensorimotor peripheral neuropathy causing paresthesias and weakness. Other neurological manifestations may occur but are less common. These include cranial nerve palsies, mononeuropathy, mononeuritis multiplex, multifocal leukoencephalopathy, and sudden deafness. Physical examination and electromyography (EMG) may be helpful in differentiating other neuropathies.

Gastrointestinal symptoms

Rarely, monoclonal IgM protein can deposit as extracellular amorphous material in the lamina propria of the gastrointestinal tract and cause severe malabsorption with diarrhoea and steatorrhea.

Diagnosis and classification

The diagnosis is based on the detection of lymphoplasmocytic lymphoma (LPL) in the bone marrow and the detection of IgM monoclonal immunoglobulin in the serum. While WM always affects the bone marrow, it less frequently affects the lymph nodes and spleen. A supporting test is the presence of the L265P mutation in the MYD88

Blood Diseases 65

gene, which is detected in approximately 90% of WM cases. However, this mutation is not specific to this disease. In addition, baseline staging in the form of a CT scan of the trunk is usually performed.

Therapy and prognosis

WM has a relatively favourable prognosis. Although the disease is not completely curable, it is an indolent disease with a long survival. 10-year survival is reported to be around 70%. However, these historical data do not reflect the introduction of new molecules into WM therapy. Given the CD20 positivity of the clone, rituximab-based regimens are preferentially used. Bruton's kinase inhibitors (ibrutinib) can then be successfully used as second-line treatment.

12 Ocular Manifestations of Waldenström's Macroglobulinaemia

The ocular manifestations of WM were first described by Waldenström in 1944 and are most often a consequence of hyperviscosity syndrome [70]. Ocular involvement is relatively common in patients with WM, with eye fundus changes in approximately 30–40% of WM patients [44]. The incidence of retinopathy ranges from 30 to 67% [44]. Central retinal artery occlusions, arteriolar changes, capillary microaneurysms, and vitreous haemorrhages are less common [42].

Clinical signs include a gradual decrease in central visual acuity and changes in visual field when the macula affects the periphery of the retina.

Objective findings

Anterior eye segment

Changes in the anterior segment include slowed or segmented blood flow through the conjunctival vessels, subconjunctival suffusion. WM may also have an autoimmune effect on the lacrimal gland, causing the development of dry eye syndrome. In some cases, conjunctival and corneal crystals and pars plana cysts may be noted [42].

Posterior eye segment

The typical manifestation of hyperviscosity retinopathy is the finding of punctate haemorrhages in the central periphery of the retina, dilatation/tortuosity of retinal veins and the development of retinal vessel occlusion. In advanced cases, optic nerve papilla oedema, neuroretinal ablation in the macula, and vitreous haemorrhage may be noted [49].

The current hypothesis of neuroretinal ablation in the macula is related to choroidal and retinal venous congestion with subsequent choroidal hyperpermeability. This, in turn, causes disruption of the blood-retina barrier, formation of RPE tears and leakage of fluid into the subretinal space [68]. Segmentation of blood flow in the perimacular region has been described as an early sign of venous congestion. As the congestion increases, haemorrhages become flame-shaped or punctate and the venous diameter increases [33].

Diagnosis

Changes in the fundus correlate with laboratory tests. With an average serum viscosity of 3.1 centipoise and an IgM level of 5442 mg/dL, the first signs of retinopathy can be noted. Symptomatic retinal changes occur at a mean viscosity of 5.6 centipoise [49]. On OCT, ablation of neuroretinas in the macula and hyperreflective deposits around photoreceptors are seen [59].

Therapy

Macular changes respond well to intravitreal injections of anti-VEGF antibodies and dexamethasone implants [74].

13 Myelodysplastic Syndrome

Myelodysplastic syndrome (MDS) is a clonal hematopoietic disease. The basic pathogenesis is a stem cell disorder in which the accumulation of genetic changes leads to a gradual increase in the number of both ineffective and blast cells. The disorder is usually multifactorial, involving both genetic and epigenetic DNA changes that are typical of MDS. Aetiological factors include previous chemotherapy and radiotherapy, but in most patients the aetiology cannot be traced. It is typically a disease of advanced age, with an average incidence of 3–5/100,000/year and increasing dramatically with age.

Clinical presentation

The clinical presentation is mainly due to peripheral cytopenia, which is typical for MDS. Usually anaemia (normocytic or slightly macrocytic, normochromic) dominates, with all the manifestations of anaemic syndrome. Bleeding occurs due to thrombocytopenia, and leukopenia is manifested by infectious complications. Neither splenomegaly nor other organomegaly is present, nor is there lymphadenopathy.

Diagnosis and classification

Diagnosis is based on blood count, where cytopenia of one or more series predominates, and bone marrow examination, usually by bone marrow. The key to dg. MDS is cytogenetics (karyotype) testing to determine chromosomal rearrangements.

Due to its relatively difficult classification, the nature of this disease is often misunderstood and misinterpreted. In fact, it is a continuous process of development of a bone marrow disorder, with clonal haematopoiesis increasing over the course of the disease until the leukaemia stage. Thus, at each time point, the number of cytopenias and the number of blasts are used to classify the disease into a given

Blood Diseases 67

clinical entity (see Table 4). The natural outcome of all types is an increase in the number of blasts and the development of acute leukaemia. However, the time horizon varies considerably, depending on the karyotype and the actual number of blasts. Currently, the WHO 2022 classification based on the number of cytopenias as well as the presence of typical genetic abnormalities is exclusively used (Table 4).

Therapy and prognosis

The prognosis of the disease is governed by several prognostic indices. The most used is the IPSS-R Index (in the Table 5), which not only allows the prognosis, but also a guide to the subsequent therapy to be estimated. The therapy of MDS represents one of the most difficult chapters of haematology. The only curative method is allogeneic stem cell transplantation, reserved for younger patients with aggressive disease. In contrast, older patients are often referred to replacement and supportive therapy (blood transfusions). New therapy includes the hypomethylating agents (azacytidine), which can delay the natural progression of the disease. The prognosis of the disease varies considerably, depending on the number of blasts and changes in the karyotype and can range from years in low-risk forms to months in aggressive forms with complex changes in the karyotype.

14 Ocular Manifestations of Myelodysplastic Syndrome

Most retinal and choroidal changes due to MDS are secondary to anaemia, thrombocytopenia or neutropenia. The prevalence of ocular complications of MDS is as follows: intraretinal haemorrhage including Rhot spots 24.4%, iridocyclitis 12.2%, hyphema 2.4%, vitreous haemorrhage 2.4%, soft exudates 2.4% [36]. Unlike acute leukaemia, MDS has platelet morphological defects that predispose to bleeding independent of platelet count [53].

The clinical presentation includes a decrease in visual acuity in the case of posterior segment involvement and red eye syndrome in acute secondary glaucoma.

Objective findings

Anterior eye segment

Angle-closure glaucoma is a rare complication of MDS [73]. Various pathological mechanisms may lead to elevated intraocular pressure in such patients. Infiltration of the iris is seen in the stroma of MDS patients near the iris root or around the sphincter, so that the iris may be thicker and brown in colour, and its incidence is around 5% of cases [39]. Intraocular pressure increases because of compression or occlusion of the trabecular meshwork by thickened iris or newly formed blood vessels. Other manifestations of MDS in the anterior segment of the eye include axial exophthalmos, iridocyclitis, and hyphema from newly formed vessels in the ventricular angle [75].

Table 4 Classification of myelodysplastic syndrome according to WHO

	Dysplastic lines	Cytopenia	Cytoses	Blasts in peripheral blood and bone marrow	Cytogenetics	Mutations
MDS with mutation *SF3B1* (MDS-*SF3B1*)	Typically ≥ 1	≥ 1	0	< 5% Bone marrow; < 2% peripheral blood	Any except isolated del(5q), − 7/del(7q), abn3q26.2, or complex	*SF3B1* (≥10%), without mutation *TP53 or RUNX1*
MDS s del(5q) [MDS-del(5q)]	Typically ≥ 1	≥ 1	Thrombocytosis is possible	< 5% BONE MARROW; < 2% peripheral blood	del(5q), with at most 1 other abnormality except − 7/del(7q)	Any except multi-hit TP53
MDS, NOS Without dysplasia	0	≥ 1	0	< 5% BONE MARROW; < 2% peripheral blood	− 7/del(7q) or complex	Any except multi-hit *TP53* or *SF3B1* (≥10% VAF)
MDS, NOS Dysplasia of 1 line	1	≥ 1	0	< 5% BONE MARROW; < 2% peripheral blood	Any except meeting the criteria for MDS-del(5q)	Any except multi-hit *TP53*; *does not meet criteria* for MDS-*SF3B1*
MDS, NOS With multilinear dysplasia	≥ 2	≥ 1	0	< 5% BONE MARROW; < 2% peripheral blood	Any except meeting the criteria for MDS-del(5q)	Any except multi-hit *TP53*; *does not meet criteria* for MDS-*SF3B1*
MDS with excess of blasts (MDS-EB)	Typically ≥ 1	≥ 1	0	5–9% BONE MARROW	Any	Any except multi-hit *TP53*

(continued)

Table 4 (continued)

	Dysplastic lines	Cytopenia	Cytoses	Blasts in peripheral blood and bone marrow	Cytogenetics	Mutations
				2–9% peripheral blood		
MDS/AML	Typically ≥ 1	≥ 1	0	10–19% bone marrow or peripheral blood	Any but AML-specific alterations	Any except *NPM1*, bZIP *CEBPA* or *TP53*

NOS not otherwise specified

Table 5 Diagnostic criteria of myeloproliferative diseases

Major criteria
1. Haemoglobin > 165 g/L in men or > 160 g/L in women or Haematocrit > 49% in men; or > 48% in women or elevated erythrocyte mass
2. Bone marrow biopsy demonstrating age-related hypercellularity with proliferation of three cell lineages (panmyelosis) including marked erythroid, granulocytic and megakaryocytic proliferation with pleomorphic, mature megakaryocytes (size differences)
3. Presence of JAK2 V617F mutation or JAK2 exon 12
Minor criterion
Subnormal serum erythropoietin level

The diagnosis of PV requires either all three main criteria or the first two main criteria and a secondary criterion

Posterior eye segment

Objective findings on the fundus consist of intraretinal haemorrhages, Rhot spots, soft exudates and vitreous haemorrhages.

Diagnosis

Diagnosis of ocular involvement in MDS is based on slit-lamp biomicroscopy and photodocumentation of the findings on the fundus.

Therapy

In the case of the development of secondary glaucoma, topical antiglaucomatous and cyclodestructive interventions are used. For long-standing vitreous haemorrhage, the treatment of choice is pars plana vitrectomy.

15 Polycythaemia Vera

Polycythaemia vera (PV) belongs to myeloproliferative disorders (MPD), which include a group of three basic entities that are grouped together due to their similar pathogenesis. They are generally referred to as Ph-(Philadelphia negative) MPDs. They are true polycythaemia (PV), primary myelofibrosis (PMF) and essential thrombocythemia (ET). The common feature of these diseases is the proliferation of the myeloid component of the bone marrow (erythrocytes and platelets share common precursors as a myeloid lineage). Thus, as seen above, the basic phenomenon is the proliferation of the cells of the respective lineage, i.e. predominantly erythrocytes in the case of PV, platelets in the case of ET and all cell lineages in the case of PMF, with a proliferation of connective tissue and loss of blood cells over time. The discovery of the JAK2 mutation, which is a kind of driver for cell proliferation through activation of the JAK/STAT pathway, has contributed to the understanding of the pathogenesis. PV is a frequent disease (10–50/100,000/year), the development of polycythaemia is

Blood Diseases   71

typical, and haemoglobin multiplication is absolute and reaches values over 200 g/L. JAK2 mutation is present in more than 95% of cases.

Clinical presentation

Symptoms are due to hyperviscosity. Hepatosplenomegaly, which is usually huge, is frequent. Typical complications include the development of thromboses (due not only to hyperviscosity, but to other mechanisms such as endothelial dysfunction). Typical symptoms include facial plethora, itching of the skin, erythromelalgia (pain in the hands or feet accompanied by erythema or, conversely, pallor), thrombosis and bleeding of various sites (often splanchnic thrombosis), visual changes (due to bleeding or hyperviscosity), and others. Abdominal pain may occur with bulky splenomegaly.

Diagnosis and classification

The diagnosis is based on bone marrow biopsy and JAK2 mutation testing. Other causes of polyglobulia (e.g. pulmonary disease) must be excluded. The final diagnosis is then made based on the criteria (Table 5).

Therapy and prognosis

The course is usually benign for many years (even decades); reversal to leukaemia is possible but rare. Treatment in most patients consists of Hb reduction (venepuncture), antiplatelet therapy (acetylsalicylic acid), or cytoreduction (hydroxyurea). More recently, JAK2 inhibitor therapy (ruxolitinib) may be used in selected patients.

16 Ocular Manifestations of Polycythaemia Vera

Hyperviscosity of the blood associated with polycythaemia is a likely cause of ocular complications. The prevalence of ocular involvement in PV is 13.6% of cases, with the vast majority of 41.2% having transient monocular blindness [76]. Clinical manifestations of PV include transient ischemic attacks in the occipital cortex, transient monocular blindness, and impaired dark adaptation [4, 58]. A cyanotic tint of the eyelids and conjunctiva can be noted on the *anterior segment* [34]. In the case of *posterior eye segment* involvement, bilateral central retinal vein occlusion is a typical finding [1]. The retinal arteries are thinned and the veins are tortuous and dilated with variable amounts of lamellar haemorrhages [64]. Other ocular manifestations of PV include occlusion of the central retinal artery [25, 56], bilateral anterior ischemic optic neuropathy [67], as well as soft exudates [2]. Venous stasis and hypercoagulable state caused by polycythaemia can result in retinal ischemia and hypoxia. The retina is one of the most metabolically active tissues. Without an adequate blood supply, oxygen demand is compensated for by neovascularisation of the retinal vessels, resulting in vitreous haemorrhage, neovascular glaucoma and tractional retinal detachment.

Diagnosis

FAG examination demonstrates delayed fluorescein filling of choroid and retina in patients with PV. The time from intravenous administration of fluorescein to the first signs of its presence in the choroid has been shown to correlate with haematocrit levels and platelet counts [76].

Therapy

In the case of the development of secondary glaucoma, local antiglaucomatous and cyclodestructive interventions are used. For long-standing vitreous haemorrhage, the treatment of choice is pars plana vitrectomy. In macular oedema with central retinal vein occlusion, anti-VEGF agents and depot dexamethasone are administered intravitreally.

17 Antiphospholipid Syndrome

Antiphospholipid syndrome (APS) is an autoimmune disease, characterised by arterial, venous or small vessel thromboembolic events and/or pregnancy complications, all in the presence of the antiphospholipid antibodies. These antibodies are a highly heterogeneous group directed against phospholipid-binding proteins. Among the most common are anticardiolipin antibodies and antibodies against beta2-glycoprotein-1. APS is either a distinct clinical entity or may accompany other systemic diseases (especially systemic lupus erythematosus). The prevalence of the disease varies between 17–50 cases per 100,000 population.

Clinical presentation

The main characteristic manifestations include venous, arterial thrombosis and/or microcirculatory thrombosis. The presence of specific pregnancy complications is also typical, especially recurrent miscarriages, pre-eclampsia or placental insufficiency. Other symptoms of APS include livedo reticularis, thrombocytopenia or transient ischemic attacks. Rarely, multiorgan failure due to small vessel thromboses occurs, a condition referred to as "catastrophic antiphospholipid syndrome". Virtually any organ can be affected because of thrombosis.

Diagnosis and classification

The diagnosis is supported by the demonstration of antiphospholipid antibodies and the presence of lupus anticoagulans (LA). LA is a laboratory phenomenon of prolonged APTT due to inhibition of the test by the antibodies present. When mixed tests are used, there is no correction of the APTT. In general, the diagnosis of APS is then made based on the presence of one or more of the above laboratory abnormalities in association with thrombosis or pregnancy complications.

Blood Diseases 73

Therapy and prognosis

Antiphospholipid syndrome is associated with increased morbidity and mortality. Survival at 10 years is estimated at 90%, with thrombotic events as the leading cause of death. Preventive measures are controversial in patients without a previous thrombotic event. Thrombosis is then managed according to generally accepted recommendations. In terms of long-term therapy, warfarin is still recommended.

18   Ocular Manifestations of Antiphospholipid Syndrome

Ocular manifestations of APS include venous and arterial occlusions on the retina, amaurosis fugax, diplopia and changes in the visual field. Extensive vaso-occlusion, neovascularisation and subsequent vitreous haemorrhage may occur. The most common ocular complication of APS is retinal vein occlusion, with an average incidence of 14–18% [22]. A proportion of patients with detectable APL will have antiphospholipid antibody syndrome (APLS). APLS is defined as vascular (arterial or venous) thrombosis or miscarriage in the presence of two positive laboratory tests performed at least 6 weeks apart [40].

Generally, APS develops in young individuals, occasionally in children, threatening their visual and life prognosis [29]. In children, diagnosis is particularly difficult, because APS can be associated with infections, autoimmune diseases, and metabolic disorders. Often well-known risk factors for APS (hypertension, atherosclerosis, smoking, etc.) cannot be identified in children. Vascular retinal thromboses are the most common, both unilateral and bilateral [63] and can develop in patients with primary and secondary APS [24]. Secondary APS is most associated with occlusion of retinal arterioles and venules and occasionally with neovascularisation.

The clinical presentation includes a decrease in visual acuity if the posterior segment of the eye is affected and problems with dry eye syndrome.

Objective findings

Anterior eye segment

The prevalence of anterior eye segment involvement ranges from 35 to 76% [50]. This includes the following manifestations: lid telangiectasia, conjunctival microaneurysms, dry eye syndrome, episcleritis, scleritis, uveitis, and keratitis [12]. Keratoconjunctivitis caused by dry eye syndrome can cause mild or severe symptoms. The most common corneal involvement in patients with SLE is punctate epithelial keratopathy. In addition, three types of changes can be found in the periphery of the cornea [35].

1. Asymptomatic, non-infectious thinning of the margins
2. Limbal infiltrates
3. Limbal ulceration with infiltration and vascularisation.

More than 45% of patients with scleritis, especially necrotising scleritis, have underlying systemic disease, including SLE, with or without APS [35].

Posterior eye segment

Approximately 80% of patients with APS have ocular manifestations on the fundus [50]. The prevalence of posterior segment involvement is as follows: retinal vasculitis 60%, vitritis 38%, retinal detachment 15%, central retinal artery occlusion 7%. In addition, posterior segment findings include tortuous and dilated veins, soft exudates, haemorrhages, zones of capillary nonperfusion, development of NVC and vitreous haemorrhage [19]. Amaurosis fugax is a frequent manifestation.

Diagnosis is based on biomicroscopy of the anterior segment of the eye and photodocumentation of the fundus.

Therapy

Panretinal laser photocoagulation is used in cases of retinal venous thrombosis and the presence of neovascularisation to prevent neovascular complications, such as neovascular glaucoma [19]. In cases of vitreous haemorrhage, PPV may be necessary.

References

1. Abu El-Asrar AM, Abdel Gader AG, Al-Amro S, et al. Hypercoaguable states in patients with retinal venous occlusion. Documenta Ophthalmol. 1998;95:133–43.
2. Ahn BY, Choi KD, Choi YJ, et al. Isolated monocular visual loss as an initial manifestation of polycythemia vera. J Neurol Sci. 2007;258:151–3.
3. Aisen ML, Bacon BR, Goodman AM, et al. Retinal abnormalities associated with anemia. Arch Ophthalmol. 1983;101:1049–52.
4. Aug Blood AM, Lowenthal EA, Nowakowski RW. Retinopathy secondary to anemia from myeloid metaplasia in polycythemia vera. J Am Optom Assoc. 1997;68:734–8.
5. Aziz HA, Peereboom DM, Singh AD. Primary central nervous system lymphoma. Int Ophthalmol Clin. 2015;55:111–21.
6. Barry RJ, Tasiopoulou A, Murray PI, et al. Characteristic optical coherence tomography findings in patients with primary vitreoretinal lymphoma: a novel aid to early diagnosis. Br J Ophthalmol. 2018;102(10):1362–6.
7. Benson DO, Fitzgibbon JF, Goodnight SH. The visual system in thrombotic thrombocytopenic purpura. Arch Ophtalmol. 1980;12:413–7.
8. Berenbom A, Davila RM, Lin HS, et al. Treatment outcomes for primary intraocular lymphoma: implications for external beam radiotherapy. Eye. 2007;21:1198–201.
9. Bertram B, Remky A, Arend O, et al. Protein C, protein S and antithrombin III in acute ocular occlusive diseases. Ger J Ophthalmol. 1995;4:332–5.

Blood Diseases 75

10. Burki E. Uber Hornhautveranderungen bei einem Fall von multiple Myelom (Plasmocytoma). Ophthalmologica. 1958;135:565–72.
11. Cassoux N, Merle-Beral H, LeHoang P, et al. Interleukin-10 and intraocular-central nervous system lymphoma. Ophthalmology. 2001;108:426–7.
12. Castanon C, Amigo MC, Banales JL, et al. Ocular vaso-occlusive disease in primary antiphospholipid syndrome. Ophthalmology. 1995;102:256–62.
13. Chan CC, Sen HN. Current concepts in diagnosing and managing primary vitreoretinal (intraocular) lymphoma. Discov Med. 2013;15:93–100.
14. Chan CC, Whitcup SM, Solomon D, et al. Interleukin-10 in the vitreous of patients with primary intraocular lymphoma. Am J Ophthalmol. 1995;120:671–3.
15. Cook WC. A case of sickle-cell anemia with associated subarachnoid hemorrhage. J Med. 1930;11:541.
16. Coupland SE, Damato B. Understanding intraocular lymphomas. Clin Exp Ophthalmol. 2008;36:564–78.
17. Coupland SE, Heimann H, Bechrakis NE. Primary intraocular lymphoma: a review of the clinical, histopathological and molecular biological features. Graefe's Arch Clin Exp Ophthalmol. 2004;242:901–13.
18. Davis JL. Intraocular lymphoma: a clinical perspective. Eye. 2013;27:153–62.
19. Demirci FY, Kucukkaya R, Akarcay K, et al. Ocular involvement in primary antiphospholipid syndrome. Int Ophthalmol. 1998;22:323–9.
20. Do DV, Dhaliwal RS, Schachat AP. Leukemias and lymphomas. In: Ryan SJ, editor. Retina. Part 2. 5th ed. Vol. 3. China: Elsevier; 2013. pp. 2359–72.
21. Doubek M, Spacek M, Pospisilova S, et al. Recommendations for diagnosis and treatment of chronic lymphocytic leukemia (CLL)—2018. Transfuze Hematol Today. 2018;24(3):208–20.
22. Durrani OM, Gordon C, Murray PI. Primary anti-phospholipid antibody syndrome (APS). Surv Ophthalmol. 2002;47:215–38.
23. Egawa M, Mitamura Y, Hayashi Y, et al. Spectral-domain optical coherence tomographic and fundus autofluorescence findings in eyes with primary intraocular lymphoma. Clin Ophthalmol. 2014;8:335–41.
24. Ermakova NA, Alekberova ZS, Reshetniak TM, et al. Retinal vascular lesions in systemic lupus erythematosus and secondary antiphospholipid syndrome. Vestn Oftalmol. 2005;121:31–6.
25. Ganesan S, Raman R, Sharma T. Polycythemia causing posterior segment vascular occlusions. Oman J Ophthalmol. 2017;10(1):33–5.
26. Ghesquieres H, Chevrier M, Laadhari M, et al. Lenalidomide in combination with intravenous rituximab (REVRI) in relapsed/refractory primary CNS lymphoma or primary intraocular lymphoma: a multicenter prospective 'proof of concept' phase II study of the French Oculo-Cerebral lymphoma (LOC) Network and the Lymphoma Study Association (LYSA)†. Ann Oncol. 2019;30(4):621–8.
27. Gill MK, Jampol LM. Variations in the presentation of primary intraocular lymphoma: case reports and a review. Surv Ophthalmol. 2001;45:463–71.
28. Goldbaum MH, Jampol LM, Goldberg MF. The disc sign in sickling hemoglobinopathies. Arch Ophthalmol. 1978;96(9):1597–600.
29. Hartnett ME, Laposata M, Van Cott E. Antiphospholipid antibody syndrome in a six-year-old female patient. Am J Ophthalmol. 2003;135(4):542–4.
30. Hashida N, Nakai K, Saitoh N, et al. Association between ocular findings and preventive therapy with onset of central nervous system involvement in patients with primary vitreoretinal lymphoma. Graefes Arch Clin Exp Ophthalmol. 2014;252:687–93.
31. Hirsh J, Guyatt G, Albers GW, et al. Executive summary: American College of chest physicians evidence-based clinical practice guidelines (8th edition). Chest. 2008;133(6):71–109.
32. Hochhaus A, Saussele S, Rosti G, et al. Chronic myeloid leukaemia: ESMO clinical practice guidelines. Ann Oncol. 2017;28(4):41–51.
33. Imhof JW, Baars H, Verloop MC. Clinical and hematological aspects of macroglobulinemia of Waldenstram. Acta Med Stand. 1959;3:349–66.

34. Jabaily J, Iland HJ, Laszlo J, et al. Neurologic manifestations of essential thrombocythemia. Ann Intern Med. 1983;99:513–8.
35. Kanski JJ. Keratitis in systemic collagen vascular disorders. Clinical ophthalmology. Oxford: Butterworth Heinemann; 2004. pp. 122–4.
36. Kezuka T, Usui N, Suzuki E, et al. Ocular complications in myelodysplastic syndromes as preleukemic disorders. Jpn J Ophthalmol. 2005;49(5):377–83.
37. Knapp AJ, Gartner S, Henkind P. Multiple myeloma and its ocular manifestations. Surv Ophthalmol. 1987;31:343–51.
38. Kuykendall A, Duployez N, Boissel N, et al. Acute myeloid leukemia: the good, the bad, and the ugly. Am Soc Clin Oncol Educ Book. 2018;38:555–73.
39. Leonardi N, Rupani M, Dent G, et al. Analysis of 135 autopsy eyes for ocular involvement in leukemia. Am J Ophthalmol. 1990;109:436–44.
40. Levine JS, Branch DW, Rauch J. The antiphospholipid syndrome. N Engl J Med. 2002;346:752–63.
41. Lewellen DR, Singerman LJ. Thrombotic thrombocytopenic purpura with optic disk neovascularization, vitreous hemorrhage, retinal detachment and optic atrophy. Am J Ophtalmol. 1980;89:840–4.
42. Lewis RA, Falls HF, Troyer DA. Ocular manifestations of hypercupremia associated with multiple myeloma. Arch Ophthalmol. 1975;3:1050–3.
43. Lobo A, Lightman S. Vitreous aspiration needle tap in the diagnosis of intraocular inflammation. Ophthalmology. 2003;110:595–9.
44. Logothetis J, Silverstein P, Coe J. Neurologic aspects of Waldenstrdm's macroglobulinemia. Arch Neural. 1960;3:564–73.
45. Mansour AM, Salti HI, Han DP, et al. Ocular findings in aplastic anemia. Ophthalmologica. 2000;214:399–402.
46. Marchese A, Miserocchi E, Giuffrè C, et al. Aurora borealis and string of pearls in vitreoretinal lymphoma: patterns of vitreous haze. Br J Ophthalmol. 2019;103:1656–9.
47. Matsuo T, Ichimura K, Ichikawa T, et al. Positron emission tomography/computed tomography after immunocytochemical and clonal diagnosis of intraocular lymphoma with vitrectomy cell blocks. J Clin Exp Hematop. 2009;49:77–87.
48. Matuskova V, Karkanova, M, Vysluzilova, D. Differential diagnosis of intraocular lymphomas—our experience. In: Collection of abstracts XIX of the CZVRA congress. Mikulov; 2019. pp. 34–5.
49. Menke MN, Feke GT, McMeel JW, et al. Hyperviscosity-related retinopathy in waldenstrom macroglobulinemia. Arch Ophthalmol. 2006;124(11):1601–6.
50. Miserocchi E, Baltatzis S, Foster CS. Ocular features associated with anticardiolipin antibodies: descriptive study. Am J Ophthalmol. 2001;131:451–6.
51. Moll A, Niwald A, Gratek M, et al. Ocular complications in leukaemias and malignant lymphomas in children. Klin Oczna. 2004;106:783–7.
52. Murray PI, Young DW, Aggarwal RK, et al. Von Willebrand factor, endothelial damage and ocular disease. Ocul Immunol Inflamm. 1993;1(4):315–22.
53. Neukirchen J, Blum S, Kuendgen A, et al. Platelet counts and hemorrhagic diathesis in patients with myelodysplastic syndromes. Eur J Hematol. 2009;83(5):477–82.
54. Orellana J, Friedman AH. Ocular manifestations of multiple myeloma, Waldenström's macroglobulinemia and benign monoclonal gammopathy. Surv Ophthalmol. 1981;26:157–69.
55. Paulusova V, Radocha J, Slezak R. Manifestations of anemia in the oral cavity. General Med. 2013;93(1):4–9.
56. Rao K, Shenoy SB, Kamath Y, et al. Central retinal artery occlusion as a presenting manifestation of polycythemia vera. BMJ Case Rep. 2016;2016:bcr2016216417.
57. Reddy SC, Jackson N, Menon BS. Ocular involvement in leukemia—a study of 288 cases. Ophthalmologica. 2003;217:441–5.
58. Rothstein T. Bilateral, central retinal vein closure as the initial manifestation of polycythemia. Am J Ophthalmol. 1972;74(2):256–60.

Blood Diseases 77

59. Roy K, Ghosh S, Kumar B, et al. Characteristic OCT Pattern in Waldenstrom Macroglobulinemia. Optom Vis Sci. 2015;92(5):e106–9.
60. Sagoo MS, Mehta H, Swampillai AJ. Primary intraocular lymphoma. Surv Ophthalmol. 2014;59:503–16.
61. Shibata K, Shimamoto Y, Nishimura T, et al. Ocular manifestations in adult T-cell leukaemia/lymphoma. Ann Hematol. 1997;74:163–8.
62. Shields JA, Shields CL. Intraocular tumors: an Atlas and textbook. 3rd ed. Philadelphia, PA: Wolters Kluwer; 2016. pp. 525–4.
63. Sobecki R, Korporowicz D, Terapinska-Pakula K. Ophthalmic signs in antiphospholipid syndrome. Klin Oczna. 2004;106:661–3.
64. Strassman I, Silverstone BZ, Seelenfreund MH, et al. Essential thrombocythemia: a rare cause of central retinal artery occlusion. Metab Pediatr Syst Ophthalmol. 1991;14:18–20.
65. Tang LJ, Gu CL, Zhang P. Intraocular lymphoma. Int J Ophthalmol. 2017;10(8):1301–7.
66. Terwilliger T, Abdul-Hay M. Acute lymphoblastic leukemia:a comprehensive review and 2017 update. Blood Cancer J. 2017;7(6):e577.
67. Tönz MS, Rigamonti V, Iliev ME. Simultaneous, bilateral anterior ischemic optic neuropathy (AION) in polycythemia vera: a case report. Klin Mon Augenheilkd. 2008;225:504–6.
68. Vasileiou V, Kotoula M, Tsironi E, et al. Bilateral vision loss in Waldenstrom's macroglobulinemia. Ann Hematol. 2020;99(1):193–4.
69. Vydra J, Cetkovsky P. Hematology in a nutshell. Young front, Prague; 2015.
70. Waldenström J. Incipient myelomatosis or "essential" hyperglobulinemia with fibrinogenopenia: a new syndrome? Acta Med Scand. 1944;117:216–22.
71. Whitcup SM, Stark-Vancs V, Wittes RE, et al. Association of interleukin 10 in the vitreous and cerebrospinal fluid and primary central nervous system lymphoma. Arch Ophthalmol. 1997;115:1157–60.
72. Williamson TH, Rumley A, Lowe GDO. Blood viscosity, coagulation and activated protein C resistance in central retinal vein occlusion:a population-controlled study. Br J Ophthalmol. 1996;80:203–8.
73. Wohlrab TM, Pleyer U, Rohrbach JM, et al. Sudden increase in intraocular pressure as an initial manifestation of myelodysplastic syndrome. Am J Ophthalmol. 1995;119:370–2.
74. Xu LT, Courtney RJ, Ehlers JP. Bevacizumab therapy and multimodal ultrawide-field imaging in immunogammopathy maculopathy secondary to Waldenström's macroglobulinemia. Ophthalmic Surg Lasers Imaging Retina. 2015;46(2):262–5.
75. Yamagami S, Ando K, Akahoshi T, et al. Exophthalmos in myelodysplastic syndrome. Acta Ophthalmol (Copenh). 1991;69:261–5.
76. Yang HS, Joe SG, Kim JG, et al. Delayed choroidal and retinal blood flow in polycythemia vera patients with transient ocular blindness: a preliminary study with fluorescein angiography. Br J Hematol. 2013;161:745–7.

Lung Diseases

**Marketa Stredova, Vladimir Koblizek, Alexandr Stepanov⊙,
Larisa Solichova, Vladimir Bartos, Vit Havel, Eva Kocova,
and Helena Hornychova**

1 Tuberculosis

Tuberculosis (TB) is a serious preventable and curable infectious disease caused by strains of *Mycobacterium tuberculosis complex*. Tuberculosis predominantly affects the lungs (pulmonary TB) but can affect any other organ in the body (extrapulmonary TB). Other (non-tuberculous) mycobacteria are opportunistic pathogens. They are referred to as non-tuberculous mycobacteria or atypical mycobacteria; their reservoir is water and soil and will be the subject of a separate chapter of the book.

M. Stredova (✉)
Eye Centre VISUS, spol. s r.o., Nemcove 738, 547 01 Nachod, Czech Republic
e-mail: marketa.stredova@gmail.com

M. Stredova · A. Stepanov
Department of Ophthalmology, University Hospital and Faculty of Medicine of Charles University in Hradec Králové, Sokolska 581, 500 05 Hradec Králové, Czech Republic
e-mail: stepanov.doctor@gmail.com

V. Koblizek · L. Solichova · V. Bartos · V. Havel · H. Hornychova
Department of Pulmonology, University Hospital and Faculty of Medicine of Charles University in Hradec Králové, Sokolska 581, 500 05 Hradec Králové, Czech Republic
e-mail: vladimir.koblizek@fnhk.cz

L. Solichova
e-mail: larisa.solichova@fnhk.cz

V. Bartos
e-mail: vladimir.bartos@fnhk.cz

V. Havel
e-mail: vit.havel@fnhk.cz

H. Hornychova
e-mail: helena.hornychova@fnhk.cz

© The Author(s), under exclusive license to Springer Nature Switzerland AG 2024
A. Stepanov and J. Studnicka (eds.), *Ocular Manifestations of Systemic Diseases*,
https://doi.org/10.1007/978-3-031-58592-0_3

Epidemiology

Tuberculosis is a worldwide disease. Countries with a higher incidence of tuberculosis include Lithuania, Moldova, Romania, Russia and Ukraine. Tuberculosis is more common in older men.

Transmission

Tuberculosis is a droplet-borne respiratory infection, so the source is predominantly an individual with the pulmonary form of tuberculosis. Persons with microscopic sputum positivity are the most infectious [9].

Theoretically, transmission can occur after contact with infected secretions of patients or by inoculation from tuberculous foci. The incubation period of tuberculosis is reported to be in the wide range of 4 weeks to 2 years after exposure. Transmission usually requires prolonged, close contact with a mycobacteria-secreting patient.

Therefore, *epidemiological anamnesis* plays an important role in the diagnostic algorithm in the case of suspected TB disease—the country of origin, stay in countries with high incidence, long-term close contact with TB should be investigated.

Aetiology

The causative agent of tuberculosis is necessarily a pathogenic mycobacterium from the *Mycobacterium tuberculosis complex* (MTB). MTBs are aerobic non-sporulating non-mobile acid-fast rods (abbreviated as ART) with a very long generation time. MTBs can survive for years in lymph nodes, in calcified foci of the lung or in other organs. The typical and exceptional characteristics of mycobacteria are mainly due to the structure of their cell walls.

Pathogenesis

The immune response to MTB is complex and involves both innate and adaptive immune populations. Alveolar macrophages and T lymphocytes play a key role in the organisation of this response. The cytokines *interferon (INF) gamma* and *tumour necrosis factor (TNF) alpha* also play an important role. After mycobacteria enter the lungs of immunocompetent persons, effective protection usually develops within 2–8 weeks. A complex reaction with the formation of specific granulomas develops. In the immunocompromised individual, there is no effective eradication of mycobacteria

---

E. Kocova
Department of Radiology, University Hospital and Faculty of Medicine of Charles University in Hradec Králové, Sokolska 581, 500 05 Hradec Králové, Czech Republic
e-mail: eva.kocova@fnhk.cz

A. Stepanov
Ophthalmology Department, Klaudian's Hospital, Vaclava Klementa 147, 293 01 Mlada Boleslav, Czech Republic

Third Faculty of Medicine in Prague, Charles University, Ruska 2411, 100 00 Prague, Czech Republic

Lung Diseases 81

and active tuberculosis develops (called *primary infection*), which is either localised (most often in the lungs) or disseminated. In the case of haematogenous dissemination with the appearance of small granulomas in various tissues, it is referred to as *miliary dissemination*, which is often seen *in the fundus*, liver, lung, and brain. Because MTB can survive in humans for decades after the initial infection, tuberculosis can manifest itself many years later when specific immunity is reduced, e.g. by certain drugs (anti-TNF-alpha drugs), diseases (HIV/AIDS) or age.

Clinical presentation

Latent tuberculosis infection

Latent tuberculous infection is defined as a state of persistent immune response to MTB antigen stimulation, without evidence of active tuberculous disease. Isolated surviving mycobacteria are beyond our usual detection capabilities, do not multiply, the person has no symptoms, and the disease cannot spread. Their presence cannot be proved by histopathology. Latent TB infection can only be detected with IGRA tests, which are performed specifically in groups at higher risk of developing active (manifest) TB. Latent TB is treated quite differently from manifest TB, so if IGRAs are positive, the findings of other investigations (e.g. imaging) must be considered very carefully in relation to possible active TB.

Manifest (active) tuberculosis—or TB

Tuberculosis is usually chronic and slow progressing. The pulmonary form of the disease (PTB) is the most common. The classic general symptoms are cough, weight loss, excessive fatigue, night sweats and subfebrile (37–37.9 °C). A chest scan or CT scan of the lungs shows a typical picture. In the case of extrapulmonary tuberculosis, the complaints may be completely nonspecific and difficult to assess; the overall symptoms may not be expressed.

If extrapulmonary TB is suspected or proven, the patient should always be referred to a pneumologist to rule out the current pulmonary form of TB, which occurs together in many patients.

Extrapulmonary tuberculosis

The term extrapulmonary tuberculosis (or extrapulmonary TB—abbreviated EPTB) refers to the involvement of organs other than the lungs. It currently accounts for about 15% of all reported cases. The diagnosis should be made based on at least one positive culture, a positive finding on histological examination (specific granuloma with or without ART) and/or a convincing clinical presentation consistent with EPTB, followed by a decision to administer (as a therapeutic test) an antituberculous treatment regimen. Positivity of IGRA test, PCR method of MTB determination may help in diagnosis. If multiple organs are affected, the case is reported according to the most clinically/prognostically severe localisation. In the case of simultaneous lung involvement, the case is always classified as pulmonary tuberculosis (PTB).

Diagnosis

Microscopic examination

Basic method of rapid detection. After special staining of the sample, it gives a result within hours. For a positive result, a high bacterial load (10^3–10^4 bacteria) in 1ml of biological material is required. Microscopic examination cannot distinguish the causative agents of tuberculosis from atypical mycobacteria (causative agents of mycobacteriosis—see separate chapter), nor does it detect their viability.

Molecular genetic methods (PCR—polymerase chain reaction)

Despite some limitations, these are other basic and rapid (within hours) methods for detecting mycobacteria. They also capture non-viable mycobacteria or fragments of mycobacteria and are less sensitive to culture. *False negative* results may therefore occur in paucibacillary tuberculosis (with minimal mycobacteria), in children and when processing small sample volumes. *False positives* are found in patients after antituberculous (AT) treatment.

Although the negativity of PCR testing does not exclude TB disease (especially in clinically and epidemiologically suspected persons), it is part of a sophisticated decision-making process.

Cultivation

It is the *gold standard* for tuberculosis diagnosis. Cultivation is the *most sensitive method of* detecting live mycobacteria and its positivity is unequivocal proof of tuberculous disease.

It is always necessary to make a clear request for mycobacterial cultivation on the application form, as special soils are used. MTBs are usually detected after three weeks at the earliest, and cultures are reported as negative after six weeks, regardless of the cultivation method used.

The whole spectrum of samples (sputum, urine, liquor, secretions, and lavage from different parts of the human body), including samples of solid tissues, can be processed microscopically, by cultivation and PCR.

Histopathology

The characteristic histopathological feature of TB is the specific granuloma. The pathologist sometimes finds a typical caseificating (with ash necrosis) epithelioid cell granuloma. However, in the early stages of TB disease or in immunocompromised persons, granulomas without caseification may also occur. In some cases, the pathologist may also detect the presence of acid-fast rods (ARRs). Histological examination can sometimes be quite non-specific and the accurate diagnosis of TB needs to be supported by other investigations.

IGRA (Interferon Gamma Release Assay) tests

IGRAs belong among the *indirect tests* that detect the production of INF gamma *in a blood sample* after contact with specific mycobacterial antigens from the test detection system. They are used to diagnose latent TB infection, or as a test to support the diagnosis of TB disease, for example in extrapulmonary TB. However, a negative IGRA test does not exclude the presence of tuberculosis. These tests are not the basis for the diagnosis of TB as a disease. IGRA tests may also be positive for a few non-tuberculous mycobacteria or after tuberculosis has been treated properly. In practice, the most used IGRA tests are the QuantiFeron (QNF) TB GOLD and the TspotTB test. QNF is usually indicated first. TspotTB is more appropriate for immunosuppressed patients and patients with indeterminate results from a previous QNF test.

Tuberculin skin test

It is a "historical" indirect test showing only non-specific delayed hyperreactivity to antigens of various mycobacteria. It is gradually being replaced by IGRA tests and is now performed by only a few pneumology outpatient clinics.

Therapy

Antituberculosis treatment for pulmonary and extrapulmonary TB is initiated and managed by a pulmonologist, who also performs the initial and follow-up mandatory reporting of TB and works closely with the specialist performing organ-specific treatment.

The mainstay of treatment for pulmonary and extrapulmonary tuberculosis is pharmacological therapy for six months for both variants. In some cases of EPTB, treatment is prolonged or supplemented with glucocorticoids or organ-specific therapy. The initial phase of treatment usually takes place in an inpatient facility, with further treatment occurring in the outpatient setting. The main antituberculosis drugs used for treatment are isoniazid (H), rifampicin (R), pyrazinamide (Z) and ethambutol (E).

Drugs have several adverse and side effects that need to be monitored. From an ophthalmic point of view, *ethambutol* is the riskiest drug, and initial and regular eye examinations should be performed for the possibility of retrobulbar neuritis, colour defects and impaired visual acuity. The changes may be irreversible. Drug-resistant tuberculosis is a serious condition that requires highly specific treatment for more than 1 year.

Dispensary care

All newly diagnosed active pulmonary and extrapulmonary tuberculosis cases are subject to mandatory reporting. Reporting is done by the physician/department initiating treatment. If treatment is not initiated, reporting is done by the physician who diagnoses the disease. The patient is then dispensed to the appropriate Pneumology outpatient clinic according to the place of residence.

2 Ocular Manifestations of Tuberculosis

Eye involvement in TB occurs by various mechanisms, which can be broadly divided into exogenous, endogenous (haematogenous) and secondary infection of the eye by direct infection from another infectious focus. The most common route of infection is the haematogenous route, which mainly affects the uvea due to its high blood supply. A rarer form of TB transmission is the exogenous route, where the site of entry of infection is usually the anterior segment of the eye (eyelids, conjunctiva, cornea, sclera, lacrimal sac). Secondary infection of the eye by the direct route can occur, for example, by contamination of the sputum itself [2].

Clinical manifestations and objective findings

Orbit

Tuberculosis of the orbit is more common in children, and very rare in adults. Symptoms can be diverse. Clinically, decreased vision, epiphora, eyelid swelling, conjunctival chemosis, pathological Marcus-Gunn type pupillary reactions and proptosis may be present [10]. Pathological orbital contents can be detected on imaging in some cases.

Eyelids

The skin of the eyelids has typical manifestations of the cutaneous form of tuberculosis in the form of red-brown nodules. The involvement of the eyelids in tuberculosis is usually in the form of a cold abscess or a chalazion-like lesion [2].

Conjunctiva

In primary conjunctival TB infection, the conjunctiva is congested (hyperaemia), mucopurulent secretion and eyelid swelling are present. In a chronic course, the tissues may scar. In some cases, localised enlargement of lymphatic nodes is also present [2, 10].

Cornea

There are two forms of corneal involvement in TB: *interstitial keratitis* or *phlyctenular keratoconjunctivitis* [10].

Interstitial keratitis in tuberculosis is a unilateral peripheral vascularised infiltrate of the stroma. Phlyctenular keratoconjunctivitis arises from hypersensitivity and is characterised by a small pink formation at the limbus, called a phlyctenule. It is manifested by tearing, with a foreign body sensation and photophobia [2].

Sclera

Scleral involvement in TB is heterogeneous. The available case reports describe cases with a circumscribed dark red area of the sclera with chronic granulomatous inflammation and necrosis, which may lead to scleromalacia, and a form of scleral ulcer or nodule has been described [2].

Uvea

Tuberculous uveitis can be unilateral or bilateral. They are divided according to the affected structure into anterior and posterior, with anterior uveitis being more common [35]. Anterior uveitis is further divided into granulomatous or non-granulomatous according to the nature of the inflammation. The granulomatous form is more common, when speckled precipitates are observed on the cornea, and Koeppe's or Busacca's nodes may be present on the iris. On the other hand, in the non-granulomatous form, the iris is free of nodules and the corneal precipitates are whitish. Anterior uveitis may also manifest as isolated iritis or iridocyclitis. We may find a cellular reaction in the anterior chamber with hypopyon and posterior synechiae. Posterior uveitis, i.e. choroiditis, also exists in many clinical forms, manifesting for example as choroidal tuberculoma, the most common form of ocular tuberculosis, or choroiditis masking serpiginous choroidopathy [2].

Retina

Tuberculous retinitis tends to be focal or diffuse. Typical are grey-white lesions and vasculitis, which may be complicated by neovascularisation or vascular occlusions (Figs. 1 and 2). Retinal involvement most commonly occurs by the haematogenous route [2].

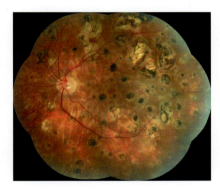

Fig. 1 Disseminated tuberculous chorioretinitis, remission

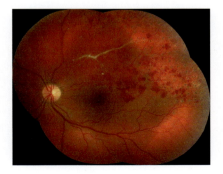

Fig. 2 Occlusive vasculitis in a patient with TB

Diagnosis

The key to diagnosis is the demonstration of the pathological agent, which can be done from a smear or biopsy (for example, in conjunctival involvement), microbiologically or histopathologically; the Mycobacterium tuberculosis genome can also be detected in intraocular fluid using PCR (polymerase chain reaction). In phlyctenular keratoconjunctivitis, a tuberculin skin test is used to immunologically assess the presence of active and latent mycobacterial infection [2]. Imaging methods are also helpful, specifically ultrasonographic examination of the eye to detect tuberculomas, or fluorescence angiography to evaluate choroidal lesions and the status of the retinal vasculature.

Differential diagnosis

- Sarcoidosis
- Syphilis
- Leprosy
- Sympathetic ophthalmia
- Herpes simplex and herpes zoster
- Vogt-Koyanagi-Harad disease
- Cryptococcal infection
- Toxoplasmosis
- Mycotic infections

Therapy

Treatment of the ocular form of tuberculosis is carried out according to the same standards as the treatment of active TB of other organs. Corticosteroids or cycloplegics are used to control ocular manifestations.

3 Non-tuberculous Mycobacterioses

Mycobacterioses are relatively rare diseases caused by non-tuberculous mycobacteria (NTM), sometimes called atypical mycobacteria or Mycobacteria Other Than Tuberculosis (MOTT), which do not belong to the Mycobacterium tuberculosis complex. NTM cause chronic infections—in adults with pre-existing lung disease, in children (even healthy ones), peripheral lymphadenitis, and, in immunocompromised people, the disease is disseminated. Purely localised forms (cutaneous, ocular, bone, etc.) often occur in association with disruption of the skin cover and direct inoculation of mycobacterium into tissue. Mycobacterioses have a similar clinical presentation to tuberculosis and the tools for diagnosis are also identical. Because of the natural resistance of nontuberculous mycobacteria to a variety of antituberculosis drugs, mycobacterioses are relatively difficult and time-consuming to treat. It is a notifiable disease (like tuberculosis) and initial isolation of patients (unlike tuberculous disease) is not necessary.

Lung Diseases

Epidemiology

Non-tuberculous mycobacteria are opportunistic pathogens that occur worldwide. Their main reservoirs are various water bodies, water pipes, wells, aquariums, whirlpools, humidifiers, and inhalers; they are also present in soil, dust, feathers, fur and animal secretions. The incidence and prevalence of non-tuberculous mycobacterioses are gradually increasing in many areas of the world, particularly in countries with declining tuberculosis prevalence. The virulence of the different types of mycobacteria varies considerably, from downright pathogenic species (e.g. *M. abscessus*) to species of minimal clinical significance (e.g. *M. gordonae*). Of the total number of mycobacterioses reported, one-third were extrapulmonary. *M. avium* and *M. kansasii* were the most frequently isolated.

Aetiology

Non-tuberculous mycobacteria (like MTB) are aerobic, acid-fast rods with other typical characteristics that divide them into several groups. The division most used is according to growth rate on culture medium into fast- versus slow-growing non-tuberculous mycobacteria [40].

Transmission

Mycobacteria are transmitted by inhalation of infectious aerosol, transfer of agents to mucous membranes, contact with skin abrasions, traumatically (penetrating trauma, rinsing with contaminated water), inoculation during medical and aesthetic procedures (contaminated tattoo ink, rinsing with contaminated water, contamination of surgical field, instruments (pedicure, manicure), etc.). Interpersonal transmission has been described in only a few cases so far and is not considered relevant in the immunocompetent population. Animal-to-human transmission is also not described. Particularly susceptible are patients with chronic lung disease and/or immunocompromised individuals (HIV+, post-transplant, on immunosuppressive therapy including biologic therapy), or the elderly and individuals with significant chest wall deformities (kyphoscoliosis). Local (especially cutaneous) forms of mycobacteriosis may affect otherwise healthy, immunocompetent individuals.

The incubation period for non-tuberculous mycobacteriosis is reported in the literature to be between 2 and 10 weeks, most commonly around 3 weeks.

Diagnosis

A problem in identifying the causative agent of disease is the ubiquitous occurrence of many mycobacterial species, which can lead to difficulty in distinguishing sample contamination from the capture of the disease-causing agent. For this reason, repeated sampling of biological material is usually necessary.

Microscopic examination

NTMs stain identically to tuberculous mycobacteria and cannot be distinguished in the microscope (they are like MTB acid-fast rods or ART). A relatively high bacterial load (at least 10^3-10^4 bacteria/ml of biological material) is required for a positive microscopic result.

Cultivation

NTM usually grow well on MTB culture media. If some specific species are suspected, the growing conditions need to be adapted. For laboratory purposes, it is therefore advisable to indicate on the application form that NTM are suspected.

Molecular genetic methods

These methods are widely used to determine the specific type of NTM. In some cases, an already fixed and stained slide can be examined.

Histopathology

It demonstrates the finding of a granulomatous lesion similar to tuberculosis.

Indirect tests

The tuberculin test is not useful for the diagnosis of NTM. The IGRA test can differentiate tuberculosis but can also be positive in cases of infection with *M. marinum, M. szulgayi* and *M. kansasii.*

Clinical symptoms are not specific—the disease is often creeping, and conventional treatment fails in the long term. Personal and medical anamnesis is important—diseases leading to immunodeficiency and/or immunosuppressive therapy increase the risk of mycobacteriosis. Epidemiological anamnesis is also essential—reservoirs, risk environment, anamnesis of medical, aesthetic and health procedures, mechanism of trauma, including skin damage. Repeated collection of material for microscopy, cultivation, PCR, or histology are always appropriate. To assess the presence of mycobacteriosis, imaging studies (skiagram, ultrasound and CT scan, or others) are appropriate, and all patients with suspected disseminated or pulmonary involvement require a comprehensive review by a pulmonologist who makes a diagnosis of pulmonary NTM according to the recommended algorithm.

Therapy

The basis is long-term (usually longer than one year) combined pharmacotherapy with antituberculosis drugs and antibiotics, initially empirically, then targeted according to the specific causative agent. Long-term pharmacotherapy consisting of drugs from different groups is burdened with many side effects. In addition, many patients do not have good adherence to long-term therapy, the immediate effect of which is often not obvious. There are recommended drug combinations for most NTM (e.g. for MAC and *M. xenopi*, clarithromycin + ethambutol + rifampicin, and for *M. kansasii*, which is also common, isoniazid + ethambutol + rifampicin). For rapidly growing NTM (e.g. *M. fortuitum, M. gondii* and others), treatment is not clearly established and is based on specific drug sensitivity results. In vitro susceptibility testing for antituberculosis and mycobacteria may not be consistent with in vivo response.

Surgical treatment is used adjunctively and in localised, persistent pulmonary and extrapulmonary forms of mycobacteriosis. It is always performed under pharmacotherapeutic cover.

The effect of treatment of mycobacteriosis is evaluated according to the clinical condition, the dynamics of findings on imaging methods and bacteriological examination. For example, diseases caused by *M. kansasii* have *a good prognosis*, *a serious* prognosis can be observed in disseminated forms of MAC (*M. avium +intracelular*) infection, while *a very serious or even fatal* prognosis can be observed in *M. abscessus* infection.

Dispensary care

The dispensary care is similar to that of TB. It is carried out at the catchment Pneumophthalmology unit according to the place of residence. The disease is subject to a mandatory reporting system, similar to TB. Reporting is done by the physician who first detected the disease, in collaboration with the locally competent outpatient Pneumophthysiology facility.

4 Ocular Manifestations of Atypical Mycobacterioses

Predisposing factors for ocular infection with atypical mycobacteriosis include a history of previous ocular surgery or trauma. Early diagnosis and initiation of treatment are needed to achieve good visual outcome.

Objective findings

Eyelids and periocular area

On the eyelids and in the periocular region, atypical mycobacteriosis is manifested by solitary or multiple nodules with purulent contents, usually located in the vicinity of a previous surgical or traumatic wound. The area around the nodules is oedematous, and in some cases, cellulitis may be present [21].

Tear ducts

Tear tract involvement is manifested by redness and swelling of the eyelids, with a maximum around the tear points, from which purulent secretions may ooze [21].

Conjunctiva

Isolated conjunctival involvement is rather rare; cases of conjunctivitis have been described in immunocompromised patients, contact lens wearers or after surgery. It is usually manifested by a marked prominent mass of conjunctival tissue conditioned by granulomatous inflammation [21].

Cornea

The cornea is the most frequently affected ocular structure in atypical mycobacteriosis. As a rule, mycobacterial keratitis occurs in patients after LASIK (laser in situ keratomileusis), pterygium ablation and keratoplasty, or after trauma with the presence of a foreign body. Other predisposing factors include the use of topical steroids or contact lens wear [21].

The clinical findings are dominated by superficial infiltrates of irregular margins with a "broken glass" appearance. There is *minimal stromal* infiltration [21], ulcers may extend deeper into stroma [45].

A complication may be the development of endophthalmitis or corneal perforation.

Keratitis caused by atypical mycobacteria can cause a severe decrease in visual acuity [21].

Sclera

Scleral involvement is manifested by nonspecific pain, secretion and chronic redness of the eye [21]. In a chronic course, it can also lead to thinning of the sclera and the development of defects, nodules or abscesses. Unfortunately, a frequent consequence is a significant visual deterioration [21].

Uvea

Atypical mycobacteriosis may affect the anterior uvea, choroid, or manifest itself as panuveitis in isolation. Choroidal involvement manifests as multifocal choroiditis, which is characterised by small yellowish lesions, located under the retinal pigment epithelium (RPE) and may be accompanied by an inflammatory reaction in the anterior chamber or vitreous [21], optic nerve atrophy and retinal haemorrhages.

Endophthalmitis

The typical objective finding in endophthalmitis caused by atypical mycobacteria is hypopyon and inflammatory reaction in the vitreous. Granulomatous precipitates are found on the cornea. If the endophthalmitis is due to a previous cataract operation, pathological material is also found on the artificial intraocular lens [21].

Orbit

Infection of the orbit with atypical mycobacteriosis is uncommon. It is manifested by limited motility of the eyeball, its protrusion and cellulitis. Osteomyelitis of the surrounding bones may be a complication [21].

Diagnosis

Diagnosis is based on the detection of infectious agents by various methods—culture, PCR (polymerase chain reaction), or histopathological examination, which is characterised by the finding of granulomatous inflammation with necrosis and mycobacteria [21].

Lung Diseases 91

Differential diagnosis

- Mycotic keratitis
- Herpetic keratitis
- Corneal inflammation caused by bacteria of the genus Nocardia or Corynebacterium
- Nocardia uveitis
- Ocular lymphoma

Therapy

Treatment of ocular atypical mycobacteriosis consists of local and total administration of ATBs, often in combination. The most used ATBs are macrolide and quinolone series preparations, amikacin, gentamycin, kanamycin; in some cases, a combination of several series is administered. Depending on the findings, surgical therapy is usually indicated, usually incisions, excisions, debridement; in the case of significant thinning of the bulb wall, e.g. in scleritis, patches are applied. In the case of development of the disease after previous implantation of foreign material, its removal is necessary. In extreme cases, evisceration or enucleation of the eye bulb is performed [21].

5 Sarcoidosis

Sarcoidosis is a multisystem inflammatory disease of unknown aetiology, with granuloma formation in affected tissues and organs. The extent of involvement in individual organs and tissues varies from patient to patient, therefore the clinical manifestations can be highly variable. Often the disease may be asymptomatic, rarely resulting in organ failure.

Epidemiology

Sarcoidosis occurs globally, in all races and age groups, although the incidence varies in different populations, particularly by race (highest incidence in black, followed by white, Hispanic and lowest in Asian populations) and latitude (increasing incidence from the equator to the poles). The disease affects women more often than men. Women are most likely to become ill around the age of 50, while men usually acquire the disease at a younger age (between 35 and 40 years); the disease is rare in children [29]. Familial occurrence is described in about 4% of cases. Sarcoidosis is considered the most common interstitial lung disease. The mortality rate for sarcoidosis tends to be low (the highest is 0.8/100,000 in American blacks, while, in American whites, it is only 0.07/100,000) [6]. The lethality rate in cohorts ranges from 1 to 8%.

Clinical presentation

Sarcoidosis can be *asymptomatic* in many patients (about 1/3 to 2/5 of patients) and the diagnosis is made based on incidental findings, especially during chest radiological examination for other reasons. Extrapulmonary forms of sarcoidosis may also be asymptomatic. Symptomatic patients may present with *nonspecific symptoms*, as opposed to symptoms based on organ involvement. Nonspecific symptoms of sarcoidosis include fatigue, malaise, fever to febrile, weight loss, and impaired mental and psychological function. Like sarcoidosis, symptoms may be acute or chronic, and may resolve spontaneously or return. *Symptoms from organ involvement* are the same as in other diseases affecting the organ.

When the *lungs and intrathoracic lymph nodes* are affected (more than 90% of sarcoidosis patients are affected), a cough, usually dry, often asthma-like discomfort, varying degrees of dyspnoea, chest discomfort to pain, and rarely haemoptysis may occur. Auditory findings on physical examination tend to be normal. Clubbing fingers and crepitus audible basally is a rare finding. In acute sarcoidosis, the most common clinical presentation is Lofgren's syndrome, manifested by fever, joint pain (talocrural joint most affected), erythema nodosum (EN) (most commonly on the tibia) + typical pattern of bilateral hilar lymphadenopathy (BHL) on chest X-ray and negative skin tuberculin test. Acute forms usually have a good prognosis and often undergo spontaneous remission, more rarely progressing to the chronic phase of the disease. What is called the "sarcoid" in the scar (reddening to brownish-red papules and swelling of old scars) is also considered an acute manifestation of sarcoidosis. On the other hand, in chronic sarcoidosis (i.e. disease lasting more than two years), the onset of symptoms is gradual and subtle, with respiratory and other organ symptoms, to which the patient often partially adapts. In addition to the lung parenchyma itself, the *airways* (larynx, trachea, bronchi, bronchioles) may also be affected, leading to bronchial obstruction and bronchiectasis. Airway hyperresponsiveness with cough is present in more than 1/5 of patients.

Sarcoidosis of peripheral lymph nodes and spleen is relatively common (about 1/3 of patients).

The nodules are mostly painless, mobile, without fluctuation, without fistulas, without redness. Their enlargement is often accompanied by splenomegaly, which is usually asymptomatic, rarely manifested by hypersplenism or abdominal pain.

Skin involvement is described in about 1/4 of patients. In acute sarcoidosis there is EN-sensitive, oozing, reddened subcutaneous tissue (histologically non-granulomatous type of inflammation), usually on the tibiae; the finding is more often symmetrical, more rarely affecting EN upper limbs. Among the forms of cutaneous sarcoidosis (histologically with evidence of granulomatous inflammation) is the formation of reddish infiltrates, papules in old scars, called sarcoids in the scars. In chronic cutaneous sarcoidosis, various skin manifestations can be seen, most often subcutaneous small- or large-eye sarcoidosis, especially on the face, arms, and trunk, usually reddish-brown in colour, non-itching, usually painless. Rarely, lupus pernio is seen in our population—induced red-brown plaques, most commonly affecting the nose, forehead, lips, and auricles with destructive development (usually in the black population).

Sarcoidosis of *the musculoskeletal system* is described in 25–40% of patients, especially arthralgia in granulomatous periarthritis or, less often, arthritis (usually non-erosive and non-deforming).

Sarcoidosis of *the liver* is a typical case of high detection of granulomas on biopsy (up to 80% of patients), while hepatomegaly can be demonstrated sonographically in about 1/5 patients, but liver failure, portal hypertension or death from liver failure is rare.

Central and peripheral *nervous system* (CNS, PNS) involvement is clinically demonstrated in 5–15% of cases. It can be a focal involvement of the brain, spinal cord, involvement of the cranial nerves, especially the *n. facialis* (VII.) when infiltration changes the base of the skull.

Sarcoidosis of *the heart* is clinically evident in 5–10% of sarcoidosis patients, but accounts for up to one-half of sarcoidosis deaths. It is most manifested by arrhythmias (from benign extrasystoles to atrioventricular blockade, ventricular tachycardia with sudden death), more rarely by granulomatous infiltration to myocardial fibrosis with impaired cardiac function and heart failure, and rarely by valvular involvement.

Affections of *other organs* such as gastrointestinal tract, urinary and genital system, endocrine glands, ENT manifestations are uncommon.

Diagnosis

Diagnosis of sarcoidosis is based on compatible clinical and radiological findings, histological evidence of epithelioid noncaseating granulomas, and especially on simultaneous exclusion of other diseases with similar clinical manifestations and histological findings. The presence of granulomas in one organ is not sufficient for diagnosis. The optimal diagnostic and therapeutic considerations include not only the diagnosis itself, but also the determination of the extent and severity of organ involvement and the assessment of disease activity (inactive, persistent, progressive).

Laboratory examination is nonspecific and makes only a limited contribution to the diagnosis. As a rule, it shows increased erythrocyte sedimentation and C-reactive protein (CRP) in the acute stage.

Imaging methods are the main auxiliary methods in the diagnosis and monitoring of sarcoidosis. The basis is still the native chest X ray, on which more than 90% of patients have pathological findings. It still determines the stages of intrathoracic sarcoidosis. There are five stages of sarcoidosis according to the findings on the chest X ray: Stage 0—completely normal findings on the chest X ray. The patient has an extrapulmonary form of sarcoidosis or a nodular form of sarcoidosis, which is not visible on the chest X-ray and is only revealed by chest CT. Stage I—bilateral hilar lymphadenopathy (BHL)—usually symmetrical polycyclic enlargement of the hilar lymph nodes + enlargement of the mediastinal nodes (Fig. 3).

In chronic stages, calcifications—rarely shell-shaped, appear in the nodes. Stage II—bilateral hilar lymphadenopathy persists on imaging, but there is also involvement of the lung parenchyma, usually in the nature of nodules, especially perihilarly in the middle and upper lung fields (Fig. 4).

Sometimes a transition from Stage I to Stage II can be observed over time, when the progressively enlarged lymph nodes become smaller and, conversely, changes in the lung parenchyma become more prominent—this is referred to as the "escape of sarcoidosis into the lung". Stage III—at this stage, changes are seen

Fig. 3 Sarcoidosis stage 1 chest X ray, posteroanterior view: lungs expanded, no congestion. Bilateral hilar symmetrical enlargement of lymph nodes. Lung parenchyma with normal findings

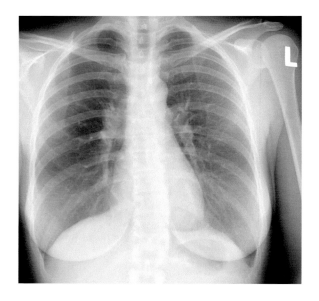

Fig. 4 Sarcoidosis stage 2 chest X ray, posteroanterior view: lungs expanded, no congestion. Bilateral hilar symmetrical enlargement of lymph nodes. In the lung parenchyma, bilateral small nodules mainly centrally, bilaterally in the upper lung fields (on HRCT of the lung typical conglomerates of small nodules in perilymphatic distribution)

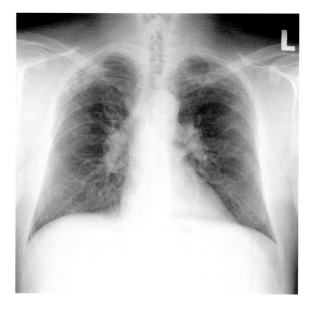

only in the lung parenchyma without enlargement of the intrathoracic lymph nodes, reticulonodulation predominates, without significant fibrotic changes (Fig. 5).

Stage IV—changes in the lung parenchyma are characterised by reticulations with predominance in the upper lung fields, pulmonary fibrosis, apicalisation of the hilum

Lung Diseases

Fig. 5 Sarcoidosis stage 3 chest X ray, posteroanterior view: lungs expanded, mediastinum and pulmonary hila without enlargement. Bilateral findings of small pulmonary nodules, especially in the upper and middle lung fields

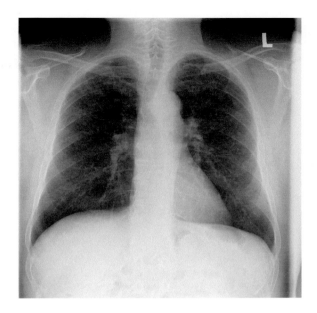

and enlargement of the mediastinum, bullae formation, disfiguring of vessels and confluent opacities (Fig. 6).

Fig. 6 Sarcoidosis stage 4 chest X ray, posteroanterior view: lungs expanded, bilateral traction of the hila apically with numerous reticulations extending from the hila towards the periphery of the lungs, without clear nodules

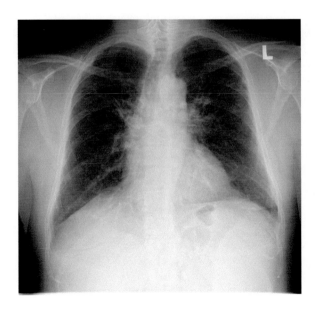

In addition to the typical changes described, large to tumour-forming nodules, atelactases with compression of the bronchi by nodules, migrating infiltrates, etc. may occur.

High-resolution computed tomography (HRCT) is nowadays the basic examination in the diagnosis and assessment of the type of lung involvement, localisation of sarcoidosis, evolution over time, allows the assessment of the activity, but also the resolution into Stages III and IV, also allows detailed imaging of lung nodules, mediastinum, and lung hilum (even those not visible on the native chest image). The most typical reversible manifestations in the lung parenchyma are multiple small nodules located centrilobularlly and subpleurally, so in perilymphatic distribution and less typical increased density—ground glass opacities. The irreversible changes include signs of fibrosis, distortion of vessels and bronchi, traction bronchiectasis and, more rarely, honeycomb-like lung remodelling. CT scanning should always be performed at the time of diagnosis and further at follow-up if there are unclear developments on the native chest radiograph (Figs. 7, 8, 9, 10, and 11) [49].

Magnetic resonance imaging (MRI) is mainly used in suspected neurosarcoidosis (brain, spinal cord, optic nerve), sarcoidosis of the musculoskeletal system (muscles, bones, joints) and heart.

Sonographic examination is mainly used in the examination of the abdomen (hepatosplenomegaly, sarcoidosis of the renal parenchyma, nephrolithiasis, etc.), in the imaging of nodal syndrome in the neck, axillae and groin and in the examination of the heart.

Positron emission tomography (PET/CT) is increasingly being used and allows a comprehensive assessment of the extent of pulmonary and extrapulmonary involvement, and at the same time allows the activity of the process even in chronic lesions to be assessed (Figs. 12 and 13).

Examination of lung function is important to assess pulmonary limitation due to sarcoidosis.

The impairment of lung function increases in the higher stages of the disease.

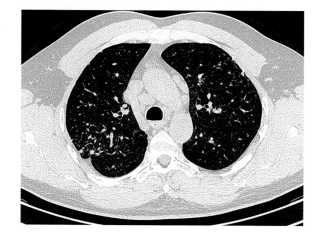

Fig. 7 Sarcoidosis stage 2 HRCT of the lungs, transversal scan, lung window: bilaterally multiple nodules in the lung parenchyma in typical perilymphatic distribution (nodules centrilobularly, but also on fissures and subpleurally) with a maximum centrally in the upper lobes

Lung Diseases

Fig. 8 Sarcoidosis stage 2 native CT of the lungs, transversal scan, mediastinal window: massive symmetrical hilar lymphadenopathy, lymphadenopathy subcarinally

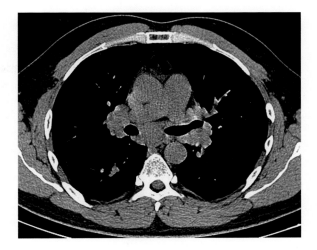

Fig. 9 Sarcoidosis stage 3 HRCT of the lungs, transversal scan, lung window: multiple small-nodular lung involvement in perilymphatic distribution, mainly centrally in the upper lobes

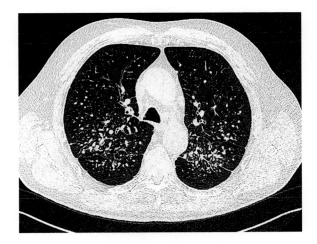

The basic examination in the diagnosis of sarcoidosis includes *bronchoscopy*. Macroscopically on examination, the endoscopic findings on the mucous membranes may be normal, but often irregularities or yellowish nodules-granulomas can be seen on the mucous membranes, and blunted carinae due to oppression by enlarged nodules are usually evident. Puncture of enlarged nodes can also be performed, optimally under ultrasound guidance (EBUS examination) (Figs. 14, 15, and 16).

Therapy

The treatment of sarcoidosis is based on two important facts: one is that the aetiology of the disease remains unknown, and the second is that the disease often resolves spontaneously. Therefore, treatment is approached only after an individual

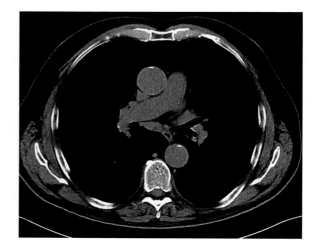

Fig. 10 Sarcoidosis stage 3 native CT of the lungs, transversal scan, mediastinal window: without significant mediastinal or hilar lymphadenopathy

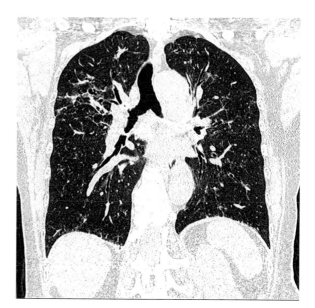

Fig. 11 Sarcoidosis stage 4 HRCT of the lungs, coronal reconstruction, lung window: traction of the lung hila apically with prominent traction bronchiectasias extending from the lung hila apically. Numerous reticulations in the upper lobes especially centrally. Occasional small lung nodules bilaterally centrally in the perilymphatic distribution

assessment of the extent of the disease, the severity of symptoms, the risk of progression, but also after consideration of the expected side effects of treatment. In practice, about one-half of the patients are treated. There is no need to treat asymptomatic cases of Stages 0 and I. Progressive or symptomatic forms (dyspnoea, cough, chest pain) of Stages II, III and IV are considered a clear indication [5]. *Corticosteroids* are the mainstay of treatment for pulmonary and extrapulmonary sarcoidosis, usually administered orally (rarely topically), in low and medium doses, only in high doses for life-threatening forms. If their effect is inadequate or failing, if the

Lung Diseases

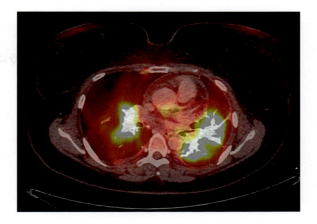

Fig. 12 PETCT before treatment, transverse scan: bilateral hilar lymphadenopathy, FGD avid and conspicuous perihilar FDG avid pulmonary nodule conglomerates

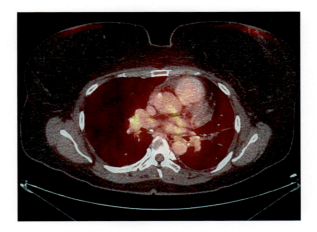

Fig. 13 PETCT after treatment, transverse scan: clear regression of FDG avid lymphadenopathy and FDG avid nodular lung involvement

disease relapses, if serious side effects occur, or when it is necessary to administer higher doses of corticosteroids to maintain disease control, they are combined with or replaced by other immunosuppressive agents (methotrexate, hydroxychloroquine, azathioprine, leflunomide, mycophenolate, cyclophosphamide). In refractory forms of sarcoidosis, patients may also be given antiTNF alpha biologics (infliximab, adalimumab, golimumab) or rituximab [4]. In patients where, despite these treatments, progression of findings and development of pulmonary fibrosis occurs, antifibrotic drugs (pirfenidone, nintedanib) may be considered. Non-pharmacological treatment is also part of the treatment of patients with sarcoidosis.

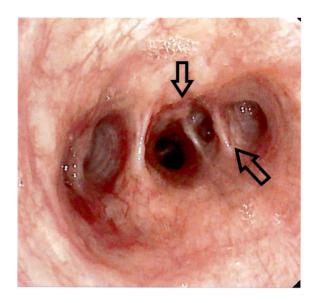

Fig. 14 Bronchoscopic image of sarcoidosis affecting the airway mucosa, histological sampling of the arrows, confirmed sarcoid bronchitis (granulomatous inflammation in the airway mucosa)

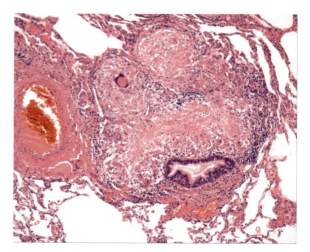

Fig. 15 Histological picture of sarcoidosis of the lung—advanced pulmonary sarcoidosis with fibrosis (haematoxylin eosin, magnification 200 times)—specific granulomas without necrotising (epithelioid cells, multinucleated cells, central fibrosis) in the bronchovascular bundle

6   Ocular Manifestations of Sarcoidosis

Sarcoidosis is a granulomatous inflammatory disease affecting almost any ocular structure [28]. It is referred to as the "great imitator" due to its nonspecific manifestations that can mimic other diseases. Eye involvement is often its first symptom [50].

Fig. 16 Histological picture of sarcoidosis in the lymph node—relatively early changes in the lymph node in sarcoidosis—specific granulomas without necrotising (epithelioid cells, multinucleated cells, central fibrosis in granulomas), still relatively well preserved original lymph node parenchyma

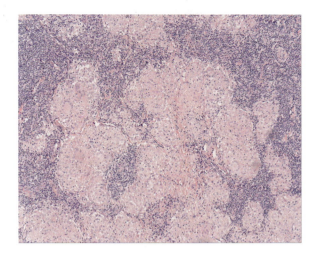

Risk factors

- HIV co-infection
- Age—the highest prevalence is in patients aged 55 years.

Clinical symptoms and objective findings

Orbit

Sarcoidosis of the orbit is manifested by pain, redness, decreased vision, proptosis of the eyeball or ptosis of the eyelids. A complication may be occlusion of the central retinal artery caused by external oppression by the orbital mass [28].

Eyelids

Sarcoidosis of the eyelids is manifested by their oedema and redness of various extent and clinical appearance—from small papules and nodules to large masses. It can also lead to scarring of the eyelids, with their subsequent deformities or to eyelid retraction when the m. tarsalis superior Mülleri is affected [28].

The lacrimal system

The lacrimal gland is affected by sarcoidosis relatively often [50]. It can be asymptomatic or lead to the development of dry eye syndrome with discomfort and irritation. Palpation can detect its enlargement, and homogeneous enhancement is present on CT. If the lacrimal ducts are affected, the consequence is often their obstruction and epiphora [28].

Cornea

Corneal involvement may be manifested as superficial punctate, interstitial, or peripheral ulcerative keratitis. The most common is keratitis punctata superficialis, with typical subepithelial calcium deposits in Bowman's layer. Corneal disease may also occur secondary to involvement of the lacrimal gland by sarcoidosis, leading to keratoconjunctivitis sicca or involvement of the central nervous system by sarcoidosis with paresis of the *n. facialis* and lagophthalmos leading to exposure keratopathy or to poorly therapeutically manageable corneal ulceration [28].

Conjunctiva

Manifestations of sarcoidosis on the conjunctiva may be in the form of whitish deposits, hyperaemia and follicular reaction, or conjunctival granulomas. In a chronic course, scarring and symblepharon formation may occur [28]. Very often, however, sarcoidosis of the conjunctiva is asymptomatic [50].

Sclera

Scleral involvement in sarcoidosis is rare [50]. It manifests as anterior diffuse, anterior nodular or posterior scleritis [28].

Uvea and fundus

Uveitis due to sarcoidosis can take the form of anterior, intermediate, posterior or panuveitis [50].

The objective findings of anterior uveitis are dominated by corneal greasy precipitates, inflammatory reaction in the anterior chamber, with eventual secondary elevation of intraocular pressure. Hypopyon is rarely found in these cases. In more severe inflammations, nodules on the iris and posterior synechiae are also encountered [28].

In intermediate uveitis, vitreous opacities are found, with the appearance of snowballs or a string of pearls, and neovascularisation may be present on the optic disc and retina. Cystoid macular oedema is diagnosed on OCT [28].

Posterior uveitis is usually bilateral, although the findings tend to be asymmetric. They may present as multifocal choroiditis or by the presence of solitary or multiple choroidal granulomas, leading to decreased vision if centrally located or to retinal detachment if the granulomas are larger in size [28].

Vasculitis with yellow-white exudates along the veins is also a frequent manifestation of sarcoidosis and may be complicated by venous occlusion. In some cases, epiretinal membrane development also occurs [28].

Nonspecific symptoms of anterior uveitis include photophobia, pain and redness of the eye, and decreased vision. In intermediate uveitis, complaints of impaired vision with opacities in the visual field predominate [28].

Optic nerve

When the optic nerve is affected, atrophy or oedema of its disc can be observed, possibly granulomas and nodules are present [28]. Visual impairment, defects in the visual field and abnormal pupillary reactions occur [28].

Lung Diseases

Diagnosis

The diagnosis of ocular sarcoidosis is based on biomicroscopic examination, supplemented by fluorescence angiography.

Four levels of certainty of diagnosis and their diagnostic criteria:

(1) *Definite ocular sarcoidosis*—presence of uveitis with typical symptoms, corresponding biopsy.
(2) *Presumed ocular sarcoidosis*—presence of uveitis with typical symptoms, finding of bilateral hilar lymphadenopathy, without biopsy.
(3) *Probable ocular sarcoidosis*—presence of at least 3 ocular symptoms, positivity of 2 laboratory tests, no hilar lymphadenopathy on the X-ray, no biopsy.
(4) *Possible ocular sarcoidosis*—presence of at least 4 ocular symptoms and positivity of 2 laboratory tests, negative result of lung biopsy [17, 28].

Differential diagnosis

- Tuberculous uveitis
- Scleritis in rheumatoid arthritis

Therapy

Local ocular treatment consists of the application of corticosteroids (including intravitreal administration) [50] and cycloplegics. In scleritis, the first-choice drugs are non-steroidal antiphlogistic drugs [28]. In the case of orbital involvement, surgical intervention is considered. Local treatment is usually supplemented by systemic treatment, which consists of corticosteroids or immunosuppressants [50].

Complications include the occurrence of complicated cataract, secondary glaucoma, epiretinal membrane and macular oedema.

7 Superior Vena Cava Syndrome, Generalised Pulmonary Malignancies and Malignancies Generalised to the Lungs

Malignant lung disease is most often of primary bronchopulmonary origin—bronchogenic carcinoma. The incidence in women is approximately 50% as high. Bronchogenic carcinoma (by external oppression of the tumour on the vein, by direct penetration into the venous lumen or sometimes in conjunction with a hypercoagulable state with formation of venous thrombosis) is the most common cause of a group of symptoms resulting from reduced or even completely stopped flow (towards the right atrium) of blood through the superior vena cava, called *superior vena cava syndrome* (or VCS syndrome).

Generalised lung malignancies (Stage IV) unfortunately account for more than one-half of all new cases of bronchogenic carcinoma in the Europe. The other one-quarter are patients with locally advanced bronchogenic carcinoma (Stage III).

The lung is also the second most frequently affected organ *by tumour metastases*. The following types of neoplasms metastasise most frequently to the lungs: breast tumours, tumours from other parts of the lung, tumours of the digestive tract, tumours of the kidney, thyroid, head and neck, lymphomas, sarcomas, malignant melanoma, and prostate cancer. In many tumours, the presence of clinically evident metastases is rarely encountered, but they are found at autopsy (Table 1).

Clinical presentation

Clinical manifestations of *bronchogenic carcinoma are late*. This is why most patients (in the EU) present late, already at the time of loco-regionally advanced (Stage III) or generalised (Stage IV) disease. Manifestations of *generalised lung cancer* include nonspecific complaints (fatigue, weight loss, night sweats, subfebrile, inappetence) and respiratory distress (cough, haemoptysis, dyspnoea, unspecified chest pain), or signs of generalisation (to the skeleton—pain, to the liver—pain, dyspepsia, to the brain—paresis of the limbs, epileptic paroxysms, psychological changes in frontal lobe involvement, etc.).

The main manifestations of *VCS* are swelling of the face, neck and upper extremities, with visible dilatation of the coiled veins in the subcutaneous tissue of the neck and upper chest. Patients may cough and experience impaired breathing. Hoarseness, a swollen and congested throat, mouth and nasal mucosa, epistaxis, swelling around the eyes, conjunctival redness, headache, fatigue, exhaustion, dizziness, haemoptysis, and nonspecific chest pain are other manifestations of advanced VCS. The most severe forms of VCS syndrome are airway stenosis and cerebral oedema due to reduced venous blood outflow.

Table 1 Incidence of lung metastases (clinically clear or sectionally proven)

Location of the primary tumour	Incidence of the primary tumour in the Czech Republic (according to ÚZIS, data 2016)	Incidence of lung metastases during treatment (%)	Incidence of lung metastases found during autopsy (%)
Colon + rectum	7610 (M 4582, F 3028)	< 5	25–40
Prostate	M 7305	5	15–50
Breast	F 7220	4	60
Lungs	6782 (M 4478, F 2304)	30	40
Kidneys	3202 (M 2000, F 1202)	20	50–70
Pancreas	2243 (M 1165, F 1078)	< 1	25–40
Melanoma	2609 (M 1404, F 1205)	5	66–80
Bladder	2099 (M 1559, F 540)	7	25–30
Uterus (outside the cervix)	F 2012	< 1	30–40
Ovary	F 998	5	10–25
Cervix	F 822	5	10–25

M males, F females

Lung Diseases

Pulmonary metastases remain asymptomatic for a relatively long time and are usually found: (a) during the *initial* staging of newly diagnosed tumours or (b) during regular follow-up of cancer patients. Symptomatic patients are then characterised by the following symptoms: (c) cough with/without haemoptysis and dyspnoea—central localisation in the trachea and large bronchi, (d) pleural chest pain when peripherally localised metastases penetrate the parietal pleura, or persistent pain when pulmonary metastases penetrate the skeleton (ribs, sternum, vertebrae). A severely symptomatic form of metastatic involvement manifested by worsening dyspnoea and hypoxaemia (easily detected by a fall in SpO2) is carcinomatous lymphangitis (tumour involvement of lymph nodes and pathways).

Diagnosis

The diagnosis of bronchogenic carcinoma and lung metastases relies on imaging. The basic diagnostic method is the native summative postero-anterior chest scan. A more detailed view of the lung parenchyma, mediastinum and pleura is of course possible with modern CT of the chest (possibly with contrast medium administration).

Bronchoscopic examination helps to determine the morphological structure of central endobronchial lesions or assists in morphological diagnosis by transbronchial lung biopsy or cryobiopsy of peripheral lesions, or biopsy of extraluminal lesions targeted by endobronchial ultrasound (linear for central biopsies, radial for peripherally located biopsies). Lesions adjacent to the oesophagus can be verified by transoesophageal endoscopy—the EUS. However, some peripheral lesions still escape the above-mentioned techniques. Therefore, to obtain specimens for morphological verification, transrectal puncture of the lesion navigated by chest CT is indicated. Histological verification of metastatic involvement of mediastinal lymph nodes or larger peripheral lesions is possible by thoracic surgery (mediastinoscopy or wedge-shaped lung resection). Soon, it may be possible to use endobronchial robotic systems (now available in the USA) for precise sampling of small peripheral lesions beyond the reach of current technical capabilities.

Patients with VCS syndrome (Stage III or IV bronchogenic carcinoma) usually experience symptoms 2–4 weeks before diagnosis. VCS syndrome is not infrequently the first manifestation of bronchogenic carcinoma. The basic examination is a native summative posterior chest scan finding the presence of tumour-induced shadowing insistent from the right on the mediastinum in the region of the superior vena cava. A CT scan of the chest offers a more refined view. In all cases of VCS syndrome, another common cause, lymphoma, must be excluded.

Therapy

Generalised lung cancer is treated according to the type and stage of the tumour, the patient's health status determined by the presence/absence of comorbidities and his/her current physical status. The primary modality for chemosensitive type of bronchogenic carcinoma (small cell carcinoma) is chemotherapy. The primary modality for painful skeletal involvement or haemoptysis is radiotherapy. Surgical treatment, with some exceptions, is not reserved for clinical Stage III or IV; it has a role in individual cases. New therapeutic options for non-small-cell bronchogenic carcinoma are provided by biological therapy directed at a specific molecular target confirmed in a patient-specific tumour tissue sample and immunotherapies administered also in a specific group of preselected patients.

Therapy of VCS syndrome includes treatment targeted at the specific type of bronchogenic carcinoma in Stage III or IV and treatment of possible thrombosis (thrombolysis, anticoagulation) of the superior vena cava.

In the treatment of lung metastases from other tumours, the treatment of the primary tumour is crucial. Chemosensitive primary tumours can be favourably affected by chemotherapy. Metastases from tumours with available biological therapy or tumours with a favourable response to immunotherapy can be relatively successfully eliminated.

If the lung metastasis is solitary (i.e. a single metastasis in one lung) and the patient's condition allows surgery, the first line of treatment is surgical resection of the lung metastasis—i.e. metastasectomy.

8 Ocular Manifestations of Superior Vena Cava Syndrome

The superior vena cava syndrome is a condition in which there is obstruction and restriction of blood flow in the v. cava superior, most commonly due to thoracic neoplasia, hilar lymphadenopathy, or aortic aneurysm [42]. Due to the venous drainage of the eye, venous hypertension can also be manifested here [3]. The ocular and general symptoms worsen in the horizontal position of the patient [3]. The severity and extent of symptoms depend on the location of the obstruction and the rate of development of the condition [42].

Clinical symptoms and objective findings

Patients may experience blurred vision, but often do not report any subjective ocular abnormalities.

In the objective findings, eyelid oedema, conjunctival oedema and injection, enlargement of periorbital, episcleral and conjunctival veins may be present on the *anterior eye segment* [3].

As the intraocular fluid drains into the venous system, elevation of intraocular pressure is also a common symptom.

In some patients, the intraocular tension is normal in the sitting position, in others it is elevated, but in the supine position there is always an elevation. Bulb protrusion to exophthalmos may be present [3].

Peripapillary retinal oedema, increased venous filling or pulsation of the central retinal vein on the optic disc margin can be observed at the *posterior eye segment* [3].

The optic disc may have indistinct margins or be oedematous [3].

At the same time, however, pathological exsanguination of the optic disc or visual field disturbances at the perimeter are not present [3].

Lung Diseases

Diagnosis

Among the eye examinations, measurement of intraocular pressure and exophthalmometry in sitting and lying position are essential.

Differential diagnosis

- Thrombosis of the central retinal vein
- Episcleritis and scleritis

Therapy

The therapy of ocular symptoms in v. cava superior syndrome is primarily to address the primary cause of its occurrence. Topically applied pilocarpine is used to reduce intraocular pressure [3]. Cases where secondary glaucoma has been addressed surgically have also been described [18].

9 Tuberous Sclerosis and Lymphangioleiomyomatosis A

Tuberous sclerosis complex (TSC) is an autosomal dominantly inherited multisystem disease, characterised by the development of multiple benign tumours that most commonly affect the skin, brain, eyes, lungs, and kidneys. The disease is caused by a congenital or de novo germline or somatic *mutation in* the *TSC1* or *TSC2* genes, which encode the hamartin and tuberin proteins. It is a relatively rare disease, with an incidence of 1:5000–10,000 individuals worldwide.

Clinical presentation

The disease leads to the development of multiple benign tumours, which can affect many organs, but most commonly the skin, brain, lungs, kidneys, and eyes. Almost all patients with TSC have some form of skin changes, and most suffer from neuropsychiatric symptoms, particularly epilepsy and cognitive dysfunction. Renal and pulmonary involvement is prognostically serious but less common.

Skin manifestations

The cutaneous manifestation of TSC includes several morphological entities. Characteristic changes include hypopigmented macules, facial angiofibromas, periungual fibromas and shagreen skin. Hypopigmented macules are the earliest cutaneous feature of TSC. Angiofibromas are the most striking manifestation of TSC. These are pink to brownish papules, symmetrically localised in the midface. Periungual fibromas also occur in about 3/4 of patients and usually arise in the second decade of life. About one-half of the patients have what is called shagreen skin. These are pink to yellowish-brown raised skin plaques with an uneven surface, located most often in the lumbar region and on the back, which usually arise in the first decade of life.

Neurological manifestations

The extent of nervous system involvement is highly variable and about 50% of patients have no neurological symptoms. 80–90% of symptomatic patients develop epilepsy, often within the first two years of life. Intracranial lesions are classified into four categories. Cortical glioneuronal hamartomas (tubercles) occur in up to 95% of patients. These are multiple, most often frontally localised lesions that may contain calcifications. Subependymal nodules (SN) are also found in almost all patients. They occur along the walls of the third cerebral ventricle and lateral ventricles and often contain calcifications. Subependymal giant cell tumours (SGCT) are benign slow-growing tumours in the periventricular region that usually arise from subependymal nodules (Fig. 17). They occur in about 10–20% of patients. Dysplastic white matter changes represent the last group.

Cardiological manifestations

The typical manifestation of TSC in the heart is multiple rhabdomyomas, benign tumours that are very rare outside the association with TSC. They are usually asymptomatic but can cause heart failure or arrhythmias.

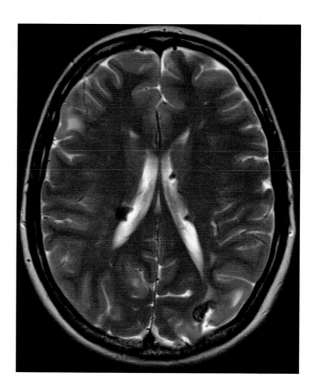

Fig. 17 Subependymal tumours in a patient with tuberous sclerosis

Fig. 18 Multiple pulmonary cysts in a patient with sporadic LAM

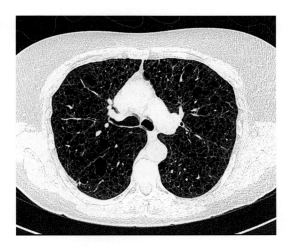

Pulmonary impairment

The most common pulmonary manifestation of TSC is lymphangioleiomyomatosis (LAM). It occurs in about 40% of women with TSC and very rarely in men. Its prevalence increases with age, and it is one of the late manifestations of TSC. It is characterised by the formation of multiple bilateral thin-walled pulmonary cysts that compress healthy lung parenchyma and, if the visceral pleura is perforated, can cause pneumothorax (Fig. 18).

An asymptomatic course or only a mild degree of exertional dyspnoea is common, but rarely respiratory failure can occur. The diagnostic method of choice is HRCT of the lungs, which should be performed in every patient with newly diagnosed TSC, even in the absence of respiratory symptoms. The presence of more than ten, but usually hundreds of bilateral thin-walled cysts ranging in size from a few millimetres to 2 cm is the typical picture of LAM.

Renal impairment

Renal manifestations of TSC include angiomyolipoma, cysts and renal cell carcinoma. The most common renal manifestation of TSC is angiomyolipoma (AML), a benign slow-growing mesenchymal tumour caused by clonal proliferation of perivascular epithelioid cells in which both alleles of the TSC gene have been mutated (Fig. 19).

Most angiomyolipomas are asymptomatic, but they can cause haemorrhage or, less commonly, compression of surrounding tissues with the development of secondary hypertension, haematuria, lumbar pain, or renal insufficiency. Multiple renal cysts are the second most common renal manifestation of TSC.

Diagnosis

The revised diagnostic criteria defined by the International Tuberous Sclerosis Complex Conference in 2012 are currently in force. To make a diagnosis of definite

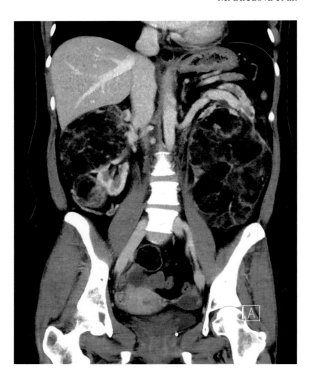

Fig. 19 Bilateral large renal angiomyolipomas in a patient with TSC

TSC based on clinical symptoms, 2 main, or 1 main and 2 secondary criteria must be met. Diagnosis of possible TSC requires meeting 1 major or 2 or more minor criteria.

TSC can also be diagnosed by identifying pathological mutations in the TSC 1 and 2 genes.

Therapy

The treatment of TSC is mainly focused on the neurological, pulmonary and renal manifestations of the disease. In addition to symptomatic treatment and organ-specific treatment of complications arising from TSC, many cases are now treated with m-TOR inhibitors that target the deregulated signalling cascade.

10 Ocular Manifestations of Tuberous Sclerosis

It is a neurocutaneous syndrome with autosomal dominant inheritance, although more than 75% of cases are due to a de novo mutation [48]. Due to the multi-organ involvement, the overall clinical presentation is highly variable. Regarding the ocular

Lung Diseases

manifestations, retinal hamartomas are most found in patients with tuberous sclerosis. This disease is classified as a phakomatosis.

Clinical symptoms and objective findings

Eyelids

Angiofibromas, or adenoma sebaceum, are a typical cutaneous manifestation of TSC, and their occurrence has also been described on the skin of the eyelids [30]. These are purple macules that later develop into red to brownish papules due to the multiplication of the fibrous component.

Retina

Astrocytic retinal hamartomas are the most common ocular manifestation of TSC and are therefore included in its diagnostic criteria [32]. They occur both unilaterally and bilaterally.

Morphologically, there are three types: a smooth flat lesion of greyish colour, a white mulberry-shaped opacity, and a third type which is a combination of the two types [36].

Hamartomas may be associated with the development of neovascularisation.

An association with the finding of vascular endothelial growth factor expression on the surface of tubers in other organs is suggested [32].

Cases of extensive vitreous haemorrhage have also been described [48].

However, retinal lesions in TSC rarely have a negative effect on visual function.

In TSC, besides hamartomas, pigmentary changes in the sense of hyper- and hypopigmentation can be found on the back of the eye [36].

Neuro-ophthalmological manifestations

Neuro-ophthalmological manifestations in TSC include optic nerve hamartomas, optic disc oedema at higher intracranial pressure, visual field defects and 3rd, 4th and 6th cranial nerve palsies [48].

In superficially located astrocytic hamartomas of the optic nerve, it is always necessary to exclude optic nerve oedema, which they may mimic in appearance. However, hamartomas are typically unilateral and asymptomatic [48].

Defects in the visual field can occur as a result of a failure in any part of the visual pathway, i.e. also secondary to CNS involvement, but rarely also due to retinal hamartomas or during treatment with vigabatrin used in paediatric patients to therapeutically affect epiparoxysms [48].

Disruption of the function of the *n. oculomotorius* is rare, occurring when it is oppressed by an aneurysm of the a. communicans posterior [48]. Complete paresis of the 3rd cranial nerve is manifested by ipsilateral ptosis, mydriasis, hypotropia and exotropia [48].

Paresis of the *n. abducens* occurs mainly due to intracranial hypertension [48].

Diagnosis

Includes examination of the anterior eye segment using biomicroscopy, posterior eye segment using fundus photography. Additional examination methods—perimetry to exclude scotomas, and OCT to confirm the presence of macular oedema.

Differential diagnosis

Retinal hamartomas—choroidal osteoma, amelanotic melanoma, retinitis pigmentosa, haemangioma, neurofibromatosis, retinoblastoma, or choroidal metastases [32].

Hamartomas of the optic nerve—oedema and drusen of the optic nerve [48].

Therapy

In general, treatment of TSC is symptomatic, with an attempt to maintain proper function of the affected organ (Portocarrerro et al. 2018).

In asymptomatic retinal hamartomas, no therapy is needed. Patients are treated if there is a decrease in visual acuity.

In the presence of subretinal fluid, according to the literature, various modalities have been used to promote its absorption, such as laser photocoagulation, photodynamic therapy, or intravitreal anti-VEGF injection. In the case of vitreous haemorrhage without spontaneous absorption, pars plana vitrectomy is resorted to [32].

In the case of optic nerve hamartomas, no intervention is required due to the typical absence of symptoms [48].

11 Chronic Obstructive Pulmonary Disease

Chronic obstructive pulmonary disease (COPD) is a common respiratory disease of adults characterised by a fixed airflow obstruction that is not reversible after inhaled bronchodilators. The main cause of COPD is the prolonged inhalation of harmful substances, most commonly cigarette smoking and/or occupational or environmental pollutants. All this in a genetically susceptible individual. Spirometry with salbutamol administration, appropriately supplemented by other methods: chest imaging, sputum examination (culture), blood analysis (eosinophils, alpha-1-antitrypsin) and ECG, are essential to confirm the diagnosis of COPD and exclude alternative diagnoses. The most common clinical manifestations of COPD are shortness of breath, reduced exercise tolerance, fatigue, cough with/without mucus production. Long-term treatment consists of eliminating the inhalation challenge and administering long-acting inhaled bronchodilators. A minority of patients benefit from inhaled glucocorticosteroids or oral azithromycin, mucoactive drugs (erdotein or acetylcysteine) or roflumilast. Some patients may benefit from bronchoscopic techniques, surgery, or oxygen therapy or non-invasive ventilatory support. All patients benefit from regular pulmonary rehabilitation or influenza, pneumococcal and COVID-19 vaccination.

Definitions

The Global Initiative for Chronic Obstructive Lung Disease (GOLD) 2023 defines COPD as "a heterogeneous lung disease characterised by chronic respiratory symptoms (dyspnoea, cough, sputum production, exacerbations) due to airway abnormalities (chronic bronchitis, chronic bronchiolitis) and/or alveolar destruction (emphysema) resulting in persistent, often progressive airflow obstruction [1].

Chronic bronchitis is defined as chronic productive cough for at least three months in each of two consecutive years in an individual in whom other causes of chronic cough have been excluded. Chronic bronchitis may precede the development of airflow limitation.

Emphysema describes the enlargement of the airspaces distal to the terminal bronchioles; it is associated with destruction of the alveolar architecture without significant pulmonary fibrosis. Emphysema may be present in patients without airflow limitation.

Airflow limitation is an abnormally reduced ability to exhale properly and efficiently. The presence and severity of airflow limitation is determined by spirometry. The term airflow limitation is sometimes replaced by bronchial obstruction [34].

Epidemiology

Chronic obstructive pulmonary disease (COPD) had an estimated prevalence of 175 million people with about 3.2 million deaths worldwide [38]. In the EU, the overall prevalence of COPD has increased in women between 2001 and 2019, but continues to decrease in men, and in some countries the prevalence in women now exceeds that in men. There are currently more than 36 million Europeans with COPD. Overall, COPD mortality in the EU has decreased slightly between 2001 and 2019, but this decrease is not universal. In 2019, median age-standardised mortality in Europe reach 24/100,000 for men and 12/100,000 for women [38].

Aetiology

The most common risk factor is chronic cigarette smoking (at least 10 pack years); other influences include exposure to harmful fumes, smoke and dust in work, public and home environments. Other risks include repeated respiratory infections in childhood, the presence of HIV or premature birth. Presence of a genetically determined increased susceptibility to the disease in every patient with COPD [34]. This is most obvious in the case of alpha-1-antitrypsin deficiency (more severe forms of the deficiency significantly accelerate the development of emphysema).

Diagnosis

Four conditions must be met to confirm a diagnosis of COPD: (a) the presence of pulmonary symptoms (dyspnoea, cough or sputum production); b) the appropriate risk context (chronic cigarette smoking or other risk exposure); (c) clear evidence of airflow limitation on postbronchodilator spirometry; (d) absence of alternative explanations for the symptoms and airflow limitation [12]. Spirometry detects two main parameters necessary to confirm airflow limitation: reduced forced expiratory volume in one second (FEV1) and reduced FEV1/FVC ratio below 0.7. However, as the FEV1/FVC ratio decreases with age, the European Respiratory Society has proposed (in 2021) the use of the 5th percentile (or a z-score of -1.645) of the FEV1/FVC ratio rather than the simple universal value (0.7) mentioned above [43]. Unlike asthma, airflow limitation in COPD does not disappear completely after bronchodilator (salbutamol) treatment, so spirometry before and after bronchodilator treatment is needed to confirm the diagnosis of COPD.

Differential diagnosis

It should be noted that the presence of respiratory symptoms, long-term inhalation risk exposure and airflow limitation on spirometry is not specific. Therefore, alternative diagnoses (especially asthma) should always be excluded at the time of diagnosis. In practice, it is sometimes not possible to make a complete distinction between bronchial asthma and COPD, in which case it is referred to as asthma and COPD overlap (ACO) or COPD with asthma (COPD-A). Other chronic diagnoses with persistent airflow limitation include bronchiectasis, constrictive bronchiolitis, diffuse panbronchiolitis, left-sided heart failure, sarcoidosis and lymphangioleiomyomatosis.

Clinical presentation

The three main symptoms of COPD are breathlessness, chronic cough and sputum production. The most common and early symptom is dyspnoea on exertion. Less common symptoms include fatigue, wheezing and chest tightness [12]. All these symptoms can occur independently. Most people report that symptoms vary throughout the day or week, with mornings typically being the worst time of day.

The stable course of COPD can be interrupted by episodes of sudden clinical worsening (exacerbations). It is usually associated with an acute increase in the intensity of the main symptoms (more coughing, more sputum production, more breathlessness) beyond the usual day-to-day variation. An COPD exacerbation leads to a change in treatment (more medication or a new medication).

Physical examination findings vary with the severity of COPD: (a) In mild stages, the physical examination may be normal. Subtle clues include prolonged expiratory time and faint end-expiratory wheezing on forced expiratory manoeuvres; (b) As the severity of airflow obstruction increases, the physical examination may reveal lung hyperinflation: increased resonance to chest percussion, diminished breath sounds, expiratory wheezing and increased chest volume (barrel chest) and depressed diaphragm (Fig. 20); (c) Patients with end-stage COPD may adopt postures that relieve breathlessness—leaning forward with arms outstretched and weight supported on the palms and elbows (Fig. 21).

In addition, these patients may use accessory respiratory muscles of the neck and shoulder girdle, prolonged pursed-lip expiration and paradoxical retraction of the lower interspaces during inspiration [12]. Central cyanosis, asterixis of the upper

Lung Diseases

Fig. 20 Emphysema in chronic obstructive pulmonary disease, HRCT of the lungs

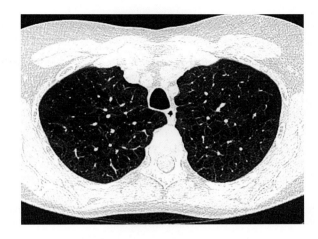

Fig. 21 Severe predominantly lower lobe emphysema in chronic obstructive pulmonary disease. HRCT of the lungs

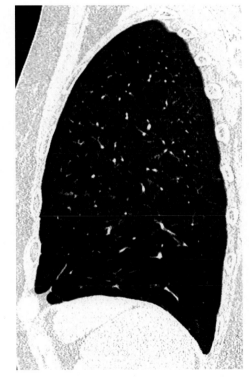

extremities, enlarged tender liver and distention of the neck veins may be observed due to right heart failure in advanced COPD individuals.

Classification and prognosis

Several strategies have been developed to classify everyone with COPD: (a) the GOLD 2023 categories (A or B or E) use a multidimensional approach with symptom monitoring (mMRC dyspnoea scale or COPD Assessment Test—CAT) and exacerbation history to guide basic pharmacological management; (b) the BODE index calculates body mass index, airflow limitation, dyspnoea and exercise capacity (six-minute walk distance) to estimate prognosis [1].

Therapy

The initial treatment of newly diagnosed COPD patients is based on a GOLD 2023 category [1]. Pharmacotherapy is stepwise. At follow-up visits, the next treatment is adjusted based on symptoms (mainly dyspnoea) and exacerbation history. The basic components (long-acting bronchodilators) of COPD medication are administered by inhalation. All patients should be advised to stop smoking to reduce other inhaled risks and be educated about optimal inhaler technique. Seasonal influenza vaccination and COVID-19 vaccination should be recommended for all patients. Pneumococcal vaccination should be given to those with non-mild COPD or a higher comorbidity burden. In addition to inhaled bronchodilators (the mainstay of COPD therapy), the modern drug portfolio includes inhaled glucocorticoids, oral roflumilast, azithromycin and erdosteine. The above drugs are designed for specific types of patients (COPD phenotype-targeted therapy).

Pulmonary rehabilitation and regular physical activity (walking, gardening, etc.) is a basic therapeutic non-pharmacological intervention. It is reasonable to aim for a normal or slightly overweight body mass index with a generally healthy diet. Long-term oxygen therapy should be given to all COPD patients with chronic resting hypoxaemia ($PaO2 < 7.3$ kPa) [12]. Selected people with advanced COPD may benefit from home non-invasive ventilation, bronchoscopic and surgical intervention or lung transplantation.

12 Ocular Manifestations of Chronic Obstructive Pulmonary Disease

In COPD, peripheral airway obstruction and parenchymal destruction occur, and pulmonary vascular abnormalities reduce the gas exchange capacity of the lungs, with subsequent development of hypoxaemia and later hypercapnia, secondary erythrocytosis and leukocytosis, which contribute to hyperviscosity and increased risk of thrombosis. These factors lead to ocular complications, such as central and branch retinal vein occlusion and non-arteritic anterior ischaemic optic neuropathy.

Clinical symptoms and objective findings

Anterior eye segment

Severe hypoxaemia and hypercapnia in COPD lead to a variety of metabolic, circulatory, respiratory, enzymatic, endocrine, and haematological disorders. The faces of patients with severe COPD acquire a polyglobular, plethoric and cyanotic appearance. Conjunctival hyperaemia, exophthalmos, swelling and sweating of the face, and a peculiar weeping appearance of the patient called "frog face" appear. In addition, chronic pulmonary diseases, including COPD, bronchial asthma, postoperative lung cancer, and pulmonary fibrosis are associated with a decrease in corneal endothelial cell density below 2,000 cells/mm^2 [19], therefore, patients with COPD are more prone to develop corneal endothelial dysfunction after cataract surgery.

Posterior eye segment

Hypoxia and chronic inflammation in COPD cause pulmonary arterial hypertension, increased intrathoracic pressure and decreased venous return. Reduced venous return and increased vascular resistance lead to diastolic and systolic dysfunction of the left ventricle and concomitant dilation of peripheral veins, including those in the eye fundus [51]. Thus, chronic hypoxaemia causes mild retinal changes that manifest as segmental dilation and tortuosity of large retinal vessels [24].

The interactive action of hypoxaemia and hypercapnia causes moderate retinal changes (retinal haemorrhage). In the case of severe hypoxaemia and hypercapnia, optic nerve and macular oedema develop in parallel with the formation of retinal haemorrhages and an increased risk of retinal vessel thrombosis [13].

Optic nerve oedema in patients with COPD due to pulmonary emphysema was first described by Cameron in 1933 [7]. Factors leading to optic nerve papilla involvement may include increased intravenous pressure and polycythaemia in addition to hypoxaemia and hypercapnia.

Patients with COPD also experience thinning of RFNL in all segments, but most markedly in the lower quadrants [47]. Chronic systemic inflammation and hypoxia given by the underlying disease induce the production of oxidative stress compounds and a disruption in the balance between dangerous oxidants and antioxidant stores [11], with subsequent axonal nerve loss and ganglion cell death [27]. The decrease in RNFL thickness leads to scotomas in the visual field and a decrease in visual acuity [15].

Another manifestation of COPD in the posterior eye segment is dilatation of the retinal veins and an increase in choroidal thickness. Hypoxia and chronic inflammation in COPD cause pulmonary arterial hypertension, increased intrathoracic pressure and decreased venous return. Decreased venous return and increased vascular resistance in turn lead to diastolic and systolic dysfunction of the left ventricle and concomitant dilation of peripheral veins, including vessels in the eye fundus [51].

Differential diagnosis

- Decrease in corneal endotheliocyte density—Fuchs endothelial dystrophy
- Optic nerve oedema—optic nerve drusen, intraocular optic neuritis
- Macular oedema—Irvin-Gass syndrome

Diagnosis

Includes examination of the anterior eye segment using slit lamp, posterior eye segment using fundus photography. Additional examination methods—perimetry to exclude scotomas and OCT to show possible optic nerve and macular oedema.

Therapy

The fundamental goal is to compensate for the overall COPD disease with the help of multidisciplinary collaboration. In the case of development of macular oedema due to retinal vein thrombosis, the treatment of choice is intravitreal administration of anti-VEGF agents or corticosteroids.

13 Cystic Fibrosis

Cystic fibrosis is a multisystem disorder and the most common inherited disease affecting Caucasians in the EU, North America and Australia/New Zealand [37]. Patients treated with newly available medicines are surviving into middle and old age. New treatment options have completely changed the fate of new patients in developed countries. However, the problem of previously treated or untreated people with CF remains.

The main complications and consequences of untreated or inadequately treated CF are chronic, often resistant, respiratory infections, including mycobacterial infections, haemoptysis, respiratory failure, malabsorption, cirrhosis, diabetes mellitus, osteopathy, and infertility. The diagnosis, monitoring and treatment of all patients with CF is beyond the scope of the general practitioner. Each CF patient requires an experienced multidisciplinary team to follow the patient from infancy to adulthood. An optimal team includes paediatrician, pulmonologist, microbiologist, radiologist, physiotherapist, dietician, diabetologist, specialist nurses, clinical pharmacist and psychologist.

Definition

Cystic fibrosis (CF), an autosomal recessive disease, is the most common inherited disease in Caucasians. CF occurs in slightly lower numbers in non-Caucasian ethnic groups.

The gene on the long arm of 7th chromosome encodes a multifunctional protein, the cystic fibrosis transmembrane conductance regulator (CFTR), which is active at the apical membrane of respiratory epithelial cells. CFTR functions as a chloride channel and regulates the epithelial sodium channel (ENaC).

Five classes of mutations have been described [37]. Classes I, II and III represent multiple disease-causing mutations in the CFTR gene associated with pancreas-insufficient CF, whereas those with milder disease-causing mutations (classes IV and V) are pancreas-sufficient. The combination of maternal and paternal CFTR genes results in a specific genotype. However, there is a poor correlation between the genotype and the pulmonary clinical manifestations of the disease. The most common mutation in the EU is Phe508del.

Epidemiology

Recent registry analyses show a mean prevalence of 7.37/100,000 in the 27 EU countries, which is similar to the 7.97/100,000 in the United States, with only one outlier, the Republic of Ireland (29.8/100,000) [23]. In contrast, CF is rare in Asians. In some parts of the world, CF is under-diagnosed due to poor access to healthcare, misdiagnosis, high infant mortality, and low life expectancy. These include Latin America, Africa, and India.

Diagnosis

The diagnosis of CF is based on compatible clinical findings in one or more organ systems (upper and/or lower respiratory tract, pancreas, liver and other parts of the gastrointestinal tract, reproductive system) with biochemical and genetic confirmation. An elevated sweat chloride test (> 60 mmol/L) is essential for routine laboratory confirmation. Abnormal nasal transepithelial potential difference (NPD), tests for specific genetic mutations (>1800 variants are currently described), immunoreactive trypsinogen (IRT), faecal fat content and pancreatic enzyme secretion (faecal elastase) may also be useful in some cases.

Non-paediatric physicians will encounter CF patients in two ways: (a) referral from a paediatric unit of an already diagnosed case, more common in developed countries; (b) new diagnosis in adulthood, often in mild "atypical" cases of CF [23].

Clinical presentation

The abnormal transport of chloride, sodium and bicarbonate due to CFTR gene mutations leads to thick, viscous secretions in the upper/lower airways, lungs, pancreas, liver, intestines and reproductive tract, and increased salt content in the skin secretions of the sweat glands. The typical CF patient gradually develops multisystem disease affecting several or all the above-mentioned organs.

Some CF cases present with hyperechogenic and dilated bowel or absent gallbladder on routine antenatal ultrasound. CT may be associated with preterm birth and/or low birth weight. Children with CF have typically been diagnosed because of: (a) meconium ileus (immediately after birth); (b) respiratory symptoms due to sinus/nasopharyngeal/lung disease; (c) failure to thrive due to malabsorption/malnutrition due to pancreatitis, bowel or liver impairment.

In adulthood, the manifestations of CF are as follows: (a) intermittent/persistent productive cough, rales, wheezing and/or rhonchi, dyspnoea as a result of chronic bronchitis and/or bronchiectasis and/or recurrent chronic respiratory infections and/or pneumonia (*Staphylococcus aureus*, *Haemophilus influenzae*, later *Pseudomonas aeruginosa*, *Stenotrophomonas maltophilia*, *Burkholderia cepacia*, Aspergillus species, non-tuberculous mycobacteria such as *M. abscessus* or *M. avium* complex); (b) rhinorrhoea, nasal congestion/obstruction, epistaxis, hyposmia/anosmia, ageusia, snoring, obstructive sleep apnoea, headache secondary to chronic rhinitis with/without nasal polyps and/or chronic pansinusitis; (c) steatorrhoea, poor weight gain, cachexia, oedema, anaemia, coagulopathy, diabetes as a result of progressive exocrine and endocrine pancreatic insufficiency. These patients also suffer from deficiencies of fat-soluble vitamins (A, D, E, K) and electrolyte abnormalities; (d) more than 95% of CF men are infertile due to defects in sperm transport, CF women are less fertile than healthy women [37], (e) Increased risk of fractures due to osteopenia and osteoporosis, clubbed fingers and toes due to hypertrophic osteoarthropathy; (f) Kidney pain, kidney infection, microscopic/macroscopic haematuria due to nephrolithiasis/nephrocalcinosis. Some people with CF suffer from repeated episodes of deterioration (called CF exacerbations similarly to COPD exacerbation) [37]. In addition, spontaneous pneumothorax and haemoptysis are recognised complications of CF, particularly in advanced stages of lung damage (Figs. 22 and 23).

Differential diagnosis

Symptoms of the following disorders may mimic CF: (a) primary immunodeficiencies; (b) primary ciliary dyskinesia; (c) non-CF bronchiectasis; (d) alpha-1-antitrypsin deficiency; (e) advanced COPD.

Therapy

CF therapy has undergone a revolution in recent years. All patients (six years and older) with CF should undergo CFTR genotyping to determine if this carries one of the CFTR gene mutations approved for CFTR modulator therapy [31]. A highly effective CFTR modulator combination (elexacaftor-tezacaftor-ivacaftor) has become the mainstay of therapy for some mutations. In some patients, we use a dual tezacaftor-ivacaftor combination or ivacaftor monotherapy. This new class of drugs (in mono, dual or triple forms) that modulate (compensate) the function of the congenitally defective CFTR protein is indicated for most CF patients [31].

Other CF treatments include drugs that liquefy viscous respiratory secretions/mucus in the airways. These include inhaled DNase and inhaled hypertonic saline.

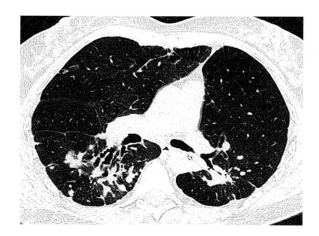

Fig. 22 Cystic fibrosis, transverse view, HRCT of the lungs

Fig. 23 Cystic fibrosis, HRCT of the lungs

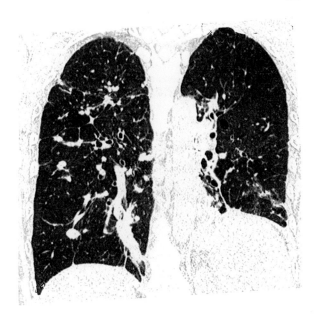

For each patient, chest physiotherapy methods aimed at airway clearance (effective expectoration) are effective. Inhaled bronchodilators (especially sympathomimetics) play an important role in the treatment of bronchial obstruction. Annual influenza, pneumococcal and COVID-19 vaccinations are essential. Antibiotics (oral azithromycin or inhaled tobramycin or antibiotics against bacterial, mycobacterial, and fungal infections) also have their place, although less than before CFTR modulation therapy. Oral ibuprofen has been shown to have an anti-inflammatory effect in people with less severe lung involvement. In patients with impaired exocrine pancreatic function, we provide adequate oral replacement therapy, fat-soluble vitamins and compensate for nutritional deficiencies. Some patients need insulin therapy, osteoporosis drugs and a range of other medications.

Prognosis

Lung disease remains the leading cause of death in CF worldwide. Recent advances in treatment, including the use of CFTR modulators (see above), have dramatically improved the survival prognosis for people with CF. In addition, many people with CF achieve sustained relief from chronic respiratory and digestive symptoms. In addition, CFTR modulator therapy appears to improve fertility rates and other clinical outcomes.

14 Ocular Manifestations of Cystic Fibrosis

CF is caused by mutations in the cystic fibrosis transmembrane conductance regulator (CFTR) gene on chromosome 7 [20]. Although several studies have confirmed the presence of CFTR in the eyes of CF patients (corneal and conjunctival epithelium, corneal endothelium and RPE), the aetiology of ocular changes in CF patients is still not well understood [46].

Clinical symptoms and objective findings

Anterior eye segment

The most common manifestation of CF in the anterior segment of the eye is tear film disruption [14]. Meibomian glands are modified sebaceous holocrine glands on the lid margin. Their main function is the production of an essential lipid component of the tear film that protects the cornea against microbes and evaporation of the aqueous component (called tear film stabiliser). Tear film disorder in CF patients leads to the subsequent development of evaporative dry eye syndrome and secondary blepharitis [22]. Other manifestations of CF in the anterior eye segment include oculosympathetic paresis and the development of complicated cataracts [8]. There are also reports of vitamin A malabsorption and conjunctival xerosis in patients with CF [26]. Vitamin A causes lysosomal membrane lability, resulting in the release of hydrolytic enzymes into the ciliary epithelium and activation of ascorbate transport into the ventricular fluid [25]. Low concentrations of vitamin A in the ventricular fluid also alter mucopolysaccharide metabolism. The consequence is the stabilisation of the acid hydrolytic enzyme containing lysosome-8 and the development of ciliary body oedema.

Posterior eye segment

The most common ocular manifestations of CF in the posterior eye segment include nyctalopia, due to the malabsorptive vitamin A deficiency, decreased contrast sensitivity, retinal vein occlusion, and optic nerve involvement [8, 41, 44].

Mutations in the cystic fibrosis transmembrane conductance regulator in CF patients are thought to lead to activation of pro-inflammatory cellular pathways and subsequent increases in fibrinogen and other inflammatory markers [39]. The rise in fibrinogen levels is associated with an increased risk of retinal vascular abnormalities, including CRVO and BRVO [33]. The cause of optic nerve changes is the toxic effect of chloramphenicol treatment in CF [16].

Another complication of CF is a significant decrease in the thickness of the peripapillary retinal nerve fibre layer in the inferior quadrant, which is similar to the finding in early glaucoma [14].

Differential diagnosis

- Decrease in the thickness of the peripapillary nerve fibre layer—chronic open-angle glaucoma
- Optic nerve impairment—toxic impairment due to methanol use

Diagnosis

Diagnosis consists of anterior segment biomicroscopy, including BUT test and ophthalmoscopy of the posterior eye segment. Additional investigative methods include OCT of the optic nerve and perimetry to confirm a decrease of the peripapillary nerve fibre layer. OCT of the macula is used to rule out CME in retinal venous occlusions.

Therapy

When complicated cataract occurs, the treatment of choice is phacoemulsification, followed by implantation of an artificial intraocular lens. In the case of development of macular oedema, intravitreal injections of anti-VEGF agents or corticosteroids are used.

References

1. Agustí A, Celli BR, Criner GJ, et al. Global Initiative for Chronic Obstructive Lung Disease 2023 Report: GOLD Executive Summary. Eur Respir J. 2023;61(4):2300239.
2. Albert DM, Raven ML. Ocular tuberculosis. Microbiol Spectr. 2016;4(6):10.
3. Alfano JE, Alfano PA. Glaucoma and the superior vena caval obstruction syndrome. Am J Ophthalmol. 1956;42(5):685–96.
4. Baughman RP, Grutters JC. New treatment strategies for pulmonary sarcoidosis: antimetabolites, biological drugs, and other treatment approaches. Lancet Resp Med. 2015;3:813–22.
5. Baughman RP, Judson MA, Wells A. The indications for the treatment of sarcoidosis: Wells Law. Sarcoid Vasc Dif Lung Dis. 2017;34:280–2.
6. Bradley B, Branley HM, Egan JJ, et al. Interstitial lung disease guideline: the British Thoracic Society in collaboration with the Thoracic Society of Australia and New Zealand and the Irish Thoracic Society. Thorax. 2008;63(11):1–58.
7. Cameron AJ. Papilloedema in pulmonary emphysema. Br J Ophthalmol. 1933;17:167.
8. Castagna I, Roszkowska AM, Fama F, et al. The eye in cystic fibrosis. Eur J Ophthalmol. 2001;11(1):9–14.
9. Churchyard G, Kim P, Shah NC, et al. What we know about tuberculosis transmission: an overview. J Infect Dis. 2017;216(6):629–35.
10. De Benedetti ZME, Carranza LB, Gotuzzo HE, Rolando CI. Tuberculosis ocular [Ocular tuberculosis]. Rev Chilena Infectol. 2007 Aug;24(4):284–95. Spanish. https://doi.org/10.4067/s0716-10182007000400004. Epub 2007 Aug 20. PMID: 17728915.
11. Domej W, Oettl K, Renner W. Oxidative stress and free radicals in COPD—implications and relevance for treatment. Int J Chron Obstruct Pulmon Dis. 2014;9(1):1207–24.
12. Duffy SP, Criner GJ. Chronic obstructive pulmonary disease: evaluation and management. Med Clin North Am. 2019;103(3):453–61.
13. Fisher OA, Romanchikov I, Ignateva L. Effect of local revasularization of choroid on ocular tissues and lipid peroxidation in experimental atherosclerotic chorioretinopathy. West Oftalmol. 1998;114(4):32.

14. Giannakouras P, Kanakis M, Diamantea F, et al. Ophthalmologic manifestations of adult patients with cystic fibrosis. Eur J Ophthalmol. 2021;8:11206721211008780.
15. Gunes A, Demirci S, Umul A. Vision loss and RNFL thinning after internal carotid arter occlusion and middle cerebral artery infarction. Acta Inform Med. 2014;22(6):413–4.
16. Harley RD, Huang NN, Macri CH, et al. Optic neuritis and optic atrophy following chloramphenicol in cystic fibrosis patients. Trans Am Acad Ophthalmol Otolaryngol. 1970;74:1011–31.
17. Herbort CP, Rao NA, Mochizuki M, et al. International criteria for the diagnosis of ocular sarcoidosis: results of the first International Workshop On Ocular Sarcoidosis (IWOS). Ocul Immunol Inflamm. 2009;17(3):160–9.
18. Ho YJ, Yeh CH, Lai CC, et al. ExPRESS miniature glaucoma shunt for intractable secondary glaucoma in superior vena cava syndrome—a case report. BMC Ophthalmol. 2016;16:125.
19. Ishikawa A. Risk factors for reduced corneal endothelial cell density before cataract surgery. J Cataract Refract Surg. 2002;28:1982–92.
20. Kerem B, Rommens JM, Buchanan JA, et al. Identification of the cystic fibrosis gene: genetic analysis. Science. 1989;245(4922):1073–80.
21. Kheir WJ, Sheheitli H, Abdul Fattah M, et al. Nontuberculous mycobacterial ocular infections: a systematic review of the literature. Biomed Res Int. 2015;2015: 164989.
22. Khurana AK, Moudgil SS, Parmar IP, et al. Tear film flow and stability in acute and chronic conjunctivitis. Acta Ophthalmol (Copenh). 1987;65(3):303–5.
23. Klimova B, Kuca K, Novotny M, et al. Cystic fibrosis revisited—a review study. Med Chem. 2017;13(2):102–9.
24. Liu X, Wang W, Wang AR, et al. Pathogenesis of retinal neovascularization in a rat model of oxygen fluctuations-induced retinopathy. Zhonghua Er Ke Za Zhi. 2007;45(1):7.
25. Mehra A, Umar A, Dubey SS, et al. The effect of vitamin A and cortisone on ascorbic acid content in the aqueous humor. Ann Ophthalmol. 1982;14:1013–5.
26. Neugebauer MA, Vernon SA, Brimlow G, et al. Nyctalopia and conjunctival xerosis indicating vitamin A deficiency in cystic fibrosis. Eye. 1989;3:360–4.
27. Palombi K, Renard E, Levy P, et al. Non-arteritic anterior ischaemic optic neuropathy is nearly systematically associated with obstructive sleep apnoea. Br J Ophthalmol. 2006;90(7):879–82.
28. Pasadhika S, Rosenbaum JT. Ocular sarcoidosis. Clin Chest Med. 2015;36(4):669–83.
29. Pastorova B, Kolek V, Zurkova M, et al. Age-related aspects of sarcoidosis. Stud Pneumol Pthisol. 2018;78:107–11.
30. Portocarrero LKL, Quental KN, Samorano LP, Oliveira ZNP, Rivitti-Machado MCDM. Tuberous sclerosis complex: review based on new diagnostic criteria. An Bras Dermatol. 2018 Jun;93(3):323–331. https://doi.org/10.1590/abd1806-4841.20186972. PMID: 29924239; PMCID: PMC6001077.
31. Rafeeq MM, Murad HAS. Cystic fibrosis: current therapeutic targets and future approaches. J Transl Med. 2017;15(1):84.
32. Rajasekaran NM, Horo S, Kuriakose T. Primary ocular presentation of tuberous sclerosis—a case report. Indian J Ophthalmol. 2019;67(3):433–5.
33. Risse F, Frank RD, Weinberger AW. Thrombophilia in patients with retinal vein occlusion: a retrospective analysis. Ophthalmologica. 2014;232(1):46–52.
34. Ritchie AI, Wedzicha JA. Definition, causes, pathogenesis, and consequences of chronic obstructive pulmonary disease exacerbations. Clin Chest Med. 2020;41(3):421–38.
35. Rodriguez A, Calonge M, Pedroza-Seres M, Akova YA, Messmer EM, D'Amico DJ, Foster CS. Referral patterns of uveitis in a tertiary eye care center. Arch Ophthalmol. 1996 May;114(5):593–9. https://doi.org/10.1001/archopht.1996.01100130585016. PMID: 8619771.
36. Rowley SA, O'Callaghan FJ, Osborne JP. Ophthalmic manifestations of tuberous sclerosis: a population-based study. Br J Ophthalmol. 2001;85(4):420–3.
37. Savant AP, McColley SA. Cystic fibrosis year in review 2016. Pediatr Pulmonol. 2017;52(8):1092–102.
38. Segal LN, Martinez FJ. Chronic obstructive pulmonary disease subpopulations and phenotyping. J Allergy Clin Immunol. 2018;141(6):1961–71.

39. Slobodianik NH, Feliu MS, Perris P, et al. Inflammatory biomarker profile in children with cystic fibrosis: preliminary study. Proc Nutr Soc. 2010;69(3):354–6.
40. Solovic I, Vasakova M, et al. Tuberculosis in facts and figures. Praha: Maxdorf; 2019.
41. Spaide RF, Diamond G, D'Amico RA, et al. Ocular findings in cystic fibrosis. Am J Ophthalmol. 1987;103(2):204–10.
42. Stankova Y, Vasutova I, Skrickova J. Superior vena cava syndrome: definition, etiology, physiology, symptoms, diagnosis and treatment. Intern Med. 2007;53(11):1211–4.
43. Stanojevic S, Kaminsky DA, Miller MR, et al. ERS/ATS technical standard on interpretive strategies for routine lung function tests. Eur Respir J. 2022;60(1):2101499.
44. Starr MR, Norby SM, Scott JP, et al. Acute retinal vein occlusion and cystic fibrosis. Int J Retina Vitreous. 2018;4:26.
45. Turner L. Atypical mycobacterial infections in ophthalmology. Trans Am Ophthalmol Soc. 1970;68:667–729.
46. Turner HC, Bernstein A, Candia OA. Presence of CFTR in the conjunctival epithelium. Curr Eye Res. 2002;24(3):182–7.
47. Ugurlu E, Pekel G, Altinisik G, et al. New aspect for systemic effects of COPD: eye findings. Clin Respir J. 2018;12(1):247–52.
48. Wan MJ, Chan KL, Jastrzembski BG, et al. Neuro-ophthalmological manifestations of tuberous sclerosis: current perspectives. Eye Brain. 2019;11:13–23.
49. Weclawek M, Ziora D, Jastrzebski D. Imaging method for pulmonary sarcoidosis. Adv Respir Med. 2020;88:18–26.
50. Yang SJ, Salek S, Rosenbaum JT. Ocular sarcoidosis: new diagnostic modalities and treatment. Curr Opin Pulm Med. 2017;23(5):458–67.
51. Zangiabadi A, De Pasquale CG, Sajkov D. Pulmonary hypertension and right heart dysfunction in chronic lung disease. BioMed Res Int. 2014;2014: 739674.

Gastrointestinal Diseases

Alexandr Stepanov⑩, Marcela Kopacova, Ilja Tacheci, Marie Burova, and Petr Hulek

1 Inflammatory Bowel Diseases

Inflammatory bowel disease (IBD) primarily consists of two units: Crohn's disease (CD) and ulcerative colitis (UC). While UC affects only the mucosa of the colon, CD can affect any part of the digestive tract from the oral cavity to the anus and occupies the entire wall of the intestinal wall. Both units have their own pathological and clinical characteristics, but they significantly overlap [37]. Sometimes it is not possible (especially at the onset of the disease and diagnosis) to classify a colon disease unambiguously and it is then called IBD colitis. The incidence of both diseases is increasing worldwide [45].

A. Stepanov (✉)
Department of Ophthalmology, Klaudian's Hospital, Vaclava Klementa 147, 293 01 Mlada Boleslav, Czech Republic
e-mail: stepanov.doctor@gmail.com

Third Faculty of Medicine in Prague, Charles University, Ruska 2411, 100 00 Prague, Czech Republic

A. Stepanov · M. Burova
Department of Ophthalmology, University Hospital and Faculty of Medicine of Charles University in Hradec Králové, Sokolska 581, 500 05 Hradec Králové, Czech Republic
e-mail: marie.burova@fnhk.cz

M. Kopacova · I. Tacheci · P. Hulek
Department of Gastroenterology, University Hospital and Faculty of Medicine of Charles University in Hradec Králové, Sokolska 581, 500 05 Hradec Králové, Czech Republic
e-mail: marcela.kopacova@fnhk.cz

I. Tacheci
e-mail: ilja.tacheci@fnhk.cz

P. Hulek
e-mail: petr.hulek@fnhk.cz

© The Author(s), under exclusive license to Springer Nature Switzerland AG 2024
A. Stepanov and J. Studnicka (eds.), *Ocular Manifestations of Systemic Diseases*,
https://doi.org/10.1007/978-3-031-58592-0_4

Fig. 4.1 **a** Normal endoscopic image of the jejunum, mucosal thinning into regular circular (Kerckring) folds, villi clearly visible in water immersion. **b** Endoscopic image of normal colon, shiny pink mucosa with vascular pattern

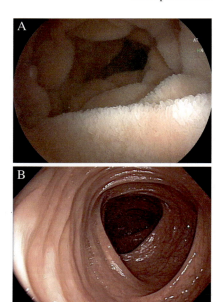

Normal endoscopic findings in the small bowel and colon are shown in Fig. 4.1a, b.

Aetiopathogenesis

The aetiopathogenesis of IBD is not fully understood, suspected factors are:

Genetic influences—data confirming the influence of genetic factors on the development of IBD have been obtained mainly from studies on twins, suggesting that the influence of genetics is clearly more severe in CD compared to UC [5, 11]. Children whose parents both have IBD have a 33% risk of developing IBD by age 30. The clinical manifestations and behaviour of the disease also show genetic features [19, 21].

Geographic factors—the incidence and prevalence of the disease is geographically stratified. It is lower in Asia and the Middle East, but also varies with the industrialisation of developing countries. In general, with the development of industry and urbanisation, the number of IBD diseases in the population is increasing.

Demographic influences—the development of IBD usually occurs between the ages of 15 and 30.

The influence of race and ethnicity is evident in the increased occurrence in the Jewish population.

Gastrointestinal Diseases

Risk factors

Smoking is a risk factor for CD, but not for UC. Nicotine and other products used for smoking can directly affect the mucosal immune response, smooth muscle tone, intestinal permeability, and microcirculation.

Physical activity is associated with a reduced risk for CD, but not for UC. Some data suggest a reduction in activity of CD due to the participation in physical activities by patients.

Dietary influences—fibre intake reduces the risk of developing CD, but not UC. Increased intake of animal fat and polyunsaturated fatty acids is associated with increased incidence of both UC and CD. Conversely, increased intake of ω-3 fatty acids is associated with a lower risk of CD. Vitamin D and sun exposure deficiency lead to a higher incidence of IBD.

Microbial factors—infection and immune response probably play a role in the pathogenesis of IBD [24].

Medications—antibiotics are associated with the development of CD, but not UC. NSAIDs are also associated with a higher risk of CD and UC, probably because of their ability to disrupt the mucosal barrier. Oral contraceptives and hormone replacement lead to a higher risk of UC.

Stress can lead to the exacerbation of symptoms in patients with IBD.

1.1 Crohn's Disease

CD is a transmural inflammation of the intestinal wall that affects any part of the digestive tract. Typical is the non-continuous involvement of the digestive tract; the disease has a segmental character, with the omission of certain sections of the intestine that have a normal appearance [41]. The most common location is the area of the terminal ileum and ileocaecal junction. The small intestine is affected in most patients with CD. Isolated colitis is reported significantly less frequently, in about 20% of cases. One-third of patients have perianal involvement. Only about 5% suffer from gastroduodenal or oral diseases. Involvement of the oesophagus and the oral part of the small intestine is less common.

As the involvement is transmural, it can lead to fibrotic changes on the digestive tract with scarring and stenosis (obstructive form), or to the formation of microperforations and the development of fistulas (perforating form).

CD is classified according to characteristics including age at the time of diagnosis of the disease, the location of the involvement and the behaviour of the disease—whether stenoses or fistulas are formed. There are several classification schemes, but, in practice and for study purposes, the Montreal Classification is most used [37].

Clinical symptoms

The main symptoms are usually abdominal pain, diarrhoea (admixture of blood and mucus in the stool), fatigue and weight loss (or inability to gain weight), and growth retardation in children [41].

Pain is usually localised in the area of the ileocaecal junction to the right iliac fossa, and can mimic appendicitis. Patients with the stenosing form present with colicky pain and ileus (Figs. 4.2 and 4.3a, b).

Causes of diarrhoea include excessive fluid secretion and impaired fluid absorption when the mucosa is affected by inflammation, malabsorption of bile acids when the terminal ileum is affected, steatorrhoea in severe impairment of the enterohepatic circulation of bile salts, and, in some patients, intestinal shunts due to interstitial fistulation with subsequent bacterial overgrowth and appendicular syndrome. All

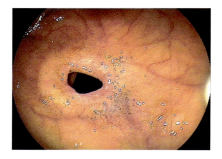

Fig. 4.2 Postinflammatory fibrous stenosis of the jejunum in a patient with Crohn's disease. The diameter of the stenosis is 3 mm, the bowel is dilated prestenotically, without Kerckring's folds

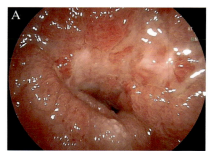
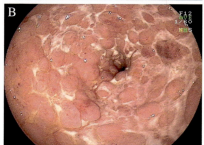

Fig. 4.3 a Florid inflammatory stenosis of the jejunum, fibrin-covered ulcerations evident. **b** Mucosal hyperregeneration between ulcerations, disappearing villi

Gastrointestinal Diseases

these mechanisms, including scarring and loss of intestinal surface area, lead to manifestations of malassimilation in severe disease.

Fatigue is a common finding caused by frequent diarrhoea, decreased food intake with impaired absorption and malnutrition, blood loss and anaemia.

Fever occurs less frequently. It is a symptom of a complicating disease, often in intestinal perforation with the formation of intra-abdominal abscesses. *Fistulas* form a communication between two organs with an epithelial lining, usually from the intestine to the bladder, to the skin, to another part of the intestine or to the vagina. Fistulation into the retroperitoneum may produce abscesses in the psoas area with associated symptoms, possibly ureteral obstruction and hydronephrosis. Phlegmon can also be a complication of the perforating form. Up to one-fifth of patients with CD develop perineal involvement with abscess formation, fistulas, and subsequent scarring (Fig. 4.4).

Inflammation of the intestinal wall can vary in expression, from small aphthous lesions to deep ulcers with a fibrinous lining and hyperregeneration of the surrounding mucosa, inflammatory polyps or relief called "cobblestone", where individual hyper-regenerative regions form post-inflammatory polyps macroscopically impressive as cobblestones (Fig. 4.5).

The manifestation of the disease in other localisations depends on the part of the gastrointestinal tract affected; in the mouth, painful aphthous lesions of the oral

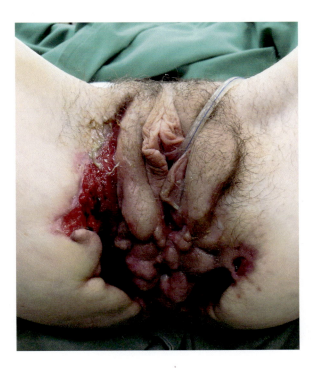

Fig. 4.4 Severe devastation of the perineal region in fistulating Crohn's disease

Fig. 4.5 Post-inflammatory mucosal hyperregeneration of cobblestone pattern

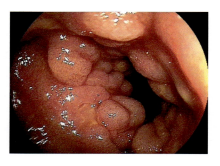

mucosa and gums, in the oesophagus it may manifest as odynophagia or dysphagia, in the gastroduodenum as epigastric pain, nausea or vomiting. The manifestations in this area are identical with gastroduodenal ulcer disease or obstruction of the gastric outlet. Affection of the oral part of the small intestine is usually accompanied by *malassimilation*, especially malabsorption. If more than 100 cm of terminal ileum is resected, the enterohepatic circulation of bile acid salts is disturbed and hepatic regulation of bile acid production is inadequate. The resulting condition is fat malabsorption.

Complications

In addition to the intestinal complications mentioned above (fistulation, intraabdominal abscesses, stenosis, diarrhoea, and malassimilation), extraintestinal manifestations of CD are also observed.

Arthropathy is the most common extraintestinal complication, affecting 20–30% of CD patients. Axial and small joints can be affected, sacroiliitis or ankylosing spondylitis can also be found.

Skin involvement is observed in 10% of patients, usually erythema nodosum and pyoderma gangrenosum. Fortunately, vulvar involvement with pain, redness, swelling and ulceration with subsequent scarring is rare.

Primary sclerosing cholangitis is found in 5% of patients with CD.

Nephrolithiasis and metabolic bone disease are common complications, especially of long-standing CD; glucocorticoid treatment, impaired absorption of vitamin D and calcium are involved in its development. Nephrolithiasis is also promoted by dehydration during diarrhoea and metabolic acidosis.

Infectious complications are common in immunocompromised patients; cytomegalovirus infection should be considered.

Secondary amyloidosis is fortunately a rare complication of CD.

Lymphoproliferative disease is increased threefold compared to the healthy population in patients treated with anti-TNF agents (non-Hodgkin's lymphoma), but these

Gastrointestinal Diseases   133

patients are usually also treated with thiopurines. There is also a higher risk of developing *malignant melanoma*.

For *ocular manifestations* see below.

Diagnosis

Clinical symptoms (pain, diarrhoea, fatigue, malaise, and weight loss) lead to the suspicion of CD. On routine laboratory examination, we often find anaemia, leucocytosis, mineralabnormalities including iron deficiency, increased inflammatory markers and vitamin B12 and D deficiency. Intestinal inflammatory markers (faecal calprotectin and CRP) are examined.

Endoscopic methods with the possibility of sampling for histology are the gold standard for CD examination. Imaging examinations (abdominal ultrasound, CT and magnetic resonance imaging) are valuable for assessing the general condition, GIT involvement and extra-abdominal complications.

Differential diagnosis

The spectrum of diseases that need to be differentiated is quite broad, due to the clinical manifestation of the disease: abdominal pain, diarrhoea, and weight loss.

Infectious colitis should be excluded, especially in patients with acute course and diarrhoea. *Ulcerative colitis* is sometimes difficult to distinguish from CD at the onset of the disease, but the diagnosis of UC is unlikely in patients with small bowel involvement, focal or segmental bowel involvement (especially rectal involvement), perianal involvement, fistulation, and malnutrition. *Diverticulitis* with inflammatory involvement of the diverticulum and its surroundings, or formation of a periappendicular abscess or fistulation. *Coeliac disease* can also be accompanied by inflammatory mucosal involvement with ulcerations and malnutrition, diarrhoea, and abdominal pain. *Irritable bowel syndrome* also often presents with abdominal pain and diarrhoea, but these patients do not develop an inflammatory response and mucosal involvement. *Lactose intolerance* and other food intolerancies also have similar symptoms to CD—i.e. diarrhoea, abdominal pain and bloating.

In other diseases is necessary distinquish appendicitis, ischaemic colitis, diseases causing perforation or obstruction of the intestine (benign tumours, carcinoma), common variable immunodeficiency (CVID), or cryptogenic multifocal ulcerative stenosing enteritis (CMUSE).

Therapy

In the treatment of IBD, corticosteroids are used in the first line, then immunosuppressants (especially thiopurines), antibiotics, 5-ASA preparations and, in more severe diseases, biological therapy (anti-TNFs, anti-integrin and anti-interleukin drugs). Mesenchymal stem cell therapy appears to be promising for the treatment of the fistulating form.

1.2 Ulcerative Colitis

Inflammation in ulcerative colitis affects the lining of the colon. The normal mucosa of the colon is compact, glossy, pink with a well-defined vascular pattern (Fig. 4.1b). In inflammation, the mucosa becomes edematous, erythematous, the vascular pattern disappears, and the mucosa is fragile, often with fibrin exudates, erosions, or ulcerations (Fig. 4.6). The disease typically affects young people aged 30–40 years.

Clinical symptoms

The clinical presentation is dominated by diarrhoea, often with blood and mucus or gas. Rectal syndrome, i.e. repeated painful urging to defecate, accompanied by a feeling of inadequate defecation and passing small amounts of usually liquid stool, is common. Unlike Crohn's disease, the involvement is continuous, but the extent of the affected mucosa varies. There are three types of disability: (1) rectum only (30–60%), (2) rectum, sigma and descending colon—left-sided colitis (16–45%), or (3) involvement extending beyond the lienal flexure—extensive type (14–35%) [44].

Diagnosis

The basis of diagnosis is endoscopic examination of the colon, i.e. coloscopy with sampling for histology. Other laboratory and imaging methods are similar to CD. In UC, however, there are no manifestations of malnutrition.

Differential diagnosis

Differentially, we must differentiate infectious colitis (bacterial, viral and mycotic), ischaemic, post-radiation, drug-induced colitis and "IBD-like" colitis in immunodeficient patients.

Complications

The local complication is *fulminant colitis*, with the risk of developing *toxic megacolon*. Distension of the colon in this complication can lead to a *perforation episode*. Another complication is *bleeding* into the colon. The development of *colorectal cancer* is a serious local complication, whose risk factors are the duration of the

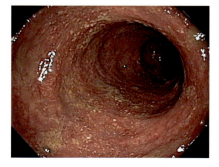

Fig. 4.6 Inflammatory altered mucosa of the colon in ulcerative colitis

Gastrointestinal Diseases

disease (after 20 years 3%, after 30 years 7%), the extent of colonic involvement (especially extensive involvement is risky), persistent disease activity and coexistence with primary sclerosing cholangitis.

As with CD, systemic complications include *thromboembolic* events and other *malignancies* (non-Hodgkin's lymphomas and skin tumours).

Therapy

In the treatment, a similar spectrum of medicines is used as in Crohn's disease. In both diseases, endoscopic and surgical therapy form an essential part of the treatment; psychotherapy and drug therapy for anxiety and depression are also an important part of the treatment. Increasingly, with the development of treatment options, understanding of pharmacokinetics, the use of biomarkers, and a deeper understanding of the pathophysiology of IBD, subpopulations of patients can be identified who are likely to respond to specific treatments. This personalised medicine appears to be the future in combatting idiopathic intestinal inflammation.

2 Ocular Manifestations of Inflammatory Bowel Diseases

The incidence of ocular complications in CD and UC ranges from 3.5 to 43% and is more common in CD than UC [18]. These include conjunctivitis, episcleritis, scleritis, marginal keratitis, anterior uveitis, retinitis, retinal vascular occlusive disease, optic neuritis, and orbital involvement [25]. Ocular manifestations may precede or follow systemic manifestations of inflammatory bowel disease (IBD). Several factors are associated with an increased risk of ocular manifestations. Patients with colitis and ileocolitis have a higher risk of ocular impairment compared to patients with ileitis. Affection of other organs also increases the risk. Especially in patients with CD and arthralgia, the risk of ocular involvement increases to 33%. Episcleritis occurs in 29% of cases and is an indicator of disease activity. Scleritis occurs in 18% of cases and anterior uveitis in 17% of cases [31].

The pathophysiology of extraintestinal manifestations of IBD is not well known but is most probably related to the inflammatory nature of the disease. Current theories include the presence of circulating antigen–antibody complexes or the production of autoantibodies against cellular antigens of the colon and extraintestinal organs. Inflammation causes damage to the epithelium of the intestinal mucosa, subsequently allowing proteins or microorganisms to pass through the intestinal barrier and cause a reactive response of the lymphoid tissue. This in turn leads to the production of antibodies or antigen–antibody complexes that circulate in the body and cause systemic inflammation. This immune response to colonic antigen may explain why ocular manifestations may occur more frequently with colitis and ileocolitis than with small bowel involvement alone. Genetic factors may also play a role in the ocular manifestations of IBD. Patients with extraintestinal manifestations of CD have a higher prevalence of HLA-B27 leukocytes than the healthy population.

Risk factors

- HLA-B27 positivity
- Immunosuppressive state
- Associated connective tissue diseases.

Clinical symptoms and objective findings

Ocular complications can be divided into primary, secondary and related. Primary complications are temporarily associated with exacerbations of IBD and tend to regress after initiation of systemic therapy. These include keratopathy, episcleritis and scleritis. Secondary complications arise from primary complications and include the development of steroid cataracts, scleromalacia due to scleritis, and dry eye syndrome due to hypovitaminosis A following bowel resection. Associated complications are common in the general population and cannot be correlated with IBD alone.

Orbit

Inflammatory diseases of the orbit have a variety of clinical manifestations, depending on several factors—the primary affected structures, an increase in orbital pressure and direct compression. Common findings include conjunctival injection, chemosis, eyelid swelling, proptosis, diplopia, pain on eye movement, ophthalmoplegia and decrease of the visual acuity [33]. Differential diagnosis includes malignancy, orbital cellulitis and trauma. Associations of systemic inflammatory diseases with orbital involvement include autoimmune thyroid disease, sarcoidosis, granulomatosis with polyangiitis, systemic lupus erythematosus and other connective tissue diseases. Dacryoadenitis is the rarest form of ocular adnexal involvement in IBD and usually presents with unilateral upper eyelid swelling, erythema and pain.

The pathophysiological mechanisms of orbital involvement in IBD are not clearly understood and require further investigation. Proposed pathogenetic autoimmune mechanisms include genetic predisposition, antigenic effect of Ig, and immunopathogenic autoantibodies against organ-specific cellular antigens shared by the colon and extraintestinal organs. The immune response to the colon antigen may explain why ocular manifestations are more common in colonic involvement.

Anterior eye segment

Keratopathy

Corneal involvement is a rare manifestation of IBD. Subjectively, the patient reports eye pain, foreign body sensation, eye irritation and, in severe cases, a decrease of the visual acuity. Corneal complications associated with IBD manifest as subepithelial keratopathy with two forms. The first is described as epithelial or subepithelial small grey dots located in the anterior layers of the cornea. The second has been described as deeper lamellar subepithelial infiltrates or corneal scarring. The involvement is usually bilateral and symmetrical, with infiltrates located 2–3 mm from the limbus. The pathophysiology of the formation of these infiltrates is unknown. Corneal involvement can also arise secondary to scleritis.

Episcleritis

Episcleritis is the most common ocular manifestation of IBD. Objective findings include episcleral injection, either sectoral or diffuse, which disappears after local administration of phenylephrine drops or after impression. There is no decrease of the vision, changes in pupillary response to light, corneal involvement, or photophobia. Mild to moderate eye pain and tenderness to touch are typical. Episcleritis is associated with active CD and can be considered as an indicator of the activity of IBD. Systemic treatment of IBD is usually sufficient to relieve ocular symptoms.

Scleritis

Scleritis is a rarer complication of IBD that can lead to severe eye impairment. Objective findings include deep conjunctival injection, which does not disappear following administration of phenylephrine and manifests itself with more pain in the eye than in the case of episcleritis. In rare cases, scleritis may be associated with peripheral stromal infiltrates of the cornea. Scleritis, unlike episcleritis, is not always associated with active IBD and can occur in patients in remission. Recurrent scleritis can result in scleromalacia perforans, an extensive thinning of the sclera that can lead to perforation (Fig. 4.7).

Up to 50% of patients with scleritis have an accompanying systemic disease, so a thorough examination of the patient's general condition is recommended [36]. Distinguishing between scleritis and episcleritis can sometimes be difficult. In general, scleritis occurs in older patients, is more painful and may show a characteristic bluish tint of the affected area of the sclera. In contrast, episcleritis usually occurs in a younger age group and is less painful. Under the dilated vessels, the normal shade of the sclera is preserved.

Anterior uveitis

Patients' subjective complaints consist of blurred vision and headaches. Although IBD can present with posterior uveitis or even panuveitis, the typical manifestation is a nongranulomatous form of acute anterior uveitis, which usually does not correlate

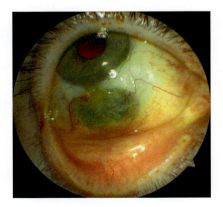

Fig. 4.7 Scleromalacia in a patient with Crohn's disease

with active intestinal disease. It may occur during the resting or active period of inflammatory bowel disease and may precede the diagnosis of IBD. Often, ocular manifestations are associated with skin findings of erythema nodosum and arthralgia. An association between CD, sacroiliitis and acute iritis has been demonstrated. These patients are often HLA-B27 positive.

It should be noted that asymptomatic uveitis was found in a significant percentage of patients with IBD. Similarly, some patients with uveitis have reported clinically quiescent colonoscopic findings associated with IBD, as have patients with spondylarthropathy [31]. Long-term complications of uveitis include the development of complicated cataracts, the formation of posterior and anterior synechiae, which can lead to secondary glaucoma. Secondary macular oedema may also occur. Treatment of uveitis includes cycloplegics and topical steroids and often requires systemic steroids and immunosuppressants.

Posterior eye segment

Retinal vasculitis

Although systemic vasculitis can be a complication of IBD affecting different parts of the body (skin, eyes, brain and lungs), retinal vasculitis is not very common. One possible pathogenic mechanism is inflammatory microvascular occlusion associated with vasculitis. The pathogenesis in Crohn's disease may include vascular damage, focal arthritis, fibrin deposition and arterial occlusion or neovascularisation. Granulomatous inflammation is associated with focal destruction of the vessel wall, adhesion of chronic inflammatory cells to the luminal surface of the lesion and fibrin deposition.

Associated ocular complications

Cataracts and open-angle glaucoma are complications of long-term intraocular inflammation or long-term use of corticosteroids. Some ocular manifestations are related to the medicines used in the treatment of IBD, such as corneal infiltrates and diffuse retinopathy related to adalimumab, anterior ischaemic optic neuropathy, and retinal vein thrombosis developing after infliximab [25]. Cyclosporine may cause a rare optic neuropathy. Methotrexate levels in tears approach serum levels after short-term use, which can lead to chronic irritation of the conjunctiva, cornea, and eyelids.

The use of biological therapy (anti-TNFs) may be complicated by the development of secondary uveitis, which has been described with etanercept, infliximab, adalimumab and rifabutin.

Neurological side effects of drug therapy can cause visual impairment without direct damage to the eye. For example, optic nerve damage can occur because of damage to optic nerve tissue due to inflammation and/or ischaemia, intracranial hypertension, and the secondary effect of anti-TNF therapy.

After bowel resection in the context of IBD, short bowel syndromes and malabsorption can lead to vitamin A deficiency, which can lead to nyctalopia and keratoconjunctivitis sicca. There is also a known association between the use of latanoprost

Gastrointestinal Diseases

drops in the treatment of glaucoma and the recurrence of IBD, where systemic absorption of a prostaglandin analogue induces an increase in intestinal inflammation.

Diagnosis

Diagnosis of ocular manifestations of IBD includes biomicroscopic examination, digital fundus photography, CT or MRI of the orbit to detect inflammatory changes or optic nerve involvement.

Differential diagnosis

- Rheumatoid arthritis
- Granulomatosis with polyangiitis (formerly Wegener's granulomatosis)
- Systemic lupus erythematosus
- Reactive arthritis
- Herpes zoster ophthalmicus
- Syphilis
- Gout
- Tuberculosis.

Therapy

Corticosteroids are the first-line treatment for most ocular complications of IBD. Local or subtenon administration of steroids is used in cases of scleritis and anterior uveitis. If ocular findings are refractory to topical treatment, systemic administration should be considered. Another option is the administration of systemic NSAIDs. A third option is the use of cytotoxic immunosuppressants such as azathioprine. This treatment is particularly effective in HLA-B27-positive patients. An alternative to immunosuppressive agents is biological therapy, such as the administration of infliximab, monoclonal antibodies to TNF-α.

3 Familial Adenomatous Polyposis

Familial adenomatous polyposis (FAP) is an autosomal dominantly inherited disease caused by a germline mutation of the tumour suppressor gene APC (Adenomatous Polyposis Coli), localised on chromosome 5q. The disease occurs worldwide, in both sexes, with a prevalence of 2–3 per 100,000 people [15]. The abnormal gene may be acquired from the affected parent (risk is 50%) or may arise as a new mutation (in about 25% of patients) [39]. Clinically, different localisations of mutations within the gene manifest as classic or attenuated FAP [13, 34]. Benign retinal lesions (congenial hypertrophy of the retinal pigment epithelium) occur in mutations localised between codons 463–1444.

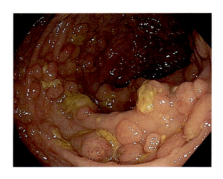

Fig. 4.8 Familial adenomatous polyposis, classic form. Hundreds of small colonic adenomas on colonoscopic examination of a patient before colectomy (25-year-old). Colonoscopy

Clinical symptoms

The fundamental manifestation of the disease is the presence of multiple colonic adenomas (Fig. 4.8). It is an important cancer predisposition syndrome, responsible for approximately 1% of colorectal cancers. The disease tends to be asymptomatic for a long time; the first manifestation may be a malignant tumour.

Classic form of FAP

In classic form of FAP, the first polyps of the colon appear in adolescence (12–17 years) [7]. Diffuse (carpet-like) polyposis of the colon (hundreds to thousands of polyps) occurs after the age of 20 (Fig. 4.9). Colorectal cancer (more often left-sided) arises in all patients with adenomas around the age of 40. Other (extracolonic) malignancies are also more common.

Attenuated FAP

This form is characterised by a lower number of colorectal polyps (up to 100) (Fig. 4.10), localised more in the right colon, at an older age (about 20 years later compared to classic form of FAP). Approximately one-fifth of the affected patients survive without developing cancer, and 10–30% of patients have no known APC mutation [23].

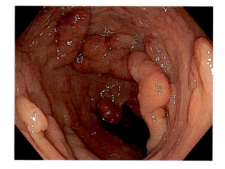

Fig. 4.9 Familial adenomatous polyposis, classic form. Advanced adenomas of the colon (adenomas with high-grade dysplasia) in a patient before colectomy (23-year-old). Colonoscopy

Gastrointestinal Diseases

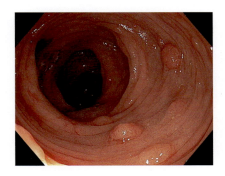

Fig. 4.10 Familial adenomatous polyposis, attenuated form. Dozens of colonic adenomas on colonoscopic examination in a 45-year-old patient

Extracolonic polyps

Gastrointestinal polyps occur relatively frequently in FAP outside the colon (30–100% of patients). The most common are gastric polyps (multiple, sessile polyps from cystic dilatation of the fundic glands: Fig. 4.11a, b).

Isolated gastric adenomas are rarer. Furthermore, adenomas of the duodenum are more common (Fig. 4.12a, b), especially in and around the papilla of Vater [38]. These polyps are the second most common precancerous lesion in patients with FAP after colonic adenomas (lifetime risk of cancer ranges from 4 to 12%).

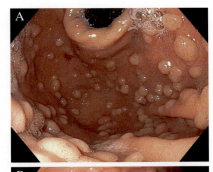

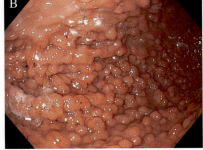

Fig. 4.11 a Familial adenomatous polyposis, gastroscopy. **b** Fundic gland polyps of the stomach, gastroscopy

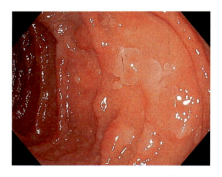

Fig. 4.12 Severe duodenal adenomatosis in a 38-year-old patient with familial adenomatous polyposis after colectomy. Gastroscopy

Other clinical manifestations

Patients with FAP have a higher incidence of various other malignant (thyroid, brain, liver, pancreatic, desmoid tumours) and benign diseases (fibromas, odontomas, osteomas, epidermoid cysts, adrenal adenomas).

Turcot syndrome is a historical term referring to the combination of familial colorectal cancer and brain tumours (FAP and medulloblastoma or CNS gliomas). *Gardner's syndrome* refers to concomitant polyposis of the colon and extracolonic manifestations (desmoid tumours, epidermoid skin cysts, lipomas, fibromas, dental malformations, osteomas of the jaw, CHRPE) [9, 22].

Desmoid tumours occur in up to 20% of FAP patients, more often in women of child-bearing age (hormonal influences) and after intra-abdominal surgery (including colectomy). Histologically, they are of mesenchymal origin, arising more often in the abdominal wall and in the mesentery. The tumours do not metastasise and may manifest locally as aggressive growth with abdominal pain, disorders of intestinal patency, vascular supply, or bleeding. Diagnosis and surveillance are based on CT or MRI scans. In treatment, there are some efficacy data for antioestrogens (tamoxifen), non-steroidal anti-inflammatory drugs (celecoxib). Chemotherapy (doxorubicin) and radiotherapy (due to side effects) are reserved for patients with inoperable findings. Some biologics (imatinib) have also shown efficacy in studies. Surgical treatment is reserved for patients with complications; the risk of recurrence is high.

Diagnosis

The gold standard of diagnosis is colonoscopy with histological examination of biopsy specimens or resected polyps. The disease is suspected in patients with more than 10 colorectal adenomas, or in combination of adenomas and FAP-associated diseases (CHRPE, duodenal adenomatosis, desmoid tumours, etc.). As part of the initial examination, it is necessary to obtain a family anamnesis (autosomal dominant type of inheritance of polyposis and occurrence of associated diseases). The detection of germline mutations in the APC gene is diagnostic (however, the absence of mutations—especially in patients with an attenuated colonic phenotype—does not exclude FAP). The patient's first-degree relatives are offered genetic testing and

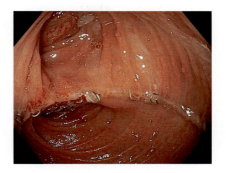

Fig. 4.13 Endoscopic examination of the pouch in a patient after proctocolectomy with ileo-pouch anal anastomosis

colonoscopy (from the age of 12) [28]. The patient undergoes further colonoscopic examination (with endoscopic resection of adenomas larger than 5 mm) until colectomy. Lifelong endoscopic surveillance of the retained rectum or pouch (depending on the type of surgery) is necessarily performed after colectomy [39, 43]. For attenuated FAP, colonoscopy with resection of high-risk colonic adenomas is a possible alternative to surgery. Regular upper endoscopies associated with careful examination of the duodenum and removal of high-risk adenomas are also a standard part of APC surveillance program.

Therapy

The basic treatment is colectomy as prevention of colorectal cancer. Only some forms of attenuated FAP can be treated by repeated endoscopic resection of polyps > 5 mm. In the classic form of FAP, on the other hand, colectomy is necessary, the only question is its correct timing and the type (extent) of the procedure. Colectomy with ileorectal anastomosis can be considered (instead of proctocolectomy with ileo-pouch anal anastomosis (IPAA) or colostomy) in cases of relatively milder rectal involvement (Fig. 4.13).

The patient's personal preferences, pregnancy planning, personal and family anamnesis (including an anamnesis of carcinoma or desmoid tumours) also play an important role in deciding on the type of colectomy. In general, total proctocolectomy with IPAA can be considered a more radical solution, with the risk of reducing the fecundity of female patients. Although there are data on some effect of chemoprevention (some non-steroidal anti-inflammatory drugs: sulindac, celecoxib) on the development of adenomas, its use is still controversial, and considered on an individual basis, not replacing colectomy in the prevention of cancer. After the surgery, the patient undergoes surveillance for life. Not only lower (retained rectum, pouch) and upper (stomach, duodenum) endoscopy with resection of larger polyps is performed, but also other examinations, with the aim of early detection of FAP-associated malignancies (regular physical examinations including thyroid, abdominal ultrasound). An initial eye examination is recommended.

4 Ocular Manifestations of Familial Adenomatous Polyposis

A variant of FAP with extraintestinal manifestations is referred to as Gardner's syndrome. A highly specific symptom is congenital hypertrophy of the retinal pigment epithelium (CHRPE), manifested in about 80–90% of cases [13, 22, 26, 32, 34, 40, 43].

Clinical symptoms

Most patients are asymptomatic—CHRPE does not affect the patient's visual acuity [14, 40, 42]. Rare formation and growth of orbital osteoma can cause exophthalmos, diplopia and eventually a decrease in vision [26, 42]. A decrease in vision can also be caused by papillary congestion in intracranial hypertension in Turcot syndrome. Epidermoid cysts of the eyelids can cause cosmetic problems, sometimes even mechanical ptosis [22, 42].

Objective findings

In Gardner's syndrome, congenital hypertrophy of the RPE is found, manifested by multiple pigmented foci, chaotically scattered throughout the retina bilaterally [8]. The lesions have a size of up to 0.5 PD, ovoid shape, irregular margins. One of the edges can often have the appearance of a depigmented "fishtail". Some lesions may be surrounded by a depigmented halo. Larger lesions sometimes show depigmented lacunae [9, 14]. This bilateral multifocal congenital RPE hypertrophy is a highly specific marker in patients with FAP, occurring in about 80–90% of cases [13]. However, it must be distinguished from benign CHRPE, which has 2 forms [9, 22].

Solitary

- Flat, dark grey or black, round or oval lesion, clearly demarcated
- May have hypopigmented lacunae in the centre or may be flanked by a depigmented halo
- The size of the lesion usually varies between 100 μm and several PD.

Multiple

- Multifocal lesions scattered on the fundus (often in one quadrant) have the appearance of "bear tracks"—one larger lesion is surrounded by several smaller ones (Fig. 4.14).

Other ocular manifestations such as orbital osteoma and epidermoid cysts of the eyelids are rarely found in Gardner's syndrome [34, 42]. Oedema of the optic disc is described in Turcot syndrome because of intracranial hypertension caused by a brain tumour [22].

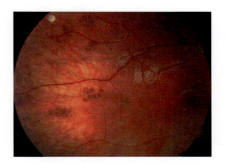

Fig. 4.14 RPE hypertrophy in a patient with familial adenomatous polyposis. *Note* Used with permission of Bohdan Kousal, MD, Ph.D.

Diagnosis

Hypoautofluorescence of lesions is typical, due to high melanin content [14]. FAG does not show fluorescein leakage. On examination, blockage of choroidal fluorescence is observed, except in depigmented lacunae (where we see hyperfluorescence of window defects) and halo (normal fluorescence). OCT examination reveals thinning of the neuroretina and loss of photoreceptors in the lesion, and absent RPE in the lacunar area [14].

Differential diagnosis

- Benign CHRPE
- Choroidal nevus
- Choroidal melanoma
- Melanocytoma
- Reactive hyperplasia of the RPE (following injury)
- Pigmented lattice degeneration of the retina
- Chorioretinal scar (after chorioretinitis, e.g. toxoplasmosis, toxocariasis, after trauma, after laser photocoagulation)
- Hamartoma of the RPE.

Therapy

Ocular manifestations usually do not require treatment.

5 Wilson's Disease

Wilson's disease combines two etiopathogenetic factors: a genetic defect and an environmental factor—copper, which accumulates in the brain, liver, eyes, and other organs.

The mechanism of tissue damage by copper, which is an essential element and serves as a cofactor in many enzymes involved in energy metabolism, is conditioned by a deficiency of the copper-transporting ATP-ase, which causes impaired excretion of copper into the bile and its accumulation in the brain, liver, and many other organs [1].

Clinical presentation

The clinical presentation of Wilson's disease is very heterogeneous. The disease is a disease of the younger age. Only rarely does it begin before the age of 5 or after the age of 50 [12]. The peak incidence falls in the second to third decade of life, specifically in the period 13–25 years of age [3]. The disease is slightly more common in men.

According to the prevailing symptomatology, we distinguish the forms:

- Neuropsychiatric form
- Hepatic form
- Other forms.

Neuropsychiatric form

The disease often begins with inconspicuous symptoms—slight tremor, speech impairment, micrographia. In the developed stage of the disease, dysarthria, dystonia, rigidity, tremor, hyperkinesis predominate. Speech is affected in almost all patients. Psychiatric symptomatology is almost always present—personality changes, irritability, as well as severe depression requiring psychiatric hospitalisation also being possible [10]. Untreated, the disease progresses rapidly and completely immobilises the patient.

Almost invariably, full-blown, clinically silent, liver cirrhosis is present in these patients.

The severity of neurological impairment is most often assessed by using what is called the "WD rating scale".

Hepatic form

Wilson's disease may present only as liver disease, without any clinically detectable neurological symptomatology. Liver disease can manifest in five clinical and morphological forms. The picture of hepatic steatosis does not have a characteristic clinical presentation, consisting mainly of histological changes, therefore it is not discussed separately [17].

Acute hepatitis

The picture is identical to viral hepatitis. The disease may occur several years before the manifestation of the underlying disease. It usually regresses spontaneously and adjusts to the norm.

Chronic active hepatitis

Clinical and laboratory symptomatology is pronounced. Icterus may be present, severe coagulation disorder, marked elevation of aminotransferases, hepatosplenomegaly, and sometimes ascites are very common. Ceruloplasmin is often only insignificantly reduced. It is currently the most common form of

Gastrointestinal Diseases

hepatic manifestation. The disease has a marked tendency to progress with severe haemocoagulation disorders and a tendency to bleeding.

Fulminant hepatic failure

This is an extremely severe form of Wilson's disease. Fulminant liver failure is found either at the beginning of the disease in young individuals or in patients who discontinue treatment for a long time. The interval from discontinuation to disease manifestation is between five months and five years.

Without liver transplantation, fulminant liver failure always ends in death.

Liver Cirrhosis

If the hepatic form of the disease manifests itself only at the stage of liver cirrhosis, the manifestation is usually turbulent with a picture of liver failure. Untreated patients have rapidly progressive liver cirrhosis, almost always with significant coagulation disorders and portal hypertension.

Other forms of manifestation

Rarer forms of Wilson's disease are possible—renal, bone and joint, cardiac, endocrine, haemolytic attacks [29].

Diagnosis

Biochemical changes

The basic screening test is the determination of serum ceruloplasmin levels. Urinary copper excretion greater than 1.5 μmol/24 h (100 μg/24 h) is a constant finding in the symptomatic form of Wilson's disease [30]. Recently, less emphasis has been placed on the penicillamine "stress" test, which consists of inducing urinary copper excretion with penicillamine.

Copper in the liver

The copper content of the liver is the most accurate diagnostic parameter and establishes the diagnosis of Wilson's disease. Normal levels of copper in liver tissue are low at 25–50 μg Cu/g of dry liver tissue. The upper limit for heterozygotes of Wilson's disease is 250 μg Cu/g dry liver tissue. Values in patients with Wilson's disease most often range between 450 and 1200 μg Cu/g.

Genetic Examination

Genetic testing is particularly useful in families with a proven anamnesis of Wilson's disease—when screening siblings of patients.

Diagnosis in the asymptomatic phase is more difficult, with normal serum ceruloplasmin and copper levels, as well as normal urinary copper excretion; the Kayser-Fleischer ring is also almost always absent [4]. However, a significant increase in liver copper content is present in all asymptomatic patients. Values tend to be higher than in patients in the symptomatic phase of the disease. The indications for testing for Wilson's disease are listed in Table 4.1.

Table 4.1 Indications for testing for Wilson's disease

Unclear liver lesion in children and young adults
Juvenile liver cirrhosis
Non-B—non-C chronic hepatitis
Hepatic steatosis
Liver disorder with hemolysis
Fulminant liver failure
Neurological-psychiatric diseases of young adults
Dystonia
Extrapyramidal syndrome
Tremor
Dysarthria
Hypersalivation
Depression
Hysteria
Psychosis
Amonoaciduria, Fanconi syndrome, nephrolithiasis, distal renal tubular acidosis
Hypouricemia
Kayser-Fleischer ring
Sanflower cataract
Siblings of affected individuals

Therapy

The purpose of the treatment is to remove the accumulated copper from the organ and to reduce its toxicity.

Penicillamine

The drug of first choice is still penicillamine (beta-beta dimethyl cysteine), which forms a chelate with copper that is excreted in the urine. In addition, it could reactivate enzymes containing sulfhydryl groups. Penicillamine treatment is a lifelong treatment and should not be discontinued for an extended period.

Undesirable effects: adverse reactions, mostly minor, are reported in up to 20% of patients.

Zinc

Zinc is now the most common alternative to penicillamine treatment.

Liver Transplantation

Liver transplantation is the only possible treatment for the fulminant form of Wilson's disease, with excellent results. Other indications for transplantation are progressive liver failure unresponsive to medical therapy and advanced cirrhosis with portal hypertension and complications.

Gastrointestinal Diseases

Prognosis

Until the discovery of an effective therapy, the prognosis was not favourable. Patients died within one to six years after the manifestation of clinical symptoms. This is still the prognosis of undiagnosed patients today.

Penicillamine fundamentally changed the prognosis of the disease. If treatment is started in the asymptomatic phase, it is possible to completely prevent the manifestation of the disease. Treatment can significantly improve even very advanced cases. The prognosis of Wilson's disease patients with hepatic cirrhosis with portal hypertension is ten times better than that of similarly advanced liver cirrhosis of other aetiologies. Wilson's disease is not a contraindication to pregnancy.

5.1 Ocular Manifestations of Wilson's Disease

Clinical symptoms

Problems in Wilson's disease are caused by liver, kidney, or neuropsychiatric disorders [3, 4, 10]. Subjective eye complaints are usually not present. Vision decline and colour vision disorder can very rarely be caused by optic neuropathy. Other rarer symptoms, such as night blindness and squinting, are described in the literature [6, 16, 27, 35].

Objective findings

The most typical ophthalmological manifestation of Wilson's disease is the Kayser-Fleischer ring, which is caused by copper deposition in the periphery of the cornea at the level of Descemet's membrane. It first appears in the upper part of the cornea, then copper deposits are seen at the lower edge of the cornea, and only later does a full circle form, which is separated from the limbus by a clear zone [16]. The KF ring is usually found bilaterally, its width is 1–3 mm. Sometimes it can be seen with the naked eye, but usually to rule it out or confirm it, we need to examine the patient on a slit lamp [10]. The Kayser-Fleischer ring is observed in about 80–95% of patients with the neurological form of the disease, while its incidence in patients with the hepatic form is about 50–65%. The KF ring usually does not interfere with vision. It is brown to golden in colour but can sometimes be green [2, 12, 27].

Sunflower cataract is another specific symptom of Wilson's disease. This is a clouding of the lens under its anterior and posterior capsule, caused by copper deposition at this point. The formation of sunflower cataract does not significantly affect the visual acuity of the patient [2].

Conjunctival icterus—yellow discoloration of the conjunctivae caused by hyperbilirubinaemia in patients with hepatic impairment [6].

Rare ocular manifestations of Wilson's disease include eye movement abnormalities, decreased blink frequency, night blindness, and optic neuropathy [20, 35].

The intensity of ocular symptoms may decrease with the initiation of pharmacological treatment or after liver transplantation, sometimes completely disappearing [2, 6, 12].

Diagnosis

Gonioscopy reveals copper deposits in the periphery of Descemet's membrane, which may be visible before being observed on the slit lamp [35]. OCT of the anterior segment helps to show the hyperreflectivity of copper accumulation at the level of Descemet's membrane [16].

Differential diagnosis

The false Kayser-Fleischer ring can be observed in chronic cholestatic liver diseases of other aetiologies (e.g. primary biliary cirrhosis, chronic active hepatitis, alcoholic cirrhosis, cryptogenic cirrhosis, progressive intrahepatic cholestasis). Deposition of deposits in Descemet's membrane in these pathologies is probably due to a secondary defect in the copper metabolism. The level of ceruloplasmin is usually normal [2].

Chalcosis is another cause of a false KF ring. It occurs in intraocular bodies containing copper, which is deposited in Descemet's membrane, under the anterior lens capsule and other intraocular basement membranes. Thus, we can also observe sunflower cataract in chalcosis. It should be mentioned that copper has a toxic effect on the retina. If the foreign body contains more than 85% copper, a severe inflammatory reaction or even necrosis of the intraocular structures can occur. The patient usually has a anamnesis of penetrating trauma to the eye [2].

Hereditary hyperferritinaemia with congenital cataract (hereditary hyperferritinaemia cataract syndrome)—an autosomal dominant hereditary pathology, characterised by elevated serum L-ferritin levels and the development of cataracts at an early age. Cataracts are caused by ferritin deposition and have a characteristic sunflower-like appearance [2].

Therapy

The ocular manifestations of Wilson's disease usually do not require special treatment.

References

1. Ala A, Walker AP, Ashkan K. Wilson's disease. Lancet. 2007;369(9559):397–408.
2. Amalnath DS, Subrahmanyam DK. Ocular signs in Wilson disease. Ann Indian Acad Neurol. 2012;15(3):200–1.
3. Bruha R, Marecek Z, Martasek P, et al. Wilson's disease. Time Medicine. 2009;148:544–8.
4. Bruha R, Marecek Z, Pospisilova L, et al. Long-term follow-up of Wilson disease: natural history, treatment, mutations analysis and phenotypic correlation. Liver Int. 2011;31(1):83–91.
5. Cho JH. The Nod2 gene in Crohn's disease: implications for future research into the genetics and immunology of Crohn's disease. Inflamm Bowel Dis. 2001;7(3):271–5.
6. Chou LT, Horkey D, Slabaugh M. Acute-onset optic neuropathy in Wilson's disease. Case Rep Ophthalmol. 2018;9:520–5.

Gastrointestinal Diseases

7. Cohen S, Gorodnichenco A, Weiss B, et al. Polyposis syndromes in children and adolescents:a case series data analysis. Eur J Gastroenterol Hepatol. 2014;26:972–7.
8. Coleman P, Barnard NA. Congenital hypertrophy of the retinal pigment epithelium:prevalence and ocular features in the optometric population. Ophthalmic Physiol Opt. 2007;27:547–55.
9. Deibert B, Ferris L, Weishaar P. The link between colon cancer and congenital hypertrophy of the retinal pigment epithelium (CHRPE). Am J Ophthalmol Case Rep. 2019;15:100524.
10. Drohobecka O, Balaz M, Rektorova I. Acute neuropsychiatric symptoms of Wilson's disease, treatment and the issue of non-compliance:case report of a young patient. Neurol Pract. 2012;13(3):135–9.
11. Duerr RH. The genetics of inflammatory bowel disease. Gastroenterol Clin North Am. 2002;31(1):63–76.
12. Dusek P, Bruha R, Burgetova A, et al. Wilson's disease. Czech Slov Neurol. 2013;109(5):539–49.
13. Falt P, Fojtik P, Kliment M. Gastrointestinal polyposis syndromes. General Med. 2009;11(12):558–60.
14. Fung AT, Pellegrini M, Shields CL. Congenital hypertrophy of the retinal pigment epithelium: enhanced-depth imaging optical coherence tomography in 18 cases. Ophthalmology. 2014;121(1):251–6.
15. Galiatsatos P, Foulkes WD. Familial adenomatous polyposis. Am J Gastroenterol. 2006;101(2):385–98.
16. Goel S, Sahay P, Maharana PK, et al. Ocular manifestations of Wilson's disease. BMJ Case Rep. 2019;12:e229662.
17. Hammad SC, Arayamparambil CA. Wilson disease. Treasure Island (FL): StatPearls Publishing; 2020.
18. Hopkins DJ, Horan E, Burton IL, et al. Ocular disorders in a series of 332 patients with Crohn's disease. Br J Ophthalmol. 1974;58(8):732–7.
19. Hugot JP, Laurent-Puig P, Gower-Rousseau C, et al. Mapping of a susceptibility locus for Crohn's disease on chromosome 16. Nature. 1996;379(6568):821–3.
20. Ingster-Moati I, Bui Quoc E, Woimant F. Ocular motility and Wilson's disease: a study on 34 patients. J Neurol Neurosurg Psychiatr. 2007;78(11):1199–201.
21. Karban A, Eliakim R, Brant SR. Genetics of inflammatory bowel disease. Isr Med Assoc J. 2002;4(10):798–802.
22. Katsanos KH, Syrrou M, Tsianos EV. The value of ophthalmic examinations in familial adenomatous polyposis syndrome screening. Ann Gastroenterol. 2003;16(4):287–99.
23. Kennedy RD, Potter DD, Moir CR, et al. The natural history of familial adenomatous polyposis syndrome: a 24-year review of a single center experience in screening, diagnosis, and outcomes. J Ped Surg. 2014;49:82–6.
24. Kleessen B, Kroesen AJ, Buhr HJ, et al. Mucosal and invading bacteria in patients with inflammatory bowel disease compared with controls. Scand J Gastroenterol. 2002;37(9):1034–41.
25. Knox DL, Schachat AP, Mustonen E. Primary, secondary and coincidental ocular complications of Crohn's disease. Ophthalmology. 1984;91(2):163–73.
26. Kuchynka P. Ophthalmology. 2nd, revised and supplemented edition. Prague: Grada; 2016.
27. Kunimoto DY, Kanitkar KD, Makar M. The Wills eye manual: office and emergency room diagnosis and treatment of eye disease. Lippincott Williams & Wilkins; 2004.
28. van Leerdam ME, Roos VH, van Hooft JE, et al. Endoscopic management of polyposis syndromes: European Society of Gastrointestinal Endoscopy (ESGE) guideline. Endoscopy. 2019;51(9):877–95.
29. Marecek Z, Bruha R. Wilson's disease, chapter 12 in the book hepatology. 3rd edition. Prague: Grada; 2018.
30. Marecek Z. Wilson's disease. Galen; 1996.
31. Mintz R, Feller ER, Bahr RL, et al. Ocular manifestations of inflammatory bowel disease. Inflamm Bowel Dis. 2004;10(2):135–9.
32. Munden PM, Sobol WM, Weingeist TA. Ocular findings in Turcot syndrome (glioma-polyposis). Ophthalmology. 1991;98(1):111–4.

33. Petrelli EA, McKinley M, Troncale FJ. Ocular manifestations of inflammatory bowel disease. Ann Ophthalmol. 1982;14(4):356–60.
34. Plevova P, Stekrova J, Kohoutova M, et al. Familial adenomatous polyposis. Clin Oncol. 2009;22:16–9.
35. Saiduzzafar H, Ansari Z, Kumar M. Wilson's disease with special reference to ocular manifestations (a case report). Indian J Ophthalmol. 1978;26:37–9.
36. Salmon JF, Wright JP, Murray AD. Ocular inflammation in Crohn's disease. Ophthalmology. 1991;98(4):480–4.
37. Satsangi J, Silverberg MS, Vermere S, et al. The Montreal classification of inflammatory bowel disease: controversies, consensus, and implications. Gut. 2006;55:749–53.
38. Spigelman AD, Williams CB, Talbot IC, et al. Upper gastrointestinal cancer in patients with familial adenomatous polyposis. Lancet. 1989;2:783–5.
39. Syngal S, Brand RE, Church JM, et al. ACG clinical guideline: genetic testing and management of hereditary gastrointestinal cancer syndromes. Am J Gastroenterol. 2015;110:223.
40. Tiret A, Taiel-Sartral M, Tiret E, et al. Diagnostic value of fundus examination in familial adenomatous polyposis. Br J Ophthalmol. 1997;81:755–8.
41. Torres J, Mehandru S, Colombel JF, et al. Crohn's disease. Lancet. 2017;389(10080):1741–55.
42. Traboulsi EI. Compendium of inherited disorders and the eye. New York: Oxford University Press; 2005.
43. Trna J, Stiburek O, Klimova K, et al. Familial adenomatous polyposis—recommendations for screening and dispensary. General Med. 2010;12(3):145–7.
44. Ungaro R, Mehandru S, Allen PB, et al. Ulcerative colitis. Lancet. 2017;389(10080):1756–70.
45. Zboril V. Idiopathic intestinal inflammation. Prague: Young Front; 2018.

Metabolic and Endocrine Diseases

Jan Studnicka, Marta Karhanova, Filip Gabalec, Alexandr Stepanov, Vladimir Blaha, Martina Lasticova, Jana Kalitova, and Jan Schovanek

1 Diabetes Mellitus

Diabetes mellitus (DM) is a heterogeneous group of chronic diseases with abnormal glucose metabolism, characterised by the presence of hyperglycaemia. It is associated with a relative and/or absolute deficiency of insulin secretion and varying degrees of insulin resistance. In addition to hyperglycaemia, other disorders of carbohydrate, lipid and protein metabolism are present. Hyperglycaemia is then associated in all types of diabetes with the risk of developing chronic complications.

Based on the pathophysiological mechanism, diabetes is classified into several categories:

1. Type 1 DM—caused by autoimmune β-cell destruction with absolute insulin deficiency
2. Type 2 DM—caused by progressive impairment of insulin secretion by the β-cell, often in the terrain of insulin resistance
3. Gestational DM—diabetes diagnosed in pregnancy

J. Studnicka · A. Stepanov
Department of Ophthalmology, University Hospital and Faculty of Medicine of Charles University in Hradec Králové, Sokolska 581, 500 05 Hradec Králové, Czech Republic
e-mail: jan.studnicka@ocni-visus.cz

J. Studnicka
Eye Centre VISUS, spol. s.r.o., Nemcove 738, 547 01 Nachod, Czech Republic

M. Karhanova · J. Kalitova · J. Schovanek
Department of Ophthalmology, 3rd Department of Internal Medicine – Nephrology, Rheumatology and Endocrinology, University Hospital and Faculty of Medicine of Palacky University in Olomouc, Zdravotníků 248/7, 771 47 Olomouc, Czech Republic
e-mail: marta.karhanova@fnol.cz

J. Kalitova
e-mail: jana.kalitova@fnol.cz

© The Author(s), under exclusive license to Springer Nature Switzerland AG 2024
A. Stepanov and J. Studnicka (eds.), *Ocular Manifestations of Systemic Diseases*,
https://doi.org/10.1007/978-3-031-58592-0_5

4. Other specific types of diabetes—resulting from other specific causes, e.g. monogenic diabetes, exocrine pancreatic disease, conditions after pancreatectomy, endocrine diseases (hyperthyroidism, acromegaly, glucagonoma, pheochromocytoma), drug-induced (glucocorticoid treatment, after organ transplantation).

In addition to DM, there are also conditions associated with impaired glucose metabolism, referred to as borderline disorders of glucose homeostasis or prediabetes. Prediabetes is usually associated with abdominal obesity, dyslipidaemia with high triglycerides and/or low HDL-cholesterol and arterial hypertension [3].

Epidemiology

Globally, an estimated 537 million adults are living with diabetes, according to the latest 2019 data from the International Diabetes Federation [48]. Diabetes is the 9th leading cause of mortality globally in 2020, attributing to over 2 million deaths annually due to diabetes directly and kidney disease due to diabetes [31].

Risk factors

Type 1 DM:

- Family history—first-degree relative with type 1 DM
- Age—more likely to occur in childhood, adolescence and young adulthood

Type 2 DM:

- Prediabetes
- Age
- Overweight/obesity
- Lack of physical activity
- Family history—more pronounced genetic predisposition than in type 1 diabetes

---

J. Schovanek
e-mail: jan.schovanek@fnol.cz

F. Gabalec · V. Blaha · M. Lasticova
3rd Department of Internal Medicine – Metabolic Care and Gerontology, University Hospital and Faculty of Medicine of Charles University in Hradec Králové, Sokolska 581, 500 05 Hradec Králové, Czech Republic
e-mail: filip.gabalec@fnhk.cz

V. Blaha
e-mail: vladimir.blaha@fnhk.cz

M. Lasticova
e-mail: martina.lasticova@fnhk.cz

A. Stepanov (✉)
Ophthalmology Department, Klaudian's Hospital, Vaclava Klementa 147, 293 01 Mlada Boleslav, Czech Republic
e-mail: stepanov.doctor@gmail.com

Third Faculty of Medicine in Prague, Charles University, Ruska 2411, 100 00 Prague, Czech Republic

Metabolic and Endocrine Diseases

- Polycystic ovary syndrome
- Anamnesis of gestational diabetes
- Medication—glucocorticoids, thiazide diuretics, atypical antipsychotics, statins

Clinical presentation

Type 1 diabetes mellitus

The basis of type 1 diabetes is autoimmune destruction of pancreatic β-cells and subsequent absolute insulin deficiency. It manifests itself with classic symptoms— thirst, polydipsia, polyuria, nocturnal urination, weight loss with normal appetite and fatigue. Often, very acute ketoacidosis with acetone breathing develops, eventually leading to alteration of mental status and even coma. In adulthood, there is a slower loss of insulin secretory capacity and patients suffer symptoms of hyperglycaemia for longer periods before a diagnosis of diabetes is made [79].

Type 2 diabetes mellitus

Hyperglycaemia in type 2 diabetes is caused by progressive impairment of insulin secretion by the β-cell in the terrain of insulin resistance. Most patients are asymptomatic at the time of diagnosis and hyperglycaemia is usually detected incidentally on laboratory examination. Less frequently, type 2 diabetes is diagnosed based on hyperglycaemic symptoms. Occasionally, type 2 diabetes manifests as a hyperosmolar hyperglycaemic state with marked hyperglycaemia, severe dehydration, and possibly impaired consciousness, without ketoacidosis [79].

Diagnosis

For the diagnosis of DM, *fasting plasma glucose, random glucose* testing and *oral glucose tolerance test (OGTT)* are used.

The OGTT consists of administering 75 g of glucose, with glycaemic testing being performed before glucose administration, after 60 minutes (for the diagnosis of gestational diabetes), and 120 minutes after glucose administration.

Normal fasting glycaemia values are in the range of 3.9–5.5 mmol/l; glycaemia in a healthy person is up to 7.8 mmol/l 2 hours after the OGTT.

In the case of *symptomatic hyperglycaemia*, when the patient presents with the classic symptoms of hyperglycaemia (thirst, polydipsia, polyuria, weight loss), a diagnosis of diabetes is made at glycaemic values of 11.1 mmol/l and above.

Asymptomatic hyperglycaemia is usually found in type 2 diabetes. Here the diagnosis of diabetes is made as follows:

- Fasting glycaemia $\geq$ 7.0 mmol/l (in the absence of symptoms of hyperglycaemia, this must be confirmed by a repeat test performed on another day)
- Glycaemia at minute 120 of OGTT $\geq$ 11.1 mmol/l

Prediabetes (borderline disorders of glucose homeostasis)

Values that are not normal, but do not meet the criteria for a diagnosis of diabetes, identify an individual with borderline impairment of glucose homeostasis. The criteria for their diagnosis are as follows:

- Increased fasting glycaemia—fasting glycaemia values from 5.6 to 6.9 mmol/l
- Impaired glucose tolerance—glycaemia at minute 120 of OGTT from 7.8 to 11.0 mmol/l

Other laboratory tests to clarify the diagnosis of diabetes

Determination of C-peptide fasting and after meal stimulation helps to determine the secretory capacity of β-cells and the degree of insulin deficiency. Low to zero values are found in type 1 diabetes.

Autoantibody testing is important for the diagnosis of type 1 diabetes. These include islet cell autoantibodies (ICA), insulin autoantibodies (IAA), glutamic acid decarboxylase (GAD) and protein tyrosine phosphatase (IA2) antibodies.

Glycated haemoglobin (HbA1c) is produced by non-enzymatic glycation of haemoglobin and reflects the average glycaemia over the 6–8 weeks prior to the test. Elevated values correlate with increased risk of complications and are used as a parameter to assess long-term glycemic control.

In diabetic patients, we also investigate *glycosuria*, which is currently of only indicative importance in the context of self-monitoring of glycaemia, and *ketonuria* and *ketonemia* in type 1 diabetic patients when ketoacidosis is suspected [3].

Differential diagnosis

Other causes of hyperglycaemia

Transient hyperglycaemia may occur in severe acute illness in non-diabetic patients. It is referred to as "stress hyperglycaemia" and its development is associated with increased serum concentrations of stress hormones (cortisol, catecholamines, glucagon, growth hormone), resulting in increased gluconeogenesis, glycogenolysis and insulin resistance [3].

Therapy

Chronic hyperglycaemia in diabetes results in macrovascular (atherosclerotic) and microvascular complications (diabetic retinopathy, nephropathy and neuropathy). In patients with type 1 DM, a lower incidence of microvascular complications (diabetic retinopathy, nephropathy and retinopathy) and a slower progression of microvascular complications with tight glycemic control were demonstrated in the Diabetes Control and Complications Trial (DCCT) [30, 68]. Its extension, the DCCT/EDIC (Epidemiology of Diabetes Interventions and Complications Study) also demonstrated a reduction in cardiovascular risk [67].

The UKPDS (United Kingdom Prospective Diabetes Study) and ADVANCE (Action in Diabetes and Vascular Disease: preterax and diamicron—MR Controlled Evaluation) trials in patients with type 2 DM showed a similar effect on reducing the risk of microvascular complications in patients with more intensive treatment and tighter diabetes control. The effect of tight glycaemic control on cardiovascular risk in patients with type 2 DM has not been demonstrated; risk reduction appears to be achievable if tight glycaemic control is reached as soon as possible after onset, and in patients with a longer history of chronic hyperglycaemia, cardiovascular risk is no longer substantially reduced [77, 102, 112]. Conversely, intensive treatment

Metabolic and Endocrine Diseases

in patients with long-standing DM or high cardiovascular risk may have negative consequences, as shown by the ACCORD (Action to Control Cardiovascular Risk in Diabetes) [24], VADT (Veterans Affairs Diabetes Trial) and ADVANCE studies. Reduction of morbidity and mortality in diabetic patients is achieved by intervention of other atherosclerotic risk factors—hypertension, dyslipidaemia, smoking [97].

Treatment objectives

The basic principle of treatment is to set target values for glycaemia and glycated haemoglobin. Patient performs self-monitoring of blood glucose, and values obtained are useful in adjusting treatment, especially in patients on insulin treatment. Other important methods of monitoring glycaemia are flash glucose monitoring (FGM) and continuous glucose monitoring (CGM).

The setting of treatment goals must be individualised, based on the needs of the individual. The treatment goals should reflect on the one hand, the desire to prevent or slow the progression of microvascular complications, and on the other hand, the risk of hypoglycaemia, which may outweigh the benefit of glycaemic control for chronic complications [3].

- In most patients, the target HbA1c values are up to 53 mmol/mol.
- In some patients, assuming safe treatment without the occurrence of more severe hypoglycaemia, it is possible to set HbA1c targets of up to 47 mmol/mol.
- Less intensive target HbA1c values of up to 64 mmol/mol are acceptable for patients with a history of severe hypoglycaemia, limited life expectancy, advanced microvascular or macrovascular complications, and severe comorbidities.
- Tight glycaemic control with target HbA1c values up to 42 mmol/mol is recommended during pregnancy [3].

In the treatment of diabetes, non-pharmacological and pharmacological treatment is used. Non-pharmacological treatment focuses on lifestyle modification in terms of diet, regular physical activity and weight reduction.

Diet

Type 1 diabetic patients are not obese, so they do not require restrictions on foods other than simple carbohydrates and should be able to calculate ingested carbohydrate amounts. The principle is regulated dietary intake and they should include foods in their diet that help reduce the risk of atherosclerosis.

Most patients with type 2 diabetes are overweight or obese, and obesity is associated with the development of insulin resistance. Therefore, caloric restriction is part of the dietary recommendations. Significant limitation of simple carbohydrates, reduction of saturated fat and increase in fibre intake are appropriate.

Physical activity

In patients with type 1 DM, regular physical activity is important for maintaining muscle mass and cardiovascular fitness. Patients must be instructed to adjust insulin doses to avoid hypoglycaemia during exercise.

In the case of type 2 DM, a regular exercise regime leads to weight loss and weight maintenance, improved insulin sensitivity and has positive effect on the cardiovascular system. Regular physical activity, preferably aerobic (brisk walking, running, swimming) is recommended, 3 to 4 times a week for at least 30 minutes [20, 79].

Pharmacotherapy of diabetes

Metformin

Metformin is the drug of choice for patients with type 2 DM unless contraindicated (chronic kidney disease, advanced heart failure and other potentially hypoxemic conditions, hepatic insufficiency). The main effect is thought to be a reduction in hepatic gluconeogenesis and a reduction of insulin resistance. The advantage is the low risk of hypoglycaemia and high efficacy [3, 112].

Insulin secretagogues

Sulfonylurea derivatives and other insulin secretagogues stimulate insulin secretion and release from pancreatic β-cells. The most common side effect is hypoglycaemia. Preparations with a shorter half-life are preferable, e.g. glimepiride, glipizide, gliclazide.

Repaglinide and nateglinide are short-acting insulin secretagogues that have a similar mechanism of action to sulfonylurea derivatives. They have slightly lower efficacy.

Thiazolidinediones (glitazones)

Glitazones are antidiabetic drugs that reduce insulin resistance; they affect not only glucose metabolism, but also adipose tissue. The only representative, pioglitazone, is not suitable in patients with chronic heart failure, osteoporosis, risk of falls, and in patients with macular oedema.

Incretin treatment

Incretins are hormones released by the digestive tract after food intake. They stimulate insulin secretion in response to glycaemia, they slow gastric emptying and suppress appetite. GLP-1 receptor agonists (incretin mimetics) and DPP-4 inhibitors (gliptins), which inhibit the GLP-1-degrading enzyme dipeptidyl peptidase 4 (DPP-4), are used in treatment. DPP-4 inhibitors have a minimal risk of hypoglycaemia and other side effects. Incretin mimetics are significantly more effective. Recently, many benefits of GLP-1 RA treatment have been demonstrated, particularly on the cardiovascular system in patients with pre-existing cardiovascular disease.

SGLT2 (sodium-glucose cotransporter 2, gliflosins) inhibitors

Gliflozins block glucose reabsorption in the kidneys and cause glucosuria. They have proven benefits in patients with pre-existing atherosclerotic cardiovascular disease and in slowing the progression of chronic kidney disease.

Metabolic and Endocrine Diseases

Insulin

Insulin replacement therapy is essential in patients with type 1 diabetes mellitus. Given the absolute insulin deficiency, we try to mimic physiological insulin secretion, either by administering several daily doses of insulin using insulin applicators (pens) or by using an insulin pump.

In type 2 diabetic patients, insulin therapy is indicated after failure of treatment with non-insulin antidiabetic agents, when other antidiabetic agents are contraindicated, and in pregnancy. The development of type 2 DM involves failure of insulin production by the β-cell as its dysfunction progresses. Insulin can be administered in a single daily dose in combination with oral antidiabetic agents. Another option is to administer 2 daily doses of premixed insulin or an intensified insulin regimen as in type 1 diabetes [3, 79].

2 Ocular Manifestations of Diabetes

Diabetic retinopathy (DR) is the most common microvascular complication of diabetes and is the leading cause of vision loss in the working-age population in industrialised countries [35]. Blindness in DR is most caused by diabetic macular oedema (DME), especially in type 2 diabetics. Vision loss due to proliferative retinopathy is less common, mainly due to effective treatment (laser photocoagulation and pars plana vitrectomy).

The 2017 International Council of Ophthalmology (ICO) Conclusions for the Care of the Eye with Diabetic Changes report an incidence of diabetic retinopathy of 34.6% in patients with diabetes in Europe, USA, Australia and Asia [121]. Globally, the number of adults with DR and DME is estimated to be 103.12 million and 18.83 million in 2020, respectively, and is projected to increase to 160.5 million and 28.61 million by 2045 [111].

Pathogenesis

The basis of DR and DME is hyperglycaemia, which leads by various mechanisms to microcirculatory failure. Capillary dilatation is the first clinically significant early manifestation of retinopathy. The ongoing process is manifested on the capillaries by the disappearance of pericytes. The contact between endothelial cells and pericytes loosens and they cease to influence blood flow in the capillaries, which results in gradual involution of the vasculature. Because of the preceding changes, capillary hyperpermeability occurs with leakage of serum into the retina and the development of retinal oedema. Another underlying clinical finding in diabetic retinopathy is retinal vascular occlusion, which is followed by the development of ischaemic retinal areas with increased release of angiogenic factors [99]. Chronic inflammatory processes in the capillaries also play a role in the pathophysiology of DR. The consequence is a deepening retinal hypoxia. Hypoxia and retinal ischaemia stimulate the overproduction of angiogenic factors (e.g. vascular endothelial growth factor—VEGF), which further increase capillary permeability and, through their angiogenic effects, have a direct effect on the formation of newly formed retinal vessels. They are fragmented and prone to bleeding. High levels of inflammatory mediators correlate with the development of fibrosis in advanced stages of proliferative DR [4]. Maturation of fibrovascular membranes results in traction and, in terminal stages, tractional retinal detachment.

Risk factors

The main risk factors include the duration of diabetes, type of diabetes (we observe more frequent development of DR in type 1 DM), unsatisfactory compensation of diabetes, arterial hypertension, presence of macro- or microalbuminuria and dyslipidaemia [99]. Another established risk factor is pregnancy, which accelerates existing advanced forms of DR. Proliferative DR thus needs to be treated with laser, ideally before the onset of pregnancy. In general, however, diabetic retinopathy is not a contraindication to spontaneous delivery [121]. Individual decisions must be made in diabetic women with proliferative DR and risk of vitreous hemorrhage.

Normoglycaemic re-entry phenomenon (early worsening syndrome) occurs when treatment with an intensified insulin regimen or insulin pump is followed by a rapid fall in glycated haemoglobin (HbA1c). The higher the glycated haemoglobin level at the start of compensation and the longer the period of poor diabetes compensation, the higher the risk of developing the syndrome with worsening diabetic retinopathy after a rapid fall in HbA1c. The existence of this syndrome is not a reason to delay glycaemic compensation. However, it requires more frequent eye fundus examinations.

Diagnosis

In addition to the examinations used in ophthalmology in general, the evaluation of pathological changes in the retina is crucial. For this we use ophthalmoscopy, colour fundus photography, fluorescein angiography, OCT and OCT angiography. To document the maximum changes and status of the retinal periphery, we currently use wide-field systems.

Fluorescein angiography has been the most important method in the diagnosis and monitoring of patients with DR and DME for decades. Although it is now primarily being replaced by OCT in the diagnosis of DME, it remains essential in deciding the presence of leaking microaneurysms, differentiating IRMA from retinal neovascularisation, and determining the area of capillary nonperfusion and the extent of the foveal avascular zone (Fig. 1).

OCT is essential in the diagnosis, classification, monitoring and indication for treatment of patients with DME (Fig. 2). Findings on OCT can be biomarkers of treatment success and disease prognosis.

OCT angiography allows examination of the retinal and choroidal vasculature without the application of contrast medium. Its benefit in diabetic retinopathy is the detection of retinal disorders, with the possibility of differentiation according to

Fig. 1 Signs of proliferative diabetic retinopathy on FAG with extensive sections of capillary nonperfusion and retinal neovascularization present

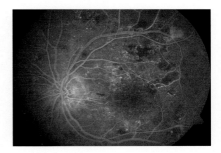

Fig. 2 Diffuse diabetic macular oedema with neuroretinal macrocysts on OCT

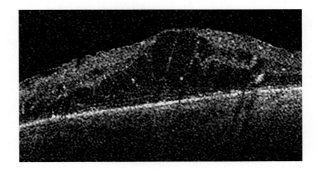

retinal layers. Changes of the deep capillary plexus are difficult to detect with conventional fluorescence angiography. In proliferative diabetic retinopathy, the presence of retinal neovascularisation can be demonstrated (Fig. 3).

Clinical presentations

In the initial stages of DR, disappearance of the capillary network is found with dilatation of the surrounding capillaries, enlargement of the foveal avascular zone and formation of microaneurysms. These changes are the result of occlusions and atrophy of the damaged capillaries and may not initially affect the diabetic's vision [103]. Continued changes are characterised by arteriolar obliteration with the formation of larger nonperfused areas. Because of damage to the vascular wall, intraretinal hemorrhages occur after rupture of microaneurysms, capillaries or venules. Their character (dot-blot, flame-shaped, cluster, diffuse, petaloid) is determined mainly by their location in different layers of the retina and the origin of the hemorrhage. Most often, when newly formed vessels rupture, preretinal hemorrhage occurs, localised between the retina and the posterior vitreous membrane. If a newly formed vessel growing from the retina into the vitreous ruptures, intravitreal hemorrhage may be observed [99].

Because of the breakdown of the inner hemato-ocular barrier of microaneurysms and capillaries, extracellular oedema with fluid accumulation in the outer plexiform layer of the retina occurs. In the case of intracellular retinal oedema, a greyish discolouration of the retina is observed. It is localised in the neural and ganglion

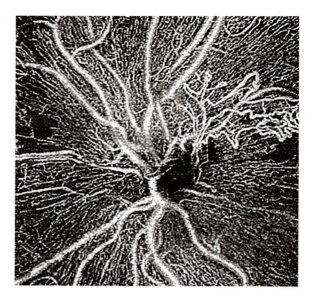

Fig. 3 Capillary network dropouts of the superficial capillary plexus and newly formed vessels arising from the optic disc demonstrated on OCT A

cell layer of the retina and is seen in more extensive zones of capillary nonperfusion [99]. Hard exudates consisting of lipoproteins and fibrin are seen in the area of leaking microaneurysms and capillaries. Particularly in the macular area, extensive plaques may form, leaving scars and defects of the retinal pigment epithelium and photoreceptors with permanent visual impairment. Another finding in DR is cotton wool spots (soft exudates), which are a manifestation of arteriolar occlusion in the retinal nerve layer and indicate focal ischaemia in that area. In advanced forms of retinopathy, venous abnormalities such as venous beading or venous loops may be seen (Fig. 4).

Intraretinal microvascular abnormalities (IRMAs) are changes in the capillary network seen on the retina [119]. Prolonged retinal ischaemia at the site of capillary and arteriolar nonperfusion is the impetus for the development and growth of retinal neovascularisation. Intraretinal neovascularisations always develop from the

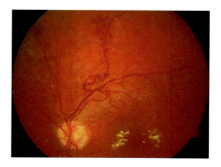

Fig. 4 Phlebopathy of the retinal veins with omega loop

Fig. 5 High-risk proliferative diabetic retinopathy

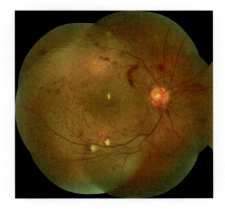

venous trunk and are most found in the post-equatorial part of the retina and in the upper temporal quadrant [99]. At the periphery of the nonperfused areas, preretinal neovascularisations are found growing through the internal limiting membrane. Their growth towards the vitreous may be followed by retinal traction. In severe retinal capillary nonperfusion, neovascularisations may develop at the optic disc (Fig. 5).

Along the newly formed vessels, fibrous tissue growth can be observed, which progressively contracts and leads to retinal traction and detachment [94] (Fig. 6).

Classification and system of controls

The basic classification of DR is into *non-proliferative* and *proliferative*. Classification of clinical findings according to the International Council of Ophthalmology [121] (Table 1).

The current basic system of classification of DME is based on OCT diagnosis and localization of the edema in relation to the center of the macula (Table 2).

Central involved DME is further divided into the state with deterioration of VA (worse than 20/32—Snellen worse than 6/9) and the state without deterioration of VA (20/32 and better—Snellen 6/9 and better) [40, 121] (Fig. 7).

A key factor in the more detailed diagnosis and classification of DME is an analysis of morphological retinal changes, the detection of precisely defined biomarkers and

Fig. 6 High-risk proliferative diabetic retinopathy with fibrovascular proliferation and tractional retinal detachment

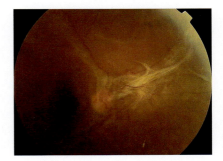

Table 1 Assessment of clinical findings according to the International Council of Ophthalmology

Diabetic retinopathy	Finding on the retina
Mild non-proliferative DR	Microaneurysms only
Moderate non-proliferative DR	Microaneurysms and other changes (punctate and mottled haemorrhages, hard exudates, cotton-wool spots) but less than in severe non-proliferative DR
Severe non-proliferative DR	Signs of moderate non-proliferative DR with at least one of the following changes: Intraretinal haemorrhage (≥ 20 in each quadrant) Phlebopathy (in 2 quadrants) Intraretinal microvascular abnormalities (in 1 quadrant) No evidence of proliferative retinopathy
Proliferative DR	Signs of severe non-proliferative DR and at least one of the following: Neovascularization Intravitreal haemorrhage Preretinal haemorrhage

Table 2 DME classification

Diabetic macular edema	Retinal findings
No DME	No increase in retinal (macular) thickness, absence of hard exudates
Non-CIDME (non-central involved DME)	Increase in macular thickness outside 1 mm diameter of the central subfoveal zone
CIDME (central involved DME)	Increase in macular thickness inside 1 mm diameter of the central subfoveal zone

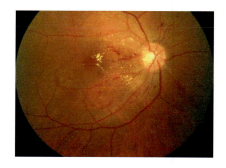

Fig. 7 Diabetic macular oedema with hard exudates in the macula

an assessment of the thickness of the subfoveal zone with a diameter of 1 mm around the center (CST—central subfield thickness). Classification parameters and main markers of DME are: retinal thickness, size of intraretinal cysts, visibility of the outer limiting membrane/ellipsoid zone in the fovea, presence of DRIL (disorganisation of the inner retinal layers), presence of subfoveal fluid, presence and number of hyperreflective intraretinal lesions—foci, and vitreoretinal status [40, 75].

Retinal examination is indicated in adult diabetics at the time of diagnosis of diabetes. In the case of children with type 1 diabetes, it is recommended to start regular monitoring 5 years after the diagnosis of diabetes mellitus. Further follow-up should be at an interval of 1–2 years in the absence of DR and DME or in mild non-proliferative DR. More frequent follow-ups are needed in diabetic patients with more advanced stages of DR, DME, during pregnancy, at the initiation of treatment with identified regimen or insulin pump, initiation of peritoneal dialysis or hemodialysis, change of classification of DM, decompensation of hypertension, and following transplant of kidney, pancreas, islets of Langerhans [69, 121].

This ideal condition is not met in a significant proportion of patients in routine practice, so high hopes have recently been placed on the involvement of artificial intelligence (AI) to analyse retinal findings.

Treatment

Influencing the underlying risk factors for DR

The need to compensate for both types of DM to reduce the risk of diabetic retinopathy has been demonstrated in several clinical studies [30, 97, 102]. Less stringent glycaemic targets are preferred in patients with a anamnesis of severe hypogly-caemia, shorter life expectancy, advanced micro- and macrovascular complications, or extensive comorbidities [97].

Achieving normal blood pressure values is also essential in both types of diabetes, as shown by the results of large studies [23, 96, 102].

Results of observational studies describe an association between serum lipids and diabetic ophthalmopathy [24, 28, 57, 122]. Elevated levels of total and LDL-cholesterol and triglycerides are associated with progression of retinopathy, proliferative retinopathy and development of macular oedema.

This knowledge has led to the assumption that a reduction in the risk of microvas-cular complications can also be achieved by treating dyslipidaemia. The results of large recent trials are convincing: two randomised, placebo-controlled trials, FIELD and ACCORD, showed that treatment with fenofibrate led to a statistically and clinically significant reduction in the risk of retinopathy [24, 57, 122].

DME and DR laser treatment

The aim of classic laser photocoagulation therapy is occlusion of leaking microa-neurysms, thermal destruction of ischaemic retina, increase of oxygen supply to the surrounding retina, reduction of proangiogenic factors and release of cytokines from RPE and Müller cells. Subsequently, visual function is stabilised, regression of present neovascularisation and prevention of new neovascularisation. In the case of subthreshold laser treatment, the goal is biological stimulation of retinal pigment epithelial cells, without their thermal coagulation and damage to the surrounding retina. Conventional laser treatment may be indicated for focal paramacular oedema to close leaking microaneurysms and capillaries [37, 91]. Subthreshold laser treat-ment may be beneficial in DME with good initial visual acuity and low CRT [91].

Fig. 8 Diabetic retinopathy treated with laser

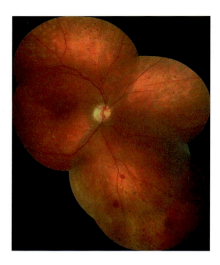

In cases of very advanced NPDR and PDR, laser treatment of the retinal periphery is performed (Fig. 8) [32, 36].

Intravitreal administration of corticosteroids in the treatment of DME

Corticosteroids have an anti-inflammatory and anti-angiogenic effect. Influence on leukostasis, inhibition of intracellular adhesion molecule (ICAM)-1 expression and levels of inflammatory (IL-6, interferon-induced protein-10, monocyte-chemoattractant protein-1, platelet-derived growth factor [PDGF]-AA) and angiogenic (VEGF) cytokines leads to a reduction in vascular hyperpermeability and subsequently to a reduction in macular oedema [91]. Corticosteroids are administered either directly into the vitreous as a solution (*triamcinolone*), or as an implant that is gradually degraded with slow release of the active ingredient (*dexamethasone posterior segment delivery system*), or permanently sutured to the sclera with gradual release of the active ingredient into the vitreous (*fluocinolone acetonide*). Treatment with triamcinolone is off-label only. Treatment with dexamethasone posterior segment delivery system (Ozurdex) is approved for patients with chronic macular oedema and pseudophakia and for patients for whom other treatments are inadequate or not suitable. The use of fluocinolone acetonide (Iluvien) is reserved for patients with chronic DME that does not respond adequately to available treatments. In phakic patients, it is important to note the high risk of developing cataracts. Patients must be regularly monitored for the risk of elevation of intraocular pressure [91].

Corticosteroids might be the better choice as first-line treatment in the case of patients who have a history of a major cardiovascular event or cerebrovascular accidents. Another group of patients who may be suitable to start corticosteroid therapy are those who are not willing to come for monthly injections at the start of treatment [91]. Patients with advanced morphological changes on OCT (persistent oedema,

Metabolic and Endocrine Diseases

presence of inflammatory biomarkers) are now also recommended to start corticosteroid therapy [40]. In nonresponders who have already been treated with anti-VEGF (after 3–6 injections, depending on the specific response of each patient), it is reasonable to switch to a steroid [91].

Intravitreal administration of VEGF blockers in the treatment of DME and DR

Factors affecting VEGF levels in DME result from microvascular abnormalities underlying chronic hyperglycaemia. Reduction of retinal flow leads to ischaemia of the inner retinal layers and subsequent increased VEGF release; another reason for its higher expression is basement membrane thickening, pericyte loss and endothelial cell damage [16, 120]. VEGF binds to the surface of endothelial cells via receptors VEGFR1 and VEGFR2. Increased binding to endothelial cells results in angiogenesis, lymphangiogenesis and the production of cytokines and proteases [42]. VEGF plays a role in the development and maintenance of vascular function. It increases vascular permeability, participates in the inhibition of thrombogenesis, inhibits apoptosis and has a pro-inflammatory effect [82, 108]. VEGF blockers prevent its binding to the appropriate receptors on vascular endothelial cells in various ways.

A non-selective VEGF A inhibitor is *ranibizumab* (Lucentis). It is a recombinant, humanised monoclonal antibody with a size of 48 kDa. By removing the original Fc (fragment crystallisable) part of the antibody, it has reduced immunogenicity and cytotoxicity. The small size of the ranibizumab molecule allows for easy permeation across the retina to the target endothelial cell receptor after intravitreal administration [14, 76].

Another VEGF blocker approved for the treatment of DME is *aflibercept* (Eylea), which is a recombinant fusion protein that consists of the VEGFR1 and VEGFR2 portions and the Fc portion of IgG. When administered intravitreally, its receptors act as a decoy for VEGF A, B and placental growth factor (PlGF), thereby preventing their action on receptors on endothelial cells of retinal and choroidal vessels [76, 101].

Brolucizumab (Beovu) is a single-chain fragment of a humanised monoclonal antibody with a molecular weight of 26 kDa that binds to all VEGF-A isoforms and thus prevents VEGF-A binding to VEGFR1 and VEGFR2 receptors. By inhibiting this binding, brolucizumab suppresses endothelial cell proliferation and reduces vascular permeability [107].

Faricimab (Vabysmo) is a novel specific anti-Ang 2/anti-VEGF antibody designed for intravitreal use. In addition to the known positive effect of VEGF blockade on reducing vessel wall permeability and vessel proliferation, it also exploits the effect on angiopoietin 2, which is manifested by a reduction in inflammation and improved vessel wall stability.

The growth factors angiopoietin 1 and 2 (Ang-1) and (Ang-2) bind to the transmembrane receptor tyrosine kinase (Tie2), which is expressed in the endothelium of blood vessels. Activation of Tie2 signalling with Ang-1 promotes vascular stability and barrier function of new and existing blood vessels, facilitating pericyte delivery and preventing vascular permeability induced by inflammatory cytokines. Under conditions such as hypoxia, hyperglycaemia, or oxidative stress, Ang-2 levels are elevated. Ang-2 binds competitively to Tie2 and inhibits Ang-1 signalling, leading to endothelial and vascular destabilisation, blood-retinal barrier breakdown, and inflammation [11, 90].

Based on the results of clinical trials, VEGF blockers are indicated as the first-line treatment for DME [91]. Repeated administration of both drugs has shown significant improvement in visual acuity in most patients over a period of several years. The efficacy of these agents has also been verified in the treatment of proliferative DR. Compared with laser retinal treatment, repeated administration of both drugs was associated with a lower need for vitrectomy for intravitreal bleeding [44, 95]. However, due to the significantly higher cost of treatment with both ranibizumab and aflibercept compared to laser treatment, laser panretinal photocoagulation is still the method of choice in the treatment of proliferative diabetic retinopathy.

Another treatment option for diabetic retinopathy is pars plana vitrectomy. Current indications include poor transparency of the optical media (intravitreal hemorrhage and vitreous opacities), vitreoretinal traction in the posterior pole of the eye and tractional retinal detachment, fibrovascular proliferation, and epiretinal membranes, pathological vitreous detachment (vitreomacular adhesions and traction), refractory diffuse diabetic macular oedema, retrohyaloid hemorrhage, and the combination of anterior segment pathology with hemorrhagic or neovascular manifestations in the posterior segment of the eye (neovascular glaucoma, iris rubeosis hyphema) [104].

Anterior eye segment manifestations in DM

Corneal diseases

Patients with DM have significantly reduced corneal sensitivity, which correlates with the severity of DR [84, 87]. The presumed cause is a decrease in the number of long nerve fibre bundles recorded in vivo by confocal microscopy. In addition, dry eye syndrome is known to occur twice as often in the diabetic population [70]. These factors are responsible for the higher incidence of bacterial and neurotrophic corneal ulcers in DM patients [39, 47]. Reduced corneal sensitivity and improper neural regulation in DM patients lead to slower healing of the corneal epithelium after trauma, frequent recurrent erosions and, at worst, permanent changes in the corneal epithelial layer, especially in contact lens wearers [47]. The therapy for most cases of dry eye syndrome is tear film replacement with artificial tears, ideally without preservatives.

Dry eye syndrome and neurotrophic keratopathy in diabetes

Insulin-dependent advanced diabetes also affects the quality of the superficial layers of the eye. Some studies have reported symptomatology consistent with sicca syndrome in up to 54% of diabetic patients [65]. Initial symptoms of dry eye are rather subjectively unpleasant, but with prolonged duration and significant disturbances in tear film production and stability, they lead to intermediate and advanced forms of epitheliopathy. Chronic epithelial defects reduce visual function and, with potential secondary infection (most often bacterial), can have devastating consequences (corneal ulceration, risk of eyeball penetration, risk of developing endophthalmitis) [103].

Metabolic and Endocrine Diseases

The most frequently cited etiologic factors for the increased incidence of dry eye in diabetes are:

1) angiopathy with involvement of the capillary network of the anterior segment of the eye and conjunctiva, leading to reduced perfusion support of the lacrimal glands and goblet cells—and thus reduced production of the aqueous and mucin components of the tear film.
2) hyperglycaemia as a source of osmotic instability of corneal and conjunctival epithelial structures—loss of osmotic balance of epithelial cells leads to desiccation and vulnerability of the epithelium.
3) diabetic neuropathy as a cause of partial denervation of the ocular surface—feedback leads to an overall reduction in the production of tear film components.

Therapy for most cases is tear film replacement with artificial tears [103].

Glaucoma

Primary open-angle glaucoma

Several studies have shown a higher incidence of primary open-angle glaucoma (POAG) in patients with DM compared to the healthy population [58, 59, 63, 66]. In the treatment of PGOU in patients with DM, it is important to note that potential side effects of beta-blockers include a decrease in glucose tolerance and masking of hypoglycaemic symptoms. Therefore, this group of drugs should be used with caution in diabetic patients.

Angle-closure glaucoma

The higher incidence of narrow-angle glaucoma (NAG) in DM patients can be explained mainly by lens swelling during hyperglycaemia due to hyperosmolarity with subsequent reduction of the anterior chamber angle.

Neovascular glaucoma

Despite the widespread use of laser panretinal coagulation, PDR remains the second most common cause of neovascular glaucoma [17]. The underlying aetiological factor is retinal ischaemia [64]. Hypoxic precincts generate increased levels of angiogenic factors, mainly VEGF, which potentiate the formation of newly formed vessels with the development of rubeosis (Fig. 9).

Subsequently, these vessels grow into the ventricular angle where a fibrovascular membrane forms. The fibrous tissue often contracts and can cause ectropion of the iris tissue and the formation of anterior synechiae. Subsequently, the chamber angle gradually closes and the IOP increases extremely, but it may be elevated early in rubeosis because of increased permeability of the vascular wall and leakage of proteins from the newly formed vessels into the intraocular fluid [125].

The therapy of neovascular glaucoma is complex and follows the evolution of the disease. In the early stages of the disease, laser treatment of the ischaemic parts of the retina and possible application of VEGF blockers should be strongly emphasised [78, 88]. Compensation for diabetes is essential. When rubeosis progresses and

Fig. 9 Iris rubeosis

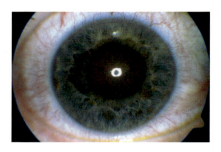

neovascularisation occurs in the still open ventricular angle, local anti-glaucomatous therapy is often effective. Carbonic anhydrase blockers and beta-blockers are preferred. Another option for the treatment of early stage neovascular glaucoma is goniophotocoagulation, where direct treatment of the pathological vessels with an argon laser is performed at the anterior chamber angle.

Surgical methods are indicated for closure and blockage of the ventricular angle. On the one hand, those that facilitate the outflow of intraocular fluid (filtering surgery, drainage implants), on the other hand, those interventions that reduce the production of intraocular fluid (cyclophotocoagulation/cryo-destruction of the ciliary body). The success rate of filtering surgery in neovascular glaucoma is higher when using 5-fluorouracil or mitomycin C.

In the terminal phases of the disease, the focus is usually only on alleviating subjectively unpleasant sensations—mostly chronic pain. Chemical retrobulbar denervation (alcohol), irradiation of the eyeball with gamma rays from Leksell's gamma knife or removal of the eye (evisceration, enucleation) are options.

Glaucoma associated with obturation of the trabecular meshwork

Glaucoma associated with blood cells clogging the trabeculae is not a rare finding in diabetics. In vitreous haemorrhage, erythrocytes are not resorbed in the vitreous and turn into "ghost cells", which then migrate across the anterior hyaloid membrane and around the zonule of the lens into the anterior chamber of the eye and, after several weeks, block the outflow of intraocular fluid through the trabecular meshwork at the chamber angle [19]. In the anterior chamber, these cells can be clearly seen on slit-lamp examination. In severe cases, true hypopyon based on uveitis or endophthalmitis must be distinguished from pseudohypopyon, which is typical of ghost-cell glaucoma.

Another clinical entity is haemolytic glaucoma, where macrophages that have engulfed erythrocytes clog the trabeculum. Since this condition is self-limiting, in most cases only local hypotensive treatment is sufficient [41]. Exceptionally, anterior chamber lavage should be performed.

Hemosiderosis glaucoma was first described in 1960 and is caused by obstruction of the outflow tract by iron deposition, with subsequent degeneration and accompanying inflammation [114]. This type of glaucoma has a later onset than ghost-cell glaucoma, and so in most cases arises a year or more after vitreous haemorrhage [19].

Metabolic and Endocrine Diseases

Refractive errors

Transient swelling of the lens in diabetics often causes *"diabetic myopia"*. The cause is thought to be the accumulation of sorbitol, the product of glucose reduction, which has a marked osmotic effect. Its action causes the lens to become more spherical, thus increasing its refractive power [13]. Transient hyperopic shift is often seen in patients with hyperglycaemia after plasma glucose compensation [74].

Cataract

Diabetes mellitus is a common risk factor for cataract in the developed world. There is a three- to fourfold increased prevalence of cataract in patients with diabetes under the age of 65 years and a twofold increased prevalence in those over 65 years of age [60]. There is a direct association between duration of diabetes, DM compensation and cataract incidence. Diabetic cataract is usually not morphologically different from age-related cataract, but it occurs 20–30 years earlier. Young diabetic patients often develop snowflake-shaped posterior subcapsular cataracts with superficial vacuoles that progress rapidly [105].

Hyperglycaemia is the driver of cataract development in diabetes. The enzymatic conversion of glucose to sorbitol and its intracellular accumulation skews the osmotic balance of the lens and more fluid is absorbed into the lens through the increased permeability of the capsule. These changes cause lens masses to liquefy, disorganisation of the fibres, and thus opacity formation and apoptosis of lens epithelial cells [99].

Optic nerve involvement

Diabetic papillopathy

In the case of diabetic papillopathy, unilateral or sometimes bilateral transient optic disc oedema occurs in patients with long-term decompensated DM. It is usually associated with a mild decrease in visual acuity and physiological findings at the perimeter. Exceptionally, enlargement of the blind spot or arcuate scotoma may occur [105]. The typical finding on FAG is diffuse leakage from the optic nerve papillae, gradually grading over time. In approximately 50% of cases, the oedema occurs bilaterally [6]. In cases of bilateral involvement, optic nerve oedema may be caused by malignant arterial hypertension or be a manifestation of increased intracranial pressure (papilledema).

Non-arteritic form of anterior ischaemic optic neuropathy

It is a common cause of optic nerve oedema, especially in elderly patients. Risk factors for the development of this entity include coronary artery disease, hypercholesterolaemia and DM.

Ischaemic optic neuropathy in patients with DM is characterised by a sudden severe decline in visual acuity, dyschromatopsia, optic nerve oedema, a marked relative afferent pupillary defect and an altitudinal hemianopic loss of the lower or upper part of the visual field at the perimeter (Fig. 10).

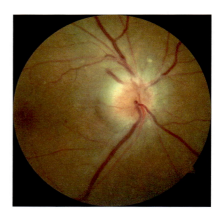

Fig. 10 Ischemic optic disc oedema in anterior ischemic optic neuropathy

Optic nerve atrophy

This can occur in patients with DM because of diabetic optic nerve oedema or after AION. Other possible causes include such complications of diabetic retinopathy as ischaemia of the neuroretinal nerve fibre layer and ganglion cell involvement (Fig. 11).

Cranial nerves involvement

Patients with DM may have isolated paresis of the cranial nerves (III, IV or VI) due to focal occlusion of small vessels supplying the nervous tissue with subsequent ischaemic demyelination. The differential diagnosis includes transient ischaemic attack, stroke, occlusive vasculitis, previous CNS trauma, and compressive brain lesions [105]. The pathology of the cranial nerves mainly occurs in patients over 50 years. Rucker mentions the presence of DM in 15.4% of patients with paresis of the abducens nerve, in 20% of patients with lesions of the oculomotor nerve, and in 4.5% of patients with paresis of the eye muscles [86]. Paresis of the eye muscles in

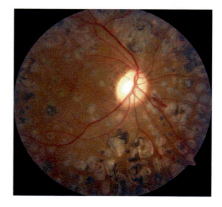

Fig. 11 Optic disc atrophy

Metabolic and Endocrine Diseases

diabetes usually occur quickly, they are usually unilateral and are often accompanied by pain in the temporal region [71].

Greco et al. published the results of a 10-year retrospective study of diabetic patients. A total of 6765 patients were hospitalized, and ophthalmoplegia was found in 27 patients (0.4%). Isolated lesion of the III cranial nerve was observed in the majority of patients (59.3%), and paresis of the VI cranial nerve occurred in 29.6% of patients and was observed more frequently than lesions of all oculomotor nerves (11.1%) [43].

The lesion typically occurs in patients with non-severe diabetes and often in latent diabetes. The prognosis is favorable enough, with remission usually occurring within a few weeks to 4 months, but cases of recurrence can also be observed [71].

Pupillary reaction disorders

Disorders of the pupillary reaction are manifested by Argyll Robertson like pupils, an isolated violation of reaction to the accommodation, uneven pupils and a weak response to drugs that dilate the pupils. According to various authors, the frequency of these disorders in patients with diabetic polyneuropathy is between 9 and 24% [71].

3 Hyperlipoproteinaemia and Dyslipidaemia

Hyperlipoproteinaemia and dyslipidaemia are a group of metabolic diseases characterised by elevated plasma lipid and lipoprotein levels. They result from increased synthesis and/or decreased breakdown of plasma lipoproteins. Depending on the cause, they are divided into primary (genetically determined), and secondary, resulting from another underlying disease. In most patients, it is a combination of genetic factors and environmental influences, especially lifestyle. *According to the EAS* (European Atherosclerosis Society), they are divided into three groups according to the concentration of basic lipoproteins in the plasma:

- Hypercholesterolaemia (elevated total and LDL (low density lipoprotein) cholesterol)
- Mixed (combined) hyperlipoproteinaemia (with elevation of both cholesterol and triglycerides)
- Hypertriglyceridaemia (elevated triglycerides contained in VLDL (very low-density lipoprotein))

The primary causes are monogenic or polygenic disorders. These include:

- Familial hypercholesterolaemia (FH)
- Congenital LDL-cholesterol disorders other than FH
- Familial combined hyperlipidaemia
- Familial dysbetalipoproteinaemia (hyperlipoproteinaemia Type III)
- Familial hyperlipoproteinaemia Type I
- Familial hypertriglyceridaemia

174 J. Studnicka et al.

- Familial hyperlipoproteinaemia Type V
- Polygenic hypercholesterolaemia
- Familial combined hyperlipidaemia (FKH)

Secondary hyperlipoproteinaemias are the result of an underlying disease in which lipid and lipoprotein metabolism is altered (Table 3).

This may be an isolated increase in cholesterol, an isolated hypertriglyceridaemia, or an increase in cholesterol and triglycerides simultaneously. Some primary and secondary hyperlipoproteinaemias are common and may occur together, e.g. there may be a simultaneous coincidence of hyperlipoproteinaemia and diabetes mellitus.

Hypercholesterolaemia, particularly elevated plasma LDL-cholesterol levels, is one of the most important risk factors for the development of atherosclerosis and cardiovascular disease. HDL-cholesterol is protective—the higher its concentration, the lower the risk of cardiovascular disease. Severe hypertriglyceridaemia is a significant risk factor for acute pancreatitis [22].

Epidemiology

Hyperlipoproteinaemias are very common, affecting tens of percent of the adult population. The prevalence may vary, depending on the target lipid profile parameters set. In familial hypercholesterolaemia, the prevalence of the heterozygous form is reported to be around 1:250 individuals worldwide. The homozygous form is rare,

Table 3 Secondary hyperlipoproteinaemia

Hypercholesterolaemia
Acute intermittent porphyria
Mental anorexia
Hypertriglyceridemia
Diabetes mellitus
Uraemia
Obesity
Alcoholism
Treatment with certain beta-blockers
Systemic lupus erythematosus
Dysgammaglobulinaemia
Glycogenosis type 1
Lipodystrophy
Combined hyperlipidaemia
Hypothyroidism
Nephrotic syndrome
Acromegaly
Treatment with diuretics
Corticosteroid treatment

Metabolic and Endocrine Diseases

originally predicted to occur in 1 case in 1 million individuals, but recent data show a higher prevalence of 1:160,000–300,000 individuals [12, 72].

Risk factors

- Genetically determined
- Obesity
- Diabetes mellitus
- Thyroid disease (hypothyroidism)
- Kidney disease (nephrotic syndrome, end-stage renal disease, kidney transplantation)
- Alcohol consumption
- Drugs (thiazides, cyclosporine, anabolic steroids, glucocorticoids, oestrogens, beta-blockers, tegretol)

Clinical manifestation

Hyperlipoproteinaemias may be asymptomatic or result in symptomatic cardiovascular disease. The development of atherosclerotic cardiovascular disease (coronary artery disease, peripheral artery disease, cerebral atherosclerosis) is associated with high LDL-cholesterol levels. The relationship with the level and duration of high LDL-cholesterol levels is important. Individuals with familial hypercholesterolaemia (both homozygous and heterozygous forms) have high LDL-cholesterol levels from birth, whereas in hypercholesterolaemia developed in adulthood, high LDL-cholesterol concentrations are of shorter duration and therefore there is a lower risk of premature development of atherosclerotic cardiovascular disease. With high LDL-cholesterol levels, eyelid xanthelasmas, arcus lipoides corneae, and tendon xanthomas over the Achilles tendon, elbow, knee joints, and over the metacarpophalangeal joints may develop. In addition to the above findings, patients with the homozygous form of familial hypercholesterolaemia may also have cutaneous xanthomas. In patients with severe hypertriglyceridaemia, eruptive xanthomas (small yellow-white papules) can be seen on the trunk, elbows, buttocks, knees. Patients with rare dyslipoproteinaemia may have palmar and tuberous xanthomas. Extremely high lipid levels give the plasma a chylous character [22].

Diagnosis

Hyperlipoproteinaemias are diagnosed by measuring serum lipids. However, in some patients with characteristic physical findings, they can be assumed. Routine examination includes the determination of total cholesterol, triglycerides and HDL-cholesterol (lipid profile). LDL-cholesterol can be measured directly by enzymatic methods or by ultracentrifugation, but in clinical practice its value is often calculated using the Friedewald formula:

$$LDL\text{-}c = TC - HDL\text{-}c - (TG/2.2) \text{ in mmol/l}$$

It is also possible to calculate the atherogenic index, the ratio of total to HDL-cholesterol.

In selected groups of patients, apolipoproteins A1, B and lipoprotein(a) are examined.

Traditionally, fasting lipid profile testing has been recommended. However, recent studies have shown that the differences for most lipid parameters in fasting and non-fasting samples are small. Lipid spectrum testing is not performed during acute illness (triglycerides increase and cholesterol levels decrease in inflammatory conditions).

In a patient diagnosed with hyperlipoproteinaemia, we also perform measurement of TSH, glycaemia and CK (creatine kinase) and liver function tests before starting drug therapy. We also look for signs of atherosclerosis—on physical examination palpation and auscultation of the carotid and femoral arteries and pulsations in the arteries of the lower extremities. Among auxiliary methods, ultrasonography of the carotid arteries, lower limb arteries, ankle brachial index (ABI) and examination using non-invasive cardiology and angiology methods are used. An important part of the examination is to search for other risk factors for atherosclerosis (smoking, diabetes mellitus, hypertension).

Genetic testing can be added in individuals with a clinical diagnosis of familial hypercholesterolaemia (testing for mutations in genes for LDL receptor, ApoB, PCSK9). However, this is not necessary and it will not change the approach to treatment in affected individuals [110].

Differential diagnosis

The differential diagnosis of hyperlipoproteinemia involves the classification of the individual types and the possible detection of a secondary cause of hyper-lipoproteinemia. Familial hypercholesterolaemia is characterised by extreme LDL-cholesterol levels and early development of atherosclerotic cardiovascular disease. In homozygotes, the disease manifestation in childhood is typical [22].

Therapy

Recommendations from the European Society of Cardiology and the European Atherosclerosis Society emphasise an individualised approach to the treatment of hyperlipoproteinaemias, based on overall cardiovascular risk. Based on cardiovascular risk, patients can be divided into four categories: very high risk, high risk, intermediate risk, and low risk (Table 4). The latest version of guidelines was published in 2021 [115].

Setting treatment goals is also useful in physician–patient communication. The main goal is LDL-cholesterol reduction; the greater the absolute reduction in LDL-cholesterol, the more pronounced the reduction in cardiovascular risk. Reducing LDL-cholesterol to the lowest possible levels is important, at least in patients at high cardiovascular risk, and it is therefore recommended that LDL-cholesterol levels be reduced to at least 50% of baseline values (Table 5) [110].

Metabolic and Endocrine Diseases

Table 4 Cardiovascular (CV) risk categories

Very high risk
Documented atherosclerotic CV disease
Clinically—previous ACS, stable angina, coronary revascularization, ischaemic stroke, TIA, ischaemic PAD
Imaging—significant atherosclerotic plaque on coronary angiography/CT/USG of carotid arteries
Diabetes mellitus with organ involvement, or at least 3 RF, or DM1 lasting > 20 years
Severe CKD (eGFR < 30 ml/minutes)
Calculated SCORE $\geq$ 10% per 10-year risk of fatal CV event
High risk
Significantly elevated individual RF: TC > 8 mmol/l, LDL-c > 4.9 mmol/l, BP $\geq$ 180/110
FH without other significant RFs
DM without organ involvement with duration of DM $\geq$ 10 years or another additional RF
Moderate CKD (eGFR 30–59 ml/minutes)
Calculated SCORE $\geq$ 5% per 10-year risk of fatal CV event
Moderate risk
Diabetes mellitus at younger age (DM1 < 35 years, DM2 < 50 years) with DM duration < 10 years without additional RF
Calculated SCORE > 1% and $\leq$ 5% per 10-year risk of fatal CV event
Low risk
Calculated SCORE < 1% per 10-year risk of fatal CV event

ACS—acute coronary syndrome, TIA—transient ischaemic attack, iPAD—ischaemic peripheral artery disease, RF—risk factor, CKD—chronic kidney disease, eGFR—estimated glomerular filtration rate, SCORE—systematic coronary risk evaluation, DM1—type 1 diabetes mellitus, DM2—type 2 diabetes mellitus, TC—total cholesterol, LDL-c—LDL-cholesterol

Table 5 The goals of treatment of hyperlipoproteinemia in cardiovascular prevention

LDL-c (primary target)
Very high risk: LDL-c reduction of $\geq$ 50% versus baseline and LDL-c $\leq$ 1.4 mmol/l
High risk: LDL-c reduction of $\geq$ 50% versus baseline and LDL-c $\leq$ 1.8 mmol/l
Medium risk: LDL-c $\leq$ 2.6 mmol/l
Low risk: LDL-c $\leq$ 2.6 mmol/l
Non-HDL-c (secondary target)
< 2.2, 2.6 and 3.4 mmol/l for very high, high and moderate risk
Triglycerides
< 1.7 mmol/l is an indicator of low risk
Diabetes mellitus
HbAc < 53 mmol/mol

HbA1c—glycated haemoglobin, HDL-c—HDL-cholesterol

Non-pharmacological treatment

The treatment of hyperlipoproteinemia is based on non-pharmacological measures—diet, weight reduction in overweight or obese patients, and lifestyle modification (physical activity, smoking cessation, or educational activities in the field of lifestyle modification).

Diet

Dietary recommendations are aimed at affecting serum lipid levels, but also hypertension and weight reduction. The results of epidemiological studies show that the risk of cardiovascular events is reduced in individuals who have a diet rich in low-starch vegetables, fruits, legumes, fish, vegetable oils, whole grains and a reduced intake of red and processed meats and refined carbohydrates. Reducing cardiovascular risk can be achieved by replacing animal fats, including milk fat, with vegetable sources and polyunsaturated fatty acids. In patients with hypertension, reduction of salt intake is recommended.

Physical activity

Regular aerobic physical activity can increase HDL-cholesterol levels and lead to weight loss. For example, brisk walking 25–30 km per week (or its equivalent—running, cycling, swimming, rowing) is recommended. Regular physical activity for at least 30 minutes a day improves the patient's general physical condition and quality of life, has a preventive effect in terms of preserving muscle and bone mass, especially in older patients, and is also important in patients who are not overweight or obese [110].

Pharmacological treatment

Statins

Statins reduce endogenous cholesterol synthesis in the liver by inhibiting the enzyme HMG-CoA reductase. HMG-CoA (3-hydroxy-3-methylglutaryl-coenzyme A) is a key enzyme in cholesterol biosynthesis. Reduction of intracellular cholesterol results in increased expression of the LDL receptor on the surface of the hepatocyte, leading to increased uptake of LDL-cholesterol from the blood and decreased plasma concentrations of LDL- and other ApoB-containing lipoproteins, including triglyceride-rich particles.

LDL-cholesterol reduction is dose-dependent and varies from statin to statin. The more potent statins include atorvastatin, rosuvastatin and pitavastatin. Their other effects include a modest rise in HDL-cholesterol, anti-inflammatory and antioxidant effects.

If the patient does not tolerate the recommended dose of statin due to side effects or does not achieve the target values at the maximum tolerated dose of statin, the addition of another non-statin hypolipidemic drug is recommended.

Statins are generally well tolerated, but sometimes adverse effects on muscles or glucose homeostasis can occur. The most common side effect is myopathy, which

Metabolic and Endocrine Diseases

occurs most often because of drug interactions. These include drugs metabolised by cytochrome P450 3A4, such as some antimicrobial drugs (itraconazole, ketoconazole, erythromycin, clindamycin), calcium antagonists (verapamil, diltiazem, amlodipine), and others (cyclosporine, amiodarone, gemfibrozil, grapefruit juice). The most severe form of muscle damage is rhabdomyolysis, in which severe muscle pain, muscle necrosis, and myoglobinuria occur and can cause renal failure and death. It is accompanied by a marked elevation of CK—more than 10 times the upper limit of normal values. Sometimes muscle symptoms occur with statin treatment, with muscle pain and tenderness, but no rise in CK. Sometimes a slight rise in ALT (alanine aminotransferase) can be seen in statin-treated patients (more often with high-dose statins), but this is not a sign of hepatotoxicity or impaired liver function. Progression to liver failure is extremely rare. Statin therapy can lead to impaired glucose metabolism and the development of type 2 diabetes mellitus, again with high doses of statins being risky, in elderly patients and in the presence of other risk factors for diabetes (overweight, insulin resistance) [85, 110].

Cholesterol absorption inhibitors

Ezetimibe inhibits the absorption of cholesterol in the intestine without affecting the absorption of fat-soluble nutrients. As a result of its action, the amount of cholesterol that reaches the liver is reduced, leading to an increase in LDL receptor expression and an increase in the uptake of LDL-cholesterol from the blood. Ezetimibe slightly lowers triglycerides and leads to a slight increase in HDL-cholesterol. The dual inhibition (combined treatment with a statin and ezetimibe) reduces LDL-cholesterol levels by 15% more than statin monotherapy. Treatment with ezetimibe is well tolerated, and hepatic failure is extremely rarely described with ezetimibe monotherapy or in combination with a statin.

Bile acid sequestrants

Cholestyramine, colestipol, and colesevelam are not absorbable from the gastrointestinal tract. They act in the intestine, where they interrupt the enterohepatic bile acid cycle. In the liver, depletion of bile acids results in their synthesis from cholesterol, increased expression of the LDL receptor and a decrease in circulating LDL-cholesterol. Because they are not absorbed, they are safe for women of childbearing age and children. Their use is limited by frequent adverse effects in the gastrointestinal tract (flatulence, obstipation, dyspepsia, nausea). They may increase circulating triglycerides in some patients, and decreased absorption of fat-soluble vitamins has been reported [110].

PCSK9 inhibitors (proprotein convertase subtilisin/kexin type 9)

Proprotein convertase subtilisin kexin-9 is involved in the intracellular and extracellular regulation of LDL receptor expression. The target of action of PCSK9 inhibitors is this protein. Interaction of PCSK9 with the LDL receptor triggers intracellular degradation of the LDL receptor. Degradation of the LDL receptor in the liver appears to be essential for lowering LDL-cholesterol when treated with PCSK9 inhibitors, which block the interaction between PCSK9 and the LDL receptor. Treatment with PCSK9 inhibitors increases the number of functional LDL receptors on the cell surface and leads to a reduction in circulating LDL-cholesterol levels. Evolocumab and alirocumab are currently available in clinical practice; they are monoclonal antibodies that reduce plasma PCSK9 levels. They are administered by injection, subcutaneously, once or twice a month. The best effect is seen when combined with a statin [110].

Inclisiran

Inclisiran is a small interfering RNA (siRNA), that acts as an inhibitor of a proprotein convertase, inhibiting translation of the protein PCSK9. Reduced circulating PCSK9 decrease circulating LDL-cholesterol due to decreased degradation of LDL receptor. It is administered subcutaneously once per 3–6 months. An advantage is that no specific serious adverse events were observed.

Bempedoic acid

Bempedoic acid is a first-in-class oral small molecule that inhibits cholesterol synthesis by inhibiting the action of ATP citrate lyase, a cytosolic enzyme upstream of HMG-CoA reductase. In monotherapy, bempedoic acid reduces LDL-c levels by ~ 30% and by about 50% in combination with ezetimibe.

Lomitapide

Lomitapide is an MTP (microsomal triglyceride transfer protein) inhibitor, used in combination with a statin to treat homozygous familial hypercholesterolaemia. MTP inhibition disrupts the transfer of triglycerides and phospholipids from the endoplasmic reticulum to ApoB, thereby reducing VLDL formation in the liver and chylomicrons in the intestine.

Fibrates

The mechanism of action of fibrates is the activation of PPAR-α (peroxisome proliferator-activated receptor-α), thereby affecting transcription factors that, among other things, regulate various steps in lipid and lipoprotein metabolism. Fibrates effectively reduce triglyceride and triglyceride-rich lipoprotein levels and increase HDL-cholesterol levels. They are well tolerated, with a small percentage of patients reporting gastrointestinal symptoms and skin exanthema. The most common side effects are myopathy, rise in liver transaminases and cholelithiasis. Gemfibrozil inhibits statin metabolism by the glucuronidation pathway and significantly increases plasma statin levels. Fenofibrate has different pharmacokinetics and a much lower risk of myopathy when combined with a statin.

Omega-3 fatty acids

In pharmacological doses, Omega-3 fatty acids lead to a reduction in triglycerides. The mechanism of action is unclear, partly explained by their ability to interact with PPAR receptors [110].

Metabolic and Endocrine Diseases 181

4 Ocular Manifestations of Hyperlipoproteinaemia and Dyslipidaemia

Hyperlipoproteinaemia and dyslipidaemia are manifested by involvement of the periocular region (xanthelasmas of the eyelids) and the anterior segment of the eye (arcus senilis, lipid keratopathy and crystalline stromal dystrophy) [15]. Clinical manifestations in the posterior segment of the eye are quite rare and include the finding of cholesterol crystals on the retina.

Clinical symptoms and objective findings

Periocular region

Xanthelasma palpebrarum

Xanthelasma palpebrarum, or simply xanthelasma, is a yellow plaque-like skin lesion arising from the medial parts of the upper and lower eyelids [26]. They may be soft, semi-solid or solid, often occurring in multiple, symmetrical patterns, and adjacent lesions may merge. Xanthelasmas are caused by infiltration of the eyelid skin by xanthoma cells, which are histiocytes that store lipids in cytoplasmic vacuoles. The main lipid associated with xanthelasma is cholesterol, usually esterified to unsaturated fatty acids. A probable hypothesis for the development of xanthelasmas is leakage of lipids from the plasma due to some form of vascular trauma [56]. Xanthelasmas are more common in women than in men (prevalence 1.1% vs. 0.3%) and, as with arcus senilis, their prevalence tends to increase with age.

Anterior eye segment

Arcus lipoides corneae, arcus senilis

Arcus lipoides corneae is described as a grey-white ring that is separated from the limbus by a clear zone 0.3–1 mm wide. Initially, the upper and lower periphery of the cornea is affected, and, with the passage of time, a complete intermediate ring is formed. This finding was first described by Canton in 1850 [20]. It is caused by extracellular lipid deposition in the peripheral cornea. The deposits are composed of cholesterol, cholesterol esters, phospholipids, and triglycerides. Fatty acids that make up many of the deposited lipid molecules include palmitic, stearic, oleic, and linoleic acids. Lipids are deposited in the cornea of healthy individuals, but it is thought that aging increases their amount, which can lead to the development of arcus senilis. The estimated prevalence is 8% in people aged 40–49 years, 45% in people aged 50–59 years and 75% in people aged 70–79 years. In general, arcus senilis is more common in men than in women. In most cases, both eyes are affected. The highest incidence is seen in African American males, followed by females of the same race, then Caucasian males, followed by females. The early development of corneal arcus is a manifestation of hyperlipoproteinaemia, mainly due to excess LDL [93]. Hyperlipoproteinaemia types IIa and IIb, which are not familial, are the most likely findings in individuals who develop corneal arcus before the age of 50 years. The most common familial cause of corneal arcus is type IIa hypercholesterolaemia.

Biomicroscopy of the anterior segment of the eye reveals extensive involvement of Bowman's membrane, corneal stroma and Descemet's membrane.

Lipid keratopathy

Lipid keratopathy was first described by Cogan and Kuwabara [25]. Its cause is lipid deposition in the corneal stroma, which is always associated with pathological corneal vascularisation. The finding may be mono- or bilateral. Lipid deposition is increased when concomitant ocular disease is present, or in situations where blood flow and vascular permeability are increased. Lipid keratopathy is much more common in women than in men, in a ratio of 70:30. Such an association is thought to be related to higher HDL levels in premenopausal women. The finding of hypercholesterolaemia (total cholesterol greater than 8 mmol/l) is the most common blood abnormality with which lipid keratopathy is associated.

Central crystal dystrophy

Schnyder's central crystalline dystrophy is bilateral, and predominantly axial and paraxial lipid deposition in the anterior corneal stroma. Cholesterol was identified as a histologic component of opacity crystals as early as 1934 [113]. Familial hypercholesterolaemia, familial hypertriglyceridaemia, and familial dysbetalipoproteinaemia are the most common types of abnormalities associated with this disease.

Posterior eye segment

Intraocular complications are rarely observed and include the finding of cholesterol crystals in the retina.

Differential diagnosis

- Lipoid proteinosis (Urbach-Wiethe disease)
- Lichen sclerosus et atrophicus

Diagnosis

Diagnosis of ocular manifestations of hyperlipoproteinaemia and dyslipidaemia includes biomicroscopy of the anterior segment and digital fundus photography to detect possible involvement of the posterior segment of the eye.

Therapy

In the case of finding eyelids affected by xanthelasmas, surgical excision is the first-choice method. Findings in the anterior segment and intraocular structures do not require ocular treatment but do require compensation for hyperlipoproteinaemia and dyslipidaemia.

Metabolic and Endocrine Diseases

5 Thyroid Eye Disease

Thyroid eye disease (TED), also known as Thyroid-associated orbitopathy (TAO) or simply Graves orbitopathy (GO), is a severe chronic eye disease associated with autoimmune thyroid disease (ATD) [18, 116]. It most commonly affects patients with Graves-Basedow (GB) disease, the most common cause of hyperthyroidism, especially during the florid phase of the disease. However, it can also affect patients with other types of ATD, especially chronic autoimmune thyroiditis, also in hypofunctioning or eufunctioning (about 10%) states or in patients without detectable thyroid disease. Ocular symptoms of varying severity can be detected in approximately 40% of patients at the beginning of GB disease, 3–5% of whom are at risk of progression to severe forms of TED.

Epidemiology

TED is a relatively rare disease. The incidence is 19–42/100,000 inhabitants/year. It is more common in women, as is GB hyperthyroidism. The female/male ratio for mild TED is 9.3, for moderate TED 3.2 and for severe TED 1.4 [9, 118]. Thus, it can be said that when TED manifests itself in men, they are at increased risk of a more severe disease course.

There are two peaks in the disease incidence depending on age of the patients. Women are most often affected at the age 40–44 years and 60–64 years, and men at the age 45–49 years and 65–69 years [46]. Data on prevalence are lacking and are only estimated at about 90 cases per 100,000 population. Moderate to severe TED occurs in 1 in 20 (5%) patients with Graves-Basedow disease. GB disease has an annual incidence of 20–50/100,000 people, with a peak incidence between 30 and 50 years of age. GB disease has an annual incidence of 20–50/100,000 people, with a peak incidence between 30 and 50 years of age [118].

Pathogenesis

TED is classified as an autoimmune disease, but the exact aetiopathogenesis of this disease is still unknown. A cross-reactive autoimmune inflammatory reaction against antigens shared by the thyroid and orbital soft tissues is suspected. Autoantibodies (thyroid-stimulating immunoglobulins) targeting the thyrotropin receptor drive hyperthyroidism in Graves' disease, but data indicate that additional autoantigens and antibodies are involved in the development of thyroid eye disease. The insulin-like growth factor I receptor (IGF-IR), which is overexpressed by orbital fibroblasts and B and T cells in Graves' disease and thyroid eye disease, plays a central role (Fig. 12).

Thyrotropin receptors and IGF-IRs form physical and functional complexes that cause thyroid eye disease, including hyaluronan accumulation and cytokine expression, resulting in inflammation, oedema, and expansion of extraocular muscle and adipose tissue [34]. The effect of released cytokines results in an acceleration of glycosaminoglycan production with excess hyaluronic acid and collagen formation paralleling infiltration of the orbital muscles and the fat body. Therefore, overall,

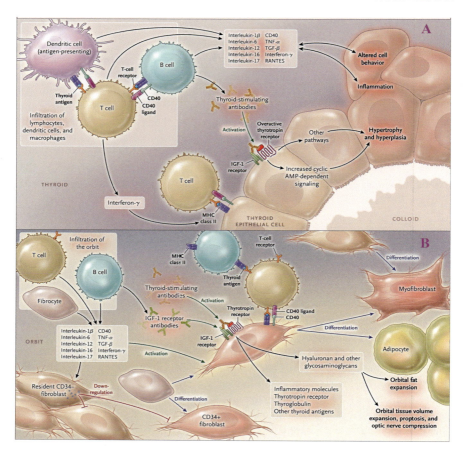

Fig. 12 Pathogenesis of Graves-Basedow disease and endocrine orbitopathy (loosely based on Smith and Hegedus [98]). Panel A shows a theoretical model of Graves' disease. Thyroid-stimulating immunoglobulins (TRAK), through the TSH receptor, provoke overproduction of thyroid hormones, thus bypassing the normal regulatory role of TSH. In addition, B and T lymphocytes and antigen presenting cells produce interleukins 1β, 6, and 12; interferon-γ; tumour necrosis factor α; CD40 and other cytokines. These cytokines activate and maintain inflammation in the thyroid gland. Panel B shows a theoretical model of the pathogenesis of endocrine orbitopathy. The orbit is infiltrated by B and T lymphocytes and CD34+ fibrocytes. Fibrocytes further differentiate into CD34+ fibroblasts, which further differentiate into myofibroblasts or adipocytes. These fibroblasts are in orbit also with CD34—fibroblasts. These cells may produce additional cytokines depending on signals in the microenvironment (interleukins 1β, 6, 8, and 16; tumour necrosis factor α (TNF-α); RANTES (regulated on activation, normal T-cell expressed and secreted); and CD40). These cytokines activate fibroblasts that express low levels of the TSH receptor, thyroglobulin, and other thyroid antigens. TRAK also activates the IGF-1 receptor complex, which leads to the expression of inflammatory molecules and the synthesis of glycosaminoglycans or the production of hyaluronate. This leads to further expansion of orbital tissues

Metabolic and Endocrine Diseases

there is an increase in the volume of the orbital adipose and the connective tissue and orbicularis oculi. However, the ratio of orbital muscle and orbital fat/connective tissue involvement can be highly variable. In patients younger than 40 years of age, the preferential involvement of adipose tissue is described more often, while in the older patients the involvement of the orbicularis oculi is more prevalent. Infiltration of connective tissue leads to increased volume and exophthalmos, while infiltration of the oculomotor muscles leads first to oedema and later to fibrotisation and restriction of the mobility of these muscles, resulting in diplopia [5, 124].

Risk factors

- Smoking (active and passive)
- Stress
- Male sex
- Higher age
- DM
- Possible influence of genetic factors: current evidence points to the role of five genes: CD40, cytotoxic T lymphocyte antigen-4 (CTLA-4), protein tyrosine phosphatase-22 (PTPN-22), HLA-MHC and X chromosome-associated genes.

Several possible risk factors for TED are still being studied. A higher frequency of partial polymorphisms in the genes for IL-1α and IL-1RA has been found in patients with GB thyrotoxicosis and TED, compared to patients with GB thyrotoxicosis without TED. However, the risk of TED is believed to depend more on environmental factors than genetic factors. Smoking is currently considered the most important modifiable risk factor for the development and progression of TED. Smokers have a higher risk of a more severe disease course and are more likely to experience disease progression and poor response to treatment [38, 100]. Smokers with TED are also more likely to undergo orbital decompression and restrictive strabismus surgery. Older men with DM also have a higher risk of progression to more severe forms of TED [62].

Clinical presentation and objective findings

General symptoms of hyperthyroidism

Graves-Basedow disease (GB) causes hyperthyroidism, a syndrome characterised by excessive secretion of thyroid hormones and their effects on peripheral tissues. The spectrum of symptoms affects the entire organism. However, it also depends on the patient's age, severity, and duration. The most common symptoms, which occur in > 50% of patients, are fatigue, weight loss, heat and sweating intolerance, tremor, and palpitations. For a simplified view, see Fig. 13.

Eye symptoms

Since TED affects all orbital structures (orbital connective and adipose tissue, orbital septum, external orbicularis oculi, and lacrimal gland), the clinical presentation can be highly variable. Therefore, the first symptoms can be overlooked or treated as

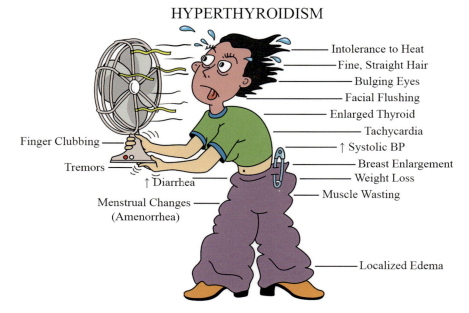

Fig. 13 Hyperthyroidism (with permission of Grada Publishing a.s.)

a different diagnosis. Patients most often complain of light-headedness, dry eye, swelling of the eyelids, or pressure behind the eyes. Sometimes they themselves notice (or are alerted by others) a change in appearance due to eyelid retraction or exophthalmos [117].

Eyelid symptoms are by far the most common initial manifestation of TED. Eyelid *retraction* occurs in up to 90% of patients at some stage of TED and can be unilateral or bilateral. Retraction of the upper eyelid is a condition in which the edge of the upper eyelid does not overlie (or touch) the corneal limbus when viewed anteriorly (Fig. 14A).

We describe the lower eyelid retraction when the lower eyelid does not touch the limbus. If looking forward, a strip of the sclera is seen between the limbus and the upper eyelid, and this is *Dalrymple's sign*. The slight retraction of the upper eyelid can often be masked by swelling of the eyelids, which is typical of active TED. The swelling is usually most noticeable in the morning and is always confined to the orbital part of the eyelids, ending at the orbital septum—*Enroth's sign* (Fig. 15).

Therefore, any patient with suspected TED should always be examined in the downward view when the retraction of the upper lid is more apparent. If the eyelid is lagging behind the globe in a downward gaze, i.e., there is no eyelid-bulb alignment, this is *Graefe's sign* (Fig. 14B).

The typical lid symptoms of TED are summarised in Table 6 [55].

In the active phase of the disease, an *injection (congestion) of the conjunctiva* is often found. Typical of TED is the localisation of congestion on the attachments of

Metabolic and Endocrine Diseases

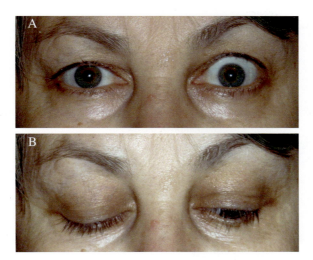

Fig. 14 A Female patient with marked upper eyelid retraction on the left. In the forward view, Dalrymple's sign is evident—an exposed strip of sclera between the limbus and the retracted eyelid. B Female patient with marked upper eyelid retraction on the left. In the downward view Graefe's sign—upper eyelid lacking movement

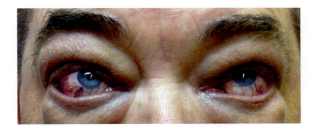

Fig. 15 Patient in the active phase of endocrine orbitopathy with marked bilateral upper and lower lid oedema, conjunctival injection accentuated mainly over the eyelid muscle attachments, and a congested caruncle and incipient conjunctival chemosis (oedema) are also seen. With a relatively small exophthalmos, the oculomotor muscles are markedly dilated—bilateral optic neuropathy is present

the external oculomotor muscles. When there is a significant overpressure in the orbit, chemosis of the conjunctiva and caruncle engorgement (lacrimal gland) may then be found (Fig. 15). However, if the conjunctiva is markedly reddened, especially in the upper part of the globe, then this is very likely to be *upper limbal keratoconjunctivitis* (inflammation of the cornea in the limbus and conjunctiva), which is typical of TED. Conjunctival hyperaemia and exposure keratopathy (corneal involvement due to corneal drying) can also contribute to *lagophthalmos* (inability to close the eye), which is most often due to a combination of marked exophthalmos and lid retraction.

Table 6 Eyelid symptoms of endocrine orbitopathy

Dalrymple	Looking forward, a strip of sclera is visible between the limbus and the retracted eyelid
Graefe	Lack of upper eyelid alignment in downward gaze
Enroth	Preseptal eyelid oedema
Kocher	Accentuation of upper eyelid retraction during fixation (e.g. during photography)
Jellinek	Abnormal brown pigmentation of the eyelids
Rosebach	Slight trembling of the closed eyelids
Boston	Saccadic movement of the upper eyelid when looking down
Stellwag	Less frequent blinking
Gifford	Upper eyelid eversion is difficult to impossible

TED is also often associated with "dry eye"—keratoconjunctivitis sicca. The aetiology of TED is multifactorial—thyroid dysfunction, use of general medications, and the disease itself (the inflammatory process affects all orbital compartments, including the lacrimal gland). Typical subjective complaints include a sensation of sand and tearing in the eye.

Exophthalmos is another very typical symptom of TED. It can be unilateral (Fig. 16) or bilateral (Fig. 17), symmetrical, or asymmetrical.

It is caused by the increased volume of orbital fat and orbicularis oculi muscles. Patients with significant exophthalmos are at risk for serious corneal complications with concomitant lagophthalmos (Fig. 18).

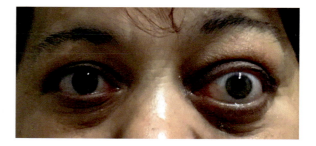

Fig. 16 Female patient with significant left-sided exophthalmos due to endocrine orbitopathy

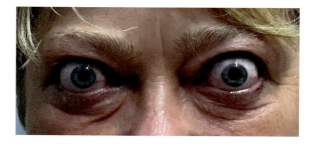

Fig. 17 Female patient with significant bilateral exophthalmos due to endocrine orbitopathy

Fig. 18 Patient with very severe endocrine orbitopathy—on the right already with corneal complications due to a combination of prominent exophthalmos and lagophthalmos (non-opening of the eye)

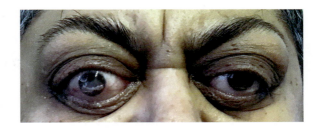

Fig. 19 Patient with restrictive strabismus in endocrine orbitopathy, as a result of the involvement of mainly the inferior and internal rectus muscles, the left bulbus is turned nasally and downward

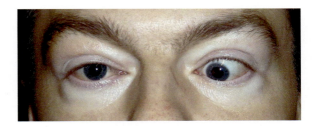

Repeated subluxations of the globe (e.g. in the case of inadvertent eye movements), where the eyelids become trapped on the globe equator, are no exception.

Diplopia (double vision) due to *eye movement disorders* in TED is often a severe problem for patients and significantly reduces their quality of life. This occurs in 30–50% of patients with TED, who might eventually need subsequent strabismus surgery (9–15% of patients). In the first stage, the motility of the eyeball is limited only due to inflammatory oedema in the muscle—thus, diplopia tends to be intermittent (after awakening, during fatigue, in extreme gaze directions). With further progression of the disease, fibrosis occurs in the muscle, and diplopia is also seen in the primary position. Gradual scarring leads to eye deviation, with the bulbus often curling down or converging in the final stage (Fig. 19).

Dysthyroid Optic Neuropathy (DON) is a serious condition requiring immediate therapeutic intervention. Late diagnosis can lead to blindness. DON affects approximately 3–5% of patients with TED. DON results from compression of the optic nerve and its vascular supply, due to an increase in the volume of orbital tissue and marked enlargement of the orbicularis oculi muscles near the orbital apex (Fig. 15). Symptoms of optic neuropathy may be subtle at first, like slightly blurred vision or loss of perception of colour saturation. On examination, central visual acuity may be reduced (but not necessarily), and defects in the visual field (paracentral or central scotomas) may be diagnosed. In about half of the cases, oedema of the optic disc is found. Patients with a relatively low degree of exophthalmos and markedly dilated eye muscles are at greater risk.

Increases in intraocular pressure are also relatively common in patients with TED. It is caused by a combination of several factors. The thickening of the orbicularis oculi muscles and the increased volume of adipose tissue and connective tissue in the orbit will cause an increase in episcleral venous pressure and limit the venous flow from the orbit. In addition, there is an increased accumulation of glycosaminoglycans in the trabecular meshwork, resulting in an increased outflow resistance. In patients with an affected inferior rectus muscle, there may then be a "pseudoglaucoma"—an increase in intraocular pressure due to the pincer mechanism in the affected eye when trying to fixate in the primary position [88].

Diagnosis

The diagnosis of EO is based on clinical, laboratory, and imaging findings. Close interdisciplinary collaboration between ophthalmologists, endocrinologists, and radiologists is a must.

Endocrinological examination

The endocrine examination aims to evaluate the thyroid gland function (TSH, fT3, fT4), possible thyroid autoimmune disease (set of antibodies), and thyroid gland structure (ultrasound). The determination of antibodies against TSH receptors (anti-rTSH, TRAK, TSI) is essential and should be performed repeatedly during TED treatment, as they are partially correlated with disease activity. It is also advisable to investigate autoantibodies against thyroglobulin (anti-Tg) and thyroid peroxidase (anti-TPO). Among imaging examinations, thyroid ultrasound is the method of choice to help detect nodules in the thyroid gland. If autonomic nodule or polynodous goitre is suspected, thyroid scintigraphy is added.

Ophthalmological examination

It consists of taking a detailed medical anamnesis, careful examination of the ocular adnexa, visual acuity, eye motility, anterior and posterior segment on a slit lamp, and measurement of intraocular pressure. Bulb protrusion (exophthalmos) is measured using a Hertel exophthalmometer (Fig. 20). Based on the examinations performed (and with the aid of imaging) [33], the ophthalmologist then determines the severity and activity of the disease.

Imaging

Initially, a sonographic examination (ultrasound) of the orbit and orbicularis oculi is performed most often. This is a relatively accessible, fast, and minimally burdensome method. The orbicularis oculi's width, internal structure, and reflectivity are assessed. However, ultrasound does not allow good visualisation of the posterior third of the orbit and the orbital apex. In typical cases, no further imaging is needed. In the case of

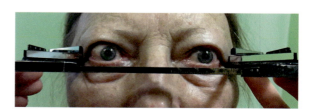

Fig. 20 Examination of the degree of exophthalmos using the Hertel exophthalmometer

an atypical clinical presentation, absence of antibodies, and in the case of markedly asymmetric involvement, other diseases or malignancies (diff. dg meningioma of the orbit, orbital pseudotumour or myositis, carotid-cavernous fistula, orbital lymphoma) should be excluded. In this diagnosis, we prefer MRI over CT, not only due to the low radiation burden, but also because of the possibility of assessing the disease activity (presence of oedema). On the other hand, CT provides good imaging of bony structures before planned orbital decompression in the case of suspected optic neuropathy, which is inexpensive, accessible, and fast. The disadvantage is the radiation burden, which is not suitable for routine monitoring or in children [55, 73].

Assessment of activity, severity, and quality of life

Several phases characterise the natural course of TED. Recognition of these phases, particularly the distinction between the degree of disability (severity of the disease) and its activity, is crucial for successful treatment.

In the initial phase of TED, there is typically a gradual worsening of the clinical signs of the disease. This is followed by a plateau phase with gradual stabilisation of the condition, and, in the last stage of the disease, its activity is gradually eliminated. The functional and cosmetic abnormalities that then persist are permanent. However, the duration of each phase of the disease is highly variable and difficult to predict. The *activity* of the disease attempts to assess the degree of the ongoing inflammatory process (highest in the initial phase of TED). On the contrary, the *severity* of the disease describes the degree of functional or cosmetic deficit at any stage of TED. The hypothetical relationship between activity and disease severity during the natural course of TED is demonstrated by the Rundle curve (Graph 1).

The sooner therapy is started after the first signs of activity appear, the lower the risk of permanent sequelae.

Evaluation of the severity and activity requires considerable investigator experience, especially given the highly variable initial manifestations of TED. The severity

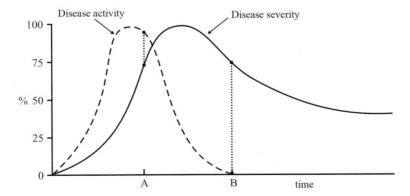

Graph 1 The so-called the Rundle curve depicts the relationship between activity and disease severity during the natural progression of endocrine orbitopathy

of TED can be assessed using different classifications. The European Group on Graves' Orbitopathy (EUGOGO) is the most used classification, which divides TED into three grades: mild, moderate, and severe (Table 7).

TED activity is most assessed using the Mourits clinical activity score (CAS) [61]. A slightly modified formulation is currently used, where a total of 7 points (Table 8) are assessed.

The first 2 points are scored by the patient, the next points by the physician. For each present symptom, 1 point is assigned. A CAS score ≥ 3 is significant for *active* disease. Other severity and activity classifications used include the NO SPECS or VISA classifications. According to the latest recommendations, when making treatment decisions, it is also advisable to assess the impact of the disease on the patient's daily life (Quality of Life questionnaire) for each patient.

Table 7 Assessment of severity of endocrine orbitopathy according to the European Group on Graves' orbitopathy (EUGOGO)

Mild form of TED	Patients in whom TED has only a minimal impact on normal daily activities and administration of conventional immunosuppressive therapy is therefore not indicated • Eyelid retraction < 2 mm • Mild soft tissue involvement • Exophthalmos < 3 mm for a given race and sex (for most of the European population, exophthalmos up to 23–24 mm) – No diplopia or intermittent diplopia (intermittent, with fatigue)
Moderate form of TED	Patients who are not at risk of vision loss, but whose TED significantly affects their ability to perform normal daily activities and the administration of immunosuppressive therapy (active form) or surgical management (inactive forms) is therefore indicated • Eyelid retraction ≥ 2 mm • Moderate or severe soft tissue involvement • Exophthalmos ≥ 3 mm for a given race and sex – Diplopia non-constant (outside the primary position of the eyeball) or constant (in the primary or reading position of the eyeball)
Severe form of TED	Patients at risk of vision loss • Dysthyroid optic neuropathy – Corneal involvement (exposure keratopathy)

The presence of at least one of the symptoms determines the severity of EO

Table 8 Clinical activity score (CAS)—the European Group on Graves' Orbitopathy (EUGOGO) assessment of endocrine orbitopathy activity

Pain or pressure behind the eye
Pain when moving the eye (up, down or sideways)
Erythema of the eyelids
Redness of the conjunctiva
Chemosis
Eyelid oedema
Inflammatory oedema of the caruncle

Therapy

The chances of a patient with TED being completely cured without permanent consequences (both cosmetic and affecting visual function) are significantly increased by early diagnosis of TED in its acute phase and the corresponding sufficiently aggressive treatment [81]. The treatment of TED is always complex, often long-term, and requires close multidisciplinary cooperation between the ophthalmologist and endocrinologist, possibly the surgeon, otorhinolaryngologist, and radiologist. The choice of treatment and its success depends mainly on a correct assessment of the disease activity (CAS), its severity (EUGOGO), and the impact of the disease on the patient's daily life (QoL questionnaire) [10, 18, 49]. An integral part of the whole process is then sufficient instruction and motivation of the patient, who must consistently follow the regimen [92]. A schematic representation of the TED treatment is shown in Graph 2.

The essential lifestyle modification for all TED patients, in general, is immediate and complete smoking cessation. It is also necessary to avoid any exposure to cigarette smoke (passive smoking). Furthermore, excess mental and physical stress must be eliminated, infections should not be left untreated and sufficient rest should be taken. *Topical therapy* is rather symptomatic and is guided by an ophthalmologist—most often, lubricants in drops, gels, or ointments are recommended.

The cornerstone of successful treatment of TED is *achieving and maintaining stable thyroid function.* Both hypo and hyperfunction of the thyroid gland worsen

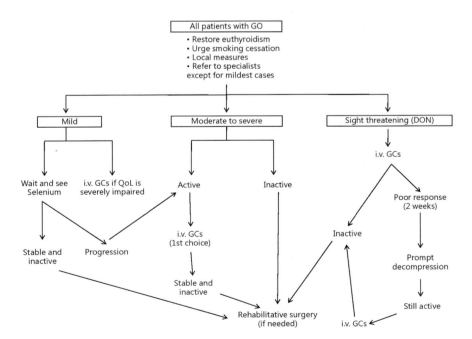

Graph 2 Treatment of endocrine orbitopathy, adapted from Bartalena et al. [7]

the course of orbitopathy. In the case of hyperthyroidism (thyrotoxicosis), thyrostatic therapy (methimazole) is the first line of treatment, with the aim of normalising thyroid hormone levels as soon as possible (normalisation of fT4 occurs first, TSH later). If this therapeutic strategy is unsuccessful (relapse of thyrotoxicosis with gradual dose reduction, significant side effects in terms of hepatopathy or leukopenia), total thyroidectomy (TTE) is indicated in the calming phase [9]. The decision on the individual steps, including the indication for TTE, is entirely in the hands of the endocrinologist. In the case of active TED, thyroidectomy is often preceded by pulse administration of methylprednisolone. Thyroid ablation with iodine 131 (RAI) is another possible modality for the treatment of hyperthyroidism but is associated with a slightly increased risk of exacerbation or de novo TED [8]. RAI is the treatment modality used in the USA, rather than in Europe, in adult patients without active or moderate or severe TED.

Immunosuppressive therapy of TED is indicated for moderate and severe forms of the disease in the active phase. In the inactive stage of the disease, if permanent fibrotic changes have already occurred, immunomodulatory therapy will be ineffective and unnecessarily burdensome for the patient.

The most common treatment strategy for mild forms is the "wait-and-see" method or the consideration of selenium replacement or pentoxifylline. After euthyroid and smoking cessation, spontaneous calming of TED occurs very often. Only if even a mild form of TED significantly affects the patient's quality of life, should it be reclassified as moderate and treated as such.

Immunosuppressive therapy is most effective only in the early stages of the disease. *Corticosteroids* can be administered orally or intravenously, while intravenous administration is considered more effective with a lower incidence of adverse effects [7]. Therefore, oral corticosteroids are no longer recommended as a part of first-line treatment. In Europe, the EUGOGO developed the most followed treatment protocols, giving high importance to minimising the side effects and therefore reduced the previously used high doses of iv. Methylprednisolone. Currently, there are two possible first-line treatments for moderate to severe TED (A) 0.5 g of methylprednisone once weekly for six weeks and 0.25 g in the following six weeks (cumulative dose 4.5 g); alternatively, higher cumulative doses not exceeding 8 g can be used as monotherapy in most severe cases and constant/inconsistent diplopia. (B) Combination of i.v. methylprednisolone (same regimen as above) plus *mycophenolate sodium* (or *mofetil*) orally daily. This drug combination has moved into first-line treatment based on the MINGO study, demonstrating the efficacy and safety of combining i.v. methylprednisolone with low-dose mycophenolate per os. The risk–benefit ratio of low-dose mycophenolate, either as monotherapy or in combination with i.v. glucocorticoid treatment in active moderate-to-severe GO is highly favourable, given its reassuring safety profile and promising efficacy [51, 123].

Before initiating therapy, liver function and viral liver hepatitis markers, liver ultrasound, and glycaemia are recommended. Arterial hypertension and diabetes should be compensated [10]. The success rate of treatment is about 75 to 80%. Contraindications are severe cardiovascular disease, psychiatric illness, acute or recent viral

Metabolic and Endocrine Diseases

hepatitis, and elevated liver function tests. Treatment should be administered in facilities with sufficient experience in this treatment and with the adequate provision and monitoring of adverse effects. During treatment (at least every other pulse), it is recommended to check glycaemia, liver tests, mineral panel, ECG and BP. During treatment, it is recommended to administer proton pump inhibitors and consider the prevention of thrombosis. Bisphosphonates are recommended in patients with multiple risk factors for osteoporosis.

In approximately 20–30% of patients, intravenous methylprednisone therapy is ineffective, or the treatment effect is only short-term, with subsequent rapid reactivation of the inflammatory process in the orbit. This refers to the cortico-resistant TED, in which the most appropriate second-line therapy must be carefully considered. Several options have been suggested as a second-line treatment: administration of another series of corticoid therapy (if the cumulative dose of 8 g of methylprednisone has not already been exceeded), a combination of oral corticosteroids with either cyclosporine or azathioprine, orbital radiotherapy combined with oral or i.v. glucocorticoids, rituximab, and tocilizumab. It is also possible to choose a "wait and see" strategy, i.e. to wait for spontaneous extinction of the activity, but this is associated with a risk of the worsening of possible permanent changes.

Teprotumumab (TEP)

Antibodies against IGF-1 have shown efficacy in reducing inflammatory symptoms and disease relapse. TEP is the newest agent applied to the management of TED and, paradoxically, is the only drug approved by the Food and Drug Administration (FDA) for the treatment of TED for patients ≥ 18 years of age. Teprotumumab has recently been adored as the possible first-line treatment for TED, in countries where available, by the consensus statement of the American Thyroid Association and the European Thyroid Association. EMA approval is expected [18].

Rituximab is a humanised chimeric monoclonal antibody against CD20 that blocks the activation and differentiation of B lymphocytes. Because the autoimmunity in Basedow's disease is primarily mediated by B-cell autoimmunity. Based on the available data, rituximab is a valid second-line treatment option. However, it should not be used in long duration orbitopathy or where the optic nerve is compromised (risk of DON) [106].

Tocilizumab is a humanized monoclonal antibody against the interleukin (IL)-6 receptor, its use for TED is off-label it may be considered as a second-line treatment for moderate-to-severe and active glucocorticoid-resistant GO.

Radiotherapy of the orbits is another treatment option, but generally less used [109]. The standard treatment is 20 Gy divided into ten doses. The treatment can then be combined with corticoid therapy.

The most serious manifestation of severe forms of TED is Dysthyroid Optic Neuropathy (DON), which requires immediate therapeutic intervention to prevent visual impairment. In early signs of optic nerve compression, the first choice is vigorous immunosuppressive therapy. In cases of clearly expressed optic nerve damage due to optic nerve compression or when corticosteroids have an insufficient effect, surgical decompression of the orbit is the method of choice.

Surgical decompression of the orbit consists of the surgical removal of one or more walls of the orbit (medial, lateral wall, or base of the orbit). It is also possible to remove extraocular and intraconal fat, alone or simultaneously with the bony part of the orbit. Several procedures have been described. At present, endoscopic techniques are preferred, as they have a perfect effect and a relatively low risk of complications. The medial wall of the orbit can be removed by this route, often in combination with the inferior wall. Indications for orbital decompression are compressive optic neuropathy or marked exophthalmos with exposure keratopathy. Exceptionally, the procedure can also be indicated from a cosmetic point of view in the inactive stage of TED, e.g. in the case of marked asymmetric exophthalmos.

Topical therapy

For all forms of TED lubrication therapy in the form of drops, gels or ointments are recommended. In lagophthalmic keratopathy, a contact lens may be applied for intensive lubrication and ATB coverage to improve healing, or temporary lid tarsorrhaphy may be considered. Topical application of corticosteroids in drops or ointments has no effect, even supportive, on soothing the TED itself, but subjectively may bring the temporary patient relief from some of its manifestations. In the case of a significant elevation of intraocular tension due to increased episcleral pressure, the use of topical antiglaucoma agents is appropriate. In disruptive diplopia, full or sectoral semitransparent occlusion in front of the non-dominant eye on the glass of dioptric or sunglasses has proven useful. For minor deviations, diplopia can be eliminated with prismatic spectacle correction.

In the case of permanent changes in the orbital tissues despite the therapy, corrective surgical procedures can be performed in the inactive phase of the disease (at least one year after the activity extinction). These include unilateral or bilateral orbital decompression (in the case of marked or asymmetric exophthalmos, drying of the anterior segment of the eyes from lagophthalmos), restrictive strabismus surgery (in the case of diplopia) [53, 54] or eyelid retraction surgery (in the case of cosmetically distracting asymmetry, lagophthalmos).

6 Multiple Endocrine Neoplasia

Multiple endocrine neoplasia syndromes (MEN), which are inherited in an autosomal dominant manner, are characterized by the presence of two or more tumours in a patient, of which there are four main types (MEN1-4).

Genetic testing should be offered to patients with MEN and their first-degree relatives. Individuals with the mutation who are at risk of developing tumours should undergo regular clinical, biochemical and radiological screening for early detection and treatment of tumours.

Treatment of patients with MEN, which aims to minimize disease-related morbidity and mortality while preserving quality of life, requires a multidisciplinary approach [2].

Metabolic and Endocrine Diseases

Multiple endocrine neoplasia I (Wermer's syndrome)

The syndrome is caused by a mutation in the tumour suppressor gene MEN1 on chromosome 11 (a protein called menin). 80% of cases manifest by the age of 40, affecting both sexes and occurring at all ages. It affects about 1 in 30,000 people.

Clinical presentation

MEN1 is characterised by the appearance of neuroendocrine tumours of the parathyroid glands, the anterior pituitary and the duodenum, and pancreas, and occasionally carcinoids of the anterior colon and adrenal glands. The majority (85%) are first with parathyroid tumour and associated primary hyperparathyroidism; the rest are insulinomas or prolactinomas [2].

Diagnosis

MEN1 is suspected if a person has at least two of the above most common tumours.

Therapy

Most of these tumours are treated by surgery, or by taking drugs that suppress the growth or function of the tumour. Parathyroid tumours, which are almost always benign, should be surgically removed. There are challenging treatment issues associated with the removal of neuroendocrine tumours of the pancreas. In addition to its role in normal digestion, the pancreas regulates blood glucose levels through insulin production. Removal of the pancreas will cause diabetes mellitus, and, at the same time, pancreatic enzyme supplements will need to be taken to aid digestion. Doctors must balance the benefits of removing the pancreas in a person with MEN1, such as preventing cancer, with the risks of developing diabetes. Patients with a neuroendocrine pancreatic tumour that has spread to the liver can be treated with a somatostatin analogue or a drug that regulates signalling in pancreatic islet cells, everolimus. Other neuroendocrine tumours are usually removed surgically, and further treatment may be recommended [27]. Pituitary tumours producing the hormone prolactin are most treated with dopamine agonists. Tumours producing growth hormone or adrenocorticotropin hormone or non-functioning tumours are most often treated with surgery [80].

Multiple endocrine neoplasia 2 (formerly 2A)

The syndrome is caused by a mutation in the RET proto-oncogene on chromosome 10.

Clinical presentation

MEN2 is characterised by the occurrence of medullary thyroid carcinoma (MTC), pheochromocytomas and parathyroid tumours. MEN2 includes variants MEN2A with Hirschsprung's disease, MEN2A with cutaneous lichenoid amyloidosis and familial MTC only.

Diagnosis

It includes calcium, phosphorus, and PTH levels for primary hyperparathyroidism, as well as thyroid ultrasound and serum calcitonin in medullary thyroid carcinoma, and plasma or urinary metanephrines in pheochromocytoma.

Therapy

The optimal solution in most cases is surgery. Medullary thyroid carcinoma is mild to moderately aggressive. Prophylactic total thyroidectomy is recommended early for children who carry the MEN2A mutation, depending on the type of mutation. MEN2 (2A) carriers should be screened for pheochromocytoma and medullary thyroid carcinoma before any surgical intervention [89].

Multiple endocrine neoplasia type 3 (formerly MEN 2B)

The syndrome is also caused by a germline mutation of the RET proto-oncogene.

Clinical presentation

MEN3 is characterised by the presence of MTC and pheochromocytomas in association with the marfanoid habit (75% of cases), mucosal neuromas (more than 90% of cases), medullary corneal fibres and intestinal ganglioneuromatosis. Patients may also have skeletal abnormalities (87%) and delayed puberty (43%).

Diagnosis and therapy

Optimally, surgical solution, as in the previous types. Medullary thyroid carcinoma is aggressive and manifests at an early age. Therefore, early genetic screening must be performed in children whose parents have MEN3 (2B), and in children who carry the ret proto-oncogene mutation, total thyroidectomy must be performed prophylactically at a very early age. Again, depending on the type of mutation [21].

Multiple endocrine neoplasia type 4 (MEN 4)

A tumour syndrome caused by germline mutations in the tumour suppressor gene CDKN1B on chromosome 12p13 and encodes a protein known as CK1P27kip1 (p27) [29, 45].

Clinical presentation

MEN4 patients are particularly susceptible to parathyroid adenomas (80%), pituitary adenomas (less aggressive than MEN1), neuroendocrine pancreatic tumours and adrenal tumours. Unlike MEN1 patients, MEN4 patients are also susceptible to kidney cancer, testicular cancer, neuroendocrine carcinoma of the cervix and primary ovarian failure.

Therapy

Surgical treatment of the tumour is the first choice. In the case of inoperability or hyperfunction, pharmacological treatment can be used similarly to MEN1, see above.

Ocular manifestations of MEN syndromes

The most common ocular manifestations of MEN syndromes include defects in the visual field, such as bitemporal hemianopsia due to the presence of pituitary adenomas (see Pituitary Adenomas). Attention should also be paid to the examination of the ocular adnexa. Patients with MEN2 may have prominent eyebrows and, in MEN3, rarely, with mucinous neurinomas of the eyelid and conjunctiva, which can cause eyelid thickening and irregularities of the eyelashes. More prominent nerves can also be seen on the cornea in patients with MEN2 and 3 [52].

7   Wolfram Syndrome

Wolfram syndrome (WFS) is a rare genetic cause of juvenile diabetes mellitus, characterised by pancreatic β-cell destruction and concomitant optic nerve atrophy. WFS syndrome is also known as DIDMOAD syndrome (i.e. Diabetes Insipidus, Diabetes Mellitus, Optic Atrophy, and Deafness) due to its association with other symptoms. It may present with various other neurological findings (e.g. peripheral neuropathy, ataxia and cognitive impairment), or other systemic findings (e.g. renal abnormalities, gonadal atrophy and psychiatric disorders). It is an autosomal recessively inherited disease, caused by mutations in the WFS1 gene, which encodes the transmembrane protein tungstate. Classically, WFS is associated with mutations in the WFS1 gene; however, other mutations at different loci have been shown to cause similar syndromes [83].

Clinical presentation and objective findings

WFS is a slowly progressive neurodegenerative process and there is also selective destruction of pancreatic beta cells. Diabetes mellitus with onset in childhood is usually the first manifestation. Optic atrophy follows early in the second decade, and later in the second decade, diabetes insipidus and deafness appear. Finally, neurological and genitourinary problems appear on average in the third decade. Diabetes mellitus and optic atrophy are present in all cases, but the expression of other features varies. The duration of diabetes is associated with the development of microvascular complications.

The usual associated neurological manifestations of WFS are trunk ataxia, peripheral neuropathy, and cognitive impairment. However, other neurological symptoms include anosmia, gag reflex, myoclonus, epilepsy, nystagmus, and autonomic neuropathy (including orthostatic hypotension, gastroparesis, and resting tachycardia). Psychiatric findings are prevalent in patients with WFS1, but occur later in the course of the disease, with anxiety and depression being the most common. However, severe depression, psychosis, impulsivity, and verbal and physical aggression may also occur. Genitourinary symptoms vary considerably; bladder instability or atony can cause urge or overflow incontinence. Structural abnormalities include hydroureteronephrosis and sphincter abnormalities that predispose patients to recurrent urinary tract infections. Hypogonadism is also common, with erectile dysfunction in men, irregular menstrual cycles in women, and impaired fertility in both sexes. Patients with WFS1 may also have a short stature due to growth hormone (GH) deficiency and hypothyroidism. Other manifestations of this disease include structural heart abnormalities, such as pulmonary valve stenosis and cardiomyopathy, anaemia, and limited joint mobility [50].

Diagnosis

Most patients do not experience all four symptoms that are part of the name "DID-MOAD". Therefore, the diagnosis of WFS can only be made based on the simultaneous presence of DM and optic atrophy, ideally at an early age. It is essential to suspect WFS in the presence of DM and optic atrophy, especially if antibodies to glutamic acid decarboxylase and islet cell antibodies, which are commonly found in Type 1 diabetes mellitus, are negative. If a patient with DM develops optic nerve atrophy, the physician should suspect WFS. Molecular genetic testing allows confirmation of the disease, genetic counseling and screening in high-risk, asymptomatic individuals with a significant family anamnesis.

Therapy

Emphasis should be placed on optimising glycaemic control, with insulin therapy according to standard guidelines for insulin-dependent diabetes mellitus. Exogenous replacement may be necessary for specific hormonal deficiencies, e.g. desmopressin for DI, growth hormone for pathological short stature and levothyroxine for hypothyroidism. Treatment of urological complications [1].

Ocular manifestations of Wolfram syndrome

Optic atrophy is the primary criterion for diagnosing WFS and the main ocular manifestation. Clinically, it is manifested by a reduction in central visual acuity, colour defects, defects in the visual field, optic disc pallor, and nerve fiber layer thinning (RNFL). Symptoms usually appear around the age of 11 and are mild at first. Gradual progression of the disease leads to a blindness on an average of 8 years from the diagnosis of optic atrophy. Other neuro-ophthalmological manifestations include nystagmus and strabismus, which tend to be associated with more severe systemic complications. Other ocular findings described include cataract, glaucoma and pigmentary maculopathy or retinopathy [50].

References

1. Abreu D, Urano F. Current landscape of treatments for wolfram syndrome. Trends Pharmacol Sci. 2019;40(10):711–4.
2. Al-Salameh AG, Cadiot A, Calender P, et al. Clinical aspects of multiple endocrine neoplasia type 1. Nat Rev Endocrinol. 2021;17(4):207–24.

Metabolic and Endocrine Diseases

3. American Diabetes Association. Standards of medical care in diabetes-2020. Abridged for primary care providers. Clin Diabetes. 2020;38(1):10–38.
4. Amoaku WM, Ghanchi F, Bailey C, et al. Diabetic retinopathy and diabetic macular oedema pathways and management: UK Consensus Working Group. Eye (Lond). 2020;34(Suppl 1):1–51.
5. Bahn RS. Current insights into the pathogenesis of Graves' ophthalmopathy. Horm Metab Res. 2015;47(10):773–8.
6. Barr CC, Glaser JS, Blankenship G. Acute disc swelling in juvenile diabetes: clinical profile and natural history of 12 cases. Arch Ophthalmol. 1980;98:2185–92.
7. Bartalena L, Baldeschi L, Boboridis K, et al. The 2016 European Thyroid Association/European Group on Graves' Orbitopathy guidelines for the management of Graves' orbitopathy. Eur Thyroid J. 2016;5(1):9–26.
8. Bartalena L, Macchia E, Marcocci C, et al. Effects of treatment modalities for Graves' hyperthyroidism on Graves' orbitopathy: a 2015 Italian Society of Endocrinology Consensus Statement. J Endocrinol Invest. 2015;38(4):481–7.
9. Bartalena L, Pinchera A, Marcocci C. Management of Graves' ophthalmopathy: reality and perspectives. Endocr Rev. 2000;21(2):168–99.
10. Bartalena LG, Kahaly J, Baldeschi L, et al. The 2021 European Group on Graves' Orbitopathy (EUGOGO) clinical practice guidelines for the medical management of Graves' orbitopathy. Eur J Endocrinol. 2021;185(4):43–67.
11. Benest AV, Kruse K, Savant S, et al. Angiopoietin-2 is critical for cytokine-induced vascular leakage. PLoS ONE. 2013;8(8): e70459.
12. Benn M, Watts GF, Tybjaerg-Hansen A, et al. Familial hypercholesterolemia in the danish general population: prevalence, coronary artery disease, and cholesterol-lowering medication. J Clin Endocrinol Metab. 2014;99(12):4758–9.
13. Benson WE, Brown GC, Tasman W. Diabetes and its ocular complications. Philadelphia: WB Saunders Co.; 1988. p. 27–34.
14. Blick SK, Keating GM, Wagstaff AJ. Ranibizumab. Drugs. 2007;67(8):1199–206.
15. Blodi FC, Yarbrough JC. Ocular manifestations of familial hypercholesterolemia. Am J Ophthalmol. 1963;55:714–8.
16. Boyer DS, Hopkins JJ, Sorof J, et al. Anti-vascular endothelial growth factor therapy for diabetic macular edema. Ther Adv Endocrinol Metab. 2013;4(6):151–69.
17. Brown GC, Magargal LE, Schachat A, et al. Neovascular glaucoma: etiologic considerations. Ophthalmology. 1984;91:315–20.
18. Burch HB, Perros P, Bednarczuk T, et al. Management of thyroid eye disease: a Consensus Statement by the American Thyroid Association and the European Thyroid Association. Eur Thyroid J. 2022;11(6): e220189.
19. Campbell DG, Schertzer RM. Ghost cell glaucoma. In: Ritch R, Shields MB, Kurpin T, editors. The glaucomas. 2nd ed. St Louis: CV Mosby Co.; 1996. p. 1277–85.
20. Canton E. Observation on the arcus senilis or fatty degeneration of the cornea. Lancet. 1850;55(1393):560–2.
21. Castinetti F, Moley J, Mulligan L, et al. A comprehensive review on MEN2B. Endocr Relat Cancer. 2018;25(2):29–39.
22. Ceska R, et al. Cholesterol and atherosclerosis, treatment of dyslipidemia. Triton; 2012.
23. Chaturvedi N, Sjolie AK, Stephenson JM, et al. Effect of lisinopril on progression of retinopathy in normotensive people with type 1 diabetes. The EUCLID Study Group. EURODIAB controlled trial of Lisinopril in insulin-dependent diabetes mellitus. Lancet. 1998;351:28–31.
24. Chew EY, Ambrosius WT, Davis MD, et al. Effects of medical therapies on retinopathy progression in type 2 diabetes. N Engl J Med. 2010;363(3):233–44.
25. Cogan DG, Kuwabara T. Lipid keratopathy and atheroma. Circulation. 1958;18(4):519–25.
26. Crispin S. Ocular lipid deposition and hyperlipoproteinaemia. Prog Retin Eye Res. 2002;21(2):169–224.

27. Dai M, Mullins CS, Lu L, et al. Recent advances in diagnosis and treatment of gastroenteropancreatic neuroendocrine neoplasms. World J Gastrointest Surg. 2022;14(5):383–96.
28. Davis MD, Fisher MR, Gangnon RE, et al. Risk factors for high-risk proliferative diabetic retinopathy and severe visual loss. Early treatment diabetic retinopathy study report 18. Invest Ophthalmol Vis Sci. 1998;39:233–52.
29. De Herder WW, Hofland J. Multiple endocrine neoplasia type 4. In: Feingold KR, Anawalt B, Blackman MR, et al., editors. Endotext [internet]. South Dartmouth (MA): MDText.com, Inc.; 2000. Available from: https://www.ncbi.nlm.nih.gov/books/NBK578575/
30. Diabetes Control and Complications Trial Group. The effect of intensive treatment of diabetes on the development and progression of long-term complications in insulin-dependent diabetes mellitus. N Engl J Med. 1993;1993(329):977–86.
31. Diabetes WHO. Available at: www.who.int, 16 Sept 2022
32. Diabetic Retinopathy Study Research Group. Preliminary report on effects of photocoagulation therapy. Am J Ophthalmol. 1976;81(4):383–96.
33. Dickinson AJ, Perros P. Controversies in the clinical evaluation of active thyroid-associated orbitopathy:use of a detailed protocol with comparative photographs for objective assessment. Clin Endocrinol (Oxf). 2001;55(3):283–303.
34. Douglas RS, Kahaly GJ, Patel A, et al. Teprotumumab for the treatment of active thyroid eye disease. N Engl J Med. 2020;382(4):341–52.
35. Duh E, et al. Diabetic retinopathy and systematic complications. In: Duh E, editor. Diabetic retinopathy. New Jersey: Humana Press; 2009. p. 465–85.
36. Early Treatment Diabetic Retinopathy Study Research Group. Early photocoagulation for diabetic retinopathy. ETDRS report number 9. Ophthalmology. 1991;98(5 Suppl):766–85.
37. Early Treatment Diabetic Retinopathy Study Research Group. Photocoagulation for diabetic macular edema. ETDRS report number 1. Arch Ophthalmol. 1985;103:1796–806.
38. Eckstein A, Quadbeck B, Mueller G, et al. Impact of smoking on the response to treatment of thyroid associated ophthalmopathy. Br J Ophthalmol. 2003;87(6):773–6.
39. Eichenbaum JW, Feldstein M, Podos SM. Extended-wear soft contact lenses and corneal ulcers. Br J Ophthalmol. 1982;66:663–6.
40. Ernest J, Němčanský J, Vysloužilová D, et al. Diabetic macular edema—diagnostics and treatment guidelines. Čes. a slov. Oftal. 2023; 79(5):225–35.
41. Fenton RH, Zimmerman LE. Hemolytic glaucoma:an unusual cause of acute openangle secondary glaucoma. Arch Ophthalmol. 1963;70:236–9.
42. Ferrari N, Gerber HP, LeCouter J. The biology of VEGF and its receptors. Nat Med. 2003;9:669–76.
43. Greco D, Gambina F, Maggio F. Ophthalmoplegia in diabetes mellitus: a retrospective study. Acta Diabetol. 2009;46(1):23–6.
44. Gross JG, Glassman AR, Jampol LM, et al. Panretinal photocoagulation vs intravitreous ranibizumab for proliferative diabetic retinopathy: a randomized clinical trial. JAMA. 2015;314(20):2137–46.
45. Halperin R, Arnon L, Nasirov S, et al. Germline CDKN1B variant type and site are associated with phenotype in MEN4. Endocr Relat Cancer. 2022;30(1): e220174.
46. Hrda P, Novak Z, Sterzl I. Endocrine orbitopathy. Prague: Maxdorf; 2009. p. 109.
47. Hyndiuk RA, Kazarian EL, Schultz RO, et al. Neurotrophic corneal ulcers in diabetes mellitus. Arch Ophthalmol. 1977;95:2193–6.
48. International Diabetes Federation. IDF diabetes atlas. 10th ed. Brussels, Belgium; 2021. Available at: https://www.diabetesatlas.org
49. Jiskra J. Management of Graves ophthalmopathy—2022 update. J Czech Phys. 2022;161(5):198–206.
50. Kabanovski A, Donaldson L, Margolin E. Neuro-ophthalmological manifestations of Wolfram syndrome: case series and review of the literature. J Neurol Sci. 2022;437: 120267.
51. Kahaly GJ, Riedl M, König J, et al. European Group on Graves' Orbitopathy (EUGOGO). Mycophenolate plus methylprednisolone versus methylprednisolone alone in active, moderate-to-severe Graves' orbitopathy (MINGO): a randomised, observer-masked, multicentre trial. Lancet Diabetes Endocrinol. 2018;6(4):287–98.

Metabolic and Endocrine Diseases

52. Kamboj A, Lause M, Kumar P. Ophthalmic manifestations of endocrine disorders-endocrinology and the eye. Transl Pediatr. 2017;6(4):286–99.
53. Karhanova M, Kalitova J, Vlacil O, et al. Conservative management options for thyroid disease induced diplopia. Cesk Slov Oftalmol. 2013;69(5):220–4.
54. Karhanova M, Vlacil O, Sin M, et al. Adjustable versus non-adjustable sutures in strabismus surgery in patients with thyroid ophthalmopathy. Cesk Slov Oftalmol. 2012;68(5):207–13.
55. Karhanova M. Endocrine orbitopathies from an ophthalmologist's point of view. Med Pract. 2013;10(2):68–71.
56. Kavoussi H, Ebrahimi A, Rezaei M, et al. Serum lipid profile and clinical characteristics of patients with xanthelasma palpebrarum. An Bras Dermatol. 2016;91(4):468–71.
57. Keech AC, Mitchell P, Summanen PA, et al. Effect of fenofibrate on the need for laser treatment for diabetic retinopathy (FIELD study): a randomised controlled trial. Lancet. 2007;370:1687–97.
58. Klein BE, Klein R, Jensen SC. Open-angle glaucoma and older-onset diabetes: the Beaver Dam Eye Study. Ophthalmology. 1994;101:1173–7.
59. Klein BE, Klein R, Moss SE. Intraocular pressure in diabetic persons. Ophthalmology. 1984;91:1356–60.
60. Klein BE, Klein R, Moss SE. Prevalence of cataracts in a population-based study of persons with diabetes mellitus. Ophthalmology. 1985;92:1191–6.
61. Mouritz MP, Koornneef L, Wiersinga WM, et al. Clinical criteria for the assessment of disease activity in Graves' ophthalmopathy: a novel approach. Br J Ophthalmol. 1989;73:639–644.
62. Le Moli R, Muscia V, Tumminia A, et al. Type 2 diabetic patients with Graves' disease have more frequent and severe Graves' orbitopathy. Nutr Metab Cardiovasc Dis. 2015;25(5):452–7.
63. Leske MC, Podgor MJ. Intraocular pressure, cardiovascular risk variables, and visual field defects. Am J Epidemiol. 1983;118:280–7.
64. Little HL, Rosenthal AR, Dellaporta A, et al. The effect of pan-retinal photocoagulation on rubeosis iridis. Am J Ophthalmol. 1976;81:804–9.
65. Manaviat MR, Rashidi M, Afkhami-Ardekani M, Shoja MR. Prevalence of dry eye syndrome and diabetic retinopathy in type 2 diabetic patients. BMC Ophthalmol. 2008;8:10.
66. Mitchell P, Smith W, Chey T, et al. Open-angle glaucoma and diabetes: the Blue Mountains eye study, Australia. Ophthalmology. 1997;104:712–8.
67. Nathan DM, Cleary PA, Backlund JY, et al. Intensive diabetes treatment and cardiovascular disease in patients with type 1 diabetes. N Engl J Med. 2005;353(25):2643–53.
68. Nathan DM, Genuth S, Lachin J, et al. The effect of intensive treatment of diabetes on the development and progression of long-term complications in insulin-dependent diabetes mellitus. N Engl J Med. 1993;329(14):977–86.
69. Němčanský J, Studnička J, Vysloužilová D, et al. Diabetic retinopathy and diabetic macular edema—screening. Čes. a slov. Oftal. 2023;79(5):250–5.
70. Nepp J, Abela C, Polzer I, et al. Is there a correlation between the severity of diabetic retinopathy and keratoconjunctivitis sicca? Cornea. 2000;19:487–91.
71. Nesrullayeva N. Oculomotor disorders in patients with diabetes. Arch Neurol Neurosci. 2018;1(5). https://doi.org/10.33552/ANN.MS.ID.000524
72. Nordestgaard BG, Chapman MJ, Humphries SE, et al. Familial hypercholesterolaemia is underdiagnosed and undertreated in the general population: guidance for clinicians to prevent coronary heart disease: consensus statement of the European Atherosclerosis Society. Eur Heart J. 2013;34:3478.
73. North VS, Freitag SK. A review of imaging modalities in thyroid-associated orbitopathy. Int Ophthalmol Clin. 2019;59(4):81–93.
74. Okamoto F, Sone H, Nonoyama T, et al. Refractive changes in diabetic patients during intensive glycaemic control. Br J Ophthalmol. 2000;84:1097–102.
75. Panozzo G, Cicinelli MV, Augustin AJ, et al. An optical coherence tomography-based grading of diabetic maculopathy proposed by an international expert panel: The European School for Advanced Studies in Ophthalmology classification. Eur J Ophthalmol. 2020;30(1):8–18.

76. Papadopoulos N, Martin J, Ruan Q, et al. Binding and neutralization of vascular endothelial growth factor (VEGF) and related ligands by VEGF Trap, ranibizumab and bevacizumab. Angiogenesis. 2012;15(2):171–85.
77. Patel A, MacMahon S, Chalmers J, et al. Intensive blood glucose control and vascular outcomes in patients with type 2 diabetes. N Engl J Med. 2009;358(24):2560–72.
78. Pavan PR, Folk JC, Weingeist TA, et al. Diabetic rubeosis and panretinal photocoagulation. Arch Ophthalmol. 1983;101:882–4.
79. Pelikanova T, Bartos V, et al. Practical diabetology. 6th updated and supplemented ed. Maxdorf; 2018.
80. Pieterman CRC, Valk GD. Update on the clinical management of multiple endocrine neoplasia type 1. Clin Endocrinol (Oxf). 2022;97(4):409–23.
81. Prummel MF, Bakker A, Wiersinga WM, et al. Multi-center study on the characteristics and treatment strategies of patients with Graves' orbitopathy: the first European Group on Graves' Orbitopathy experience. Eur J Endocrinol. 2003;148(5):491–5.
82. Qaum T, Xu Q, Joussen AM, et al. VEGF-initiated blood-retinal barrier breakdown in early diabetes. Invest Ophthalmol Vis Sci. 2001;42:2408–13.
83. Rigoli L, Caruso V, Salzano G, et al. Wolfram syndrome 1: from genetics to therapy. Int J Environ Res Public Health. 2022;19(6):3225.
84. Rogell GD. Corneal hypesthesia and retinopathy in diabetes mellitus. Ophthalmology. 1980;87:229–33.
85. Rosolova H. Current state of hypolipidemic treatment in our country. Interv Akut Kardiol. 2016;15(2):81–4.
86. Rucker CW. The causes of paralysis of the third, fourth, and sixth cranial nerves. Am J Ophthalmol. 1966;61:1293–8.
87. Saito J, Enoki M, Hara M, et al. Correlation of corneal sensation, but not of basal or reflex tear secretion, with the stage of diabetic retinopathy. Cornea. 2003;22:15–8.
88. Samkova K. Secondary glaucoma, Mladá fronta; 2016.
89. Saravana-Bawan B, Pasternak JD. Multiple endocrine neoplasia 2: an overview. Ther Adv Chronic Dis. 2022;13:20406223221079250.
90. Sharma A, Kumar N, Kuppermann BD, et al. Faricimab: expanding horizon beyond VEGF. Eye (Lond). 2020;34(5):802–4.
91. Schmidt-Erfurth U, Garcia-Arumi J, Bandello F, et al. Guidelines for the management of diabetic macular edema by the European Society of Retina Specialists (EURETINA). Ophthalmologica. 2017;237:185–222.
92. Schovanek J, Cibickova L, Karhanova M. Endocrine orbitopathy and new recommendations. General Med. 2017;19(5):246–50.
93. Segal P, Insull W, Chambless LE, et al. The association of dyslipoproteinemia with corneal arcus and xanthelasma. The lipid research clinics program prevalence study. Circulation. 1986;73(2):108–18.
94. Silva PAS, Cavallerano JD, Sun JK, et al. Proliferative diabetic retinopathy. In: Ryan SJ, editor-in-chief. Retina, vol. II, 5th ed. Saunders, an imprint of Elsevier Inc.; 2013, p. 969–1000
95. Sivaprasad S, Prevost AT, Vasconcelos JC, et al. Clinical efficacy of intravitreal aflibercept versus panretinal photocoagulation for best corrected visual acuity in patients with proliferative diabetic retinopathy at 52 weeks (CLARITY):a multicentre, single-blinded, randomised, controlled, phase 2b, non-inferiority trial. Lancet. 2017;389(10085):2193–203.
96. Sjolie AK, Klein R, Porta M, et al. Effect of candesartan on progression and regression of retinopathy in type 2 diabetes (DIRECT-Protect 2): a randomised placebo-controlled trial. Lancet. 2008;372:1385–93.
97. Skyler JS, Bergenstal R, Bonow RO, et al. Intensive glycemic control and the prevention of cardiovascular events: implications of the ACCORD, ADVANCE and VADT: a position statement of the American Diabetes Association and a scientific statement of the American College of Cardiology Foundation and the American Heart Association. Diabetes Care. 2009;39:187–92.
98. Smith TJ, Hegedus L. Graves' disease. N Engl J Med. 2016;375(16):1552–65.

Metabolic and Endocrine Diseases

99. Sosna T, et al. Diabetic retinopathy, 2nd revised ed. Prague: Axonite CZ; 2016.
100. Stan MN, Bahn RS. Risk factors for development or deterioration of Graves' ophthalmopathy. Thyroid. 2010;20(7):777–83.
101. Stewart MW, Rosenfeld PJ. Predicted biological activity of intravitreal VEGF-trap. Br J Ophthalmol. 2008;92:667–8.
102. Stratton IM, Cull CA, Adler AI, et al. Additive effects of glycaemia and blood pressure exposure on risk of complications in type 2 diabetes: a prospective observational study (UKPDS 75). Diabetologia. 2006;49:1761–9.
103. Studnicka J, Nemec P. Eye complications in diabetes. Postgrad Med. 2018;20(1):80–7.
104. Studnička J, Němčanský J, Vysloužilová D, et al. Diabetic retinopathy—diagnostics and treatment guidelines. Čes. a slov. Oftal. 2023;79(5):238–47.
105. Studnicka J, Stepanov A. Ocular complications of diabetes. In: Rozsival P, editor. Trends in contemporary ophthalmology, vol. 12, 1st ed. Prague: Galen; 2019. p. 129–53.
106. Supronik J, Szelachowska M, Kretowski A, et al. Rituximab in the treatment of Graves' orbitopathy: latest updates and perspectives. Endocr Connect. 2022;11(12): e220303.
107. Tadayoni R, Sararols L, Weissgerber G, et al. Brolucizumab: a newly developed anti-VEGF molecule for the treatment of neovascular age-related macular degeneration. Ophthalmologica. 2021;244(2):93–101.
108. Takahashi H, Shibuya M. The vascular endothelial growth factor (VEGF)/VEGF receptor system and its role under physiological and pathological conditions. Clin Sci (Lond). 2005;109:227–41.
109. Tanda ML, Bartalena L. Efficacy and safety of orbital radiotherapy for Graves' orbitopathy. J Clin Endocrinol Metab. 2012;97(11):3857–65.
110. Task Force Members. ESC National Cardiac Societies; ESC Committee for Practice Guidelines (CPG): 2019 ESC/EAS guidelines for the management of dyslipidaemias: lipid modification to reduce cardiovascular risk. Atherosclerosis. 2019;290:140–205.
111. Teo ZL, Tham YC, Yu M, et al. Global prevalence of diabetic retinopathy and projection of burden through 2045: systematic review and meta-analysis. Ophthalmology. 2021;128(11):1580–91.
112. UK Prospective Diabetes Study (UKPDS) Group. Effect of intensive blood-glucose control with metformin on complications in overweight patients with type 2 diabetes (UKPDS 34). Lancet. 1998;352:854–65.
113. Vanghelovici M. Structure of cholesterol. J Chem Technol Biotechnol. 1934;53:998–1006.
114. Vannas M, Teir H. Hemosiderosis in eyes with secondary glaucoma after delayed intraocular hemorrhages. Acta Ophthalmol (Copenh). 1960;38:254–67.
115. Visseren FLJ, Mach F, Smulders YM, et al. ESC Guidelines on cardiovascular disease prevention in clinical practice. Eur Heart J. 2022 Nov 7;43(42):4468.
116. Wagner LH, Bradley EA, Tooley AA, et al. Thyroid eye disease or Graves' orbitopathy: what name to use, and why it matters. Front Endocrinol (Lausanne). 2022;13:1083886.
117. Wiersinga W, Kahaly G. Graves' orbitopathy: a multidisciplinary approach—questions and answers. Karger; 2010.
118. Wiersinga WM, Bartalena L. Epidemiology and prevention of Graves' ophthalmopathy. Thyroid. 2002;12(10):855–60.
119. Wiley HE, Ferris FL III. Nonproliferative diabetic retinopathy and diabetic macular edema. In: Ryan SJ, editor-in-chief. Retina, vol. II, 5th ed. Saunders, an imprint of Elsevier Inc., 2013, p. 940–68.
120. Witmer AN, Vrensen GF, Van Noorden CJ, et al. Vascular endothelial growth factors and angiogenesis in eye disease. Prog Retin Eye Res. 2003;22:1–29.
121. Wong TY, Sun J, Kawasaki R, et al. Guidelines on diabetic eye care: the international council of ophthalmology recommendations for screening, follow-up, referral, and treatment based on resource settings. Ophthalmology. 2018;125(10):1608–22.
122. Wright AD, Dodson PM. Medical management of diabetic retinopathy: fenofibrate and ACCORD Eye studies. Eye. 2011;25(7):843–9.

123. Ye X, Bo X, Hu X, et al. Efficacy and safety of mycophenolate mofetil in patients with active moderate-to-severe Graves' orbitopathy. Clin Endocrinol (Oxf). 2017;86(2):247–55.
124. Zhang P, Zhu H. Cytokines in thyroid-associated ophthalmopathy. J Immunol Res. 2022;2022:2528046.
125. Zirm M. Protein glaucoma—overtaxing of flow mechanisms? Preliminary report. **Ophthalmologica**. 1982;184:155–61.

Rheumatic Diseases

Jan Nemcansky, Petr Bradna, and Veronika Kolarcikova

Rheumatology is a branch of internal medicine that includes a diverse group of diseases with a common feature of musculoskeletal disorders. In most rheumatic diseases, the underlying mechanism is inflammatory, although, as in the case of osteoarthritis, there may be local inflammatory mechanisms, and the usual overall markers of inflammation (increased erythrocyte sedimentation rate, CRP, and other acute phase proteins) are absent.

Here we pay particular attention to systemic connective tissue diseases, which are diseases of the whole organism, where the musculoskeletal system is one of the affected systems and the eye is often affected organ [26]. The eye examination is therefore an important part of the diagnosis of most systemic diseases and provides very valuable information for diagnosis, assessment of activity and effect of treatment.

J. Nemcansky (✉) · V. Kolarcikova
Department of Ophthalmology, University Hospital and Faculty of Medicine of Ostrava University, 17. Listopadu 1790/5, 708 00 Ostrava, Czech Republic
e-mail: jan.nemcansky@fno.cz

V. Kolarcikova
e-mail: veronika.kolarcikova@fno.cz

P. Bradna
Department of Rheumatology Diseases, University Hospital and Faculty of Medicine of Charles University in Hradec Králové, Sokolska 581, 500 05 Hradec Králové, Czech Republic
e-mail: petr.bradna@fnhk.cz

© The Author(s), under exclusive license to Springer Nature Switzerland AG 2024
A. Stepanov and J. Studnicka (eds.), *Ocular Manifestations of Systemic Diseases*,
https://doi.org/10.1007/978-3-031-58592-0_6

1 Rheumatoid Arthritis

Rheumatoid arthritis is a systemic disease affecting joints, extra-articular structures of the musculoskeletal system and many other organs and systems outside the locomotor system (cardiovascular system by accelerated atherogenesis, lungs by interstitial fibrosis, serous surfaces by pleurisy and pericarditis, bone by osteoporosis and others). The disease affects about 1% of the population of developed countries and leads to significant impairment of quality of life and, in some patients, to disability, especially cardiovascular consequences leading to shortened survival.

Pathogenesis

The pathogenesis of rheumatoid arthritis is driven by autoimmune mechanisms with the formation of typical autoantibodies [rheumatoid factors, antibodies to modified-citrullinated (ACPA) or carbamylated proteins and several other autoimmune features]. Current theory is based on an abnormal response to altered proteins, leading to autoimmune reactions, and triggering of mediators of inflammation (cytokines, interleukins and others) that lead to the manifestation of inflammation of joints and other affected structures and their irreversible damage.

Clinical presentation

The typical manifestation is polyarthritis, affecting mainly the small joints of the hands and feet, but in principle any joint in the body (Fig. 1).

The affected joints are painful, swollen, and stiff, especially in the morning, for a long time (30 min to several hours). The function of the affected joint is impaired, and all its components are damaged (synovitis with excessive joint fluid production, formation of an aggressive infiltrate (pannus) that destroys the articular cartilage (narrowing of the joint space) and subchondral bone (erosions). Morphological changes (X-ray, ultrasound, MRI) occur over months to years of disease progression. In an unfavourable case, the destructive process can lead to loss of its function or even ankylosis of the involved joint [6].

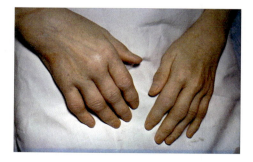

Fig. 1 Hands in rheumatoid arthritis. Swelling of the PIP, MCP and wrist joints

Diagnosis is based on evidence of joint swelling, increased signs of inflammation and the presence of typical autoantibodies [1]. The detection of the disease at its earliest stage, i.e. within months of the onset of joint swelling, is of paramount importance. Early treatment significantly reduces the risk of joint destruction and can prevent it in some patients.

Differential diagnosis

The differential diagnosis should distinguish other systemic connective tissue diseases, osteoarthritis, spondyloarthritis including reactive, paraneoplastic, or crystal-induced arthritis. A serious acute differential diagnostic possibility is septic arthritis. Among extra-articular manifestations, acceleration of atherogenesis with risk of cardiovascular events (myocardial infarction, stroke) should be mentioned. A long-term inflammatory reaction probably plays a role. A common extra-articular manifestation is secondary Sjögren's syndrome, an autoimmune disorder of the lacrimal and salivary glands leading to xerophthalmia and swallowing difficulties. On chest ultrasound, pleural and/or pericardial effusion, fortunately mostly subclinical, can be observed. The lungs may be affected by interstitial fibrosis, and AA amyloidosis may occur with prolonged activity. In seropositive patients (rheumatoid factors), what are called rheumatoid nodules occur, more often on the extensor side of the joints (Fig. 2).

Therapy

Successful therapy is based on catching the disease at its earliest stage, when the administration of disease-modifying drugs (DMARDs), such as methotrexate (caution, given in one dose per week) or leflunomide or sulfasalazine (if methotrexate is contraindicated), can prevent subsequent destructive changes. Symptomatic therapy includes analgesics and non-steroidal antirheumatic drugs. Corticosteroid therapy may be useful in the short term (overlapping time to effect of DMARDs); given the severe side effects, administration should be as short as possible, with

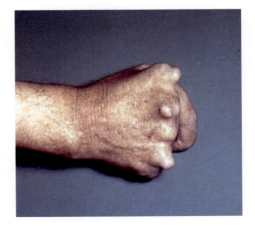

Fig. 2 Rheumatoid nodules in rheumatoid arthritis are usually located on the extensor side of the joint

gradual reduction and discontinuation optimally within 3 months. If treatment with conventional synthetic DMARDs does not result in disease remission, biological therapy (bDMARDs) blocking proinflammatory cytokines or other components of the inflammatory cascade is considered [34]. Currently, targeted synthetic therapy (tsDMARDs) can also be used, blocking the transmission of the inflammatory signal to the nucleus of the effector cell. The effect is equivalent to biologics, with the advantage of a rapid onset of effect and an oral form of administration.

The goal of treatment should be to achieve and maintain remission of the disease [9]. Of the non-pharmacological treatments, long-term physical therapy is essential, preferably under the supervision of a physiotherapist, balneotherapy is also effective. The use of suspensory splints, orthoses is important in the prevention of deformities. Physical methods also have an analgesic effect. A prerequisite for successful treatment is the active cooperation of an informed patient [24].

2 Ocular Manifestations of Rheumatoid Arthritis

In rheumatoid arthritis, the eyes are affected by dry eye syndrome (DES) in about 10–35% of patients (the most common ocular manifestation in RA) [26]. Reduced tear secretion and altered tear composition are caused by lymphocytic infiltration and subsequent tear gland fibrosis. Symptoms of DES usually do not correlate with the severity of arthritis, whereas other manifestations such as episcleritis and scleritis occur in very active and long-lasting cases. The cause of the necrotising form without inflammation (called scleromalacia perforans) tends to be severe cases of RA. Other ocular manifestations of RA include peripheral thinning of the cornea, acute stromal keratitis, and peripheral corneal ulceration (*peripheral ulceral keratitis, PUK*). Anterior uveitis is rare, more often in association with keratitis or scleritis. Vasculitis can occur secondary to scleritis in the form of peripheral retinal vasculitis; retinal vasculopathy is rare and is not occlusive.

Risk factors

- The presence of certain autoantibodies (rheumatoid factor, antibodies to citrullinated peptides)
- Higher number of affected joints
- Persistently high acute phase reactants (CRP, sedimentation)
- The presence of certain genetic factors (called the "shared epitope")

Clinical presentation

DES is characterised by fluctuations in symptoms during the day, week, or season, as well as depending on the environment (windy weather, air conditioning, visually demanding activities). The most common symptoms are dryness, cutting, burning, foreign body sensation, photophobia, fluctuations in vision, pain, feeling of pressure behind the eye, increased reflex tearing. In episcleritis and scleritis, what is called

Fig. 3 Scleromalacia perforans—scleral tissue spacing without accompanying inflammation, through which the dark choroid shines

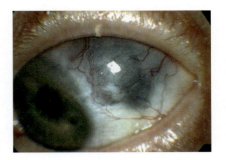

the "red eye" is observed; patients experience increased sensitivity to pain in the eye, which is particularly persistent in scleritis and may even wake them from sleep. In contrast, pain is absent in the necrotising form without inflammation, and the patient can often be alerted to the symptoms of the disease by his surroundings. Corneal affections and anterior uveitis are accompanied by red eye, pain and photophobia.

Objective findings

In SSO, we observe hyperaemia to conjunctival injection, decrease to absence of the tear meniscus, folds of the bulbar conjunctiva (LIPCOF classification), conjunctival and corneal epitheliopathy, cellular detritus on the ocular surface and corneal filaments (in advanced conditions). The findings in episcleritis and scleritis are described in Sect. 12. In the necrotising form of scleritis without inflammation, which is caused by arteriolar obliteration, yellowish or greyish scleral nodules are visible at the beginning, in which necrosis is manifested by spacing of scleral tissue without accompanying inflammation. The dark choroid shines through these openings and uveal prolapse may emerge if there is an increase in intraocular pressure (Fig. 3).

Spontaneous perforation is rare, but the bulbus is at risk of traumatic perforation. The findings in PUK are described in Sect. 11. In stromal keratitis, stromal infiltration occurs without epithelial disruption and is accompanied by the presence of newly formed vessels. In the resting stage, stromal scarring with eventual thinning of the cornea and emptied vessels are found. Complications of PUK, episcleritis and scleritis are described in Sect. 12.

Diagnosis

The examination of the anterior segment and the fundus is based on a slit-lamp biomicroscopy. In the diagnosis of SSO, basic examinations include staining of the ocular surface with fluorescein or lissamine green, measurement of TBUT (tear break-up time), Schirmer's test I and II and measurement of tear film osmolarity. In recent years, modern imaging devices have been used increasingly, which allow not only tear film analysis, but also photo- and video-documentation and monitoring of parameters over time and with the use of neural networks. Using specialised illumination (transillumination, infrared light) and observation techniques, it is possible to observe the morphology of meibomian glands in vivo, an examination called meibography. Contact meibography using a special light probe (which is applied to the eyelid from the skin side and illuminates it) has recently been increasingly replaced by techniques using an infrared light source (not touching the eyelid) and an infrared video camera—non-contact meibography. Other possible techniques are laser confocal meibography and OCT meibography.

Differential diagnosis

- Anterior uveitis or PUK of other aetiology
- Episcleritis and scleritis of other aetiologies
- Idiopathic vasculitis

Therapy

Treatment of DES is symptomatic. The mainstay of treatment is tear supplementation with drops, preferably without preservatives; tear outflow can be reduced by temporary or permanent tear duct closures (collagen or silicone plugs, tear point coagulation); in severe forms with filaments, a contact lens can be applied to mechanically protect the surface of the eye. Biological tear substitutes (autologous serum from whole blood or platelet concentrate) and topical anti-inflammatory drugs (corticosteroids, cyclosporine A) are available. In the treatment of anterior segment affections, corticosteroids, NSAIDs, are applied topically according to the type and severity of inflammation, and antibiotics in keratitis. In the treatment of episcleritis and scleritis, local steroid treatment is sufficient in non-necrotising forms or NSAIDs in general. Combined immunosuppressive therapy should be used for necrotising forms, biological therapy for refractory forms (rituximab), see Sect. 11 for more details.

Cave: application of corticosteroids periocularly can lead to the development of necrosis. General treatment is in collaboration with a rheumatologist.

3   Juvenile Idiopathic Arthritis

Juvenile idiopathic arthritis (JIA) is the most common systemic inflammatory disease of childhood [44]. It can begin at any age in childhood, usually after 6 months of life. There is a preponderance of affected girls.

The aetiology of the disease is unknown. Genetic associations, especially in the HLA region, and genes affecting pro-inflammatory cytokine production can be traced in different forms of the disease; a common genetic basis is lacking.

Clinical presentation

The clinical presentation is varied, and according to the Edmonton classification, the following forms can be distinguished:

- Systemic arthritis (Still's disease)
- Oligoarthritis form
- Polyarthritis RF seropositive and seronegative

Rheumatic Diseases

- Arthritis with enthesitis
- Psoriatic arthritis
- Undifferentiated form

The systemic form of the disease has recently been classified as a kind of autoinflammatory disease.

Fever with transient cutaneous exanthem, hepato- and splenomegaly, non-specific lymphadenopathy is common. Arthritis is common and may be delayed after the onset of systemic manifestations. The disease may have one or more attacks of systemic symptoms that may persist into adulthood. In addition to peripheral and axial arthritis, some sufferers have short stature (premature closure of the growth fissures), a receding mandible (micrognathia) when the temporomandibular joint is affected and shortening of the phalanges of the fingers.

In some severe cases, macrophage activation syndrome with febrile lung damage, liver lesions, coagulation disorders and cytopenia may occur. This is a life-threatening complication, often requiring intensive care with life support.

Arthritic forms of JIA most often affect the knee joints with swelling, impaired function, and pain; prognostic implications may include inflammation of the hip joint. In the hands, proximal as well as distal interphalangeal joints are affected. Together with growth disorders, they lead to the picture of brachydactyly (pawed hand). Affection of the peripheral joints leads to deformities and the development of severe functional disorders up to ankylosis. At the patella, JIA is characterised by cervical involvement, and inflammatory involvement of the C1–2 region may lead to instability with manifestations of cervical myelopathy with life-threatening consequences (attention during preoperative preparation—intubation).

Inflammatory involvement of the eye can accompany all forms of JIA, but most often the enthesitic form with more frequent HLA B27 positivity.

Diagnosis

Diagnosis is based on clinical findings, supplemented by laboratory evidence of inflammatory activity; the disease is usually seronegative, and the positivity of antinuclear antibodies (ANA), rheumatoid factors (RF) and antibodies to citrullinated proteins (ACPA) help to clarify the type of disease. In the systemic form, serum ferritin levels tend to be markedly elevated, especially in the setting of the macrophage activation syndrome.

In some patients, the activity of joint and systemic manifestations decreases with adolescence, but others develop a picture consistent with rheumatoid arthritis or spondyloarthritis.

Therapy

Therapy includes non-steroidal antirheumatic drugs; the use of glucocorticoids, if necessary, should be as short-term as possible due to the adverse effects on the developing organism. In active arthritis, local application to the inflamed joint is preferable. The primary disease-modifying drug is methotrexate, also in JIA, but the dosage is calculated per body surface area.

Biological therapy represents a significant advance in the treatment of JIA and is used especially in severe, refractory forms of the disease. Tumour necrosis factor blockers are mainly used, alternatively biologics with other mechanisms of action. In the systemic form, the IL-1 receptor blocker anakinra or interleukin 6 blockers are used. In addition to its disease-modifying effect on joint disability, biological therapy can antagonise growth impairment and the development of typical deformities [30]. It has been successfully used also in JIA with ocular complications.

4 Ocular Manifestations of Juvenile Idiopathic Arthritis

A common and serious extra-articular manifestation of juvenile idiopathic arthritis is uveitis, the incidence of which varies from one form of JIA to another; in the oligoarticular form in 20%, in the polyarticular form in 5%, and in the systemic form the ocular involvement is rare [21]. The onset of uveitis is usually 5–7 years after the onset of joint disease, the course is biphasic, with a second phase of activity at the onset of puberty [20]. Chronic uveitis occurs primarily in the oligoarticular form with ANA positivity, requires regular follow-up and aggressive therapy, and may occur before the onset of arthritis. It has a relapsing and remitting course in 60% of patients and is bilateral in more than one-half of children [18]. There is no correlation between the degree of eye and joint inflammation, and ocular manifestations may persist even after remission of arthritis. Uveitis in psoriatic arthritis occurs in children with early onset disease and ANA positivity. Acute symptomatic uveitis occurs mainly in children with HLA B27 positivity, usually does not lead to major complications and often relapses. It also occurs in patients with arthritis with enthesopathy and in patients with psoriatic arthritis. In contrast, episcleritis and DES are rare in children.

Risk factors

- Female sex (but boys have a worse prognosis)
- Oligoarticular form
- Presence of circulating antinuclear antibodies (ANA), presence of HLA B27 antigen
- Low age of first manifestation of the disease
- Advanced changes in the anterior segment of the eye at the first follow-up are a risk factor for the development of further complications, regardless of treatment
- Earlier onset of uveitis than arthritis

Clinical presentation

Ocular symptoms are variable, and chronic uveitis can be asymptomatic for a long time. Decreased vision is more often the result of complications. In acute uveitis, patients suffer from photophobia, eye pain and redness of the eye.

Objective findings

Chronic uveitis often occurs in the pale eye, is of the non-granulomatous type, usually bilateral (up to 70%) with an asymmetric course [4]. Small to medium precipitates are present on the endothelium, with cells and flare in the anterior chamber. The latter may not even be markedly evident and yet induces the formation of synechiae. In a long-term course with the development of complications, we observe zonular keratopathy on the cornea, posterior synechiae on the iris, development of cataracts on the lens, cystoid macular oedema (CME) on the fundus, and more rarely, optic disc oedema. In less frequent acute anterior uveitis, we see a picture of serous uveitis with the presence of cells or fibrin in the anterior chamber, rarely a hypopyon may form in HLA B27 positive patients [14].

Due to the often-asymptomatic course of ocular inflammation, regular ophthalmologic dispensation is necessary in paediatric patients with JIA. The frequency of follow-up depends on risk factors (age of first manifestation of JIA, presence of ANA antibodies, type of JIA). Screening is not necessary in the systemic form, but in the polyarticular and oligoarticular forms, depending on ANA positivity and disease duration, we plan to check every 2–6 months, and once a year after the age of 12 years. Patients who have completed long-term systemic therapy are followed every 2 months for the first 6 months, after which there is a return to standard screening.

Complications

In chronic uveitis, iris-lens adhesions are a common complication (called posterior synechiae, Fig. 4).

Cataracts are caused either by the action of inflammatory mediators directly on the lens by changing the composition of the aqueous humour or because of long-term corticosteroid treatment. Secondary glaucoma is a serious complication, occurring in up to 40% of patients with ocular manifestations of JIA; in addition to uveitis, long-term steroid therapy contributes to pressure elevation [18]. It is often refractory to local therapy and therefore early surgical management is often necessary. Zonular keratopathy is caused by the deposition of calcium salts in Bowman's layer, starting from the periphery and gradually forming a band extending through the centre

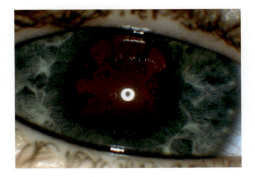

Fig. 4 Posterior iris synechiae in a patient with chronic uveitis in JIA

of the cornea that can significantly affect vision. CME is a potentially irreversible complication in chronic uveitis, with subsequent permanent visual impairment.

Diagnosis

Diagnosis relies primarily on a very careful slit-lamp examination of the anterior segment, focusing on the presence of cells and flare in the anterior chamber. We also regularly examine the fundus. FAG and OCT contribute to the early diagnosis of CME and to monitoring its changes in response to treatment.

Differential diagnosis

- Sarcoidosis
- Lyme disease
- Reactive arthritis, uveitis associated with idiopathic intestinal inflammation
- Herpetic anterior uveitis
- Idiopathic chronic anterior uveitis
- Neonatal multisystem inflammatory disease

Therapy

The first step in the treatment of uveitis is administration of topical cycloplegics (4% homatropine) and corticosteroids (dexamethasone) in the form of drops, in dosage according to the inflammatory reaction, sometimes in the beginning up to every hour, ointment at night. Topical and systemic antiphlogistics have only a supportive effect. If the inflammatory activity persists despite intensive topical therapy or a long-term resolution of signs of inflammation (especially flare) cannot be achieved repeatedly after reduction of topical corticosteroid therapy, we proceed to total immunosuppressive therapy. We approach total corticosteroid therapy for ocular indications in uveitis complications such as CME or papillary oedema because of their rapid onset of effects; in some cases, pulsed therapy may be preferred. Corticosteroids in general can be used in the short term, even in severe uveitis as a bridging therapy until the onset of action of methotrexate. If immunosuppressive therapy fails, treatment with anti-TNFα antibodies (especially adalimumab or infliximab) is effective from an ophthalmic point of view. Overall therapy is carried out in collaboration with paediatric rheumatologists. ANA-positive patients with chronic anterior uveitis without inflammatory joint activity should be treated as patients with JIA-associated uveitis. Early treatment of CME is necessary to prevent progression to irreversible changes in the macula and is an indication to initiate treatment or to augment existing therapy. Treatment of zonular keratopathy involves dissolution of salts by chelation with EDTA or photoablation with an excimer laser. An interval of at least three months without signs of inflammation is recommended before possible cataract surgery, and it is not uncommon to perform anterior and posterior capsulotomy during surgery. Primary IOL implantation in children with JIA is controversial and often debated, depending on age, laterality, and severity of inflammation. In antiglaucoma therapy,

Rheumatic Diseases

beta-blockers are the drug of choice, or in combination with carbonic anhydrase inhibitors. Opinions differ on the use of prostaglandin analogues because of their possible reversible side effects such as uveitis and CME, yet they tend to be administered mainly because of their good effect on pressure reduction. In the case of failure of local therapy, early surgical treatment (peripheral iridectomy, trabeculectomy) is indicated, or the use of drainage implants. Total therapy is performed in accordance with rheumatologists and other specialists involved in long-term treatment.

5 Spondyloarthritis

Spondyloarthritis refers to a group of rheumatic diseases with several common features in pathogenesis and clinic. Similar symptoms are as follows:

- Binding with the HLA B27 antigen
- Involvement of the axial and peripheral skeleton
- Occurrence of extra-articular musculoskeletal disorders (enthesitis, dactylitis)

Classification

- Ankylosing spondylitis
- Non-radiographic axial spondyloarthritis
- Arthritis in intestinal inflammation
- Reactive arthritis
- Psoriatic arthritis

Furthermore, the group of spondyloarthritis includes undifferentiated spondyloarthritis and other subtypes, which will not be discussed here. While the first four entities are classified as axial spondyloarthritis with predominant involvement of the spine and SI joints, psoriatic arthritis has predominantly peripheral involvement.

5.1 Ankylosing Spondylitis

Ankylosing spondylitis is historically called Bechterev's disease after the Russian military doctor V.M. Bechterev, who described it as a peculiar disease.

Aetiology

As in most rheumatic diseases, is complex, with the involvement of genetic predispositions and environmental influences. Ankylosing spondylitis is a disease with one of the closest links to the HLA antigen. HLA B-27 is present in 92–97% of patients. However, a small proportion of patients who test negative for HLA-B27 do not differ clinically or in prognosis from positive patients. In contrast to rheumatoid arthritis, where the predominance of inflammatory and destructive changes occurs in the synovial joint environment, the primary affected structure in ankylosing spondylitis

Fig. 5 Sacroiliitis in ankylosing spondylitis. The joint space is uneven, of varying width, with bone bridges in some places. The subchondral bone is sclerotic

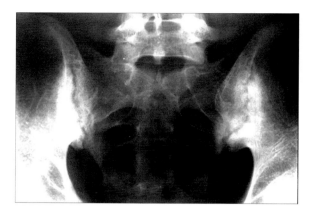

is the tendon attachment (enthesis). Histological findings have shown continuous development of enthesitis to ectopic calcification, enthesophyte or spinal syndesmophyte. The spine and SI joint are the predilection locus of change and the process generally progresses from the SI joint in an ascending fashion (Fig. 5).

Even ankylosing spondylitis is a systemic disease and can affect the respiratory system (interstitial lung changes), or the cardiovascular system (accelerated atherogenesis, AV block, aortic root dilatation with aortic insufficiency). The kidneys can be affected by amyloidosis as the result of chronic inflammation.

Clinical presentation

Clinically, ankylosing spondylitis is manifested by inflammatory pain in the lower back, with marked stiffness. The difficulty radiates to the buttocks and worsens at rest, so that it interferes with sleep over the morning, when it forces the patient to walk to stir up the stiffness. Movement relieves the difficulty, unlike the mechanical cause of back pain, which is aggravated by movement. Gradually, stiffening of the spinal compartments occurs with ascending progression. Initially, enthesitic changes progress to osteoplastic changes (syndesmophytes), leading to complete spinal stiffness with a radiographic picture of a "bamboo rod". Increasing thoracic kyphosis leads to the typical forward-bending posture, where the patient is unable to look in front of him or to the side due to the involvement of the cervical spine. When the root joints of the limbs (hips, shoulders) are affected, the patient may become completely immobilised, requiring large joint replacements or vertebrosurgical adjustment of the head position. Arthritis mainly affects the joints of the lower limbs. Typical manifestations are tendon pains in various localisations, most often in the Achilles tendon attachment to the heels—their recurrence should lead to suspicion of the possibility of spondyloarthritis. Other frequently affected tendons include the plantar aponeurosis tendon attachment to the heel, the tendon attachments to the patella, the pelvis, and the sternocleidomastoid junction. Sonography demonstrates inflammatory activity; X-ray later presents osteoplastic changes—enthesophytes.

Diagnosis

The diagnosis is based on spinal mobility disorder, radiographic findings of sacroiliitis and enthesophytes or syndesmophytes with HLA B27 positivity (New York criteria). The disadvantage is that the diagnosis can be made only in the case of advanced morphological changes, usually after years of subjective complaints. Therefore, to initiate early treatment, the signs of non-X-ray axial Spondyloarthritis have recently been looked for, when the X-ray is still normal but there are already changes on MRI of the SI joint [31] A proportion of patients with non-radiographic axial Spondyloarthritis will eventually develop a typical AS picture.

Differential diagnosis is especially guided against very common mechanical back pain, where a good history can usually distinguish between these two pathogenetically different situations.

The final diagnosis is then made by a rheumatologist. Repeated attacks of uveitis, especially in HLA B27-positive patients, may also be a reason for referral to rheumatologist.

Therapy

In ankylosing spondylitis, despite all pharmacological methods, regular targeted exercise, ideally under the supervision of a physiotherapist, is an essential treatment measure. It has a significant effect on the limitation of spinal mobility. Patients with ankylosing spondylitis should exercise daily, and group activities within a patient self-help organisation, which organises reconditioning and rehabilitation activities, are beneficial.

Drug therapy starts with the administration of non-steroidal antirheumatic drugs (NSAIDs), which are usually very effective and, in some cases, sufficient in the long term. The effect of NSAIDs on slowing down osteoplastic changes is discussed. Corticosteroids are suitable locally, especially for enthesitis, but per os administration, especially long-term, is not indicated. Synthetic disease-modifying drugs are ineffective on axial skeletal involvement. Sulfasalazine may be effective for peripheral arthritis. Enthesitis and dactylitis [swelling of the entire finger in a combination of tendon, joint and soft tissue inflammation—"sausage finger" (Fig. 6)] are usually unaffected by this treatment.

Biological treatment represents the next step after the failure of the current procedure. Tumour necrosis factor alpha blockers are used. Monoclonal antibodies are more effective in preventing uveitis recurrences than soluble receptor. Biologic drugs acting on a different substrate that are used in RA have proven ineffective in axial Spondyloarthritis. Only interleukin 17A-blocking agents have shown good efficacy on both axial and peripheral manifestations of AS, including peripheral enthesitis and dactylitis. A retarding effect on morphological changes with the biologic drugs used so far has been demonstrated only after four years of therapy. The efficacy of Janus kinase inhibitors is currently being investigated, with promising results [28].

Fig. 6 Dactylitis in psoriatic arthritis. Dactylitis is a swelling of the entire finger involving arthritis, tenosynovitis and inflammatory swelling of the subcutaneous tissue. See the first digits bilaterally and second digit of the right lower limb

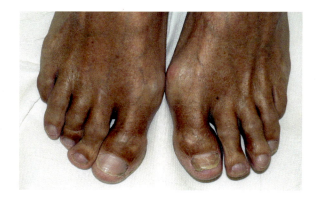

5.2 Non-radiographic Axial Spondyloarthritis

Inflammatory lower back pain usually precedes the X-ray changes typical of ankylosing spondylitis by years. Moreover, some patients do not fulfil the criteria for AS diagnosis even in the long term. A breakthrough in this respect was the introduction of MRI examination of the SI joint, which showed the presence of inflammatory changes (bone marrow oedema) in many such patients. Yet, in terms of difficulties, impairment of quality of life and, as it turned out, even the effect of treatment, these patients did not differ from patients with X-ray sacroiliitis.

For this reason, a new unit was introduced—non-radiographic axial Spondyloarthritis—and a set of classification criteria was created, which allowed the start of treatment to be significantly delayed to the onset of clinical difficulties. In a proportion of patients, non-radiographic Spondyloarthritis can be an early stage in the development of ankylosing spondylitis (within two years, 12% of patients developed typical X-ray findings for AS), but a significant proportion of patients remain in the non-radiographic phase.

5.3 Spondyloarthritis in Intestinal Inflammation

The association between impaired intestinal permeability and spondyloarthritis is evident in most spondyloarthritis diseases. Histological and endoscopic studies demonstrate intestinal disorders in up to one-half of ankylosing spondylitis patients. Musculoskeletal involvement in non-specific intestinal inflammation, i.e. Crohn's disease, ulcerative or undifferentiated colitis, is referred to as enteropathic arthritis.

Clinical presentation

It manifests either as peripheral oligoarthritis, often with hand joint involvement, or as symptoms of axial spondyloarthritis, including SI joint involvement. HLA B27 is more common in the axial form, but the association is not nearly as tight as in

Rheumatic Diseases

ankylosing spondylitis. Like other spondyloarthritis, enteropathic arthritis may be accompanied by ocular inflammation, most commonly anterior uveitis, sometimes recurrent or episcleritis.

Somewhat outside the group of enteropathic arthritis are two disease entities combining gastroenterological and musculoskeletal disorders.

Arthritis in coeliac disease affects more often the large joints, but it can also be axial. As a rule, it is non-erosive. Signs of coeliac disease should be looked for, failure to thrive, tendency to diarrhoea, anaemia may not be pronounced. Laboratory diagnosis of the presence of antibodies to transglutaminase and gliadin and histological evidence at endoscopy will assist.

The introduction of a gluten-free diet is usually sufficient in therapy.

Whipple's disease is a rare disease caused by an intestinal infection with the microorganism Trophorhyma whipplei. Diarrhoea is the main manifestation; arthritis occurs in up to 80% of patients and may precede gastroenterological symptoms. The evidence is histological from endoscopy. Treatment is antibiotic.

5.4 Ocular Manifestations of Ankylosing Spondylitis

The typical ocular manifestation of ankylosing spondylitis is acute anterior serofibrinous uveitis. It affects 25–30% of patients [14], and 90% are positive for the HLA B27 antigen [35]. It is usually clinically uncorrelated with inflammatory joint activity. It presents as a unilateral inflammation that alternately affects both eyes. Acute exacerbations of anterior uveitis may be relatively rarely replaced by chronic, usually bilateral uveitis with complications such as vitritis, papillary oedema, anterior optic nerve ischaemia, CME, and epiretinal membrane. Other ocular manifestations include scleritis, episcleritis, keratitis and mechanical ptosis.

Risk factors

- HLA B27 antigen positivity
- Male gender

Clinical presentation

Patients complain of pain (worsening on accommodation), pupillary constriction with inflammation affected iris, impaired vision, photophobia, and redness of the eye.

Objective symptoms

In uveitis, mixed injection is seen on the bulb, tyndallisation is evident in the anterior chamber, not infrequently severe fibrinous reaction (Fig. 7), hypopyon formation is frequent, the iris is congested, and there is a marked tendency to form posterior synechiae.

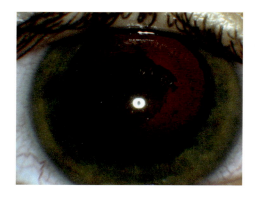

Fig. 7 Acute anterior uveitis in an HLA B27 positive patient—pupil in artificial mydriasis, residual posterior synechiae in the lower part, fibrin mesh resorbing in the pupil

Diagnosis

Diagnosis is based on slit-lamp examination of the eye. OCT examination reveals the presence of CME and is used to monitor the effect of treatment, OCT is also used to diagnose and monitor optic nerve changes in possible glaucoma. The perimeter is used to assess the extent of visual field damage in glaucoma.

Differential diagnosis

- Other HLA B27 positive uveitis
- BN, endogenous endophthalmitis, masking syndromes
- Syphilis, borreliosis

Complications

Complications of inflammation can be persistent anterior and posterior synechiae, development of cataract and secondary glaucoma, CME, and rarely optic disc oedema.

Therapy

The treatment of uveitis requires the use of topical corticosteroids with a strong anti-inflammatory effect (dexamethasone) and cycloplegics (4% homatropine), according to the severity of the inflammation. Steroids initially every 30 min to every 1 h, ointment at night, with gradual reduction, according to the decline of inflammation. Repeated administration of mydriatics in the Outpatient Clinic, along with application of local heat (e.g. applying a surgical glove filled with warm water) may be used to agitate the synechiae. In severe forms, corticosteroids can be administered subconjunctivally. When intraocular pressure elevates, beta-blockers and carbonic anhydrase inhibitors are applied. Overall, NSAIDs can be given when there is significant inflammatory activity; oral corticosteroids are usually not necessary and can be given in lower doses in CME. The use of anti-TNF drugs in systemic rheumatological indications also significantly reduces the incidence of uveitis recurrences.

Rheumatic Diseases

5.5 Reactive Arthritis

It is synovitis induced by an immunological reaction to a previous infection, most often of the urogenital tract (*Chlamydia*) or intestine (*Salmonella, Shigella, Campylobacter*).

After a latency period of several weeks, joint inflammation occurs, most often oligoarthritis of the joints of the lower limbs, sometimes of the joints of the upper limbs. The association with the presence of HLA B27 is relatively close (above 50%).

Clinical presentation

Inflammatory changes of tendons and joints with swelling of the fingers, i.e. dactylitis, enthesitis and skin lesions resembling psoriasis are quite common.

Diagnosis

Nucleic acid grafts of the causative organism can be detected in synovial fluid by sensitive methods, but this is never a complete microorganism.

Therapy

In most reactive arthritis, antimicrobial therapy is unsuccessful, but in chlamydial reactive arthritis, the data are not clear.

The prognosis of the disease is usually good, even with symptomatic treatment, but the disease can relapse, and, in some patients, it can progress to chronic arthritis similar to rheumatoid arthritis even with similar therapy.

5.6 Ocular Manifestations of Reactive Arthritis

The best-known ocular manifestation of reactive arthritis is the triad (called Reiter's syndrome): conjunctivitis, urethritis, and arthritis. Urethritis is usually the first to appear, followed by bilateral mucopurulent conjunctivitis after about 2 weeks, and arthritis is the last to appear. However, up to 20% of patients may also have acute iridocyclitis [4, 21] and, more rarely, bilateral chronic uveitis, keratitis, episcleritis, scleritis, intermediate uveitis are observed, and, very rarely, optic neuritis or occlusive retinal vasculitis.

Risk factors

HLA B27 antigen positivity.

Clinical presentation

Patients complain of photophobia, decreased vision, pain, and redness of the eye.

Objective findings

The most common finding is papillary conjunctivitis, which is bilateral, with mucopurulent secretion, usually resolving spontaneously after a week. Keratitis is characterised by subepithelial infiltrates and small epithelial lesions, occurring in isolation or with conjunctivitis. Anterior uveitis is acute, with mixed injection, with small precipitates on the endothelium, cells in the anterior chamber, serofibrinous inflammation is uncommon, hypopyon forms rarely, but posterior synechiae may occur.

Complications

Possible complications are CME, cataract and optic disc oedema.

Diagnosis

Diagnosis is based on slit-lamp examination of the eye. OCT examination reveals the presence of CME.

Differential diagnosis

- HLA B27 positive acute anterior uveitis without systemic disease
- BN, endogenous endophthalmitis, masking syndromes
- Syphilis

Therapy

Ocular manifestations respond well to local treatment with corticosteroids, which can be supplemented with NSAIDs and mydriatic agents, depending on the severity of inflammation. NSAIDs can also be administered generally, while treatment with oral corticosteroids is usually not necessary for ocular indications. Treatment of the general disease is guided by a specialist in the field.

5.7 Psoriatic Arthritis

In epidemiological studies, psoriasis is accompanied by musculoskeletal symptoms in up to one-third of cases. Other systemic manifestations, including accelerated atherogenesis, are also very common, so that the disease is referred to as psoriatic disease.

Clinical presentation

Arthritis most often affects peripheral joints (DIP joints of the hands, knees), so psoriatic arthritis is classified as peripheral spondyloarthritis. However, involvement of the axial skeleton with sacroiliitis, parasyndesmophytes of the spine and increased HLA B27 is also quite common. Movement disability usually begins years after the onset of cutaneous psoriasis, but, in a minority of cases, psoriatic arthritis may precede psoriasis. According to the CASPAR criteria, the presence of cutaneous psoriasis

Rheumatic Diseases

in close blood relatives is also a classification criterion for psoriatic arthritis [37]. Onychopathy is a frequent manifestation, especially when distal joints are affected. It includes changes, ranging from onychomycosis-like nail plate delamination to relatively subtle manifestations such as grooves or dimples in the nail plate.

Diagnosis

The typical radiographic manifestation is a combination of destructive and osteo-plastic changes in the peripheral and axial skeleton (enthesophytes, parasyndesmo-phytes). In the borderline case, it can lead to complete destruction of the hand skeleton, called mutating arthritis. Enthesitis and dactylitis (sausage finger) are common.

Therapy

In psoriatic arthritis, methotrexate (as in rheumatoid arthritis) is successfully used as a first-line disease-modifying treatment. For severe enthesitis and dactylitis, the EULAR recommendations allow biological treatment immediately after failure of non-steroidal antirheumatic drugs. TNF alpha, interleukin 17 or 12/23 blockers or a phosphodiesterase 4 inhibitor (apremilast) are effective. IL-6 blockers and other drugs with alternative mechanisms of action have not been successful in spondyloarthritis. Janus kinase inhibitors are currently in clinical trials and may be considered as an alternative according to EULAR [10, 22]. Biological therapy is indicated by a rheumatologist or dermatologist according to the prevailing clinical presentation.

5.8 Ocular Manifestations of Psoriatic Arthritis

In psoriatic arthritis, uveitis is the ocular manifestation in about 5% of patients [4], usually as mild, unilateral, recurrent acute anterior uveitis, more rarely as bilateral chronic anterior uveitis.

Risk factors

- Axial skeletal disability
- HLA B27 antigen positivity

Clinical presentation

Patients complain of photophobia, decreased vision, pain and redness of the eye.

Objective findings

Anterior uveitis is acute, with mixed injection, with small precipitates on the endothe-lium, with the presence of cells in the anterior chamber of varying intensity, posterior synechiae may arise.

Diagnosis

Diagnosis is based on slit-lamp examination of the eye, including the fundus. OCT examination is used to diagnose and evaluate changes in CME.

Differential diagnosis

- HLA B27 positive acute anterior uveitis without systemic disease
- JIA and uveitis

Complications

Possible complications are CME, cataract and optic disc oedema.

Therapy

In the treatment of uveitis, topical corticosteroids and cycloplegics are used, according to the intensity of inflammation, NSAIDs locally and overall. Administration of total corticosteroids usually does not affect the activity and recurrence of uveitis. Total treatment is guided by a specialist in the field.

6 Systemic Lupus Erythematosus

Systemic lupus erythematosus is a chronic autoimmune disease, affecting practically any organ or system of the body.

The disease is characterised by the production of several autoantibodies, especially against cell nucleus antigens. Vitally, the most serious are involvement of kidney, central nervous system, and haematological disorders.

The aetiology of the disease is still not fully understood. Genetic predisposition plays an important role; several predispositions have been demonstrated, especially in genes affecting immune reactions. It is likely that the disposition is due to a complex influence of several factors.

The role of apoptosis disorders, the interplay of T and B lymphocytes and the cytokine network is considered in the pathogenesis; it is certain that B-lymphocytes are activated, producing organ-non-specific autoantibodies, which are then deposited in the form of immune complexes in the blood vessels of various organs and impair their function.

Clinical presentation

The clinical presentation of systemic lupus erythematosus (SLE) is typically very varied and practically individually expressed in each patient, which complicates the diagnosis and monitoring of the therapeutic effect [41].

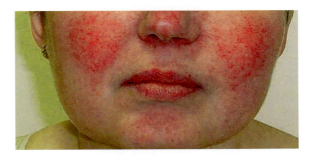

Fig. 8 Butterfly-like exanthem in systemic lupus erythematosus

Skin impairment

It occurs in up to 80% of patients. Classic butterfly exanthema affecting the central parts of the cheeks and the back of the nose can be encountered (Fig. 8); dermatitis can affect the skin of the entire head and trunk. On the skin of the trunk, we may see the discoid exanthema with a red border and a faded centre.

Paralysis of subcutaneous blood vessels can lead to the image of livedo reticularis, a reticular pattern especially on the lower limbs. Involvement of subcutaneous structures may lead to panniculitis with possible necrosis. Increased photosensitivity of the skin can often be demonstrated, which can lead also to systemic exacerbation after UV exposure.

Joint and muscular impairment

The typical disability in SLE is non-erosive arthritis. On the hands, it can lead to a picture of what is called Jaccaud's arthropathy with Z-deformity of the thumbs and flexion deformities of the fingers. In bone involvement, a picture is seen of aseptic osteonecrosis in the femoral neck, knee joints or humeral head. Osteoporosis is common (also due to treatment). Muscle lesions are usually manifested by myalgias, weakness or feelings of muscle tension.

Renal impairment

Before the introduction of effective therapy, SLE used to be the most common fatal manifestation. Proteinuria, microscopic haematuria, sometimes leukocyturia are found in the urine. Nitrogen catabolites rise as a manifestation of advanced renal damage, earlier glomerular filtration rate decreases. The type of glomerulonephritis is specified by renal biopsy, the finding is decisive for the choice of treatment. Current therapy has significantly improved the prognosis of renal involvement. SLE patients with terminal renal failure are indicated for transplantation. Arterial hypertension is a frequent finding, often in association with nephropathy.

Impairment of the cardiovascular system

A relatively common finding is exudative pericarditis, but rarely clinically manifest. More severe is valvular involvement (Libmann-Sacks endocarditis), which may be an indication for surgical management. As a result of involvement of small intracardiac vessels, dispersive myocardial fibrosis occurs, which may manifest as signs of heart failure or arrhythmias.

SLE significantly accelerates atherogenesis, and coronary events can occur even at a very young age. Cardiac involvement has become the leading cause of late mortality in patients after the prognosis of the acute phase of the disease has improved, especially renal involvement.

Of the vascular disorders, a procoagulant state in the presence of antiphospholipid antibodies is dangerous. Arterial or venous thromboses in almost any localisation and thromboembolic events can occur. Raynaud's syndrome or livedo reticularis may occur.

Impairment of the nervous system

Changes in nervous structures occur in the course of the disease in most patients. The spectrum of manifestations ranges from thrombotic strokes, dispersive white matter involvement with cognitive deficits, and asymmetric polyneuropathy with peripheral nerve involvement (mononeuritis multiplex). Epileptic seizures may be a relatively frequent and sometimes initial manifestation, less frequent is a manifestation of psychosis. The frequency of less noticeable cognitive changes, mood changes, etc. depends on the definition used and the examination method. In the vast majority, these are not consequences of vasculitis, but disruption of the blood–brain barrier is common. Persistent headache is among the classification criteria of SLE.

Impairment of the lungs

Inflammatory changes on serous surfaces are common in SLE. The most common is the demonstration of pleural effusion; pleuritic disorders are less common. Lupus pneumonitis can be encountered in lung parenchyma. A serious complication with a high mortality is the syndrome of diffuse alveolar haemorrhage due to vasculitis of the alveolar vessels. It manifests with rapidly developing respiratory distress (haemoptysis is present only in a minority of cases), extensive opacification of both lung fields on CT and anaemia. It is an emergency condition requiring immediate hospitalisation in an ICU. In some cases, it requires temporary ventilatory support. The mortality rate depends on the speed of initiation of treatment and varies between 20 and 90% in different reports for severe cases in the ICU. Chronically, pulmonary interstitial fibrosis with development of respiratory insufficiency or pulmonary arterial hypertension with vital risk may occur.

Haematological manifestations

Cytopenia can be a manifestation of disease activity. Thrombocytopenia occurs as part of the antiphospholipid syndrome. In addition to anaemia of chronic diseases, haemolysis with Coombs test positivity and sideropenia from minor losses to the GIT are the main contributors to anaemia.

Antiphospholipid syndrome is characterised by the presence of antibodies against phospholipids, beta2glycoprotein 1 and/or the presence of a lupus anticoagulant—this will result in a prolongation of the partial thromboplastin time—although the

Rheumatic Diseases

finding represents a significant procoagulant risk. Clinically, it is manifested by arterial (heart, brain) and venous thromboses, and in women it leads to recurrent spontaneous abortions. Patients with primary antiphospholipid syndrome partially develop systemic lupus erythematosus over time. Rare but prognostically very serious is the catastrophic antiphospholipid syndrome, when multiple systems are affected simultaneously or in a short time.

Autoantibodies

Antinuclear antibodies (ANA, ANF) are almost standard in SLE patients (about 95% at the time of activity). The examination serves as a screening test. ANA-negative SLE is very rare, but in disease remission the antibodies may temporarily disappear.

Antibodies against native double-stranded DNA (dsDNA) are present in most patients with active SLE (40–90%). They are virtually specific for the disease. However, there is no direct association between dsDNA Ab titre and disease activity.

Antibodies to soluble nuclear antigens (ENA) target a wide range of antigenic substrates. Specific for SLE are anti-Sm antibodies. The presence of U1 RNP antibodies is common in mixed connective tissue disease.

Antiphospholipid antibodies should always be tested in SLE patients due to thrombotic risks—see above. ACl anti-cardiolipin antibodies in the IgM and IgG class and the presence of lupus anticoagulants (LAK) are tested. The risk of thrombosis increases with positive findings, the highest in the case of triple positivity (aCl IgM + aCl IgG + LAK). Coombs antibodies—in a positive case (about 30%), it is necessary to look for signs of haemolysis.

Diagnosis

Diagnosis is difficult due to the highly variable manifestations of the disease; therefore classification criteria can be used. Several sets of classification criteria have been proposed over time, the most recent being those proposed by a team of European and North American experts in 2019—see Table 1 [3].

Therapy

General recommendations

- Avoid sunlight or other sources of UV radiation. High-filter (30–50) sunscreens are recommended
- Anti-atherosclerotic diet
- Possibly vitamin D3 and calcium supplementation
- No smoking
- Fitness movement
- Before starting immunosuppression, immunise against influenza (repeat even during treatment) and pneumococcus
- Ban on live vaccines
- Consultation of hormonal contraception

Table 1 SLE classification criteria

Baseline criterion: Positive ANA, if not, do not classify as SLE

Clinical involvement		Immunological criteria	
Constitutional		Antiphospholipid antibodies	
Fever (>38.3)	2	Antiphospholipid antibodies aCl or B2GP-1 or LAK	2
Haematology		**Complement**	
Leukopenia < 4 × 10^9	3	Reduced C3 or C4 levels	3
Thrombocytopenia < 100 × 10^9	4	Reduced C3 and C4 levels	4
Autoimmune haemolysis	4	**SLE specific antibodies**	
Neuropsychiatric		antidsDNA or antiSm	6
Delirium	2		
Psychosis	3		
Generalized or partial convulsions	5		
Mucocutaneous			
Alopecia without scaring	2		
Ulcers in the mouth	2		
Subacute cutaneous or discoid lupus	4		
Acute cutaneous lupus (facial or generalized)	6		
Serious			
Pleural or pericardial effusion	5		
Acute pericarditis	6		
Musculoskeletal			
Joint disability	6		
Renal			
Proteinuria >0.5 g/24 h	4		
Biopsy evidence of class II or V lupus nephritis	8		
Biopsy evidence of lupus nephritis class III or IV	10		

Classify as SLE when score ≥ 10 and ≥1 clinical criterion

- Pregnancy is possible, but it is necessary to contact the rheumatologist in advance, check whether SLE is in remission, adjust medication, treatment of antiphospholipid syndrome, monitor as a risk pregnancy (higher risk of pre-eclampsia, special treatment of hypertension)

Rheumatic Diseases

Pharmacotherapy

- *Non-steroidal antirheumatic drugs,* considering the possible effect on hypertension and renal function
- *Antimalarials,* (hydroxychloroquine) indicated in most patients unless contraindicated
- *Glucocorticoids,* rapid effect, relapse after reduction or discontinuation. Serious side effects, hence more recently a move away from chronic treatment. Essential in high disease activity
- *Azathioprine,* the primary drug for the maintenance phase of treatment. At higher doses, control of TPMT (thiopurine methyltransferase) mutation with slow elimination of azathioprine metabolites, increase a risk of overdose [8]. Do not combine with allopurinol
- *Methotrexate,* an alternative to antimalarials, doses as for rheumatoid arthritis (lx per week!)
- *Cyclophosphamide,* with high activity and damage to vital organs. After control of activity, switch to maintenance therapy
- *Mycophenolate mofetil,* can be used in the induction and maintenance phase or after induction with Cyclophosphamide or Rituximab

Biological treatment

- *Rituximab* (monoclonal Ab against B-lymphocytes (CD20)) is an alternative to the administration of Cyclophosphamide [7]. After the induction phase, switch to maintenance therapy
- *Belimumab,* moderately to highly active SLE except for severe renal and CNS involvement [8]

7 Ocular Manifestations of Systemic Lupus Erythematosus

Ocular involvement occurs in about 30% of patients with systemic lupus, and ocular manifestations occur mostly in patients with already diagnosed underlying disease in its active phase [14]. The finding is highly variable. When the ocular adnexa are affected, we observe ptosis or oedema of the eyelids, which may be affected by discoid cutaneous lupus; when the anterior segment is affected, we observe madarosis (loss of eyelashes), dry eye syndrome (the most common symptom), peripheral ulcerative keratitis, episcleritis or scleritis, and rarely anterior uveitis (more often associated with PUK). In SLE, involvement of the posterior segment of the eye is one of the most serious manifestations of the disease, often sight threatening. Retinal vasculopathy or vasculitis is quite often associated with signs of CNS involvement, is considered an important criterion of the severity of the overall disease, and may indicate an exacerbation of SLE. The prevalence is currently reported to be around 3% [18]. Microangiopathy is caused by deposition of immune complexes in the vessel wall with subsequent vasculitis, endothelial damage, and vascular thrombosis. Occlusions of the retinal arteries have been observed (Fig. 9), rarely of the veins,

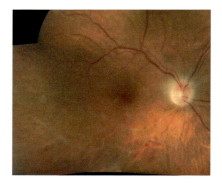

Fig. 9 Status post branch arterial occlusion in a patient with SLE—arteries with a "silver wiring" appearance

and in some cases severe vaso-occlusive retinopathy with development of retinal neovascularisation (NVE).

When central artery occlusion occurs in young individuals, SLE should be thought of in the differential diagnosis. Lupus choroidopathy is characterised by retinal detachment or retinal pigmented epithelium. Choroidal infarcts are another complication, probably due to immunodeposits in choroidal vessels. Cranial nerve damage occurs in 5–42% of cases [20]. Optic neuropathy affects about 1% of patients and may present as acute retrobulbar neuritis or ischaemic neuropathy [21].

Ocular manifestations associated with lupus anticoagulants are amaurosis fugax (short-term, transient visual impairment), occlusion of retinal veins or arteries, and anterior optic ischaemia (AION).

Risk factors

- Female gender
- The Asian race and African Americans
- The presence of antiphospholipid antibodies as a predictor of thrombosis risk
- Nephropathy, hypertension

Clinical presentation

The clinical presentation of SSO is described in detail in Sect. 1. In the case of anterior segment involvement, painful symptoms predominate, photophobia and "red eye" appear, while, in the case of cranial nerve involvement, patients report diplopia, complain of visual acuity impairment, colour vision disturbances, reduced contrast sensitivity or visual field disturbances. Vascular occlusions are accompanied by varying degrees of decrease in visual acuity and visual field disturbances. Sometimes patients are asymptomatic.

Objective findings

When the eyelids are affected, oedema or ptosis may be evident; the manifestations of episcleritis, scleritis and PUK are mentioned in the ocular manifestations of GPA; the symptoms of SSO are discussed in Sect. 1. Arteritis is associated with

Fig. 10 Cotton wool spots in the macula of a patient with SLE

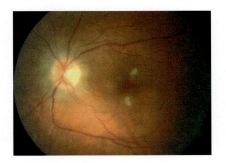

capillary leakage, with manifestations of arterial sheathing, retinal and preretinal haemorrhages and retinal ischaemia. The classic manifestation is cotton wool spots (Fig. 10).

Vasculopathy (more common in renal involvement) is manifested by narrowing of the arteries, flame-shaped haemorrhages, retinal exudations to papillary oedema. In arterial occlusion, positive RAPD of varying degrees, the affected retina is pale, oedematous, with macular involvement, a cherry spot is seen in the centre, the arteries are narrow, segmentation of the blood column may be seen. Venous occlusion is accompanied by dilatation and tortuosity of the veins, retinal oedema, deep or superficial retinal haemorrhages, cotton wool spots, hard exudates, and macular oedema, and, in central occlusion, optic disc oedema. The ischaemic form leads to neovascularisation. In cranial nerve damage, there are oculomotor disturbances, ptosis, or disturbances of pupillary reactions. In optic ischaemia, the optic disc oedema is found, usually with subsequent atrophy.

Diagnosis

Diagnosis includes examination of the anterior segment and fundus in the artificial mydriasis on a slit lamp. Dry eye tests may be included. Perimeter examinations are used to determine the extent of visual field dropouts and to monitor for changes (e.g. altitudinal or arcuate dropouts in AION). Disturbances of capillary perfusion (corresponding to cotton wool spots) and late-stage dye leakage in possible NVE are well visualised on FAG. FAG also has applications in vascular occlusions. ICG reveals zones of nonperfusion at the site of choroidal infarcts. OCT examination of the macula is used to monitor cystoid oedema in venous occlusions and to monitor changes in the optic nerve papilla.

Differential diagnosis

- Dry eye syndrome from another cause
- Idiopathic vasculitis

Complications

A complication of vascular occlusions may be the development of neovascularisation and secondary neovascular glaucoma. Oedema of the optic disc often progresses to atrophy with permanent visual impairment.

Therapy

Local therapy for dry eye is described in the RA chapter. In manifestations of anterior eye inflammation in lupus erythematosus, topical corticosteroids, NSAIDs are applied and, in the case of keratitis, antibiotics. In secondary glaucoma, permanent antiglaucoma therapy is necessary. In the presence of more extensive ischaemia and NVE, laser photocoagulation of the retina is indicated. Intravitreal application of anti-VEGF agents or administration of a slow-release steroid implant is effective in the treatment of cystoid oedema in venous occlusions. Overall therapy is guided in collaboration with a rheumatologist and nephrologist. Pulse therapy with methylprednisone with cyclophosphamide is used in choroidopathy, and remission occurs in 82% of patients. In neuro-ophthalmic involvement, treatment consists of systemic administration of corticosteroids, together with immunosuppressants such as cyclophosphamide or methotrexate. The visual prognosis after optic neuropathy is unfavourable. Anticoagulants as thrombosis prevention can be used, especially in the presence of antiphospholipid antibodies.

In APS in acute thrombosis, treatment is initiated with heparin, more commonly fractionated forms of LMWH (low molecular weight heparin). Warfarin is started concomitantly with heparin to achieve therapeutic levels according to INR 2–3. In pregnant women, warfarin is contraindicated and LMWH is given. Acetylsalicylic acid in low doses (50–100 mg daily) is more commonly used in patients with secondary APS secondary to SLE or other diseases.

8 Systemic Scleroderma

Scleroderma is a heterogeneous group of diseases with a common picture of fibrotic changes of the skin and internal organs (interstitial pulmonary fibrosis, GIT involvement), vascular involvement (Raynaud's phenomenon, pulmonary hypertension, myocardium) [39]. It is a rare disease; epidemiological data are poor and very variable, with recent data from Sweden showing a prevalence of 20 cases per million population.

Clinical presentation

Fibrosis with stiffening of the skin occurs especially predictively on the acral parts of the limbs and face (Fig. 11).

Localised forms (morphea) without organ involvement occur; systemic forms of the disease are the subject of rheumatological care.

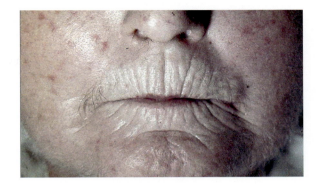

Fig. 11 Face in systemic scleroderma. The skin is stiff, non-flexible, smooth, there are telangiectasias (dilated blood vessels on the cheeks), there are radial lines around the mouth, the mouth is reduced due to fibrotic changes of the subcutaneous tissue

Systemic scleroderma (SD, systemic sclerosis) occurs mainly in two variants—a skin-limited and a diffuse form—differing in symptoms, presence of autoantibodies and tendency to systemic involvement.

Skin-limited form

Skin involvement mainly of acral parts and face, Raynaud's phenomenon (whitening of acral parts of limbs with subsequent cyanosis, cold provocation) is common, defects on finger acres (digital ulceration), occasionally subcutaneous calcinosis (known as CREST syndrome), oesophageal involvement, pulmonary arterial hypertension. Anticentromere antibodies are usually present in the laboratory picture.

Diffusion form

The progression of skin changes affects not only the acral parts, but also the trunk. Tenosynovitis is the source of palpable tremors over the tendons. There is a greater tendency to affect internal organs. The laboratory picture shows antibodies to topoisomerase (Scl-70).

Scleroderma sine scleroderma

A rare form of the disease, corresponding to the organ manifestations of systemic scleroderma, but without skin involvement.

Overlappings

With other systemic connective tissue diseases are common. A proportion of patients with a picture of undifferentiated systemic connective tissue disease develop systemic scleroderma during time.

Impairment of individual systems

Kidneys

One of the rarer but life-threatening systemic manifestations is scleroderma renal crisis. It is a rapidly progressive renal failure, accompanied by severe arterial hypertension. It is more common in the early phase of the disease, more so in the cutaneous diffuse form of SD. The risk is increased by treatment with higher doses of glucocorticoids or the presence of antibodies against RNA polymerase III. It is one of the important causes of mortality. As an acute complication, it requires intensive treatment, may lead to the need for dialysis treatment and kidney transplantation. The possibility of renal crisis is indicated by a rise in BP and creatinine, headache, visual disturbances. The presence of milder signs of renal lesions in the form of proteinuria and decreased renal function is described in up to 25% of SD patients.

Lungs

Clinically, it manifests itself as shortness of breath, dry cough, and auditory crepitations during pulmonary bass. The underlying cause is involvement of the lung interstitium in the form of non-specific interstitial pneumonia (NSIP), or usual interstitial pneumonia (UIP). Classification is clarified by HRCT of the lungs and functional examination, and biopsy when uncertain. It leads to respiratory insufficiency with subsequent right heart congestion. Interstitial pulmonary fibrosis is one of the most common organ involvements in SD.

Heart

In the myocardium, dispersive fibrosis occurs because of repeated ischaemia and reperfusion (similar to Raynaud's syndrome). The consequence is impaired contractility with systolic and diastolic myocardial dysfunction, ectopic arrhythmias, and impulse conduction disturbances. Valvular involvement is present in more than 1/3 of patients, mostly subclinical. Pericarditis is common, up to 20% of cases are symptomatic, but most of the time it is a subclinical sonographic finding of effusion.

Pulmonary arterial hypertension

It is one of the most serious life-threatening complications of SD. The underlying cause is the sclerodermic involvement of the pulmonary vasculature. It may not be associated with significant pulmonary fibrosis. It is more common in the limited form of scleroderma, but also occurs in the diffuse form of SD. Clinically, it manifests with exertional dyspnoea (shortening of the 6-min walk test) and signs of right ventricular heart failure.

Digital ulcerations

Occur on the acral parts of the extremities, usually together with Raynaud's phenomenon. Scleroderma skin is easily vulnerable and minor injuries take a long time and are difficult to heal. Sometimes dimpled scars on the fingertips can be observed without a preceding trauma, which will assist in differentiating it from primary Raynaud's syndrome. Non-healing defects may lead to the need for amputation of the finger article, but then poor stump healing can be expected. Even without surgical intervention, SD can lead to shortening of the finger phalanx or more. Facial telangiectasias may lead to the diagnosis along with skin changes.

Digestive tract

The most common manifestation is impaired lower oesophageal sphincter motility with swallowing difficulties and gastroesophageal reflux. The impairment can be demonstrated at a subclinical stage, which may contribute to early diagnosis. Sicca syndrome may also be involved in swallowing difficulties. In the stomach, dilatation of blood vessels (watermelon stomach) with anaemia may occur. Frequent is bowel involvement, with bacterial overgrowth and motility disturbances, rarely leading up to ileus and bowel perforation.

Musculoskeletal disability

It is common and manifests itself in arthralgias, stiffness, tenosynovitis with frictional murmur over the tendons, occasionally arthritis. Restriction of thoracic mobility may contribute to respiratory insufficiency, oppression of n. medianus may lead to carpal tunnel syndrome.

Diagnosis

Clinical presentation supplemented by examination of target systems. Capillaroscopy of the nail bed is useful in early diagnosis. Laboratory examination shows typical autoantibodies and signs of target system involvement. Periodic screening of pulmonary hypertension by sonography (min. once per year) is necessary.

The 2013 Euro-American classification criteria (Table 2) may be helpful in diagnosis, although they were developed for classification purposes for clinical trials [38].

Table 2 Classification criteria for systemic scleroderma

Symptom	Characteristics	Points
Thickening of the skin of both hands extending proximally beyond the MCP joints	Sufficient for diagnosis	9*
	Oedematous finger infiltration*	2*
	Sclerodactyly proximal to PIP, distal to MCP*	4*
Defects on acres of fingers	Ulceration	2*
	Dimpled scars	3*
Teleangiectasias		2
Abnormal capillaroscopy	Typical for SD	2
Pulmonary arterial hypertension or interstitial lung involvement		2
Raynaud's phenomenon		3
Specific antibodies	Centromeres, Scl-70, RNA polymerase III*	3

*The highest value in the category is counted

Therapy

The approach to therapy of systemic scleroderma is determined by the presence of systemic manifestations.

The procedure for individual manifestations is summarised in the recommendations of the European League Against Rheumatism (EULAR), last modified in 2017 [19]. Skin and vascular manifestations can sometimes be favourably influenced by treatment with calcium channel inhibitors. In the development of renal crisis, early administration of an ACE inhibitor is the main treatment, but it is not recommended to be administered prophylactically. Higher doses of glucocorticoids are not recommended, due to the risk of facilitating renal crisis.

From immunomodulatory drugs, methotrexate is used, significant activity of a disease, especially pulmonary impairment, is treated cyclophosphamide or mycophenolate mofetil. Azathioprine is used as maintenance therapy.

Recently, the treatment options for pulmonary arterial hypertension (prostanoids, endothelin receptor blockers, phosphodiesterase 5 inhibitors) have significantly expanded, demonstrably increasing survival and quality of life of patients. More recently, the growth factor receptor blocker nintedanib has been introduced in the treatment of interstitial pulmonary fibrosis [5]. Patients with systemic scleroderma should be followed and treated in an experienced rheumatology department with the possibility of multidisciplinary collaboration.

Prognosis

The prognosis of patients with systemic scleroderma is mainly influenced by organ involvement, the most important in terms of mortality are the consequences of pulmonary arterial hypertension, interstitial pulmonary fibrosis, eventual renal crisis or severe GIT and myocardial involvement. 10-year survival is around 65–80%. Further improvement can be expected with the introduction of effective methods of treatment of organ manifestations.

9 Ocular Manifestations of Systemic Scleroderma

Scleroderma can result in atrophy of the eyelid skin and telangiectasia, a dry eye syndrome. Rarely, there is a reduction of the conjunctival fornix and vascular changes of the conjunctiva and nodular episcleritis. Glaucoma (including normotensive glaucoma) is more frequently encountered. Enophthalmos due to atrophy of the orbital contents has been described. Retinal vasculitis is rare, vasculopathy is more frequently described.

Risk factors

- Male sex—prognostically unfavourable
- Cutaneous diffuse form

Rheumatic Diseases 239

- Age over 65 years
- Decrease in renal function, visceral organ involvement (lung, heart, GIT), anaemia and thrombocytopenia

Clinical presentation

Dry eye is manifested by burning, cutting, discomfort and hyperaemia of the conjunctiva. In more severe cases, patients have impaired vision.

Objective findings

In atrophy of the eyelids, the skin is thinned with eventual enlargement of blood vessels; in nodular episcleritis, one or more sensitive nodules are found, usually in the eye slit, which fade after injection of adrenaline or 10% epinephrine. The finding in DES is described in the RA chapter. In vasculopathy, haemorrhages and cotton wool spots and numerous zones of choroidal nonperfusion are found.

Diagnosis

The type and extent of ocular involvement is determined by examination of the anterior segment and fundus in mydriasis on a slit lamp, with DES using diagnostic tests. FAG may be indicated to determine the extent of zones of nonperfusion.

Differential diagnosis

Vasculitis or vasculopathy in malignant masking syndromes.

Therapy

Local therapy of DES is in the RA chapter. Treatment of episcleritis with mild manifestations is not necessary, e.g. local application of corticosteroids is usually effective; NSAIDs, e.g. meloxicam or ibuprofen, can be added for several weeks. Medical treatment of any glaucoma is necessary. Total immunosuppressive treatment is based on the systemic disease.

10 Sjogren's Syndrome

Sjögren's syndrome (SjS) is a chronic autoimmune inflammatory disorder, affecting mainly the exocrine glands, especially the lacrimal and salivary glands, but also other organ involvement. Other systemic manifestations include arthralgia, arthritis, autoimmune thyroiditis, interstitial lung involvement, tubulointerstitial nephritis, tubular disorders, neurological involvement (polyneuropathy), erythema annulare, and cutaneous vasculitis [25].

SjS can accompany other systemic connective tissue diseases (secondary SjS), most commonly rheumatoid arthritis. Patients with SjS have a higher risk of lymphoproliferation, especially non-Hodgkin's lymphoma from B lymphocytes.

The aetiopathogenesis is not fully elucidated, genetic predisposition is assumed to be involved and infectious influences, especially viral ones. Primary and secondary SjS have statistically different HLA DR predispositions (DR3 versus DR4).

Clinical presentation

Involvement of the lacrimal and salivary glands leads to the picture of "sicca syndrome" manifested by burning eyes, sensation of a foreign body, swallowing disorders with the need to washing down food, lead to worsened caries of teeth, periodontitis, taste disorders. Tear secretion disorder can be objectified (Schirmer's test), reduced salivation is confirmed by Skach's test. For histological confirmation, a biopsy of the labial salivary gland is used. Sjogren's syndrome accounts for a minority of patients with sicca syndrome (about 10%).

Involvement of the exocrine glands of the respiratory system leads to dry irritant cough. Impairment of secretion of vaginal glands in women can lead to dyspareunia. Objectively, swelling of the salivary glands can be observed.

Extraglandular manifestations

Skin—scaling, itching of the skin occurs in one-quarter to one-half of patients. Raynaud's syndrome occurs in up to one-third of patients. Cutaneous vasculitis is described in about 10% of patients, usually without systemic involvement, and erythema annulare mainly affects the upper trunk in about one-tenth of patients.

Arthralgias occur in about 50% of cases; arthritis is rarer, is non-erosive, more often involving hands, wrists, or knees.

Pulmonary involvement in the form of interstitial fibrosis occurs in about one-tenth of the cases; clinically it is less pronounced, dry cough can also be a consequence of bronchial gland involvement; functional examination and HRCT of the lungs will help in differentiation.

Cardiovascular involvement—pregnant women with anti-Ro or anti-La antibodies positivity, a typical immunological finding in SjS, may develop intrauterine foetal carditis, leading to congenital AV block—therefore, pregnancies of women with these antibodies must be monitored as high-risk with more frequent foetal echocardiography. A higher atherogenic risk has been described for SjS in adulthood.

Dyspeptic disorders are partly related to impaired exocrine secretion, with oesophageal motility disorder to oesophagitis and atrophic gastritis being more common.

Interstitial nephritis occurs in 5–10% of patients, most commonly as renal tubular acidosis or interstitial cystitis with dysuria.

Lymphoproliferative risk – can manifest itself most often as extranodular B-cell non-Hodgkin's lymphoma with localisation in the affected glands, most often salivary, but also in the GIT or respiratory system. Clinically, it may manifest itself by sudden swelling of the gland during the disease, appearance of monoclonal protein, disappearance of Ro and La autoantibodies. Sonography of the salivary glands with targeted biopsy will help in the diagnosis. Megaloblastic anaemia may occur in atrophic gastritis.

Diagnosis

It is based on the evidence of involvement of the lacrimal and salivary glands and immunological findings (anti-Ro and anti-La antibodies). Recently, increased emphasis has been placed on histological findings and imaging methods, especially sonography.

The current classification criteria for Sjögren's syndrome were published in 2017 (Table 3).

A score ≥4 is required to meet the classification criteria. The entry criterion is ocular or oral symptomatology, and the exclusion criterion is a history of head and neck actinotherapy, active hepatitis C infection, AIDS, sarcoidosis, amyloidosis, graft versus host reaction or IgG4 disease [32].

Laboratory findings

- Acute phase proteins tend to be elevated or normal
- Typical is the positivity of autoantibodies anti-Ro and anti-La, synonyms of SSA and SSB
- Swollen salivary and lacrimal glands, with absence of autoantibodies may be a manifestation of IgG4 disease
- Other autoantibodies may be present, especially rheumatoid factors, various antinuclear antibodies (ANA) or antibodies to thyroid antigens

Therapy

The treatment consists of substitution of the missing secretion (artificial tears, stimulation of tear and saliva production), and symptomatic therapy. Topical ocular, mucolytics, and possibly lubricants for dyspareunia can also be used.

In active systemic manifestations of SjS, a general treatment can be used according to the predominant manifestations. Non-steroidal antirheumatic drugs, low-dose glucocorticoids for the necessary period, possibly immunomodulants: methotrexate, hydroxychloroquine, may be considered. For severe systemic manifestations, cyclophosphamide or rituximab may be used [29]. Therapy should always be guided by a multidisciplinary team (rheumatologist, ophthalmologist, dentist, haematologist, and others).

Table 3 Classification criteria for Sjögren's syndrome

		Points
1	Focal lymphocyte sialoadenitis in the labial salivary gland with the focus score ≥1	3
2	Anti SSA/Ro positivity	3
3	Evidence of dry keratoconjunctivitis OSS ≥ 5 or van Bijsterveld score ≥4 in at least 1 eye	1
4	Schirmer test ≤ 5 mm in at least 1 eye	1
5	Unstimulated sialometry ≤0.1 ml/min	1

Prognosis

The prognosis of SjS patients ranges from mild disability requiring only symptomatic therapy and not affecting morbidity or mortality (most cases) to prognostically severe disability (risk factors include renal involvement, purpura, cryoglobulinemia) and risk of lymphoproliferative diseases.

11 Ocular Manifestations of Sjogren's Syndrome

Sjogren's syndrome is an autoimmune disease in which there is lymphocytic infiltration and subsequent fibrosis of the lacrimal gland and salivary glands, but other exogenous glands in the body may also be functionally affected. The presence of rheumatoid factor, anti-SSA antibodies, anti-SSB antibodies or antinuclear antibodies and hypergammaglobulinaemia are characteristic. In primary SjS, xerostomia and xerophthalmia are present; in addition, other connective or collagen tissue diseases such as rheumatoid arthritis, scleroderma or SLE are detected in secondary SjS. SjS more commonly affects women.

90% of patients with SjS have keratoconjunctivitis sicca (KCS) [21]. The reduced tear secretion and the change in tear composition are caused by the involvement of the lacrimal gland. In the early stages, diagnosis may be difficult, because the lacrimal gland reflexively produces enough tears [21].

Risk factors

- Female gender
- The presence of systemic connective tissue disease

Clinical presentation

The most common symptoms are dryness, cutting or burning of the eyes, foreign body sensation, light-headedness, fluctuation of vision, pain, feeling of pressure behind the eye. It is also typical for symptoms to fluctuate during the day, week, or season, possibly depending on the environment (windy weather, air conditioning, visually demanding activity).

Objective findings

In KCS, hyperaemia or conjunctival injection are observed, a decrease to absence of the tear meniscus, t-t folds of the bulbar conjunctiva, epitheliopathy of the conjunctiva and cornea, cellular detritus on the surface of the eye and corneal filaments (in advanced conditions).

Diagnosis

The examination of the anterior segment of the eye is based on a slit lamp. The position and condition of the eyelids are also assessed, the condition of the tear meniscus on the lower eyelid margin (the norm is 0.2 mm) is measured, the condition of the

Rheumatic Diseases 243

conjunctiva and cornea is assessed, and the LIPCOF (lid parallel conjunctival folds) classification is used—the number and height of conjunctival folds in relation to the height of the normal tear meniscus. For this, we use $10\times$ magnification and a narrow beam of lamp light; we classify from grade 0: no folds to grade 4: multiple folds higher than the normal tear meniscus.

We use diagnostic tests to assess the quantity and quality of the tear film. Schirmer tests measure the aqueous component and the reflective production of tears. The Schirmer I test is used to measure total tear secretion. We do not administer anaesthetic to the eye before the test. A 35 mm strip of filter paper is folded to 5 mm and inserted externally behind the lid margin. The patient can blink. After 5 min, the readings are taken. Normal values are above 15 mm, initial deficiency is 10–15 mm, advanced deficiency is 5–10 mm, severe deficiency is below 5 mm. The same test can be used to determine basal tear secretion after excluding reflex tearing. The procedure is the same, but the test is performed after application of local anaesthetic to the eyes and in a darkened room. The Schirmer II test is used to determine reflex tear secretion. The procedure is the same as for Test I, but after introducing the strips into the eyes, the surface of the conjunctiva is irritated with a cotton swab (no topical anaesthetic is given). The break-up time test (BUT) measures the stability of the tear film. We stain the surface of the patient's eye with fluorescein without the use of anaesthesia. We examine on a slit lamp with a blue filter, while avoiding blinking by the patient, and observe when the stained film on the corneal surface breaks. Normal values are 15 s, 5–10 s indicates shortening and less than 5 s significant shortening.

The diagnosis includes staining the surface of the eye with fluorescein (the dye penetrates the surface defects of the epithelium) or staining with Bengal red or Lissamine green (the desquamated epithelium of the conjunctiva and cornea is stained).

We are also increasingly using modern automatic tear film analysers for tear film investigation, photo- and video-documentation and development over time.

Differential diagnosis

- Other causes of dry eye syndrome
- Eyelid position disorder—e.g. lagophthalmos, endocrine orbitopathy
- Blepharitis
- Skin diseases—e.g. pemphigoid, Stevens-Johnson syndrome
- Chemical and physical damage
- Vitamin A deficiency
- Age-related decreased secretion, neurogenic hyposecretion
- Certain drugs—e.g. antidepressants, neuroleptics, cytostatics, hormonal contraceptives
- Epitheliopathy—corneal dystrophies, corneal scars, corneal anaesthesia

Complications

Permanent disruption of the tear film layer can lead to increased susceptibility of the eye to infections (conjunctivitis and corneal inflammation), minor corneal injuries (erosions), impaired wound healing, and corneal scarring.

Therapy

Treatment of KCS is symptomatic. Modification of the external environment can be recommended—limitation of stay in a smoky, dusty, but also air-conditioned space, as well as modification of the daily regime—enough sleep and fluids, limitation of time in front of a monitor, TV, phone screen or tablet. It is also advisable to limit the wearing of contact lenses for a long time.

The basis of treatment is mainly tear supplementation with drops, preferably without preservatives. For each patient, it is necessary to find the most suitable preparation and frequency of dripping.

The lacrimal gland can be stimulated locally with eledoisin or with total pilocarpine, but these options are severely limited due to frequent side effects. Biological tear substitutes (autologous whole blood serum or platelet concentrate) or topical anti-inflammatory drugs (corticosteroids, cyclosporine A) are available for the treatment of severe KCS. Tear outflow can be reduced by temporary or permanent tear duct closures (collagen or silicone plugs). In severe forms with filaments, a contact lens can be temporarily applied to mechanically protect the surface of the eye.

In severe cases, treatment is guided by an ophthalmologist specialising in corneal and ocular surface diseases.

Systemic treatment is guided by a rheumatologist.

12 Systemic Vasculitis

The classification of systemic vasculitis is based on the size of the affected arteries according to the Chappel-Hill 2012 consensus [17]. Vasculitis affecting *large vessels* include Takayasu's arteritis and giant cell vasculitis. *Medium vessel* translucency is affected by polyarteritis nodosa and Kawasaki arteritis. The group of vasculitis affecting *small vessels* is broad. According to the presence of ANCA antibodies, they are divided into:

ANCA-associated vasculitis:

- Granulomatosis with polyarteritis (formerly Wegener's)
- Eosinophilic granulomatosis with polyarteritis (formerly Churg-Strauss syndrome)
- Microscopic polyangiitis

Rheumatic Diseases

Immunocomplex vasculitis:

- Anti-GBM vasculitis
- Cryoglobulinemic vasculitis
- IgA vasculitis (Henoch-Schönlein)
- Anti-C1q vasculitis (hypocomplementemic urticarial vasculitis)

Vasculitis in Behçet's and Cogan's syndrome affects blood vessels of different diameters.

From another aspect, vasculitis can be divided into diseases affecting one organ (e.g. cutaneous leukocytoclastic vasculitis or primary CNS vasculitis), vasculitis associated with systemic disease and vasculitis with probable aetiology, e.g. in hepatitis B, C, pollen, paraneoplastic and others. Here, we only discuss diseases with significant ocular symptomatology.

12.1 Giant Cell Arteritis

The synonym is temporal arteritis according to the typical localisation of involvement, or also Horton's disease. It is the most common primary vasculitis in persons over 50 years of age. The incidence has a geographical gradient peaking northward (Europe, America). The prevalence in the North American population is 223/100,000 inhabitants (Olmsted, Minnesota). A significant proportion of patients also have symptoms of rheumatic polymyalgia.

Aetiopathogenesis is unknown, genetic basis is considered (DRB 1*), pathogenetic relation to aging is not clear, influence of some infections is considered.

Morphologically, it is a segmental panarteritis, with infiltration of the vessel wall by a mixed infiltrate with CD4+ T-lymphocytes and typical giant multinucleated cells. Proinflammatory signalling of IL-1, IL-6, IL-17/23 is activated. Thrombosis may be involved in arterial occlusion.

The typical location is the carotid basin; more recent work, especially using positron emission tomography (PET), shows that, in a significant proportion of patients, other large vessels (aorta, a. subclavia, axillaris, abdominal arteries) are also affected.

Clinical presentation

Non-specific symptoms consist of sub- to febrilia in half of the patients, weakness, lack of appetite, weight loss.

- A prominent symptom is a *headache* in the temporal region or generalised. Up to one-half of patients report palpatory tenderness of the scalp
- *Jaw claudication* (34–42% of patients) during chewing, due to ischaemia of the masticatory muscles is a relatively specific problem in this type of vasculitis
- *The pulsation of the a. temporalis* is weakened or even disappears. Often a stiff, tender band is palpable over the a. temporalis

A vascular murmur may be heard over involved artery (carotid, abdominal aorta).

- *Visual impairment* may be the first manifestation in up to one-fifth of patients with untreated temporal arthritis
- Other neurological manifestations can include *confusion, hearing loss and even stroke*

Involvement of the great arteries may lead to limb claudication, the finding on the a. temporalis may be negative in such a case. Aortitis can lead to aortic insufficiency in the presence of aortic root enlargement, coronary artery involvement, aneurysm, or dissection, especially in the thoracic segment.

Physical findings show weakening or loss of pulse in the affected artery, vascular murmur, thickening and painfulness of the course of the affected (temporal) artery. Sonography may show disappearance of blood flow along the wall of the affected vessel (halo sign). Blood pressure in the extremities may vary laterally to the point of being unmeasurable on the affected side.

The most common musculoskeletal symptom is pain and weakness of the brachial plexus muscles; arthralgia and synovitis may occur, especially in the shoulder and pelvis (demonstrable by sonography or PET/CT scan).

Diagnosis

Laboratory findings are not typical, significant elevation of laboratory signs of inflammation (SE, CRP) is common, but not mandatory. Antibodies are not typical [27]. The gold standard of diagnosis is temporal artery biopsy, recently considered not necessary in the presence of positive ultrasound findings. Extracranial involvement is demonstrated by Doppler sonography of the great vessels, MRI angiography, but activity is best captured by PET/CT scanning.

Therapy

For the risk of vision loss, active temporal arteritis is an established rheumatological emergence. Early initiation of treatment can prevent blindness; untreated, the condition is highly likely to affect both eyes. High-dose glucocorticoids with gradual detraction dominate therapy, with parenteral pulse therapy with intravenous methylprednisolone when vision loss is imminent. Do not wait for complete results to start treatment! The amaurosis already formed is usually irreversible.

Given the need for prolonged use of higher doses of glucocorticoids, the risks of side effects, including osteoporotic vertebral fractures, should be kept in mind, and appropriate treatment should be monitored and initiated in a timely manner. Corticosteroid treatment should last for at least 2 years, in some cases long term at low dose.

In refractory or relapsing disease, administration of IL-6 blockers is indicated.

Rheumatic Diseases

12.2 Takayasu's Arteritis

It is a granulomatous panarteritis affecting mainly the aorta and its branches, synonyms are as follows: aortic arch syndrome, pulseless disease.

The aetiology is unclear. T-cell mediated cytotoxicity seems to be involved in the pathogenesis.

In the wall of the affected vessel, there is an inflammatory mixed infiltrate in the media and adventitia, granulomatous inflammation mainly affects the media, intima-media hyperplasia leads to stenosis. Segmental involvement more rarely leads to aneurysms.

Clinical presentation

In the first phase of the disease, general symptoms dominate; Takayasu arteritis (TA) is one of the possible causes of fever of undetermined origin (FUO) syndrome. Fatigue, weight loss, night sweats, and arthralgia are common.

In the further course, symptoms of vascular involvement, pain or palpation tenderness (e.g. carotidodynia syndrome) may be present, followed by the consequences of ischaemia in the territory of the affected artery:

- *a. subclavia*, claudication pain in the arms, weakening to disappearance of the pulse on the wrist, pressure difference on the limbs
- *aorta*, valve insufficiency in aortic root enlargement, renovascular arterial hypertension, claudication on the lower limbs
- *carotids*, visual disturbances, CNS ischaemia
- *coronary vessels* in up to 25% of patients
- *a. vertebralis*, dizziness, headache, syncope

The classification criteria are as follows:

- Onset by the age of 40
- Claudication of the limbs
- Weakening of pulsations on the brachial arteries
- Difference in systolic BP on both HCs more than 10 torr
- Murmur over the arteria subclavia or abdominal aorta
- Evidence of stenosis or occlusion of the aorta, its main branches, or proximal arteries of the extremities

In the presence of ≥ 3 criteria, the sensitivity is 90.5% and the specificity 97.8% [16].

Latest criteria ACR/EULAR from 2022 gets along from different score of 10 clinical and imaging findings, conditions are age over 60 and imaging sign of vasculitis [11].

Diagnosis

Laboratory signs of inflammation tend to be elevated, there is anaemia of chronic disease and hypergammaglobulinaemia. There are no typical antibodies. Of the imaging examinations, sonography of the vessels to assess progression (acceleration of the flow), MRI or CT angiography to detect wall thickening, stenoses or aneurysms are useful. In addition, PET/CT will show current activity, which is particularly useful in dg of early involvement. Classic angiography is the gold standard but represents a greater burden for the patient.

Therapy

In the acute phase, high-dose glucocorticoids, alternatively together with methotrexate; in refractory states, the Il-6 blocker tocilizumab. Surgical reconstructive procedures, if needed, should be performed in remission of the disease. Treatment by inhibitors of IL-6 or TNF can be used in refractory or relapsing disease [15].

12.3 Ocular Manifestations of Giant Cell Arteritis and Takayasu's Arteritis

About 50% of patients with giant cell arteritis develop ocular symptoms, sometimes as the first manifestation of the disease [26]. Anterior ischaemia of the optic nerve, called arteritic, is typical (AAION). Rarely, posterior ischaemic optic neuropathy occurs. If treatment is not initiated in time, one-third of patients develop involvement of the other eye within a week [4]. Up to one-half of untreated individuals go blind [21]. AION may be preceded by transient visual disturbances (amaurosis fugax). AION may be combined with occlusion of the cilioretinal artery or central retinal artery. It may be accompanied by transient or permanent diplopia in the presence of ischaemia of oculomotor muscles or nerves or cortical blindness.

Visual disturbances occur in about 30% of TA cases and take the form of blurred vision, diplopia or transient unilateral amaurosis (amaurosis fugax), episcleritis and iritis [20].

Risk factors

- Age over 60 for giant cell arteritis
- Smoking, low body mass index and early menopause may be independent risk factors for giant cell arteritis
- Female gender at TA

Clinical presentation

Patients may suffer from blurred vision, diplopia, or transient unilateral vision loss (amaurosis fugax). In anterior optic ischaemia, a unilateral, rapid, and painless decrease in vision of varying degrees, usually marked, is typical. It may be accompanied by periocular pain.

Objective findings

AAION in giant cell arteritis is characterised by pale oedema of the papilla of the optic nerve (Fig. 12) due to impaired perfusion in the posterior ciliary arteries.

The edges of the target are wiped off, and there are splinter-shaped haemorrhage at its margins. The retinal arteries may be narrowed with irregularly translucent lumen, ischaemic cotton wool spots may be seen. This then results in atrophy of the optic nerve papillae with excavation (Fig. 13).

Altitudinal depressions of the visual field (upper or lower half) are typical.

Hypertonic retinopathy is a common finding in TA. Microaneurysms, venous dilatation and haemorrhage resemble diabetic retinopathy. Late sequelae are optic nerve atrophy, retinal detachment, and vitreous haemorrhage. The ocular findings in TA are classified into four grades according to Uyama and Asayama. Grade 1: enlargement of the retinal veins. Grade 2: formation of microaneurysms. Grade 3: formation of arteriovenous anastomoses. Grade 4: presence of complications such as cataract, proliferative vitreoretinopathy, and vitreous haemorrhage [20]. Ocular ischaemic syndrome is diagnosed when ischaemic features are present simultaneously in the anterior (neovascularisation of the iris, neovascular glaucoma) and posterior segment of the eye (AION), or in the orbit. Exudative retinal detachment has also been described [20].

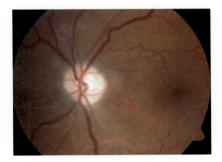

Fig. 12 Optic disc oedema in AION

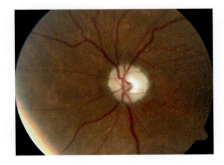

Fig. 13 Optic disc atrophy after AION

Diagnosis

In OBA, the diagnosis of optic disc oedema and its subsequent atrophy is based on biomicroscopic examination of the fundus on a slit lamp. We observe a relative afferent pupillary defect (RAPD) in the affected eye. We also complete a perimetric examination to assess the visual field. On FAG examination, optic nerve hyperfluorescence is seen in the late phase, with slowed or absent perfusion with possible concomitant retinal artery occlusion. OCT examination can be used to monitor the size of the optic disc oedema and its changes over time, including the transition to atrophy. In the laboratory, high sedimentation rates (often over 100/h) and elevated CRP levels dominate, and their levels are used to monitor the effects of treatment. Histological examination of the arteria temporalis biopsy will confirm the diagnosis, but the affected segment should be examined. A negative biopsy result with typical clinical findings does not exclude the diagnosis of OBA. Biopsy is performed before starting corticosteroid therapy. If a biopsy cannot be performed urgently, the introduction of treatment takes precedence.

In TA, the diagnosis is based on an examination of the anterior segment of the eye, including gonioscopy (examination of the ventricular angle) on a slit lamp and biomicroscopic examination of the fundus. The exact extent of retinal changes is refined by FAG examination. There is a high erythrocyte sedimentation rate in the laboratory.

For both diseases, arterial ultrasonography is an available non-invasive examination of large vessels. Other methods are PET, MRI, echocardiography, or angiography.

Differential diagnosis

- Non-arteritic anterior optic nerve ischaemia (NAION)
- Central retinal vein occlusion
- Neuritis optica
- Central retinal artery occlusion

Complications

Complications of corticosteroid treatment include steroid cataract and steroid glaucoma. Optic atrophy leads to permanent visual impairment. Neovascular glaucoma may develop because of ischaemia. Complications include vitreous haemorrhage and vitreoproliferative changes.

Therapy

Corticosteroids are the drug of choice for OBA, and treatment should be started as soon as possible to prevent the development of a stroke or loss of vision. The initial dose is 40–60 mg of prednisone daily. If there is a risk of serious ischaemic complications (amaurosis fugax, blindness in one eye, incipient signs of visual impairment in the other eye), initiate treatment with methylprednisolone infusion 500–1000 mg per day for 3 consecutive days and then continue with oral prednisone (60 mg per day). After about 2–4 weeks, i.e. after the inflammation indices have decreased and the symptoms have subsided, the dose can be gradually reduced after 1–2 weeks (by 10 mg every 2 weeks to 20 mg daily, then by 2.5 mg every 2 weeks to 10 mg, then by 1 mg at monthly intervals) [20]. Supplementation of calcium, vitamin D, administration of proton pump blockers is necessary. Treatment must be long- term, maintenance dose is usually at least one year. In AAION, however, even high doses of corticosteroids do not sufficiently ensure improvement of visual function, the prognosis is poor. The purpose of treatment is to prevent blindness in the other eye. If the effect of corticosteroids is insufficient or as a means of reducing steroid treatment, other immunosuppressive drugs—e.g. methotrexate—can be used with caution.

In TA, prednisone is also the drug of choice at an initial dose of 0.5–1 mg/kg/day. Therapy is long- term with sedimentation control and PET after several months. If the steroid dose cannot be reduced, cyclosporine A, pulses of cyclophosphamide or azathioprine should be added. More recently, methotrexate is given. Blood pressure compensation is part of the treatment.

12.4 Granulomatosis with Polyangiitis

It predictively affects the respiratory tract (granulomatous sinusitis, chronic rhinitis, destruction of the nasal skeleton—saddle nose, hoarseness, stridor (Fig. 14).

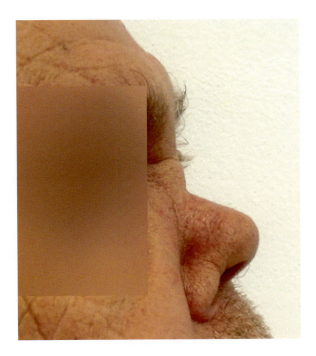

Fig. 14 Nasal bones involvement with typical saddle-shaped deformity in granulomatosis with polyangiitis

Pulmonary involvement with cough, dyspnoea, cavitary granulomas, development of respiratory insufficiency. Relatively common is the syndrome of diffuse alveolar haemorrhage, caused by alveolar vasculitis, with a picture of rapidly developing respiratory failure, often with the need for ventilatory support and significant anaemia. It is often associated with acute renal failure (pulmonary-renal syndrome). It is a condition with a high acute mortality, if not recognised and treated promptly.

Non-specific symptoms are common. Renal involvement manifests as rapidly progressive necrotising glomerulonephritis and may lead to irreversible renal failure within days. Neurological involvement usually manifests as mononeuritis multiplex (dispersive asymmetric vasculitis vasa nervorum). On the skin, there is palpable purpura or livedo reticularis from involvement of subcutaneous vessels.

Therapy of ANCA-associated vasculitis consists of high-dosed glucocorticoids immunosuppressive drugs, quite often is necessary intensive care in acute situations [2, 23, 42].

12.5 Ocular Manifestations of Granulomatosis with Polyangiitis

Depending on the localisation of inflammation, all ocular structures may be affected in granulomatosis with polyangiitis; ocular symptoms may be the first manifestations of the disease [14]. Ocular manifestation is reported to be between 16 and 58% in GPA [21]. Orbital changes occur in up to one-third of cases and result from direct spread of inflammation from adjacent paranasal sinuses. Eyelid involvement is uncommon, heterogeneous, and may be associated with tear duct obstruction. The extraocular muscles and lacrimal gland may be affected. Changes in the anterior segment of the eye are very common. Isolated anterior uveitis is rare, more often associated with scleritis and PUK. Posterior segment involvement is reported in 16% [21] and may present with vitritis, vasculitis and retinal vessel occlusion.

Risk factors

Presence of autoantibodies against neutrophil cytoplasm (c-ANCA).

Clinical presentation

Patients' problems can be variable, depending on the location of the disability. They complain of symptoms of dry eye in lacrimal gland disorders, red eye (when the anterior segment and the orbit are affected), pain (behind the eye when the orbit is affected, increasing seizure-like in scleritis, pressure in episcleritis, foreign body sensation in corneal involvement), photophobia, diplopia, visual disturbance of varying degrees.

Objective findings

In orbital involvement, protrusion of the bulb, chemosis of the conjunctiva, ophthalmoplegia, retinal vascular congestion and optic disc oedema are found. In PUK,

Fig. 15
Episcleritis—diffuse surface congestion in a patient with GPA

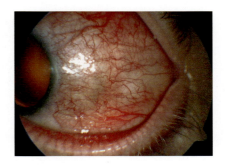

corneal infiltration along the limbus is typical, spreading circumferentially and deeply, gradually thinning to a deep defect that may end in perforation. Conjunctival hyperaemia is present and may sometimes be subtle. In episcleritis (Fig. 15), a sectorial diffuse redness is seen, usually within the extent of the palpebral fissure, or the presence of a tender nodule moving against the base.

In scleritis, a deep redness is visible, usually starting in the upper temporal quadrant, which does not disappear even with instillation of epinephrine or 10% phenylephrine; a scleral nodule immobile against the base may be seen; in the necrotising inflammatory form, solitary or multiple avascular whitish foci lined by hyperaemic sclera are seen; the necrotic sclera becomes translucent, revealing dark areas of choroid. Obliteration of blood vessels is the cause of necrosis. In posterior scleritis, an elevated lesion on the posterior segment of the eye and diffuse thickening of the sclera on ultrasound examination are observed; it may be accompanied by impaired mobility and protrusion of the globe. In retinal vasculitis, cotton wool spots and intraretinal haemorrhages, manifestations of vasculopathy and neovascularisation are differentiated. Vasculopathy, neovascularisation and retinal haemorrhage are the most common manifestations. Optic nerve neuritis to bulb protrusion may occur, due to involvement of the retrobulbar space by granulomatous inflammation.

Diagnosis

The diagnosis is based on the examination of the anterior segment of the eye and the fundus on a slit lamp. OCT examination of the anterior segment can be used to monitor changes in corneal thickness, OCT of the papilla to monitor optic disc oedema, OCT of the macula to evaluate possible CME. USG examination helps in the diagnosis of posterior scleritis (thickening of the sclera, and what is called the T-sign—fluid collection in the subtenon space around the optic nerve). The FAG shows leakage of dye from vessels and areas of nonperfusion at the site of occlusions. When the orbit is affected, a Hertel exophthalmometer is used to assess the degree of eyeball protrusion, and, in the case of oculomotor disorders, it is supplemented with a detailed examination of oculomotor balance, including a Lancaster screen. In case of orbital impairment, a CT scan can also be used. In the laboratory, sedimentation is consistently elevated, and immunocomplexes and CRP are usually elevated. An important diagnostic criterion is the c-ANCA level, which fluctuates with disease activity, but fluctuations in levels may not be related to ocular activity. Histological examination of the affected tissue may confirm the diagnosis.

Differential diagnosis

Depending on the ocular manifestations:

- *Corneal ulceration*—infectious ulcer, marginal keratitis in chronic blepharitis, Terrien's marginal degeneration, Mooren's ulcer
- *Posterior sclerites*—a tumour process, degenerative process, metabolic and genetic diseases affecting the sclera
- *Panuveitis/scleritis idiopathic* or associated with another systemic disease or vasculitis (SLE, BN, polyarteritis nodosa, sarcoidosis, EGP)
- *Panuveitis of infectious origin* (TB, syphilis, ARN, CMV retinitis, toxoplasma retinitis)

Complications

Corneal involvement can lead to loss of transparency, neovascularisation, and perforation of the cornea, while scleral involvement can lead to thinning of the sclera and perforation with loss of bulb integrity. Scleritis can be complicated by corneal involvement, cataract, and secondary glaucoma. Posterior scleritis can be complicated by uveitis, exudative retinal detachment, choroidal ablation, CME, optic disc oedema, secondary glaucoma, and cataract. Long-term optic nerve compression can result in optic nerve atrophy, with visual acuity loss of varying intensity. The damage to the retina and optic disc is often irreversible, with a permanent decline in visual function.

Therapy

The treatment of DES is described in Sect. 1. Local anti-inflammatory therapy (corticosteroids or NSAIDs) will reduce the inflammatory manifestations in the anterior segment but has little effect without general treatment. *Cave:* Periocular application of corticosteroids may contribute to scleral perforation [14]. Artificial tears may be applied in an adjunctive fashion, and antibiotics prophylactically for corneal infiltrates. Recurrent episcleritis responds favourably to long-term treatment with oral NSAIDs. In non-necrotising anterior scleritis, we administer NSAIDs in general, exceptionally in severe and unresponsive inflammation, prednisone orally. In the case of necrotising anterior scleritis with inflammation, systemic corticosteroids or in combination with other immunosuppressants, cyclosporine A (2.5–5 mg/kg/day) in a double or triple combination (methotrexate, azathioprine) are used. Mycophenolate mofetil (2 g/day) is also effective, and cyclophosphamide (2.5 mg/kg/day) is the drug of choice for GPA. The treatment of posterior scleritis is identical to that of the anterior necrotising form with inflammation. Orbital involvement in GPA is an indication for general treatment. Surgical therapy is possible in the treatment of peripheral corneal ulceration or necrotising scleritis to preserve the integrity of the globe (implantation of preserved or lyophilised sclera, synthetic materials such as Gore-Tex using tissue glue, corneal and scleral implants, amniotic membrane, lamellar eccentric keratoplasty).

The overall treatment is in the hands of the specialist and has two goals: to achieve remission with aggressive combined immunosuppression and to prevent relapse with maintenance therapy. To induce remission, prednisone at an initial dose of 1 mg/kg/day together with cyclophosphamide 2 mg/kg/day for the generalised form (also intravenous for the rapidly progressive or fulminant form), or methotrexate for the early systemic form, are used as first-choice drugs. For life-threatening conditions or organ function, methylprednisolone 1 g/day in an infusion for 3 consecutive days is added. In refractory forms, high doses of intravenous immunoglobulins or repeated plasmapheresis are added. Because of adverse effects, cyclophosphamide cannot be given long-term; in the maintenance phase, corticosteroids are combined with azathioprine, methotrexate, cyclosporine A; alternatively, mycophenolate mofetil or tacrolimus can be given. Of the biologics, infliximab and rituximab can be administered.

12.6 Eosinophilic Granulomatosis with Polyangiitis

Eosinophilic granulomatosis with polyangiitis is associated with bronchial asthma and peripheral eosinophilia. The lung involvement is similar to that of GPA, but the infiltration is variable or occurs under the picture of eosinophilic pneumonia. Eosinophilic inflammation can also occur in other organs (oesophagus, stomach, etc.) A serious complication is eosinophilic myocarditis and coronary vasculitis with life-threatening cardiac events even in young patients. Vasculitis can also occur on mesenteric arteries, then leading to an ischaemic bowel event.

Diffuse alveolar haemorrhage is less common than in GPA. Laboratory findings include p-ANCA directed against myeloperoxidase and eosinophilia in the differential blood picture.

12.7 Ocular Manifestations of Eosinophilic Granulomatosis with Polyangiitis

Ocular manifestation is present in EGP in less than 5% of cases [26]. It is usually a neuro-ophthalmological complication of intracranial involvement (oculomotor nerve palsy), or ischaemic neuropathy similar to giant cell arteritis. A small number of cases of uveitis have been described, usually in association with optic nerve papilla oedema or neurological complications. Episcleritis or scleritis, peripheral ulcerative keratitis may be present. Arterial and venous occlusions have also been described.

Risk factors

Presence of autoantibodies against neutrophil cytoplasm (mostly p-ANCA, less c-ANCA).

Clinical presentation and objective findings

Clinical symptoms, objective findings, complications, diagnosis, differential diagnosis of episcleritis, scleritis, peripheral ulcerative keratitis in Sect. 12, ischaemic neuropathy in Sect. 12.3.

Therapy

The overall therapy is in the hands of a specialist in the field. Corticosteroids are sufficient for milder forms. For more severe forms or when corticosteroids are contraindicated, azathioprine, methotrexate, or mycophenolate mofetil are added. In multiorgan manifestations, they are combined with cyclophosphamide in the form of pulses. In the most severe forms with renal involvement, treatment is initiated with pulses of methylprednisolone up to a total dose of 3 g. For resistant forms, interferon alpha is an alternative treatment.

12.8   Microscopic Polyangiitis

Microscopic polyangiitis is characterised by predilection of the kidney involvement (> 80%). The diagnosis is confirmed by renal biopsy. Lung involvement is less common, but diffuse alveolar haemorrhage and pulmonary-renal syndrome may occur. The neurological and cutaneous manifestations are similar to those of GPA. p-ANCA antibodies are more frequently demonstrated than c-ANCA. The therapeutic approach is specified in the 2016 joint recommendation of EULAR and the European Nephrology and Dialysis Transplant Association (ERA-EDTA) [42]. For very severe conditions, treatment in the acute phase is guided by massive doses of glucocorticoids with gradual detraction, cyclophosphamide, or rituximab. With rapid renal failure, a series of plasmapheresis is appropriate. In maintenance therapy, the safer azathioprine or mycophenolate mophetil is used. In less severe situations, glucocorticoids with methotrexate used.

12.9   Polyarteritis Nodosa

Polyarteritis nodosa is a rare form of vasculitis of mainly medium-sized vessels. It does not affect the kidneys and is ANCA-negative. It is characterised by skin involvement (necrotic lesions on the extremities, livedo reticularis), GIT involvement with a sudden abdominal episode with intestinal ischaemia; mononeuritis multiplex type is common. Orchitis in men is characteristic. Typical findings on angiography of the

Rheumatic Diseases

viscera include multiple stenoses, aneurysms and vessel occlusions. Similar findings may be present in the cerebral arteries. Definitive confirmation of the diagnosis is a biopsy of the affected organ, affecting all layers of the vascular wall.

12.10 Ocular Manifestations of Polyarteritis Nodosa

Polyarteritis nodosa (PAN) is a rare necrotising inflammatory vascular disease, affecting medium-sized and small arteries and leading to end-organ infarcts. Men are affected three times more often than women. The eyes are affected in about 10–20% of patients with PAN [18]. Necrotising scleritis, peripheral ulcerative keratitis (usually bilateral), anterior uveitis (with or without scleritis), retinal and choroidal vasculitis with ischaemia are possible [18]. The small and medium choroidal and retinal arteries are affected by inflammation in about 10% of cases. Hypertensive retinopathy is a secondary manifestation of renal involvement in PAN, leading to the development of hypertension. Neuro-ophthalmological manifestations include cranial nerve paresis, amaurosis fugax, homonymous hemianopsia, Horner's syndrome, and optic atrophy.

Risk factors

Male gender.

Clinical presentation

Inflammatory manifestations on the anterior segment of the eye are accompanied by "red eye", pain, photophobia, decrease in vision. With peripheral localisation of vasculitis, patients are initially without ocular symptoms. Later, in the case of the development of vitreous haemorrhage and opacities in the vitreous, a decrease in vision occurs. With central vasculitis, they complain of blurred vision and rapidly deteriorating vision.

Objective findings

The ocular findings in PUK and necrotising scleritis are described in Sect. 12. Hypertensive angiopathy is characterised by changes in the blood vessels (narrowing of arteries, crossing phenomena), haemorrhages, cotton wool spots, or star-shaped arrangement of hard exudates in the macula, up to oedema of the papilla of the optic disc [40]. Affection of the posterior ciliary arteries and choroidal vessels causes choroidal infarcts and exudative retinal detachment. Occlusions of predominantly retinal arteries are a frequent manifestation of the disease and are associated with retinal ischaemia to necrosis, cotton wool spots, Roth spots, and retinal infiltrates. In the chronic stage—neovascularisation forms.

Diagnosis

Diagnosis relies primarily on slit-lamp examination of both the anterior segment and the fundus in artificial mydriasis biomicroscopically. FAG examination demonstrates dye leakage in the inflamed vessel and zones of nonperfusion at the site of vascular occlusions. Perimeter examination is used to determine the extent of the dropouts in the field of view and to monitor changes in the field of view. OCT examination of the macula is used to monitor the development of CME and changes in the optic nerve papilla (oedema, atrophy).

Differential diagnosis

- Corneal ulceration—infectious ulcer, marginal keratitis in chronic blepharitis, Terrien's marginal degeneration, Mooren's ulcer
- Vasculopathy
- Arterial and venous occlusions of non-inflammatory origin
- Panuveitis/scleritis idiopathic or associated with another systemic disease or vasculitis (SLE, BN, GPA, sarcoidosis, EGP)
- Vasculitis of infectious origin
- Masking syndrome

Complications

Complications of PUK and necrotising scleritis are described in Sect. 12.5. Complications of vasculitis are the formation of neovascularisation, which can lead to vitreous haemorrhage. Oedema of the papilla may progress to atrophy with permanent visual impairment.

Therapy

In the case of vasculitis, general therapy is necessary, which is guided by a rheumatologist. Aggressive immunosuppressive therapy is often lifesaving [18]. PPV is indicated in non-resorbable vitreous haemorrhage.

13 Behçet's Disease

Behçet's disease is classified as a vasculitis affecting blood vessels of varying size. The characteristic triad is aphthous ulcerations, perigenital ulceration and uveitis. Geographically, the maximum incidence is in the Mediterranean region, the incidence follows the ancient Silk Road. European prevalence is 1–9/100,000 population. The association with the HLA B51 allele points to a possible genetic basis; elevation of pro-inflammatory cytokines (IL-17, IL-21, TGF-β) may be involved in the pathogenesis but may also be a consequence.

Clinical presentation

Oral aphthae occur in most patients, are significantly painful, heal spontaneously, but recur. Ulcerations on the external genitalia are present in 60–90% of patients, are torpid and may scar. The vascular involvement includes vasculitis of vessels of different size and its sequelae. Thrombophlebitis and deep vein thrombosis are common. Aneurysms of pulmonary arteries can cause fatal haemorrhage. CNS

Rheumatic Diseases 259

involvement is manifested by aseptic meningitis, lesions, and cognitive impairment (up to 30% of patients). Musculoskeletal involvement is manifested by monoarthritis of the middle joints, non-deforming but recurrent.

Diagnosis

The diagnosis is based on the presence of a typical triad of impairments [33]. A specific method of examination is the pathergy phenomenon—after subcutaneous injection of a needle, a papule or pustule develops at the injection site within 48 h.

Therapy

Skin lesions and arthritis respond to colchicine therapy. More severe ocular involvement, GIT involvement, neurological lesions, deep vein thrombosis or arterial involvement require glucocorticoids and immunosuppressive therapy, possibly biologic therapy with TNF blockers, ustekinumab, IL-6 or IL-17 blockers [43].

14 Ocular Manifestations of Behçet's Disease

Ocular manifestations in Behçet's disease may be one of the first manifestations of the disease. They are described in 60–85% of cases [21]. Ocular involvement is almost always bilateral, but individual attacks are usually unilateral or asymmetrical. Blindness due to ocular involvement in BN is described in 25% of cases [21]. A more favourable prognosis is described in women and in the form affecting the anterior segment, where remissions are longer than 6 months and the overall manifestations of BN are not numerous. The number and severity of recurrences in the first five years are crucial for irreversible ocular disability [21]. It is a severe sight-threatening inflammation, requiring the deployment of combined immunosuppressive therapy [14].

Risk factors

- HLA B51 antigen (more severe course of the disease)
- The appearance of neurological symptoms and disability (increased mortality)
- Geographical occurrence: Japan, Eastern Mediterranean, USA, Middle East; Turkey and Southeast Asia have a higher incidence and severity of uveitis

Clinical presentation

Patients' ocular symptoms can be variable and include a decrease in visual acuity of varying intensity, depending on the manifestations of inflammation, eye pain and photophobia.

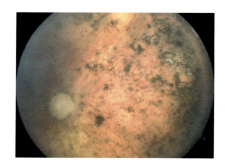

Fig. 16 Advanced findings in a patient after repeated attacks of posterior uveitis in BN—papillary atrophy, thinning to obliteration of vessels, diffuse chorioretinal scars

Objective findings

The main finding is recurrent serous anterior uveitis, sometimes with hypopyon formation. Uveitis often recurs. Signs of granulomatous inflammation (presence of mutton-fat precipitates on the endothelium, nodules on the iris or in the pupil) exclude BN [35]. Isolated anterior uveitis can also occur with minimal symptoms (known as cold hypopyon) or be completely asymptomatic. The intensity of vitritis may vary, and the fundus is dominated by the finding of retinal vasculitis affecting both arteries and veins, not infrequently occlusive with marked retinal ischaemia. The vessels are dilated, tortuous, accompanied by loose yellowish exudates and haemorrhages. Hypoxia due to vascular occlusions leads to retinal and optic disc neovascularisation, which tends to cause vitreous haemorrhages. Other manifestations are greyish white or yellowish uncircumscribed deposits in the retina and choroid. If ischaemia affects the optic nerve, oedema of the papillae occurs, with subsequent atrophy. In the case of recurrences, thinning, fibrotisation and occlusion of blood vessels may be noted, as well as the formation of chorioretinal scars (Fig. 16).

Vitreoretinal pathology is a rare cause of retinal hole formation and its subsequent detachment. Less common manifestations may include conjunctivitis, conjunctival ulceration, episcleritis, scleritis and ophthalmoplegia in neurological involvement. A papilledema has also been described as a sign of intracranial hypertension in cerebral vein thrombosis or dural sinus.

Diagnosis

For diagnosis, the anterior segment and fundus are examined biomicroscopically in a slit lamp. FAG examination is used to assess the activity of vasculitis, the exact extent of areas of non-perfusion after vascular occlusions and the extent of neovascularisation. OCT is used to view and monitor the extent of CME and ERM.

Differential diagnosis

- Anterior uveitis in HLA B27-positive patients
- Lens-induced anterior uveitis
- Mycotic and bacterial uveitis
- Retinopathy in SLE, syphilis
- Masking syndromes

Complications

Complications include posterior synechiae, neovascular glaucoma, cataract, vitreous opacification and haemorrhage, retinal vessel sheathing (up to silver wiring appearance), retinal neovascularisation, cystoid macular oedema, ERM, and papillary atrophy.

Therapy

In anterior uveitis, intensive therapy with corticosteroids (every hour) and mydriatics in the form of drops is necessary initially, gradually in a decreasing dose for 6–8 weeks. If therapy fails, corticosteroids can be applied peribulbarly. Non-steroidal antiphlogistic drugs have analgesic and anti-inflammatory effects. In the treatment of glaucoma, beta-blockers and carbonic anhydrase inhibitors are deployed.

BN is considered an absolute indication for immunosuppressive therapy. Posterior uveitis is treated with total corticosteroid administration (at the beginning of pulse therapy, in combination with additional immunosuppressive therapy. Corticosteroids alone are effective only at the onset of the disease; they are ineffective when administered in monotherapy for a long time, and the inflammation becomes resistant. Cyclosporine A (2–5 mg/kg/day) and azathioprine (2.5 mg/kg/day) are good immunosuppressive agents; mycophenolate mofetil and pulse therapy with cyclophosphamide may be additional drugs. Biological therapy that has proven effective includes interferon alfa and infliximab, which are well tolerated, provide better control of ocular inflammation, and reduce recurrences. Rituximab is effective for retinal vasculitis. Therapy must be long-term, and drug doses must be adjusted (increased or decreased) according to the activity of the inflammation. Surgical treatment (surgery for cataract, vitreoretinal complications, or secondary glaucoma) should be performed in patients without signs of inflammatory activity and with sufficient immunosuppressive therapy. Treatment of neovascularisation with retinal laser photocoagulation is possible, but some uveologists warn against it because of the risk of possible exacerbation of the disease.

15 Cogan Syndrome

Cogan's syndrome is a rare vasculitis affecting blood vessels of the eyes, vestibular apparatus and with systemic vasculitis, especially of the aorta. Inner ear involvement is manifested by dizziness, nausea, tinnitus, and hearing loss, usually bilateral, up to complete loss. Aortitis occurs in about one-tenth of patients and may lead to aortic insufficiency or manifestations of myocardial ischaemia. The disease has no specific test; inflammatory laboratory markers may be elevated.

The diagnosis is based on the clinical presentation, there are no broadly used classification criteria for the rarity of the condition [13].

Therapy is mainly guided by the severity of the ocular involvement or other serious organ lesions and includes a broad spectrum, ranging from topical glucocorticoids to systemic immunosuppressive therapy with cyclophosphamide [36]. Reports on the effect of biological therapy are still controversial (tocilizumab, rituximab, TNF-alpha blockers) [12].

16 Ocular Manifestations of Cogan Syndrome

Cogan syndrome is a rare disease, affecting mainly young adults, both sexes equally often, but children can also acquire the disease. Typically, it involves interstitial keratitis associated with vestibulocochlear disease, most manifested by sudden hearing loss (50% of cases) and other symptoms such as tinnitus, vertigo, nausea, and vomiting. Hearing loss can be permanent. The syndrome may occur alone or in association with systemic vasculitis in up to 30% of cases (polyarteritis nodosa, RA, GPA) [4]. Vasculitis explains systemic symptoms, most commonly headache, arthralgia, temperature and aortitis. The ocular involvement in typical Cogan syndrome includes interstitial keratitis, accompanied by conjunctival hyperaemia, sometimes suffusion, and anterior uveitis; in atypical Cogan syndrome, exophthalmos, tenonitis, conjunctivitis, episcleritis, scleritis, posterior uveitis, vitritis, papillitis, and occlusive vasculitis may be encountered.

Risk factors

- Unknown

Clinical presentation

Patients complain of "red eye", tearing, photophobia and eye pain. The decrease in visual acuity depends on the degree of corneal involvement.

Objective findings

Keratitis is usually bilateral, only sometimes unilateral. We see keratitis of varying degrees on the cornea of the eye, typically starting in the periphery in the anterior stroma, then progressing deeper and more centrally, leaving opacities in the cornea that may be accompanied by varying degrees of pathological vascularisation.

Diagnosis

From an ophthalmic point of view, it relies on the examination of the anterior segment on a slit lamp. ENT examination, NMR of the head and other examinations according to the general symptoms are indicated.

Differential diagnosis

Interstitial keratitis of other aetiology, which may be associated with deafness (TB, chlamydial and viral infections, RA).

Complications

A complication is scarring of the cornea, leading to deterioration of visual acuity.

Therapy

In ocular topical therapy, corticosteroids or mydriatic agents in keratitis are used. In the acute phase, local therapy is supported by systemic corticosteroid therapy in moderate to high doses to prevent hearing loss [21]. Overall long-term therapy is based on systemic symptoms and any systemic vasculitis detected.

References

1. Aletaha D, Neogi T, Silman AJ, et al. Rheumatoid arthritis classification criteria: an ACR/EULAR collaborative initiative. Ann Rheum Dis. 2010;69:1580–8.
2. Almaani S, Fussner LA, Brodsky S, et al. ANCA-associated vasculitis: an update. J Clin Med. 2021;10(7):1446.
3. Aringer M, Costenbader K, Daikh D, et al. European league against rheumatism/American College of Rheumatology classification criteria for systemic lupus erythematosus. Ann Rheum Dis. 2019;78:1151–9.
4. Bowling B. Kanski's clinical ophthalmology. 8th ed. Amsterdam: Elsevier; 2016.
5. Bukiri H, Volkmann ER. Current advances in the treatment of systemic sclerosis. Curr Opin Pharmacol. 2022;64:102211.
6. England BR. Clinical manifestations of rheumatoid arthritis. Up to date www.uptodate.com ©2023 UpToDate, Inc.
7. Fanouriakis A, Kostopoulou M, Alunno A, et al. 2019 update of the EULAR recommendations for the management of systemic lupus erythematosus. Ann Rheum Dis. 2019;78(6):736–45.
8. Fanouriakis A, Kostopoulou M, Cheema K, et al. Update of the Joint European League Against Rheumatism and European Renal Association-European Dialysis and Transplant Association (EULAR/ERA-EDTA) recommendations for the management of lupus nephritis. Ann Rheum Dis. 2020;79(6):713–23.
9. Felson DT, Smolen JS, Wells G, et al. American College of Rheumatology/European League against rheumatism provisional definition of remission in rheumatoid arthritis for clinical trials. Ann Rheum Dis. 2011;70:404–13.
10. Gossec L, Baraliakos X, Kerschbaumer A, et al. EULAR recommendations for the management of psoriatic arthritis with pharmacological therapies: 2019 update. Ann Rheum Dis. 2020;79:700–12.
11. Grayson PC, Ponte C, Suppiah R, Robson JC, Gribbons KB, Judge A, Craven A, Khalid S, Hutchings A, Danda D, Luqmani RA, Watts RA, Merkel PA; DCVAS study group. 2022 American College of Rheumatology/EULAR classification criteria for takayasu arteritis. Arthritis Rheumatol. 2022 Dec;74(12):1872–1880. https://doi.org/10.1002/art.42324. Epub 2022 Nov 8. PMID: 36349501.
12. Greco A, De Virgilio A, Ralli M, et al. Behçet's disease: new insights into pathophysiology, clinical features and treatment options. Autoimmun Rev. 2018;17:567–75.
13. Greco A, Gallo A, Fusconi M, et al. Cogan's syndrome: an autoimmune inner ear disease. Autoimmun Rev. 2013;12(3):396–400.
14. Heissigerova J. Ophthalmology: for undergraduate and postgraduate study. Prague: Maxdorf s.r.o; 2018.
15. Hellmich B, Agueda A, Monti S, et al. Update of the EULAR recommendations for the management of large vessel vasculitis. Ann Rheum Dis. 2020;79:19–30.

16. Hunder GG, Bloch DA, Michel BA, et al. The American College of Rheumatology 1990 revised criteria for the classification of giant cell arteritis. Arthritis Rheum. 1990;33:1122–8.
17. Jennette JC. Overview of the 2012 revised international Chapel hill consensus conference nomenclature of vasculitides. Clin Exp Nephrol. 2013 Oct;17(5):603–606. https://doi.org/10.1007/s10157-013-0869-6. Epub 2013 Sep 27. PMID: 24072416; PMCID: PMC4029362.
18. Jones N. Uveitis. 2nd ed. London: JP Medical; 2013.
19. Kowal-Bielecka O, Fransen J, Avouac J, Becker M, Kulak A, Allanore Y, Distler O, Clements P, Cutolo M, Czirjak L, Damjanov N, Del Galdo F, Denton CP, Distler JHW, Foeldvari I, Figelstone K, Frerix M, Furst DE, Guiducci S, Hunzelmann N, Khanna D, Matucci-Cerinic M, Herrick AL, van den Hoogen F, van Laar JM, Riemekasten G, Silver R, Smith V, Sulli A, Tarner I, Tyndall A, Welling J, Wigley F, Valentini G, Walker UA, Zulian F, Müller-Ladner U; EUSTAR Coauthors. Update of EULAR recommendations for the treatment of systemic sclerosis. Ann Rheum Dis. 2017 Aug; 76(8):1327–1339. https://doi.org/10.1136/annrheumdis-2016-209909. Epub 2016 Nov 9. PMID: 27941129.
20. Kozak I, Rovensky J, Stvrtinova V, et al. Ophthalmorheumatology. Prague: Galen; 2017.
21. Kuchynka P. Ophthalmology. 2nd ed. Prague: Grada Publishing a.s; 2016.
22. Kvist-Hansen A, Riis Hansen P, Skov L. Systemic treatment of psoriasis with JAK Inhibitors: a review. Dermatol Ther (Heidelb). 2020;10:29–42.
23. Merkel PA. Overview of and approach to the vasculitides in adults. Up to date www.uptodate.com ©2023 UpToDate, Inc.
24. Moreland LW, Canella A. General principles and overview of management of rheumatoid arthritis in adults. Up to date www.uptodate.com ©2023 UpToDate, Inc.
25. Negrini S, Emmi G, Greco M, et al. Sjögren's syndrome: a systemic autoimmune disease. Clin Exp Med. 2022;22(1):9–25.
26. Pavelka K. Rheumatology. 2nd revised. Prague: Galen; 2010.
27. Ponte C, Grayson PC, Robson JC, et al. 2022 American College of Rheumatology/EULAR classification criteria for giant cell arteritis. Ann Rheum Dis. 2022;81:1647–53.
28. Ramiro S, Nikiphorou E, Sepriano A, et al. ASAS-EULAR recommendations for the management of axial spondyloarthritis: 2022 update. Ann Rheum Dis. 2023;82:19–34.
29. Ramos-Casals M, Brito-Zerón P, Bombardieri S, et al. EULAR recommendations for the management of Sjogren's syndrome with topical and systemic therapies. Ann Rheum Dis. 2020;79:3–18.
30. Ringold S, Angeles-Han ST, Beukelman T, et al. American College of Rheumatology/Arthritis Foundation guideline for the treatment of juvenile idiopathic arthritis: therapeutic approaches for non-systemic polyarthritis, sacroiliitis, and enthesitis arthritis. Care Res. 2019;71:717–34.
31. Rudwaleit M, van der Heijde D, Landewé R, et al. The Assessment of SpondyloArthritis International Society classification criteria for peripheral spondyloarthritis and for spondyloarthritis in general. Ann Rheum Dis. 2011;70(1):25–31.
32. Shiboski CH, Shiboski SC, Seror R, et al. 2016 American College of Rheumatology/European League Against Rheumatism classification criteria for primary Sjögren's syndrome. Ann Rheum Dis. 2017;76:9–16.
33. Smith EL, Yazici Y. Clinical manifestations and diagnosis of Behçet syndrome. Up to date www.uptodate.com ©2023 UpToDate, Inc.
34. Smolen JS, Landewé RBM, Bergstra SA, et al. EULAR recommendations for the management of rheumatoid arthritis with synthetic and biological disease-modifying antirheumatic drugs: 2022 update. Ann Rheum Dis. 2023;82:3–18.
35. Svozilkova P. Uveitis in case reports. Prague: Maxdorf; 2016.
36. Tayer-Shifman OE, Ilan O, Tovi H, et al. Cogan's syndrome—clinical guidelines and novel therapeutic approaches. Clinic Rev Allerg Immunol. 2014;47:65–72.
37. Taylor W, Gladman D, Helliwell P, et al. Classification criteria for psoriatic arthritis: development of new criteria from a large international study. Arthritis Rheum. 2006;54:2665–73.
38. van den Hoogen F, Khanna D, Frensen J, et al. Classification criteria for systemic sclerosis: an ACR-EULAR collaborative initiative. Arthritis Rheum. 2013;65:2737–47.

Rheumatic Diseases

39. Varga J. Clinical manifestations and diagnosis of systemic sclerosis (scleroderma) in adults. Up to date www.uptodate.com ©2023 UpToDate, Inc.
40. Vazquez-Romo KA, Rodriguez-Hernandez A, Paczka JA, et al. Optic neuropathy secondary to polyarteritis nodosa, case report, and diagnostic challenges. Front Neurol. 2017;8:490.
41. Wallace DJ, Gladman DD. Clinical manifestations and diagnosis of systemic lupus erythematosus in adults. Up to date www.uptodate.com ©2023 UpToDate, Inc.
42. Yates M, Watts RA, Bajema IM, et al. EULAR/ERA-EDTA recommendations for the management of ANCA-associated vasculitis. Ann Rheum Dis. 2016;75:1583–94.
43. Yazici Y. Management of Behcet syndrome. Curr Opin Rheumatol. 2020;32:35–40.
44. Zaripova LN, Midgley A, Christmas SE, et al. Juvenile idiopathic arthritis: from aetiopathogenesis to therapeutic approaches. Pediatr Rheumatol. 2021;19:135–49.

Skin Diseases

Marketa Stredova, Miloslav Salavec, and Andrea Bartlova

1 Epidermal Necrolysis

Stevens-Johnson syndrome (SJS) and toxic epidermal necrolysis (TEN) are diseases within the spectrum of severe cutaneous adverse reactions (SCAR) affecting the skin and mucosal membranes. They are most often caused by a hypersensitivity reaction to certain drugs (antibiotics, anticonvulsants or non-steroidal anti-inflammatory drugs, see below), more rarely by parainfection in *Herpes simplex* and *Mycoplasma pneumoniae* infections, in malignant tumours and in connection with vaccination in children. They occur with relatively high frequency in immunosuppressed patients, especially HIV-positive persons [7]. Stevens-Johnson syndrome without skin involvement (mucous membranes, eyes) is called Fuchs syndrome. This spectrum of SCAR diseases includes other clinical entities differing in clinical manifestations, prognosis and aetiology, such as erythema multiforme majus (EMM) or the bullous form of erythema multiforme.

SJS and TEN are characterised by skin erythema with formation of blisters of various extent, haemorrhagic erosions of mucosal membranes, with manifestations

---

M. Stredova (✉)
Eye Centre VISUS, spol. s r.o., Nemcove 738, 547 01 Nachod, Czech Republic
e-mail: marketa.stredova@gmail.com

Department of Ophthalmology, University Hospital and Faculty of Medicine of Charles University in Hradec Králové, Sokolska 581, 500 05 Hradec Králové, Czech Republic

M. Salavec · A. Bartlova
Department of Skin and Sexually Transmitted Diseases, University Hospital and Faculty of Medicine of Charles University in Hradec Králové, Sokolska 581, 500 05 Hradec Králové, Czech Republic
e-mail: miloslav.salavec@fnhk.cz

A. Bartlova
e-mail: andrea.bartlova@fnhk.cz

© The Author(s), under exclusive license to Springer Nature Switzerland AG 2024
A. Stepanov and J. Studnicka (eds.), *Ocular Manifestations of Systemic Diseases*,
https://doi.org/10.1007/978-3-031-58592-0_7

of stomatitis, balanitis, colpitis, severe conjunctivitis and blepharitis. The first symptoms of the disease are often fever and fatigue, which may persist or even increase after the appearance of mucocutaneous lesions [7].

The classification published by Bastuji-Garin in 1993 is based on the type of individual lesions and the extent of blister formation and erosions in relation to the overall skin surface (*B*ody *S*urface *A*rea, BSA) [4].

Skin changes in these severe skin reactions are classified based on the type of individual lesions and the proportion of BSA involvement. They are typically disc-like with a regular round shape, well circumscribed and showing at least three distinct concentric zones: a purpuric central disc with or without blistering, an oedematous intermediate ring with infiltration and an erythematous outer ring.

In contrast, atypical, infiltrated discs present with only two zones and poor demarcation, whereas atypical flat discs are characterised by a vesicular or bullous lesion in the centre, and these vesicular lesions may blend.

Typical or atypical infiltrated discs are characteristic of erythema multiforme majus (EMM). They appear mainly on the limbs, sometimes also on the face and trunk, especially in children. On the other hand, spreading, often confluent purple macules or atypical flat disc-like lesions, predominantly occurring on the trunk, are among the cutaneous characteristics of SJS. In both units, different mucosal areas are also severely affected. As only small blisters appear in the disc-like lesions of most EMM cases, the extent of skin shedding is usually limited—often to 1–2% of BSA, whereas in SJS these values are higher but do not exceed 10%. The diagnosis of TEN requires the detection of skin detachment in more than 30% of the BSA, which represents the entire trunk excluding the buttocks. Disseminated macules and atypical disc-like lesions, such as those found in SJS, precede epidermal detachment in most cases (TEN with macular changes). However, cases of TEN arising from larger erythema without evidence of confluent macules and with an extent of detachment slightly greater than 10% (TEN without macular changes, also called TEN with extensive erythema) may also be found. SJS and TEN are sometimes very difficult to distinguish between, because, even with less extensive skin shedding, SJS may show signs of extensive skin necrosis typical of TEN [20]. A direct Nikolsky sign and an indirect Nikolsky sign (displacement of an existing blister) are known characteristics of this phenomenon. However, recently the use of the terms "wet" and "dry" Nikolsky signs have been discussed to describe the base of the blister and thus the level of epidermal separation. Haemorrhagic erosions present on at least one of the mucosal membranes are diagnosed in EMM, SJS and in the "overlap" of SJS/TEN but may be absent in some cases of TEN. The summarised characteristics of these units are presented in Table 7.1.

While SJS, "overlap" SJS/TEN and TEN with present macular changes are considered as a single entity of varying severity, EMM differs in both clinical characteristics and aetiology [25].

Epidemiology

The average annual incidence of TEN worldwide ranges from 0.4–1.3 cases/million population. For unknown reasons, women are affected at higher rates (1.5:1 ratio). TEN occurs in all age groups; however, the average age of patients is reported

Skin Diseases

Table 7.1 Characteristics of different types of SCAR (Severe Cutaneous Adverse Reactions)

SCAR type	SJS	SJS/TEN overlap	TEN	EMM
Extent of disability according to BSA	3–10%	10–30%	> 30% (TEN on the basis of erythema > 10%)	1–2%
Morphology of skin lesions	Spreading, often confluent purpuric macular lesions, atypical flat disc lesions, haemorrhagic blisters	Lesions of both types of SCAR	Initially disseminated confluent maculae and typical disc lesions, less frequently TEN on the background of extensive erythema without macular lesions	Typical convex disc lesions, smaller vesicles
Localization of disability	Especially on the trunk Mucosal involvement (haemorrhagic erosions)		Haemorrhagic erosions are sometimes not present	Especially the extremities, on the trunk and face especially in children Mucosal involvement NO
Nikolsky's sign	Positive	Positive	Positive	Negative
CRP	High values	High values	High values	Low values
Aetiology	Drug induction	Drug induction	Drug induction	Parainfectious

(SJS: Stevens-Johnson syndrome; SJS/TEN overlap: transitional type of Stevens-Johnson syndrome and toxic epidermal necrolysis; TEN: toxic epidermal necrolysis; EMM: erythema multiforme majus; BSA: body surface area; CRP: total reactive protein)

to be between 46–63 years of age. Possible mechanisms od inducing skin lesions are immunopathways resulting in keratinocyte apoptosis in TEN in adults (Table 7.2), whereas parainfectious aetiology is more common in children [13]. Older people have a higher risk of developing the disease, also due to the numerous medications indicated.

Clinical presentation

SJS and TEN are characterised by skin erythema with formation of blisters of various extent, haemorrhagic erosions of mucosal membranes with manifestations of stomatitis, balanitis, colpitis, severe conjunctivitis and blepharitis. The first symptoms of the disease are often fever and fatigue, which may persist or even increase after the appearance of mucocutaneous lesions. It is sometimes very difficult to distinguish between SJS and TEN. Because, even with less extensive skin shedding (as in SJS), SJS may also show signs of extensive skin necrosis typical of TEN.

Table 7.2 Drug groups associated with SJS/TEN

Antibiotics	Chemotherapeutics
Aminoglycosides Chloramphenicol Macrolides (Erythromycin) Penicillins Sulphonamides Tetracyclines Quinolones (Ciprofloxacin, Trovafloxacin) Gyrase inhibitors	Antituberculotics Nitrofurans
Analgesics, antiphlogistics, antirheumatics **Anticonvulsants, hypnotics, sedatives (NSAIDs)**	**Anticonvulsants, hypnotics, sedatives**
Phenylbutazones, Oxybutazones Diclofenac Ibuprofen Indomethacin Salicylic acid Piroxicam, Tenoxicam Phenacetin Pyrazonolone derivatives Benoxaprofen	Phenobarbital Phenytoin Phenothiazine derivatives Carbamazepine Derivatives of hydantoin Valproic acid Lamotrigine
Antifungals	*Antineoplastic chemotherapeutics*
Griseofulvin Fluconazole Terbinafine	Chlorambucil Cyclophosphamide Methotrexate
Antiuratics	*Betablockers*
Allopurinol Colchicine	Atenolol Propranolol
Diuretics	
Chlorthalidone Benzothiazidine derivatives	

For these reasons, a transitional group of SJS/TEN diseases characterised by blisters and erosions between 10–30% of BSA was also defined and labelled as "SJS/TEN overlap". A positive Nikolsky sign for SJS, TEN and the overlap group is present. Haemorrhagic erosions present on at least one of the mucosal membranes are diagnosed in EMM, SJS and in the "overlap" of SJS/TEN but may be absent in some cases of TEN. While SJS, "overlap" SJS/TEN and TEN with present macular changes are considered as a single entity of different severity, erythema multiforme majus (EMM) is different both in clinical characteristics and aetiological factors.

1.1 *Stevens-Johnson Syndrome*

Classification

Skin Diseases

As suggested above, skin changes in the disease are classified based on the type of individual lesions and the proportion of BSA involvement. Stevens-Johnson syndrome, "overlap" SJS/TEN and TEN with macular changes present are essentially considered as a single entity of varying severity.

Clinical presentation

The course of the disease varies individually. Onset of skin changes does not cause subjective discomfort initially, except for some pruritus. Patients report fatigue and headaches, and dissemination of skin eruption is often accompanied by haemorrhages and blistering. The oral, ocular, genital mucosa are affected. However, bronchitis, pneumonia, kidney involvement with haematuria and high fever may also occur. Renal failure in tubular necrosis and toxic circulatory failure are also rare.

Examinations

In the clinical presentation of SJS, spreading, often confluent purpuric macules or atypical flat target lesions are found, predominantly arising on the trunk. Various mucosal regions are also severely affected (Figs. 7.1 and 7.2).

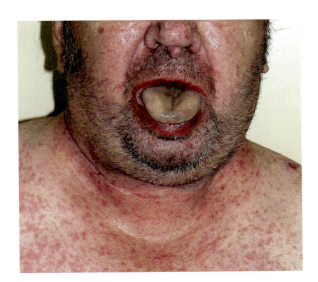

Fig. 7.1 Skin and mucosal manifestations in a patient with SJS

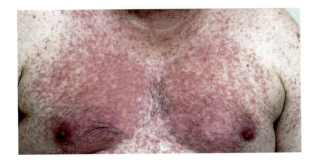

Fig. 7.2 Torso involvement in a patient with SJS

The extent of skin shedding is usually limited—often from 3 to 10% of the BSA (higher for the SJS/TEN overlap unit and TEN) [21]. Haemorrhagic erosions present on at least one of the mucosal membranes tend to be present in SJS, as in EMM, in the SJS/TEN "overlap".

Differential diagnosis

It is necessary to differentiate foot and mouth disease, when blistering occurs in the palms of the hands and on the mucous membrane of the oral cavity. The problems may also be *Pemphigus vulgaris* with manifestations limited to the mucous membranes (especially the oral cavity), or the multiform character of bullous pemphigoid in the acute phase of the disease (differentiated according to the age structure of those affected). A similar picture can be presented by *vasculitis allergica* or *dermatitis herpetiformis*. Flat blisters on the palms and dorsal sides of the hands and painful involvement of the oral mucosa without involvement of the lips may be present in *hand, foot and mouth disease* (Coxsackie A16, A5, A10 viruses). It is important also to remember *morbus Kawasaki*. Finally, even the initial phase of TEN can mimic the picture of SJS.

Diagnosis

Histopathological examination in Stevens-Johnson syndrome shows vasodilatation, with an infiltrate consisting mainly of lymphocytes in the upper corium with a tendency to exocytosis.

Therapy

In all SCAR clinical entities, therapy must be tailored to the severity and extent of disability in the individual patient. Given the circumstances of the ambiguous pathogenesis of SJS/TEN, therapy is based on non-specific and symptomatic agents. Symptomatic therapy will be important in patients with extensive skin surface shedding, requiring intensive care in specialised centres [41]. In addition, the aim of therapy is to prevent serious consequences, such as strictures of mucosal membranes and the development of symblepharon.

Specialised care is critical when mucosal surfaces are affected. The severity of mucosal involvement is often inconsistent with the extent of skin surface shedding, and the neglect of mucosal lesion care can lead to lifelong problems.

Immunomodulatory and systemic therapy

- Immunomodulatory therapies are also indicated in the treatment of SJS/TEN. The increased number of infections, the risk of suppression of septicaemia symptoms, delayed re-epithelialisation and prolonged duration of hospitalisation, as well as higher mortality rates argue against the use of systemic corticosteroids. IVIG, which has been documented as an effective treatment for TEN, based on the hypothesis that human immunoglobulin antibodies block Fas-mediated keratinocyte necrosis in vitro, is still controversial. The SCORTEN score is used to evaluate the prognosis of individual patients (Table 7.3) [11]. Despite all these controversies, experts consider it most important to stop the administration of all drugs potentially triggering the development of the disease.

Contraindications to the administration of corticosteroids are sepsis, mycotic affections, peptic ulcers, and pulmonary oedema.

Skin Diseases

Table 7.3 SJS/TEN score: SCORTEN (Severity-of-illness score for TEN), 1 point for each positive item

Evaluated items	Points	0 points	1 point/1 item
Age of those affected		< 40 years	> 40 years
Heart rate		< 120/min	> 120/min
History of malignancy		No	Yes
BSA—% of total body surface area affected		< 10%	> 10%
S-urea		< 10 mmol/L	> 10 mmol/L
S-HCO$_3^-$		> 20 mmol/L	< 20 mmol/L
S-glucose		< 14 mmol/L	> 14 mmol/L
		Minimum 0 points, maximum 7 points	

1.2 Toxic Epidermal Necrolysis (Lyell's Syndrome)

Classification

It is the same clinical entity as SJS, differing in the extent and severity of the disability. The specific drugs administered are most often in the background.

Clinical presentation

The course of the disease is more severe, due to the larger extent of the disease compared to SJS.

Examinations

The extent of disability is reported to be more than 30% of the BSA. In these cases, typical disc-like lesions and disseminated macular, gradually confluent eruption with predominantly skin involvement are found.

Diagnosis

The diagnostic methods are identical to those described above for SJS.

Therapy

In general, all the therapeutic schemes outlined above apply, with an emphasis on supportive care and interdisciplinary collaboration [8, 17, 33, 42].

Prognosis

The prognosis of the disease tends to be worse compared to SJS, due to the extent and severity of TEN.

1.3 SJS/TEN Overlap

Classification

The transitional type of SJS/TEN is characterised by a range of disability from 10–30% BSA.

Clinical presentation

The course of the disease is identical to that described above for SJS. Due to the greater extent of involvement of the total BSA, a higher number of ensuing complications can be expected.

Examinations

In the clinical presentation, we find changes that correspond to typical lesions of both SJS and TEN. Thus, the presence of spreading, often confluent, purpuric macules, atypical flat disc-like lesions, as well as disseminated confluent erythematous foci with typical disc-like lesions are found. Nikolsky phenomena are often positive. Various mucosal regions are also affected, where we find haemorrhagic erosions. Skin shedding ranges from 3–10% BSA.

Diagnosis

Histopathological examination in this type shows similar findings to those described for SJS above. The cellular infiltrate composed of T-lymphocytes is more abundant compared to SJS. Signs of vacuolar degeneration in the epidermis may also be detected.

Therapy

Topical and systemic therapy are identical to the data mentioned above. Due to the definition of a transitional state, the need for intensive supportive care increases.

Prognosis

Transitional states are characterised by a higher incidence of complications, possibly serious consequences. These complications otherwise correspond to the complications mentioned above.

2 Ocular Manifestations of Stevens-Johnson Syndrome

Ocular involvement in Stevens-Johnson syndrome (SJS) is relatively common. Its extent and severity in the acute phase may not correlate with the degree of skin involvement [40]. SJS is a skin and mucous membrane blistering disease; in the case of the eyes, the eyelids, conjunctiva, and cornea are affected. Due to the possible gradual progression of symptoms, daily ophthalmological examination is necessary, to provide adequate care for the prevention of the development of irreversible consequences of scarring [22].

Chronic complications occur in up to one-half of patients.

Clinical symptoms

Patients most often suffer from severe eye discomfort, decreased visual acuity and photophobia.

Objective findings

Eyelids

In the acute phase, eyelid oedema occurs, eventually compromising the integrity of the eyelid skin with typical desquamation [26]. In the chronic phase, scarring of the eyelid margins follows, i.e. the orifices of the Meibomian glands and the eyelid margins have an uneven surface [10] . Abnormalities of the eyelashes or pathological position of the eyelids are also found.

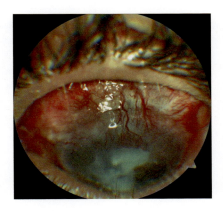

Fig. 7.3 Anterior segment findings in a patient with SJS. Symblepharon, conjunctivalisation and corneal scarring

Conjunctiva

In milder affections, the manifestation of SJS on the conjunctiva is only in the form of its congestion, with possible mucous secretion or chemosis. In more severe cases, membranous conjunctivitis or disruption of epithelial integrity develops [35]. The size of the lesion determines the severity of the condition. In the chronic phase, the development of symblepharons and shortening of fornixes is typical.

Cornea

The manifestations of SJS on the cornea have a wide spectrum. In the acute phase, we find punctate keratopathy or epithelial defects, depending on the severity of the involvement; later a corneal ulcer or corneal perforation may develop (Fig. 7.3) [35].

If the limbal stem cells are damaged, this causes conjunctivalisation and corneal scarring [2]. Irregular astigmatism, corneal bulging and uneven corneal surface are other causes of visual acuity loss in the chronic phase of the disease [32].

Diagnosis

From the ophthalmological point of view, the basic examination of the anterior ocular segment after fluorescein staining to assess the integrity of the ocular surface is crucial.

Differential diagnosis

- Erythema multiforme major
- Acute cutaneous form of lupus erythematosus similar to toxic epidermal necrolysis
- Bullous dermatosis with linear deposits of IgA in the dermo-epidermal junction
- Type 1 immunopathological reaction to the drug

Therapy

Topical antibiotics, cyclosporine, corticosteroids, and artificial tears are administered for ocular manifestations of SJS. In severe dry eye syndrome in the chronic phase, serum drops are prescribed [40]. Scleral and therapeutic contact lenses are also used. Among the surgical interventions used in this diagnosis, amniotic membrane transplantation is essential; its early performance (within 7–10 days) serves to prevent long-term scarring sequelae in more severe cases with conjunctival staining over 1 cm in diameter [10]. When symblepharons occur, they are loosened. Tear point occlusion is considered in chronic dry eye syndrome. Other procedures in SJS include corneal replacement with keratoprosthesis, limbal cell transplantation or mucosal membrane graft to replace scarred tarsal conjunctiva [40]. Standard corneal transplantation (*penetrating keratoplasty,* PKP) is doomed to failure [35].

3 Atopic Dermatitis

Atopic dermatitis (AD), syn. *prurigo Besnier, neurodermatitis atopica,* is a common itchy chronic or chronically relapsing non-infectious, hereditary disease [28]. It usually starts in infancy. The clinical presentation is characterised by a triad of manifestations: dermatitis, xerosis and pruritus. Alternating periods of remission and exacerbation of symptoms are typical. It is often associated with a positive personal or family anamnesis of allergic rhinitis, conjunctivitis and bronchial asthma.

Epidemiology

AD is a disease predominantly of infancy and childhood. Most cases of AD manifest by the age of 3 years—called the "early-onset" form. In approximately 70% of children, spontaneous remission occurs before reaching adulthood [28]. AD can first manifest in adulthood—known as the "late-onset" form.

Aetiopathogenesis

AD is a multifactorial disease and the aetiopathogenesis is very complex. It is a genetically complex disease, resulting both from the interaction between the genes themselves and between the genes and the external environment. The skin barrier disorder is considered to be primary and is related both to a disorder of keratinisation, but also to a reduced number of ceramides. Furthermore, morphological abnormalities of Odland's lamellar bodies and impaired exocytosis into the extracellular matrix were described. This is related to the reduced ability of atopic skin to bind water (excessive water leakage and the typical dryness of atopic skin). Because of the barrier disorder, the skin is more susceptible to colonisation by *Staphylococcus aureus* strains, both in areas with eczema and in areas of clinically "healthy" skin (in 90% of patients with AD) [28]. Staphylococci produce what are called "superantigens" (enterotoxins A and B, toxin TSST-1—toxic shock syndrome toxin 1, etc.), which themselves can induce inflammation by their toxic effects and also significantly activate T-lymphocytes (Th2 type of inflammation) and macrophages.

Clinical presentation

The first and obvious symptom is pruritus. The manifestations of AD are highly variable and change, depending on the age of the patient [3].

Several forms of AD can be distinguished according to age:

Infant form—begins, as a rule, in the first months of life. Manifestations are usually localised symmetrically on the cheeks and forehead; progression to the whole face, neck, scalp or earlobes and dissemination to the diaper localisation are possible [12]. Morphologically, they are itchy papules and vesicles, with a tendency to merge into erythematous plaques. Wetting is typical and the surface of the lesions is covered with

Fig. 7.4 Atopic eczema, Dannie-Morgani infraorbital eyelash

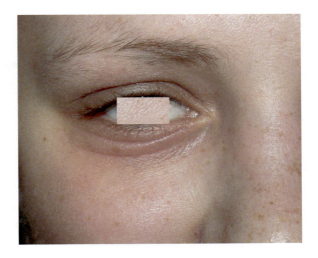

yellow crusts after drying. The manifestations are severely itchy, leading to scratching and impetiginisation of the lesions with regional lymphadenitis. The child tends to be tearful and sleeps poorly. The skin is dry, peels gently, and rhagades may form in the folds. In exceptional cases, erythroderma may occur. Deterioration of AD tends to be related to infections. Definitive healing is possible within a year, but symptoms often return within two years of age and persist even longer in some patients.

Paediatric form—in children from toddler age to 14 years. The character of eczematous manifestations changes, exudation subsides and the process becomes chronic. In addition to the face, the neck, flexor limbs, backs of hands, ankles, buttocks, back of thighs, lips, onychodystrophy may occur. Lichenification and distinctive deep skin lines are typical. Again, there is often an impetiginisation of the symptoms. The skin of the eyelids is darker and thickened and there is a double fold under the eyes (Dannie-Morgani infraorbital lash, Fig. 7.4).

Cheilitis tends to be non-allergic. Exacerbation of eczema typically occurs in spring and autumn. Staying in the sun is beneficial, cold makes the symptoms worse. Inhalant allergens and stress as exacerbating factors (e.g. testing at school) are added to the provoking factors. Other atopic diseases can include bronchial asthma, hay fever and allergic conjunctivitis. There is a greater susceptibility to otitis media. There are alternating remissions and exacerbations, with a tendency towards a decrease in symptoms. By the age of 9 years, AD symptoms resolve in about 80% of patients. Infectious complications include eczema herpeticatum (superinfection with herpes simplex virus), more rarely eczema verrucatum (HP viruses) or moluscatum (molluscum viruses MCV1 and 2). Erythroderma in childhood is rare, it is called *erythrodermia atopica Hill.*

AD in adolescents—cases of AD persisting from childhood into adolescence. Deterioration in girls occurs during menstruation, nervous instability appears. The clinical presentation of AD in adolescents is increasingly characterised by lichenification, typically symmetrical, flexural localisation (elbow and popliteal fossae),

Fig. 7.5 Atopic eczema, lichenification

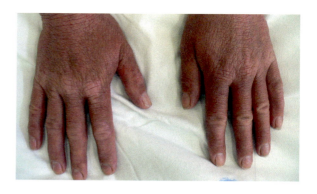

wrists, ankles, neck. The manifestations are accompanied by excoriations. Dissemination may occur. The colour of atopic skin changes to a dirty brownish-grey, which is especially accentuated around the eyes. The lateral part of the eyebrows (Herthoghe's sign) disappears. The hair is dry, lacking shine, sometimes even thinning. Nails tend to be shiny due to constant scratching. Asthma attacks and spring hay fever increase in intensity, while skin symptoms usually subside when asthma worsens and vice versa.

AD in adults—may occur as the first manifestation of the disease, even in patients who have not previously suffered from eczema. However, it usually precedes the infant and childhood form or asthma. The clinical presentation may be identical to that of adolescents, or limited to certain localisations (frustum form of atopic eczema)—eczema on the eyelids, hands, or only on the pads of the fingers and plantar aspects of the toes (*pulpitis sicca*), follicular hyperkeratosis on external surfaces of the arms (*keratosis pilaris*), atopic cheilitis, eczema of the nipples, vulva, etc. The scalp may also be affected. The skin of adult patients is more lichenified (Fig. 7.5) and the pruritus is more intense.

The pruriginous form of AD is part of adult AD, characterised by severe itching, which can clinically sometimes mimic scabies. AD in adults can vary in severity, including generalisation and erythroderma. In women, it often worsens before menstruation, while in pregnancy, eczema often disappears. Contact sensitisation occurs more frequently than in the general population, due to a broken skin barrier (nickel is the most common allergen, like non-atopics).

Classification

There are two basic forms of AD:

- *allergic (extrinsic)*—constitutes 80% of patients with AD, IgE elevation, sensitisation to environmental allergens (food, inhalants) and often other atopic diseases—*bronchial asthma*, rhino-conjunctivitis are typical [28].
- *non-allergic (intrinsic)*—constitutes approximately 20% of patients with AD, IgE is normal, they are not sensitised to exogenous allergens; *bronchial asthma* or rhino-conjunctivitis are not present.

Examinations

bacteriological examination (culture examination of a skin swab, where up to 90% of golden staphylococcus aureus is found), focal infections (throat swab, ENT or dental examination, gynaecological examination in women), internal examination, eye examination, or stool examination for parasites.

Diagnosis

A careful family and personal anamnesis, a typical clinical presentation, white dermographism, IgE elevation, and histological verification in the case of uncertain diagnosis, are important.

Differential diagnosis

It is necessary to distinguish other forms of eczema (contact allergic eczema, nummular and microbial eczema, asteatotic, dyshidrotic eczema, irritant dermatitis), pyoderma, mycoses, *scabies, lichen planus* or *verrucosus*, psoriasis, *prurigo, dermatitis herpetiformis Duhring*, drug exanthemas, *mycosis fungoides*, actinitic reticuloid.

Therapy

Treatment of AD must be complex. Preventive measures, identification and elimination of provoking factors, patient education are essential. The therapeutic approach is individual, depending on the current severity of AD.

Topical therapy

It is the basis of AD treatment. The means of treatment are chosen according to the stage of eczema. The appropriate galenic form of the product must be selected accordingly [3].

Emollients are essential in the care of dry atopic skin (they restore the broken skin barrier, moisturise, adjust pH). With regular use of emollients, their corticoid-sparing effect is proven. They are also used in the form of baths (oil, herbal, colloidal—bran).

Local corticosteroids play an indispensable role in the treatment of AD, especially in the acute phase. They are chosen as the first line of anti-inflammatory treatment. Fourth-generation corticosteroids with a better safety profile are preferred.

Local calcineurin inhibitors are another option for topical treatment of eczema. They have anti-inflammatory effects (about as effective as moderate corticosteroids). They have a strong antipruritic effect and do not have the side effects of corticosteroids (their application does not lead to skin atrophy), so they can be administered continuously for a long time.

Local antibiotics and antiseptics are suitable in impetiginised cases, especially in massive colonisation of the skin with golden staphylococcus.

Systemic therapy

Antihistamines are a very important part of the treatment of AD, especially to affect pruritus and related sleep disorders.

Systemic antibiotics are indicated for impetiginisation, often accompanied by lymphadenitis and lymphangitis, increased laboratory signs of inflammation and alteration of the patient's condition.

Systemic antiviral drugs are administered in *eczema herpeticatum*.

Systemic antifungals may be considered in severe AD with head and neck involvement in patients with colonisation of *Malassezia* yeast (preferably M. sympodialis).

Systemic corticoids are only used for short periods of time for acute conditions (they are completely unsuitable for long-term treatment).

Among systemic immunosuppressants, cyclosporine A is the only approved drug in this case.

Biological therapy. In 2018, dupilumab (a fully human monoclonal antibody against the common receptor subunit for IL-4 and IL-13) was approved for the treatment of moderate and severe AD in adults [5].

4 Ocular Manifestations of Atopic Dermatitis

AD is a chronic skin disease, with possible manifestations on the eyes, most often in the form of blepharitis and keratoconjunctivitis. There is also a higher risk of developing keratoconus, glaucoma, cataracts at a younger age or retinal detachment [16].

Clinical symptoms and objective findings

Eyelids

When eyelids are affected by AD, their redness, slight swelling and small fissures and scaling of the skin may be present [30, 31]. The most common subjective complaints of patients with atopic blepharitis include itchy eyelids and a foreign body sensation.

Conjunctiva and cornea

The typical manifestation of AD on the anterior segment of the eye is atopic keratoconjunctivitis, which occurs in up to 40% of patients [16]. The conjunctiva is infiltrated with mast cells, eosinophils and lymphocytes, may be hypertrophic and fibrotic changes may be found on biopsy of the tarsal conjunctiva [12, 16]. Corneal involvement is usually in the form of punctate epitheliopathy or more extensive epithelial defects, which in a chronic course can lead to irreversible scarring complications with decreased visual acuity. Here too, patients suffer from significant ocular discomfort with itching and redness of the eyes.

At the same time, AD patients have a higher risk of developing keratoconus with an incidence of 0.5–39% [14]. Its incidence increases if the SCORAD (Severity Scoring of Atopic Dermatitis) index is higher, i.e. the course of AD is more severe [31]. At the same time, patients who rub their eyes due to atopy have a much higher risk of developing keratoconus.

Lens

Up to one-quarter of AD patients develop cataracts at a young age, with rapid progression [16, 24]. Chronic use of corticosteroids locally and in general, eye rubbing, and disruption of the haemato-retinal barrier are considered risk factors.

Retina

Retinal detachment occurs in up to 20% of AD patients. The presumed predisposing factor is also eye rubbing, which can lead to the formation of tears in the periphery of the retina [27, 37].

Optic nerve

Chronic use of corticosteroids in the facial area to relieve atopic symptoms may result in secondary steroid glaucoma [16]. This must be kept in mind, so that visual functions are not irreversibly damaged. At the same time, atopic glaucoma patients in a study by Takakuwa et al. showed increased levels of inflammatory cytokines in the ventricular fluid, specifically IL (interleukin) 8 and CCL (chemotactic cytokine) 2, and abnormalities in the trabecular meshwork [38].

Diagnosis
Diagnosis is based on the clinical presentation.
Differential Diagnosis

- Conjunctivitis of other aetiologies
- Rosacea

Therapy
In blepharitis, emphasis is placed on eyelid hygiene. Locally, weak corticosteroids, calcineurin inhibitors, antibiotics if necessary, are administered. In keratoconjunctivitis, topical antihistamines and mast cell stabilisers are administered—corticosteroids or calcineurin inhibitors in the short term, and cyclosporine in the long term. Therapeutic contact lenses are applied for the subjective relief of corneal impairment. In patients with keratoconus, the refractive error is corrected, and corneal crosslinking may be considered. Cataract and retinal detachment are treated surgically, while glaucoma is treated with antiglaucomatous drugs. However, prevention is also key, especially by warning patients not to rub their eyes and to be careful when taking corticosteroids [16].

5 Rosacea

Rosacea is a common chronic, non-infectious, inflammatory, recurrent disease of the pilosebaceous unit, with localisation on the face (especially in the middle part). The aetiology is multifactorial. Typical symptoms include facial erythema, chronic inflammation, and fibrosis, but the clinical presentation is very diverse [3].

Epidemiology
The global prevalence of rosacea ranges from 5–22% [3, 29]. It occurs mainly in persons of the Celtic phenotype with fair skin, blue eyes and fair or black hair (phototype I and II). It affects people in the age range of 30–60 years, with the highest frequency after the age of 50.

Clinical presentation
Rosacea is characterised by a range of clinical manifestations—erythema of varying intensity, telangiectasia, inflammatory manifestations to permanent phymatous changes. Secondarily, burning and stinging in the face, oedema, dry skin, phyma, peripheral flushing and ocular manifestations may occur [3, 29].

Classification

In 2002, The National Rosacea Society's Expert Committee on the Classification and Staging of Rosacea identified four subtypes of rosacea—erythematotelangiectatic, papulopustular, phymatous and ocular [29].

Subtype 1: Erythematotelangiectatic rosacea (syn. erythrosis, couperosis, rubeosis) is characterised mainly by flushing and persistent centrofacial erythema.

Subtype 2: Papulopustular rosacea is characterised by persistent centrofacial erythema, often with oedema and transient formation of papules and pustules (not only centrofacially, but also periorbitally, perinasally and periorally).

Subtype 3: Phymatous rosacea (Figs. 7.6, 7.7) is characterised by thickening and roughness of the skin, oedema, and irregularly shaped nodosities in the convex areas of the face, causing a cauliflower-like appearance and enlargement of the affected areas.

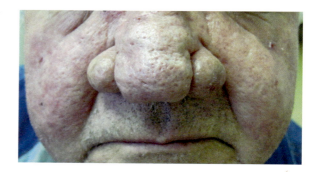

Fig. 7.6 Phymatous rosacea

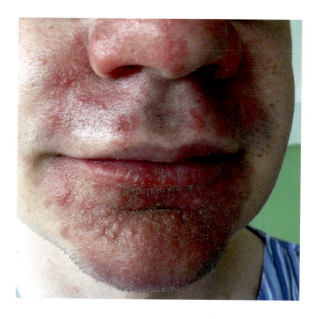

Fig. 7.7 Rosacea (gnatophyma)

Skin Diseases

Subtype 4: Ocular rosacea may not be associated with skin manifestations and in about 20% of cases it precedes skin symptomatology. It often causes chronic inflammation of the eyelids and cornea. It is closely associated with dysfunction and inflammation of the Meibomian glands, causing an abnormal lipid composition of the tear film, with subsequent dryness of the surface of the eye (usually the first symptom).

Other variants and special forms of rosacea

Granulomatous (lipoid) rosacea is a chronic form of the disease. Typical signs are stiff, yellowish-brownish, or red papules or nodules 3–5 mm in size, which may lead to scarring. Manifestations are localised on the cheeks, eyelids, under the eyes, around the mouth and neck and rarely accompanied by bilateral eyelid swelling.

Rosacea fulminans affects mostly women in adulthood, mostly between 20–30 years of age. It is manifested by the sudden appearance (within days to weeks) of papules, pustules, large nodules, fistulas, and deep abscesses on the face. Manifestations are accompanied by pronounced erythema and oedema.

Conglobate rosacea. The clinical presentation is characterised by intensely reddened skin with haemorrhagic nodular abscesses and induced plaques. It is clinically like *acne conglobata* and is chronic in nature.

Gram-negative rosacea is caused by gram-negative microbes (Klebsiella, Proteus, Escherichia coli, Pseudomonas, etc.). The clinical presentation corresponds to subtypes 2–3 of rosacea. Prolonged systemic antibiotic therapy is often necessary according to sensitivity.

"Halogen" rosacea may occur after systemic administration of iodide or bromide. Clinically, it resembles the conglobate form of rosacea.

Persistent oedematous rosacea has a chronic course and is characterised by persistent swelling, which may be caused by a chronic inflammatory process accompanied by increased permeability of capillary walls and obstruction of lymphatic vessels or fibrosis caused by mast cells. Fixed swelling is found mainly on the forehead, between the eyebrows, symmetrically on the eyelids or upper parts of the cheeks and on the nose.

Diagnosis and examinations

Diagnostic criteria include primary manifestations and symptoms (transient or persistent flushing, papules, pustules, telangiectasia) and secondary manifestations and symptoms (pinching, burning, elevated and reddened plaques without changes in the surrounding skin, dry skin appearance, oedema, ocular involvement, peripheral localisation of manifestations, phymatous changes). The "guidelines" for the diagnosis of rosacea require the presence of one or more primary and secondary manifestations and symptoms.

Differential diagnosis

Includes *acne vulgaris, seborrheic dermatitis, perioral dermatitis, demodicosis, chronic discoid lupus erythematosus,* contact allergic dermatitis, sarcoidosis, *dermatomyositis, polycythemia vera, facies mitralis,* syphilis, tuberculosis, carcinoid, Hajer's syndrome (rare familial rosaceiform genodermatosis).

Therapy

Rosacea requires long-term treatment due to its chronicity. Therapy depends on the intensity of the clinical manifestations and the subtype. Before starting therapy, provocative factors of rosacea must be identified. Local therapy leads to an improvement in the *stratum corneum* barrier function, reduces irritation and reactivity of the skin, which leads to a reduction in inflammatory manifestations [3, 29]. Systemic therapy is indicated mainly in severe forms and in less severe forms of the disease, where combined local therapy has not led to the expected improvement.

6 Ocular Manifestations of Rosacea

Ocular involvement in rosacea occurs in up to 70% of cases and often appears before skin symptoms. This disease primarily affects the blood vessels and pilosebaceous units, and as far as the ocular manifestation is concerned, it manifests bilaterally and non-specifically, which makes early and correct diagnosis difficult [43].

Clinical symptoms

Due to the involvement of the anterior segment of the eye in patients with ocular manifestations of rosacea, the subjective discomfort associated with dry eye syndrome is typical, i.e. the sensation of a foreign body, burning, itching and watery eyes, or a decrease in visual acuity in corneal involvement [3, 43].

Objective findings

Eyelids

The most common finding on the eyelids is dysfunction of the Meibomian glands, with dilatation of their orifice at the eyelid margin, increased secretion, and foamy tear film. Recurrent chalazia and hordeola, anterior or posterior blepharitis and eyelid margins with irregular margins are also common [3, 43].

Conjunctiva

Chronic inflammation of the conjunctiva results in hyperaemia and papillary reaction. Teleangiectasia of blood vessels, cicatricial changes or fibrous remodelling of conjunctival tissue are also considered typical manifestations [43].

Cornea

Typical manifestations of rosacea on the cornea are superficial keratitis and epithelial erosion [43]. Triangular corneal infiltrates can also be found, initially at the limbus and centrally as the disease progresses (Fig. 7.8).

Corneal ulcers can lead to perforation [3]. Corneal thinning can also occur in rosacea, leading to high astigmatism and decreased visual acuity.

Rosacea can also manifest itself in the form of iritis, episcleritis and scleritis.

Diagnosis

The diagnosis of rosacea is based on clinical findings. There is no specific diagnostic test [43]. Schirmer's test and TBUT (tear break-up time) examination are used to assess the degree of dry eye syndrome.

Differential diagnosis

- Seborrheic blepharokeratoconjunctivitis

Fig. 7.8 Corneal infiltrate at the limbus in a patient with acne rosacea

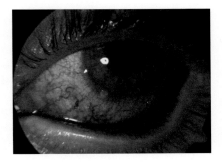

- Blepharokeratoconjunctivitis of staphylococcal aetiology
- Carcinoma of the sebaceous gland

Therapy

For ocular manifestations of rosacea, artificial tears are administered [3, 43]. To relieve inflammation of the lacrimal gland with a subsequent improvement in its function, cyclosporine is administered. Eyelid hygiene and the application of warm compresses are also important. Other local preparations include antibiotics or short-term corticosteroids. If the course of the eye disease is moderate, general antibiotic treatment (tetracyclines, doxycycline or azithromycin, erythromycin) is indicated. In severe dry eye syndrome, tear point occlusion is often considered. In the case of thinning or perforation of the cornea, the choice is to suture the amniotic membrane or conjunctival flap or to apply tissue adhesives [43].

7 Mucous Membrane Pemphigoid

Mucosal membranous pemphigoid (MMP), a unit also described as scarring pemphigoid, is a group of rare chronic autoimmune blistering diseases, with predominant involvement of mucosal membranes including conjunctivae and occasionally the skin [1, 19]. If skin manifestations are present, then development of tense blisters and erosions, often localised on the head, neck or at sites of trauma. Mucosal lesions often heal by scarring—hence the name "scarring pemphigoid". The disease leads to decreased vision, blindness and supraglottic stenosis, with manifestations of hoarseness or airway obstruction (laryngeal and oesophageal stenosis). The first international consensus on mucocutaneous membranous pemphigoid was published in 2002 by Chan [6]. Classification of patients with mucocutaneous membranous pemphigoid is difficult, because many other autoimmune blistering dermatoses can affect mucous membranes, e.g. bullous pemphigoid, *epidermolysis bullosa acquisita*, *anti p-200 pemphigoid*, etc. The clinical manifestation of this disease is also heterogeneous—sometimes involvement of the ocular mucosa, sometimes oropharyngeal lesions are found. Differences in clinical manifestations do not seem to be associated with heterogeneity of target antigens.

Epidemiology

According to studies conducted in France and Germany, the incidence of MMP is estimated at 2 cases/1 million inhabitants. There is no known racial predilection. The disease affects women more often in a ratio of 2:1. The majority of those affected are elderly, with an average age of between 62 and 66 years.

Aetiopathogenesis

It is an autoimmune blistering disease. Like other autoimmune diseases, genetic susceptibility and environmental factors lead to the development of antibody production.

Clinical presentation

Patients with MMP typically have persistent painful erosions of mucosal membranes. Clinical manifestations depend on the location of the lesion. Most patients have oral mucosal involvement, including erosions and manifestations of desquamative gingivitis. Impairment of the lacrimal glands and ducts leads to reduced production of tears and mucus, and reduced tear formation leads to dry eye and other trauma [34]. The result is known as "pacification" and blindness. Some patients with ocular involvement may have MMP without the development of oropharyngeal, skin or other mucosal changes. Patients with purely ocular involvement form a specific subtype of MMP patients, differing from classic BP by low frequency of IGG and C3 immunoglobulin in direct immunofluorescence. In addition, they are usually negative when tested for circulating antibodies by indirect immunofluorescence. The oral mucosa is affected in the form of recurrent painful erosions. The gums are most often affected, followed by the palatal and buccal mucosa. However, a blister can form anywhere on the oral mucosa. Oropharyngeal involvement is manifested by hoarseness or dysphagia. Changes in the pharyngeal region are associated with MMP, with the presence of anti-laminin-332 antibodies. Progressive scarring leads to oesophageal stenosis (requiring dilatation procedures). Involvement of the supraglottic region may lead to airway obstruction requiring tracheostomy. Involvement of the nasal mucosa manifests as epistaxis, crusting of the nasal mucosa. The perianal or genital area (clitoris, labia, glans, penis) may also be affected. Skin lesions occur in approximately one-third of MMP patients and present as tense vesicles or bullae with clear or haemorrhagic contents. Healing leaves scars or milia. Affection of the scalp can lead to alopecia. Pruritus may be present at the site of blisters but can also be generalised. The cutaneous form of MMP with head and neck involvement without mucosal involvement is called the Brunsting-Perry variant of localised bullous pemphigoid (Fig. 7.9).

Patients are predominantly elderly males and present with recurrent vesiculobullous eruptions of the head and neck, healing with atrophic scars. Histological, immunofluorescence and immuno-electron microscopic findings are similar to other patients with MMP.

Classification

In addition to the classic forms of MMP involving the eyes, oral and nasal mucosa, the following terms are known from the literature:

Fig. 7.9 Cutaneous form of membranous pemphigoid

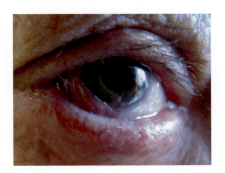

- *Brunsting-Perry pemphigoid*—the disease is considered a localised form of scarring pemphigoid without mucosal involvement, or one of the forms of *epidermolysis bullosa acquisita*. According to some authors, it should be classified as a separate clinical entity distinct from MMP (this would also apply to the following form).
- Disseminated *Provost type*—is characterised by blister development and scarring; the manifestations are disseminated, but limited to the skin, not the mucous membranes.

Examinations

- Routine laboratory tests are not helpful for the diagnosis of MMP. Most haematological values are within the reference range, while the following parameters may be elevated: immunoglobulins, erythrocyte sedimentation rate and CRP.
- Direct immunofluorescence (DIF)—linear deposits of IgG, IgA autoantibodies (in 20%) in the dermo-epidermal junction.
- Immunoelectron microscopy—binding of autoantibodies mainly in the lamina lucida.
- Circulating autoantibodies in 10%, maximum 20% of patients in low titres (1:10 to 1:20).
- Salt-split substrate (salt-split-skin)—for MMPs with BP180 antigen reactivity binding to the epidermal part; for MMPs with laminin-332 reactivity binding to the dermal part.
- Immunoblot (Western blot), immunoprecipitation and immunoelectron microscopy—used to better identify target antigens.
- ELISA tests using recombinant target antigens—characterise autoantibody reactivity.
- CT, X-ray with contrast in upper respiratory tract, oesophagus or as part of tumour screening in anti-laminin-332 MMP.

A summary of target antigens is presented in Table 7.4.

Diagnosis

- Typical clinical presentation as described above (involvement of mucous membranes in various locations and skin).

Table 7.4 Target antigens in MMP

Identified target antigens in MMPs	
Recognised antigens	
Bullous pemphigoid antigen 1 BP230	
Bullous pemphigoid antigen 2 BP180	
Laminin 5	
Laminin 6	
Collagen type VII	
Beta 4 integrin subunit	
Unrecognised antigens	
168-kd epithelial protein	
120-kd epithelial protein*	
Uncein	
*The 120-kd epithelial protein described by Sarret et al. and Chan et al. may in fact be a hidden ectodomain of the BP180 antigen	

- Laboratory tests—see the description in the Examinations section.

The diagnostic criteria are summarised in Table 7.5.

Differential diagnosis

- Lichen planus
- Stevens-Johnson syndrome
- Erythema multiforme
- Pemphigus vulgaris
- Paraneoplastic pemphigus
- Bullous pemphigoid
- Linear IgA bullous dermatosis with dominant skin involvement
- *Epidermolysis bullosa acquisita* with predominant skin involvement
- Bullous disease in dialysis patients
- Drug-induced bullous diseases

Therapy

Table 7.5 Diagnostic criteria for mucocutaneous membrane (scarring mucosal) pemphigoid

Type of examination	Findings
Clinical examination	Erosion and ulceration of mucous membranes with scarring
Histology	Subepidermal graft (blister) + sparse, mixed inflammatory leukocytic infiltrate
DIF	Linear IgG and C3 deposits in the DEJ
IIF using salt-split-skin substrate	Binding of IgG or IgA autoantibodies on both epidermal and dermal sides of graft
ELISA/Imunoblot	BP180-, laminin 332, $\alpha6\beta4$ integrin-specific IgG/IgA autoantibodies

Skin Diseases 289

The goal of MMP therapy is to suppress extensive blistering, promote healing and prevent scarring. The lowest doses of immunosuppressive drugs should be used to suppress disease activity, minimising the risk to patients. Treatment of the disease is extremely difficult. Even with optimal disease control, further blisters may develop. The risks and benefits of therapy must be assessed individually for each patient.

8 Ocular Manifestations of Mucous Membrane Pemphigoid

The ocular form of MMP affects up to 70% of patients with this disease [9]. The median age is 65 + years, although MMP can occur at any age. There are several classifications of ocular cicatricial pemphigoid (OCP), the most well-known being the Foster classification and the Mondino and Brown classification. Foster distinguishes 4 stages: 1. Subconjunctival scarring and fibrosis, 2. Fornix shortening, 3. Symblepharon, 4. Ankyloblepharon. Mondino and Brown base their classification on the change in depth of the inferior fornix: Stage 1—reduction of the depth of the lower fornix by 0–25%, 2. By 25–50%, 3. By 50–75%, 4. By 75–100% [9, 36].

Clinical symptoms

Initially, the symptoms are non-specific, which is why the diagnosis is often made late. Patients with OCP suffer mainly from bilateral eye redness, tearing and burning. As the disease progresses, symptoms pathognomonic for the ocular form of MMP develop.

The problems tend to be chronic with exacerbations [44].

The disease can also present as acute conjunctivitis and limbitis, with rapid progression of the disease and scarring of the conjunctiva [9].

Objective findings

Eyelids

Ocular scarring pemphigoid usually manifests on the eyelids in the form of blepharitis, entropion, trichiasis and keratinisation of the lid margins; ankyloblefaron may develop in the final stage [9].

Conjunctiva

The manifestations of conjunctival disease vary according to its duration. At the beginning of the disease, hyperaemia and papillary reaction of the conjunctiva are observed.

Subsequently, due to chronic inflammation, fibrosis develops subconjunctivally with shortening of the inferior fornix [9]. The last phase of the disease is characterised by symblepharon formation and keratinisation of the conjunctiva.

Cornea

On the cornea, exposure keratopathy, punctate epithelial keratitis, small corneal erosions, and infiltrates in the periphery with pathological vascularisation are observed [9, 36]. Later, persistent epithelial defects to corneal ulcers may form, which may be complicated by corneal perforation. In some cases, conjunctivalisation and keratinisation of the cornea occur [18].

Tear film

In the later stages of ocular cicatricial pemphigoid, all three components of the tear film are disrupted [9]. Due to the loss of conjunctival goblet cells, the mucous component of tears is negatively affected; scarring in the area of the Meibomian gland orifice is the cause of insufficient lipid component, and the aqueous component of tears also decreases.

Diagnosis

Diagnosis is based on histological examination of a skin sample and blood sampling, in addition to clinical findings. On haematoxylin–eosin staining, typical subepithelial detachment and inflammatory infiltrate are found [44]; on direct immunofluorescence, linear deposits of immunoglobulin (Ig) G/C3/A are present along the basement membrane. Using indirect immunofluorescence, circulating antibodies can be detected in the blood [36].

Differential diagnosis

- Rosacea
- Graft versus Host Disease
- Stevens-Johnson syndrome
- Sebaceous cells carcinoma
- Atopic keratoconjunctivitis
- Trachoma
- Pemphigus vulgaris

Therapy

Eye treatment includes dry eye therapy, i.e. artificial tears without preservatives, serum drops or vitamin A. Corticosteroids or cyclosporine are administered if secondary inflammation of the eye develops based on keratoconjunctivitis sicca [15]. Secondary bacterial infection is treated with antibiotics. In blepharitis, emphasis is placed on eyelid hygiene. If necessary, scleral or conventional contact lenses are applied. General therapy for ocular indications includes administration of tetracyclines to relieve the symptoms of blepharitis, or oral antivirals for viral superinfection [9]. Dapsone is a promising and useful agent in patients with autoimmune mucocutaneous blistering diseases, especially in MMP [39]. Biologic forms of management with the use of rituximab are also used [23]. An interdisciplinary approach in management has great importance in the treatment of MMP.

As far as surgical treatment is concerned, tarsorrhaphy, amniotic membrane transplantation, and possibly tissue glue can be applied in the case of a persistent epithelial defect [9]. In the case of lagophthalmos or entropion with exposure keratopathy, and in the case of the necessity to wear contact lenses, reconstruction of fornixes using buccal mucosa or amniotic membrane is possible. In trichiasis, electro epilation of aberrant eyelashes may be indicated; in severe dry eye, tear point occlusion is considered.

References

1. Amber KT, Bloom R, Hertl M. A systematic review with pooled analysis of clinical presentation and immunodiagnostic testing in mucous membrane pemphigoid: association of anti-laminin-332 IgG with oropharyngeal involvement and the usefulness of ELISA. J Eur Acad Dermatol Venereol. 2016;30(1):72–7.
2. Araki Y, Sotoyono C, Inatomi T. Successful treatment of Stevens-Johnson syndrome with steroid pulse therapy at disease onset. Am J Ophthalmol. 2009;147(6):1004–11.
3. Barankin B, Guenther L. Rosacea and atopic dermatitis. Two common oculocutaneous disorders. Can Fam Physician. 2002;48:721–4.
4. Bastuji-Garin S, Rzany B, Stern RS, et al. Clinical classification of cases of toxic epidermal necrolysis, Stevens-Johnson syndrome, and erythema multiforme. Arch Dermatol. 1993;129:92–6.
5. Brodska P. Treatment of moderate and severe atopic eczema in adult patients. Dermatol Practice. 2019;13(1):9–12.
6. Chan LS, Ahmed AR, Anhalt GJ, et al. The first international consensus on mucous membrane pemphigoid: definition, diagnostic criteria, pathogenic factors, medical treatment, and prognostic indicators. Arch Dermatol. 2002;138(3):370–9.
7. Cohen V, Jelinek SP, Schwarz RA. Toxic epidermal necrolysis: background, pathophysiology, etiology. Update Oct 21 (2015). http://emedicine.medscape.com/article/229698-overview.
8. Faye O, Roujeau JC. Treatment of epidermal necrolysis with high-dose intravenous immunoglobulins (IVIg) clinical experience to date. Druha. 2005;65(15):2085–90.
9. Georgoudis P, Sabatino F, Szentmary N, et al. Ocular Mucous Membrane Pemphigoid: current state of pathophysiology. Diagnostics and Treatment Ophthalmol Ther. 2019;8(1):5–17.
10. Gregory DG. New grading system and treatment guidelines for the acute ocular manifestations of Stevens-Johnson Syndrome. Ophthalmology. 2016;123(8):1653–8.
11. Guégan S, Bastuji-Garin S, Poszepczynska-Guigné E, et al. Performance of the SCORTEN during the first five days of hospitalization to predict the prognosis of epidermal necrolysis. J Invest Dermatol. 2006;126(2):272–6.
12. Guglielmetti S, Dart JK, Calder V. Atopic keratoconjunctivitis and atopic dermatitis. Curr Opin Allergy Clin Immunol. 2010;10:478–85.
13. Halevy S, Ghislain PD, Mockenhaupt M, et al. Allopurinol is the most common cause of Stevens-Johnson syndrome and toxic epidermal necrolysis in Europe and Israel. J Am Acad Dermatol. 2008;58(1):25–32.
14. Harrison RJ, Klouda PT, Easty DL, et al. Association between keratoconus and atopy. Br J Ophthalmol. 1989;73:816–22.
15. Heiligenhaus A, Bonsmann G, Heinz C, et al. Diagnostic and therapeutic recommendations for mucous membrane pemphigoid of the eye. Klin Monbl Augenheilkd. 2005;222(9):689–703.
16. Hsu JI, Pflugfelder SC, Kim SJ. Ocular complications of atopic dermatitis. Cutis. 2019;104(03):189–93.
17. Kardaun SH, Jonkman MF. Dexamethasone pulse therapy for Stevens-Johnson syndrome/toxic epidermal necrolysis. Acta Derm Venereol. 2007;87(2):144–8.
18. Kirzhner M, Jakobiec FA. Ocular cicatricial pemphigoid: a review of clinical features, immunopathology, differential diagnosis, and current management. Semin Ophthalmol. 2011;26(4–5):270–7.
19. Lazarova Z, Yancey K. Cicatricial pemphigoid: immunopathogenesis and treatment. Derm Ther. 2002;15:382–8.
20. Liss Y, Mockenhaupt M. Erythema exsudativum multiforme majus versus Stevens-Johnson syndrome: differences in clinical pattern and etiology. J Invest Dermatol. 2006;126:106.
21. Lonjou C, Borot N, Sekula P, et al. A European study of HLA-B in Stevens-Johnson syndrome and toxic epidermal necrolysis related to five high-risk drugs. Pharmacogenet Genomics. 2008;18(2):99–107.
22. López-García JS, Rivas JL, García-Lozano CI, et al. Ocular features and histopathologic changes during follow-up of toxic epidermal necrolysis. Ophthalmology. 2011;118:265–71.

23. Maley A, Warren M, Haberman I. Rituximab combined with conventional therapy versus conventional therapy alone for the treatment of mucous membrane pemphigoid (MMP). J Am Acad Dermatol. 2016;74(5):835–40.
24. Matsuo T, Saito H, Matsuo N. Cataract and aqueous flare levels in patients with atopic dermatitis. Am J Ophthalmol. 1997;124(1):36–9.
25. Mockenhaupt M. Severe cutaneous adverse reactions. In: Burgdorf WHC, Plewig G, Wolff HH, Landthaler M, editors. Braun-Falco's Dermatology (3rd Edition). Germany: Springer Medizin Verlag, Heidelberg; 2008. p. 473–83.
26. Morales ME, Purdue GF, Verity SM, et al. Ophthalmic Manifestations of Stevens-Johnson syndrome and toxic epidermal necrolysis and relation to SCORTEN. Am J Ophthalmol. 2010;150(4):505-10.e1.
27. Nakatsu A, Wada Y, Kondo T. Retinal detachment in patients with atopic dermatitis. 5year retrospective survey. Ophthalmologica. 1995;209:160–4.
28. Nevoralova Z. Atopic eczema—theory and practical advice. Pediatrician Practice. 2015;16(2):89–95.
29. Rosacea PR. Dermatol For Practice. 2017;11(1):6–11.
30. Papier A, Tuttle DJ, Mahar TJ. Differential diagnosis of the swollen red eyelid. Am Fam Physician. 2008;77(11):1505.
31. Pietruszyńska M, Zawadzka-Krajewska A, Duda P, et al. Ophthalmic manifestations of atopic dermatitis. Postepy Dermatol Alergol. 2020;37(2):174–9.
32. Saeed HN, Kohanim S, Le HG, et al. Stevens-Johnson syndrome and Corneal Ectasia: management and a case for association. Am J Ophthalmol. 2016;169:276–81.
33. Schneck J, Fagot JP, Sekula P, et al. Effects of treatments on the mortality of Stevens-Johnson syndrome and toxic epidermal necrolysis: a retrospective study on patients included in the prospective EuroSCAR study. J Am Acad Dermatol. 2008;58(1):33–40.
34. Scully C, Carrozzo M, Gandolfo S, et al. Update on mucous membrane pemphigoid: a heterogeneous immune-mediated subepithelial blistering entity. Oral Surg Oral Med Oral Pathol Oral Radiol Endod. 1999;88(1):56–68.
35. Sotozono C, Ueta M, Koizumi N, et al. Diagnosis and treatment of Stevens-Johnson syndrome and toxic epidermal necrolysis with ocular complications. Ophthalmology. 2009;116(4):685–90.
36. Szabo E, Palos M, Skalicka P. Ocular cicatricial pemphigoid—a retrospective study. Cesk Slov Oftalmol. 2016;72(1):283–92.
37. Takahashi M, Suzuma K, Inaba I, et al. Retinal detachment associated with atopic dermatitis. Br J Ophthalmol. 1996;80(1):54–7.
38. Takakuwa K, Hamanaka T, Mori K, et al. Atopic Glaucoma: clinical and pathophysiological analysis. J Glaucoma. 2015;24(9):662–8.
39. Tavakolpour S. The role of intravenous immunoglobulin in treatment of mucous membrane pemphigoid: a review of literature. J Res Med Sci. 2016;21:37.
40. Thong BY. Stevens-Johnson syndrome/toxic epidermal necrolysis: an Asia-Pacific perspective. Asia Pac Allergy. 2013;3(4):215–23.
41. Torres-Navarro I, Briz-Redón Á, Botella-Estrada R. Systemic therapies for Stevens-Johnson syndrome and toxic epidermal necrolysis: a SCORTEN-based systematic review and meta-analysis. J Eur Acad Dermatol Venereol. 2021;35(1):159–71.
42. Valeyrie-Allanore L, Wolkenstein P, Brochard L, et al. Open trial of ciclosporin treatment for Stevens-Johnson syndrome and toxic epidermal necrolysis. Br J Dermatol. 2010;163:847–53.
43. Vieira AC, Höfling-Lima AL, Mannis MJ. Ocular rosacea—a review. Arq Bras Oftalmol. 2012;75:363–9.
44. Xu HH, Werth VP, Parisi E, Sollecito TP. Mucous membrane pemphigoid. Dent Clin North Am. 2013;57:611–30.

Sexually Transmitted Diseases

Jan Nemcansky, Miloslav Salavec, Sabina Nemcanska, Dominika Linzerova, and Pavel Bostik

1 HIV/AIDS

It is a viral disease of fatal course due to immune failure. It was first described in 1981 in the USA, but HIV had been circulating for at least two decades before that in the Central African region. AIDS (*A*cquired *I*mmunodeficiency *S*yndrome) is undoubtedly an STI (Sexually Transmitted Infections), but its clinical manifestations in the genital tract are minor. Despite major efforts by health professionals and researchers 40 years after the first cases were discovered, HIV infection remains a problem that is proving difficult on all fronts—pathogenesis, therapy and possible vaccination [32]. Untreated HIV infection is a progressive and multisystemic disease that can lead to death in many cases due to immune system failure. The nature of the disease, i.e. an infection attacking the immune system and leading to its gradual

---

J. Nemcansky (✉) · S. Nemcanska · D. Linzerova
Department of Ophthalmology, University Hospital and Faculty of Medicine of Ostrava University, 17 Listopadu 1790/5, 70800 Ostrava, Czech Republic
e-mail: jan.nemcansky@fno.cz

S. Nemcanska
e-mail: sabina.nemcanska@fno.cz

D. Linzerova
e-mail: dominika.linzerova@fno.cz

M. Salavec
Department of Skin and Sexually Transmitted Diseases, University Hospital and Faculty of Medicine of Charles University in Hradec Králové, Sokolska 581, 50005 Hradec Králové, Czech Republic
e-mail: miloslav.salavec@fnhk.cz

P. Bostik
Department of Microbiology, University Hospital and Faculty of Medicine of Charles University in Hradec Králové, Sokolska 581, 50005 Hradec Králové, Czech Republic
e-mail: pavel.bostik@fnhk.cz

© The Author(s), under exclusive license to Springer Nature Switzerland AG 2024
A. Stepanov and J. Studnicka (eds.), *Ocular Manifestations of Systemic Diseases*,
https://doi.org/10.1007/978-3-031-58592-0_8

disablement, is critical for all therapeutic efforts, especially as there is only a very limited reliance on the body's own immune mechanisms when a positive response to therapy occurs. At the same time, however, the development of therapeutic options is currently changing the disease picture in developed countries, with a decreasing proportion of treated patients with the "classic" course of the disease as described here, but instead some rarer disabilities may begin to occur that were previously limited due to the shorter survival of infected patients.

Epidemiology

In terms of transmission, the categories of MSM (men who have sex with men) and bisexual individuals dominate. According to the World Health Organization (WHO), as of 2021, HIV/AIDS has killed approximately 40.1 million people, and approximately 38.4 million people are infected with HIV globally [46]. Of these 38.4 million people, 75% are receiving antiretroviral treatment [46].

Aetiology and Pathogenesis

The virus that causes immunodeficiency (HIV 1,2) belongs to the group of retroviruses. Monitoring the amount of $CD4+/mm^3$ allows the severity of the disease to be evaluated according to the decrease; the monitoring is also based on the division of stages, phases or categories of the disease.

After 6–8 weeks, most people infected with HIV begin to form antibodies to various viral proteins. This reaction occurs in almost 100% of those affected within 3 months of infection. The role of antibodies in the immune response in HIV-1 infection is still discussed. In the initial stages of infection, antibodies are induced, but they are not neutralising. It is only in the later stages of the disease that neutralising antibodies appear, which are usually specific for a given viral variant.

Whatever the host's response, the development of HIV infection is primarily influenced by the intensity of viral replication. Some HIV strains have a higher cytopathogenic potential and multiply more rapidly. Infection in this case predetermines the unfavourable course of the disease. In general, HIV-1 infection has a less favourable prognosis than HIV-2 infection.

HIV can be found in blood, semen, vaginal secretions, saliva, synovial fluid, breast milk, tears, urine, serum, cerebrospinal fluid and bronchoalveolar fluid. However, to date, only transmission through blood and blood products, semen, cervicovaginal secretions and breast milk has been detected. HIV is not transmitted through normal domestic and social contact or insect bites, nor are dried bloodstains dangerous.

Transmission in MSM is particularly risky with anogenital contact. The passive partner is particularly at risk, as microtrauma and trauma to the rectal mucosa facilitate the transmission of infection, and the thickening function of the rectum is also involved. Orogenital and oroanal contacts seem to pose less risk.

Heterosexual transmission of HIV is possible in both directions. It is easier to transmit from male to female than vice versa. Transmission of the virus is greatly facilitated by genital ulcers (the risk is 400–800% higher), and inflammation.

HIV transmission is possible among healthcare workers. Cases have been reported following accidental infected needle injuries.

Sexually Transmitted Diseases

An infant can be infected from the mother mostly by the transplacental route, then during birth or during breastfeeding. The risk of transmission is estimated at 30–65%.

Transmission through blood and blood derivatives contributed to the spread of the HIV pandemic, especially in the early years.

Adult HIV transmission is usually sexual, with more than 80% in developed countries and probably much higher in developing countries [32]. In this case, infection requires an impairment of the skin or mucosal surface to allow the virus to contact with CD 4 cells. Langerhans cells of the skin are important: once infected, they migrate from the skin to the peripheral lymph nodes and infect CD4 lymphocytes and monocytes, which are the main targets of the virus.

Clinical Presentation

With prolonged untreated HIV infection, there is a gradual destruction of the immune system and consequently an increased risk of infection with other pathogens, known as "opportunistic infections" (OIs) [32]. The name itself suggests that these are infections that occur in an environment of immunological suppression. The progression of HIV infection is usually monitored by monitoring the CD4 lymphocyte count. A drop below 500 CD4 lymphocytes/μL usually characterises disease progression and a certain level of immunosuppression. A drop below 200/μL indicates a serious risk of OI and is itself (in the case of HIV positivity) a defining criterion for AIDS. In this context, it is important to note the difference between HIV infection and AIDS [32]. HIV infection can persist for varying lengths of time, without manifesting the clinical symptoms that define AIDS. Untreated HIV infection is chronic and progressive. It occurs in three stages—primary infection, chronic latent infection, and clinically manifest AIDS.

After transmission of the virus into the body, the acute, primary infection phase occurs. It is bounded on one side by the moment of infection and on the other side by the moment of induction of detectable antibodies. Most patients at this stage experience symptoms of varying intensity described as "seroconversion disease" (see below). Typical symptoms, which can last from days to weeks, include fatigue, lymphadenopathy, headache, rash, joint pain, anorexia, nausea, vomiting, diarrhoea, and, in some patients, opportunistic infections (OI) symptoms such as mucosal candidiasis, probably from transient immunosuppression [30]. Neurological manifestations such as meningitis, encephalitis, peripheral neuropathies and myelopathy are also possible.

After the initial "eclipse" phase, when the virus replicates locally and is undetectable in the blood, there is a phase of massive viral replication in the lymphoid organs until "peak viremia" is reached. This results in a rapid depletion of CD4 T lymphocytes, which, however, eventually return to normal, although they often do not reach pre-infectious values. From a diagnostic point of view, it is important to note that, during the eclipse, the infection is not detectable by any available means. Subsequently, it is possible to detect viral RNA, but the antibodies are still negative and it is only towards the end of the acute phase that antibodies can be detected by standard tests (Fig. 1).

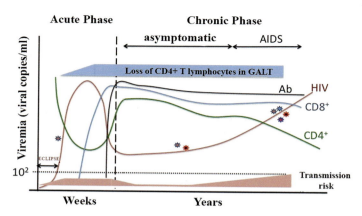

Fig. 1 Course of immunological and virological parameters in HIV infection

While the primary infection phase is relatively well-defined, the subsequent latency phase has an individual course in the order of units to decades, with a median of about 10 years. At the beginning of this period, there is a kind of balance between viral replication and the immune system, which is then slowly or more rapidly disrupted. This is manifested by a gradual decrease in CD4 lymphocyte levels and a gradual increase in viral replication.

The moment the immune system is so impaired that symptoms typical of AIDS, as defined by the CDC, begin to manifest, the AIDS phase of the disease begins (Table 1).

AIDS is defined as HIV positivity and the presence of at least one other AIDS-defining disease or, as mentioned above, HIV positivity and a CD4 cell count below 200/μL (or less than 14% of lymphocytes), which are themselves AIDS-defining criteria even in the absence of any other symptoms [32]. A further clinical classification of AIDS into stages based on the observation of clinical symptoms in the absence of laboratory tests is shown in Table 2.

Diagnosis and Laboratory Examinations

In addition to clinical symptoms, which are very varied over time, laboratory tests (diagnosis and monitoring of the disease) are also available.

ELISA tests are used to detect the presence of antibodies in serum against viral particles. Today, kits are used to detect both HIV-1 and HIV-2 and are highly sensitive but can give false positive results. Therefore, all "reactive samples" are verified by confirmatory methods. In this case, it is mainly the Western Blot. Only based on this result can it be confirmed that the patient is seropositive. Other important tests include PCR, virus typing (HIV-1, HIV-2), viral load monitoring (detecting the amount of HIV in the blood, i.e. above 50 copies of HIV RNA/mL), antiviral drug resistance tests (genotypic and phenotypic), and tests for drug levels in the blood.

Sexually Transmitted Diseases

Table 1 Diseases/syndromes characterising AIDS (according to CDC 1993)

Pathogen/clinical entity	Characteristics/location
Candidiasis	Bronchial, tracheal, pulmonary
	Oesophageal
Herpetic viruses	CMV disease (other than liver, spleen, lymph nodes)
	CMV retinitis
	HSV: chronic ulcerations (>1 month), bronchitis, pneumonitis, esophagitis
Coccidiomycosis	Disseminated
Cryptococcosis	Extrapulmonary
Cryptosporidiosis	Chronic intestinal (>1 month)
Histoplasmosis	Disseminated
Isosporiasis	Chronic intestinal (>1 month)
Pneumocystis jiroveci	Pneumonia (PCP)
Salmonella	Recurrent sepsis
Toxoplasma	Encephalitis, cerebral involvement
Mycobacterium	M. avium complex or disseminated M. avium disease
	M. tuberculosis disease, any site
	Disseminated disease by other species
Neoplasms	Invasive cervical carcinoma
	Kaposi's sarcoma
	Burkitt's lymphoma
	Immunoblastic lymphoma
	Primary cerebral lymphoma
Other syndromes	Recurrent pneumonia
	Progressive multifocal leukoencephalopathy (PML)
	HIV "wasting" syndrome
	HIV encephalopathy
Syndromes defining AIDS in children	Multiple recurrent bacterial infections
	Interstitial pneumonia

Clinical cutaneous signs of HIV infection are considered an important "monitor" of infection. These are multiple and can be schematically divided into infectious, neoplastic and non-specific:

(a) *Infectious.*

I. Viral: Herpes simplex in the form of primo-infection usually has a severe course, with fever accompanied by pain. Dissemination of the virus to the skin, blood and internal organs can sometimes be fatal. Recurrent herpes simplex is also difficult to heal, the bases of the vesicles often undergo necrosis. Shingles often

Table 2 Categorisation of stages of HIV infection according to clinical symptoms (according to CDC 993)

Category A One or more symptoms in an HIV-positive individual over 13 years of age in the absence of a cat. B and C	Asymptomatic HIV infection
	Chronic generalized lymphadenopathy (PGL)
	Acute HIV infection with symptoms of "seroconversion" disease, or history of acute HIV infection
Category B One or more symptoms in an HIV-positive individual over 13 years of age in the absence of cat. C	Symptoms that are related to HIV infection or indicate a defect in cellular immunity
	Diseases whose course or therapy is complicated by HIV infection
	E.g. Persistent and recurrent oral and vaginal candidiasis; general symptoms—prolonged fever or diarrhoea; recurrent or extensive shingles, listeriosis, pelvic inflammatory disease, "hairy" leukoplakia, etc.
Category C	Yeast infections (Candida)—oesophageal, tracheal, bronchial, pulmonary
	Cryptococcosis—extrapulmonary
	CMV—extrahepatic, splenic and nodal; retinitis
	Chronic intestinal isosporiasis (>1 month)
	Mycobacterium-disseminated or extrapulmonary disease
	Cryptosporidiosis with diarrhoea > 1 month
	Coccidiomycosis
	HSV disease with prolonged cutaneous symptoms, or with lung or oesophageal involvement
	PCP
	PML
	Recurrent bacterial pneumonia
	HIV encephalopathy
	Salmonella—recurrent sepsis
	Invasive cervical cancer
	Lymphoma—Burkitt's, immunoblastic, or primary cerebral
	Kaposi's sarcoma
	CNS (central nervous system) toxoplasmosis
	"Wasting" syndrome

Sexually Transmitted Diseases 299

affects more than one location, with numerous blisters on the skin outside the respective innervation zone (aberrant vesicles). Mollusca contagiosa in HIV patients tend to relapse and spread. Viral warts are also difficult to treat, whether vulgar verrucae or *condylomata acuminata* (called "pointed spots") [32]. Hairy leukoplakia of the tongue, caused by the Epstein-Barr virus, is manifested by whitish, wrinkled stripes on the sides of the tongue. This is typical of HIV infection and is also an unfavourable prognostic sign, as it is a criterion of stage IV C 2 (Table 2).

II. Bacterial: Staphylococcal skin infections are common. In syphilis infection, the serology may be false negative, due to immunodeficiency and the course is atypical with interspersed stages.

III. Parasitic: Most of these are scabies, often with an atypical course (*scabies norvegica*).

IV. Fungal: Yeast diseases of the oral cavity are present in the early stages of HIV infection. Genital candidiasis is also common. *Pityrosporum ovale* and *Trichophyton rubrum* cause folliculitis.

(b) *Tumours*

Kaposi's sarcoma is the most common tumour seen during HIV infection. It occurs mainly in the upper half of the body and on mucous membranes. Clinically, it begins as small macules or papules, barely palpable, and pink in colour. During development, infiltration occurs and regular smooth elevations are formed. They are usually smaller than in classic Kaposi's sarcoma and often oval. Over time, they can become confluent, darkening the surface, which becomes keratotic. Of the internal organs, Kaposi's sarcoma mostly affects the gastro-intestinal tract and respiratory tract, where it causes mainly haemorrhagic complications and death occurring by haemorrhage [36]. Aggressive forms of basocellular carcnomas (BCC) and spinocellular carcinomas (SCC) are also reported.

(c) *Non-specific*

During HIV infection, seborrheic dermatitis is often observed, which can progress to erythroderma. Generalised pruritus associated with dry skin is not uncommon. Drug induced exanthems are common, mostly after cotrimoxazole (Biseptol® tablets).

Therapy

Therapy belongs entirely to the field of infectiology and tends to be concentrated in HIV-AIDS centres. The goal of antiretroviral therapy is to achieve the most effective virological and immunological response. Specific antiretroviral therapy focuses on inhibiting individual phases of the viral replication cycle. It either interferes with key HIV enzymes (reverse transcriptase, proteinases, integrity), or prevents the virus from entering the cell (entry inhibitors, fusion inhibitors) [32].

Within each category, there are currently multiple antivirals that can be used. However, the basis of current therapy is the use of combinations of drugs from different groups, which leads to the inhibition of the viral cycle at multiple sites.

This approach especially prevents the emergence and selection of viral mutants resistant to individual antivirals. This combination therapy was called Highly-Active-AntiRetroviral-Therapy (HAART), or more recently cART (combination-AntiRetroviral-Therapy).

Potent antiretroviral therapy (ART) leads to restoration of the immune system and improved overall clinical status, including a decrease in the frequency of opportunistic infections and improved mortality parameters [17]. Up to 90% of patients survive longer than 10 years, thanks to the introduction of cART therapy.

2 Ocular Manifestations of HIV/AIDS

HIV infection causes a gradual destruction of the immune system. It usually takes many years from HIV infection to the onset of full-blown AIDS. For this reason, the ocular manifestations and clinical symptoms can be very diverse and variable, depending on the stage of the disease—similar to the overall symptoms [15].

Ocular manifestations, which accompanied about 70–80% of HIV-positive patients before the introduction of antiretroviral therapy, affect the adnexa, anterior and posterior segment of the eye [24]. They can be caused by the HIV virus itself (microangiopathy, retinitis, neuroretinal disorder), as well as by opportunistic infections and tumours (Kaposi's sarcoma, lymphoma) at a severe stage of immunodeficiency [1, 10, 17]. The clinical course of the ocular manifestations can be influenced by antiretroviral therapy, as well as modified in case of their coincidence. Many of them develop rapidly and have devastating consequences. However, they are very amenable to treatment, so early diagnosis is very important [1].

Manifestations Unrelated to Opportunistic Infections

The pathogenesis of these findings is not clearly explained. Impaired perfusion, infection of HIV endothelial cells, deposition of circulating immunocomplexes, and toxic effects of treatment leading to vessel wall damage, ischaemia caused by small vessel occlusions, and, in the case of the retina, disruption of the haematoretinal barrier, are all suspected [1, 17, 22, 39].

HIV microvasculopathy and HIV retinopathy are the most common ocular complications of HIV infection. They occur in up to 70% of AIDS patients and 40% of patients in stage B HIV infection. They are rarely identified in patients in the early stages of infection (less than 1%). They affect the conjunctiva, retina and optic nerve. On the conjunctiva, tortuous dilated vessels are found, with interrupted blood column and microaneurysms (Figs. 2 and 3).

A characteristic finding on the retina is cotton wool spots caused by infarcts in the nerve fibre layer. In addition, microaneurysms, haemorrhages (punctate, splinter, clematis haemorrhages) and telangiectasia are observed (Fig. 4).

More rarely, cystoid macular oedema may occur. As a result of microvascular occlusion, decolouration and atrophy of the optic nerve target can occur [1, 4, 22].

Fig. 2 HIV microvasculopathy – tortuosity of blood vessels, intermittent blood column

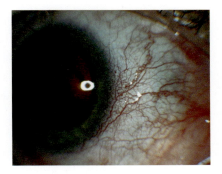

Fig. 3 HIV microvasculopathy of the conjunctiva – detail

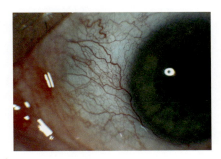

Fig. 4 HIV retinopathy – haemorrhage, cotton-woolly deposits

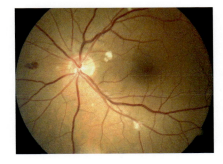

HIV microvasculopathy and retinopathy are not sight-threatening findings. In most cases, they are asymptomatic, picked up as an incidental finding on examination of the fundus. Larger lesions may be perceived by patients as minor visual disturbances. Treatment is not necessary. The presence of HIV retinopathy usually indicates disease progression and may signal treatment failure [1, 20].

Direct exposure to HIV virus is also implicated in neuroretinal dysfunction, which is manifested by abnormalities in the visual field, decreased contrast sensitivity, changes in colour vision, and decreased visual acuity in the absence of optic media transparency and ocular opportunistic infection. This disorder correlates with a reduction in the thickness of the nerve fibre layer. Risk factors include a decrease in

CD4 + lymphocyte levels and high viral load. The symptoms can be alleviated by antiretroviral therapy [3, 10, 22].

Manifestations Related to Opportunistic Infections

These are caused by microorganisms with low virulence, that cause disease only in immunodeficient individuals. Viruses, bacteria, fungi and parasites are typical opportunistic pathogens [29].

Cytomegalovirus

Human cytomegalovirus (CMV) from the herpesvirus group is the cause of the most common and most serious ocular opportunistic infection in HIV-positive patients—cytomegalovirus retinitis [1, 17, 20].

This clinical entity occurs at the stage of profound immunodeficiency, when CD4+ lymphocyte levels fall below $100/\mu L$ [37]. Currently, its incidence has fallen below 5% [17, 20], due to more frequent detection of HIV infection and early initiation of treatment. However, it remains the most common cause of vision loss in AIDS patients [20, 21, 37]. Its occurrence is bilateral with lateral asymmetry [1, 4, 17].

Recurrence of the disease is very common and usually occurs at the margins of old lesions. In typical cases, on ophthalmological examination, variously sized, irregular, vaguely demarcated yellow-white foci of infiltrated retina are found, accompanied by haemorrhage, usually starting in the periphery and gradually spreading along the retinal vessels to the posterior pole of the eye (Figs. 5 and 6).

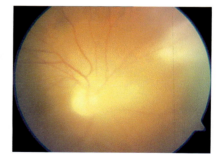

Fig. 5 Cytomegalic retinitis – optic nerve target obscured by vitreous opacities, inflammatory retinal deposits in the right upper quadrant

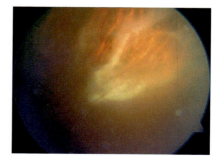

Fig. 6 Cytomegalic retinitis – retinal detachment and partial resolution of vitritis

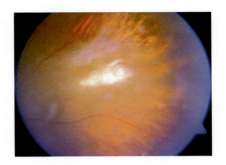

Fig. 7 Cytomegalic retinitis – regression of retinal deposits, transformation into choroidal scar

Accompanying vitritis or anterior uveitis is usually mild due to the weakened immune response of the organism. The damaged retina becomes necrotic and, in its place, partially pigmented, scarred, atrophic foci form, which represent the locus minoris resistentiae for the development of retinal detachment (Fig. 7) [1, 6, 17, 20].

Due to the frequent peripheral localisation of the initial stage, CMV retinitis is asymptomatic in more than 50% of cases. With continued findings, patients complain of blurred vision, decreased visual acuity, flying flies and defects in the visual field [1, 14, 31].

The diagnosis is based on ophthalmological findings. In case of ambiguity, it can be complemented by detection of viral DNA in blood or vitreous by PCR. Because of the decline in immune function and the "morbidity" of the population, the determination of antibodies in serum is usually inconclusive [1, 30].

The basis of treatment is antiretroviral therapy to restore immune functions, together with systemic virostatic therapy (oral valganciclovir, ganciclovir, foscarnet and intravenous cidofovir), combined with the administration of intravitreal implants with ganciclovir, or PPV. Despite early therapy, the prognosis of the disease is very poor and ends in permanent vision loss. Regular screening ophthalmological examination remains a preventive measure [4, 6, 20, 21, 31].

Varicella Zoster Virus

Infection caused by varicella zoster virus (VZV) manifests as herpes zoster ophthalmicus, with involvement of the eyelids, conjunctiva, and cornea, accompanied by subsequent scarring or postherpetic neuralgia, or, conversely, corneal anaesthesia with the development of neurotrophic keratopathy, or possibly neurotrophic keratopathy. The development of anterior and posterior uveitis, retrobulbar neuritis and paresis of oculomotor muscles, or as a rare but very severe progressive retinal necrosis (PORN) [1, 17].

Herpes zoster ophthalmicus is characterised by a vesicular rash along the ophthalmic branch of the trigeminal nerve, preceded by several days of severe neuralgic pain, itching and burning. In 50% of cases 1–3 weeks after cutaneous efflorescence, anterior uveitis (iridocyclitis) develops in the form of focal or diffuse inflammation with formation of endothelial precipitates, inflammatory reaction in the anterior chamber, hyperaemia, iris leakage and formation of posterior synechiae, accompanied by elevation of intraocular pressure. The incidence is 15–25 times higher in HIV-positive patients, and, if shingles occurs in young individuals, it may be an early manifestation of HIV infection [1, 4, 6, 17].

It also often occurs in immunodeficient patients in a disseminated fashion with involvement of multiple dermatomes. Skin lesions tend to be large, deep and haemorrhagic, and heal with a depigmented scar with a residual skin defect [1].

Subjectively, sufferers complain of blurred vision, redness, and pain in the eye. General symptoms include fatigue, fever, nausea, and headache [1].

The diagnosis is based on the clinical presentation. Rarely, it must be confirmed by PCR examination of swollen skin lesions or ventricular fluid. Therapy consists of local application of steroids, mydriatics or cycloplegics. In general, antivirals are administered—acyclovir. Beta-blockers or carbonic anhydrase inhibitors are used to reduce intraocular pressure [1, 4, 6, 31].

Progressive outer retinal necrosis (PORN) manifests as a sudden, unilateral loss of vision with pain and photophobia. The course of the disease is very rapid and its prognosis is very poor. In more than one-half of the cases, despite adequate and timely treatment, the loss of luminosity results. It is characterised by the presence of multiple homogeneous yellow-whitish foci of retinal necrosis, usually without accompanying haemorrhage, which gradually merge and spread from the periphery to the centre with frequent macular involvement. There are no or minimal signs of anterior uveitis, vitritis and vasculitis. At a later stage, scarring and "shredded" disintegration of the retina occurs, which is accompanied by frequent retinal detachment and optic nerve atrophy. In up to 75% of cases, retinal involvement is preceded by seeding of skin efflorescence [1, 4, 6, 31].

The diagnosis is again based on the clinical presentation, or the detection of viral DNA in vitreous or ventricular fluid by PCR. Therapy consists of combined antiretroviral therapy, together with aggressive systemic antiviral therapy (acyclovir, foscarnet) initially administered intravenously, then orally with long-term maintenance therapy to prevent recurrence.

More rarely, the causative agent in this case may be the herpes simplex virus [1, 4, 6, 31].

Toxoplasma

The ocular form of toxoplasmosis, caused obligatorily by the intracellular parasitic protozoan Toxoplasma gondii, is one of the other opportunistic infections in HIV-positive patients, in which it presents as a progressive, more often bilateral recurrent, multifocal, necrotising, chorioretinal infection leading to retinal destruction. On the eye fundus there are round, whitish, oedematous lesions accompanied by mild anterior uveitis, vitritis, vasculitis, less often papillitis. Older lesions are bordered by a hyperpigmented rim with central atrophy. In late stages, it can be complicated by proliferative vitreoretinopathy, retinal detachment, neovascularisation, and glaucoma [1, 4, 31].

Subjective symptoms are eye pain with visual disturbance, photophobia. In 10–40% of cases, neurological symptoms related to associate CNS involvement are present [1, 4, 31].

The diagnosis is confirmed by the clinical presentation, detection of antibodies and detection of parasite DNA in intraocular fluids. Serological testing tends to be unreliable. The imaging methods that can assist in the diagnosis are OCT, which shows oedema of the optic nerve target, and fluorescence angiography, which shows a hyper fluorescent active lesion [1, 4, 31].

It is important to note that HIV-positive patients do not have a self-limiting disability. Treatment is performed by an infectious disease specialist. Currently, a combination of the following drugs is used: pyrimethamine, sulfadiazine, folic acid together with the antibiotics azithromycin or clindamycin [1, 4, 31].

Herpes Simplex Virus

Infection caused by herpes simplex virus (HSV) can lead to eruption of skin efflorescence on the eyelids, keratoconjunctivitis, iritis, or rarely to acute retinal necrosis (ARN) [17].

Herpes simplex keratitis is manifested by painful, often recurrent corneal ulcerations with characteristic dendritic branching, visible on slit-lamp examination, often associated with corneal scarring. Treatment consists of topical application of virostatics (acyclovir, ganciclovir) and cycloplegics. Total administration of oral acyclovir reduces the risk of recurrence by up to one-half [1, 4, 6, 31].

Acute retinal necrosis (ARN) is a rare form of posterior uveitis that manifests as fulminant inflammation of the peripheral retina with sudden loss of vision, pain and photophobia. About 30% are at risk of the other eye being affected. The prodromal stage is a flu-like illness. In addition to HSV, varicella zoster virus can also cause this disease [4, 6, 17, 31].

ARN presents with granulomatous uveitis of varying intensity, accompanied by the presence of cells and tingling in the anterior chamber. Large mutton-fat precipitates are found on the endothelium. Vitritis often reaches such intensity that it can obscure changes in the eye fundus. On the retina, rapidly spreading, yellow-whitish necrotic lesions with retinal haemorrhages are found. All this is accompanied by elevation of intraocular pressure. A common complication is retinal detachment, with proliferative vitreoretinopathy requiring surgical intervention [1, 4, 31].

Diagnosis is based on the clinical presentation, supported by viral analysis of ocular fluids by PCR or retinochoroidal biopsy. Therapy is initiated by intravitreal administration of acyclovir for 10–14 days, followed by oral administration for 4–6 weeks with gradual reduction to a maintenance dose. The total treatment time takes many months, sometimes years [1, 4, 31].

Other opportunistic pathogens include cryptococci, pneumocystis, candida, atypical mycobacteria, microsporidia, pneumococci, listeria, papillomaviruses, etc. [4, 17, 29].

Tumour Ocular Manifestations

Kaposi's sarcoma, a highly vascularised red–purple nodule, is the most common cancer in HIV-positive patients. It occurs in 30–35% of patients in the AIDS stage. In the ocular localisation, it occurs mainly on the eyelids, conjunctivae, occasionally also in the orbit. It is a relatively aggressive tumour with frequent dissemination to the gastrointestinal tract, liver and lungs. Treatment options include cryotherapy, surgical excision, radiotherapy and chemotherapy [1, 4].

Malignant lymphoma is 100 times more common in HIV-positive patients than in the healthy population. It can be localised intraocularly, intraorbitally and intracranially. The following symptoms are related to the localisation: vitritis, peripapillary infiltration, optic nerve target oedema, subretinal deposits, accompanying stripes along the vessels and vascular occlusions in intraocular localisation, eyelid ptosis and bulb protrusion in intraorbital localisation.

The diagnosis is confirmed by pars plana vitrectomy with sampling for cytological examination. The treatment is radiation and chemotherapy [4].

Neuro-ophthalmological Symptomatology

Non-infectious optic nerve involvement can occur in up to 40% of AIDS patients as a manifestation of CNS and optic pathway involvement. It includes optic nerve target oedema, anterior optic ischaemia, optic nerve atrophy, impaired pupillary responses, retrobulbar neuritis, visual field deficits, and oculomotor muscle paresis. The cause may be the virus itself in the advanced stage of the disease, intracranial hypertension in primary or secondary CNS involvement (non-Hodgkin's lymphoma, metastasis of Kaposi's sarcoma) or CNS involvement by opportunistic infections (toxoplasma encephalitis, cryptococcal meningitis) [1, 4].

Differential Diagnosis

HIV retinopathy must be differentially diagnosed from diabetic retinopathy, hypertensive angiopathy, incipient CMV retinitis, chorioretinitis caused by toxoplasma and VZV. Cotton wool spots on the retina may also be present in patients treated with interferon alfa [1, 20, 21, 30].

Early recognition of CMV retinitis, acute retinal necrosis, progressive outer retinal necrosis and toxoplasma chorioretinitis is also crucial, due to the different aetiological agents and thus different treatment management [1, 4, 6, 31].

With the development of effective treatment for HIV infection, a new clinical entity of cytomegalovirus eye involvement, IRIS—immune reconstruction inflammatory syndrome (or IRU—immune recovery uveitis), has emerged. It is a special form of violent pathological reaction after the initiation of antiretroviral therapy as a process of immune restoration of the organism. Its incidence is approx. 10% of cases of ocular involvement and is significantly more common in patients with advanced immunodeficiency (CD4+ lymphocytes < 100/μL) with high VL who have not been treated with ART. Clinically, it is manifested by anterior uveitis, marked vitritis and papillitis. Complications, such as epiretinal membranes, CME, cataracts and, in rare cases, neovascularisation and vitreoretinal proliferation may occur. The association of initiation of ART with a good immunological response and negative CMV detection in intraocular fluid is important for the diagnosis. Treatment of IRIS consists of continuing antiretroviral therapy, in combination with systemic administration of corticosteroids, which are otherwise contraindicated in AIDS patients [6, 20, 21, 30, 31].

Sexually Transmitted Diseases

3 Syphilis

A chronic, worldwide infectious disease, transmitted mainly by sexual contact caused by the spirochete *Treponema pallidum* subsp. pallidum (belonging to the family Spirochaetaceae, genus Treponema). It affects various organs, including the skin, eyes, cardiovascular, musculoskeletal, and central nervous systems. It is called the "disease monkey" (simia morborum) for its ability to mimic a variety of diseases. The modern name comes from Girolamo Francastor, who published the poem "*Syphilis sivé morbus gallicus*" in Verona in 1530. In the poem, he praises the shepherd Syphilus, punished by Apollo with disease for building altars, not to the gods, but to his king.

Aetiology and Pathogenesis

Any area of the skin and mucous membranes can be a gateway to infection, but it is usually the genital area or oral cavity. The incubation period is most commonly 21 days, with a range of 9–90 days, but up to 110 days has been reported. It can be prolonged due to infectious diseases or the effect of antibiotics. Only early syphilis is highly infectious; infectiousness decreases with disease progression. Transmission of the infection occurs by penetration of spirochetes through mucosal membranes and abrasions of epithelial surfaces, most often by sexual contact (in more than 95% of cases); the non-venereal mode of transmission is very rare—intrauterine (transplacental transmission from mother to child), blood transfusion or infected needle injuries—rarely professional chancres of doctors and midwives, or laboratory accidents (*syphilis insontium*—syphilis of the innocent) [7]. Indirect contamination (toilet seats, glasses) is practically non-existent. With infection in the infected birth canal, *syphilis connatalis* develops.

The incidence of disease reflects social change. A significant decrease in incidence was observed after the introduction of effective penicillin treatment for this disease. The most common age group affected is between 15 and 30 years. For the development of the disease, as for other sexually transmitted diseases, risk factors include unprotected sex, promiscuity, drug addiction, etc.

It is a disease that has a systemic character from the beginning of the infection. Untreated syphilis persists for decades and can lead to death.

Clinical Presentation, Course and Differential Diagnosis in Individual Stages

Syphilis is divided into acquired or congenital forms. Acquired syphilis is divided into early, i.e. infectious (according to WHO within 2 years of infection) and late. Early syphilis is divided into primary, secondary and early latent. Late syphilis is divided into latent and tertiary. In principle, latent syphilis does not pose an epidemiological risk, but the infection can be transmitted to the foetus even at this stage.

(a) *Acquired syphilis—Syphilis acquisita*

The incubation period is usually 3 weeks. The time until the first symptoms appear is called the "first incubation period". Currently, there are no clinical signs of the disease.

Syphilis primaria

The first incubation period ends with the appearance of the primary affect. It is usually single, usually asymmetrically localised, subjectively painless (can be completely overlooked by the patient) [9]. The size of the primary affect varies, as does the degree of induction (usually "playing card consistency"). Morphologically, an erosive chancre is found (the surface is slightly eroded) or *hard ulcer*—defined as a small bowl-shaped ulcer, which differs from a chancroid by the absence of an undermined margin. The base and rim are rigid and infiltrated (Fig. 8).

A special form is *oedema indurativum* (more common in women). It occurs on the labium, in the foreskin and occasionally on the scrotum as a stiff swelling caused by an inflammatory reaction of the lymphatic vessels of the affected area. Primary affections occur most often in the genital area (90%)—in men, in the *glans penis* (*ulcus durum*) and in the *sulcus coronarius* (chancre), possibly on the inner leaf of the foreskin (this may be called an "imprint ulcer"). In women, the occurrence is most often observed on the cervix, in the labia majora and minora, or in the posterior commissure. The *clitoris* and urethral orifice (chancre) may also be affected. Extragenital lesions are localised perianally and intrarectally (MSM individuals individuals) and in the oral cavity and periorally, (affections on the lips are common) [9]. The areola of the nipple may also be affected by syphilitic manifestation.

The ulcer goes unnoticed in up to 30% of cases. It most often appears as an induced erosion with a palpable, pinkish-red, shiny base. The typical *ulcus durum* (hard ulcer) is a circular excavation up to 2 cm in diameter, with sessile (i.e. unsupported, unlike *ulcus molle*) induced margins and a firm red base with typical serous exudation on compression (Fig. 8). However, there are several atypical clinical presentations [14]. Uninduced erosion often affects the mucous membranes. An untreated ulcer heals within 6 weeks, treated within 1–2 weeks, healing mostly without a scar, lymphadenopathy subsides for months.

Syphilitic bubo (*lymphadenitis specifica*)—an indolent swelling of the lymph nodes in association with primary affection, which appears in the catchment area of the lymphatic drainage. Patients may experience increased fatigue, headache, fever,

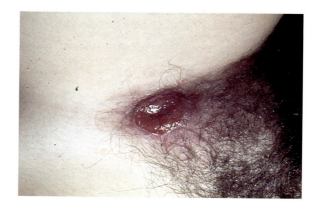

Fig. 8 Syphilis primaria, ulcus durum

Sexually Transmitted Diseases

scratchy throat, and joint pain. In men, the inguinal lymph nodes swell unilaterally when the primary affection is located on the external genitalia. Depending on the localisation of the primary affect, the submental, retromandibular, axillary, intra-abdominal nodes, etc. may be affected. Bubo involves more pronounced swelling of the nodes, compared to *polyscleradenitis* in secondary syphilis. With treatment, regression occurs.

Therefore, diagnosis of *syphilis primaria* is established:

- *Based on suspicious history, presence of primary infection and swollen regional lymph nodes*
- *By detection of Treponema pallidum by dark-field microscopy, direct immunofluorescence or PCR*
- *By serologic tests*—see below, (classification into *syphilis primaria seronegativa* and *seropositiva,* according to the onset of antibody activity within the primary stage).

Syphilis secundaria

It usually begins at Week 9 (3–12 weeks) after infection, with the appearance of exanthema (which is often not noticed by the patient) and is an expression of haematogenous dissemination of the infection. In the beginning, a primary ulcer or scar may still be present, and there is persistent confluent lymphadenopathy. General prodromal "flu-like" symptoms (increased temperature, fatigue, arthralgia, myalgia, cephalgia, generalised painless lymphadenopathy) may be present before the onset of exanthema. The clinical presentation is very varied, with skin and mucous membrane involvement in 80% [9]. The cutaneous manifestations of initial exanthema are usually itchy, symmetrical, disseminated eruptions of manifestations containing Treponemas beginning on the trunk. Different types of exanthems are described:

- Maculous (*roseola syphilitica*)
- Papulous, papulosquamous
- Pustular.

The most common manifestation of secondary syphilis is *syphilis maculosa* (*roseola syphilitica*, Fig. 9), which is characterised by a symmetrical seeding of monomorphic, oval, pink, sometimes hardly noticeable, non-peeling macules, 2–4 mm in size, affecting the embolising localisation, i.e. mostly the lateral parts of the trunk and abdomen, on the limbs' more flexor parts, pubic area and inner thighs.

Exanthema is not usually localised in the face and scalp. It becomes more pronounced by congestion when the patient is allowed to bend over several times. Lesions contain few Treponemas. The symptoms subside within 2 weeks.

Syphilis papulosa et papulosquamosa is manifested by seeding of maculopapular manifestations in the embolisation localisation. These are semirigid, sharply demarcated, red-brown, flat, shiny (lichenoid) papules, sometimes with a collar of desquamation on the periphery. Later, desquamation becomes more pronounced (mimicking psoriasis), with hyperkeratosis forming on the palms and backs of the hands. The

Fig. 9 Syphilis secundaria, macular exanthema

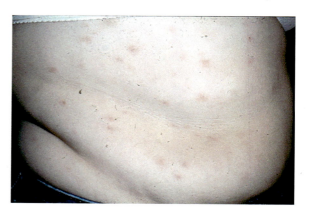

involvement of the palms and sols of the feet significantly supports the diagnosis of syphilis (Figs. 10 and 11).

Papules can form at the interface between the hairy part of the head and the forehead (*corona veneris*). Manifestations last for weeks to months (disappearing within 1 year).

Syphilis condylomatosa represent wet papular lesions in the intertriginous spaces (at the sites of wet patches). These manifestations are very abundant in Treponemas. When present perianally and peri-genitally, they are referred to as *condylomata lata* (Fig. 12). These are flat, pink, slightly elevated papules covered with a fuzzy coating with abundant Treponemas (very infectious).

Syphilis pustulosa is a very rare form of different appearance (acneiform, varioliform, etc.).

Leucoderma syphiliticum arises after resolution of exanthema in the form of ill-defined, irregular macules 3–5 mm in diameter. The most common locations are the

Fig. 10 Syphilis secundaria, exanthema in the palms of the hands

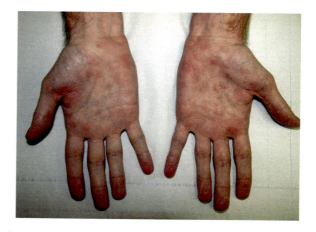

Sexually Transmitted Diseases

Fig. 11 Syphilis secundaria, plantar localisation of exanthema

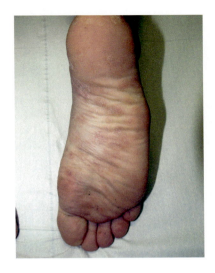

Fig. 12 Syphilis secundaria, condylomata lata

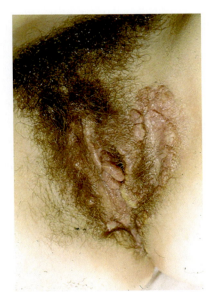

lateral neck ("Venus necklace"), the neckline, and the anterior axillary lashes [9]. Less frequently, dark brown hyperpigmentation resembling *lichen planus* occurs.

Alopecia syphilitica occurs around the 9th week after the onset of the secondary stage, usually at the site of the preceding exanthema in two forms. The first is *alopecia syphilitica diffusa* with thinning of the scalp, which may have a yellow-red colour indicative of ongoing inflammation. *Alopecia syphilitica areolaris* (microareolaris) is manifested by multiple, small, irregular, confluent, yellow-red spots. Spontaneous recovery occurs.

Mucosal symptoms in the oral cavity are present in one-third of patients and consist of an enanthema of erythematous macules and papules, which soon become covered with a yellow-white coating. On the dorsum of the tongue, there are smooth fused flat muzzles which may resemble the shell of a turtle. *Papulae rhagadiformes* may be present in the corners of the mouth. *Angina syphilitica* is manifested by swelling and redness of the tonsils (associated with generalised lymphadenopathy) with painful swallowing, later with the formation of greyish plaques on their surface. Hoarseness accompanies *pharyngitis et laryngitis syphilitica*.

Systemic symptoms include fever, inappetence, fatigue, there may be mild meningeal symptoms suggestive of early neurosyphilis (up to 50% cephalgia, neck stiffness), arthralgia, myalgia, long bone pain, rarely signs of hepatitis, glomerulonephritis, uveitis [19].

Syphilis secundaria latens (also early latent syphilis) is a period of secondary syphilis, when symptoms usually resolve, serology is positive, and the untreated patient is infectious. After 2 years from the infection (however, this limit is artificially set), the patient passes into the *syphilis latens* phase. Recurrent exanthema of *syphilis secundaria* occurs within 2 years of the initial exanthema and affects about 25% of patients. It may be the reappearance of an ulcer or exanthema. The exanthemas are smaller in size and are often limited to the oral and anogenital region, taking on an annular configuration.

Morphologically, there is a loss of symmetrical localisation over time in the secondary stage. Thus, lesions symmetrically arranged in groups characterise the late secondary stage. In the case of complete loss of symmetry, we speak of transition to tertiary stage.

Secondary syphilis lasts 2–3 years. Currently, a specific allergy develops and there is a tendency to develop syphilitic granulomas.

Syphilis tertiaria (Late Form)

It develops over a period of 3–7 years, the lesions are asymmetrical, in groups, with a tendency to fuse and heal to form atrophic scars. We do not find Treponemas in the lesions, they are not infectious and the causative agent cannot be identified by dark-field examination. At this stage, it is a specific granulomatous inflammation with necrosis and development of syphilitic granulomas. Both non-specific and specific (treponemal) serological tests are positive at this stage.

Type IV cellular reaction, according to Coombs and Gell, is required for the development of *syphilis tertiaria*. Syphilitic antigens are behind the formation and development of typical syphilitic granulomas—gummata. As the disease progresses further, a state of anergy may develop. This is likely to lead to late neurosyphilitic manifestations, such as *tabes dorsalis* and progressive paralysis (parenchymatous syphilis). Allergy and anergy cannot stand simultaneously side by side in the body. If *syphilis tertiaria* with allergy is present, manifestations of parenchymatous syphilis cannot arise. Tertiary syphilis develops 3–7 years or more after the secondary stage as granulomatous inflammation, which can be classified as interstitial diffuse (parenchymatous) or localised with gum formation. Organ involvement may also be affected by syphilitic endarteritis. Treponemas are very rarely present, demonstrable by PCR, but the patients are not infectious. Approx. 30% of patients have negative non-treponemal tests, while treponemal tests remain positive throughout life.

Cutaneous manifestations consist of papules, nodules and gummata. Most often it is a cluster of red-brown papules or nodules that heal by atrophy with pigment shifts in the centre and spread further in the periphery. Often, they acquire various arrangements (annular, serpiginous, polycyclic) and form even morbid areas, or they may be covered with scales—*syphilis tuberoserpiginosa (noduloulcerative syphilis)*. Sometimes small vesicles with crusting and necrotic base form in them—*syphilis tuberoulceroserpiginosa*.

Gummata begin in the skin as a subcutaneous painless red–purple nodule, which softens in the centre; necrosis occurs with the formation of a fistula or ulcer, often kidney-shaped, with rolled steep edges, up to several centimetres in size, from which oozes a viscous yellowish fluid resembling *gumi Arabici* (hence the name). It heals within weeks to months, with a whitish scar with a hyperpigmented rim.

In the oral region, gum can lead to destruction and deformation of the soft and hard palate, nasal septum, tongue (Fig. 13), tonsils, and uvula. Interstitial glossitis, if superficial, leads to scarring of the surface; deep glossitis after transient macroglossia leads to scarring with the formation of a ragged tongue—*lingua lobata*.

In the late form of the disease, organ systems are also affected. It is mainly a painful affection of bones (*osteomyelitis, periostitis*, sclerosing osteitis, *osteochondritis*) and muscles. Cardiovascular syphilis manifests itself 15–30 years after infection and mainly affects the ascending aorta (mesaortitis) with outlying coronary vessels, with aneurysms and risk of rupture, valvular and coronary artery insufficiency. The liver and other organs may also be affected.

Neurosyphilis

Neurosyphilis develops 5–35 years after infection (not in the congenital form), with positive serology and usually findings in cerebrospinal fluid. Meningeal

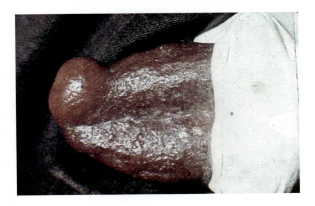

Fig. 13 Syphilis tertiaria, gumma tongue

neurosyphilis is characterised by symptoms of meningitis with cerebral, cranial nerve or spinal symptoms.

Meningovascular neurosyphilis is caused by endarteritis with stroke symptomatology. Meningovascular symptomatology appears, as a rule, 5–10 years after the second stage.

Parenchymatous syphilis is related to a reduced immune response, occurs 15–20 years after secondary syphilis and has two forms (clinical entities): *paralysis progressiva* and *tabes dorsalis*. *Paralysis progressiva* shows psychiatric symptoms (cognitive function, personality changes, psychotic changes and progressive dementia) and neurological symptoms, in the sense of progressive to complete paralysis, leading to death within 2.5 years. *Tabes dorsalis* (*ataxia locomotoria*) arises from damage to the posterior cords and spinal roots, characterised initially by attacks of shooting, stabbing visceral pain and paraesthesia, later by ataxia with the typical gait of a parade march, positive Romberg's sign (loss of stability when eyes are closed and standing with the feet together), positive Argyll-Robertson's sign (preserved pupillary reaction to accommodation, but disappearing to light), trophic ulcerations on the legs, etc. It usually ends in severe disability.

(b) *Syphilis congenital—congenital form*

Congenital syphilis is usually the result of transplacentally acquired infection of the developing foetus from the 4th month of gestation [35]. Foetal infection can occur during any stage of maternal syphilis. However, the manifestation is determined by the stage of maternal syphilis, the adequacy and timing of maternal treatment and the immunological reactions of the foetus [16]. The disease should be seen as extremely serious—it leads to premature births, miscarriages, congenital infection or even death of newborns [33].

It is generally stated that the longer the time elapses since the primary maternal infection, the less likely the infection is to be transmitted to the foetus. The risk is reported to range from 70 to 100% during primary maternal syphilis, 9% during secondary maternal syphilis and approx. 30% if the mother is in the latent syphilis stage. The outcome of untreated infection in the foetus is extremely variable. Approximately 25% of infections result in intrauterine death, with a further 25–30% of untreated babies dying perinatally [13]. One- third of live-born babies with congenital syphilis show clinical signs of syphilis at the time of birth. Foetal treponemal infection occurs in the 4th to 5th month of gestation after the completion of placental development. The earlier the stage of the disease in the mother, the more severe the consequences for foetal development.

Maternal infection before or during the first trimester will not appear in the foetus if syphilis is diagnosed early and treated correctly. If the mother is infected at conception and the infection is not treated, massive infection of the placenta occurs in the early syphilitic phase and, in the 4th to 5th month, *Treponema pallidum* penetrates the placenta directly into the foetal blood. The placenta is enlarged, inflamed and oedematous. The villi contain syphilitic granulomatous tissue (Fränkel granulomas). The foetus is poorly nourished and remains small. In the 7th to 8th month, syphilitic miscarriage occurs.

Sexually Transmitted Diseases

If the mother's infection is of an earlier date (late secondary syphilis), the placenta is less affected (less Treponemas), the mother gives birth to a live infant with clinical signs of congenital syphilis. In the case of maternal infection of a very old date (late syphilis), the mother may give birth to a healthy baby. If the mother is infected just a few weeks before delivery, a healthy baby can be born, but there is also the possibility of infecting the baby with florid infectious lesions during delivery. The latter is an isolated case of *acquired syphilis* with the development of primary affection at the site of inoculation (*syphilis connatalis*).

Clinical Classification of Syphilis congenita

The congenital form of syphilis can be divided into 2 basic units—*Syphilis congenita recens* and *syphilis congenita tarda*. The recent form arises in older maternal infection or in maternal infection in the second half of pregnancy. The late form arises in latent maternal infection, with manifestations noticeable after the 5th year of life and peaking at puberty. *Syphilis praenatalis* refers to the form of maternal infection at the time of conception, resulting in miscarriage or premature stillbirth (skin maceration, interstitial changes of the liver and lungs, and bone changes).

Syphilis Congenita Recens

Skin lesions may not be noticeable in children with congenital syphilis, but the skin tends to be pale and rough (senile appearance). Affected children are usually underweight. Early syphilitic rhinitis (*coryza syphilitica*), lung involvement (*pneumonia alba*), liver involvement (interstitial hepatitis), splenomegaly, anaemia, encephalomeningitis with hydrocephalus and syphilitic osteochondritis (*epiphyseolysis*, Parrot's pseudoparalysis) are detected. On the skin, infiltrates are detected on the heels ("varnished feet"), as well as macular, papular and papulopustular exanthemas, *condylomata lata* and focal alopecia. Polyscleradenitis is regularly detected. Periorally localized papular rash with progression to flat induction of the lip skin is detected. The induced tissue gives rise to deep radial furrows (3rd to 7th week of life)—known as "Parrot's furrows" (scars). These are a persistent stigma of congenital syphilis. In some patients, blistering lesions are found in the palms and soles of the feet, forearms, and shins—*pemphigus syphiliticus*.

Diagnosis is based on serological examination, direct detection of *Treponema pallidum* (Table 3) and clinical examination (Table 4).

Syphilis congenita tarda

Late manifestation of congenital syphilis occurs after two years of age and is the result of untreated early systemic disease. These changes can be prevented by treating children before three months of age.

Persistent stigmata in congenital syphilis are divided into three groups:

1. Reliable stigmata

The typical finding is a saddle-shaped nose (Fig. 14), the nasal mucosa is red and swollen, diffuse.

Table 3 Syphilis—clinical manifestations and diagnosis

Stage of syphilis	Main clinical manifestations	Diagnosis	Infectivity
Primary	Ulcus durum, regional lymphadenopathy	Microscopy in the background, serological tests 1–4 weeks after the onset of the ulcer, PCR	Yes
Secondary	Skin exanthemas, generalized lymphadenopathy, mucosal enanthemas, condylomata lata, alopecia, recurrent exanthema	Serology PCR, Possibly dark field microscopy	Yes
Early latent	Not present	Serology	Low
Late latent	Not present	Serology	Low
Tertiary	Gummata, neurological, cardiovascular manifestations	Dark field microscopy, serology, PCR	Low

Table 4 Clinical findings in syphilis congenita

Syphilis congenita recens	Syphilis congenita tarda
	Short maxilla
Abortus	Saddle nose
Inflammatory changes of the placenta (enlargement, focal proliferative inflammation of the villi, endovascular proliferation, relative immaturity of the villi)	Protruding mandible
Non-immune hydrops	Gothic high arched palate
Intrauterine growth retardation	Hutchinson's teeth
Hepatosplenomegaly $\pm$ icterus	Mulberry molars
Generalized lymphadenopathy	Perioral fissures
Bone abnormalities (diaphyseal periostitis, osteochondritis, Wimberger's sign—bilateral tibial findings)	Higoumenaki's sign
Skin and mucosal changes (mucosal deposits, pigmented macules, seeding of blisters, erythema of palms and soles, persistent seeding in the diaper area)	Interstitial keratitis
Persistent rhinitis	Neurological abnormalities (mental retardation, deafness n. VIII, hydrocephalus)
Nephrotic syndrome	Scapular changes
Pneumonia alba	Clutton's joints
Neurological abnormalities (pseudoparalysis)	Sabre-shaped tibiae

Fig. 14 Syphilis congenita, saddle nose

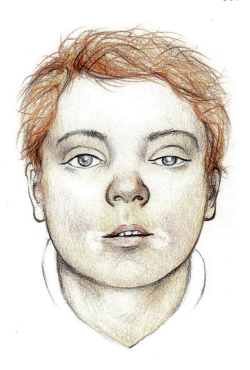

Hyperplastic changes are followed by ulcerations, the septum is destroyed by a gummy process. Another sign is Parrot's furrows—a scar-like structure, periorally but also perianally. The development of what is called the Hutchinson's triad can also be noted: Hutchinson's incisor (barrel-shaped teeth, narrow at the incisal surface with a semilunar notch in the bite line), interstitial keratitis (*keratitis profunda*) and vestibular deafness [33].

2. *Less reliable stigmata*

Osteochondritis syphilitica with degenerative changes of cartilage and hyperostosis resulting in changes of caput quadratum, Olympian forehead, sabre shape of the tibiae. Another sign is the Higoumenakis sign – thickening of the sternal end of the clavicle.

3. *Unreliable stigmata*

This includes high placental weight, gothic palate (narrow and high) and Dubois sign—shortened little finger.

Diagnosis

Examination for syphilis is part of the examination procedures for donors, blood, tissues, organs and semen, part of the examination in pregnancy (prenatal care), basic new-born screening (postnatal care), examination of hospitalised patients and in the preoperative preparation of patients (see recommendations below).

Direct detection of *Treponema pallidum* is performed microscopically using a "dark-field microscopy" with a paraboloid condenser (only the rays reflected by the observed object penetrate the objective). Examination of mucosal manifestations (oral, anal) is difficult, due to the presence of non-pathogenic spirochetes (e.g., *Treponema microdentium*), which have more lively movements and irregular coils. If the lesions have been treated or one microscopic examination was negative, saline compresses are applied to the ulcer and the examination is repeated after 1–2 days. In the case of an enlarged sentinel node, the nodal punctate can also be examined microscopically. Microscopic examination can also be performed by direct immunofluorescence (DFA-TP). Molecular genetic methods (PCR, LCR—polymerase and ligase chain reaction) can also be used for direct detection.

An important part of the diagnosis is the indirect detection of antibodies in the serum. However, antibodies do not guarantee immunity. The individual is immune to reinfection only during early syphilis. Serological tests are divided into specific, treponemal tests (determining antibodies against specific antigens of *Treponema pallidum*), which are positive around the 3rd–4th week after infection (a week earlier in the IgM class), and non-specific, non-treponemal tests (against cardiolipin released during tissue destruction from mitochondria), which are positive around the 5th–6th week after infection [27]. Of the non-treponemal tests, the VDRL reaction is now most used (*V*enereal *D*isease *R*esearch *L*aboratory *T*est) and RRR (*R*apid *R*eagin *R*eaction) using cardiolipin with lecithin and cholesterol as antigen.

The treponemal tests include: TPHA (*Treponema pallidum* haemagglutination assay) and its variant MHA-TP (micro haemagglutination assay), FTA-ABS (fluorescent treponema antibody absorption test), 19S-IgM FTA-ABS, 19S-IgM SPHA (Solid Phase Haemagglutination Test). In special cases, the Nelson TPI test can be used (Treponema Pallidum Immobilisation test).

The tests are further divided into screening tests for routine use, which are used in the first line, and confirmatory tests, which confirm the detected positivity [47]. Activity monitoring tests are useful to assess the effectiveness of treatment.

False positivity of specific and non-specific tests can be observed in autoimmune diseases, HIV infection, pregnancy, other spirochete infections (Borrelia, Leptospira), leprosy, infectious mononucleosis, malaria, and is indistinguishable from endemic treponematoses (bejel, yaws, pinta).

False negativity can be seen in HIV infection (all facts see Tables 5, 6, 7).

Table 5 False negative serological tests

False negative tests
Malignant syphilis
Mothers of children with congenital syphilis
Zonal phenomenon
HIV infection

Sexually Transmitted Diseases

Table 6 Causes of false (non-specific) positive results in non-treponemal tests

Acute	Chronic
Hepatitides	Autoimmune diseases
Parotitis	/SLE, thyroiditis, RA,../
Varicella	Leprosy
Infectious mononucleosis	Drug abuse
Viral infections /HSV, VZV, CMV/	Cachexia
Extensive myocardial infarction	Immunoglobulin abnormalities
Extensive tissue damage	Malignant diseases
/Crash syndrome, burns/	Old age
Malaria	Other trapanematoses
Toxoplasmosis	/Yaws, pinta, bejel/
Morbus Weili Typhus recurrens Trypanosomiasis Vaccination Pregnancy Poisoning/lead, chloroform, ether/ Electroshock Sulphonamide therapy	

Table 7 Causes of false-positive reactions in treponemal tests

Acute	Chronic
Hepatitides	Autoimmune diseases
Borreliosis	Immunoglobulin abnormalities
Infectious mononucleosis	Other treponematoses
Malaria	(framboesia tropica, pinta)
Vaccination	Malignant diseases
Drug abuse	
Idiopathic	

Course of serological reactions: non-treponemal tests can be negative in about 30% of patients without treatment and usually disappear gradually after treatment. If they persist after treatment, we speak of a serological scar. Treponemal tests remain positive for life in 90% of patients after proper treatment (patients treated in the primary stage remain negative for up to 3 years), whereas IgM tests remain negative for up to 1 year after treatment (Fig. 15) [27].

Cerebrospinal fluid is investigated when neurosyphilis is suspected and when it is excluded from the register by the same tests as in serum. VDRL can be up to 70% negative, but positivity is indicative of neurolues. Simultaneous negativity of FTA-ABS and TPHA excludes neurosyphilis. Routinely, a standard examination of

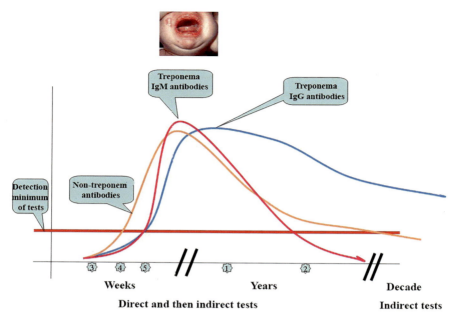

Fig. 15 Course of seroreactions in syphilis

the liquor is performed to determine the number of cells and proteins. When in doubt, Western blotting, PCR or IgM antibodies can assist.

Therapy

The drug of first choice is *parenteral penicillin*, to which no resistance has been observed in over 70 years of use. To cure, a blood penicillin concentration of 0.03 IU/mL must be maintained for 7 days. Neurosyphilis is treated with crystalline penicillin 12–24 mil. IU IV/day for 10–21 days; the alternative is doxycycline 200 mg/day PO for 28 days. In pregnant women with penicillin allergy, azithromycin 500 mg/day PO 10 days, ceftriaxone 250–500 mg IM 10 days [38, 42].

4 Ocular Manifestations of Syphilis

The eye is not a common site of syphilitic infection. Ocular involvement is relatively rare yet may be the first sign of previously unrecognised lues. The ocular form of syphilis accompanies both congenital and acquired forms of syphilis in all their stages (primary, secondary, latent, and tertiary). It can be caused either by direct invasion of spirochetes into ocular tissue, or because of an immune reaction in tissues sensitised by the pathogen. Treponema usually enters the eye through the bloodstream. The disease can affect almost all structures of the eye, including the eyelids, conjunctiva,

Sexually Transmitted Diseases

sclera, cornea, lens, uveal tract, retina, retinal vessels, optic nerve, pupillomotor pathway and cranial nerves [6, 11, 14].

Acquired syphilis

Ocular manifestations of acquired lues occur mainly in the secondary and tertiary stages of the disease. In the primary stage, a painless hard ulcer (*ulcus durum*) may occur on the eyelids or conjunctiva, accompanied by enlargement of the regional lymph nodes. It usually heals spontaneously within 2–6 weeks.

In the *secondary stage*, non-specific conjunctivitis is diagnosed on the anterior segment of the eye. The course is usually chronic and is characterised by diffuse papillary reaction, conjunctival injection and chemosis. If the conjunctiva is the gateway to infection, *Parinaud's oculoglandular syndrome* develops, manifested by unilateral granulomatous conjunctivitis with unilateral painful lymphadenopathy (preauricular and submandibular). The diagnosis is confirmed by conjunctival biopsy, which shows the presence of spirochetes [4, 6, 28].

Episcleritis usually occurs in the secondary stage of syphilis, scleritis more in the tertiary stage. Its course is basically no different from any other purulent infectious scleritis. However, it is characterised by its prolonged course, unresponsive to conventional therapy [11].

The most common ocular complication of acquired syphilis is *anterior uveitis* in up to 56%. It is often the first manifestation of the latent form of syphilis. In 71% it occurs under the picture of granulomatous or nongranulomatous iridocyclitis. In 50% of cases, the finding is bilateral. It is characterised by the presence of dilated iris capillaries (iris roseata) and multiple papules (iris papulosa). Inflammatory nodules (iris nodosa), which are found at the edge of the pupil, gradually turn into atrophic depigmented iris [6, 11, 14].

Less frequently, uveitis is secondary to intermediate uveitis, posterior uveitis or panuveitis, usually in the late stages of the infection. When the posterior segment of the eye is affected, vitritis, necrotising retinitis, chorioretinitis, retinal vasculitis and optic neuritis can be observed. The most common of these manifestations is chorioretinitis, which is characterised by multifocal lesions that may merge and mimic ARN, are characterised by early hypofluorescence and late saturation on fluorescein angiography, and often spread from the posterior pole to the periphery (unlike ARN). Chorioretinitis is also accompanied by vitritis, with small whitish opacities and flat secondary retinal detachment.

We can also encounter acute posterior placoid chorioretinopathy (APPC) with typical yellowish round lesions with raised edges in the macular area.

In vasculitis, arterioles are more often affected; it is not infrequently occlusive and the appearance of "ground glass" is typical.

In 1–2% of patients in the secondary stage, meningitis occurs, which in intracranial hypertension can manifest as optic nerve target oedema. Other neuro-ophthalmological manifestations may include optic neuritis, neuropathy and what is called Argyll-Robertson pupillary aneurysm (disappearance of the direct and consensual reaction in the affected eye, preservation of the reaction in near vision, possible presence of miotic pupils, anisocoria) [6, 11, 14, 28].

The *tertiary stage* of syphilis is characterised by the formation of granulomatous lesions healing by scarring, known as gummata. These are found on the skin of the eyelids, in the tear ducts (dacryoadenitis, dacryocystitis). In the orbital region, bilateral periostitis is the most common. Other manifestations in this stage include blepharitis with madarosis, keratitis, iridocyclitis, vasculitis, chorioretinitis, vaso-occlusive disease, choroidal effusions, and neuro-ophthalmological manifestations similar to those in the secondary stage; in addition, paralysis of the oculomotor nerves are observed, and defects in the visual field when the brain is affected [11, 14, 15, 28].

Congenital syphilis

It is an infection of the foetus or newborn by a spirochete transmitted from an infected mother intrauterine (transplacentally) or at birth. The risk of transmission is highest in the primary and secondary stages of the disease (up to 50%). Ocular symptomatology develops slowly in children. Ocular manifestations of congenital lues include anterior uveitis, interstitial keratitis, dislocated or subluxated lens, cataract, optic neuropathy, pigmentary retinopathy, and Argyll-Robertson pupil [4, 6].

Interstitial keratitis

The initial symptoms of interstitial keratitis (IK) can manifest themselves as early as a few weeks after birth, but most often develop between 5 and 25 years of age. In 80% of cases, both eyes are affected sooner or later [11]. Interstitial keratitis is characterised by acute pain and a marked decrease in visual acuity caused by stromal oedema. Cellular infiltration of the cornea starts from the limbus to the centre. It is associated with deep vascularisation and opacification. After a few months, as the inflammation subsides, the cornea begins to clear from the periphery, but centrally a degree of cloudiness persists. Healing is characterised by the formation of nonperfused—emptied—blood vessels ("ghost vessels"), deep scarring of the stroma, thinning of the cornea, development of astigmatism and keratopathy.

Pigmentary Retinopathy of the "Salt-and-Pepper" Type

This is the first sign of involvement of the posterior segment of the eye caused by perinatal chorioretinitis. Chorioretinitis takes the form of bilateral multifocal inflammation, when the initially active grey-white foci transform into pigmented districts scattered among the whitish foci of the atrophic retina. The result is retinal pigmentary changes, resembling a salt-and-pepper image, located predominantly along blood vessels, less often juxtapapillary or centrally [28].

Diagnosis

The diagnosis of ocular syphilis is established from the clinical presentation by a complete ophthalmological examination, consisting of pupil examination, anterior segment slit-lamp examination and biomicroscopic examination of the fundus in artificial mydriasis. These objective tests are complemented by a series of serological tests (VDRL, RRR, TPHA, FTA-ABS, ELISA, EIA, TPI). With proper diagnosis and prompt antibiotic treatment, most ocular symptoms of syphilis can be successfully treated.

Sexually Transmitted Diseases

Differential Diagnosis

- TORCH (toxoplasmosis, varicella, rubella, CMV, herpes simplex virus)
- Retinitis pigmentosa
- Multifocal chorioretinitis
- Uveitis (anterior, scraping, posterior, panuveitis)

Therapy

The diagnosis of syphilis is subject to mandatory reporting. Its treatment is also compulsory by law. All current and previous sexual partners of the infected person, who have been in contact with the infected person in the last six months, must also be tested and treated. Systemic antibiotics, topical and systemic steroids, and surgical removal of necrotic tissue for easier penetration of drugs are used to treat syphilis. Penicillin antibiotics (benzathine–penicillin, procaine–benzylpenicillin, penicillin G) have remained the drug of first choice since 1947. In patients with penicillin allergy, doxycycline, azithromycin, and ceftriaxone are used as alternatives. Systemic corticosteroids are an appropriate adjunctive treatment for more severe posterior uveitis, scleritis and optic neuritis.

5 Chlamydial Urogenital Infections

Urogenital infection caused by *Chlamydia trachomatis* serotype D-K is the most common bacterial STI in Europe and the USA. In women, up to 80% are asymptomatic and can lead to serious late complications, including pelvic inflammatory disease (PID), infertility, tubal sterility, and ectopic pregnancy [2]. In men, the infection is symptomatic in 50–75% of cases and is characterised by urethral discharge, dysuria, possibly symptoms of epididymitis and prostatitis [5]. It is often associated with gonorrhoea or manifests itself as a persistence of difficulties after its treatment (postgonococcal urethritis). It is always necessary to examine and treat sexual partners. Chlamydia infection increases the risk of HIV infection.

Epidemiology, Aetiology and Incubation Period

The refinement of diagnostic methods and the introduction of new molecular genetic methods into routine practice have led to the recognition that chlamydial infections are one of the most serious global health problems. Chlamydial infections are a sexually transmitted disease and are more common than gonococcal infections (2–4 times) and are often combined with them. The contact type of infection may only be relevant in chlamydial conjunctivitis. It is estimated that they account for about 50% of all urogenital infections in industrialised countries [25].

The frequency of male-to-female and female-to-male transmission is the same at approx. 68%. The spread of infection depends on the degree of sexual promiscuity of the population. Young people are the most at-risk group. The risk of infection increases with the number of sexual partners. Newborns born to mothers with cervical chlamydial infection have a 60–70% chance of being infected with conjunctivitis or pneumonia.

The incubation period lasts 7–21 days. Half of chlamydial infections in women and one-third in men are clinically inapparent.

Clinical Presentation

Chlamydial Infection in Women

Complications are mostly asymptomatic (up to 80% in women), infection with transition to chronicity. Clinical symptoms very often appear only because of a fibroproductive process that results in inflammatory changes. Primary chlamydial infection in women occurs in the monolayer cylindrical epithelium of the cervix and paraurethral glands and may also affect the rectal mucosa [26]. Chlamydial infection should be thought of with purulent or mucopurulent discharge from the cervix, which is oedematous and may bleed on contact. Women may complain of menstrual difficulties, pain in the lower abdomen during sexual intercourse, vaginal discharge, or pruritus. Increased sedimentation with normal leukocyte counts in the blood count are found. *C. trachomatis* has been isolated from the urethra of women with dysuria, where it may be responsible for acute urethral syndrome, and is one of the most important pathogens involved in pelvic inflammatory disease (PID). Infection of the lower genital tract can pass to the endometrium, fallopian tubes, as well as to the abdominal cavity, and can cause an adhesive process up to the form of Fitz-Hugh-Curtis syndrome (adhesions in the small pelvis, perisplenitis, perihepatitis). The most serious consequences of upper genital tract infection include tubal sterility and ectopic pregnancy. Chlamydial infection is implicated in obstetric complications, and its impact on preterm birth and recurrent miscarriages is discussed. Infection in newborns of mothers with cervicitis occurs in 20–50% under the picture of conjunctivitis, which appears within 3 weeks after birth and may disappear spontaneously. 10–20% of newborns show a picture of pneumonia, which significantly worsens the postpartum course in preterm infants.

Chlamydial Infection in Men

It may be symptomatic (about 50% in men), or present as urethritis with mucous or mucopurulent urethral discharge, itching and dysuria. In MSM (men who have sex with men), it causes proctocolitis, which has a milder course than infections caused by the more invasive *Ch. trachomatis* biovar, lymphogranuloma *venereum*. Among the consequences and complications of the infection, epididymitis (intracanalicular spread, a less pronounced finding compared to gonorrhoea) and orchitis, with a possible negative effect on fertility (epididymitis can result in adhesions and thus obstruction of the epididymal ducts, which can cause *oligozoospermia*, and *azoospermia* in less common bilateral epididymitis.)

Young men may be affected by Reiter's syndrome, characterised by arthritis, urethritis and conjunctivitis. It is sometimes accompanied by plantar hyperkeratosis (*keratodermia blenorrhagica*).

Sexually Transmitted Diseases 325

Extragenital Manifestations of Chlamydial Infection

Chlamydial Proctitis

Chlamydial proctitis in a male is the result of passive anal intercourse. Up to 15% of proctitis in MSM population is caused by Chlamydia trachomatis. In a female, chlamydial proctitis, based on anatomical facts, may be a manifestation of the spread of genital infection to the rectum.

The clinical presentation includes an asymptomatic course to anorectal pain, mucopurulent discharge and itching, as well as secondary anal eczema [41]. Proctoscopic examination reveals red, swollen and vulnerable mucosa, with mucopurulent secretion and very rarely erosive changes. Deeper ulcerations require further differentiation.

Chlamydial Infection in the Newborn

If the mother has chlamydial cervicitis, the causative organism can be transmitted to the newborn during delivery by contact with infected secretions, or even by aspiration. The probability of such vertical transmission is approximately 60–70%. 35–50% of new-borns then develop conjunctivitis and 11–20% develop pneumonia [43].

Diagnosis

A urethral or endocervical swab is sent for examination, possibly a urine sample, or a conjunctival swab in conjunctivitis. The result of the test depends on the correct collection, storage and transport of the sample. The removal must be sufficiently vigorous due to the need to obtain the necessary amount of epithelium. Direct detection involves detection of the antigen by direct immunofluorescence or ELISA. Specific stretches of DNA can be detected by molecular genetic methods—amplification method (PCR, LCR) or hybridisation [8, 18]. The sensitivity of amplification methods is estimated at 90–98%. Chlamydia can be cultured on tissue cultures and the sensitivity of this method is approx. 70–75%. Indirect detection of antibodies by serological methods is less informative; the demonstration of a significant increase in antibody titre is important. Antibodies can persist for a long time, making it difficult to distinguish between current and past infections. Serology is mainly important in the detection of chlamydial pneumonia during primo-infection in new-borns, where we detect IgM.

Direct and indirect evidence of the causative agent in chlamydial urogenital infections are summarised in Tables 8 and 9.

Table 8 Indirect serological evidence of *Ch. trachomatis* in urogenital infections

Methodology		Material	Sensitivity	Pathogen
Genus-specific antibodies	ELISA	Serum		Ch.trach Ch. pneum
Species-specific antibodies	MIF, ELISA	Serum		Ch.trach Ch.pneum Ch. psittaci

Table 9 Direct serological evidence of *Ch. trachomatis* in urogenital infections

Methodology		Material	Sensitivity (%)	Pathogen
Cultivation		Swab	60–80	Ch. trach
Detection of Ag	ELISA	Swab	50–80	Ch. trach
	MIF	Swab	50–80	Ch. trach
Detection of DNA	Without amplification	Swab	50–80	Ch. trach
	With amplification	Swab, urine, puncture	92–99	N. gonorrh Ch. trach

Recommendations for the diagnosis of urogenital and selected extragenital forms of infection in men and women are summarised in Tables 10, 11 and 12.

Therapy

In adults, macrolide antibiotics (especially azithromycin) and tetracyclines are used; fluorinated quinolones can also be used. Treatment of sexual contacts is necessary. The causative agent is not sensitive to penicillin or cephalosporins. The therapy is summarized in Tables 13 and 14. For neonatal infections, a macrolide antibiotic in

Table 10 Recommendations for dg. genitourinary infections in women

NAAT of endocervical sample, possibly urine

NK hybridization test: Gen-Probe PACE 2, Digene Hybrid Capture II

EIA or DFA of endocervical sample

Culture of endocervical sample

Amplification tests (NAATs—nucleic acid amplification tests)

Table 11 Recommendations for dg. genitourinary infection in men

NAAT of urethral sample, possibly urine

NK hybridization test: Gen-Probe PACE 2, Digene Hybrid Capture II

EIA or DFA of urethral sample

Culture of urethral specimen

Amplification tests (NAATs—nucleic acid amplification tests)

Table 12 Recommendations for the diagnosis of extragenital *Ch. trachomatis* infections

Culture of the specimen with MOMP staining

DFA of specimen with MOMP staining

DFA—monoclonal fluorescent antibodies, not suitable for asymptomatic patients—small amount of the causative agent in the samples), direct detection method, urine can also be tested
MOMP—major outer membrane protein, on the cell surface, prevents binding of immunoglobulins

Sexually Transmitted Diseases 327

Table 13 Basic therapy for chlamydial infections

Uncomplicated acute infections	Complicated infections
Doxycycline 2 × 100 mg PO, 7 days	Doxycycline 4 mg/kg PO 10–14 days
Doxycycline 200 mg 1 × d PO, 7 days	Doxycycline 200 mg PO for 3 weeks
Azithromycin 1 g PO	Azithromycin 1 g PO weekly to a total dose of at least 10–12 g

Table 14 Alternative therapies for chlamydial infections

Uncomplicated acute infections	Complicated infections
Ofloxacin 200 (300) mg PO 2 times daily for 7 days	Roxithromycin 150 mg PO 2 times daily for 3 weeks
Clarithromycin 500 mg PO 2 times daily for 7 days	Clarithromycin 500 mg PO 2 times daily for 3 weeks
Levofloxacin 500 mg PO 2 times daily for 7 days	Ofloxacin 200 mg PO 2 times daily for 3 weeks
Roxithromycin 150 mg PO 2 times daily for 7 days	Ciprofloxacin 500 mg PO 2 times daily for 3 weeks
Erythromycin 500 mg PO 4 times daily for 7 days	

the dosage form of syrup is recommended for 5 days, according to the weight of the new-born [25].

6 Ocular Manifestations of Chlamydial Urogenital Infections

Eye disease is caused by *Chlamydia trachomatis* serotypes A-K. Serotypes A, B, Ba and C cause trachoma and serotypes D-K cause adult conjunctivitis. In the neonatal period, acute conjunctivitis can be caused by *C. trachomatis* or *C. pneumoniae*.

6.1 Trachoma

Trachoma is a chronic infectious, sight-threatening eye disease, resulting from recurrent chronic conjunctivitis caused by *C. trachomatis* serotypes A, B, Ba and C. It occurs mainly in economically less developed areas of North Africa, the Middle East, India, Central Australia and Central and South America. According to the World Health Organization, it remains the leading infectious cause of blindness and the leading cause of blindness that can be eliminated by prevention [45]. Worldwide, the number of people blind due to trachoma is 3%, 8 million people have irreversible visual impairment, and 84 million cases are registered with active disease [40]. The Alliance for the Global Elimination of Blinding Trachoma (GET 2020) at WHO was established to eliminate trachoma by 2020, mainly by implementing the SAFE (Surgery, Antibiotics, Face cleaning, Environment) strategy. This strategy includes measures for surgical treatment of advanced complications of Trachoma, early antibiotic treatment of active disease, hygienic measures focusing mainly on facial cleanliness and improved environmental conditions in endemic areas, such as access to drinking water and disinfectants, separation of livestock from living areas, improved sanitation facilities, etc. [34, 40, 44].

Risk Factors

Transmission of chlamydia usually occurs through insects, direct contact or indirectly through contaminated objects—clothes, towels, etc. In Trachoma endemic areas, the main problems are poverty, overcrowding, low levels of hygiene, lack of access to cleaning and disinfecting agents, inadequate and often completely absent sources of safe water and close cohabitation between people and livestock, including sharing of living quarters. Too many people living in households is also a well-documented risk factor. In fact, the largest reservoir of infection is the group of household caregivers who are extremely susceptible to infection. The correlation of occurrence with epidemic or bacterial conjunctivitis of other aetiologies in endemic areas (especially Haemophilus, Pneumococcus, Moraxella sp.) has also been described [34, 40].

Trachoma is known as a "low-grade infection"—repeated contact is needed for the outbreak of the disease, which is why it spreads so well in crowded dwellings and through repeated contact with flies.

Clinical Symptoms

In the early phase, which usually takes place in early childhood, the disease has an uncomplicated course, often with only mild tearing, foreign body sensation, itching and redness of the eyes, or is completely asymptomatic. It may occasionally be accompanied by painful lymphadenopathy. After primo-infection, transient immunity occurs, but also sensitisation to reinfection, which later leads to a stronger inflammatory response of the organism to the new presence of the antigen [4, 6]. For this reason, vaccination is not a suitable means of preventing the spread of Trachoma. In the late and chronic phase, a chronic inflammatory reaction occurs, a cell-mediated late type of hypersensitivity to the sudden repeated presence of chlamydial antigen – Type IV reaction. Gradually progressive scarring changes are manifested by trichiasis pain, foreign body sensations, photophobia, corneal ulcer pain [4,](Bowling 2016). In the final stage, a vascularised and scarred cornea is a leading symptom of visual impairment at the level of blindness. At the same time, the infection closes the outlets of the lacrimal gland, which is the cause of dryness of the eye, and which further aggravates all the symptoms, along with a change in the quality of tears, destroying the fairy cells [4, 6].

Sexually Transmitted Diseases

Objective Findings

Primo-infection occurs most often in preschool children [44]. It presents as acute mucopurulent conjunctivitis with conjunctival hyperaemia, papillary and later follicular reaction on the tarsus, lacrimation, usually without corneal involvement or with epithelial keratopathy, pannus may be present. Overall, swelling of the preauricular nodes can be observed.

After reinfection, the disease progresses in intermingled acute inflammatory and chronic scarring phases. Chronic stages of Trachoma occur in middle age, proceeding according to the current stage under the image of early reinfection, with a pronounced follicular reaction on the tarsal conjunctiva, through diffuse conjunctivitis to scarring changes accompanied by the disappearance of cup cells, the formation of linear and star-shaped scars, more on the upper tarsal conjunctiva, healing of follicles with the formation of the Herbert's pits on the limbus, Arlt's lines on the tarsus, trichiasis and subsequently the development of corneal ulcers and opacities with corneal vascularisation are seen in the late stage of Trachoma.

Classification

Worldwide, two classification systems are used to determine the different stages of the disease.

McCallan's Classification

- Stage I—Initial Trachoma with follicular reaction on the tarsal conjunctiva, often with preauricular lymphadenopathy
- Stage II—Follicular and papillary reaction to tarsus—according to the predominant type of reaction, it is divided into Stage IIa (follicular) and IIb (papillary)
- Stage III—Tarsal conjunctival scarring
- Stage IV—Trichiasis, conjunctiva without follicles, healing Trachoma

WHO classification (more commonly used today) [45]:

- TF follicular inflammatory reaction, at least five follicles are present on the upper tarsus
- TI deepening of the inflammatory reaction with thickening of the tarsus, overlapping more than half of the deep tarsal vessels
- TS scarring, presence of white Arlt's lines on the upper tarsal conjunctiva
- TT trichiasis, eyelashes are turned against the surface of the eye
- CO corneal opacity in front of the pupil, in the optical axis

Diagnosis

In diagnostics, conjunctival swabs and subsequent culture, PCR examination and, finally, cytological examination with Giemsa staining (and detection of perinuclear inclusion bodies) are used. Histological examination can also be used in the case of diagnostic confusion.

Differential Diagnosis

In the acute phase, any conjunctivitis of other aetiology (viral, bacterial, chemical) is considered.

In the late stage of chronic conjunctivitis, other infections, ocular scarring pemphigoid, Stevens-Johnson syndrome, post-burn and burn conditions are ruled out.

Therapy

In total, Azithromycin is administered in a single dose of 20mg/kg in children, 1g in adults, in pregnancy Erythromycin 500 mg twice daily for two weeks. Therapy is administered to all members of the same household, repeated once a year.

Topically, 1% tetracycline ointment is used twice daily for six weeks.

Late complications require surgical management (eyelid surgery, corneal transplantation is difficult and does not have a good prognosis, amblyopia from anopsia is often present, secondary complications are common) [4, 6]. Treatment of Trachoma is one of the priorities of the WHO programme. Simple eyelid surgery for trichiasis is very helpful, so nurses are trained to perform these procedures, which greatly reduces the incidence of blindness due to repeated corneal damage from eyelid malposition [44].

6.2   Inclusion Conjunctivitis in Adults

Chlamydial infections caused by *Ch. trachomatis* serotypes D-K are one of the most common sexually transmitted diseases. This is an inclusive adult conjunctivitis, occurring mainly in economically developed countries, where it affects 5–20% of sexually active adults, unlike Trachoma [4, 6, 34].

Risk Factors

Transmission of the agent to the conjunctiva occurs by direct contact with contaminated secretions between sexual partners or, more commonly, by autoinoculation. Various diagnostic methods have detected concomitant genital chlamydial infection in 40–90% of persons with acute inclusion conjunctivitis, with eye-to-eye transmission occurring in 10% [4, 6, 34].

Clinical Symptoms and Objective Findings

Acute inclusion conjunctivitis presents as mixed papillary-follicular conjunctivitis (Figs. 16 and 17).

It may be accompanied by mild discomfort, eyelid swelling and foreign body sensation, mucopurulent secretion, conjunctival redness, punctate keratopathy and painful preauricular lymphadenopathy. Even without treatment, it is usually self-limiting, but then a recurrent course of the disease is possible with a transition to

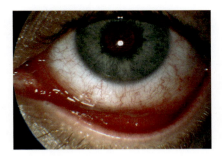

Fig. 16 Chlamydial inclusion conjunctivitis in adults – mucopurulent secretion, pseudomembrane formation

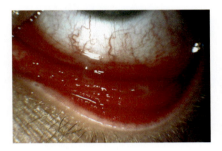

Fig. 17 Chlamydial inclusion conjunctivitis in adults – follicular reaction, mucopurulent secretion

chronicity and the development of scarring changes, usually limited to the peripheral parts of the cornea [4, 6, 34].

Complications

If antibiotic therapy is not initiated, a transition to a chronic course lasting up to years, with the development of scarring changes in the peripheral parts of the cornea is possible.

CAVE—it is advisable to consider testing for the presence of other sexually transmitted diseases.

Persistence of conjunctival follicles and corneal infiltrates after treatment is not a sign of persistent infection, but of hypersensitivity to chlamydial antigen. It is advisable to repeat the smear, serology.

Diagnosis and Differential Diagnosis

Conjunctival swabs or better scraping spatula for culture are used, and PCR examination, direct immunofluorescence and antigen detection by EIA. In the differential diagnosis, granulomatous follicular conjunctivitis with lymphadenopathy (Parinaud's syndrome) and conjunctivitis of other aetiologies—mainly viral—are considered. Examination and treatment of sexual partners are important.

Therapy

Overall, treatment with Azithromycin is used, 1 g once or repeat 2–3 times after a week. Doxycycline 100 mg twice daily for 10 days can also be used. In pregnant women, Erythromycin, or Ciprofloxacin, Amoxicillin, is administered. It is always necessary to recommend examination and possibly treatment of sexual partners.

Topical tetracycline ointment 1% is administered 2–3 times daily, in combination with general treatment to accelerate the onset of action.

7 Gonorrhoea

Acute or chronic purulent inflammation transmitted almost exclusively by sexual intercourse, primarily affecting the mucous membrane of the urogenital tract, caused by the gram-negative bacterium *Neisseria gonorrhoeae*. It can also cause inflammation of the conjunctiva, rectum and rarely the mucous membranes of the nose, mouth, and pharynx. It can also cause diseases of the musculoskeletal system, endocardium, and cornea. The name is derived from the Greek words *gonos*—seed, *rhoein*—to flow. Complicated diseases affect reproductive health (miscarriages, premature births, ectopic pregnancies, infertility). At birth, the new-born could be infected by the sick mother, with the possible consequence of blindness. Similarly to other inflammatory diseases of the urogenital tract, there is increased susceptibility to HIV infection. It is often combined with *Chlamydia trachomatis* urogenital infection.

Aetiology

The causative agent is a gram-negative diplococcus, *Neisseria gonorrhoeae* (*N. gonorrhoeae*) belonging to the family *Neisseriacae*, genus *Neisseria*. It is most often found intracellularly in leukocytes, and extracellularly (coffee-bean shape) in the early phase of infection.

Pathogenesis

Gonorrhoea is almost exclusively transmitted by sexual intercourse, through direct contact with infected mucous membranes. The only carrier is man. Exceptionally, transmission is possible by soiled linen, bedding, etc., in poor hygienic conditions (in young girls, the vaginal mucosa is not completely covered by the squamous epithelium). The highest risk group is those under 25 years of age with multiple sexual partners. Prevalence is higher in urban populations and within minorities. The risk of transmission in a single sexual encounter from an infected male to an uninfected female is 50–60%, and from an infected female to an uninfected male is 20%. Women and men with asymptomatic urethritis are a significant source of infection, with asymptomatic infections being much more common in women than in men. Oropharyngeal infection is more commonly diagnosed in women and homosexual men after fellatio. Anorectal infection is symptomatic in 18–34% of MSM individuals.

The incubation period is 2–6 days. In men, acute symptoms usually appear between Days 2–5. In adult women, the disease is often oligo- or asymptomatic.

Clinical Presentation

The clinical presentation is basically divided into two groups according to gender:

Male gonorrhoea

The incubation period is usually 2–6 days, with a range of 1–14 days. Symptoms usually are urethritis with whitish-yellow urethral discharge (Fig. 18), reddened urethral orifice, *dysuria* (burning and cutting during urination), *pollakisuria*, or *balanoposthitis*.

In about one-quarter of infections, it manifests itself only as a "morning drop" (*"goutte de bonjour"*); in 10% of men it is asymptomatic, which is the cause of the spread of the disease. At the site of the periurethral glands, paraurethral lacunae, bulbourethral Cowper's glands, inflammations to abscesses may arise, which may perforate into the urethra or externally. Ascending spread is the cause of *prostatitis, epididymitis, spermatocystitis*. Acute prostatitis is manifested by fevers, abdominal pain during defecation and urination, painful pollutions. Per rectum examination will reveal an enlarged painful prostate. In epididymitis, which is the most serious complication of gonorrhoea, there is a unilateral, painful reddened swelling of the scrotum. Male infertility arises because of obstruction of the ducts of the epididymis, sperm duct or spermatic cord.

Female gonorrhoea

Early symptoms of gonorrhoea in women are symptoms of urethritis with frequent urging to urinate and burning sensation during urination. Symptoms of urethritis and cervicitis can be overlooked or confused with another gynaecological diseases. Classically, purulent, or mucopurulent discharge from the cervix, from the urethra or anus could be present. The cervix is reddened, oedematous with contact bleeding. Profuse discharge from the cervix may be accompanied by *vulvitis* and *dermatitis* in the external genital area and thighs.

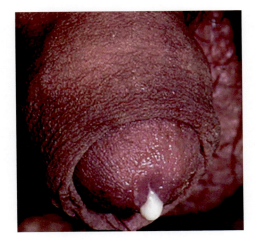

Fig. 18 Discharge in gonorrhoea

In women, the infection can spread to Skene's periurethral glands and Bartholini's glands on the labia, where a unilateral abscess can form, painful when walking and sitting. Without treatment, the infection spreads, ascending, and endometritis develops. Clinical manifestations depend on the phase of the cycle in which gonococci have penetrated the endometrium. In the middle of the cycle, the symptoms of endometritis are minimal; during menstruation the endometrial lining separates and the inflammation can heal spontaneously. When the infection penetrates during or just after menstruation, the inflammation also affects the uterine musculature, resulting in *endomyometritis*. The patient has lower abdominal pain, temperature and abnormal bleeding. The infection spreads, ascending to the fallopian tubes, pelvic peritoneum, and ovaries (Fig. 19).

Pelvic inflammatory disease (PID) is accompanied by *salpingitis, perisalpingitis, oophoritis, periophoritis*, circumscribed peritonitis (Fitz-Hughes syndrome), rarely diffuse peritonitis, tubo-ovarian abscess and Douglas abscess. The result of the inflammation is damage to the fallopian tubes and the formation of adhesions, with subsequent infertility, pelvic pain, and the risk of ectopic pregnancy.

Extragenital Forms of Gonorrhoea

Pharyngeal gonorrhoea is usually asymptomatic and not accompanied by sore throat. Anorectal gonorrhoea usually occurs in women by perineal transmission (autoinoculation), rather than anal intercourse, and is usually asymptomatic, with rare bleeding,

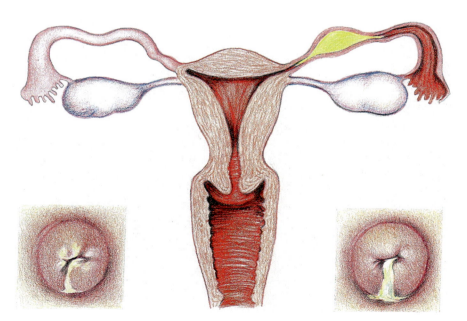

Fig. 19 Ascending spread of gonorrhoea and image of cervical landscape with discharge in gonorrhoea and chlamydial infection of the cervix in gonorrhoea

Sexually Transmitted Diseases

pain, burning and discharge from the anus. In MSM individuals, it arises because of anal intercourse.

Conjunctivitis is either a disease of newborns (*blenorrhoea neonatorum*) or adults [23]. A newborn is infected during childbirth, an adult by dirty fingers. Untreated infection could lead to *keratitis*, corneal ulcer, corneal perforation, and blindness. Prophylaxis of neonatal gonorrhoeal conjunctivitis is the routine application of an antibacterial agent, such as Septonex®, into the conjunctival sac just after birth (formerly silver nitrate solution-Credé method, neonatal creep).

Disseminated gonorrhoea affects about 0.5–3% of patients. It is accompanied by fever. A trio of symptoms – *polyarthralgia, tendosynovitis* and *dermatitis* ("arthritis-dermatitis syndrome"), with purulent arthritis without skin symptoms – are possible manifestations. The exanthema is vesicular, pustular, or haemorrhagic, usually localised on peripheral parts of the extremities, histologically with signs of leuco-cytoclastic vasculitis. Hyperkeratotic conical papules with an inflammatory rim or diffuse hyperkeratotic foci form on the hands and feet. Polyarthritis is most likely reactive, monoarthritis is a true infection. Usually one joint is affected, most often the knee. Exceptionally, several small joints are affected, they are usually swollen, red, painful. *N. gonorrhoeae* can be cultured from joint aspirate. Rare cases of menin-gitis and endocarditis have been described. In uveitis, painful, red eyes and irregular pupils are found.

Diagnosis

For a correct diagnosis, adequate sampling is necessary, which, in women, is performed from the endocervix and urethra. Samples can also be taken from the rectum, pharynx, conjunctivae, nose, and possibly also from skin lesions. Sampling of the cervix during menses, when an exacerbation of an asymptomatic infection may occur, is also appropriate.

The focus of infection detection is direct diagnosis. Microscopic examination is standardly performed in Gram staining (gonococci are phagocytosed in polymor-phonuclear cells or localised extracellularly in the early phase of the disease); it is considered as an indicative test (morphological match of representatives of the genus Neisseria, possible confusion with e.g. *Neisseria meningitidis*).

Culturing is the basis of standard diagnostics and allows accurate biochemical identification of the aetiological agent (sugar utilisation, cytochrome oxidase reac-tion, etc.) and ***determination of antibiotic susceptibility*** (worldwide increase in resistency), including beta-lactamase detection.

DNA-hybridisation or PCR detection allows the detection of nucleic acids of a microbe with high sensitivity (especially PCR as an amplification method—98.8%), even in borderline situations, and with forensic accuracy. Nevertheless, even these procedures are burdened with problems complicating clinical practice. These include the inability to test for antibiotic susceptibility (although there are approaches to detect resistance genes), the capture of DNA from dead gonococci after treatment, and false cross-positivity with some species of oral Neisseria and lactobacilli.

Differential Diagnosis

In the differential diagnosis, it is necessary to distinguish mainly infections with other microorganisms causing discharge (*Chlamydia trachomatis, Trichomonas vaginalis, Candida albicans, herpes simplex* virus, etc.).

Therapy

Treatment is mandatory for all infected persons. Due to the short generation time of gonococcus (15 min), uncomplicated forms of the disease can be treated with a single application of antibiotics. Antibiotics with high tissue penetration and high serum concentrations are suitable for single administration. For the treatment of gonorrhoea, cephalosporin, macrolide, and fluoroquinolones are used [47].

8 Ocular Manifestations of Gonococcal Infections

Gonococcus or *Neisseria gonorrhoeae*, the causative agent of gonorrhoea, can cause severe purulent conjunctivitis, with a hyperacute course and potentially devastating effects. Although gonorrhoea repeatedly ranks as one of the leading STD in the Europe, even with an increasing trend in the last 10 years, the occurrence of gonococcal conjunctivitis is fortunately very rare, especially in developed countries [12]. Infection occurs through transmission of contaminated genital secretions (during childbirth) or urine from a sexual partner or through autoinoculation [4, 6].

Risk Factors

Infection occurs through contact between the surface of the eye and contaminated secretions from a sexual partner or through autoinfection.

Symptoms and Objective Findings

Pain, swelling of the eyelids, dense purulent secretion, hyperaemia and chemosis of the conjunctiva, pseudomembranes on the tarsal conjunctiva, punctate epitheliopathy of the cornea are observed; preauricular lymphadenopathy is the rule in severe conjunctivitis. *N. gonorrhoeae* has a high affinity for corneal tissue, which it penetrates very easily, which is why this infection is so dangerous to the eye. The onset of difficulties is within hours of transmission. Very often, ocular symptoms are accompanied by urogenital complaints and the patient should be referred for investigation [4, 6, 12].

Complications

Keratitis with ulceration and perforation of the cornea or marginal ulcer under the lacunes filled with pus may develop; in severe cases, endophthalmitis may occur.

Sexually Transmitted Diseases

Diagnosis and Differential Diagnosis

A conjunctival swab for culture on chocolate agar, PCR examination, slide smear and Gram staining are performed. In the differential diagnosis, most often another bacterial conjunctivitis is excluded.

Therapy

Ceftriaxone 1 g IM or crystalline penicillin G 100,000 IU/kg/day IM for 5–7 days is administered, or Ciprofloxacin 500 mg PO in one dose, Ofloxacin 400 mg PO in one dose (fluoroquinolones are contraindicated in children under 8 years and pregnant and lactating women).

Topical fluoroquinolones, third-generation cephalosporins, gentamicin or chloramphenicol every 1–2 h in drops are administered. Hygienic measures – repeated conjunctival lavage with Betadine 1:10 solution and evacuation of pus are also important. There is a high risk of contamination of attending staff when forcibly opening the swollen eyelids, under which the secretion accumulates under pressure. For this, the use of a face shield is necessary.

If corneal complications develop, Ceftriaxone 1 g IV is administered every 12 h. When gonococcal conjunctivitis is suspected, treatment must be started promptly, without waiting for the result of the culture.

9 Chlamydial and Gonococcal Infections of the Eye in New-Borns

In new-borns of mothers with gonococcal or chlamydial genital disease, contamination of the conjunctival sac may occur during passage through the birth canal. In the first days or weeks after birth, acute conjunctivitis, ophthalmia neonatorum, develops. As prevention, disinfection of the conjunctival sac with various agents (povidone-iodine 2.5%, topical silver nitrate, erythromycin) can be performed in new-borns. Untreated conjunctivitis can progress to general infectious complications in the new-born, including pneumonia in the case of chlamydia [4, 6, 12].

Clinical Symptoms and Objective Findings

Mild conjunctivitis is very common in new-borns. In conjunctivitis with early onset and peracute course, the presence of gonococcal aetiology should be suspected. Gonococcal conjunctivitis manifests itself as early as 2–4 days after delivery, with board-like swelling of the eyelids, impressive as preseptal orbitocellulitis, purulence, hyperaemia and chemosis of the conjunctiva; formation of pseudomembranes is possible. It is essential to examine the cornea for the threat of early formation of a perforating ulcer [4, 6, 12].

Chlamydial conjunctivitis usually develops between Days 4–10 as lid swelling, diffuse hyperaemia and conjunctival chemosis, and a sanguineous discharge may be present [4, 6, 12].

Complications

Improperly or late treated neonatal ophthalmia can be complicated by very early corneal complications, including perforation and endophthalmitis. In chlamydial conjunctivitis, there is a risk of developing general complications, including otitis and pneumonia.

Diagnosis

Culture examination by conjunctival swab is used—it is conclusive in gonococcal conjunctivitis; in chlamydial conjunctivitis, PCR examination or cytology with Giemsa staining is more reliable. The clinical presentation and medical anamnesis are also important.

Therapy

Overall, for chlamydial conjunctivitis, Erythromycin 25 mg/kg is administered twice daily for 2 weeks; for gonococcal infection, Ceftriaxone 25–50 mg/kg in one dose, maximum 125 mg.

Locally, in gonococcal infections, fluoroquinolones or Gentamicin is administered every 1 h; frequent conjunctival lavages with saline or boric acid are performed in the meantime.

References

1. Ahmed I, Ai E, Chang E, et al. Ophthalmic manifestations of HIV. HIV insite knowledge base chapter [online]. USA, San Francisco: University of California; 2005. Available at http://hiv insite.ucsf.edu/InSite?page=kb-04-01-12
2. Bartonickova K. What a urologist should know about chlamydial infections—overview of the current state. Urol Pract. 2003;3:94–8.
3. Bartsch DU, Kozak I, Grant I, et al. Retinal nerve fiber and optic disc morphology in patients with human immunodeficiency virus using the Heidelberg Retina tomography 3. PLoS One 2015;10(8):e0133144.
4. Boguszakova J, et al. Eye and general diseases. In: Kuchynka P, et al., editors. Ophthalmology. Prague: Grada; 2016. p. 859–61.
5. Bostikova V, Prasil P, Kuca K, et al. Current view of chlamydial infections. Med Practice. 2016;13(5):234–7.
6. Bowling B. Kanski's clinical ophthalmology. Elsevier; 2016.
7. Braun-Falco O, Plewig G, Wolff HH. Dermatology and venereology. 4th ed. Berlin Heidelberg New York: Springer-Verlag; 1996.
8. Butcher R, Houghton J, Derrick T, et al. Reduced-cost Chlamydia trachomatis-specific multiplex real-time PCR diagnostic assay evaluated for ocular swabs and use by trachoma research programmes. J Microbiol Methods. 2017;139:95–102.
9. Centers for Disease Control and Prevention (CDC). Primary and secondary syphilis—United States, 2003–2004. MMWR Morb Mortal Wkly Rep. 2006;55(10):269–73.
10. Chiotan C, Radu L, Serban R, at al. Cytomegalovirus retinitis in HIV/AIDS patients. J Med Life. 2014;7(2):237–40.
11. Chiquet C, Khayi H, Puech C, et al. Ocular syphilis. Fr Ophtalmol. 2014;37(4):329–36.

Sexually Transmitted Diseases

12. Costumbrado J, Ng DK, Ghassemzadeh S. Gonococcal conjunctivitis. [Updated 2022 Sep 12]. In: StatPearls [Internet]. Treasure Island (FL): StatPearls Publishing; 2023. Available from: https://www.ncbi.nlm.nih.gov/books/NBK459289/
13. de Lissovoy G, Zenilman J, Nelson KE, et al. The cost of a preventable disease: estimated U.S. national medical expenditures for congenital syphilis, 1990. Public Health Rep. 1995;110(4):403–9.
14. Dourmishev L, Dourmishev A. Syphilis: uncommon presentations in adults. Clin Dermatol. 2005;23(6):555–64.
15. Gupta M, Sareen A, Sareen V. Ocular changes in sexually transmitted diseases: review of literature. JMSCR. 2017;5(3):18896–904.
16. Humphrey MD, Bradford DL. Congenital syphilis: still a reality in 1996. Med J Austral. 1996;165(7):382–5.
17. Jilich D, Kulirova V, et al. HIV infection—current trends in diagnosis, treatment and nursing. Prague: Young Front; 2014. p. 173.
18. Johnson RE, Newhall WJ, Papp JR, et al. Screening tests to detect Chlamydia trachomatis and Neisseria gonorrhoeae infections—2002. CDC MMWR (Morb Mort Weekly Rep). 2002;51(15):1–38.
19. Kiss S, Damico FM, Young LH. Ocular manifestations and treatment of syphilis. Semin Ophthalmol. 2005;20(3):161–7.
20. Kozner P, Machala L, Filous A, et al. Overview of the development of ocular opportunistic infections in HIV-positive patients. Czech Slovak Ophthalmol. 2009;65(1):36–8.
21. Kozner P, Machala L, Rozsypal H, et al. HIV retinopathy. Clin Microbiol Infect Med. 2009;15(5):183–4.
22. Kraus H. Eye and general diseases. In: Kraus H. Compendium of ophthalmology. Prague: Grada; 1997.
23. Kumar P. Gonorrhoea presenting as red eye: rare case. Indian J Sex Transm Dis AIDS. 2012;33(1):47–8.
24. Linzerova D, Stepanov A, Nemcansky J. Ocular manifestations in patients with HIV. Cesk Slov Oftalmol. 2019;74(6):234–9.
25. Matouskova M, Hanus M. Chlamydia trachomatis – a threat to the urology clinic? Urol Pract. 2009;10(2):60–4.
26. Porsova M. Urogenital chlamydial infection. Postgrad Med. 2011;1;77.
27. Resl V. Methodological recommendations for the serological investigation of syphilis. Czech Derm. 2001;76(4):210–4.
28. Rihova E. Uveitis. Prague: Grada; 2009.
29. Rozsypal H. AIDS Clinical presentation and treatment. Prague: Maxdorf; 1998. p. 236.
30. Rozsypal H. Health complications of human immunodeficiency virus (HIV) infection. In: Rozsypal H, editor. Basics of infectious medicine. Prague: Karolinum; 2015. p. 393–401.
31. Ruiz-Cruz M, Alvarado-de la Barrera C, Ablanedo-Terrazas Y, et al. Proposed clinical case definition for cytomegalovirus-immune recovery retinitis. Clin Infect Dis. 2014;59(2):298–303.
32. Salavec M, Bostikova V, Bostik P. HIV infection—history, pathogenesis, clinical manifestations. Czech-Slov Derm. 2011;86(2):67–81.
33. Salavec M, Resl V. Syphilis congenita. Czech-Slov Derm. 2001;76(2):90–8.
34. Satpathy G, Behera HS, Ahmed NH. Chlamydial eye infections: Current perspectives. Indian J Ophthalmol. 2017;65(2):97–102.
35. Schultz K, Murphy KF, Patamasucon P. Congenital syphilis Chapter 67. In: Holmes K King, Mardh PA, Sparling FP, et al. Sexually transmitted diseases. New York: McGraw-Hill inf Services Comp; 1990. p. 821–42.
36. Stankova M, Maresova V, Vanista J. HIV infection. In: Stankova M, Maresova V, Vanista J, editors. Repetitorium of infectious diseases. Prague: Triton; 2008. p. 139–43.
37. Stepanov A, Feuermannova A, Hejsek L, et al. Cytomegalovirus retinitis in a patient with acquired immunodeficiency syndrome. Czech Slovak Ophthalmol. 2014;70(4):132–7.
38. Stork J, et al. Dermatovenereology, 1st ed. Prague: Galen; 2008.

39. Tan S, Duan H, Xun T, et al. HIV-1 impairs human retinal pigment epithelial barrier function: possible association with the pathogenesis of HIV-associated retinopathy. Lab Invest. 2014;94:777–87.
40. Taylor J. Trachoma: still a major cause of blindness. Afr Health. 1995;17(3):17–8.
41. Torsova V. Urogenital chlamydial infection:still an actual problem. Practice Gynecol. 2004;4:53–7.
42. Velcevsky P, Kuklova I. Treatment of sexually transmitted diseases. Czech Slov Derm. 2008;83(3):123–35.
43. Wagenlehner FM, Weidner W, Naber KG. Chlamydia infection in urology. World J Urol. 2006;24:2–12.
44. WHO Alliance for the Elimination of Blinding Trachoma by 2020. Wkly Epidemiol Rec 2012;87(17):161–8.
45. WHO Simplified Trachoma Grading System. Commun Eye Health. 2004;17(52):68.
46. World Health Organization. HIV/AIDS Factsheet, HIV data and statistics. Retrieved 6 March 2022. Available online at www.who.int
47. Zakoucka H, Kuklova I. Diagnostics of classical venereal diseases. Czech Slov Derm. 2007;82(2):65–74.

Cancer Diseases

Veronika Matuskova, Jiri Petera, Ondrej Kubecek, and Ahmed Youbi Zakaria

1 Metastasis of Solid Tumours to the Eye

Epidemiology

Metastases of solid tumours can theoretically affect any part of the eye. As a result of the absence of the lymphatic system in the eye, intraocular metastases arise by haematogenous dissemination and occur in the most vascularised parts of the eye, including the structures of the uvea, which is most frequently affected by metastases. Among the components of the uvea, the choroid is the most frequent site of metastasis (88% of all cases), especially around the macula which exhibits the densest vascularisation [1]. This is followed by the iris (9%) and the ciliary body (2%).

In most patients with intraocular metastases, the location of the primary tumour is already known. Especially breast and lung cancer can metastasise early to the eye, again preferentially to the uvea. In some cases, intraocular metastases are the first manifestation of tumour dissemination, and the diagnosis of generalised malignancy is primarily made by the ophthalmologist. The incidence of intraocular metastases

---

V. Matuskova
Department of Ophthalmology, University Hospital in Brno, Jihlavská 340/20, 62500 Brno, Czech Republic
e-mail: v.matuskova@email.cz

J. Petera · O. Kubecek (✉)
Department of Oncology, University Hospital and Faculty of Medicine of Charles University in Hradec Králové, Sokolska 581, 50005 Hradec Králové, Czech Republic
e-mail: ondrej.kubecek@fnhk.cz

J. Petera
e-mail: jiri.petera@fnhk.cz

A. Y. Zakaria
Department of Radiation Oncology, Ahmad Bin Zayed Al Nahyan Center for Cancer Treatments, Tangier, Morocco
e-mail: zakaria.youbi@gmail.com

© The Author(s), under exclusive license to Springer Nature Switzerland AG 2024
A. Stepanov and J. Studnicka (eds.), *Ocular Manifestations of Systemic Diseases*,
https://doi.org/10.1007/978-3-031-58592-0_9

can only be estimated because a large proportion of cases are not diagnosed during the lifetime of patients. The prevalence of metastases in cancer patients in post-mortem studies is 4–10% [1]. The incidence is estimated to be about 20,000 cases per year in the USA and about 5000 cases per year in Germany [1]. This makes intraocular metastases the most common malignancy of the eye.

Choroidal metastases

Choroidal metastases are found at autopsy in about 8% of metastatic cancer-related deaths [2]. Choroidal metastases are associated with advanced cancer and poor prognosis. Of all uveal metastases, choroidal metastases account for 57–88% [1]. The perimacular region represents an ideal environment for the establishment and proliferation of haematogenously disseminated tumour cells due to dense vascularisation. In two-thirds of cases, bifocal tumour foci are found. Bifocal and unilateral metastases are mostly found in lung cancer, whereas breast cancer metastases are more often multifocal and bilateral. Metastatic foci are usually up to 9 mm in diameter and 3 mm thick [3].

Cancers with the greatest tendency to disseminate, i.e., lung cancer and breast cancer, metastasize most frequently to the choroid. Breast cancer metastases account for 40–53% of choroidal metastases, with the eye being the only metastatic manifestation in 8% [1]. Lung cancer is the source of 20–29% of choroidal metastases. Median survival for patients with choroidal metastasis is 21 months for breast cancer and 12 months for lung cancer.

Intraocular metastases of gastrointestinal (4%), prostate (2%), kidney (2–4%), and skin (2%) tumours are less common [1]. Metastases of thyroid, pancreatic, testicular, ovarian, neuroendocrine tumors, and sarcomas are even rarer.

In more than one-third of cases, choroidal metastases are the first manifestation of disseminated cancer, and, when searching for the primary tumour, lung cancer is found in 7% of cases, breast cancer in 35%, and no primary tumour is found in more than 50% [1]. Amelanotic melanoma, granulomas of various aetiologies, haemangiomas, osteomas and sclerochoroidal calcifications should be considered in the differential diagnosis.

Metastases to the iris and ciliary body

Intraocular metastases affect the iris and ciliary body in 10% of cases. In a study of patients with metastases to the iris or ciliary body, all metastases were unilateral [4]. Associated secondary glaucoma was present in 38% of cases. The most common sources of metastases were lung, colon, breast, kidney, and malignant melanoma of the skin [4].

Metastases to the retina

The sources of relatively rare retinal metastases are mainly breast, colon, lung, oesophageal, and cutaneous malignant melanoma. Retinitis, nerve fibre infarcts, haemangiomas, and haemorrhages must be considered in the differential diagnosis. Due to the relative rarity and differential diagnostic possibilities, there is often a delay in diagnosis and treatment.

Cancer Diseases 343

Metastases to the vitreous

Metastases to the vitreous are rare and are most often caused by melanomas of the skin; metastases from lung cancer and cholangiocarcinoma have also been described.

Most common solid tumours metastasising to the eye

1.1 Breast Cancer

Breast cancer is the most common cancer in women if non-melanoma skin tumours are not considered. Breast cancer represents a significant global health challenge: it is the most frequently diagnosed cancer in the world with an estimated 2.26 million cases recorded in 2020 and is the leading cause of cancer mortality among females—almost 685,000 deaths worldwide [5]. Thanks to earlier diagnosis and modern treatments, the mortality rate of breast cancer is decreasing slightly but steadily.

Symptomatology

Breast cancer can present with local manifestations, regional lymph node involvement and symptoms of distant dissemination.

Local symptoms are tactile resistance, pain, pressure or tension in the breast, nipple retraction, and pathological secretion from the breast. Inflammatory carcinoma, expressed as reddening of the skin, with underlying infiltration of cutaneous lymphatic vessels by malignant cells, is a special entity.

Regional nodes are axillary, supraclavicular, subclavian, and parasternal nodes. Typically, a tumour-infiltrating lymph node is of a firm to hard consistency. The union of several nodes into nodal packets represents locoregionally advanced disease.

Bone, lung, liver, and brain are the most common metastatic sites.

Diagnosis includes assessment of the locoregional extent of the disease (physical examination, mammography, ultrasound, MRI), evaluation of any distant manifestations of the disease and histopathological examination [6, 7]. The standard investigation for possible dissemination is lung X-ray, liver ultrasonography, and skeletal scintigraphy. Other investigations (e.g., CT, MRI) are optional.

Classification

Brest cancer is divided into five biological subtypes, in which histological prognostic and predictive indicators are considered (Table 1). The subtypes differ in prognosis (deteriorating in the Table from luminal type A with the best prognosis to triple negative subtype with the worst prognosis) and predict the choice of systemic cancer therapy.

Table 1 Biological subtypes of breast cancer

Luminal A	ER and PR positive, HER2 negative, grade 1–2, Ki 67 low (<20%)
Luminal B HER negative	ER positive PR negative, HER2 negative, grade 3, Ki 67 high (>20%)
Luminal B HER positive	ER positive PR any, HER2 positive, Ki 67 any
HER positive	ER or PR negative, HER2 positive
Basal like—triple negative	ER or PR negative, HER negative

Treatment

Breast cancer therapy is individualised with respect to the patient and her disease. It usually combines, in variable order, locoregional methods (surgery and radiotherapy) and systemic methods (chemotherapy, hormone therapy, and targeted therapy) [8]. Determination of the treatment strategy is decided on by a multidisciplinary team. Two main aspects are considered. The first is the patient, her age, general condition, comorbidities, previous and current therapy. The second is the tumour, its extent (staging), histopathological findings and the resulting prognostic and predictive factors.

Hormonal therapy, chemotherapy and targeted therapy are used in breast cancer, both in adjuvant setting and for inoperable or metastatic disease. Breast cancer is sensitive to systemic therapy, and, even in metastatic disease, significant regression of tumour infiltrates or remission of disease can be achieved. Radiotherapy is also an effective treatment modality for breast cancer.

1.2 Lung Cancer

Lung cancer is the most common cancer in men and the second most common cancer in women. There were more than 2.2 million new cases of lung cancer in 2020 [9]. At the time of diagnosis, the median age is approximately 70 years.

Classification

Lung cancer is divided into two basic groups:

The first group consists of non-small cell lung carcinomas (NSCLC), which are of epithelial origin and account for 80% of lung carcinomas. They are characterised by lower growth activity and a tendency to spread gradually by lymphogenous spread and only later by haematogenous dissemination.

The second group (about 20%) consists of small cell lung carcinomas (SCLC), which are of neuroendocrine origin. They are characterised by high growth activity and a tendency to early haematogenous dissemination and more frequent occurrence of paraneoplastic symptoms.

Aetiology

Smoking is considered the most important risk factor. Mechanical particles in the environment, chemical carcinogens (heavy metals, formaldehyde, and PVC production) and exposure to ionising radiation (uranium mines, radon in buildings) are also associated with increased risk of lung cancer.

Clinical presentation

Symptoms of lung cancer are divided into local (intrathoracic), advanced disease (extrathoracic metastatic) and paraneoplastic symptoms.

Local symptoms

The most common local symptom is a cough, dry, irritating, or productive. Haemoptysis of varying degrees occurs in about one-half of the patients.

Symptoms of advanced disease

In locoregional lymphogenous tumour propagation, the supraclavicular and cervical lymph nodes are affected.

The most common sites of distant metastases are the bones, central nervous system, liver, and adrenal glands. Distant metastases occur in 95% of SCLC, 80% of adenocarcinomas and 50% of squamous cell carcinomas [1].

Diagnosis

Standard investigations include medical history, physical examination, spirometry, bronchoscopy, lung X-ray, CT, PET/CT, and brain MRI in SCLC [7]. Skeletal scintigraphy is indicated for advanced NSCLC in the case of suspicious symptomatology and for SCLC [6].

Therapy

Non-small cell lung cancer (NSCLC)

In the early stages of NSCLC, surgical resection is the primary curative treatment. For tumours larger than 3 cm and in case of lymph node involvement, adjuvant chemotherapy is indicated. In the case of mediastinal lymph node involvement or in the case of micro- or macroscopic residue, radiotherapy is added. In locally advanced stages, surgery is combined with pre- or postoperative (radio)chemotherapy.

Therapy of very advanced and generalised stages is individual, depending on the patient's overall condition [8].

Small cell lung cancer (SCLC)

Patients diagnosed at early stages—i.e., those with the tumor confined to one side of the chest that can be treated with a single radiation field (limited disease)—are treated with either surgery or concurrent chemoradiotherapy. In more advanced cases (extensive disease), the treatment of choice is systemic chemotherapy which can be combined with immunotherapy in selected cases [10].

1.3 Other Tumours

Metastases from tumours other than breast and lung cancer account for less than 10% of intraocular secondary tumours.

Colorectal cancer is one of the most common malignancies in general. With almost 2 million new cases and 1 million deaths worldwide in 2020, colorectal cancer ranks as the third and the second most frequent cause of cancer incidence and mortality, respectively [11]. For early tumours, the basic treatment is radical surgery. Modern chemotherapy and targeted therapy have significantly prolonged the survival of patients with metastatic disease.

Oesophageal and gastric tumours are common. Metastatic disease is relatively sensitive to systemic therapy and radiosensitivity is also very good.

Prostate tumours are currently the most common malignancy in men, if non-melanoma skin tumours are not considered. The mainstay of treatment is either radical prostatectomy or radical radiotherapy.

Therapy

The treatment of intraocular metastases depends on the extent of dissemination of the primary tumour, its type, the general condition of the patient, the number, localisation and laterality of ocular involvement and the functional status of the eyes. Treatment options include systemic chemotherapy, immunotherapy, hormonal therapy, external beam radiotherapy, brachytherapy, transpupillary thermotherapy, and photodynamic therapy (PDT) [8].

Systemic treatment

Many tumours metastasizing to the eye respond very well to systemic treatment. Breast cancer and prostate cancer are sensitive to hormonal treatment, testicular, breast and ovarian cancer to chemotherapy, kidney cancer and melanoma to targeted therapy or immunotherapy. After the use of systemic treatment, significant and sometimes complete regression of intraocular metastases can occur.

Local treatment

Radiotherapy

Radiotherapy techniques include external beam radiotherapy, proton beam radiotherapy, brachytherapy, and stereotactic radiotherapy. Lung cancer metastases are less radiosensitive than breast cancer metastases. Side effects of radiotherapy may include cataract, iris neovascularisation with subsequent neovascular glaucoma, radiation retinopathy, and optic neuropathy. External beam radiotherapy can also cause skin erythema, madarosis, conjunctivitis, and keratopathy.

External radiotherapy

External beam radiotherapy is the most used form of radiotherapy for the treatment of ocular metastases. It allows preservation of the eyeball in 98% and improvement of vision in 43% of cases [12]. The target volume includes the whole eye with lens

Fig. 1 Varian Linear Accelerator, USA

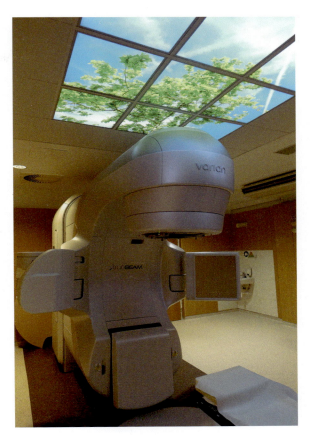

and corneal shielding. A linear accelerator (Fig. 1) with a photon beam energy of 6 MeV or electron beam energy of 15–18 meV is used as the radiation source.

Modern technologies, such as three-dimensional external beam radiotherapy or intensity-modulated radiotherapy are used (Fig. 2).

The recommended dose is 30–40 Gy in 10–20 individual fractions of 2–3 Gy. The total duration of radiation is 2–4 weeks. For patients in unfavourable general condition and with poor prognosis, a hypofractionated regimen, e.g. 25 Gy in 5 fractions, may be used [12].

Brachytherapy

Brachytherapy means irradiation from a short distance. It has the advantage of a sharp dose fall-off to the surrounding area and maximum sparing of healthy tissues. Its disadvantages are its applicability limited to small lesions and the invasive insertion of applicators. It is used for highly targeted irradiation. Applicators for brachytherapy of the eye are discs containing miniature radioisotope emitters, most commonly iodine-125 (^{125}I), ruthenium-106 (^{106}Ru), or palladium-103 (^{103}Pd) (Fig. 3). The

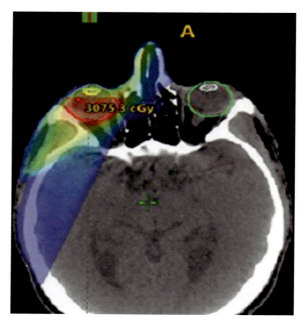

Fig. 2 Intensity modulated radiotherapy (IMRT) for choroidal metastasis

doses applied are 45–70 Gy over 3–4 days. Long-term regression of the metastatic lesion can be achieved in 94% of patients.

Proton therapy

The property of a proton beam is to deposit a high localised dose at a certain depth below the surface, which depends on the energy of the proton (Bragg peak).

Stereotactic radiotherapy and radiosurgery

Stereotactic radiotherapy and radiosurgery use multiple, precisely focused beams of radiation to irradiate a target volume with a high dose per fraction. The term radiosurgery is used for irradiation in a single fraction; irradiation in multiple fractions is referred to as stereotactic radiotherapy. High single doses have a destructive radiobiological effect on the tumour and its vasculature and are referred to as stereotactic ablative radiotherapy (SABR). Stereotactic irradiation can be achieved with a Leksell Gamma Knife, CyberKnife or a linear accelerator equipped with an adequate collimation system and an image-guided radiotherapy (IGRT) device. Figure 4A and B present choroidal metastasis of malignant melanoma before and after Gamma Knife treatment in an 85-year-old female patient with local control achieved 2.5 years after radiation.

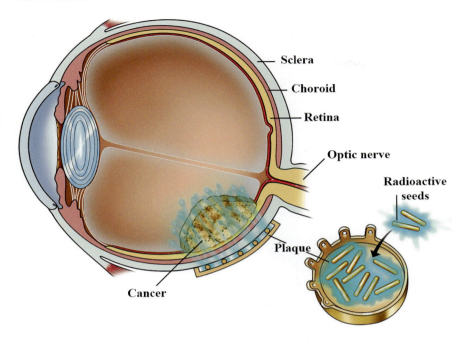

Fig. 3 Brachytherapy of uvea tumours. (With permission of Grada Publishing a.s.)

Transpupillary thermotherapy

Transpupillary thermotherapy uses infrared light with a wavelength of 810 nm to destroy tissue, which leads to a temperature increase to 60 °C. The laser targets the choroid and retinal pigment epithelium. Heating leads to induction of vascular thrombosis, thermal inhibition of angiogenesis, induction of fibrosis and tumour necrosis. Regression of small metastases after the use of transpupillary thermotherapy alone has been documented [13]. Complications include thermal damage to the surrounding retina. This method is receding into the background due to its lower efficacy.

Photodynamic therapy

On the other hand, photodynamic therapy with Visudyn (verteporfin), which is administered intravenously at a dose of 6 mg/m^2 of the body surface area, is increasingly used. Verteporfin is taken up on LDL receptors, which are present in large amounts in tumour vessels. Fifteen minutes after the start of the infusion, the lesion is irradiated with a diode laser that emits red light (689 nm). Activation of verteporfin molecules picked up in the tumour vessels leads to singlet oxygen generation and intravascular microthrombus formation, with subsequent ischaemic necrosis of the tumour [14, 15]. Another mechanism of action of photodynamic therapy is the induction of a local inflammatory response, which leads to an increase in macrophage and dendritic cell activity and phagocytosis of tumour cells. Photodynamic therapy has been used to

Fig. 4 A Choroidal metastasis before gamma irradiation. B Choroidal metastasis two years after gamma irradiation

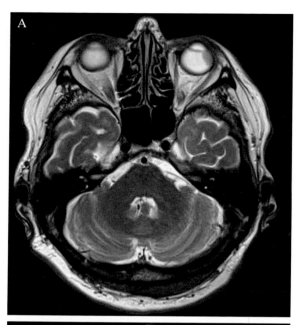

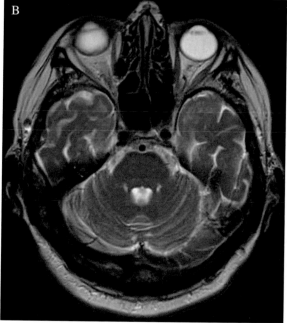

Cancer Diseases

treat small choroidal metastases with promising results. Complete tumour regression has been achieved in about 80% of cases [8, 14, 16].

Intravitreal anti-angiogenic agents

Small case series have recently demonstrated regression of intraocular metastases after intravitreal administration of bevacizumab, an anti-VEGF monoclonal antibody that inhibits tumour neoangiogenesis [13, 17]. However, this treatment was ineffective in some patients [18].

Surgical procedures

Local resection is rarely indicated. Quite rarely there are reports of successful transscleral local resection of large choroidal radioresistant metastases. Vitrectomy with retinectomy has been described in case series of retinal metastases [1, 19–21].

Prognosis

Survival for patients with intraocular metastases is generally short. Median overall survival from diagnosis of choroidal metastasis is usually only 6 months. Survival is shorter in patients with lung cancer than in patients with breast cancer. Survival worsens in the presence of additional, extraocular metastases. Patients with retinal and vitreous metastases have a particularly poor prognosis [1].

Response to local treatment is good in choroidal metastases. In general, regression of tumour intraocular infiltrates can be expected in 94% of patients and preservation of vision is possible in 75%. However, recurrences occur in about 12% of cases. After treatment of unilateral metastatic involvement, the second eye is affected in approximately 15–20% of patients [1].

2 Intraocular Metastases of Solid Tumours

Clinical symptoms

The main clinical symptoms of intraocular metastasis include a decrease in central visual acuity, metamorphopsia, photopsia or visual field loss in the case of exudative detachment. About 10–20% of metastases may be asymptomatic. Pain occurs in cases of secondary glaucoma or uveitis in metastases to the iris or ciliary body and is more common in patients with lung cancer [22].

Objective findings

Metastasis to the iris manifests as solitary or multiple small yellow-white or pink nodules in the stroma (Fig. 5).

The metastasis of the ciliated body has the character of a solitary mass. Pressure on the lens may induce the development of astigmatism. Both types may manifest secondary glaucoma. The typical picture of choroidal metastasis is a rapidly growing, slightly prominent whitish or whitish-yellowish placoid lesion, usually about 10 mm

Fig. 5 Metastasis of prostate cancer to the iris stroma

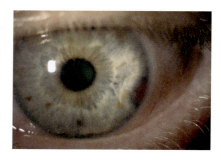

in diameter and 3 mm thick. It is most localised at the posterior pole along the temporal arcades (Fig. 6).

Only quite rarely does the metastasis break through Bruch's membrane and is mushroom-shaped. Multifocal lesions are present in one-third of patients, especially in patients with breast cancer. Retinal pigment epithelial changes "leopard spots") may be present on the fundus (Fig. 7).

Metastases are accompanied by exudative retinal detachment, more marked than in malignant choroidal melanoma. In rare cases, choroidal ablation can be observed. Signs of inflammation in the vitreous are almost never present.

Fig. 6 Choroidal metastasis

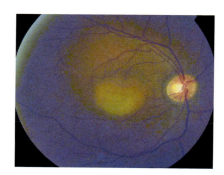

Fig. 7 Choroidal metastasis with significant RPE changes

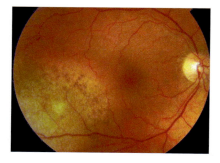

Fig. 8 Metastasis of carcinoid tumours

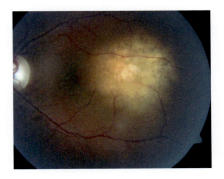

Cutaneous melanoma metastases may be grey or brown in colour, whereas carcinoid, thyroid and renal metastases may be orange (Fig. 8).

Extremely rare retinal metastases may mimic vasculitis in appearance. Vitreous metastases may resemble intraocular lymphoma [1, 2, 4].

Diagnosis

The basic diagnostic method is biomicroscopy of the fundus; digital fundus photography is used to monitor the development of the disease. Ultrasonography plays a very important role in the differential diagnosis of amelanotic melanoma (Fig. 9), choroidal haemangioma (Fig. 10) and metastasis.

On ultrasonography, metastasis is characterised by moderate to high intrinsic inhomogeneous reflectivity of the lesion on the A scan; on the B scan, we see an acoustically solid lesion of flatter dome shape, slightly prominent, with an irregular surface (Fig. 11).

Malignant melanoma, on the other hand, is characterised by a dome-shaped lesion with low homogeneous reflectivity; the A scan shows a high amplitude of the first echo and a subsequent decrease in echoes (Fig. 12).

The above differences on the ultrasonographic image are due to the different lesion structures. Metastasis, especially of breast cancer, has solid deposits of epithelial cells or glandular structure, which are the interfaces that lead to the formation of echoes,

Fig. 9 Amelanotic melanoma

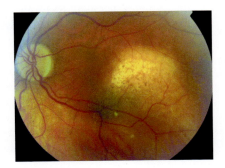

Fig. 10 Haemangioma of choroid plexus

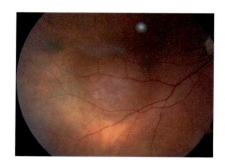

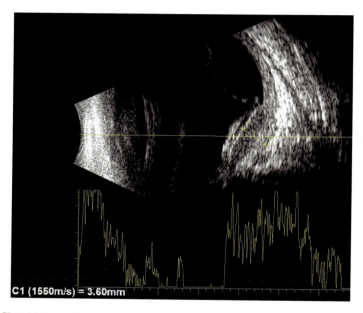

Fig. 11 Choroidal metastasis – ultrasound

forming a high reflectivity and irregular internal structure in the ultrasonographic image. Melanoma, on the other hand, has a dense cellular structure, with only a small or medium vasculature, causing a low or medium reflectivity lesion image with a regular internal structure (unless necrosis is present) [23, 24].

The pattern of growth in the choroid is also different in melanoma and metastasis. Metastases diffusely infiltrate the normal choroidal tissue and are therefore rather flat and irregular in shape. Melanoma, on the other hand, grows nodularly, thickens the choroid, and eventually perforates Bruch's membrane (this may be the cause of the secondary retinal emboli), and has a higher height-to-base ratio of the lesion (0.6) than metastasis (0.18). Another typical feature of melanoma is choroidal excavation (Fig. 13) [24].

Cancer Diseases

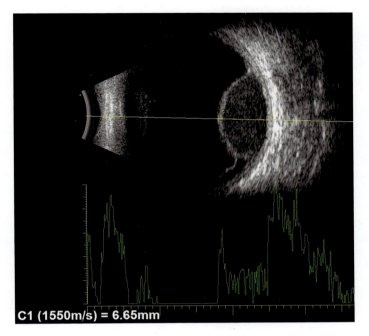

Fig. 12 Malignant melanoma of choroid – ultrasound

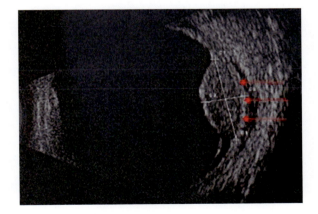

Fig. 13 Choroidal excavation in malignant melanoma of choroid – ultrasound

This is an ultrasonographic picture that results from the difference in reflectivity between the abnormal melanoma tissue that replaces the choroid and the normal choroid tissue. Choroidal excavation occurs in only one-fifth of choroidal metastases, but in two-thirds of malignant melanomas. It may be present in half of choroidal haemangiomas. The differential diagnosis of small lesions is most problematic; the ultrasonographic picture of melanoma and metastasis may be very similar [23–25].

Optical coherence tomography may be an auxiliary method in this case. In the ultrasound diagnosis of the lesion, Doppler methods showing blood flow are also used. For choroidal metastasis, hypervascularity without a dominant vessel is typical, for melanoma, hypovascularity and a dominant central vessel [6, 26].

Fluorescence angiography is an auxiliary but not decisive method in the diagnosis of metastases. On fluorescence angiography, there is a distinct block of fluorescence in the lesion area in the early phase, heterogeneous hyperfluorescence in the middle phase, and diffuse late venous hyperfluorescence (later than in melanoma), and sometimes more distinct leakage points are seen (Fig. 14 A–C).

There is never a picture of double circulation. In contrast, indocyanine angiography has a very important role in the diagnosis of metastases. A hypofluorescent lesion is seen at all stages of angiography [27, 28]. The area of hypofluorescence is

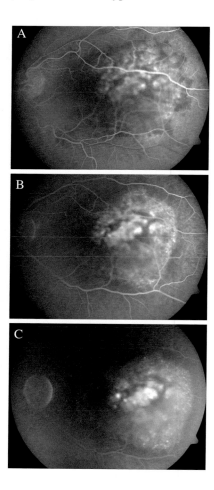

Fig. 14 A Choroidal metastasis to FA in early stage. B Choroidal metastasis to FA in intermediate stage. C Choroidal metastasis to FA in late stage

larger than the extent of the lesion seen on ophthalmoscopy. There is hypo- and hyperautofluorescence on autofluorescence, probably due to RPE changes [29]. Melanoma and haemangioma show a similar pattern [30].

Optical coherence tomography (OCT), especially enhanced depth imaging (EDI-OCT), is important for the diagnosis of small lesions in the posterior pole and for monitoring changes over time, typically after treatment. On examination, OCT will show subretinal fluid, with small hyperreflective dots in most metastases (Fig. 15).

These are likely to be the outer segments of photoreceptors, with protruding photoreceptors visible at the inner line of neuroretinal ablation. The lesion typically has a lumpy bumpy surface (in contrast to melanoma). The proportion of fibrous tissue in the metastasis increases during treatment and the internal reflectivity increases on OCT. On EDI-OCT, choroidal metastasis shows a low mean reflectivity (hyporeflectivity) of the lesion, with visible compression of the choriocapillaris and enlargement of the suprachoroidal space (Fig. 16).

EDI-OCT is even able to detect choroidal metastases that are not clinically apparent. OCT angiography shows no blood flow at the site of metastasis, and the outer retinal layers are free of pathologic blood flow (Fig. 17).

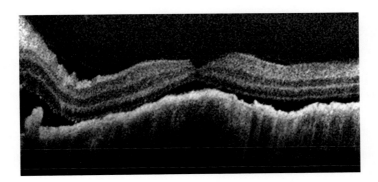

Fig. 15 Choroidal metastasis – OCT

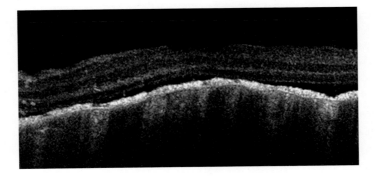

Fig. 16 Choroidal metastasis – EDI OCT

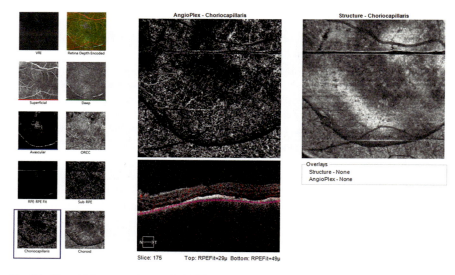

Fig. 17 Choroidal metastasis – angio OCT

In melanoma or haemangioma, dense irregular vasculature within the tumour is seen, and sometimes increased flow in the outer retinal layers [26, 31, 32].

Imaging methods, such as magnetic resonance imaging (MRI) and computed tomography (CT), are rarely used in the diagnosis of ocular metastases. On MR, the metastasis has well-defined borders and is isointense in T1 and hypointense in T2-weighted images. Thin-walled biopsy (FNAB) is also used abroad [33].

Differential diagnosis

- Amelanotic melanoma (rupture of Bruch's membrane, intrinsic vasculature on FAG, smooth surface without irregularities, only minimal exudative detachments)
- Choroidal osteoma (very flat, wavy edges, slow growth)
- Choroidal haemangioma—sometimes similar to carcinoid metastases, may be similar to findings on ultrasound, fluorescence and indocyanine angiography should be performed (hyperfluorescence is typical for haemangioma in the initial stages on ICG and gradually fluorescence decrease is observed, the wash-out phenomenon)
- Posterior scleritis [3]

Metastases of carcinoma

Carcinomas can metastasise to the orbit, eyelids, conjunctiva or intraocularly. Intraocular metastases are discussed in detail in the previous chapter.

Cancer Diseases   359

3 Metastases to the Eyelids

Metastases to the eyelids are very rare. They affect 1% of patients with metastatic involvement. The most common are metastases from breast cancer or lung cancer. Metastases of gastric, thyroid and parotid carcinoma are described only in rare cases. In addition to carcinomas, cutaneous melanoma may metastasize to the eyelids [22].

Risk factors

Metastases of carcinoma in another site.

Clinical symptoms

Metastases of carcinoma is manifested by a lesion on the eyelid.

Objective findings

Metastasis of carcinoma manifests as a solid subcutaneous nodule. It is usually a solitary lesion that can mimic a chalazion. Compared to chalazion, metastasis has less inflammatory reaction, but a higher growth rate and a tendency to ulceration. Breast cancer metastases may be indistinctly circumscribed and diffusely infiltrate the eyelid and may resemble blepharitis [30, 34].

Diagnosis

The examination of the eyelids by visual inspection is crucial for diagnosis. It is important to remember the targeted anamnestic questioning for oncological disease. In the case of a well-accessible lesion, biopsy and histological examination can be considered. In some cases, such as renal cell carcinoma, histological findings are typical. In some biopsies, metastases to the eyelids are poorly differentiated and the primary localisation cannot be determined. In breast cancer metastases, marked histiocytosis can sometimes be confusing [35, 36].

Differential diagnosis

- Chalazion
- Blepharitis

Therapy

Small enlarging lesions can be removed by local excision. For larger lesions, it is advisable to first take a small sample for histological examination. If the patient is treated with systemic chemotherapy, the eyelid metastases can only be monitored. Only in rare cases of large lesions that cannot be removed surgically and that do not respond to systemic treatment may radiotherapy be considered [3].

4 Metastases to the Conjunctiva

Metastases to the conjunctiva are rare. They are most often metastases from lung or breast cancer.

Risk factors

Metastases of carcinoma in another localisation.

Clinical symptoms

Metastases of carcinoma is manifested by a lesion on the conjunctiva.

Objective findings

Metastasis of carcinoma to the conjunctiva manifests as a rapidly growing yellowish or pink mass. The shape may be placoid or polypoid.

Diagnosis

The anterior segment slit-lamp examination is crucial for diagnosis. It is necessary to ask a targeted question about cancer when taking a personal history. As with eyelid metastases, histological examination can be performed, but may not reveal the primary lesion.

Therapy

Small metastases can be excised. For larger lesions, it is preferable to perform a biopsy first. If the patient is treated with systemic chemotherapy, the eyelid metastases can only be monitored. For lesions that do not respond to chemotherapy, radiotherapy or brachytherapy can be performed [3, 34, 37].

5 Metastases to the Orbit

Carcinomas can metastasise via haematogenous route to the orbit. Metastases account for 1–10% of orbital tumours. Metastasis to the orbit is diagnosed in 2–5% of cancer patients. The incidence of metastases is slightly increasing, which is probably related to better imaging methods and longer survival of cancer patients. Orbital metastases are mostly unilateral. In adults, breast, prostate, lung, kidney, or gastrointestinal metastases are most common. Of the carcinoids metastasising to the orbit, those from the small intestine metastasise to the orbit, and pulmonary carcinoids metastasise to the choroid. In the case of breast cancer metastases, the primary oncological diagnosis is usually already established, unlike in the case of lung cancer or carcinoid, where metastasis to the orbit may be the first manifestation of cancer. On average, metastases to the orbit manifest 52 months after the diagnosis of the primary tumour.

Fig. 18 Orbital metastasis

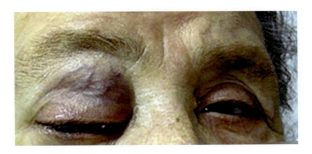

In children, orbital metastases are rare; in most cases, the primary oncological diagnosis is already known. Neuroblastoma (in neonates), Wilms tumour or Ewing sarcoma metastasise to the orbit [3, 38].

Risk factors

Metastasis of carcinoma in another localisation.

Clinical symptoms

The clinical presentation varies according to the type of primary tumour. Small metastases may be asymptomatic. Clinical symptoms include diplopia, eyeball protrusion, pain, decreased visual acuity or ptosis in almost half of the cases. In a proportion of patients there is a palpable mass in the orbit.

The presence of an orbital metastasis should be considered in all adult patients over 60 years of age without the history of cancer with a newly diagnosed symptomatic orbital mass. Metastatic origin of the lesion is proven in almost 30% [39].

Objective Findings

Typically, there is a rapidly progressive painful protrusion of the bulb with its deviation. Ptosis, as well as eyelid and conjunctival oedema, are often present (Figs. 18 and 19).

Some tumours, especially breast and gastric carcinomas (sclerosing carcinoma), may cause enophthalmos because of fibrotisation and shrinkage of the tumour. In children, neuroblastoma metastases are accompanied by bleeding into the eyelids and conjunctiva.

Diagnosis

Suspected diagnosis of orbital metastasis is made based on visual examination. In all patients, a targeted search for oncological history is needed. Imaging methods—computed tomography and magnetic resonance imaging—are important for diagnosis. Metastases are more often localised in the anterior part of the orbit. Well circumscribed, isolated intraocular lesions are contra-suggestive of the diagnosis of metastasis. Involvement of the orbicularis oculi muscles and bones is suggestive of metastasis. Metastases may also occur in the subperiosteal space.

Fig. 19 Orbital metastasis on CT

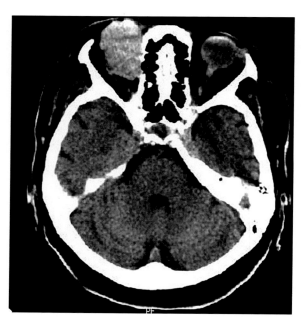

Breast cancer metastases affect more soft tissues, are diffuse and grow along the muscles and fascia. Prostate cancer metastasises to the bones of the orbit. Metastases of carcinoid or renal cell carcinoma tend to be oval and well circumscribed, resembling benign tumours of the orbit.

In all patients with orbital metastases, targeted imaging for the presence of metastases in other organs (PET/CT) is necessary [3].

Biopsy is usually performed in cases where the primary tumour is not known, usually by orbitotomy.

Differential diagnosis

- Pseudotumour of the orbit
- Benign lesions of the orbit
- Ig-G4 associated disease
- Orbital lymphoma
- Sarcoidosis

Therapy

The indication for treatment depends on the patient's overall condition and is proposed in collaboration with the oncologist. It includes radiotherapy, hormone therapy or chemotherapy. In specific cases, surgical removal may be considered, but is often limited by the location of the metastasis in the orbital tip [3].

Cancer Diseases

6 Paraneoplastic Syndromes

Paraneoplastic syndromes associated with visual impairment are rare manifestations of cancer. They are not caused by the presence of tumour cells in the affected organs, but rather the systemic effects of the tumour [40]. Although the pathogenesis of these syndromes has not been fully elucidated, an immune response induced by the tumour cells' aberrant expression of onconeural antigens is considered to be the most likely mechanism [41]. A significant proportion of patients present with visual disturbances before the primary cancer is detected, which makes diagnosing these syndromes extremely difficult [42]. In many cases, the final diagnosis is made *per exclusionem* after excluding more common eye disorder causes. Paraneoplastic syndromes associated with visual impairment include cancer-associated retinopathy (CAR), melanoma-associated retinopathy (MAR), bilateral diffuse uveal melanocytic proliferation (BDUMP) and paraneoplastic optic neuropathy (PON) [40]. Other paraneoplastic syndromes affecting the central nervous system may also manifest with visual disturbances, but their discussion is beyond the scope of this chapter.

6.1 *Cancer-Associated Retinopathy*

Cancer-associated retinopathy (CAR) is the most common paraneoplastic retinopathy, that causes bilateral and progressive vision loss and can result in blindness [43]. Cross-reactivity between the tumour and retinal cells is thought to be the main cause of the disease [44, 45]. Associations between numerous antigens and CAR have been reported. The most frequently involved antigen is a calcium-binding protein recoverin (formerly known as the CAR antigen) [40]. In addition to retinal cells, recoverin has been found in the tumour cells of small cell lung cancer (SCLC) and other lung tumours, breast cancer, and gynaecological cancers [46]. The consequence is the immune-mediated degeneration of retinal photoreceptors [40, 46]. While the exact pathogenetic mechanism has yet to be explained fully, several mechanisms—including apoptotic cell death via caspase-dependent pathways and intracellular calcium influx—have been proposed [47, 48]. The blockade of negative T-cell signalling via cytotoxic T-lymphocyte antigen 4 (CTLA-4) has been reported as a contributing factor for CAR development [49]. This may be clinically relevant, as anti-CTLA-4 antibodies are widely used in cancer therapy [50].

Risk factors

- Small cell lung cancer (SCLC)
- Non-small cell lung cancer (NSCLC)
- Breast cancer
- Tumours of the body or cervix of the uterus

- Hepatocellular carcinoma
- Lymphomas

Clinical symptoms

Patients typically report subacute visual impairment that develops over weeks to months [42]. The impairment is typically bilateral, and less often unilateral. In up to fifty percent of cases, visual disturbances may precede the diagnosis of cancer by several months [51]. Patients with dominant cone involvement tend to have photopsia, hemeralopia, loss of central visual acuity and paracentral or central scotomas. Positive visual phenomena—namely flickering and flashing lights—are typical [42]. In the case of dominant rod involvement, the most common manifestations are nyctalopia, impaired adaptation to darkness, ring scotoma or peripheral visual field loss [52]. The progressive worsening of symptoms leading to severe visual impairment is typical [40].

Objective findings

In the early stages, fundoscopic findings are normal, although vitritis may be evident. Later, a narrowing of the retinal arteries occurs, as well as slight changes in the retinal pigment epithelium. Optic disc pallor may be observed at this time [53]. Retinal phlebitis may also occur [52] (Fig. 20), although this is less common.

Diagnosis

The diagnosis is based on the history of cancer and the alteration of visual examination tests, although visual symptoms may precede the diagnosis of cancer [43]. Electroretinography (ERG) reveals a significant reduction of a- and b-wave amplitudes, even in the early stages of the disease. Both scotopic and photopic ERG are affected [40]. Increased protein and lymphocytosis can be observed in the cerebrospinal fluid [51]. Western blot examination of the serum and cerebrospinal fluid can identify antineuronal antibodies, such as those against recoverin and α-enolase [40]. In the case of a high suspicion of CAR and previously undiagnosed cancer, chest X-ray should be performed (due to the fact that lung tumours are the most common cause

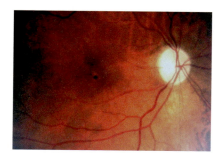

Fig. 20 Retinopathy associated with carcinoma

Cancer Diseases 365

of CAR) [54]. In the case of negative results, a CT of the chest, abdomen and pelvis, or a PET/CT, should be indicated. In women, mammography and gynaecological examinations should be conducted as well [54].

Differential diagnosis

- Retrobulbar optic neuropathy
- Toxo-nutritive or hereditary optic neuropathy
- Neuropathy of the optic nerve resulting from cytostatic treatment (especially vincristine, carmustine)
- Hereditary syndromes associated with photoreceptor degeneration (retinitis pigmentosa, cone dystrophy)
- Toxic retinopathy
- Acute zonal occult outer retinopathy (AZOOR)

Therapy

Although several drugs have been tested to treat CAR, the visual impairment associated with this syndrome typically has a poor prognosis. Treatment of the underlying cancer does not improve the ocular symptoms [55]. High doses of corticosteroids have been shown to be effective in some patients [56]. Clinical improvement has also been achieved with the use of other immunosuppressive agents, such as azathioprine, mycophenolate mofetil, cyclosporine, infliximab (anti-tumour necrosis factor α antibody) and alemtuzumab (anti-CD52 antibody) [56, 57]. Plasmapheresis and the intravenous administration of immunoglobulins (IVIg) may also have some effect [43].

6.2 Melanoma-Associated Retinopathy

Melanoma-associated retinopathy (MAR) is a very rare paraneoplastic syndrome encountered in patients with cutaneous melanoma. The disease occurs more frequently in males, with a ratio of 4.7:1 [58]. Unlike CAR, in which rods and cones are primarily affected, MAR is dominated by retinal bipolar cells [59]. The underlying cause is the production of autoantibodies against bipolar cells. Their damage then leads to impaired photoreception and signal transduction [60].

Risk factors

- Cutaneous malignant melanoma
- Male gender
- Personal or family history of autoimmune disease

Clinical symptoms

Symptoms usually appear months to years after the diagnosis of malignant melanoma, and their occurrence is often associated with disease recurrence [40, 51]. Patients typically present with nyctalopia and positive phenomena in the form of stationary or fluctuating flickering, pulsating or flashing lights, often more pronounced in bright light conditions [61]. Between four days and two months, the symptoms typically become bilateral but may remain unilateral in a minority of patients. Visual acuity and colour perception are not significantly affected, although colour discrimination may be impaired [61]. Central scotomas are unusual [42]. In contrast to CAR patients, vision is stable over a long period of time. Severe disability rarely occurs [51].

Objective findings

Fundoscopic findings are typically normal initially. Irregularities of the RPE in the form of whitish or atrophic spots or the diffuse loss of retinal pigment epithelium may be present. Advanced cases may present a granular appearance of the macula, swelling of the optic disc or a narrowing of the retinal vessels [61]. Vitritis and retinal periphlebitis have also been described [58].

Diagnosis

The following triad is typical for MAR: (1) symptoms of nyctalopia and positive visual phenomena or visual field defects; (2) the reduction of b-wave amplitudes on ERG; and (3) the presence of serum antibodies against retinal bipolar cells [62]. ERG is a very sensitive method for detecting MAR-related changes. The reduction of b-wave amplitudes associated with impaired bipolar cell function is characteristic, whereas the a-wave tends to be unchanged and exhibit preserved photoreceptor cell function [58].

Antibodies to retinal bipolar cells have been found in up to 68.8% of patients with MAR and can be used to confirm the diagnosis [62]. Several antibodies have been identified against various retinal cell antigens, such as the 35-kDa Müller glial cell protein, the 22-kDa neuronal antigen, transducin, aldolase A, aldolase C, mitofilin and titin [61].

MAR diagnosis should always lead to a search for primary malignant melanoma or relapse in the case of previously diagnosed disease. Imaging examinations (CT or PET/CT) should be performed [63]. In the case of negative findings, the search should exclude the presence of primary ocular or mucosal melanoma [61].

Differential diagnosis

- Congenital stationary night blindness
- X-linked juvenile retinoschisis
- Retinopathy associated with MEK inhibitor therapy
- Autoimmune retinopathy associated with checkpoint inhibitor therapy (anti-PD1, anti PD-L1 and anti-CTLA4 antibodies)

Therapy

Due to the rarity of the disease, there are no clear therapeutic approaches to date [40]. The treatment strategy combines two approaches: (1) cytoreduction, which involves shrinking the tumour mass to reduce the antigenic load and thus the production of autoantibodies, and (2) influencing the immune system [61, 64]. However,

Cancer Diseases

the efficacy of immunomodulatory therapy is usually limited, especially because of the irreversible retinal changes already present. Corticosteroids have not been successful in the treatment of MAR, although they may have some effect when uveitis is present [61]. A slightly greater effect can be expected with plasmapheresis and IVIg, especially in patients who do not respond to other treatments [65].

Importantly, the prognosis of malignant melanoma largely depends on the patient's immune response [66]. As such, there are concerns that using immunosuppressive therapies may increase the cancer mortality of melanoma patients [42]. While no differences have been found between treated and untreated MAR patients and melanoma patients without MAR [64], it has been suggested to avoid immunomodulating agents in patients with subclinical MAR [61, 67]. Anti-tumour immunotherapy using checkpoint inhibitors of the immune response (i.e. anti-PD1 and anti-CTLA4 antibodies) is currently the main modality to treat metastatic malignant melanoma [66]. However, these treatments can induce the development of immune-mediated adverse events (irAEs) and worsen the course of pre-existing autoimmune diseases, which may include MAR [68]. Therefore, in patients with MAR, checkpoint inhibitor therapy should be indicated on a strictly individual basis. A recent case report describes the good effect of intravitreally applied corticosteroids with concomitant systemic checkpoint inhibitor therapy [69].

6.3 Bilateral Diffuse Uveal Melanocytic Proliferation

Bilateral diffuse uveal melanocytic proliferation (BDUMP) is a rare paraneoplastic syndrome characterised by multiple benign pigmented uveal lesions, diffuse thickening of the uveal tract and rapidly progressing cataracts [70]. The age of patients tends to be in the range of 50–80 years [71]. Some authors report a slightly higher incidence in women [51, 70], while others report no gender predilection [71]. An association with tumours of the lung, ovary, body and cervix of the uterus, pancreas, gallbladder and colon has been described [51]. The most common malignancies associated with BDUMP are urogenital tract tumours in women (69%) and lung cancer in men (52%) [70]. However, in half these cases, the primary tumour is diagnosed after the onset of BDUMP [72]. The aetiopathogenesis of this syndrome has not yet been elucidated. The proliferation of benign melanocytes could be induced by trophic humoral factors produced by the primary tumour or due to a coexisting oncogenic factor [42].

Risk factors

- Lung carcinomas (SCLC, NSCLC)
- Ovarian carcinoma
- Tumours of the body and cervix of the uterus
- Pancreatic carcinoma
- Colorectal cancer

Clinical symptoms

Patients usually present with painless bilateral progressive visual loss and constricted visual fields that develop over a period of months [40, 51]. Ocular symptoms precede the manifestation of the underlying cancer by months to even years [70].

Objective findings

In approximately 85% of cases, typical lesions can be found on the fundus [71]. Gass et al. describe five dominant findings that characterise BDUMP: (1) multiple circular or oval, bland, grey-red plaques at the level of the RPE in the posterior fundus; (2) a conspicuous image on fluorescence angiography with findings of multifocal, early hyperfluorescent precincts that correspond to the presence of these plaques; (3) diffuse thickening of the uveal tract with findings of multiple mildly elevated, pigmented and non-pigmented melanocytic tumours; (4) exudative retinal detachment; and (5) rapidly progressive cataracts [73].

Other findings may include dilated episcleral vessels, pigmented precipitates on the corneal endothelium, pigmented anterior chamber cells, iris cysts or vitritis [74]. In some cases, glaucoma develops [40]. Pigmented lesions on the skin and mucous membranes can be found in roughly 25% of patients [71].

Diagnosis

Diagnosis is based on the presence of the above-mentioned findings from fundoscopy and fluorescence angiography [40]. Ultrasound examinations reveal diffuse thickening of the choroid and multiple tumour lesions. In addition to diffuse uveal tract thickening, a choroidal biopsy can detect the characteristic sparing of the choriocapillaris [75]. Moderate-to-severe loss of photopic and scotopic ERG amplitudes is present in the vast majority of patients [70]. Approximately 50% of cases present ocular symptoms before a cancer diagnosis, thus necessitating the search for the primary tumour [72, 75].

Differential diagnosis

- Diffuse choroidal melanoma
- Choroidal metastasis of malignant melanoma
- Choroidal nevi in neurofibromatosis type 1
- Congenital hypertrophy of the retinal pigment epithelium (CHRPE) in Gardner's syndrome
- Lymphomas and leukaemias
- Sarcoidosis
- Uveitis
- Scleritis
- Vogt-Koyanagi-Harada syndrome

Therapy

BDUMP prognosis is generally poor owing to the underlying malignancy with a survival rate of approximately 16 months after diagnosis [70, 72]. To date, there is

Cancer Diseases 369

no known effective therapy for this syndrome. Removal of the primary tumour may slow the progression of BDUMP [75]. In some patients, systemic corticosteroids or plasmapheresis may have an effect [70].

Complications

The syndrome is often accompanied by cataract development, which occurs in up to 73% of patients and has an unusually rapid course (development even within three months) [71]. A possible cause is the involvement of the ciliary body and the associated inadequate amount of ventricular fluid, changes in its composition or the formation of toxins [71]. BDUMP can also lead to severe neovascular glaucoma and necessitate eyeball enucleation [40].

6.4 Paraneoplastic Optic Neuropathy

Paraneoplastic optic neuropathy (PON) is a syndrome associated with acute optic nerve dysfunction. The pathophysiological mechanism of the disease is thought to be the demyelination of the optic nerve, which occurs as a result of autoantibody formation [40]. The most common tumour associated with PON is SCLC. Less common types include thyroid carcinomas, nasopharyngeal carcinomas, thymomas, renal cell carcinomas and lymphomas [76]. In children, PON has been described in neuroblastoma [77]. Researchers report no difference in the incidence of the syndrome between the sexes [78].

Risk factors

- Small cell lung cancer (SCLC)
- Thyroid carcinoma
- Nasopharyngeal carcinoma
- Thymoma
- Renal cell carcinoma
- Lymphoma

Clinical symptoms

Patients typically present with subacute, painless, progressive visual impairment, usually bilateral [78]. The symptoms may include blurred or dimmed vision, tunnel vision or visual field defects, phosphenes and dazzling vision [76]. Concomitant neurological symptomatology is often present, such as cerebellar degeneration, limbic encephalitis, sensory neuropathy or Lambert-Eaton myasthenic syndrome (LEMS) [40].

Objective findings

The initial finding is usually disc oedema, which gradually progresses to disc pallor and atrophy [40]. Retinitis and a mild cellular vitreous reaction may be present [79, 80].

Diagnosis

ERG results are usually normal [51]. Swollen optic discs are detected via ocular and optic coherence tomography examinations. These are sometimes accompanied by nerve fibre layer haemorrhages, retinitis, iritis or vitritis [76]. Cerebrospinal fluid examinations usually reveal lymphocytosis and elevated protein and oligoclonal immunoglobin bands on the electrophoresis [40]. The detection of anti-CV2 antibodies to collapsin response-mediator protein-5 (CRMP-5) in the serum or lymph is crucial [40]. Testing for other autoantibodies, such as anti-Hu, anti-Tr, anti-Yo, anti-Ri, anti-Ma2/TA7 and anti-amphiphysin, which have been shown to be associated with PON, is also recommended [78]. If even one of these autoantibodies is positive, a diagnosis of PON should be made, regardless of whether the underlying cancer has been identified [78].

Differential diagnosis

- Optic neuritis
- Toxic and nutritive optic neuropathy
- Anterior ischaemic optic neuropathy
- Pressure optic neuropathy
- Carcinomatosis meninges

Therapy

The basic therapeutic approach for PON is treatment of the primary cancer, which can improve or at least stabilise visual symptoms [81]. Immunomodulatory therapies such as corticosteroids, cyclophosphamide, plasma exchange and intravenous immunoglobulins may improve visual function in 50% of cases [82].

References

1. Konstantidinis L, Damato B. Intraocular metastases: a review. Asia Pacific J Ophthalmol. 2017;5:208–14.
2. Demirci H, Shields CL, Chao AN, et al. Uveal metastasis from breast cancer in 264 patients. Am J Ophthalmol. 2003;136:264–71.
3. Shields JA, Shields CL. Intraocular tumors: an atlas and textbook. 3rd ed. Philadelphia: Wolters Kluwer; 2016. p. 213–45, 525–54.
4. Shields CL, Shields JA, Gross NE, et al. Survey of 520 eyes with uveal metastases. Ophthalmology. 1997;104:1265–76.
5. Wilkinson L, Gathani T. Understanding breast cancer as a global health concern. Br J Radiol. 2022;95(1130):20211033.

Cancer Diseases

6. Mathis T, Jardel P, Loria O, et al. New concepts in the diagnosis and management of choroidal metastases. Prog Retin Eye Res. 2019;68:144–76.
7. Peyster RG, Augsburger JJ, Shields JA, et al. Intraocular tumors: evaluation with MR imaging. Radiology. 1988;168:773–9.
8. Bornfeld N, Biewald E, Bauer S, et al. The interdisciplinary diagnosis and treatment of intraocular tumors. Deutsches Arzteblatt Int. 2018;115:106–11.
9. Oliver AL. Lung Cancer: Epidemiology and Screening. Surg Clin North Am. 2022;102(3):335–44.
10. Dingemans C et al. Small-cell lung cancer: ESMO Clinical Practice Guidelines for diagnosis, treatment and follow-up. Ann Oncol. 2021; 32(7): 839–853. https://doi.org/10.1016/j.annonc.2021.03.207.
11. Morgan E, Arnold M, Gini A, et al. Global burden of colorectal cancer in 2020 and 2040: incidence and mortality estimates from GLOBOCAN. Gut. 2023;72(2):338–44.
12. Youbi ZA, Ciprian E, Ionela C, et al. Management of choroidal metastasis using external beam radiotherapy: a retrospective study and review of the literature. J Cancer Metastasis Treat. 2017;3:105–10.
13. Lin CJ, Tsai YY. The effect of intravitreal bevacizumab and transpupillary thermotherapy on choroidal metastases and literature review. Indian J Ophthalmol. 2015;63:37–41.
14. Ghodasra DH, Demirci H. Photodynamic Therapy for Choroidal Metastasis. Am J Ophthalmol. 2016;161:104–9.
15. Schmidt-Erfurth UM, Michels S, Kusserow C, et al. Photodynamic therapy for symptomatic choroidal hemangioma: visual and anatomic results. Ophthalmology. 2002;109(12):2284–94.
16. Kaliki S, Shields CL, Al-Dahmash SA, et al. Photodynamic therapy for choroidal metastasis in 8 cases. Ophthalmology. 2012;119:1218–22.
17. Fenicia V, Abdolrahimzadeh S, Mannino G, et al. Intravitreal bevacizumab in the successful management of choroidal metastases secondary to lung and breast cancer unresponsive to systemic therapy: a case series. Eye Lond. 2014;28:888–91.
18. Maudgil A, Sears KS, Rundle PA, et al. Failure of intravitreal bevacizumab in the treatment of choroidal metastasis. Eye Lond. 2015;29:707–11.
19. Apte RS et al. Retinal metastasis presenting as a retinal hemorrhage in a patient with adenocarcinoma of the cecum. rch Ophthalmol. 2005; 123(6): 850–3. https://doi.org/10.1001/archopht.123.6.850
20. Spadea L et al. Normal EOG values in intraretinal metastasis from cutaneous melanoma: a case report. Doc Ophthalmol. 1998; 96(4):305–9. https://doi.org/10.1023/a:1001843702335
21. Balestrazzi E et al. Local excision of retinal metastasis from cutaneous melanoma. Eur J Ophthalmol. 1995; 5(3):149–54. https://doi.org/10.1177/112067219500500301
22. Kuchynka P. Ophthalmology. 2nd ed. Prague: Grada; 2016. p. 597–8.
23. Perri P, Chiarelli M, Monari P, et al. Choroidal metastases. Echographic experience from 42 patients. Acta Ophthalmol Suppl. 1992;(204):96–8.
24. Sobottka B, Schlote T, Krumpaszky HG, et al. Choroidal metastases and choroidal melanomas:comparison of ultrasonographic findings. Br J Ophthalmol. 1998;82:159–61.
25. Verbeek AM, Thijssen JM, Cuypers MH, et al. Echographic classification of intraocular tumours. A 15-year retrospective analysis. Acta Ophthalmol (Copenh). 1994;72:416–22.
26. Demirci H, Cullen A, Sundstrom JM. Enhanced depth imaging optical coherence tomography of choroidal metastasis. Retina Phila. 2014;34:1354–9.
27. Meyer K, Augsburger JJ. Independent diagnostic value of fluorescein angiography in the evaluation of intraocular tumors. Graefes Arch Clin Exp Ophthalmol. 1999;237:489–94.
28. Shields CL, Shields JA, De Potter P. Patterns of indocyanine green videoangiography of choroidal tumours. Br. J. Ophthalmol. 1995; 79: 237–245. https://doi.org/10.1136/bjo.79.3.237
29. Ishida T, Ohno-Matsui K, Kaneko, et al. Autofluorescence of metastatic choroidal tumor. Int Ophthalmol. 2009;29:309–13.
30. Jacob P. Pathology of eyelid tumors. Indian J Ophthalmol. 2016;64(3):177–90.
31. Al-Dahmash SA, Shields CL, Kaliki S, et al. Enhanced depth imaging optical coherence tomography of choroidal metastasis in 14 eyes. Retina Phila. 2014;34:1588–93.

32. Cennamo G, Romano MR, Breve MA, et al. Evaluation of choroidal tumors with optical coherence tomography:enhanced depth imaging and OCT-angiography features. Eye Lond. 2017;31:906–15.
33. Konstantinidis L, Rospond-Kubiak I, Zeolite I, et al. Management of patients with uveal metastases at the Liverpool Ocular Oncology Centre. Br J Ophthalmol. 2014;98:92–8.
34. Bianciotto C, Demirci H, Shields CL, et al. Metastatic tumors to the eyelid: report of 20 cases and review of the literature. Arch Ophthalmol. 2009;127(8):999–1005.
35. Rodrigues MM, Font RL, Shannon GM. Metastatic mucus-secreting mammary carcinoma in the eyelid. Report of two cases. Br J Ophthalmol. 1974;58(10):877–81.
36. Shields CL, Shields JA. Tumors of the conjunctiva and cornea. Indian J Ophthalmol. 2019;67(12):1930–48.
37. Kiratli H, Shields CL, Shields JA, et al. Metastatic tumours to the conjunctiva: report of 10 cases. Br J Ophthalmol. 1996;80(1):5–8.
38. Allen RC. Orbital metastases: when to suspect? when to biopsy? Middle East Afr J Ophthalmol. 2018;25(2):60–4.
39. Shields JA, Shields CL, Scartozzi R. Survey of 1264 patients with orbital tumors and simulating lesions: The 2002 Montgomery Lecture, part 1. Ophthalmology. 2004;111(5):997–1008.
40. Alabduljalil T, Behbehani R. Paraneoplastic syndromes in neuro-ophthalmology. Curr Opin Ophthalmol. 2007;18(6):463–9.
41. Darnell RB, Posner JB. Paraneoplastic syndromes involving the nervous system. N Engl J Med. 2003;349:1543–54.
42. Ling CPW, Pavesio C. Paraneoplastic syndromes associated with visual loss. Curr Opin Ophthalmol. 2003;14(6):426–32.
43. Ramos-Ruperto L, Busca-Arenzana C, Boto-de Los Bueis A, et al. Cancer-associated retinopathy and treatment with intravenous immunoglobulin therapy. a seldom used approach? Ocul Immunol Inflamm. 2021;29:399–402.
44. Keltner JL, Roth AM, Chang RS. Photoreceptor degeneration possible autoimmune disorder. Arch Ophthalmol. 1983;101:564–9.
45. Sawyer RA, Selhorst JB, Zimmerman LE, et al. Blindness caused by photoreceptor degeneration as a remote effect of cancer. Am J Ophthalmol. 1976;81:606–13.
46. Bazhin AV, Schadendorf D, Philippov PP, et al. Recoverin as a cancer-retina antigen. Cancer Immunol Immunother. 2007;56:110–6.
47. Ohguro H, Ogawa K, Maeda T, et al. Retinal dysfunction in cancer-associated retinopathy is improved by Ca(2+) antagonist administration and dark adaptation. Invest Ophthalmol Vis Sci. 2001;42:2589–95.
48. Shiraga S, Adamus G. Mechanism of CAR syndrome: anti-recoverin antibodies are the inducers of retinal cell apoptotic death via the caspase 9- and caspase 3-dependent pathway. J Neuroimmunol. 2002;132:72–82.
49. Maeda A, Maeda T, Liang Y, et al. Effects of cytotoxic T lymphocyte antigen 4 (CTLA4) signaling and locally applied steroid on retinal dysfunction by recoverin, cancer-associated retinopathy antigen. Mol Vis. 2006;12:885–91.
50. Tang F, Du X, Liu M, et al. Anti-CTLA-4 antibodies in cancer immunotherapy:selective depletion of intratumoral regulatory T cells or checkpoint blockade? Cell Biosci. 2018;8:30.
51. Arnold AC, Lee AG. Systemic disease and neuro-ophthalmology:annual up-date 2000 (part 1). J Neuroophthalmol. 2001;21:46–61.
52. Naramala S, Ahmad J, Adapa S, et al. Case Series of Cancer-associated Retinopathy (CAR). Cureus. 2019;11: e4872.
53. Aagaard T, Reekie J, Roen A, et al. Development and validation of a cycle-specific risk score for febrile neutropenia during chemotherapy cycles 2–6 in patients with solid cancers: the (CSR) FENCE score. Int J Cancer. 2020;146:321–8.
54. Chéour M, Agrebi S, Hijazi A. Cancer associated retinopathy with periphlebitis and bilateral vitreous hemorrhage. Bull Soc Belge Ophtalmol. 2013;322:71–6.
55. Chan JW. Paraneoplastic retinopathies and optic neuropathies. Surv Ophthal. 2003;48:12–38.

Cancer Diseases

56. Espandar L, O'Brien S, Thirkill C, et al. Successful treatment of cancer-associated retinopathy with alemtuzumab. J Neurooncol. 2007;83:295–302.
57. Grewal DS, Fishman GA, Jampol LM. Autoimmune retinopathy and antiretinal antibodies: a review. Retina. 2014;34:827–45.
58. Keltner JL, Thirkill CE, Yip PT. Clinical and immunologic characteristics of melanoma-associated retinopathy syndrome: eleven new cases and a review of 51 previously published cases. J Neuroophthalmol. 2001;21:173–87.
59. Milam AH, Saari JC, Jacobson SG, et al. Autoantibodies against retinal bipolar cells in cutaneous melanoma-associated retinopathy. Invest Ophthalmol Vis Sci. 1993;34:91–100.
60. Alexander KR, Fishman GA, Peachey NS, et al. On'response defect in paraneoplastic night blindness with cutaneous malignant melanoma. Invest Ophthalmol Vis Sci. 1992;33:477–83.
61. Elsheikh S, Gurney SP, Burdon MA. Melanoma-associated retinopathy. Clin Exp Dermatol. 2020;45(2):147–52.
62. Ladewig G, Reinhold U, Thirkill CE, et al. Incidence of antiretinal antibodies in melanoma: screening of 77 serum samples from 51 patients with American Joint Committee on Cancer stage I-IV. Br J Dermatol. 2005;152:931–8.
63. Morita Y, Kimura K, Fujitsu Y, et al. Autoantibodies to transient receptor potential cation channel, subfamily M, member 1 in a Japanese patient with melanoma-associated retinopathy. Jpn J Ophthalmol. 2014;58:166–71.
64. Kellner U, Bornfeld N, Foerster MH. Severe course of cutaneous melanoma associated paraneoplastic retinopathy. Br J Ophthalmol. 1995;79:746–52.
65. Powell SF, Dudek AZ. Treatment of melanoma-associated retinopathy. Curr Treat Options Neurol. 2010;12:54–63.
66. Passarelli A, Mannavola F, Stucci LS, et al. Immune system and melanoma biology: a balance between immunosurveillance and immune escape. Oncotarget. 2017;8:106132–42.
67. Pföhler C, Haus A, Palmowski A, et al. Melanoma-associated retinopathy: high frequency of subclinical findings in patients with melanoma. Br J Dermatol. 2003;149:74–8.
68. Audemard A, de Raucourt S, Miocque S, et al. Melanoma-associated retinopathy treated with ipilimumab therapy. Dermatology. 2013;227:146–9.
69. Poujade L, Samaran Q, Mura F, et al. Melanoma-associated retinopathy during pembrolizumab treatment probably controlled by intravitreal injections of dexamethasone. Doc Ophthalmol. 2021;142:257–63.
70. Klemp K, Kiilgaard JF, Heegaard S, et al. Bilateral diffuse uveal melanocytic proliferation: case report and literature review. Acta ophthalmologica. 2017;95:439–45.
71. O'Neal KD, Butnor KJ, Perkinson KR, et al. Bilateral diffuse uveal melanocytic proliferation associated with pancreatic carcinoma: a case report and literature review of this paraneoplastic syndrome. Surv Ophthalmol. 2003;48(6):613–25.
72. Chahud F, Young RH, Remulla JF, et al. Bilateral diffuse uveal melanocytic proliferation associated with extraocular cancers: review of a process particularly associated with gynecologic cancers. Am J Surg Pathol. 2001;25:212–8.
73. Gass JDM, Gleser RG, Wilkinson CP, et al. Bilateral diffuse uveal melanocytic proliferation in patients with occult carcinoma. Arch Ophthalmol. 1990;108:527–33.
74. Murphy MA, Hart WM Jr, Olk RJ. Bilateral diffuse uveal melanocytic proliferation simulating an arteriovenous fistula. J Neuroophthalmol. 1997;17:166–9.
75. Sen J, Clewes AR, Quah SA, et al. Presymptomatic diagnosis of bronchogenic carcinoma associated with bilateral diffuse uveal melanocytic proliferation. Clin Exp Ophthalmol. 2006;34:156–8.
76. Hickman S. Paraneoplastic syndromes in neuro-ophthalmology. Ann Indian Acad Neurol. 2022;25:101–5.
77. Scott JX, Moses PD, Somashekar HR, et al. Paraneoplastic papilloedema in a child with neuroblastoma. Indian J Cancer. 2005;42:102–3.
78. Xu Q, Du W, Zhou H, et al. Distinct clinical characteristics of paraneoplastic optic neuropathy. Br J Ophthalmol. 2019;103(6):797–801.

79. Cross SA, Salomao DR, Parisi JE, et al. Paraneoplastic autoimmune optic neuritis with retinitis defined by CRMP-5-IgG. Ann Neurol. 2003;54:38–50.
80. Sheorajpanday R, Slabbynck H, Van De Sompel W, et al. Small cell lung carcinoma presenting as collapsin response-mediating protein (CRMP)-5 paraneoplastic optic neuropathy. J Neuroophthalmol. 2006;26:168–72.
81. Arés-Luque A, García-Tuñón LA, Saiz A, et al. Isolated paraneoplastic optic neuropathy associated with small-cell lung cancer and anti-CV2 antibodies. J Neurol. 2007;254(8):1131–2.
82. Cohen DA, Bhatti MT, Pulido JS, et al. Collapsin response-mediator protein 5-associated retinitis, vitritis, and optic disc edema. Ophthalmology. 2020;127:221–9.

Neurological Disorders

Zdenek Kasl, Pavel Poczos, Roman Herzig, Nada Jiraskova, Martin Matuska, and Tomas Cesak

1 Multiple Sclerosis

Multiple sclerosis (MS) is a chronic autoimmune multifactorial inflammatory disease with subsequent neurodegenerative processes. Multifocal areas of demyelination and axonal damage in the central nervous system (CNS) occur in the presence of immune cells and elevated levels of their products. The nerves' ability to conduct electrical impulses is damaged, which, depending on the location of the lesions, results in symptoms.

Z. Kasl · M. Matuska
Department of Ophthalmology, University Hospital and Faculty of Medicine in Plzen, E. Beneše 1128, 301 00 Plzen, Czech Republic
e-mail: zdenekkasl@volny.cz

M. Matuska
e-mail: matuskam@fnplzen.cz

P. Poczos (✉) · T. Cesak
Department of Neurosurgery, University Hospital and Faculty of Medicine of Charles University in Hradec Králové, Sokolska 581, 500 05 Hradec Králové, Czech Republic
e-mail: pavel.poczos@fnhk.cz

T. Cesak
e-mail: tomas.cesak@fnhk.cz

R. Herzig
Department of Neurology, University Hospital and Faculty of Medicine of Charles University in Hradec Králové, Sokolska 581, 500 05 Hradec Králové, Czech Republic
e-mail: roman.herzig@fnhk.cz

N. Jiraskova
Department of Ophthalmology, University Hospital and Faculty of Medicine of Charles University in Hradec Králové, Sokolska 581, 500 05 Hradec Králové, Czech Republic
e-mail: nada.jiraskova@fnhk.cz

© The Author(s), under exclusive license to Springer Nature Switzerland AG 2024
A. Stepanov and J. Studnicka (eds.), *Ocular Manifestations of Systemic Diseases*,
https://doi.org/10.1007/978-3-031-58592-0_10

Aetiology

The pathogenesis of MS is thought to involve a combination of genetic and environmental factors. A genetically determined immune response seems to play a primary role. Activated T lymphocytes cross the blood–brain barrier into the brain and lead to the development of a damaging inflammatory response. However, the autoimmune process also affects the grey matter of the CNS. Activated T lymphocytes in the CNS release mediators of immunity (cytokines and chemokines) triggering an inflammatory cascade, leading to the death of oligodendrocytes, destruction of the myelin sheath (enveloping nerve fibres and aiding the transmission of electrical signals) and subsequent degeneration of axons (responsible for permanent neurological deficits). Lesions are disseminated in both space and time. They can occur anywhere in the brain or spinal cord, most often in certain specific areas of the white matter. Understanding the pathophysiological processes of MS can lead not only to improved targeting of treatment, with the consequent reduction of disability progression, improved quality of life and reduced costs associated with the treatment and physical disability of patients (Valis and Pavelek 2018).

Epidemiology

It is a medically and socio-economically serious disease. It's estimated that more than 2.8 million people are living with MS worldwide according to the National Multiple Sclerosis Society [53]. Its incidence increases globally with increasing distance from the equator. The first manifestation occurs at a younger age—between 20 and 40 years, on average at about 32 years of age. The incidence is more frequent in women (about 70% of cases) [53]. MS is the most common cause of disability in young people (Valis and Pavelek 2018).

Risk factors

- Heredity (influence of the HLA system)

Over-representation of genes responsible for cellular activation, differentiation, and proliferation of helper T lymphocytes. More than 100 genetic variants have been identified—each with a low risk of developing MS.

- Race factor

The prevalence of MS varies by ethnicity. The white race has the greatest receptivity, the black race smaller, and the oriental race the least.

- Latitude gradient

Increasing prevalence with increasing distance from the equator—possible effect of hypovitaminosis D associated with less exposure to sunlight. Vitamin D is a lipophilic vitamin synthesised by the conversion of 7-dehydrocholesterol in the skin, usually by solar ultraviolet radiation. Vitamin D3 receptors play an important immune

Neurological Disorders

function—they are present on regulatory T lymphocytes. There is typical seasonal variation—in the northern hemisphere with higher activity in spring (lower serum vitamin levels) and lowest in autumn. However, dietary intake of vitamin D (fish with higher fat content, dairy products, etc.) is also important.

- Infections (viral)
- Smoking
- Stress (physical—surgery, trauma, surgery, anaesthesia; psychological) (Valis and Pavelek 2018).

Clinical presentation

Symptoms of MS are very heterogeneous and depend on the location of the lesions. They often tend to regress spontaneously, which can delay the diagnosis. In the early stages (weeks to months before the development of neurological symptoms), prolonged non-specific problems may occur—fatigue (up to 90% of patients), malaise, loss of energy, weight loss. Neurological symptoms include motor symptoms, sensory symptoms (including visual disturbances, reading disorders, pain), other ocular symptoms of MS (oculomotor disorders with diplopia, internuclear ophthalmoplegia, dissociated nystagmus), sexual and sphincter disorders, balance, and gait disturbances, neuropsychiatric (psychiatric) symptoms (emotional, mood and behavioural disturbances and cognitive dysfunction) and others. Of the sensitivity disorders, Lhermitte's symptom is common—"electrical discharges" felt when the head is bowed.

One of the most common manifestations is visual impairment of the character of retrobulbar neuritis. It is characterised by destruction of the myelin sheath and nerve fibres in the optic nerve, resulting in impaired vision that develops suddenly or over days in one eye. All qualities of visual perception are affected: visual acuity, contrast sensitivity, visual field, and color vision test. Patients often complain of pain with eye movements, localised retro- or periocularly.

Clinical forms include:

(1) *Clinical Isolated Syndrome (CIS)*

This is the first demyelinating episode. An isolated symptomatic neurological episode clinically corresponding to MS is present. More than 85% of patients with CIS progress to clinically definite MS (CDMS). About 80% of patients are monofocal (monosymptomatic), about 20% are multifocal (polysymptomatic).

(2) *Relapse Remitting (RRMS)*

It covers about 55% of cases. Clearly defined attacks and remissions are present (with complete or partial resolution, periods between relapses without progression; may last months or even years). There is a constant development of inflammatory lesions. It occurs in the early 2nd and 3rd decade, with a female to male ratio of

2:1. Initial disease activity is present in the brain (associated with cognitive deficits). It has a better prognosis, with the need for support funds averaged over 20 years. On average, most patients with RRMS will progress to another form of the disease within 19 years:

(3) *Secondary Progressive (SPMS)*

It covers about 35% of cases. Occasional relapses are present with decreasing frequency, with minimal or no remissions, plateaus. Symptoms remain constant, disability increases. There is less remyelination and more plaques leading to permanent progressive disability with less recovery.

(4) *Primary Progressive (PPMS)*

It covers approximately 9–10% of cases. From the beginning, there is a slow but sustained deterioration without relapses or remissions, with varying degrees of progression. Occasionally, plateaus or temporary minimal improvements occur. It mainly affects patients in the late 3rd and early 4th decade. Men are just as often affected as women. The initial activity of the disease is present in the spinal cord (it is associated with physical disability). It has a worse prognosis, with the need for supportive measures in about 6–7 years.

(5) *Progressive Relapsing (PRMS)*

It covers approximately 1–5% of cases. Since development, there has been a steady worsening of the disease, with clear acute relapses with or without recovery. Unlike RRMS, the periods between relapses include clinically observable ongoing disease progression.

Patients have highly variable rates of relapse and progression of disability. The typical average relapse rate is approximately 0.5/patient/year. With adequate therapy, patients achieve virtually the same life expectancy as the general population. The ability to walk is preserved in 90% of patients after 10 years and in 75% after 15 years from the onset of the disease.

Approx. 50% of patients eventually die from complications of the disease. Other causes of death are similar to the general population, but suicide rates are several times higher than in the general population and account for about 15% of MS deaths (Valis and Pavelek 2018).

Diagnosis

Early diagnosis is of paramount importance—it allows early therapeutic intervention to stop the progression of the disease.

Medical anamnesis and clinical examination

These are used to detect and diagnose attacks and disease progression. Careful anamnesis taking is very important, but MS cannot be diagnosed based on anamnesis alone,

Neurological Disorders

even in cases involving descriptions of ≥ 2 attacks affecting ≥ 2 systems, suggesting dissemination of lesions over time and space.

Magnetic resonance imaging

Magnetic resonance imaging (MRI) of the brain and spinal cord shows areas of demyelination, called plaques. They are predictively localised in the white matter of the CNS (in the brain: near the lateral ventricles and the fourth ventricle, lateral sulcus, corpus callosum, n. opticus, chiasma and tracts, corticomedullary junctions, subpial part of the brainstem; in the spinal cord: anterior fascicles, centrally from the posterior fascicles, subpial).

The McDonald criteria have been the basis of MS diagnosis since 2001 and were last revised in 2017. Their use is important for prognosis and treatment, as well as for clinical research. The four-parameter model is based on the presence of (1) lesions with enhancement after gadolinium (Gd) administration, (2) juxtacortical/ cortical lesions, (3) infratentorial lesions, and (4) at least 3 periventricular lesions (hyperintense lesions on T2-weighted images). Changes visible on MRI are much more common than clinical disease activity. Symptomatic and asymptomatic lesions on MRI may be considered sufficient to determine spatial or temporal dissemination. Lesions with enhancement after Gd administration are a likely marker of oedema/inflammation/disruption of the blood–brain barrier and are referred to as "white dwarfs". Hypointense lesions present on T1-weighted images (so-called "black holes") are probable markers of tissue damage and axonal loss. The T2-weighted images show pathologically non-specific changes, including inflammation and permanent damage; they have an unsatisfactory to fair correlation with clinical disease activity.

The term *radiologically isolated syndrome (RIS)* refers to the presence of white matter lesions resembling demyelinating disease. The neurological findings in patients with these lesions are normal and have no anamnesis compatible with MS. It is not clear whether RIS represents subclinical MS or a separate entity. However, about 33% of people with RIS will develop CIS—especially patients with spinal cord lesions.

Examination of cerebrospinal fluid

Typical is the presence of ≥ 2 oligoclonal IgG (alkaline) bands distinct from such bands present in serum and/or the presence of an increase in the IgG index. In patients with typical CIS meeting clinical or MRI criteria for spatial dissemination, their presence can be used as a proxy instead of temporal dissemination. Lymphocytic pleocytosis $\leq 50/mm^3$.

Evoked potentials

These are electrical potentials generated by the nervous system, evoked by certain short sensory stimuli. In classic demyelination, there is a slowing of conduction through the affected area up to a complete block of conduction through the demyelinated area. Visual evoked potentials (VEPs) are often abnormal in MS, even in the absence of a history of optic neuritis. Prolongation of VEP latencies is typical of optic inflammation and is most pronounced in responses to structure, especially during reversal stimulation.

Ophthalmological examination including optical coherence tomography

The impairment is usually unilateral and examination of the relative afferent pupillary defect (RAPD) is therefore very beneficial. During *ophthalmoscopy* we can observe normal appearance of the optic disc (retrobulbar neuritis) or leakage and possibly haemorrhages on the disc (intraocular neuritis). Neuritis optica is very often corrected without consequences, but often recurs. Retrobulbar optic neuritis manifests itself in later stages of subatrophy or atrophy of the optic disc. *Optical coherence tomography (OCT)* is a fast and reproducible imaging method, used to obtain a detailed image of the retina, whose pathological changes associated with MS include both the effects of optic neuritis and diffuse neurodegenerative changes. OCT can be used especially in monitoring the progression of MS and to test the effect of new drugs.

Other auxiliary examinations in the differential diagnosis

These include examination of other evoked potentials (motor, somatosensory, auditory evoked), anti-aquaporin 4 IgG antibodies (AQP-4 IgG), antiphospholipid antibodies, coagulation parameters, rheumatological screening or urological examination (Valis and Pavelek 2018).

Differential diagnosis

- Infections (viral, HIV, Lyme disease, tuberculosis, syphilis)
- Cerebrovascular accident
- Vasculitis
- Rheumatoid arthritis
- Lupus
- Other connective tissue disorders
- Sarcoidosis
- Vitamin B_{12} deficiency.

Therapy

Early treatment contributes to reducing the risk of further relapse and disability progression in MS patients. *The primary goal* of therapy is to slow the accumulation of permanent physical disability. *Other goals* are to reduce inflammation (manifested by a reduction in the frequency of clinical relapses and a reduction in the incidence of lesions both with and without enhancement on MRI—called the "lesion load"), to reduce the progression of brain atrophy, slow the accumulation of cognitive deficits and maximise quality of life. Corticosteroids are used in the *treatment of acute attack*—methylprednisolone (MP) 1 g IV for 3–5 days, followed by oral prednisone 60–80 mg/day. This is a treatment of acute exacerbation by reducing oedema and inflammation at the site of demyelination; it does not affect the final clinical status or the degree of residual neurological disability due to exacerbation. Patients with frequent relapses and treated with repeated corticosteroids are at high risk of serious side effects. The Harvard protocol, combining MP and cyclophosphamide in monthly 1 g IV pulse doses for 6 months, can be used. However, severe and frequent relapses or rapidly progressive MS pose a difficult therapeutic problem; in these cases, the use of oral azathioprine 1–2 mg/kg or a combination of immunosuppressive treatment with MP and oral azathioprine may be considered.

Significant progress *in the treatment of MS between attacks* has been achieved by the development of new drugs—called disease-modifying drugs ("DMDs"). Their use aims to reduce the frequency of relapses, slow the progression of disability, and significantly reduce the accumulation of new lesions on MRI in patients with RRMS. DMD is divided into the lines—1st line includes e.g. interferons beta, glatiramer acetate or teriflunomide; $1\frac{1}{2}^{th}$ line e.g. dimethyl fumarate, fingolimod, ocrelizumab or cladribine; 2nd line e.g. natalizumab or alemtuzumab. DMDs have different mechanisms of action, including pleiotropic effects, affecting activation of several genes (interferons, glatiramer acetate, dimethyl fumarate), reduction of cell proliferation (teriflunomide, mitoxantrone), antimigratory effect (natalizumab, fingolimod) and targeted cell depletion (alemtuzumab, ocrelizumab, cladribine). When considering the indication of individual DMDs, their efficacy and safety should always be considered. It is important not only to start treatment early, but also to escalate it early if necessary. It is important to note that axonal loss can be demonstrated as early as the preclinical stage of MS and it is therefore important to use the therapeutic window as early as possible after diagnosis, i.e. at the stage of CIS or early diagnosed CDMS/RRMS. Early initiation and escalation of therapy can prevent the development of CNS atrophy and disability. Patients whose treatment is started later do not benefit as much as patients who start therapy at the initial stage of the disease. Biological treatment should be started within 4 weeks. Two strategies can be used in therapy. In escalation therapy, treatment is initiated with safer but less effective immunomodulatory drugs, and escalation to a higher line is used if the effect is insufficient. In contrast, *induction therapy* is initiated with a highly effective drug early in the course of the disease, knowing the potential risk of serious side effects, followed by de-escalation to a safer agent once the patient is stable.

Symptomatic therapy includes treatment of the following symptoms, which can be treated with the following drugs: spasticity (stiffness, painful spasms of the flexors or extensors and clonus are the main causes of disability)—baclofen, diazepam, tizanidine, vigabatrin, botulinum toxin; intense tremor—propranolol, clonazepam; painful radiculopathies, neuralgias, painful paraesthesias—carbamazepine, gabapentin, amitriptyline; fatigue—amantadine, pemoline; sexual dysfunction—sildenafil for erectile dysfunction, lubricants for women.

Supportive treatment includes *rehabilitation* and *physiotherapy* to be used judiciously to preserve mobility, relieve spasticity, improve coordination, prevent contractures and to train patients to replace affected muscles with unaffected ones. *Occupational therapy* is important in helping patients with activities of daily living (Valis and Pavelek 2018).

2 Neuromyelitis Optica (Devic's Disease)

Neuromyelitis optica (NMO) is a severely disabling inflammatory disorder of the central nervous system of putative autoimmune aetiology that predominantly affects the optic nerves and spinal cord [54]. It is a relatively rare disease, with an incidence of 0.053–0.4/100,000, that was previously mistaken for a special type of multiple sclerosis (Ruth et al. 2013), [16, 29].

The syndrome was first published by Eugene Devic and his student Fernand Gault in 1894 [17]. In 1907, the Turkish physician Acchioté proposed naming the syndrome after Devic [1]. Up to 80% of NMO patients have positive serum NMO-Immunoglobulin G also termed aquaporin-4 antibodies [31], which has led to major advances in the differential diagnosis of demyelinating diseases. Aquaporin channels are the most numerous water channels in the central nervous system. It is now known that NMO is not the only disease caused by aquaporin receptor antibodies and therefore the manifestations of these antibodies in the central nervous system are referred to as NMO spectrum disorders [9].

An ophthalmologist should consider the diagnosis of NMO if he/she is caring for a patient who has had optic neuritis, does not have findings typical of MS on MRI, and especially if restitution of visual function is poor. In this case, the collaborating neurologist should be approached and the possible diagnosis of NMO should be pointed out. Patients also undergo magnetic resonance imaging of the spine. For ophthalmologists, this disease should be alarming, as most NMO patients develop practical blindness in at least one eye within a few years. This can only be influenced by early treatment to delay relapse of the disease. Neuromyelitis optica leads more rapidly to the development of disability in comparison to MS, causes worse pain, and is thus also associated with more frequent and deeper depression. Thus, knowledge of this clinical entity is desirable for neurologists and ophthalmologists and requires close interdisciplinary collaboration.

Risk factors

- Female gender
- Aquaporin-4 antibody positivity
- Anamnesis of other autoimmune diseases: lupus erythematosus, Sjogren's syndrome, thyroid disease, myasthenia gravis
- Pregnancy
- Patient's age around 40 years
- Genetic factors (HLA DRB1 allele).

Clinical presentation

In more than 90% of patients, NMO is a relapsing disease with attacks of optic neuritis and myelitis, or both occurring unpredictably. The previous assumption that optic neuritis and myelitis occur simultaneously or closely together in NMO has been refuted [23].

Neurological Disorders

Neuritis, which can also occur bilaterally, usually causes a major decline in central visual acuity and a perimeter dropout from the central scotoma, through nerve fibre bundle dropouts to visual field breakdown. Central visual acuity may decline during an attack to blindness of the eye. Neuritis tends to be accompanied by retrobulbar or peribulbar tenderness, accentuated by eye movement. Decline in other qualities of vision is a logical consequence of ongoing severe optic neuritis. Neuritis has a more severe course, longer restitution of visual quality and sometimes significant deterioration of visual function after the first attack. Attacks have a more dramatic course and consequences compared to the course of MS, especially in the case of untreated attacks [54]. The disease is also characterised by fatigue, weakness, pain, impaired bladder and bowel function, cognitive impairment, and depression. Currently, 5-year survival is reported for more than 90% of patients [54]. Even so, NMO is a potentially life-threatening and severely disabling disease that requires prompt and long-term immunosuppressive treatment. Death in patients with NMO is in most cases caused by severe ascending cervical myelitis or brainstem involvement leading to respiratory failure.

Objective findings

Optic neuritis in NMO occurs in a retrobulbar or intraocular form. Thus, in the ophthalmoscopic findings, a relative afferent pupillary defect is usually observed, which is generally noticeable because the attack of neuritis is deep and affects the pupillomotor fibres. On the fundus, the intraocular form is dominated by optic nerve disc oedema, while the retrobulbar form may show retinal findings without observable pathology. To objectify the findings, it is necessary to determine the central visual acuity, the extent of visual field damage, colour vision, or contrast sensitivity.

Diagnosis

In the case of the first manifestation of NMO by optic neuritis, an eye examination with the ophthalmoscopic findings described above is essential. The use of OCT in the acute phase, with retinal nerve fibre layer (RNFL) and macular thickness measurements provides input numerical values of these qualities at the time of attack onset. The regression of oedema in the intraocular form, or the expected onset of atrophy of the retinal layers, can be evaluated after both intraocular and retrobulbar forms of neuritis. The development and volume loss of the retinal layers in the macula can also be monitored. Optical coherence tomography can assist in differentiating more severe neuritis by documenting atrophy of the retinal layers of the affected eye (Fig. 1), which is more pronounced than in the first attacks of MS.

Further decrease of RNFL values in NMO is more related to disease relapses. The finding of damage to the prechiasmatic visual pathway in the context of neuritis in NMO can be further verified by examination of evoked potentials where there is a reduction in amplitudes and/or prolongation of latencies.

MRI of the brain in the case of NMO is essential. In case of a negative finding of demyelinating brain lesions, which is expected in MS and should always be the primary consideration, the neurologist complements the cerebrospinal fluid examination with laboratory testing of serum for aquaporin receptor antibodies and MRI

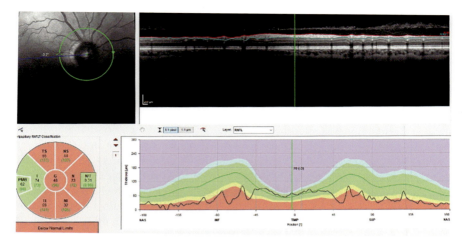

Fig. 1 State after severe neuritis of the right eye in the context of NMO, the picture shows a significant decrease in the retinal nerve fibre layer thickness of the right eye.

of the spine, where lesions typical of NMO usually affect more than three vertebral segments. However, it should be remembered that in NMO there may be both non-specific foci in the brain and foci similar to those in MS and, in some cases, may even meet the Barkhof criteria for MS. Thus, demyelinating findings on brain MRI do not exclude NMO.

Differential diagnosis

The key is to distinguish NMO from other demyelinating diseases, as the treatment of the much more common MS is different. The principal treatment for MS is immunomodulation, whereas the treatment for NMO is immunosuppressive.

Neurosarcoidosis, lymphoma, paraneoplastic syndrome, infection with neurotropic viruses, tuberculosis and Lyme disease should also be excluded. In case of severe bilateral optic neuritis, also Leber's hereditary optic neuropathy.

Therapy

The principle of NMO treatment is to delay the relapse of the disease and its severity. In the case of an acute attack, intravenous corticosteroids in high doses over several days are the first choice of treatment. There is consensus, that a prednisone taper for two to six months may be useful when recovery is slow and incomplete [32]. If the effect of corticosteroid is insufficient, plasmapheresis is under consideration.

In some cases of attacks refractory to the treatment mentioned above, intravenous immunoglobulins or cyclophosphamide can be administered [19].

In terms of long-term immunosuppressive therapy, therapy targeting B lymphocytes is used. Most commonly, patients with NMO are treated with rituximab, azathioprine, methotrexate, mycophenolate mofetil or prednisone alone, or in combination.

Neurological Disorders

Complications

From the ocular point of view, there is certainly a risk of severe neuritis with progressive loss of vision, leading in some cases to practical blindness within a few years of the disease. Gradual disability of the patient's musculoskeletal system and, finally, a strong tendency to mood decline and the development of severe depression with the need for psychiatric intervention.

3 Migraine

Migraine, together with other diseases accompanied by headache, belongs practically to the daily work portfolio of an ophthalmologist working in an outpatient clinic. This is due to the frequent proximity of the headache to the eye, the changes in vision that may precede or accompany migraine in some cases, but also to the need to exclude lesions of the eye and other tissues of the orbit as the source of the headache. Migraine is characterised by a moderate to severe headache typically affecting only one half of the head. The pain is usually throbbing and lasts from 2 hours to 72 hours. If it lasts longer than 72 hours, it is called status migrainosus. Migraines are most likely due to a combination of environmental and genetic factors. Nearly all migraine is thought to be common complex polygenic disorder [18]. Heredity plays a major role, as approximately two-thirds of cases are inherited in families. Studies conducted on twins report a 34–51% genetic influence on the likelihood of developing migraine [44]. The prevalence of chronic migraine ranges from 0.9 to 5 0.1% in general population [38]. In the prepubertal period, boys are more frequently affected, while in adulthood the ratio of afflictions reverses and women are thus afflicted with migraine two to four times more often.

The aetiology of migraine is not known yet. The brain events that initiate a migraine attack are not well understood [6]. Migraine probably originates from a vasomotor disorder and the main theory of its origin remains increased excitability of the cerebral cortex, together with abnormal function of neurons responsible for pain perception located in the trigeminal nerve in the brainstem. Serotonin levels, which are genetically influenced, are important in the pathogenesis. Serotonin raises the pain threshold and causes vasoconstriction, and its deficiency logically vasodilation and lowers the pain threshold.

Classification

Migraine is a primary headache and is divided into *six subclasses* according to the latest classification by the International Headache Society in 2004:

- Migraine without aura
- Migraine with aura
- Chronic migraine
- Complications of migraine

- Probable migraine
- Episodic syndromes that may be associated with migraine.

Some subclasses of migraines may combine with each other. It is not uncommon for a person suffering from migraine with aura also often suffer from migraines without aura.

Retinal migraine most probably has an underlying spasm of the retinal arteries, thus leading to monocular manifestations with transient visual impairment, sometimes even transient blindness of the eye. This type of migraine is difficult to classify, because in classic migraine with typical aura, there is at least impairment in both eyes with usually hemianoptic visual field involvement. Special and unusual migraines also include ophthalmoplegic migraine, where one or more oculomotor nerves develop paresis during the development of severe cephalea or hemicrania, which may persist for several weeks or even months. It first appears usually in childhood.

Risk and trigger factors

- Positive family anamnesis
- Gender according to the age of the patient—prepubertal period more often men, in adulthood more often women
- Sleep deprivation and irregular daily routine
- Stress, mental strain, fatigue and hunger

Clinical presentation

The ophthalmologist is commonly involved in the differential diagnosis of headaches. Certain types of migraines are typically accompanied by visual symptoms. Specific in terms of visual disturbances is migraine with aura. The aura is perceived by 15–30% of migraine patients. After the prodromal phase, which can precede headaches even in patients with migraine without aura and is characterised by mood changes, irritability, indigestion, and increased sensitivity to smells and noise, comes the aura phase. The aura usually lasts no longer than a few tens of minutes and is most often accompanied by a change in vision. A scintillating scotoma (a sparkly visual field defect) appears near the centre of both eyes, from which squiggly or zigzag lines often spread arcuate towards the periphery (Fig. 2). Some patients describe loss of half of the visual field, possibly image shaking and changes in colour perception.

The aura may not only be of the nature of a change in vision. Sensory auras are accompanied by tingling in the hand and arm area, sometimes spreading to the face. Speech disturbances may also occur within the aura, less common are motor difficulties within the hemiplegic migraine.

After the aura phase comes a phase of usually gradually developing unilateral, throbbing headache. The worsening of the pain is usually conditioned by physical activity. The pain may involve both halves of the head in some individuals. During the migraine, especially in the headache stage, the patient suffers from nausea and

Neurological Disorders 387

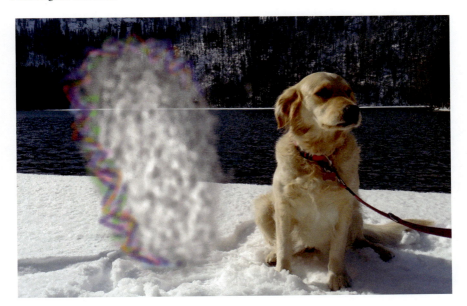

Fig. 2 Visual aura during a migraine attack

may vomit. The symptoms may be partially relieved by staying in a dark quiet area. The frequency of migraine attacks has been described as ranging from a few per week to several per lifetime, and the average migraine sufferer has approximately one attack per month.

The postdrome phase can last for several days and patients usually complain of subsiding headaches at the site of the original migraine, reduced ability to concentrate and think, and fatigue to weakness.

Diagnosis and differential diagnosis

The patient's medical anamnesis, including family anamnesis, plays a crucial role in the diagnosis of the disease. From the subjective description of the attack or recurrent conditions, we infer migraine. If the patient has a migraine with aura, then it will most often be visual, and therefore such a patient often seeks help from an ophthalmologist.

When a migraine is suspected, a pattern of 5, 4, 3, 2, 1 or 5 or more attacks (two attacks are sufficient for migraine with aura), 4 hours' to 3 days' duration, 2 or more of the following phenomena may be helpful: unilateral pain, throbbing pain, moderate to severe headache, and pain aggravated by normal physical activity. One of the following: nausea, vomiting, sensitivity to light or sound. Other diseases to consider in the case of headache include tension cephalea, neuralgia, cluster headache, intoxication, headache in vascular and extravascular disorders of the central nervous system, meningitis, headache arising from the neck, ear, tooth or ear, as well as temporal arteritis.

Therapy

The neurologist has the main role in migraine treatment and management, but the ophthalmologist should be prepared to answer the patient's questions about migraine therapy.

Preventive measures, such as lifestyle changes with sufficient regular sleep, diet together with nutritional supplements such as magnesium, coenzyme Q10 and B vitamins and medication to reduce the frequency and severity of attacks, as well as physiotherapy and chiropractic treatment, play a role in the treatment of migraine.

Agents that reduce the frequency and severity of migraine attacks include topiramate, sodium valproate, metoprolol, propranolol, tricyclic antidepressants, and beta-blockers. Other drugs include gabapentin, timolol, amitriptyline and venlafaxine.

Surgical therapy, including neurostimulator therapy, may also be considered for migraines refractory to conservative treatment.

Treatment of the migraine attack itself is most effective when given early in the attack. It usually starts with the administration of simple analgesics from the group of non-steroidal anti-inflammatory drugs, acetaminophen, acetylsalicylic acid, and caffeine. The next step in patients with migraines unresponsive to conventional analgesics may be triptans, the most used being sumatriptan, which also controls nausea well. Triptans should be avoided in patients with vascular disease, uncontrolled hypertension or hemiplegic migraine [25]. In therapy, ergotamine derivatives, dihydroergotamines are also used; on the contrary, opioids and barbiturates are not recommended.

4 Lesions of the Third Cranial Nerve

N. oculomotorius is a mixed nerve, containing parasympathetic and motor fibres. All the nuclei of the oculomotor nerve (III) are in the mesencephalon. The motor nucleus (or a group of nuclei representing individual oculomotor muscles) is located just rostral to the nucleus of n. IV. The paired *Edinger-Westphal nucleus* is located medially at the midline, and the presynaptic parasympathetic neurons emanating from it run bilaterally with the fibres of n. III. The nerve then exits the trunk at the base of the brain. In the subarachnoid space, the nerve trunk is supplied from the *a. cerebri posterior* and *a. cerebelli superior*. N. III runs through the *sinus cavernosus* (in its lateral wall, it runs rostrally from n. IV) and enters the orbit by the *superior orbital fissure* (caudally from n. IV). It motorically innervates 4 of the 6 orbicularis oculi (*m. rectus medialis* (RM), *m. rectus superior* (RS), *m. rectus inferior* (RI), and *m. obliquus inferior* (OI)) and keeps the orbital fissure open (*m. levator palpebrae superioris* (LPS)). The nuclei for RI, RM, and OI send axons only to the ipsilateral trunk of n. III, whereas the nucleus for RS sends axons only to the contralateral n. III. This anatomical arrangement makes it possible to distinguish lesions of single nuclei (*nuclear lesions*) from lesions of the nerve trunk (*fascicular lesions*) before exiting the mesencephalon, when the *nucleus ruber*, *pedunculus cerebri*, or possibly both structures are simultaneously affected. The nucleus for the RM is located most ventrally and all other nuclei send axons through this nucleus—thus, isolated involvement of this muscle is not possible. The nucleus for LPS, on the other hand, is located at the dorsocaudal edge of the nuclear complex and can thus be spared in isolation. The neurons of its inner parasympathetic branch in the orbit connect in the *ganglion ciliare* to postsynaptic neurons innervating *m. sphincter pupillae* (providing pupillary constriction) and *m. ciliaris* (mediating accommodation). When looking into near, pupillary convergence, accommodation, and pupillary response to near view occur simultaneously (Fig. 3) [2].

Aetiology

The main causes of lesions of n. III include cranial neuropathy (e.g. in diabetes mellitus), tumours of the skull base (mainly in the parasellar localisation or in the *fissura orbitalis superior*), aneurysms (on the *a. communicans posterior* or on the *a. carotis interna*), pathological processes in the area of the cavernous sinus, traumata, zoster ophthalmicus and stem lesions of various aetiology (most often vascular—ischaemia or haemorrhage, also demyelination or tumours—e.g. pinealoma) [35]. Compression of n. III also occurs in intracranial hypertension with temporal cone syndrome (*lateral tentorial herniation*) when a part of the temporal lobe (*uncus gyri hippocampi*) is pushed into the tentorial opening. Among the other possible causes of peripheral lesion of the oculomotor nerve, we should mention meningitis, temporal

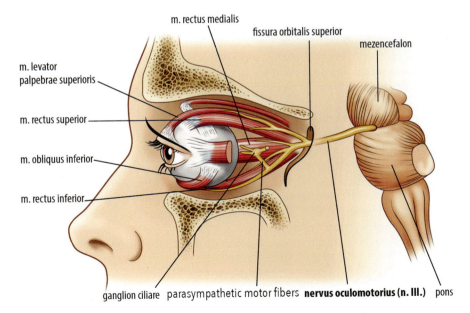

Fig. 3 Nervus oculomotorius. (With permission of Grada Publishing a.s.)

arteritis, tumours of the temporal lobe, epipharynx, small wing of the sphenoid bone, metastases, and others. In the region of the cavernous sinus, the oculomotor nerve (along with other peroneal nerves and n. V) may be affected in inflammatory thrombosis of the sinus, in carotid-cavernous fistulas, tumoural expansions, and infraclinoid aneurysms. In the region of the superior orbital fissure, n. III (along with other peroneal nerves and the 1st branch of n. V) is affected due to orbital tumours (often metastatic or secondary), trauma (stab wounds, fractures) or inflammation (periostitis). Another cause of n. III involvement may be botulism, when in the early stage there is a disorder of pupillary reaction; later, complete ophthalmoplegia develops together with bradycardia and other symptoms of a generalised disorder [2, 7].

Risk factors

These correspond to individual aetiological causes.

Clinical presentation

The general term *ophthalmoplegia* refers to the involvement of the ophthalmic nerves (n. III, n. IV and n. VI), where the lesion of n. III often dominates. If only the external muscles are affected (the pupillary function is intact), we speak of *external ophthalmoplegia*; if the internal branch is affected, we use the term *internal ophthalmoplegia*. From the quantitative point of view, ophthalmoplegia may be *complete* or *incomplete*. Complete ophthalmoplegia (total—with both branches affected) is clinically manifested by ptosis of the upper eyelid, divergent strabismus with impaired ocular motility in all directions except abduction, a wide pupil with reduced or absent photoreaction and impaired accommodation (Fig. 4).

The patient reports diplopia with horizontal and vertical disparity of images that converge only on abduction of the eye (Fig. 5).

N. oculomotorius can be disrupted anywhere in its course from the nucleus to the myoneural junction. Because the disorders caused by lesions at different sites vary in clinical expression, this can be used to make a topical and, in part, an aetiological diagnosis.

In the case of mechanical compression of n. III, the pupil is always affected since the parasympathetic fibres are located relatively superficially. In the case of ischaemic lesions of the nerve (e.g. in diabetes mellitus), the pupil may be spared.

In *nuclear disorders*, in unilateral lesions, one or more oculomotor muscles are affected, not only homolaterally but also contralaterally, whereas the LPS and especially the intraocular muscles may be spared. In a more extensive mesencephalic lesion, the nuclear lesion of n. III may be associated with vertical visual palsy and convergence or retraction nystagmus.

Fascicular lesions arise from involvement of the n. III fibres while they are still running through the brainstem and are characterised by a combination of oculomotor disturbance with other neurological symptoms. The following syndromes belong to this group:

(1) *Nothnagel's syndrome* (upper nucleus ruber syndrome)—ipsilateral lesions of n. III and contralateral cerebellar ataxia.

Neurological Disorders

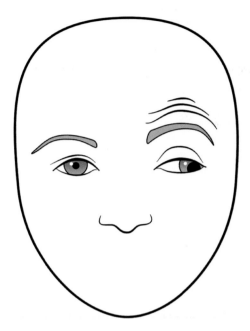

Fig. 4 Left cranial nerve III lesion with upper eyelid ptosis, divergent strabismus and mydriasis with photoreaction disorder. (With permission of Grada Publishing a.s.)

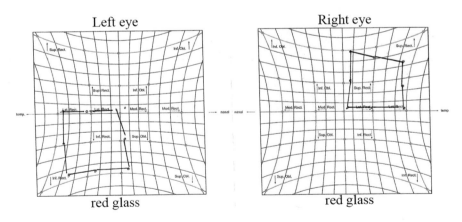

Fig. 5 Diplopia in a patient with cranial nerve III involvement

(2) *Benedict's syndrome* (lower nucleus ruber syndrome)—ipsilateral lesions n. III and contralateral *extrapyramidal hyperkinesis* and *athetosis* (*hemitremor*).
(3) *Weber's syndrome* (hemiplegia alternans superior seu oculomotorica)—homolateral lesion n. III and contralateral central hemiparesis/hemiplegia, contralateral central lesion n. VII, XII (paralysis of the muscles of the tongue without their

early atrophy, without fibrillation and fasciculations) (also contralaterally sometimes hemihypesthesia, especially dissociated for proprioception and vibratory sensation—when the lemniscus medialis is affected, and ataxia).

The *radicular lesion* arises from involvement of n. III projecting from the brainstem and the adjacent cerebellar peduncle, in which the pyramidal pathway runs. The clinical presentation is identical to Weber's syndrome. In the *fossa interpeduncularis* lesion, bilateral total lesion of n. III with quadriplegia is observed.

Basal lesions are caused by damage to n. III during its course through the subarachnoid space of the skull base. They are the most common cause of isolated peripheral n. III lesions and occur in two clinically and aetiologically distinct forms.

- The first of these has already been described in the chapter on lesions of the parasympathetic. It is a total palsy with a marked emphasis on the co-involvement of the internal (parasympathetic) branch, i.e. with a wide, unresponsive pupil. Aetiologically, we think mainly of a saccular aneurysm on *a. communicans posterior* or on *a. carotis interna* at branching of *a. communicans posterior*. The suspicion of an aneurysm is supported by the indication of previous retrobulbar and frontal pain. Lesions n. III caused by an aneurysm are poorly repaired and regenerating fibres often stray to other muscles, leading to anomalous synkinesis.

- In the second form of basal palsy, on the other hand, the internal branch is almost always spared and pupillary reactions are normal. Aetiologically, it is overwhelmingly a complication of diabetes mellitus. Recovery usually takes several weeks and is not complicated by stray reinnervation. Interestingly, impairment may not always be a manifestation of decompensated diabetes and may occur even in latent or well-compensated diabetes.

- Another valuable picture among basal lesions is what is called clivus edge syndrome (*Fisher-Brügge syndrome*), which arises when sudden pressure in the supratentorial space (e.g. subdural haemorrhage) presses n. III against the clivus edge or the margin of the tentorium by the temporal lobe (called the lateral tentorial herniation or temporal cone) [35]. Clinically, it is manifested by unilateral paralytic mydriasis, which is interpreted by the extreme sensitivity of the pupillomotor fibres to pressure in this section of the nerve. Initial miosis from irritation is usually not observed, but later paralysis of the external eye muscles may be associated.

  In the further course, n. III penetrates through the dura into the cavernous plexus and into the orbit, and its palsies associate with lesions of other oculomotor nerves and form typical syndromes according to their localisation.

- The *cavernous sinus syndrome* is manifested by a lesion (often bilateral) of all three oculomotor nerves (n. III, n. IV and n. VI), combined with an irritation-extinction lesion of one, two or all three branches of the nervus trigeminus. Other symptoms vary according to the aetiology. In inflammatory thrombosis of the sinus, eyelid oedema, chemosis and protrusion of the eye are prominent; in carotid-cavernous fistula, pulsatile exophthalmos, and intracranial murmur; in tumoural expansions and infraclinoid aneurysms, neuralgic pain in the corresponding half of the face [35].

Neurological Disorders

- In *superior orbital fissure syndrome,* only the first branch of n. trigeminus is affected in addition to the orbital nerves. Periorbital neuralgia and corneal hypesthesia are usually present. Due to the co-involvement of periarterial sympathetic fibres, the pupil is narrower rather than wider.
- *Orbital spike syndrome* is manifested by damage to all nerve structures in this localisation—n. II, n. III, n. IV, the first branch of n. V, n. VI and fibres of both autonomic systems. The complete picture includes severe visual impairment, loss of ocular motility in all directions, periorbital neuralgia, skin and corneal hypesthesia and disturbances of pupillary reactions of both afferent and efferent type. Exophthalmos (usually axial) is also present and retinal oedema or optic nerve atrophy may be observed as a sign of optic compression.
- *Painful ophthalmoplegia syndrome (Tolosa-Hunt syndrome)* is usually characterised by unilateral, either complete or incomplete, lesions of all the ophthalmic nerves (n. III, n. IV and n. VI) together with periorbital neuralgia (due to involvement of the 1st or even the 2nd branch of n. V). Internal ophthalmoplegia may also be present and sometimes visual impairment in n. II. The cause is non-specific granulomatous or non-granulomatous inflammation in the region of the anterior cavernous sinus, fissure orbitalis superior and tip of the orbit. The cause is unknown. The inflammation responds very well to corticoid therapy.

Duan's retraction syndrome is a peculiar congenital disorder of the horizontal mobility of the eye, which at first sight looks like a paralysis of the external rectus muscle, but the cause is its anomalous innervation by fibres of n. III. The disorder is not very rare, occurring mostly sporadically, is only rarely familial and then indicative of autosomal dominant inheritance with low penetrance. In the clinical presentation we find several forms of this entity: Duan syndrome I, II and III. This breadth of variation results from the pathogenesis of the disease—the innervation of the *m. rectus lateralis* by fibres of n. VI is absent and is replaced to varying degrees by fibres of n. III, destined for RM. The parts of the muscle lacking any motor innervation turn into a stiff fibrous band. The eventual treatment is surgical and is indicated only when there is a conspicuous forced posture of the head or a more pronounced strabismus in the primary position. Muscle-weakening procedures are the method of choice, as strengthening procedures may accentuate bulb retraction [2, 35].

Diagnosis

Examination of eye motility and oculomotor function (Table 1), including Hess screen.

Neuroimaging methods—especially magnetic resonance imaging and computed tomography (including angiography)—are of further benefit. In some cases, liquor examination may also be beneficial [2, 7].

Differential diagnosis

- Cranial neuropathy (e.g. in diabetes mellitus)
- Tumours (skull base—mainly in the parasellar localisation or in the fissure orbitalis superior; trunk—e.g. pinealoma; in the region of the cavernous sinus;

Table 1 The function and innervation of the extraocular muscles

Ocular muscle	Innervation	Primary function	Associated function
Medial rectus (musculus rectus int.)	III. cranial nerve	Adduction	
Lateral rectus (musculus rectus lat.)	VI. cranial nerve	Abduction	
Superior rectus (musculus rectus sup.)	III. cranial nerve	Elevation	Adduction, intorsion
Inferior rectus (musculus rectus inf.)	III. cranial nerve	Depression	Adduction, extorsion
Superior oblique (musculus obliquus sup.)	IV. cranial nerve	Intorsion	Depression, abduction
Inferior oblique (musculus obliquus inf.)	III. cranial nerve	Extorsion	Elevation, abduction

in the region of the fissure orbitalis superior; temporal lobe; epipharynx; small wing of the sphenoid bone; metastases)
- Aneurysm (on the a. communicans posterior or on the a. carotis interna, infraclinoid)
- Carotid-cavernous fistula
- Trauma
- Vascular events (ischaemia, haemorrhage) of brainstem localisation
- Inflammatory processes (zoster ophthalmicus, meningitis, temporal arteritis, inflammatory thrombosis of the cavernous sinus, periostitis)
- Demyelination
- Botulism
- Intracranial hypertension with temporal cone syndrome (lateral tentorial herniation)
- Parinaud's syndrome (dorsal mesencephalic syndrome)
- Hyperthyroidism (called 'endocrine orbitopathy' or even 'thyrotoxic exophthalmic ophthalmoplegia')
- Chronic progressive external ophthalmoplegia
- Miller-Fisher syndrome
- Horner's syndrome.

Therapy

It corresponds to individual aetiological causes.

Neurological Disorders

5 Lesions of the Fourth Cranial Nerve

N. trochlearis is a motor nerve whose nucleus lies in the mesencephalon just caudal to the motor nucleus of n. III. It is the only nerve that emerges on the dorsal side of the trunk and crosses with the contralateral nerve. It encircles the trunk and enters the *sinus cavernosus*, where it passes through the lateral wall caudal to n. III. Through the *superior orbital fissure* it enters the orbit rostrally from n. III. It innervates *m. obliquus superior*, which is the depressor (in adduction), internal rotator (in abduction), and mild abductor of the eye (Fig. 6) [2].

Aetiology

Of the known causes of n. IV involvement, closed craniocerebral injury with dorsal trunk involvement is the first. This occurs in severe trauma when, due to sudden displacement of supratentorial structures, the trunk is compressed caudally and bent dorsally. However, milder trauma can also be the cause of its involvement. To be considered are also vascular and circulatory disorders (mesencephalic ischaemia and haemorrhage, ischaemic lesions of the nerve trunk in the context of arterial hypertension or diabetes mellitus—cranial neuropathy), tumours (tectum, *sinus cavernosus*, *superior orbital fissure*), congenital lesions, postoperative lesions after surgeries in

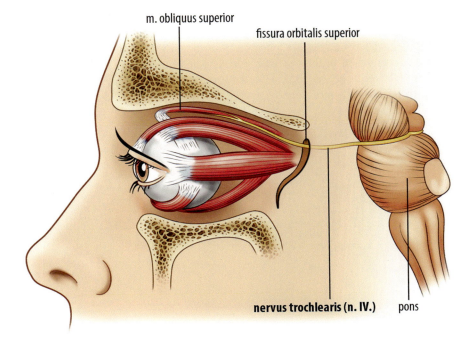

Fig. 6 *N. trochlearis*. (With permission of Grada Publishing a.s.)

the orbit, paranasal sinuses and middle cranial fossa, infections (meningitis, borreliosis, herpes zoster) and sarcoidosis [35]. Lesions can be both unilateral and bilateral, including traumatic lesions that can lead to injury of the dorsal part of the mesencephalon and both n. IV of the *tentorium cerebelli*. We think of a lesion of the nucleus in the brainstem when associated with a lesion of n. III (proximity of the nuclei) and with a bilateral lesion. About one-third of n. IV lesions remain aetiologically unresolved. Lesions in combination with n. III and n. VI lesions are listed in the chapter on *n. oculomotorius* [2, 7].

Risk factors

These correspond to individual aetiological causes.

Clinical presentation

The clinical presentation of paresis of the *n. trochlearis* is mainly characterised by the absence of deorsumvergence of the eye in adduction, and the greatest spacing of the images of the viewed object in the same direction (Fig. 7).

The lesion leads to vertical diplopia, which is maximally expressed in oblique downward and nasal views. This type of diplopia is always very disturbing for the patient and difficult to tolerate, as it causes difficulty in reading, walking downstairs, etc. The posture of the head is also characteristic, being in a forced slight forward bend and curled towards the arm of the healthy side (*torticollis ocularis*) to allow elevation and adduction of the eyeball (Fig. 8A, B).

The diagnosis is confirmed by the *Bielschowsky manoeuvre*, where the difficulty is reduced in the compensatory position described above and the hypertropia is markedly accentuated in the eye with paresis when the head is tilted towards the shoulder of the diseased side [35]. Also, the image of bilateral palsy is characteristic: it is characterised by *alternating hypertropia*, on the right when looking to the left

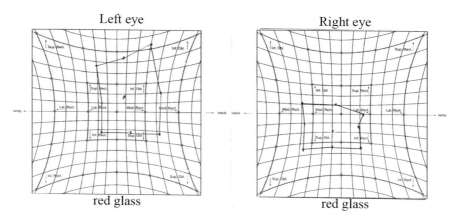

Fig. 7 Diplopia in a patient with involvement of the IV cephalic nerve

Neurological Disorders

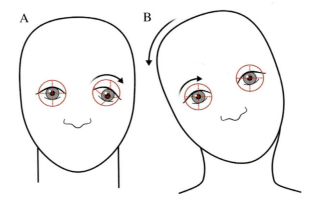

Fig. 8 A, B Lesion of the fourth cranial nerve with paresis of the m. obliquus superior on the left. (With permission of Grada Publishing a.s.). A. Deviation of the left eyeball with vertical diplopia. B. Compensatory position of the head—bowing and rotation to the arm of the healthy side and slight forward bend

and on the left when looking to the right. The lesions in the sinus cavernosus, fissure orbitalis superior and orbits have already been described in n. III [2].

Diagnosis

Examination of orbital motility and orbicularis oculi function (Table 1), including Hess' screen. Other uses include magnetic resonance imaging, computed tomography (including angiography) and liquor examination [2, 7].

Differential diagnosis of causes

- Craniocerebral trauma
- Stroke (ischaemic, haemorrhagic)
- Ischaemic lesion of the nerve trunk (in the context of arterial hypertension or diabetes mellitus—cranial neuropathy)
- Tumours
- Congenital lesions
- Postoperative lesions
- Infections (meningitis, Lyme disease, herpes zoster)
- Sarcoidosis
- (Combination with involvement of n. III and n. VI—see n. oculomotorius)
- Brown's syndrome of the m. obliquus superior tendon.

Therapy

This corresponds to individual aetiological causes.

6 Lesions of the Sixth Cranial Nerve

N. abducens is a motor nerve whose nucleus lies mediodorsally in the lower part of the *pons Varoli* and is separated from the base of the IV ventricle by the node of the *n. facialis*. n. VI ascends ventrally in the *sulcus bulbopontinus* (lateral to the *corticospinal tract*), continues rostrally through the *prepontine cistern*, passes under the *ligamentum petroclinoideum*, and, at the tip of the pyramid, passes into the lateral wall of the *sinus cavernosus* and then into the *superior orbital fissure*. It innervates the m. rectus lateralis, the function of which is abduction of the eye (Fig. 9).

In the nucleus of n. VI, large motoneurons for *m. rectus lateralis* mix with small internuclear neurons, sending axons to the contralateral *fasciculus longitudinalis medialis* and to the nucleus of n. III for the contralateral *m. rectus medialis* [2].

Aetiology

Lesion of n. VI is the most common oculomotor disorder, which is explained by its susceptibility to stretching and distortion when the nerve is long and exposed, crossing with branches of *a. basilaris*, bending at the edge of the pyramid, and, above all, traction during dislocation of the brainstem in intracranial hypertension (the susceptibility of n. VI to involvement here is due to the fixation of the nerve exit

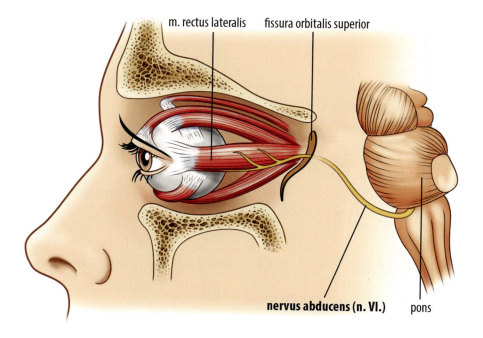

Fig. 9 *N. abducens*. (With permission of Grada Publishing a.s.)

Neurological Disorders

from the *pons* and at the point of entry under the *ligamentum petroclinoideum* at the *apex of the pyramid*).

The cause of the lesion in the subarachnoid space is usually compression by an aneurysm on *a. cerebelli anterior inferior*, *a. cerebellaris posterior inferior* or on *a. basilaris*.

An isolated lesion of n. VI is present in patients with arterial hypertension or diabetes mellitus (ischaemic lesions, cranial diabetic neuropathy). It is quite common in a carotid-cavernous fistula with pulsatile exophthalmos and more rarely accompanies dislocated fractures of the zygomaticomaxillary complex. Lesions in this region (most commonly tumours) may also produce a combination of lesions of n. VI and postganglionic sympathetic fibres, which attach to the abducens for a short distance before their connection to the first branch of *n. trigeminus*. Clinically, *Horner's syndrome* is then observed, in combination with *horizontal uncrossed diplopia*. However, an isolated n. VI lesion (uni- or bilateral) may also be a false localising sign in intracranial expansive lesions with intracranial hypertension [35]. Then, from traumatic causes, it is usually a unilateral lesion in fractures of the skull base and, more rarely, a bilateral lesion in trauma associated with a fall and head impact in the sagittal plane. An isolated lesion of n. VI may also be cryptogenic, but also a transient symptom after lumbar puncture.

Causes of nuclear and fascicular lesions may be strokes (with acute development of symptoms, usually in the elderly) or tumours of pontine localisation (with gradual development of symptoms, especially in the younger) [35].

The cause of the now very rare pyramidal apex involvement (*Gradenig's syndrome*) is usually circumscribed meningitis and pyramidal apex ostitis. The lesion in this area may also be caused by extradural inflammation of otogenic origin [2, 7].

Risk factors

These correspond to individual aetiological causes.

Clinical presentation

The clinical presentation is dominated by paralytic strabismus, when the action field of the m. rectus lateralis is impaired, the field of view is limited and the spacing of images increases. The predominance of the healthy antagonist (*m. rectus medialis* innervated by n. III) causes the eye to converge, which may eventually progress to contracture of the internal rectus muscle. Horizontal diplopia is uncrossed, as the image of the eye with paresis is always farther in the periphery when the eye is viewed in the same gaze direction (Fig. 10).

In the compensatory position, the head is rotated in the direction of function of the affected muscle (Fig. 11A, B).

With a lesion of the nucleus of n. VI, there is usually a gaze paresis in the ipsilateral direction (due to a lesion of the *m. paraabducens*) and often a lesion of n. VII, whose fibres curve around the nucleus of n. VI. In this lesion, however, the abduction of the ipsilateral eye is more affected than the adduction of the contralateral eye, and convergent strabismus is present.

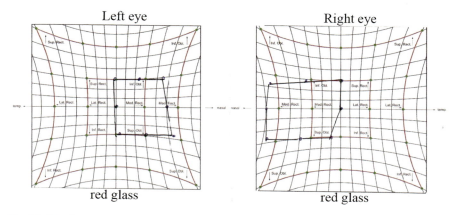

Fig. 10 Hess' screen. Diplopia in a patient with VI cranial nerve involvement

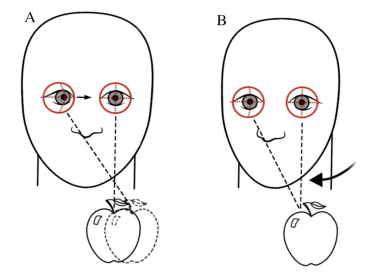

Fig. 11 A, B Lesion of the seventh cranial nerve on the right with paresis of the m. rectus lateralis on the right. (With permission of Grada Publishing a.s.). A. Deviation of the right bulb nasally from predominance of m. rectus medialis with horizontal diplopia. B. Compensatory head position—rotation to the right

In the case of a fascicular lesion of n. VI, the paralysis of *m. rectus lateralis* is accompanied by contralateral central hemiparesis or a lesion of n. V.

A lesion of n. VI is usually isolated in the subarachnoid space. In processes in the pyramidal apex, it is often associated with a lesion of n. V. (*Gradenig's syndrome*—a combination of homolateral lesion of n. VI and severe neuralgia in the first branch

Neurological Disorders

of *n. trigeminus*), or of n. VII and n. VIII. (however, when n. VII and n. VIII are affected simultaneously, it is no longer an isolated lesion of the pyramidal apex).

Nuclear and fascicular trunk lesions are manifested by the association of the lesion of n. VI with other neurological symptoms. *Foville syndrome* is caused by a lesion in the dorsal part of the brainstem and clinically is a combination of a lesion of n. VI with homolateral gaze palsy (from a lesion of the adjacent paramedian pontine reticular formation) and a homolateral lesion of n. VII. Impairment in the ventral part of the pons produces *Millard-Gubler syndrome*, manifested by a combination of a lesion of n. VI with a homolateral peripheral lesion of n. VII and contralateral central hemiplegia (in the case of a lesion of the corticospinal tract) and, possibly, a contralateral central lesion of n. XII (in the case of a lesion of the corticobulbar tract).

Lesions in the *sinus cavernosus, superior orbital fissure* and *orbits* have already been described in n. III [2].

Diagnosis

The basic diagnostic method is the strabological examination, including the examination of the position and movement of the eyeballs (Table 1) and the Hess screen. Neuroimaging methods—especially magnetic resonance imaging and computed tomography (including angiography)—are also useful. In some cases, liquor examination may also be beneficial [2, 7].

Differential diagnosis

- Intracranial hypertension
- Compression by an aneurysm (on *a. cerebelli anterior inferior, a. cerebellaris posterior inferior* or on *a. basilaris*)
- carotid-cavernous fistula
- Ischaemic lesion of the nerve trunk (in the context of arterial hypertension or diabetes mellitus—cranial neuropathy)
- Stroke (ischaemic, haemorrhagic)
- Trauma (fracture of the skull base, dislocated fracture of the zygomatomaxillary complex, trauma associated with head impact in the sagittal plane)
- Tumours
- Infections (meningitis, pyramidal apex ostitis, extradural otitis oogenousis)
- Transient symptom after lumbar puncture
- (Combination with involvement of n. III and n. IV—see n. oculomotorius)
- Möbius syndrome

Therapy

This corresponds to individual aetiological causes.

7 Lesions of the Seventh Cranial Nerve

N. facialis is a mixed nerve, which consists of two parts—about 70% are *motor nerve* fibres (supplying the muscles of the face) and the rest are *n. intermedius* (with sensory—taste fibres from the front 2/3 of the tongue, sensory and autonomic—parasympathetic) [35]. The nucleus of n. VII is in the *pons Varoli*; after exiting the trunk, the nerve runs anterolaterally through the *cerebellopontine angle* and enters the *meatus acusticus internus* (the length of this section is 23–24 mm). Nerve VIII runs laterally; *n. intermedius* is located between n. *facialis* and n. VIII. The *meatal segment* is 7–8 mm long; n. VII occupies the upper anterior part, the cochlear nerve is located caudally, the vestibular nerve dorsally. The vascular supply comes from the *a. labyrinthi*, a branch of the *a. cerebelli anterior inferior*. In pars pyramidalis, n. VII runs in the *canalis n. facialis (Fallopii)*, which is formed by three *sections*: *labyrinth* (3–4 mm long), *tympanal* (along the medial wall of the cavum tympani; 12–13 mm long), and mastoid (dorsal to the external auditory canal; 15–20 mm long). At the interface between the first and second sections is the *ganglion geniculi*, *n. petrosus superficialis major* separates here from n. VII, and, in the third section, *n. stapedius* and *chorda tympani*. Nerve VII is supplied proximally by a branch of *a. meningica media* and distally by *a. stylomastoidea*. Nerve VII exits from the *foramen stylomastoideum* and enters the *glandula parotis*. Here the nerve divides into several branches which anastomose abundantly together. The individual branches are supplied from *a. stylomastoidea, a. auricularis posterior, a. temporalis superficialis* and *a. facialis*.

N. facialis motorically innervates the mimic muscles of the midface, m. platysma, m. stapedius, m. stylohyoideus, and the venter posterior of m. digastrici (Fig. 12).

The central innervation arises from the inferior third of the gyrus praecentralis in the cortex of the frontal lobe. The fibres of the *tr. corticonuclearis* pass through the *capsula interna*, cross in the caudal pons, and terminate in the contralateral motor nucleus of n. VII. Some fibres descend caudally below the level of the nucleus of n. VII, again cross and emerge as a *Déjerin recurrent bundle* to the nucleus n. VII contralaterally (i.e. ipsilateral to the cortex). Part of the motor nucleus for innervation of the upper half of the face (*m. frontalis, corrugator glabellae*, upper part of *m. orbicularis oculi*) thus has bilateral innervation, whereas the part of the motor nucleus for innervation of the lower half of the face has innervation only contralateral to it (Fig. 13A, B).

Emotional control of the mimic muscles originates from extrapyramidal structures (frontal lobe, thalamus, and *globus pallidus*) and goes to the motor nucleus of n. VII by way of the reticular formation. The motor nucleus of n. VII is in the lower third of the pons—ventral to the nucleus of n. V and dorsolateral to the superior olivary nucleus. The fibres of the motor nucleus of n. VII project dorsally, laterally encircle the nucleus of n. VI, and return caudally between the nuclei of n. V and n. VII. They emerge caudolaterally in the pontine part and enter the cerebellopontine angle.

N. intermedius contains sensory taste fibres from the anterior 2/3 of the tongue, afferent somatic fibres from the posterior part of the external auditory canal, part of

Neurological Disorders

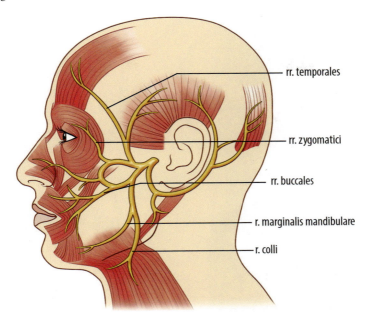

Fig. 12 *N. facialis*—motor innervation. (With permission of Grada Publishing a.s.)

the auricle and mastoid landscape, and parasympathetic fibres for the *glandula sublingualis*, *glandula submandibularis*, and for the minor glands in the nasal, paranasal sinuses, and palatine regions. Somatosensory fibres follow the path of *n. auricularis posterior* and *n. intermedius* to the sensory nucleus of the n. V in the pons. The bodies of somatosensory and gustatory neurons are in the *ganglion geniculi*. Preganglionic parasympathetic fibres begin in the *nucleus salivatorius superior* and pass through the *ganglion geniculi* without switchover. The fibres for the *glandula lacrimalis* and the minor glands follow the path of the *n. petrosus superficialis major*, recruiting the *n. petrosus profundus* containing the postganglionic sympathetic fibres, forming the *n. canalis pterygoidei*, and reconnecting to the postganglionic neurons in the *ganglion pterygopalatinum*. The preganglionic fibres for the *glandula sublingualis* and *glandula submandibularis* follow the path of the *chorda tympani* and *n. lingualis* and connect to postganglionic neurons in the *ganglion submandibulare*. Taste fibres from the anterior 2/3 of the tongue follow the path of the *n. lingualis* and *chorda tympani*, which passes through the middle ear and joins the trunk of n. VII in the *Fallopian canal*. The bodies of these neurons are in the *ganglion geniculi* and terminate in the *nucleus tractus solitarii* in the *medulla oblongata* (Fig. 14) [2].

Aetiology

The most common cause of *peripheral lesions of n. VII*, occurring in about 75% of cases, is *Bell's idiopathic palsy* [35]. Its incidence is about 23/100,000/year, with

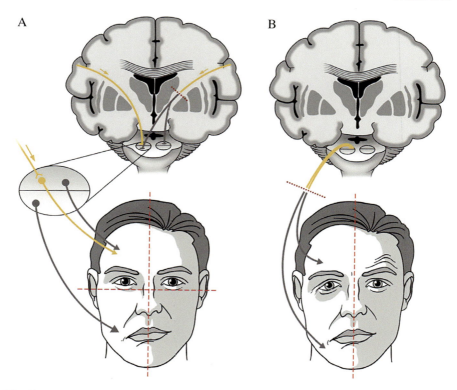

Fig. 13 Lesion of the seventh cranial nerve on the right with paresis of the facial muscles. A) Central lesion when tr. corticonuclearis is affected on the left—facial expressions in the upper face are spared. B) Peripheral lesion of n. VII. on the right—mime in the upper and lower part of the face is affected. (With permission of Grada Publishing a.s.)

equal involvement of both sexes and with the highest incidence in the age groups 15–45 and then over 80 years [35]. Recurrence occurs in about 5% of cases. The presumed cause is inflammation of *n. facialis* in the *Fallopian canal* above the *foramen stylomastoideum,* accompanied by oedema with a secondary compression of the nerve and *vasa nervorum* in the fascial sheath and ischaemia. Reactivation of herpes simplex virus 1 and 2 or herpes zoster (even without herpetic eruption) often plays a role in the aetiopathogenesis of its development. It is often preceded by exposure to cold (polio e frigore), but the association is not clear. Furthermore, possible metabolic (diabetes mellitus), vascular (arterial hypertension) or fluid retention (pregnancy) factors are considered. Depending on the intensity and extent of the inflammation, there is either reversible nerve dysfunction with demyelination (neurapraxia) or, in more severe cases, partial or complete axonal lesion (axonotmesis). In the case of *infectious or postinfectious aetiology*, in addition to herpes zoster infection (responsible for about 15% of cases of peripheral lesions of *n. facialis,* with the possible occurrence of vesicular eruption in the region of the external auditory canal, tympanic

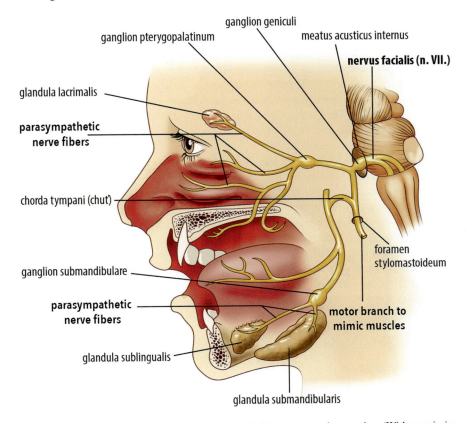

Fig. 14 *N. intermedius* efferent parasympathetic and afferent sensory innervation. (With permission of Grada Publishing a.s.)

membrane, auricle and palate in herpes zoster oticus (*Ramsay-Hunt syndrome*) with concomitant involvement of n. VIII and intense periauricular pain), Lyme disease could also apply (with possible history of tick attachment and presence of erythema migrans), Central European tick-borne encephalitis (again with possible history of tick attachment) or enteroviruses, as well as HIV and, rarely, TB, lues, diphtheria and leprosy [35].

Causes of *lesions in the canalis n. facialis* are most commonly pyramidal fractures (oblique fractures are more common, longitudinal fractures less common), acute and chronic mediootitis, mastoiditis, herpes zoster oticus (with herpetic eruption in the external auditory canal—in the Ramsay Hunt zone), cholesteatoma and Bell's palsy. Otogenic lesions with vertigo, otalgias, ear discharge, tympanic perforation, tinnitus, and hypospadias may accompany a lesion of n. VII in the labyrinthine segment of the *canalis n. facialis*.

The causes of facial lesions in the *foramen stylomastoideum* and in the section in the *glandula parotis* before the division of the nerve trunk into individual branches tend to be inflammations and tumours of the parotid, traumas of the facial skeleton and surgical interventions in this area. The causes of *lesions of the individual branches* of the *n. facialis* are again traumas and surgical interventions.

Among *tumours*, tumours of the cerebellopontine angle (schwannomas of the *n. vestibuli*, meningioma) and parotids, as well as diffuse tumour infiltration of the meninges (often leading to bilateral lesions of n. VII and, simultaneously, to lesions of other cranial nerves) are the most frequent. Primary and metastatic pontine tumours may lead to nuclear lesions of n. VII.

The causes of *bilateral lesion of n. VII*, also called *diplegia facialis*, are Guillain-Barré syndrome, sarcoidosis, Lyme disease, leukaemia, lymphomas, or pontine lesions; congenitally, it can occur in the context of Möbius syndrome with autosomal dominant inheritance and with sporadic occurrence (often simultaneously with ophthalmoplegia and other disorders of rhombencephalic development). In Melkersson-Rosenthal syndrome (multifocal granulomatous angiitis), recurrent and often bilateral lesions of n. VII occur simultaneously with swelling of the face (mainly lips, but also eyelids) and *lingua plicata*, but lesions of other cranial nerves, mononeuropathy, polyneuropathy and encephalomyelopathy may also be present. This syndrome may be genetic (mutations on chromosome 9) but can also occur in Crohn's disease and sarcoidosis [2, 7].

Risk factors

These correspond to individual aetiological causes.

Clinical presentation

The *central (supranuclear)* lesion of n. VII is characterised by preservation of motor skills in the upper part of the face (in severe central lesion, however, a slight paresis of *m. orbicularus oculi* may be present) and limitation of mimicry of the lower half of the face (especially of the perioral muscles). In a cortical lesion, isolated paresis of the mimic muscles may be present; in a subcortical lesion (e.g. in the *capsula interna*), it is usually accompanied by paresis of the limbs (on the same side). If the extrapyramidal structures providing emotional control of the mimic muscles via the reticular formation are preserved in a central (supranuclear) lesion, emotionally conditioned mimicry may be preserved, whereas free mimicry is impaired [35]. Conversely, lesions of the thalamus and mesencephalon may selectively affect the pathways providing emotional mimicry, while free mimicry remains preserved. Lesions of the *globus pallidus* and its projections are associated with partially preserved free mimicry and with bradykinesia of the mimic muscles (masked face).

In the *peripheral lesion*, there is complete paresis of the muscles in both branches (upper and lower) of n. VII.

In the case of a *nuclear lesion* in the pons, not only the motor nucleus of n. VII is affected (with ipsilateral paresis of the facial muscles in the region of both the upper and lower branches), but also *n. corticubulbaris* (with contralateral central paralysis of the muscles of the tongue) and *n. corticospinalis* (with contralateral central hemiparesis or hemiplegia). At the same time, the fibres and the nucleus of n. VI may be affected. In case of a lesion of the motor nucleus of n. VII, there is no

Neurological Disorders

impairment of lacrimal and salivary secretion, skin sensation, or taste (unless there is a concomitant lesion of the *ncl. tractus solitarii, ncl. salivatorius superior*, or sensory nucleus of n. V).

In the case of a lesion in the *cerebellopontine angle*, symptoms of a lesion of n. VIII or other structures are also present simultaneously, and because of the involvement of the fibres of *n. intermedius*, disturbances of taste on the anterior 2/3 of the tongue, lacrimal or salivary secretion and sensitivity in the innervation area of n. VII.

When the lesion is in the *canalis n. facialis* proximal to the ganglion geniculi, there are simultaneous disturbances of salivary and lacrimal secretion, hyperacusis with the absence of the stapedius reflex, disturbance of taste on the anterior 2/3 of the tongue, and usually symptoms of the lesion of n. VIII. When the lesion is in the tympanic segment, tear and salivary secretion is spared. With a lesion distal to the *n. stapedius*, hyperacusis is not present. With a lesion distal to the chorda tympani, there is no taste disturbance present.

When the lesion is in the region of the *foramen stylomastoideum* and in the section in the *glandula parotis* before the division of the nerve trunk into individual branches, there is a purely motor lesion with paralysis of the muscles of the midface. Lesions of the individual facial branches of the *n. facialis* lead to an isolated motor deficit in the respective innervation area.

In *Bell's palsy*, there is an acute development of symptoms, with an initial onset of retro- and periauricular pain (in about one-half of cases), followed by the development of paresis to plegia (at least transiently in up to 70% of cases) within hours to days [35]. Partial or complete spontaneous resolution occurs in 90% of cases. The prognosis is favourable—in the case of neurapraxia (60–80% of cases), spontaneous correction occurs within 6–8 weeks, while in axonotmesis the reinnervation process is slower, with improvement occurring between 3 and 12 months after the development of the problem and correction is never complete [35]. Residual paresis or, on the contrary, what is called postparalytic tonic or clonic spasm is often present; because of aberrant reinnervation, synkinesis or mass movements of the muscles of the whole half of the face during free or involuntary mimicry may occur. Age over 60 years, presence of diabetes mellitus, arterial hypertension, hyperacusis, and hypolacrymia (i.e. evidence of a more extensive lesion in the canal) are prognostically unfavourable factors. On the other hand, slow progression and rapid correction of the disability, especially incomplete paresis in the acute stage, are favourable prognostic factors.

The *irritative motor syndromes* include *hemispasm facialis* (with short tonic or tonic–clonic twitches, spontaneous or provoked by free contraction, stress, anxiety, fatigue or change of head position, lasting up to one minute, but possibly persisting even in sleep, initially localised usually periorbital, in the course of the disease spreading to the ipsilateral mimic muscles; simultaneous contraction of m. stapedius may lead to tinnitus and, with a prolonged course, mild paresis of the affected muscles may be present), *blepharospasm* (with bilateral synchronous contractions of the m. orbicularis oculi) and *facile myokymia* (irregular involuntary repetitive twitching of groups of muscle fibres and muscle fascicles, often spreading from one muscle to another). In the case of tics, these are rapid, stereotyped and at least partially coordinated twitches that may affect other muscle groups outside the face.

Postparalytic synkinesias are characterised by involuntary contractions of a muscle group when another group is freely activated, for example, involuntary mouth movements when the eyes are closed or vice versa in palpebral synkinesia.

"*Crocodile tears*" are characterised by unilateral lacrimation during eating [2].

Diagnosis

It is necessary to distinguish between central and peripheral lesion of n. VII and, in case of a peripheral lesion, to localise it topically depending on the above-mentioned differences in the clinical presentation.

Strabological methods

Examination of eyeball motility and oculomotor muscle function (Table 1), including Hess' screen.

Neuroimaging methods

Magnetic resonance imaging is the method of choice when a lesion is suspected in the region of the mastoid process, internal auditory canal, pontine canal or in intracranial hypertension syndrome. *Magnetic resonance angiography* is used to demonstrate compression of the nerve trunk by an aberrant vessel. In the case of lesions in the region of the *canalis n. facialis* and in traumatic lesions of the pyramid or cholesteatoma, *computed tomography* is preferable. X-ray of the pyramids is part of the ENT examination.

Electrophysiological methods

Electroencephalography can be used to diagnose Todd's postparoxysmal paresis of the facial mimic muscles or the epileptic origin of facial clonic twitches.

Electromyography and conduction studies are used to confirm peripheral lesions of the motor fibres of n. VII and to determine the degree and age of axonopathy.

Electrogustometry examination is used to differentiate the lesion of n. VII proximally and distally from the chorda tympani.

ENT examination

ENT examination, including otoneurological examination, is used to assess the presence of an n. VIII lesion and the otogenic aetiology of the problem.

Laboratory examination

Laboratory blood tests can help in the diagnosis of infection (blood count, serologic testing—e.g. for herpes viruses, Lyme disease, Central European tick-borne encephalitis, or enteroviruses), haemoblastosis (blood count), systemic autoimmune disease (autoantibody testing, sedimentation rate, rheumatologic factors), or diabetes mellitus (glycaemia, glycated haemoglobin, oral glucose tolerance test) [2, 7].

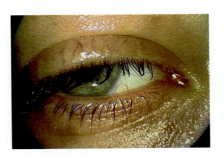

Fig. 15 Lagophthalmos in a patient with involvement of the seventh cranial nerve

Differential diagnosis

- Bell's palsy
- Diplegia facialis
- Irritative motor syndromes

Therapy

Treatment should be causal. Rehabilitation is the basis of treatment of lesion VII. Electrical stimulation can be used in the plegic muscles, but its application after the return of active mobility may lead to increased neuronal excitability and contribute to the development of post-paralytic hemifacial spasm. Short-term administration of oral corticosteroids—usually a high initial dose of prednisone (1 mg/kg) with gradual withdrawal over 7–10 days—is also considered. On the other hand, administration of antivirals (acyclovir and its derivatives) is considered controversial, even when a hypothetical mechanism of herpes virus reactivation is considered. Treatment is most effective when initiated within 3 days of the development of clinical symptoms, whereas it is no longer effective after 10 days. A very important therapeutic measure is to protect the cornea from the development of a defect or neurotrophic ulcer. The cornea is affected by both lagophthalmos (Fig. 15) and hypolacrimia (with simultaneous involvement of the n. petrosus superficialis major).

Artificial tears are applied and the cornea is covered with ointment and a bandage at night. In advanced conditions, a "wet chamber" or swimming goggles may be used. For prolonged and prognostically unfavourable conditions, surgery is performed—temporary or permanent tarsorrhaphy. The cornea can also be covered for 2–3 months by transient ptosis induced by local application of botulinum toxin to the m. levator palpebrae superioris.

The mainstay of therapy for *hemifacial spasm* is local administration of botulinum toxin to the affected muscles, which usually leads to significant functional improvement, but should be repeated at 3–6-month intervals. The efficacy of microvascular decompression, which is the method of choice in younger patients, is up to 90%, but may be complicated by lesions of n. VII or n. VIII. On the other hand, pharmacological treatment with anticonvulsants (carbamazepine, gabapentin, clonazepam) is not very effective [7].

8 Ocular Manifestations of Circulatory Disorders in the Carotid Circulation

The brain is one of the most energy-intensive organs of the human body. Although it occupies on average only 2% of the total body weight, it carries approximately 14% of the cardiac output and consumes approx. 20% of oxygen and up to 50% of glucose [13]. The brain is therefore dependent on a continuous supply of arterial blood. If the blood supply is completely interrupted, there is a loss of consciousness after only a few seconds and irreversible changes in the neurons after about 5 minutes. For this reason, the continuous blood flow through the brain is regulated at several levels, mainly by autoregulation based on the values of systemic blood pressure—when it increases, vasoconstriction of the cerebral arteries occurs and vice versa—then by metabolic regulation responding mainly to the values of partial pressure of CO_2—when it increases, vasodilation of the cerebral arteries occurs and vice versa. Another mechanism maintaining blood flow through the brain tissue are the two systems of arterial blood supply from the carotid and vertebrobasilar circulation, which are interconnected by the *Willis arterial circuit*.

Anatomy of the cerebral blood supply and relationship to the optic pathway

As mentioned above, the brain is supplied with arterial blood from two main systems, the carotid and vertebrobasilar. The *carotid system* supplies approximately 72% of the blood to the brain by way of the paired *a. carotis interna* (ACI), which arises bilaterally by bifurcation of the *a. carotis communis*. The ACI enters the intracranium through the *canalis caroticus*, and its first major intracranial branch is the *ophthalmic artery*, crucial to the visual system. This enters the orbit together with the optic nerve through the *canalis opticus* and completely nourishes the tissues of the orbit, then part of the ethmoid sinuses and facial tissues of the periocular area, where it anastomoses with branches from the *a. carotis externa*. *A. ophthalmica* after leaving the ACI, gives off another branch *a. choroidea anterior* and then branches terminally to the *a. cerebri anterior* and *a. cerebri media*, usually giving off yet another branch *a. communicans posterior* connecting the carotid and vertebrobasilar systems to the *Circle of Willis*. The *vertebrobasilar system* is formed by the paired *a. vertebralis*, which, after diverging from *a. subclavia*, passes upward through the transverse processes of the cervical vertebrae and enters intracranially through the *foramen magnum*. At the base of the skull, the two vertebral arteries then join to form the unpaired *a. basilaris*, and together in their course give off numerous branches to the brainstem, inner ear, and cerebellum, and terminate as the terminal paired *a. cerebri posterior*, which supplies blood to the medial part of the temporal and occipital lobes, including the visual cortex.

From the above anatomical overview of the blood supply to the brain, the blood supply to the optic pathway follows. The anterior portion of the visual pathway from the retina to the *corpus geniculatum laterale* is supplied with blood predominantly from the carotid circulation, while the posterior portion with the *radiatio optica* and visual cortex is supplied with blood predominantly from the vertebrobasilar

Neurological Disorders

circulation. In its central part (*tractus opticus, corpus geniculatum laterale* and anterior part of *radiatio optica*) both systems overlap considerably and the supply to the visual pathway is variable here [43]). This anatomical arrangement results in specific ophthalmic manifestations of circulatory disturbances in the different tracts (Fig. 16).

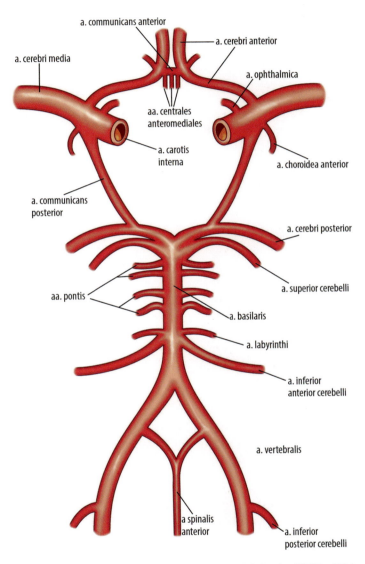

Fig. 16 Diagram of the blood supply to the brain and the arterial circuit of Willis. (With permission of Grada Publishing a.s.)

Circulatory disturbances in the carotid sinus manifest in the proximal parts of the visual pathway. When the blood supply from the retina to the optic nerve is disturbed (before the optic nerve fibres cross in the chiasm), the clinical manifestation of the lesion is always unilateral and monocular. If the interruption of blood flow affects the optic pathway from the *chiasma opticum* dorsally, the manifestation tends to be bilateral and produces typical perimetric images according to the actual arrangement of the axons of the optic pathway at the site of its involvement.

The most clinically significant manifestations of carotid circulatory disorders include:

- Amaurosis fugax
- Ocular ischaemic syndrome
- Occlusion of the arteria centralis retinae
- Anterior ischaemic optic neuropathy—AION.

Risk factors

All the above-mentioned disorders are caused by impaired blood supply to the eye, so their risk factors are virtually identical.

- Atherosclerosis
- Arterial hypertension
- Smoking
- Obesity
- Hyperlipidaemia
- Diabetes mellitus
- Older age
- Autoimmune vascular disorders (arteritis temporalis, Takayasu's arteritis).

8.1 Amaurosis Fugax

Amaurosis fugax (AF) is a transient visual impairment of various kinds, ranging from greying of the image to complete blindness of the eye. In this case, reversible vision loss is caused by a transient deterioration of the blood supply to the retina, choroid or optic nerve—a *form of transient ischaemic attack (TIA)*. Retrospective studies show that amaurosis fugax is the first clinical manifestation of significant ACI stenosis (more than 70%) in approximately 20–30% of cases and therefore an early sign of impending ictus in its basin [34]. The aetiology is most often thromboembolic from the carotid artery on the affected side; more rarely, emboli may originate from the heart in atrial fibrillation or calcification of the heart valves. Another possible cause is transient vasospasms, most often at the level of the *a. ophtalmica* or *a. centralis retinae* (retinal migraine). It is always necessary to bear in mind the autoimmune involvement of the cranial vessels—temporal arteritis.

Clinical presentation

The patient is brought to the ophthalmologist by a transient deterioration of vision. In most cases, it manifests unilaterally, but it is also possible to have bilateral difficulties represented by *homonymous hemianopsia* on the perimeter, in the case of vertebrobasilar involvement. The duration is most often seconds to minutes, but rarely the visual disturbance may last for several hours. The frequency of occurrence of the disorder is individually variable, ranging from a single attack over a prolonged period to several attacks per day. The typical feature of this affection is full reversibility of vision, i.e. after the difficulties subside, vision gradually returns to its previous state.

Objective findings

In the most common or embolisation aetiology of AF, sclerotic involvement of retinal vessels of varying degrees is seen on examination of the ocular background, and sometimes microembolism can be seen in the retinal arteries, most commonly at their junction, on ophthalmoscopy. However, the ocular findings may also be completely physiological, especially in younger individuals.

Diagnosis

Diagnosis is based on a detailed anamnesis of the disorder (frequency, laterality, triggering factor, duration, general disease), and a complete ophthalmic examination including slit-lamp fundus examination and ideally a visual field examination is always necessary. If amaurosis fugax is suspected, the ophthalmologist will indicate imaging studies—screening ultrasonography (USG) of the carotid arteries, possibly more complex CT angiography or MR angiography of the cerebral arteries. In indicated cases, USG examination of the heart should be considered to exclude cardioembolisation aetiology; when temporal arteritis is suspected, the anamnesis and clinical presentation should be considered, and blood draws with erythrocyte sedimentation rate and CRP should be performed.

Differential diagnosis

- Migraine with ocular aura
- Retinal migraine
- Obnubilations lasting a few seconds in the case of optic disc oedema
- Uhthoff's phenomenon (transient visual impairment with an increase in body temperature in patients with a history of optic neuritis).

Therapy

Any causal management of cardiovascular affection falls to the appropriate specialists (e.g. carotid endarterectomy in symptomatic significant ACI stenosis is the responsibility of a neurosurgeon or vascular surgeon). In temporal arteritis, high-dose corticosteroid therapy in collaboration with rheumatologists is initiated.

The prognosis is uncertain. Although the transient visual impairment itself is reversible, patients with significant carotid atherosclerosis are at high risk of vascular

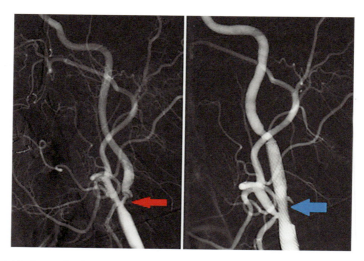

Fig. 17 Critical stenosis of the ACI. In the image on the left, digital subtraction angiography shows a marked narrowing of the ACI lumen at the point of its separation from the a. carotis communis (red arrow). On the right, the same site is improvement by a stent inserted by the interventional radiologist (blue arrow) with flow improvement of the ACI bloodstream

occlusions, either at the level of the eye or other organs, and therefore a history of AF always deserves attention (Fig. 17).

8.2 Ocular Ischaemic Syndrome

Ocular ischaemic syndrome (OIS) is a rare set of symptoms in the anterior and posterior segments of the eye, arising from chronic ischaemia of the ocular tissues, most commonly with marked atherosclerotic stenosis of the ACI, more rarely with involvement of a. ophtalmica. Epidemiologically, it occurs most often in patients over 65 years of age with a history of several cardiovascular risk factors mentioned above. Ocular ischaemic syndrome occurs only in critical ACI stenosis, when most patients have lumen narrowing greater than 90%, and complete closure of the same-sided ACI is not rare [50]. Among other rarer causes, OIS can occur in a carotid dissection or as a symptom of autoimmune vascular involvement (arteritis temporalis, Takayasu's arteritis).

Clinical presentation

Patients are most often referred to an ophthalmologist for OIS due to visual impairment or eye pain. Visual deterioration can be either acute (amaurosis fugax, anterior ischemic optic neuropathy, retinal vessel occlusion) or gradual, due to the development of cataract, secondary glaucoma, or macular oedema. Eye pain arises based on

Neurological Disorders

chronic ischaemia of ocular tissues or as a result of elevation of intraocular pressure in secondary glaucoma.

Objective findings

Approximately 2/3 of patients on slit-lamp examination show iris rubeosis and neovascularisation in the anterior segment of the eye, possibly signs of chronic anterior uveitis with cells in the anterior chamber and posterior synechiae of the iris and lens. Neovascularisation in the ventricular angle region often results in elevation of intraocular pressure and the development of secondary glaucoma. If cataract is present, it tends to be more pronounced on the affected side. On the posterior segment of the eye, sclerotic involvement of the retinal vessels is found. In 80% of patients, intraretinal haemorrhages and microaneurysms are present in the central periphery of the retina; with more pronounced ischaemia, neovascularisation of the optic nerve head and retina, macular oedema, cotton wool spots or intravitreal haemorrhages may develop.

Diagnosis

Diagnosis is based on local and general findings. Fluorescence retinal angiography is the most useful ophthalmologic diagnostic modality, with a typically prolonged interval between contrast agent injection and its appearance in the retinal vasculature. OCT examination of the macula is also useful for the diagnosis of macular oedema. Of the general examinations, the most important is the carotid examination (USG, CT AG, MRI AG); a general cardiovascular examination by an internist is also worth considering.

Differential diagnosis

- Diabetic retinopathy
- Central retinal vein occlusion

Therapy

Systemic therapy consists of compensation of the underlying internal diseases and carotid endarterectomy, indicated by the appropriate specialist based on imaging findings. In the early stages of OIS, the recanalisation of the narrowed *a. carotis* may lead to partial or complete regression of the ocular findings.

Ocular therapy focuses on minimising the consequences of secondary damage to the eye by neovascularisation. Chronic ocular ischaemia leads to increased production of VEGF (vascular endothelial growth factor), resulting in intraocular growth of newly formed blood vessels. In the anterior segment, this results in iris rubeosis and neovascularisation in the anterior chamber angle, while in the posterior segment, it results in newly formed vessels in the papilla and eventually in the retina. To reduce the oxygen demand in the eye, panretinal laser photocoagulation is the method of first choice, which reduces the overall blood supply to the eye by destroying the peripheral portion of the retinal pigment epithelium. In advanced findings with neovascularisation in the ventricular angle, this therapy is usually inadequate and the prognosis of the affected eyes aside from the visualisation is poor. To alleviate the consequences of secondary glaucoma, cyclo-destructive procedures to reduce the production of intraocular fluid or filtration surgery using drainage implants to improve its circulation are considered. Intravitreal application of depot corticosteroids and anti-VEGF agents are in the clinical trials' stage [50]. As a last resort, if the eye is already blind, evisceration or enucleation may be considered.

8.3 Central Retinal Artery Occlusion

Arteria centralis retinae (ACR) is a branch of *a. ophtalmica* that enters the optic nerve just posterior to the eyeball and enters intraocularly at the optic nerve target, where it immediately divides into superior and inferior branches and then into temporal and nasal branches for each retinal quadrant. The ACR supplies blood to the inner part of the retina, while the outer part, including the pigment epithelium, is supplied with blood from the choroid. It is a terminal artery, i.e. without collateral circulation.

The pathophysiologic basis of ACR occlusion is most often embolism of platelet and cholesterol thrombi from the ACI basin, and more rarely calcium thrombi from the calcified aortic valve. Again, the possible autoimmune aetiology of vascular occlusion in temporal arteritis must be kept in mind.

Clinical presentation

Central retinal artery occlusion is a serious ocular pathology, manifested by sudden and painless loss of vision in the affected eye, which (unlike TIA) is usually permanent. Sometimes a history is found of previous episodes of amaurosis fugax.

Objective findings

On the anterior segment, the finding is mostly without pathology, an afferent pupillary defect is usually present. On the eye fundus examination, pale ischaemic oedema is found in the basin of occluded arteries; sometimes emboli in the retinal arteries are visible, segmentation of the blood column in the vessels may be present. In ACR trunk occlusion, the entire retina is pale with a whitish tinge, contrasting with a cherry-red glowing foveola. This phenomenon is due to the anatomical structure of the retina in the foveola region, where the retina is very thin and the preserved choroidal vascular supply shines through. The extent of ischaemia depends on the localisation of the vascular occlusion—in the case of ACR trunk occlusion, the entire retina is ischaemic, but hemiretinal ischaemia is also possible when the embolus is localised in the upper or lower branch of the ACR, or local ischaemia in individual quadrants. An anatomical variant that can preserve good central vision even with ACR trunk occlusion is the presence of *a. cilioretinalis*. This is an aberrant branch present in about one-third to one-half of the population, arising from the course of the posterior ciliary arteries and usually supplying blood to the macula, including the

Neurological Disorders

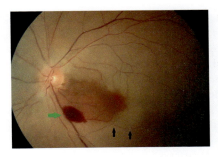

Fig. 18 Photo of the fundus of the left eye in a patient with ACR occlusion. The image clearly shows the pale ischemic oedema of the entire retina except for the central area, where the blood supply is preserved due to the presence of a. cilioretinalis. Furthermore, white emboli can be seen in the inferior temporal quadrant artery (black arrows) and preretinal haemorrhage at the inferior temporal arcade (green arrow)

maculopapillary bundle. Thus, with its presence and sufficient blood flow, the central vision of the affected eye may remains virtually intact even with ACR occlusion (Fig. 18).

Diagnosis

Slit-lamp ophthalmic examination is usually sufficient to establish the diagnosis of ACR occlusion; additional examinations include OCT of the macula to verify ischaemic oedema of the inner layers of the retina or fluorescence angiography to demonstrate non-perfusion of the affected arteries. From an overall perspective, a thorough cardiovascular examination (including sonographic examination of the carotid arteries and heart) is important to exclude the source of embolisation. In younger patients without the presence of cardiovascular risks, it is necessary to search further for a procoagulant state.

Differential diagnosis

- Amaurosis fugax
- Ocular ischaemic syndrome
- AION

Therapy

There is no single recommended procedure for ACR occlusion. None of the methods used has been shown to be significantly effective in terms of preserving vision in controlled studies [52]. Time since symptom onset is crucial in deciding whether and how to treat ACR occlusion. A time window of up to 4 hours is ideal for therapy; 24 hours from the onset of difficulty is considered an extreme time to indicate therapy. The standard therapy is to induce vasodilation with the expectation of displacing the embolus distally in the retinal artery, combined with efforts to reduce intraocular pressure, as intraocular pressure increases resistance in the retinal vasculature.

Vasodilatation is achieved by isosorbide dinitrate applied sublingually or pentoxyphylline intravenously; acetazolamide or mannitol intravenously is used to acutely reduce intraocular pressure, and attempts are made to improve perfusion eye pressure by bulb massage and surgically by paracentesis of the anterior chamber with the removal of a small amount of ventricular fluid. Invasive therapy consists of systemic intra-arterial administration of tissue plasminogen activator (tPA) to dissolve the thrombus and restore blood supply. However, even this method does not statistically significantly improve the resulting visual acuity compared to the standard approach, and it can often be complicated by serious overall adverse effects. Thus, the prognosis regarding the final visual outcome is unfavourable for ACR trunk occlusion.

8.4 Ischaemic Optic Neuropathy

The anterior part of the optic nerve is supplied with blood by sector from *aa. ciliares posteriores*; further along, the optic nerve is supplied by small branches from the basin of *a. ophtalmica*. Ischaemic optic neuropathy consists of interruption of the arterial supply to the optic nerve in its anterior part (AION—anterior ischaemic optic neuropathy) or, rarely, in its further course (PION—posterior ischaemic optic neuropathy). The clinical manifestation is usually a painless sudden loss of vision in one eye, which is most often detected in the morning after waking up.

Risk factors

These correspond to general risk factors for vascular diseases, but here it is particularly relevant to highlight the possible autoimmune aetiology in temporal arteritis. Anterior ischaemic optic neuropathy is one of the most common clinical manifestations of this autoimmune disease. Ischaemic optic neuropathy occurs in two main forms, namely *arteritic (aAION)* and *nonarteritic (nAION)*. This division is important in terms of pathophysiology, diagnosis and subsequent therapy. The significantly more common nAION usually occurs in patients over 50 years of age with the presence of cardiovascular risk factors. The main aetiological factor in its occurrence is most likely transient nocturnal hypotension which, in the terrain of pre-existing impaired blood supply to the optic nerve head, causes its temporary ischaemia with subsequent oedema and subsequent necrosis of nerve fibres. By contrast, in aAION, the cause of vessel occlusion is an ongoing autoimmune inflammation of its wall.

Clinical presentation

The typical patient with AION presents in the morning with the information that he/she has not been seeing well in the eye since morning, sometimes indicating loss of half (upper or lower) of the visual field. In aAION, other signs of ongoing temporal arteritis are usually present, i.e. temporal pain, claudication on chewing or swallowing, subfebrile, weight loss, loss of motivation, mood changes, etc.

Fig. 19
Sixty-seven-year-old man with nonarteritic anterior ischemic optic neuropathy showing optic nerve oedema in the affected eye with typical flame haemorrhage

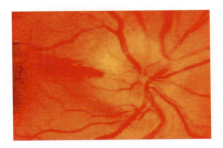

Objective findings

In both forms of AION, we usually find a relative afferent pupillary defect, with a pale ischaemic oedema of the optic nerve head on the eye fundus examination, often accompanied by flamed haemorrhages in the vicinity of the oedema (Fig. 19).

Perimetric examination of the visual field is crucial, where most often altitudinal arcuate scotomas are seen, that in most cases do not exceed the horizontal line, consistent with the vascular supply to the optic nerve disc.

Diagnosis

The diagnosis is made based on anamnesis, clinical presentation and perimeter examination (Fig. 20).

OCT measurement of the optic nerve fibre layer (RNFL) is appropriate to objectify and further monitor the development of oedema. To exclude arteritis temporalis, in which there is a risk of early involvement of the other eye, erythrocyte sedimentation rate and CRP values must always be examined in patients with AION.

Differential diagnosis

- Optic neuritis
- ACR occlusion

Therapy

In the case of aAION or temporal arteritis, it is necessary to initiate therapy with high doses of corticosteroids as early as possible, followed by gradual and careful dose reduction while controlling inflammatory parameters, especially erythrocyte sedimentation rate and CRP values. The treatment of temporal arteritis is shared between the ophthalmologist and the clinical rheumatologist or clinical pharmacologist, and it is not uncommon to leave patients on treatment for several years. By contrast, the treatment of non-arteritic AION does not have clear recommendations based on sufficient evidence-based studies and is to some extent individual to the patient, but also to the department. In the case of nAION with a shorter time history within hours to days of the development of complaints, short-term infusion therapy with corticosteroids is usually appropriate at a lower dose than in the treatment of aAION. In this case, a corticosteroid is used for its anti-oedema effect. A reduction

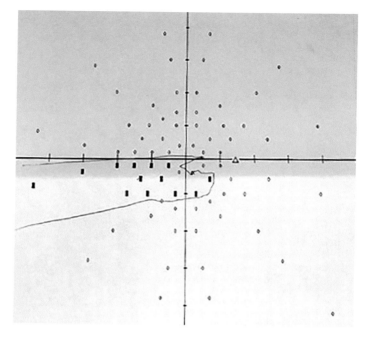

Fig. 20 On perimetric examination in the visual field, the upper or lower quadrants are typically affected in anterior ischaemic optic neuropathy and the visual field defect is usually sharply demarcated by the horizontal line—the so-called altitudinal visual field defect, shown here as an example of an incompletely developed inferior altitudinal visual field defect

in TZN swelling is attempted to be achieved, to improve the flow parameters in the affected area, thus preventing further ischaemia of the disc. Some departments opt for vasodilator therapy in a possible combination with steroids.

The prognosis is not good, aside from the improvement of the already lost part of vision or visual acuity and the affected part of the visual field, so the main goal is to prevent further ischaemic involvement of the nerve fibres of the optic nerve.

9 Circulatory Disorders in the Vertebrobasilar System

The vertebrobasilar circulation supplies blood to the entire brainstem, cerebellum, and occipital part of the cerebral cortex. Thus, the ocular manifestations of blood supply disturbances correspond to the involvement of important structures in this region. The nuclei of all the oculomotor nerves are in the brainstem, and the cortical visual centre is in the occipital lobe. However, the brainstem also contains several other vital nuclei and centres, and many nerve pathways pass through it. Therefore, in addition to ocular symptoms, blood supply disturbances are accompanied by typical

Neurological Disorders 421

general symptoms, which can be life-threatening in extreme cases. Early diagnosis of circulatory insufficiency is therefore very important, as with carotid disorders, for the overall prognosis of the patient. *Atherosclerosis* (most often thrombosis of atherosclerotic plaques) or embolism from a more proximal segment of the artery or heart (e.g. in atrial fibrillation) is the aetiology of ischaemia in the vertebrobasilar basin; other possible causes are rather rare (arterial dissection, vasospasm, coagulopathy) [37].

Risk factors

The risk factors correspond to the general risks of atherosclerosis already mentioned in the previous chapter.

Clinical presentation and objective findings

Ischaemic disorders of the vertebrobasilar circulation should be divided into two categories in terms of clinical manifestation and prognosis: *transient* (vertebrobasilar insufficiency) and *permanent* (ictus in the vertebrobasilar basin).

9.1 Vertebrobasilar Insufficiency

This is a transient and reversible disturbance of the blood supply in this area (essentially analogous to amaurosis fugax occurring in circulatory disorders of the carotid basin). In this case, however, the spectrum of clinical signs is much more varied, given the number of important nuclei and pathways occurring mainly in the brainstem [37, 45]. Episodes of difficulty usually last from tens of seconds to several minutes, and may be triggered, for example, by orthostatic hypotension or head tilt, when flow through vertebral arteries is further impaired in a pre-existing atherosclerotic terrain. The main ocular symptoms of vertebrobasilar insufficiency (VBI) include transient diplopia resulting from impaired blood supply to the nuclei of the oculocranial nerves in the brainstem, often accompanied by attacks of nystagmus and anisocoria. In addition, intermittent bilateral sudden visual deterioration is typical, usually of the character of homonymous hemianopsia or quadrantopsia. However, the ocular symptoms of VBI are accompanied by various systemic nervous disorders (nausea, vomiting, vertigo, limb paresthaesias and hemiparesis, cephalea, dysarthria, disturbances of consciousness), which are typical for the diagnosis of VBI, and their depth, frequency and specific manifestation correspond to the exact localisation of ischaemia and its severity [37].

9.2 Vertebrobasilar Ictus

From the ophthalmologist's point of view, a persistent disturbance of the blood supply to the hindbrain circulation manifests itself mainly as a visual field defect. These defects are typically of the character of homonymous contralateral hemianopsia, whether complete or partial, but always congruent (bilaterally symmetrical) and usually with sparing of the macular area. These attacks arise suddenly and may or may not be accompanied by the other brainstem symptomatology mentioned in the previous paragraph. The patient is not always aware of these visual field defects, sometimes reports impaired orientation in space with bumping into objects on the side of the defect, and often mislocalises the visual disturbance monocularly to the side of the defect in the visual field (e.g. in right-sided hemianopsia, the patient reports sudden visual impairment in the right eye). The overall clinical presentation is highly variable, depending on the localisation of the vascular occlusion. When the brainstem is involved, it is dramatic to fatal, but incidental findings of visual field disruptions indicative of vertebrobasilar ictus during perimetry for other indications are also possible. In case of involvement of the peripheral nerve nuclei, the symptoms may include transient and permanent paralytic strabismus accompanied by diplopia with manifestation, depending on the involvement of specific peripheral nerves. The visual field disturbances, as well as any oculomotor disorder, may regress at least partially over the next few months.

Diagnosis

In both above-mentioned forms of the disease, the diagnosis consists primarily of the correct evaluation of clinical symptoms, for which the patient is most often examined by a neurologist with a consultant ophthalmologist. The next step is the indication of an imaging of the vertebrobasilar vascular system. Because of the location of this vessel, it is almost impossible to assess blood flow sonographically; therefore, imaging methods with contrast agent imaging of the vessels, such as digital subtraction angiography (DSA), CT angiography, and MRI angiography, are at the forefront here (Fig. 21).

Differential diagnosis

Other possible causes of compression of the structures of the posterior cranial fossa to be considered:

- Tumours
- Aneurysms
- Cysts
- Demyelinating brainstem involvement in multiple sclerosis

Therapy

Primarily consists of a systemic approach and minimisation of risk factors; in the case of critical stenosis or even occlusion of arteries, surgical or endovascular therapeutic procedures to occlude or bypass the affected arteries may be considered. Local or systemic intravascular thrombolysis with tPA is another therapeutic option with a short history of disease manifestation. The prognosis of patients varies according to the localisation, severity, and duration of involvement. With early detection, the resulting neurological deficit may be minimal to none, whereas with severe occlusion of a. basilaris, the course is often fatal.

Neurological Disorders

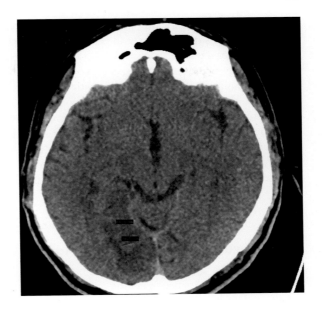

Fig. 21 Native CT of the brain showing a hypodense lesion in the right occipital lobe consistent with subacute ischaemia in the basin of the right a. cerebri posterior

10 Myasthenia Gravis

The disease is characterised by pathological progressive fatigue of the striated muscles. The cause is a block of nerve impulse transmission at the site of the neuromuscular junction, i.e. at the myoneural disc. Ocular symptoms are almost always part of the clinical presentation and, in at least one-half of cases, they are also the initial symptoms. In addition to the typical myasthenic eye and eyelid movement disorders, which are usually easy to diagnose, there are sometimes diagnostically difficult findings.

According to the **aetiopathogenesis**, myasthenia gravis (MG) is currently classified as an autoimmune disease [24]. The transmission of irritation from nerve to muscle, mediated by acetylcholine, is disrupted by antibodies probably produced in thymus cells. Myasthenic syndromes or symptomatic myasthenia are also characterised by pathological muscle fatigue, but their pathogenesis is different.

Ocular symptoms are manifested mainly as ptosis of the upper eyelid, oculomotor disorders with accompanying diplopia and insufficient closure of the palpebral fissure with possible lagophthalmos. Myasthenic ptosis is the most common and usually the first ocular symptom. It can be unilateral, bilateral and alternating, laterally symmetric or asymmetric, partial or total, often isolated at first, later usually associated with an oculomotor disorder. The basic feature of myasthenic ptosis is the variability of the function of the left upper eyelid and the position of the eyelid during the day, but also from day to day, and its dependence mainly on muscular load. Myasthenic paralysis of the eye muscles is also characterised by a variety of pictures, from paralysis of a single muscle in one eye, through various combinations that do not respect innervation patterns, to bilateral total external ophthalmoplegia [24]. Such images may mimic both peripheral and supranuclear palsies. Any atypical oculomotor disorder or combination of palsies should raise suspicion of MG. In all these cases, normal photoreactions and accommodation, typical of MG, are extremely important differential diagnostic features. In practice, paresis of the *m. orbicularis oculi* innervated by the 7th cranial nerve may be overlooked, as there is no major lagophthalmos during ptosis. However, the combination of both symptoms, in which the patient can neither open nor close the palpebral fissure properly, is typical of MG and diagnostically important. Sometimes the sphincter laxity is manifested by lower eyelid ectropion, which is accentuated towards evening ('afternoon ectropion'). Artificial tears and treatment of the underlying disease are used in therapy.

11 Subacute Sclerosing Panencephalitis

Subacute sclerosing panencephalitis (SSPE, van Bogaert, Dawson) is a very rare chronic and progressive neurodegenerative disease caused by measles virus. It typically begins approximately 7–10 years after a classic measles virus infection. Accompanying manifestations are usually behavioural changes and cognitive impairment, the disease progresses to the development of epileptic seizures, with various movement disorders and then decerebral rigidity. In the final stage of the disease, the patient is usually in a vegetative state and subsequently dies. The pathophysiological basis of the disease is direct destruction of neurons by measles virus [30]. The decline in measles vaccination rates (below 95%) has led to a loss of collective immunity and the spread of measles virus [7].

Aetiology

The pathophysiological basis of SSPE is the direct destruction of neurons by a modified measles virus that persists in the brain. This virus has a modified genome and is unable to replicate in tissue culture [7].

Epidemiology

Measles virus, which is widespread worldwide, belongs to the paramyxovirus group. The infection is spread by droplets, with maximum infectivity during the prodromal stages of the disease [7].

Risk factors

The development of SSPE occurs after measles virus infection, but the risk factors for its development are unknown.

Clinical presentation and objective findings

The development of symptoms of measles virus infection occurs after a 10-day incubation period, when fever and upper respiratory tract and conjunctival catarrh

Neurological Disorders

appear. On Day 12, white efflorescence appears on the buccal mucosa at the level of the molars (called Koplik's spots) and on Day 14, maculopapular exanthema spreads from the face to the lower limbs. The main complications of the disease are respiratory (primary viral and bacterial pneumonia) and neurological. These include *early encephalitis* in acute *disseminated encephalomyelitis (ADEM)*, then *measles inclusion body encephalitis (MIBE)* and finally *SSPE* [15].

The development of parainfectious ADEM occurs concomitantly with exanthem eruption up to 1 month (but on average 1 week) thereafter. It is a hyperergic immunopathologic reaction, occurring in an immunocompetent terrain in which diffuse involvement with cerebral oedema occurs. Clinical symptoms include paresis and disturbances of consciousness (up to coma); mortality is 5–15% [15].

The development of measles MIBE occurs 1–9 months after the development of exanthema, in immunocompromised patients who are unable to eliminate the virus. The course may be afebrile, and neurological symptoms include convulsions, development of dementia and disturbances of consciousness. Death occurs after several weeks.

The development of SSPE occurs months, but up to 7–10 years, after measles virus infection. This chronic encephalitis lasts from months to several years and affects children and younger individuals (mostly aged 2–20 years but can occur later) [15]. Unlike MIBE, the immune response is intense in SSPE. Character changes occur, mental deterioration with cognitive deterioration, myoclonia, epileptic seizures, abnormal postures, and movements. Patients die in a coma with decerebral rigidity, usually within months of the development of the first clinical signs of the disease.

Ocular manifestation is described in approximately 50% of patients and can sometimes precede the development of neurological symptoms and is thus the first sign of the disease [15]. Typical ocular symptoms are necrotising retinitis and optic nerve disc changes (edema, atrophy), and more rarely cortical blindness and other neuro-ophthalmological manifestations.

Necrotising retinitis is by far the most common ocular manifestation of SSPE [5]. The patient is usually referred to an ophthalmologist with a deterioration of visual acuity in one or both eyes. In the early stages, grey-whitish foci are found in the macula, which usually progress to necrosis of the retinal layers, including the RPE, and in some cases choroidal destruction. The foci may subsequently enlarge from the centre to the periphery, and may be associated with intraretinal haemorrhages, retinal oedema or vascular occlusions. Visual acuity tends to be impaired to varying degrees, according to the actual retinal involvement in the fovea to practical blindness. Retinitis in SSPE is characterised by quiescent findings in the vitreous and retinal vessels. Optic disc (OD) changes vary according to the stage and activity of the disease. On initial examination, there may be bilateral OD oedema with a picture of an optic disc oedema, but partial or complete OD atrophy or physiological findings are also possible [7].

Diagnosis

In the case of MIBE, specific antibodies may be detected in the serum and lymph, but only during clinical symptoms. Moreover, the changes in the lymph may be very small. EEG findings are abnormal but non-diagnostic, and CT and MRI brain findings are usually non-specific. A definitive diagnosis is only made by brain tissue biopsy (histological examination and PCR).

The diagnosis of SSPE is based on the finding of elevated levels of measles virus antibodies in the cerebrospinal fluid together with the neurological clinical presentation. Other investigations typically include electroencephalography, possibly accompanied by brain tissue biopsy or special examination of the virus genome [15]. Findings on CT or MRI of the brain tend to be non-specific and are more likely to exclude other diagnoses.

Ocular diagnosis consists of clinical examination, OCT of the macula and optic nerve and FAG of the retinal vessels. To exclude other viral retinitis, a vitreous sample from the affected eye and subsequent PCR examination may be considered. However, the clinical findings are relatively non-specific and, due to the rarity of SSPE in our setting, it is difficult to correctly classify the disease in the absence of neurological signs [7].

Differential diagnosis

Neurological

- Creutzfeldt-Jakob disease
- Other viral encephalitides
- Neurometabolic encephalopathies

Ocular

- Other viral retinitis (especially cytomegalovirus, varicella zoster and herpes simplex virus)

Therapy

In advanced disease, only symptomatic (antiepileptic drugs, antivirals in general, interferon alpha intrathecally); therefore, causal therapy is only consistent immunisation of the population with measles vaccine, which has led to the near eradication of SSPE in developed countries. Most patients die within months of the first clinical signs of the disease.

12 Phacomatoses

The term *phacomatoses* have been used since 1932 and was introduced into the literature by van der Hoeve [51]. Currently, the term *familial tumour syndromes affecting the nervous system* is also used for these *autosomal dominantly inherited neurocutaneous syndromes*. This is a group of genetically determined systemic diseases that share a common developmental mechanism. Pathological genes have high penetrance and distinct clinical variability in expression. In clinical manifestation, they are associated with the presence of neurological and cutaneous symptoms, and in

Neurological Disorders

embryonic development with abnormalities in the function and/or structure of cells formed synchronously from the neuroectodermal embryonic sheet, usually with a tendency to tumourigenesis. This includes a range of diseases, with ocular involvement occurring in *neurofibromatosis 1*, *neurofibromatosis 2* and *Von Hippel-Lindau disease* [7].

12.1 Neurofibromatosis (Recklinghausen's Disease)

The disease was first described by Von Recklinghausen in 1882 as a genetic disease with ectoderm abnormalities with a clinical manifestation of systemic progressive involvement, most commonly affecting the skin, nervous system, bones, eyes, and possibly other organs [3, 4]. Especially during the 1980s, changes in the classification of this disease occurred and, in Carey et al. [11] classified neurofibromatoses (NF) into 5 types (NF 1–5) according to clinical manifestations and genetics [11]. NF1 is clearly the most common type, comprising more than 90% of NF cases, also referred to as common or peripheral. The other four of the NF group are rare diseases, of which we mention NF2, which also has ocular involvement.

Aetiology

Both NF1 and NF2 are caused by mutations in genes that have a tumour suppressor effect in their intact form. Disruption of their function leads to increased cell growth and tumour development. In the case of NF1, the gene is located on the long arm of chromosome 17 (17q11.2). The pathological gene has almost 100% penetrance. The gene product neurofibromin is responsible for the development of the disease and experiments have shown that it plays an important role in the final differentiation of nervous and connective tissue and in the maturation of the central nervous system (CNS).

In the case of NF2, the gene is localised on the long arm of chromosome 22 (22q12) and its protein product is schwannomin (merlin).

Both NF1 and NF2 are among the diseases with the highest number of fresh mutations, with more than 50% of reported cases being sporadic.

Epidemiology

The worldwide prevalence of NF1 is estimated to be 1:2,000 to 1:3,500; NF2 is 10 times rarer [7].

Risk factors

In 50% of patients with both NF1 and NF2, the underlying genetic disability is familial (50% of cases are due to a new mutation) [12, 46]. In NF1, there is a history of tumours. NF1 progresses during periods of hormonal changes (puberty and pregnancy) [8].

Clinical presentation

The common clinical manifestations of NF are the presence of white coffee-coloured skin pigment spots ('cafe au lait') (Fig. 22), neurofibromas (Figs. 23, 24) and schwannomas and specific nodules (hamartomas) on the iris (Lisch nodules, Fig. 25) [10].

NF1 has considerable phenotypic variability. There are cafe au lait spots of larger size (at least 5 mm), multiple small pigmented spots (freckles) in the axillary and inguinal regions, skin and subcutaneous neurofibromas (these may be circumscribed, soft or hard, and sensitive to touch; a dimple may persist when pressed with a finger; plexiform neurofibromas, on the other hand, are not well demarcated, are larger and often lead to enlargement of the affected body part); patients may report itching of the skin, bone changes (including sphenoid dysplasia, scoliosis, deformities of the thoracic joints—especially the knee joints) and Lisch nodules are also present [27]. Mental subnormality is common, as are behavioural and learning disorders in

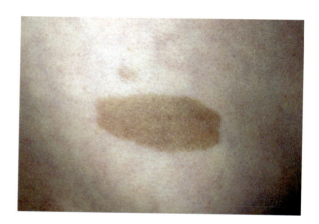

Fig. 22 Typical "cafe au lait" stain on the skin of a patient with neurofibromatosis

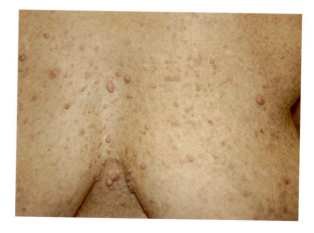

Fig. 23 Small neurofibromas on the chest of a patient with neurofibromatosis

Neurological Disorders

Fig. 24 Neurofibroma in the area behind the right ear in a young patient with Recklinghausen's disease

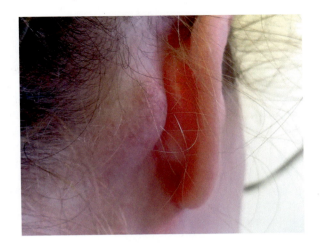

Fig. 25 Lisch nodules of the iris in a 21-year-old female patient with Recklinghausen's neurofibromatosis

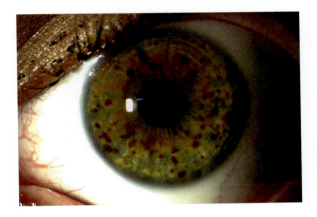

childhood, and precocious or delayed onset of puberty may occur. In terms of psychiatric illnesses, 20% of NF1 patients suffer from dysthymia and 7% from depression, and they also have increased suicidal tendencies [26]. Plexiform neurofibromas can lead to organ dysfunction. In childhood, macrocrania and macrocephaly tend to be evident.

Among the ocular manifestations of NF1, plexiform neurofibromas affecting the orbit and/or upper eyelid, which usually appear at or shortly after birth, are a problem for patients. In plexiform neurofibroma of the orbit, pulsations of the orbital contents synchronous with the pulse may be present. The upper eyelid affected by neurofibroma initially has high skin laxity, with palpable nodules in the subcutaneous tissue. With the progression of masses in the upper eyelid, pseudoptosis is evident, which gradually closes the palpebral fissure completely. The eyeball tends to be dislocated downward and the present exophthalmos is cosmetically supported by high myopia with eventual buphthalmos. The latter causes spindle-shaped thickening may affect the chiasm or both optic tracts, and may also spread further along the optic tracts, requiring repeated neuroimaging examinations of the head. Anatomical conditions and pseudoptosis of the upper eyelid arising from this basis impair visual function and put the child at risk of developing amblyopia. Strabismus ex anopsia may develop on the affected side. Patients may have pain in the orbital region, which may be further potentiated by the possible development of glaucoma. Vision may also be deprived by the growth of optic nerve gliomas or chiasmal tumours—these are clinically manifest in infancy but may remain asymptomatic.

CNS tumours may also manifest with headache or epileptic seizures. The manifestation of NF1 is highly individual; its onset can be expected in both sexes after birth and during early childhood, but it can also manifest later in life. The possibility of malignant transformation of neurofibromas into malignant peripheral nerve sheath tumours (malignant schwannomas) or neurofibrosarcomas and the coincidence of NF1 with numerous other types of neoplasms (leukaemia, pheochromocytomas) are prognostically unfavourable [28, 33]. Meningoencephalocele may develop in orbital ceiling defect with bone dysplasia at this site, with transmission of cerebral pulsation. In adulthood, vascular complications may occur based on pathological proliferation of smooth muscle and endothelium in the vessels. Other complications may include arterial hypertension and the development of pseudoarthrosis. Integration of the individual into society is hampered by frequent psychological difficulties and phobias caused by the cosmetic factor of the disease. The life expectancy of NF1 sufferers is on average 10 years shorter than that of the general population [49].

In addition to the above common symptoms, NF2 is characterised by bilateral occurrence of schwannomas of the auditory nerve; the presence of any of the following tumours: plexiform neurofibroma or neurofibroma of another type, meningioma, meningiomatosis, spinal cord ependymoma, glioma, gliohamartia or peripheral schwannoma; calcification of the brain; presenile cataract [33].

Diagnosis

The diagnosis of NF1 is based on *clinical findings* and its criteria were established in 1987 at the *National Institute of Health Conference* in Bethesda. The diagnosis of NF1 requires the presence of two or more of the following: 1) six or more café au lait spots larger than 5 mm at the site of greatest diameter in prepubertal individuals and more than 15 mm in postpubertal individuals; 2) two or more neurofibromas of any type or one plexiform neurofibroma; 3) pigmented spots in the axillae or groin; 4) glioma optica; 5) two or more iris hamartomas (Lisch nodules); 6) typical bone lesions (e.g. sphenoid bone dysplasia or cortical thinning of long bones with or without pseudoarthrosis; 7) familial occurrence of NF1 in at least one first-degree relative (parent, sibling, offspring).

X-ray examination is used to diagnose skeletal abnormalities, *magnetic resonance imaging (MRI)* or *computed tomography (CT)* to diagnose intracranial lesions.

On *ophthalmoscopy*, Lisch's nodules, or iris hamartomas, which are yellow to brown nodules protruding from the iris surface, can be found on the anterior segment of the eye.

Neurological Disorders

The diagnosis of NF2 is also based on *clinical findings* and findings on *neuroimaging*. The diagnostic criteria for NF2 are met when one of the following conditions is present: 1) bilateral 8th cranial nerve tumour; 2) a first-degree relative of NF2 and either a unilateral 8th cranial nerve tumour or two of the following: neurofibroma, meningioma, glioma, schwannoma, or juvenile posterior subcapsular opacity.

Differential diagnosis

The clinical presentation of NF is very peculiar and characteristic when the diagnostic criteria are met. However, attention should be paid to the very varied interindividual manifestations, including familial disease.

Carotid-cavernous fistula (presence of a phonendoscopically audible murmur synchronous with the heartbeat; to be excluded when the orbital ceiling is affected and subsequent meningoencephalocele develops).

Therapy

Genetic counselling, molecular genetic testing, and prenatal diagnosis play a critical role in the prevention of both NF1 and NF2. Therapy for both NF1 and NF2 is symptomatic.

12.2   Von Hippel-Lindau Disease

It is an autosomal dominantly inherited disease classified as a neurocutaneous syndrome (phakomatosis).

Aetiology

The gene, which in its intact form has a tumour suppressor effect and whose mutation is responsible for Von Hippel-Lindau disease, is localised on the short arm of chromosome 3 (3p25–26). This gene is involved in cell cycle regulation and angiogenesis.

Clinical presentation

The disease is characterised by hamartosis with multiple haemangiomas and haemangioblastomas. These are localised in the retina, cerebellum, rarely in the medulla oblongata or spinal cord, rarely supratentorial. Cerebellar haemangiomas manifest most commonly during adolescence. Multiple cysts, adenomas, and haemangiomas or haemangioblastomas of the kidney and pancreas and a marked increase in the incidence of carcinomas of these organs are serious complications of the disease. Paragangliomas may also occur.

Diagnosis

The diagnosis of tumours associated with Von Hippel-Lindau disease is mainly based on *imaging (CT and MRI)*, while retinal haemangiomas are diagnosed by *ophthalmological examination.*

Therapy

If possible, radical surgery is the method of choice for tumours. In the case of its contraindication, radiotherapy can be used (with a gamma knife for smaller lesions).

13 Metabolic Diseases of the Central Nervous System (Thesaurismoses)

Neurometabolic diseases are diseases in which a metabolic basis has been identified, often with a specified gene localisation, sometimes with a gene product, and with molecular testing options including prenatal diagnosis. There are more than 500 known genetic disorders with neurological symptoms in which an enzymatic or protein defect has been identified. The diseases can be divided into two main groups—diffuse metabolic diseases (encephalopathies) and inborn errors of metabolism and neurodegenerative diseases with predilection for certain structures of the central nervous system (CNS).

In the following, the focus is only on neurometabolic diseases with ophthalmological involvement.

Epidemiology

The incidence of storage neurometabolic disorders varies from a rare occurrence to a high-frequency clinical manifestation.

13.1 Diffuse Metabolic Encephalopathies

Peroxisomal disorders

Peroxisomes are present in virtually all cells of the body, but most abundantly in tissues with active lipid metabolism, i.e. in hepatocytes, renal tubular cells and oligodendrocytes. Peroxisomes contain dozens of enzymes involved in important anabolic and catabolic cellular processes. The functions of peroxisomes are the synthesis of plasmalogens, bile acids, cholesterol, and the degradation of hydrogen peroxide and purines or beta-oxidation of long-chain carbon fatty acids (hence the multiplication of these fatty acids), polyamines, ethanol, and others. Peroxisomes contain several antioxidant enzymes, their typical enzyme being catalase.

Neurological Disorders

The basis of peroxisomal disorders is either multiple peroxisomal enzyme deficiency (e.g. Zellweger syndrome) or deficiency of only one enzyme (e.g. adrenoleukodystrophy or its slower variant adrenomyeloneuropathy). Therefore, in diseases with multiple enzyme deficiency, in addition to neurological symptoms, skeletal deformities, craniofacial dysmorphogenesis, and disturbances of hepatic and endogenous functions are present.

Peroxisomal diseases are divided into three groups. The first group comprises diseases associated with impaired peroxisome biogenesis and includes Zellweger syndrome, neonatal adrenoleukodystrophy and infantile Refsum's disease. The second group comprises syndromes caused by the malfunction of several enzymes and is represented by rhizomelic chodrodyslasia punctata. The third group comprises diseases caused by the malfunction of a single enzyme, namely X-linked adrenoleukodystrophy and primary hyperoxaluria I. The most lethal of the above is Zellweger syndrome, in which affected individuals do not survive one year of age.

Mitochondrial encephalopathy

In mitochondrial encephalopathies, there is either a predilection for CNS involvement or a combination of myogenic and cortico-subcortical lesions, or only myogenic involvement predominates and is therefore also referred to as encephalomyopathies. They are caused by a defective mitochondrial DNA (or RNA) structure in the form of a point mutation, deletion, or duplication. Most of these disorders are maternally transmitted. Their pathogenesis involves a defect in oxidative phosphorylation, which is manifested in energy metabolism by a defect in ATP synthesis. A common biochemical marker is an increase in lactate and lactate/pyruvate ratio in serum and in liquor. Ragged-red fibres are often found in muscle biopsies.

Common clinical manifestations are short stature, hearing loss, frequent ptosis of the eyelids with lesions of the oculomotor nerves, progressive dementia, and myopathy; retinal pigmentary degeneration and cardiomyopathy may also be present. Clinical entities with ocular involvement include the following. *Kearns-Sayre syndrome (KSS)* is characterised by disease onset before the age of 20 years, impaired oculomotor innervation with ptosis of the eyelids, the presence of retinal pigmentary degeneration, and at least one of the signs of conduction heart block, cerebellar symptoms, and hyperproteinorhachia. Neuropathy with ataxia and retinal pigmentary degeneration (Neuropathy, Ataxia, Retinitis Pigmentosa; NARP) is a slowly progressive disease with manifestation in late adolescence, in which neurogenic amyotrophic syndrome, sensory neuropathy, cerebellar symptoms and retinal pigmentary degeneration are present. In addition, progressive external ophthalmoplegia (PEO) can be mentioned among the diseases of this group.

Specialised laboratory tests, including histochemical examination of muscle biopsies, immunohistochemical examination of the activity of enzymes involved in oxidative phosphorylation and molecular genetic testing, are used to refine the diagnosis of individual clinical entities.

13.2 Hereditary Errors of Metabolism

Polyodystrophies

This is a heterogeneous group of very rare, congenital, and almost exclusively autosomal recessive progressive neurometabolic diseases with predominance of cortical grey matter involvement. They are often referred to as lysosomal "storage" diseases (tesaurismoses) because their common feature is the accumulation of pathological material in cellular organelles (lysosomes). The breakdown disorder of the complex of carbohydrates, lipids, and proteins with their secondary accumulation in lysosomes results from impaired enzymatic activity or poor organelle biogenesis. Lysosomes are membrane organelles contained in animal cells, whose key function is the degradation of proteins, nucleic acids, sugars, fats, and cellular debris. In lysosomal disease, the function of hydrolases is primarily affected, and sometimes the protein hydrolase activator can also fail. In addition to CNS tissue (especially the cerebral cortex), spindle material is deposited in other tissues and damages cells by toxic influences as well as by direct mechanical pressure.

Children are usually born asymptomatic and develop symptoms within the first year of life. Subsequently, the disease manifests clinically as progressive intellectual and motor impairment with spasticity and cerebellar symptoms, as well as sensory impairment, and epilepsy is common.

Genetic, direct enzymatic and biopsy testing are used for their diagnosis.

Neuronal ceroid lipofuscinosis (Batten disease)

This is a genetically heterogeneous group of diseases with autosomal recessive inheritance.

They are caused by a lysosomal disorder with accumulation of ceroid lipopigment and lipofuscin in CNS neurons and other tissues, with their selective necrosis and atrophy.

According to the age of development and the course, we distinguish infantile, late infantile, early juvenile, juvenile and adult forms. The clinical presentation is dominated by visual impairment progressing to blindness, epileptic seizures, myoclonia, progressive motor impairment with initial ataxia and dementia. A characteristic red spot may be present on the eye fundus.

Biopsy and electroencephalography are used for diagnosis.

There is no causal treatment. Genetic counselling or prenatal diagnosis are options for disease prevention.

Niemann-Pick disease

This heterogeneous group of autosomal recessively inherited diseases is associated with the accumulation of the phospholipid sphingomyelin and non-esterified cholesterol in the cells of the reticuloendothelial system and, in some forms, in the CNS.

Neurological Disorders

Neurological impairment is particularly evident in variant C with development of the disease in childhood. The clinical presentation includes vertical gaze paresis, cerebellar symptoms with marked ataxia, dystonia, spasticity, and progressive dementia, but epileptic seizures or secondary narcolepsy-cataplexy may also occur. Adolescents may also present with psychiatric symptoms, which may dominate the clinical presentation.

On brain imaging, diffuse atrophy is usually present, but primarily affecting the cerebellum. Abdominal sonography confirms splenomegaly and often hepatomegaly. Bone marrow puncture, specific cholesterol esterification disorder test, enzymatic or molecular genetic testing are used to confirm the diagnosis. Sphingomyelinase deficiency can only be detected in a proportion of patients with neurovisceral involvement.

Therapeutic options include expensive causal replacement therapy (miglustar), hypolipidemics (but only with questionable effect) or bone marrow transplantation (with improvement of clinical presentation in visceral forms, but without improvement of neurological findings).

Alpers syndrome

This is a heterogeneous group of diseases both biochemically and genetically. The most common transmission is autosomal recessive, but recessive X chromosomally linked inheritance can also be encountered. In the aetiopathogenesis, defects in energy metabolism or selenium deficiency are involved; in some patients the metabolic defect has not been defined yet.

The disease occurs in neonatal, infantile, and juvenile forms, which differ in the speed of progression. The clinical presentation is dominated by progressive dementia and epilepsy, with several myocloniae refractory to treatment; cerebellar symptoms, dystonia, spasticity, and visual disturbance are also present. Hepatic lesions are also present.

Severe cortical atrophy is evident on brain imaging. The electroencephalographic recording is low-voltage with an abundance of fast beta-band activity and superimposed spike activity. The laboratory picture shows pathological liver tests, which may be the first sign of manifestation of the disease. Liver biopsy is used to support the diagnosis.

Selenium replacement is used for therapy in case of selenium deficiency. There is no causal treatment for other forms.

13.3 Leukodystrophies

This is a group of progressive diseases that affect the metabolism of myelin fibres.

Clinically, they present with spastic paresis (mixed type paresis if there is a peripheral component), cerebellar symptoms and, rarely, dyskinesias. Cognitive deficits, behavioural disturbances, epilepsy, and often visual and hearing impairment are associated in the course of the disease.

Demyelinating changes are detected on MRI. Enzymatic or morphological examination is used to clarify the type of leukodystrophy.

Canavan disease

This is a disease with autosomal recessive inheritance, associated with spongiform degeneration of the CNS. It arises because of aspartoacetylase deficiency.

The clinical presentation is dominated by macrocephaly, hypotonic syndrome evolving into spasticity and optic nerve atrophy. The congenital, infantile, and juvenile forms are identified.

On MRI, changes in the subcortical white matter are present symmetrically. Proteinocyte dissociation and a high concentration of N-acetylaspartate, which is also excreted in the urine and whose increased content in the brain can be demonstrated by MRI spectroscopy. Enzymatic examination is used to confirm the disease.

There is no causal treatment. Genetic prevention with heterozygote detection and prenatal diagnosis are important.

Pelizaues-Merzbacher disease

This is an X chromosomally linked orthochromatic leukodystrophy with defective formation of proteolipid (PLP), which is the basic structural protein of myelin. The disease is clinically variable, depending on the disruption of the *PLP* gene, which can be a duplication, deletion or point mutation.

The clinical presentation is characterised by striking irregular movements of the eyeballs (in the horizontal or vertical plane), resembling nystagmus and associated with oscillatory head movements, as well as psychomotor retardation, spasticity, choreoathetosis, cerebellar syndrome, optic nerve atrophy and sometimes epilepsy. Progression depends on the timing of clinical manifestation.

The MRI shows demyelinating or demyelination changes in the initial phase of the disease, which disappear later in the course of the disease, and the picture of cortical, subcortical and cerebellar atrophy predominates. The diagnosis is confirmed by molecular genetic testing.

Treatment is symptomatic. Genetic counselling and prenatal diagnosis are used for prevention.

Hypomyelination with increased N-acetylaspartyl glutamate

Clinically, it is characterised by the early development of nystagmus and epilepsy; the clinical presentation is reminiscent of Pelizaues-Merzbacher disease. The complete absence of myelin on MRI is typical.

Leukoencephalopathy with vanishing white matter changes

Manifesting in early childhood, a rapidly progressive course with ataxia, spasticity, epilepsy, and possibly optic nerve atrophy is typical. On MRI, cavities and vacuoles with variable signalling are found in the white matter of the hemispheres; MRI spectroscopy confirms elevation of lactate and glucose.

Neurological Disorders

13.4 Neurometabolic and Neurodegenerative Diseases with Predominance of Subcortical Grey Matter Involvement

This group includes several progressive diseases, often dominated by extrapyramidal syndrome. However, some of them also have ophthalmological involvement.

Primary dystonia (DYT 1)

This autosomal dominantly inherited disease with linkage to chromosome 9 with low penetrance manifests in childhood and is also referred to as torsion dystonia.

Persistent muscle contractions and repetitive movements lead to persistent abnormal limb and later axial musculature. Dyskinesias later generalise and multiple focal dystonic manifestations may be present, such as blepharospasm, oromandibular dystonia, spastic dysphonia, torticollis, or acral dystonia in the upper extremities.

The basis of diagnosis is molecular genetic testing.

Anticholinergics (in high doses) may be used in therapy, possibly in combination with benzodiazepines and antidopaminergic agents. In the case of failure of medical therapy, deep brain stimulation may be indicated.

Hallenvorden-Spatz disease (Pantothenate Kinase-Associated Neurodegeneration)

This is an autosomal recessively inherited disease with linkage to chromosome 20. The mutated gene encoding pantothenate kinase 2 is involved in neuronal damage by free radicals, with subsequent iron accumulation in the basal ganglia and in the nucleus niger.

In affected children, extrapyramidal syndrome—dystonia (with frequent equinovarous involvement in the lower limbs) combined with rigidity, oromandibular dystonia, generalised choreoathetosis—predominates. Dysarthria, progressive spasticity, sometimes retinal pigmentary degeneration, and intellectual deterioration are also present.

On CT and MRI, iron deposits are found bilaterally in the globus pallidus, creating a "tiger's eye" image.

Deep brain stimulation can be used for symptomatic therapy.

Leigh's disease (subacute necrotising encephalomyelopathy)

Mitochondrial disorders are usually the basis of this heterogeneous clinical syndrome, but some patients have autosomal recessive and X-linked inheritance without mitochondrial disorders.

The clinical presentation is characterised by ataxia, dyskinesias, changes in muscle tone and trunk dysfunction (dyspnoea, dysphagia, oculomotor disorders). The disease occurs in neonatal, infantile and juvenile forms (rare).

Necrotic foci are visible on CT and especially on T2-weighted MRI images, localised symmetrically in the basal ganglia, in the brainstem and sometimes in the white matter (including the lateral spinal cord). In most patients with mitochondrial disorder, elevated serum and lymphatic lactate and pyruvate levels are present during disease exacerbation. Mitochondrial enzyme testing is also performed.

There is no causal treatment.

13.5 Spinocerebellar Degeneration of Childhood

Friedreich's ataxia

This autosomal recessive disease with linkage to chromosome 9 is associated with amplification of the GAA triplet. The gene product is frataxin—a component of the inner mitochondrial membrane, involved in the permeability of toxic free radicals. Iron is stored in the mitochondria of cardiocytes. The prevalence of the disease in the population is 1:50,000. It is characterised by early spinocerebellar degeneration, involvement of the lateral and posterior spinal cords, skeletal deformity, and cardiomyopathy.

The severity of the disability depends on the number of GAA triplets. The manifestation of the disease occurs most often at the age of 4–15 years, rarely later. Atactic gait is predominant in the initial stages, and lower limb pain or cramps may occur after exertion. In addition, there is a neocerebellar syndrome with intrinsic tremor, nystagmus, tendon-osteal hypo- to areflexia in the lower limbs, in combination with the presence of abnormal (spastic) reflexes, dysarthria, saccadic speech, palhypesthesia. Scoliosis of the spine and what is called "Friedreich's foot" (pes excavatus with hammertoe position) develop, in most patients cardiomyopathy and in some patients impaired glucose tolerance or diabetes mellitus. Patients are usually confined to a wheelchair 15 years after the development of the disease and die between the ages of 30 and 50 (most often because of cardiomyopathy).

Diagnosis is based on EMG examination, and evoked potential testing may also be beneficial. Abnormalities on ECG (inverted T wave), echocardiography and ventricular hypertrophy on X-ray are then used to support the diagnosis. The examination of the glycaemic profile is important. Gene analysis is used to confirm the diagnosis.

Treatment is symptomatic. Medication antioxidant treatment includes coenzyme Q10, vitamins E and C, or B vitamins. A ketogenic diet is appropriate. Rehabilitation treatment is important, and surgical treatment in the case of progression of scoliosis and leg deformities.

Rarer ataxias

The rarer ataxias in childhood and adolescence are spinocerebellar syndromes associated with optic nerve atrophy, retinal degeneration, deafness, mental retardation, or hypogonadism.

Neurological Disorders

This group includes:

- *spinocerebellar degeneration associated with vitamin E deficiency*

Clinically similar to Friedreich's ataxia. It is caused by a mutation of the alpha-tocopherol transport protein (chromosome 8). It is deficient in serum vitamin E and is treatable with high doses of vitamin E.

- *abetalipoproteinaemia (Bassen-Kornzweig disease)*

Clinically, it is again similar to Friedreich's ataxia; retinal pigmentary degeneration and sometimes external ophthalmoplegia are also present. It is caused by a defect in apolipoprotein B-100 (chromosome 2), leading to malabsorption of fats and fat-soluble vitamins (A. D, E, K). Therapeutically, a diet with restriction of unsaturated fatty acids and high doses of fat-soluble vitamins is used.

Summary of ophthalmological specifics

An ophthalmologist is also involved in the process of diagnosis and supportive treatment.

Diagnosis

The most seen are corneal opacities, cataracts, pigment degeneration and pigment clumps on the retina, thinning of retinal vessels, glaucoma, and optic nerve atrophy. In X-linked adrenoleukodystrophy, vision loss occurs based on demyelination of the entire visual pathway, while the retina is spared. Early identification of these diseases, which may also be based on ocular findings, is critical for prenatal diagnosis, genetic counselling, and treatment. Vision is usually affected by corneal opacifica-tion, lens opacification, pigment epithelium disorders, and optic nerve demyelination (adrenoleukodystrophy), glaucoma and atrophy. Impaired visual function may also manifest itself as nyctalopia.

Ocular manifestations include corneal opacities and deposits in sialidosis, mucopolysaccharidosis and mucolipidosis II and III, and peroxisomal diseases. Crystal deposits in the cornea can be seen in patients with cystinosis. Bilateral cataract is the cause of decreased visual acuity in patients with peroxisomal dysfunc-tion. Many patients with mucopolysaccharidosis are hyperopic. There are several possible mechanisms to explain this phenomenon. Thickening of the sclera may lead to a reduction in the axial length of the eye and hence hyperopia [20]. Another factor may be an increase in corneal and scleral rigidity caused by the accumulation of glycosaminoglycans inducing corneal flattening and thus a reduction in optical power. Retinopathy with retinal pigmentary degeneration and associated changes on the electroretinogram may occur in the retina. Cherry spotting in the macula accompanies Tay-Sachs, Sandhoff and Niemann-Pick disease and GM1 gangliosi-dosis [36]. The histologic correlate of this retinal finding in Niemann-Pick disease is balloon-like, lipid-filled ganglion cells. Patients may have optic nerve target oedema or atrophy [14, 36]. Target oedema is common in patients with Hurler and Hurler-Scheie syndrome. Chronic oedema in mucopolysaccharidoses precedes the development of target atrophy. Thickening of the sclera and lamina cribrosa can cause deformation of the optic head and pinching of the nerve leading to atrophy. Glaucoma may occur in patients with tesaurismoses [41]. Its occurrence is related to the accumulation of masses in the extracellular matrix and softening of the anterior chamber. Anatomical changes in the ventricular angle cause impaired circulation of intraocular fluid.

The ophthalmologist can play an important role in the diagnosis of these diseases, as in some cases ocular manifestations are among the key signs of the disease [22, 48]. During ophthalmoscopy, he or she observes pathologies affecting the structures of the anterior and posterior segments of the eye and examines visual function, including the visual field, if possible. The examination of pachymetry is important, the values of which can be affected by the deposition of materials in the cornea and changes in the architecture of the tissues of the eye. Photodocumentation of the anterior and posterior segments of the eye is used to monitor development. Optic nerve oedema or atrophy and macular findings can be quantified and graphically represented using optical coherence tomography. Deterioration of retinal function is evident on the electroretinogram (ERG), where there is a reduction in the amplitude of individual waves up to complete extinction of the ERG.

Therapy

To improve the quality of life of patients with steady-state diseases, quality interdisciplinary care is needed, in which the ophthalmologist is also involved. The ophthalmic surgeon can perform perforating keratoplasty in the case of corneal opacities impairing visual acuity, and some authors recommend deep anterior lamellar keratoplasty for lower risk of rejection [20, 21], . Corneal limbal cell transplantation may also have an effect, delaying the onset of corneal opacifications. In the case of lens opacification, cataract surgery is indicated. The results of ocular surgical therapy are naturally limited by other findings in the eye, including retinal pathologies and optic nerve atrophy. It is necessary to monitor the development on the retina and optic nerve and treat any associated glaucoma.

14 Extrapyramidal Syndromes

Extrapyramidal syndromes can be characterised as a group of neurodegenerative diseases affecting the subcortical centres, especially the basal ganglia and their connections. The main function of the basal ganglia and associated structures is motor control. It follows that the impairment of these control centres causes mainly motor disturbances, but the syndromes also include disturbances of the autonomic system and cognition. Extrapyramidal diseases arise when the balance of the two main systems of neurons that produce neurotransmitters in the basal ganglia is disturbed: dopaminergic (in the substantia nigra—dopamine) and cholinergic (acetylcholine).

Neurological Disorders

A deficiency of dopamine (or an excess of acetylcholine) causes parkinsonism; an excess of dopamine (with treatment, or a deficiency of acetylcholine), on the other hand, causes mainly involuntary movements—for example, chorea. Extrapyramidal syndromes can arise on a genetic basis, but they can also occur as a complication of side effects of treatment (after first-generation antipsychotics or some neuroleptics).

Extrapyramidal disorders can be divided into two main groups. The first group are the *hypokinetic* syndromes, which restrict the patient's movement and are represented mainly by Parkinsonian syndrome. Muscle rigidity, facial hypomimicity and hypophasia to aphasia are prominent. Akinesia, or impaired initiation of free movement, and bradykinesia, or slowing of movement, are typical. Muscular rigidity is present, resisting both active and passive movement. Parkinson's syndrome is accompanied by tremor, rigidity, hypokinesia and impaired standing and walking. Parkinsonism represents a set of neurological symptoms seen in many types of extrapyramidal syndromes and other neurodegenerative diseases. The most common of these is Parkinson's disease, in which there is a loss of dopamine-producing neurons and an accumulation of Lewy body proteins in midbrain neurons. The second group, on the other hand, consists of syndromes accompanied by *hyperkinesia* or *dyskinesia*, characterised by involuntary abnormal movements. These symptomatic movements include tremor, chorea, (hemi)ballismus, dystonia, myoclonus, and tics.

In the following, we list some extrapyramidal system disorders in which the clinical presentation includes, among others, involvement of ocular structures and vision.

14.1 Progressive Supranuclear Palsy

Progressive supranuclear palsy is the most common type of atypical parkinsonism. Atypical parkinsonism is less common compared to classic parkinsonism and usually appears around the age of 60. Gait and stability are usually affected. Slowing of movement leads to a general slowing of the pace of life. Patients suffer from facial hypomimia and quite typically stare straight ahead with raised eyebrows and a wrinkled forehead. A change in speech is often present. Patients tend to be emotionally unstable, cognitively impaired and often develop dementia. Of the ocular symptoms, oculomotor disturbances especially downward gaze dominate. Diplopia appears and walking and reading can be difficult. There may be exaggerated blinking or clenching of the eye slit to blepharospasm, with difficulty in opening the eyes. There is no known effective therapy for this, yet the ophthalmologist can improve the patient's quality of life by prescribing appropriate prismatic correction. Injection of botulinum toxin into the periocular region to relieve the exaggerated blinking and blepharospasm may also be effective.

14.2 Huntington's Chorea

Huntington's chorea (HCH) is a rare, severe autosomal dominantly inherited neurodegenerative disease, affecting mainly the striatum. It is most common in middle age, but there are patients who develop their first difficulties before the age of 20, often while still at school [39]. This is a severe lethal disease. Although initially the chorea presents motorically with rather hyperkinetic involuntary movements, the motor symptoms later become hypokinetic with bradykinesia and dystonia. The typical manifestation is a jerky gait, which worsens with disease progression to a state of rigidity [40]. Initially, psychiatric disturbances and only subtle involuntary movements may be at the forefront with progressive generalisation. With further progression, impairments in memory, logic, communication, behavioural disturbances up to aggression appear and patients become demented. Ocular manifestations include impaired mobility, especially vergence, and the resulting binocular diplopia. The diagnosis is made by the physician based on clinical symptomatology, knowledge of family anamnesis with a positive parent and DNA analysis [47]. Prenatal diagnosis with amniocentesis is possible. The greatest promise in the treatment of this disease is the possibility of gene therapy. The ophthalmologist provides supportive care for related ocular complications.

14.3 Idiopathic Blepharospasm

Idiopathic blepharospasm belongs to essential blepharospasm and may be caused by a disturbance of basal ganglia function. Symptomatic blepharospasm arises as part of the eye's defence mechanisms, together with photophobia and tearing. Blepharospasm may occur as a side effect of antiparkinsonian treatment, during hormone therapy, especially during the menopause, or when benzodiazepines are abruptly discontinued. Blepharospasm is a general term for involuntary tonic or tonic–clonic spasms of the eyelid circular sphincter. The eyelid clenching comes on unexpectedly, uncontrollably, and lasts longer than a normal blink.

Idiopathic blepharospasm (also facial paraspasm, Meige's disease) appears most commonly after the age of 50 and is more common in women. Usually, the disability is bilateral and progresses from initially second isolated fleeting eyelid spasms to prolonged spasms of the mimic muscles causing grimaces to head twitches. Blepharospasm attacks can last for minutes, but can also last for several hours, causing virtual blindness in some patients with otherwise perfectly healthy visual systems. The disease thus becomes debilitating and unbearable. The trigger for an intense attack can often be a stressful situation. Diagnosis is based on the clinical presentation. Knowledge of personal and pharmacological anamnesis is essential. Treatment is dominated by topical repeated applications of botulinum toxin. Patients may take anticholinergics and tranquilizers. Despite this treatment, the disease may progress. There are also surgical treatment options, whose principle is myectomy of

Neurological Disorders

the musculus orbicularis oculi muscle fibres or neurectomy of the nerve fibres from the plexus parotideus coming to the eyelid sphincter. A very interesting supportive treatment alternative of recent years is a phenomenon based on patient experience. When the eye slit is spasmed and closed, point pressure at the temples can help to open the eyelids. The PressOpTM device, which can be mounted on the side of the spectacles, is based on this experience. This device can alleviate blepharospasm at least for a moment in an often-critical situation and at the same time free the patient's two hands. Of course, this is a supportive device, recommended as an adjunct to standard therapy.

14.4 Wilson's Disease

Wilson's disease, also called hepatolenticular degeneration, is a metabolic autosomal recessive inherited disease in which copper accumulates in the liver and damages the hepatocytes. In addition, the function of the central nervous system is impaired and haemolytic anaemia may occur. The disease is caused by a mutation in the gene of chromosome 13.

The clinical presentation consists mainly of neurological manifestations or tremor, deterioration of the patient's psychological state, speech, and motor disorders up to severe extrapyramidal syndrome. Liver involvement in the form of fibrosis followed by cirrhosis may progress to liver failure. The blood manifestation is anaemia and clotting disorders. Other manifestations include hormonal and growth disorders. Icterus may be present on the skin.

The ophthalmologist can assist in the diagnosis by observing the pathognomonic Kayser-Fleischer ring on the cornea, which is due to copper accumulation in the Descemet's membrane at the corneal limbus. On slit-lamp examination, a typical sunflower cataract can also be observed, arising from copper accumulation in the anterior capsule. The principal diagnosis is based on laboratory results with typical decreased serum ceruloplasmin and increased urinary copper excretion. The diagnosis can be confirmed by molecular genetic testing.

The treatment is lifelong and consists of a diet with restriction of copper intake, which is abundant especially in marine fish and chocolate. Application of copper chelating drugs (penicillamine) is appropriate. Reduction of copper resorption in the intestines can be achieved by regular zinc supplementation. In more advanced stages, liver transplantation should be considered.

14.5 Perinatal Encephalopathy (Cerebral Palsy)

Or more recently, cerebral palsy (CP) refers to the improper development of the motor centres of the brain or their other damage in the early developmental stage, or the impairment of central motor control and the resulting mobility disorders. The damage can occur during pregnancy, perinatally or during the first months of life. The disease usually manifests itself between the second and third year. The main clinical manifestations include delayed child development [42]. The child rolls over, climbs, sits or stands later. Cerebral palsy is divided into the most common spastic, atactic, dyskinetic and mixed.

Visual difficulties result from both eye and brain involvement. Those resulting from brain involvement are manifested by blurred vision, inability to focus on the object being viewed, visual field disturbances or impaired rapid eye movements. Children with MO often have strabismus and hypermetropia.

Cerebral palsy is not curable, but the rule of thumb is that the earlier treatment is initiated, the better the developmental disorder can be overcome. The basis of treatment is regular physiotherapy [42]. Many rehabilitation techniques are used, one of the best known being the Vojt method. Pulsed magnetotherapy can have beneficial effects, consisting mainly of a vasodilating and spasmolytic effect. Ophthalmologists can contribute to a significant improvement in the quality of life of patients with MO and help patients to integrate into the community.

References

1. Acchiote P. Sur un cas de neuromyélite subaiguë ou maladie de Devic. Bulletin officiels de la Société de neurologie de Paris. 1907;8–9:273–5.
2. Ambler Z, Bednarik J, Ruzicka E. Clinical neurology – I. general part. Prague: Triton; 2008.
3. Antônio JR, Goloni-Bertollo EM, Trídico LA. Neurofibromatosis: chronological history and current issues. An Bras Dermatol. 2013;88(3):329–43.
4. Antônio JR, Goloni-Bertollo EM, Trídico LA. Neurofibromatosis: chronological history and current issues. An Bras Dermatol. 2013;88:329–43.
5. Babu Rajesh B, Biswas Jyotirmay MS. Bilateral Macular Retinitis as the Presenting Feature of Subacute Sclerosing Panencephalitis. J Neuroophthalmol. 2007;27(4):288–91.
6. Bartleson JD, Cutrer FM. Migraine update. Diagnosis and treatment Minn Med. 2010;5:36–41.
7. Bednarik J, Ambler Z, Ruzicka E. Clinical neurology – special part II. Prague: Triton; 2010.
8. Belzeaux R, Lançon C. Neurofibromatosis type 1: psychiatric disorders and quality of life impairment. Presse Med. 2006;35:277–80.
9. Bizzoco E, Lolli F, Repice AM, et al. Prevalence of neuromyelitis optica spectrum disorder and phenotype distribution. J Neurol. 2009;256:1891–8.
10. Burris CKH, Stier MA, Salamat S, et al. Neurofibromatosis type 1: a neuro-psycho-cutaneous syndrome? Orbit. 2017;20:1–4.
11. Carey JC, Baty BJ, Johnson JP, et al. The genetic aspects of neurofibromatosis. Ann NY Acad Sci. 1986;486:45–6.
12. Cawthon RM, Weiss R, Xu GF, et al. A major segment of the neurofibromatosis type 1 gene:cDNA sequence, genomic structure, and point mutations. Cell. 1990;62:193–201.
13. Chandra A, Li WA, Stone CR, et al. The cerebral circulation and cerebrovascular disease I: Anatomy. Brain Circ. 2017;3:45–56.
14. Collins ML, Traboulsi E, Maumenee IH. Optic nerve head swelling and optic atrophy in the systemic mucopolysaccharidoses. Ophthalmology. 1990;97:1445–9.
15. Colpak Ayse I, Erdener Sefik E, Ozgen Burce et al. Neuro-ophthalmology of subacute sclerosing panencephalitis: two cases and a review of the literature. Current Opinion in Ophthalmology. 2012;23(6):466–71.

Neurological Disorders

16. Cossburn M, Tackley G, Baker K, et al. The prevalence of neuromyelitis optica in South East Wales. Eur J Neurol. 2012;19:655–9.
17. Devic E. Myélite subaiguë compliquée de névrite optique. Le Bulletin Médicale. 1894;8:1033–4.
18. Dodick DW, Gargus JJ. Why migraines strike. Sci Am. 2008;2:56–63.
19. Elsone L, Panicker J, Mutch K, et al. Role of intravenous immunoglobulin in the treatment of acute relapses of neuromyelitis optica: experience in 10 patients. Mult Scler. 2014;20(4):501–4.
20. Fahnehjelm KT, Ashworth JL, Pitz S, et al. Clinical guidelines for diagnosing and managing ocular manifestations in children with mucopolysaccharidosis. Acta Ophthalmol. 2012;90:595–602.
21. Fenzl CR, Teramoto K, Moshirfar M. Ocular manifestations and management recommendations of lysosomal storage disorders I: mucopolysaccharidoses. Clin Ophthalmol. 2015;9:1633–44.
22. Ganesh A, Bruwer Z, Al-Thihli K. An update on ocular involvement in mucopolysaccharidoses. Curr Opin Ophthalmol. 2013;24:379–88.
23. Ghezzi A, Bergamaschi R, Martinelli V, et al. Clinical characteristics, course and prognosis of relapsing Devic's neuromyelitis optica. J Neurol. 2004;251:47–52.
24. Gilhus NE. Myasthenia Gravis. N Engl J Med. 2016;375(26):2570–81.
25. Gilmore B, Michael M. Treatment of acute migraine headache. Am Fam Physician. 2011;3:271–80.
26. Gutmann DH, Aylsworth A, Carey JC, et al. The diagnostic evaluation and multidisciplinary management of neurofibromatosis 1 and neurofibromatosis 2. JAMA. 1997;278:51–7.
27. Hernández-Martín A, Duat-Rodríguez A. An update on neurofibromatosis type 1: not just café-au-lait spots and freckling. Part II. Other skin manifestations characteristics of NF1. NF1 and cancer. Actas Dermosifiliogr. 2016;107:465–73.
28. Hosoi K. Multiple neurofibromatosis (von Recklinghausen disease) with special reference to malignant transformation. Arch Surg. 1931;22:258–81.
29. Jacob A, Panicker J, Lythgoe D, et al. The epidemiology of neuromyelitis optica amongst adults in the Merseyside County of United Kingdom. J Neurol. 2013;260:2134–7.
30. Jafri SK, Kumar R, Ibrahim SH. Subacute sclerosing panencephalitis – current perspectives. Pediatric Health Med Ther. 2018;9:67–71.
31. Jarius S, Ruprecht K, Wildemann B, et al. Contrasting disease patterns in seropositive and seronegative neuromyelitis optica:a multicentre study of 175 patients. J Neuroinflammation. 2012;9:14.
32. Kimbrough DJ, Fujihara K, Jacob A, et al. Treatment of neuromyelitis optica: review and recommendations. Mult Scler Relat Disord. 2012;1:180–7.
33. Korf BR. Malignancy in neurofibromatosis type 1. Oncologist. 2000;5:477–85.
34. Kvickström P, Lindblom B, Bergström G, et al. Amaurosis fugax: risk factors and prevalence of significant carotid stenosis. Clin Ophthalmol. 2016;10:2165–70.
35. Leblanc A. The cranial nerves. Springer; 1995.
36. Libert J, Toussaint D, Guiselings R. Ocular findings in Niemann-Pick disease. Am J Ophthalmol. 1975;80:991–1002.
37. Lima Neto AC, Bittar R, Gattas GS, et al. Pathophysiology and Diagnosis of Vertebrobasilar Insufficiency: A Review of the Literature. Int Arch Otorhinolaryngol. 2017;21(3):302–7.
38. Natoli JL, Manack A, Dean B, et al. Global prevalence of chronic migraine: A systematic review. Cephalgia: An international journal of headache. 2010;10:599–609.
39. Nopoulos PC. Huntington disease: a single-gene degenerative disorder of the striatum. Dialogues Clin Neurosci. 2016;18:91–8.
40. Novak MJ, Tabrizi SJ. Huntington's disease. BMJ. 2010;340:3109.
41. Nowaczyk MJ, Clarke JT, Morin JD. Glaucoma as an early complication of Hurler's disease. Arch Dis Child. 1988;63:1091–3.
42. Oskoui M, Coutinho F, Dykeman J, et al. An update on the prevalence of cerebral palsy: a systematic review and meta-analysis. Dev Med Child Neurol. 2019;55:509–19.
43. Otravec J. Clinical neuroophthalmology. Prague: Grada; 2003.

44. Piane M, Lulli P, Farinelli I, et al. Wolff's headache and other head pain. Oxford University Press; 2001.
45. Pirau L, Lui F. Vertebrobasilar Insufficiency. StatPearls. Treasure Island (FL): StatPearls Publishing; 2020.
46. Rasmussen SA, Friedman JM. NF1 gene and neurofibromatosis 1. Am J Epidemiol. 2000;151:33–40.
47. Roos RA. Huntington's disease: a clinical review. Orphanet J Rare Dis. 2010;5:40.
48. Schumacher RG, Brzezinska R, Schulze-Frenking G, et al. Sonographic ocular findings in patients with mucopolysaccharidoses I. II and VI Pediatr Radiol. 2008;38:543–50.
49. Sorensen SA, Mulvihill JJ, Nielsen A. Long-term follow-up of von Recklinghausen neurofibromatosis. Survival and malignant neoplasms. N Engl J Med. 1986;314:1010–5.
50. Terelak-Borys B, Skonieczna K, Grabska-Liberek I. Ocular ischemic syndrome – a systematic review. Med Sci Monit. 2012;18(8):138–44.
51. Van der Hoeve J. Eye symptoms in phakomatoses (The Doyle Memorial Lecture). Trans Ophthalmol Soc. 1932;52:380–401.
52. Varma DD, Cugati S, Lee AW, et al. A review of central retinal artery occlusion: clinical presentation and management. Eye (Lond). 2013;27(6):688–97.
53. Walton C, King R, Rechtman L, et al. Rising prevalence of multiple sclerosis worldwide: Insights from the Atlas of MS, third edition. Mult Scler. 2020;26(14):1816–21.
54. Wingerchuk DM, Hogancamp WF, O'Brien PC, Weinshenker BG. The clinical course of neuromyelitis optica (Devic's syndrome). Neurology. 1999;53:1107–14.

Neurosurgical Diseases

Pavel Poczos©, Zdenek Kasl, Martin Matuska, Nada Jiraskova, and Tomas Cesak

The course of the visual pathway from the intraorbital compartment to the occipital cortex can be disrupted by a wide range of pathologies. Clinically, they are manifested not only in situations where they are localised directly in the visual pathway, but also in functionally associated areas, namely by compression due to oedema or obstruction of cerebrospinal fluid flow. The range of possible clinical manifestations is thus highly variable. In addition to the anatomically defined visual pathway, functionally important areas include the orbitofrontal cortex, brainstem nuclei, cerebellum, and some cranial nerves.

This chapter provides an overview of selected nosological entities that can attack the visual pathway, and at the same time, for which the neurosurgeon is often a major contributor to their treatment. It should be emphasised that the diagnosis and treatment of most of these pathologies require an interdisciplinary approach

---

P. Poczos (✉) · T. Cesak
Department of Neurosurgery, University Hospital and Faculty of Medicine of Charles University in Hradec Králové, Sokolska 581, 500 05 Hradec Králové, Czech Republic
e-mail: pavel.poczos@fnhk.cz

T. Cesak
e-mail: tomas.cesak@fnhk.cz

Z. Kasl · M. Matuska
Department of Ophthalmology, University Hospital and Faculty of Medicine in Plzen, E. Benese 1128, 301 00 Plzen, Czech Republic
e-mail: zdenekkasl@volny.cz

M. Matuska
e-mail: matuskam@fnplzen.cz

N. Jiraskova
Department of Ophthalmology, University Hospital and Faculty of Medicine of Charles University in Hradec Kralove, Sokolska 581, 500 05 Hradec Kralove, Czech Republic
e-mail: nada.jiraskova@fnhk.cz

© The Author(s), under exclusive license to Springer Nature Switzerland AG 2024
A. Stepanov and J. Studnicka (eds.), *Ocular Manifestations of Systemic Diseases*,
https://doi.org/10.1007/978-3-031-58592-0_11

involving not only ophthalmologists and neurosurgeons, but also radiologists, otorhinolaryngologists, pathologists, oncologists, and neurologists.

1 Selected Tumours of the CNS

Cancers represent a very diverse group of biologically distinct tumour types. Apart from *primary* tumours, the CNS may also contain *false tumours* (pseudotumours) and *secondary* brain tumours, *metastases.* The overall pooled incidence rate of primary brain tumors was found to be 10.82 per 100,000 person-years worldwide [7]. They represent 2% of all neoplasms [33]. Gliomas represent 40–50% of all intracranial tumours. Meningiomas (12–15%), secondary brain tumours (15–20%) and pituitary adenomas are also frequent, representing 10–15% of all intracranial tumours in clinical reports [25].

Brain tumours derived from tissues located under the pia mater, i.e. located inside the nervous parenchyma, are called *intra-axial. Extra-axial* tumours originate from tissues that surround the CNS externally from the pia mater (bone, hard diaper, arachnoid matter), or from formations that are anatomically clearly separated from the compact CNS mass (pituitary gland, cranial nerve sheaths, ependymal lining in intraventricular tumours).

According to anatomical localisation, brain tumours are divided into *supratentorial* (80–85%) and *infratentorial.* The latest classification of CNS tumours, updated by the World Health Organization (WHO) in 2016, uses for the first time molecular genetic characteristics (biomarkers) of tumour cells in addition to histopathological criteria [23, 33]. The description of the biological behaviour of tumours is made possible by what is called *grading.* Determination of the degree of brain tumour progression (staging) is not used. *Histological verification* based on immunohistochemistry is essential for the definitive diagnosis and correct treatment of all tumours [23]. In the hands of an experienced neuropathologist, it provides important information about the biological behaviour of the brain tumour, which is another clue for a complex treatment.

Incorrect radiological interpretation of brain *tumour-like lesions* can lead to inadequate therapy, often in the sense of over-active treatment. Such lesions include brain abscesses, cerebritis, ischaemia, intraparenchymal cerebral haemorrhages, vasculitis, demyelination, post-radiation necrosis, deposits of pathological material (amyloidoma, calcification), etc. [20].

Some *orbital tumour and non-tumour lesions* arising from structures other than the optic nerves and their sheaths, which may have a significant impact on visual function, should also be pointed out. These include metastases, angiogenic expansions (cavernomas, solitary fibrous tumour—haemangiopericytoma), peripheral nerve tumours (neurofibromas, schwannomas), mesenchymal tumours (fibrous histiocytoma), lacrimal gland tumours, inflammatory pseudotumour and others [27, 44].

Neurosurgical Diseases   449

1.1 Ocular Manifestations of Tumours of the CNS

From the ophthalmologist's point of view, the symptoms of CNS tumours can be divided into groups that depend on several factors—in particular, the location of the tumour, its size, aggressiveness, and growth rate.

Symptoms Caused by Intracranial Hypertension

Intracranial hypertension is a condition associated with an increase in intracranial pressure. Its most common causes include intracranial expansion (tumours, haematomas, cysts, abscesses), closure of the cerebrospinal fluid outflow tract with hydrocephalus, disturbance of the balance of cerebrospinal fluid production and absorption (idiopathic intracranial hypertension) or disorders of venous outflow from the brain. Symptoms arising because of increased intracranial pressure may or may not be associated with other focal neurological symptoms. The most common complaints of patients with intracranial hypertension include chronic, diffuse pressure-type headache, which may be exacerbated by coughing or the Valsava manoeuvre and sometimes by lying down. Vomiting is another symptom, and morning vomiting without previous nausea is particularly suspicious. Other general symptoms may include slowed psychomotor pace, increased fatigue, and memory impairment.

Symptoms from Optic Pathway Compression

Unlike intracranial hypertension, compressive lesions of the optic pathway often have significant localising value, because of its specific arrangement and the typical perimetric findings in affections in its various compartments. When the optic nerve is oppressed in the *prechiasmatic* part of the optic pathway before its entry into the chiasm (e.g. by intracanalicular meningioma in the optic canal or extrasellar propagation of pituitary adenoma), monocular visual field disturbances occur on the side of the lesion. In compressive *lesions of the chiasm* (most commonly pituitary adenoma, more rarely craniopharyngioma or tuberculum sellae meningioma), typical temporal visual field disruptions of bitemporal hemianopsia character arise from the lesion of the crossing fibres of the optic pathway. These defects usually start in the upper quadrants and spread to the lower quadrants and further nasally as the lesion continues to grow. Damage to the retrochiasmatic portion of the optic pathway (tractus opticus, corpus geniculatum laterale, radiatio optica, and visual cortex of the occipital lobe) is manifested by homonymous contralateral hemianopsia. The defects in the visual field of both eyes are always on the side opposite to the tumour location and their congruence (lateral symmetry) increases dorsally—when the tumour is located occipitally, the defects are congruent, whereas, in the case of optic tract compression, they may differ significantly laterally. In contrast to ischaemic lesions in the optic pathway, compressive lesions develop slowly and gradually, the patient often adapts to them spontaneously and is usually unaware of the visual field impairment to some extent.

Involvement of the Peripheral Nerves and Their Nuclei

Another possible ophthalmological manifestation of intraocular tumour is compression with involvement of the optic nerves, possibly their nuclei, and resulting paralytic strabismus, which usually causes diplopia. The compression may involve one or more oculomotor nerves and the clinical presentation and anamnesis can often be used to estimate the approximate location and biological nature of the neoplasm. When the tumour is located *infratentorially*, especially in the pontine and medulla oblongata, combined, often bilateral paresis of the optic nerve nuclei is present due to compression of the optic nerve nuclei. These pareses are often associated with other neurological symptoms caused by the compression of structures in this locality. *Supratentorial* tumours may cause paresis of the intracranial nerves, either by direct compression anywhere in their course, or indirectly by compression caused by intracranial hypertension. From a clinical point of view, paresis of n. III arising at the *temporal conus* is significant. The condition in this case is caused by significant overpressure in the supratentorial space, which displaces the base of the temporal lobe below the tentorium cerebelli. The first sign of this serious and potentially life-threatening condition is the sudden onset of homolateral mydriasis with unresponsive pupillary reaction caused by compression of the internal branch of n. III. With a further increase in pressure, complete paresis of the same-sided n. III follows; further, due to compression and dislocation of the brainstem, there is a risk of unconsciousness and death of the patient.

Direct Intraorbital Tumour Propagation

A rarer ocular manifestation of intracranial tumour is its direct growth into the orbit. In this case, the foreground of the clinical presentation is most often a progressive exophthalmos, which may be accompanied by diplopia in some visual directions by mechanical restriction of the motility of the globe or optic nerve compression at the orbital tip. This finding is most common in meningiomas (sheaths of the optic nerve, wings of the sphenoid bone) or gliomas of the optic nerve, which are typical in patients with neurofibromatosis.

Objective Findings

From the objective eye examination, the most significant finding is the *papilledema* on the eye fundus. It is a bilateral swelling of optic disc, sometimes asymmetrical, usually without associated haemorrhages in the surroundings or cotton wool spots. The clinical presentation depends on the duration of the intracranial hypertension—from images of developing oedema with blurred edges of the nasal side of the optic disc through fully developed bilateral optic disc oedema of varying prominence. The Frisen scale and disc prominence measurements are used to determine the degree of oedema. Among modern imaging methods, optical coherence tomography has contributed to ophthalmic diagnosis. Partial or complete optic nerve atrophy may develop with prolonged duration of optic atrophy. A less common ophthalmological manifestation of intracranial hypertension, which may occur alone or may also accompany the papilledema, is unilateral or bilateral paresis of n. VI. It is caused by

Neurosurgical Diseases 451

compression of the nerve by increased intracranial pressure at the predilection sites of its course. Thus, the picture of intracranial hypertension is a non-specific finding that points to intracranial pathology, but without further investigations it does not say anything about its biological nature or localisation.

1.2 Pituitary Adenomas, Rathke's Cleft Cyst

Pituitary adenomas (also known as pituitary neuroendocrine tumors - PitNETs) represent 12–17% of all primary intracranial tumours. They affect both sexes at approximately the same rate and occur most frequently in the 3rd–4th decade of life. In the population over 65 years of age, they are the *third most common intracranial neoplasm*. Their prevalence in the general population is estimated at 20 cases/100,000 person-years and the incidence varies between 1.5–2 new cases/100,000 person-years [5, 31]. The latest WHO classification of endocrine tumours remains based on immunohistochemical classification of tumours through the identification of hormones and transcription factors characteristic of each lineage of cell differentiation [36]. Pituitary adenomas are benign tumours arising from secretory cells of the adenohypophysis. In terms of hormone production, they are divided into *functional*, hormonally active, and *afunctional*, hormonally inactive. According to size, they are divided into *microadenomas* (up to 1 cm), *macroadenomas* (1–4 cm) and *giant adenomas* (over 4 cm).

Seven basic tumour subtypes are defined based on immunohistochemical examination (see below). If immunohistochemistry demonstrates the presence of hormone production without clinical response, such tumours are termed "*silent*" adenomas [36]. The most frequent type of functional adenoma is the lactotropic adenoma or *prolactinoma* (25–40%) (Fig. 1), which has a marked predominance in the female population (lit).

Somatotroph adenomas represent the second most common pituitary tumours (10–20%). The frequency of 1% places *thyrotrophinomas* (thyrotropin secreting adenomas) among very rare lesions. *Corticotroph adenomas* are more common in women, with a 5:1 ratio. It accounts for 10–15% of all pituitary tumours, as do *gonadotrophinomas* (gonadotroph adenomas) [5]. Adenomas without identifiable hormone production (known as *null cell adenomas*) have accounted for up to 25% of all cases in the past. However, in most of these cases, the presence of transcription factors corresponding to the gonadotropic lineage or, less frequently, the corticotropic lineage can be demonstrated. *Plurihormonal* and *dual adenomas* (1–3%) are characterised by the production of hormones from at least two lineages of differentiation [36]. A rare but serious cause of optic chiasm compression is *apoplexy* (Fig. 2), which is haemorrhage into the tumour or into ischaemically altered pituitary tissue.

Rathke's cleft cysts arising from embryonic remnants of Rathke's cleft in the pars intermedia of the pituitary gland are a relatively common incidental finding at autopsy in 13–26% of cases [17]. Usually, they manifest when they reach larger size. The therapeutic method of choice is surgical evacuation of the cyst.

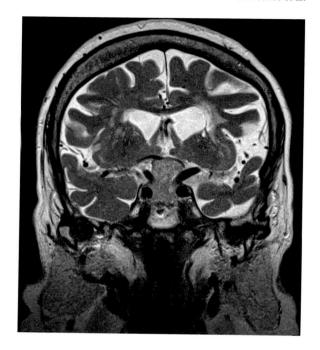

Fig. 1 Pituitary macroprolactinoma with significant suprasellar promotion. T2-weighted MRI image

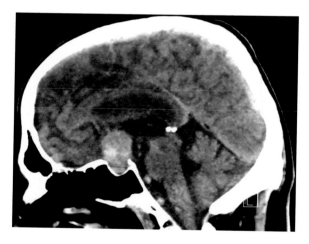

Fig. 2 Apoplexy into a null cell adenoma with evidence of transcription factors consistent with gonadotropic lineage. Native CT image

Risk Factors

- Age
- Multiple endocrine neoplasia syndrome (especially MEN-1)

Clinical Presentation

In addition to typical symptoms, such as specific hormonal and visual disturbances, it is occasionally necessary to look for symptoms of compression/invasion of the cavernous sinus (trigeminal neuralgia or retroorbital pain), hypothalamus (diencephalic syndrome) or third ventricle (obstructive hydrocephalus).

Among hormonal disorders, hyperfunction syndromes are particularly clinically striking. The time of onset of *growth hormone (STH) overproduction* predetermines the clinical manifestations. In childhood, there is a general abnormal growth with manifestations of gigantism. In adults, the term acromegaly is used. The manifestations of *hyperprolactinaemia* are disturbances of the menstrual cycle and sexual dysfunction. In males, impotence and decreased libido occur, and in both sexes, infertility. A rise in peripheral hormones originating from the adrenal medulla based on ACTH overproduction leads to *Cushing's disease.* Its manifestations include a moon-like face, fatty hump, purplish stretch marks on the abdomen, protein catabolism, increased bone resorption, psychological disorders with depression, anxiety, difficult correction of arterial hypertension, diabetes mellitus, etc. *Hyperthyroidism* is associated with weight loss, tachycardia and heat intolerance. *Increased production of gonadotropins*, luteinising (LH) and follicle-stimulating (FSH), is clinically manifested only rarely, in women by abdominal pain in ovarian hyperstimulation. Reduced hormone production by pituitary cells—hypopituitarism—results in insufficient hormone production by peripheral glands. The deficiency of individual hormones can lead to disturbances in the menstrual cycle, to a decline in the sexual sphere, nanism, inefficiency of the organism, increased fatigue, muscle weakness, etc. Pathologies of the infundibulum or posterior lobe of the pituitary gland led to insufficient production of antidiuretic hormone (ADH), which is the cause of *diabetes insipidus.*

Diagnosis

Clinical findings and *hormonal examination* often let us guess the type of pituitary adenoma. The presence of calcifications on computed tomography (CT) may help to differentiate adenoma from craniopharyngioma. *Magnetic resonance imaging* (MRI) is the method of choice in the diagnosis and monitoring of sellar pathologies (Fig. 1). It is also helpful in the evaluation of optic nerve atrophy. Rathke's cleft cysts mimic cystically degenerated pituitary adenomas. *Optical coherence tomography* (OCT) (Fig. 3) provides a well-reproducible image of a cross-section through the retina [21, 29].

It has been shown that there is a correlation between the thickness of the peripapillary retinal nerve fibre layer (RNFL) or perifoveal ganglion cell layer (GCL) and defects in the visual field due to compression of the chiasm. In addition to OCT, visual evoked potentials can also be used [32].

Differential Diagnosis

- Craniopharyngiomas, meningiomas, metastases
- Arachnoid cyst, Rathke's cleft cyst

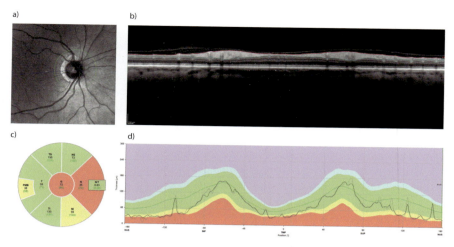

Fig. 3 OCT examination of the retina of the right eye before surgical decompression of the chiasma in a 65-year-old woman. Peripapillary RNFL measurements are along the green circle (**A**). The profile of the retinal layers along the indicated trajectory is shown in panel (**B**), which also shows the inner limiting membrane and the interface between the axonal fibre layer and the retinal ganglion cell bodies. The difference between the two profiles constitutes the thickness of the peripapillary RNFL and is shown in panel (D) as a thicker line running in the green band depicting normal values for the age group. The mean and normative values of RNFL thickness in the nasal and temporal quadrants and their superior and inferior parts, together with the global value, are shown in panel (**C**)

- Pituitary inflammation, tumours of the posterior lobe of the pituitary gland
- Pituitary hyperplasia, optic nerve glioma, apoplexy

Therapy

In prolactinoma, the treatment is primarily *pharmacological*, which consists of administration of dopaminergic agonists (bromocriptine, cabergoline). In the case of somatotroph adenoma, surgical therapy is performed in conjunction with treatment with somatostatin analogues [15]. In other tumour subtypes, the primary treatment is *surgical removal* of the lesion, especially by endoscopic transnasal approach. A third treatment option is *radiosurgery*. For small lesions without endocrinologic manifestation, *observation* is a legitimate treatment modality [5, 28, 31].

1.3 Ocular Manifestations of Pituitary Adenomas

Clinically, the picture includes endocrine and neuro-ophthalmological symptoms. Endocrine varies according to the type of tumour. The neuro-ophthalmological symptoms are mainly due to compressive lesions of the optic pathway, especially the chiasm. *Bitemporal hemianopsia* is therefore the most common symptom of pituitary

Neurosurgical Diseases

adenomas. It is usually caused by symmetrical compression of the inferior surface of the chiasm in the midline by suprasellar propagation of the adenoma. This results in a bitemporal hemianopsia with a very typical evolution. The visual excursions begin in the upper temporal quadrants and then continue into the lower temporal quadrants to complete bitemporal hemianopsia, respecting usually quite precisely the vertical meridian. About two-thirds of pituitary adenomas show this development, while, in the remaining one-third, we observe greater or lesser atypia in the perimetric findings, due either to different topographic relations of the chiasm to the saddle or pituitary or to asymmetric growth of the adenoma. Ophthalmoplegic forms of pituitary adenoma symptoms are rare and can be divided into three groups. The *first group* consists of the parasellar cavernous sinus syndrome, involving oculomotor nerve palsy associated with irritation-obliterating lesions of the trigeminal ganglion, which arise from parasellar propagation of a tumour separated from the cavernous sinus by only a thin dural wall. The lesion is usually unilateral, and the ophthalmic nerves may be affected in various combinations, ranging from isolated paresis of the abducens to total ophthalmoplegia. *The second group* is oculomotor disorders combined with chiasmatic syndrome with visual impairment. They occur in two variants. The first one, with peracute onset and usually bilateral symptomatology, is a rare pituitary apoplexy. The second, more frequent variant, with progressive development of oculomotor and visual impairment, is caused by extremely large adenomas and recurrent tumours with a tendency to infiltrative growth. *The last* diverse *group* consists of oculomotor disorders with an indirect relationship to pituitary adenoma.

Pituitary apoplexy is a relatively common finding on MRI, but clinical signs are rare. It is characterised by a peculiar picture and often very dramatic evolution, with acute life-threatening risk. It is usually triggered by the sudden rapid expansion of a necrotic or vascularised adenoma whose growth is faster than the existing blood supply. The expansion is directed laterally and upwards and oppresses not only the peripheral nerves and the optic pathway, but often also the hypothalamic vital centres at the base of the third ventricle. When it extends into the liquor pathways, a picture of subarachnoid haemorrhage emerges. The **clinical presentation** includes sudden sharp pain in the forehead or behind the eyes, collapse to coma, often with meningeal symptoms. Ocular symptoms include rapidly developing bilateral severe visual impairment and external eye muscle palsy. Blood, xanthochromia, pleocytosis and elevated protein are found in the liquor.

Treatment of pituitary tumours is divided into two groups: pharmacological and surgical. Prolactinomas overwhelmingly respond favourably to the administration of dopamine agonists. Figure 4 shows the field of view and Fig. 5 shows a CT scan of patient with prolactinomas before treatment.

After one month of treatment with Dostinex tbl. at a dose of 1 mg twice weekly with replacement therapy with hydrocortisone, thyroxine and testosterone, there was almost complete regression of the tumour portion in the suprasellar region (Fig. 6) and correction of the visual field after 5 months (Fig. 7).

Tumours that do not respond to medical therapy are indicated for surgical treatment of pituitary adenomas.

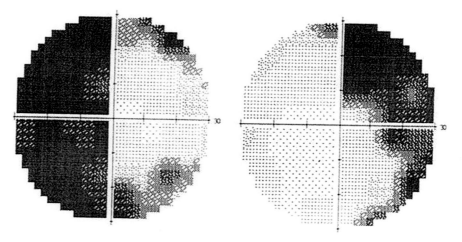

Fig. 4 Perimeter of a patient with pituitary prolactinoma before treatment

Fig. 5 CT brain of a patient with pituitary prolactinoma before treatment

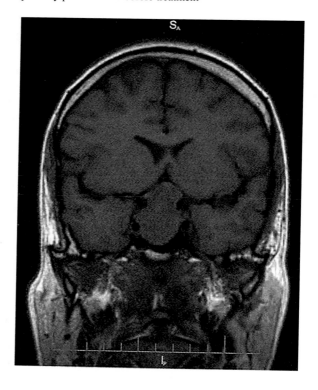

Neurosurgical Diseases

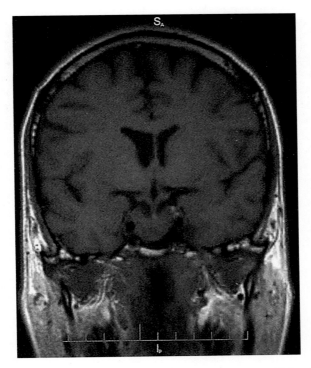

Fig. 6 CT brain of a patient with pituitary prolactinoma after treatment with Dostinex tbl

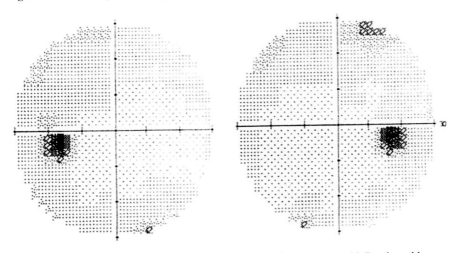

Fig. 7 Perimeter of a patient with pituitary prolactinoma after treatment with Dostinex tbl

1.4 Craniopharyngioma

Craniopharyngioma is a benign tumour that is one of the most common extra-axial tumours in childhood and adolescence (up to 10%). It represents 2–5% of all primary intracranial tumours in adults. Its incidence varies from 0.05–0.2/100,000 person-years. There are theories claiming that craniopharyngioma grows from embryonic remnants of Rathke's cleft, but others lean towards an origin from metaplastically altered adenohypophysis cells [8]. It is characterised by the formation of cystic-solid formations in the region of the Turkish chair (Fig. 8A, B), often with the presence of lumpy calcifications. There are *no* known *predisposing risk factors* for craniopharyngiomas.

Clinical Presentation

Given the location, the clinical manifestations are relatively varied. Typical visual disturbances range from sectoral visual field loss to blindness, panhypopituitarism, including diabetes insipidus, and growth retardation in children. Symptoms of intracranial hypertension are also common.

Diagnosis

The gold standard is *MRI* (Fig. 8A, B). CT is used to detect typical intralesional calcifications.

Differential Diagnosis

- Pituitary adenomas
- Chordoma, germ cell tumours, dermoid

Therapy

In the first place, radical *surgical extirpation*. The role of fractionated RT is somewhat controversial due to its numerous side effects [8]. Postoperative residuals can not only be monitored, reoperated, but also treated with *radiosurgery*.

1.5 Ocular Manifestations of Craniopharyngioma

The *clinical presentation* is very varied. In addition to the age of the patient and the localisation of the tumour, the cystic nature of the tumour is particularly important. In childhood, the clinical presentation is dominated by symptoms of intracranial hypertension due to internal hydrocephalus, in young individuals especially by endocrine disorders, and in the elderly by symptoms of chiasmal compression.

Craniopharyngioma in children is one of the most common intracranial tumours of this age. The disease begins with rapidly progressive symptoms of intracranial hypertension from internal hydrocephalus, manifested by headache with vomiting and massive congestion at the optic disc. In young children, we find characteristic

Neurosurgical Diseases

Fig. 8 A Cystoid adamantinomatous craniopharyngioma, partially vascularized, oppressive optic chiasm. T1-weighted MRI image. **B** Cystoid adamantinomatous craniopharyngioma, partially vascularized, oppressive optic chiasm. T1-weighted MRI image

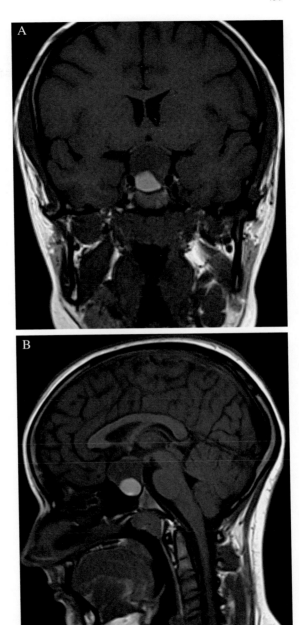

spacing of the cranial sutures. The cause is occlusion of the foramen interventriculare Monroi by suprasellar tumour promotion. The lesion, especially if not diagnosed early, seriously compromises visual function. Even in adolescents and young adults, craniopharyngioma represents the *most common* intracranial tumour. In addition to the symptoms of intracranial hypertension and chiasma compression, endocrinological signs of diencephalophysial insufficiency are prominent. Symptoms of chiasm compression are extremely varied, ranging from unilateral central scotoma to hemianopsia of various types, laterally markedly asymmetric and characterised by rapid progression. Their evolution is often fluctuating, accompanied by repeated transient improvement and new recurrence of the disorder. Craniopharyngioma in elderly individuals is characterised by bitemporal hemianopsia; endocrine signs and intracranial hypertension syndrome are often absent.

1.6 Meningiomas

Meningiomas are predominantly benign, slow-growing extra-axial tumours originated from arachnoid cells. In most cases, they are fixed to the dura mater, but there are also intraventricular meningiomas. According to histology and biological behaviour, they are divided into *meningioma* (grade I), *atypical meningioma* (grade II) and *anaplastic meningioma* (grade III) showing histologically clear signs of malignancy [2]. A description of the individual histological variants, of which there are 14, is beyond the scope of this subchapter. Meningiomas account for 14–20% of all primary intracranial tumours, with a peak incidence around the age of 45. The incidence in the population is reported to range between 2–6 cases/100,000 person-years. The incidence is higher in women [17, 48]. Approximately 1–4% of meningiomas occur in childhood and, of these, approximately one-quarter are associated with neurofibromatosis type 1 (NF1), which is also characterised by multiple localisations. The presence of, for example, *oestrogen, progesterone* and/or *androgen receptors* on tumour cells suggests that hormone therapy also may influence the development and growth of meningiomas [17].

The most common *locations* of meningiomas are *parasagittal* (21%) and *convexity* (15%). However, from an ophthalmological perspective, the *tuberculum sellae/ diaphragma sellae* (up to 13% of meningiomas) (Fig. 9), *the sphenoidal ridge* together with *the anterior clinoid process* (20–25%), and *the optic nerve sheath* are important sites of occurrence. Meningiomas localised in the cavernous sinus may grow primarily from the sinus, or the sinus may be invaded secondarily from the surrounding area. Up to 8% of meningiomas occur multifocally [2, 17].

Tuberculum sellae meningiomas (Fig. 9) often mimic suprasellar extension of pituitary tumours. In *clinoid* and *medial variants of meningiomas of the lesser wing of the sphenoid bone*, there is often invasion of surrounding anatomical structures (superior orbital fissure, orbit, and cavernous sinus), which in turn can result in a diverse range of neurological symptoms.

Neurosurgical Diseases

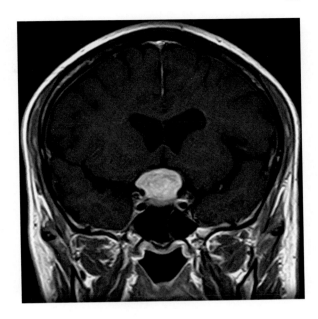

Fig. 9 Meningothelial meningioma (WHO grade I) of the tubercle of the saddle and anterior clinoid process on the right. T1-weighted MRI image after contrast agent administration

The so-called *spheno-orbital meningiomas* are characterised by dominant intraosseous involvement of the sphenoid bone wing, with intracranial propagation at a form of a flat "en plaque" soft tissue component (Fig. 10A, B). In this case, it's the optic nerve sheath are itself is not affected by the tumour.

Optic nerve sheath meningiomas account for approximately one-third of all optic nerve neoplasms, about 2% of all orbital tumours, and 1–2% of all meningiomas. Meningioma of the optic nerve sheath may occur throughout the nerve's intraorbital course. It typically spreads circumferentially around the optic nerve, which has a significant impact on its pial vascular supply and axonal transport. Up to 25% of optic nerve meningiomas occur in children, where tumour behaviour tends to be more aggressive. However, most orbital meningiomas are represented by primary intracranial tumours with secondary intraorbital propagation [1].

Risk Factors

- Female gender
- Radiation
- Hormone therapy, NF1 and 2
- Aberrations in the long arm of chromosome 22

Clinical Presentation

If meningiomas are not clinically mute, then their symptoms are non-specific. They include chronic headache, often with a sight predilection, increased fatigue, or focal deficit (see CNS neurological diseases). Bulky suprasellar spreading meningiomas are associated with visual field or pituitary or hypothalamic disorders. Exophthalmos

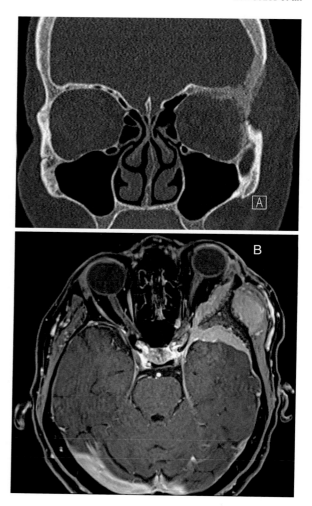

Fig. 10 A Atypical sphenoorbital meningioma (WHO grade II) on the left. CT image. **B** Atypical sphenoorbital meningioma (WHO grade II) on the left. T1-weighted MRI image after contrast agent administration

often alerts us to the presence of spheno-orbital meningiomas. The Walsh triad is pathognomonic for optic nerve meningiomas.

Diagnosis

Calcifications, typical for some meningiomas, extra-axial growth (Fig. 10A) or displacement of midline structures are readily apparent on *CT*.

"Dural tail" is a common finding. The typical tram track sign, is caused by parallel thickening and enhancement around the optic nerve, is often found in optic nerve meningiomas. *DSA* provides valuable information about the relationship to surrounding vessels and highlights the potential hypervascularisation of the process. It can also mitigate this hypervascularisation preoperatively by using embolization material to facilitate tumour resection.

Neurosurgical Diseases

Differential Diagnosis

- Various pituitary pathologies, metastases
- Gliomas of the optic nerve or hypothalamus, chordoma, epidermoid
- Bone abnormalities (chondromyxoid fibroma, osteoma)
- Vascular lesions (aneurysm, carotid-cavernous fistula).

Therapy

Surgical removal including the infiltrated dura is the treatment of choice for symptomatic meningiomas. Prognosis of the disease is influenced not only by the surgical radicality, but also by the histological character and biological behaviour of the tumour [2]. *Radiosurgery* is indicated especially for smaller, slow-growing lesions in surgically hardly accessible areas or in elderly patients. For larger processes, conventional fractionated *RT* is also used. The 5-year survival rate for benign forms varies between 70 and 90% [17].

In the case of *optic nerve sheath meningiomas*, surgical removal is indicated mainly when intracranial spread is present or when the chiasma and contralateral optic nerve are compromised. Optic nerve decompression following a longitudinal fenestration of the affected sheath often leads to further paradoxical visual deterioration. The primary treatment for optic nerve sheath meningiomas is *observation* or fractionated *radiosurgery* [1, 17].

1.7 Ocular Manifestations of Meningiomas

Meningioma of the sheath of the optic nerve can arise at any distance behind the bulb. In most cases, the nerve regrows circumferentially, or the dural sheath may become perforated and form an exophytic nodule. It may gradually fill the entire space of the muscular cone and penetrate the orbital wall. In the *clinical presentation*, the main symptom is a very slowly increasing axial exophthalmos. In late stages, visual impairment or oculomotor disorders may occur. The optic nerve disc is often swollen.

Canalicular meningiomas are rare dwarf tumours located in the optic canal. The only symptom is a slowly progressive loss of visual functions. Even with current diagnostic possibilities, the tumour is often not correctly diagnosed and is only detected during exploratory craniotomy.

Meningioma tuberculi sellae is one of the major suprasellar tumours that pushes the chiasm upward and backward. In the clinical presentation, the first, and often for a long time the only, symptom is usually a decrease in visual acuity in one eye due to central scotoma, which slowly but steadily progresses. Unfortunately, the slow progression of the disorder is often not even noticed by the patient himself and he sees a doctor only when the vision of the other eye deteriorates. At this stage, the characteristic finding is blindness of one eye and temporal hemianopsia of the other eye. On the fundus of the eye there is mostly simple optic disc atrophy, unilateral or laterally asymmetric. Endocrine or other neurological signs are usually absent, the saddle is not enlarged, but there is usually a distinct hyperostosis of the saddle hump and possibly of the planum sphenoideum.

Meningioma of the lesser wing or sphenoid rim is much more common and its neuro-ophthalmological symptomatology more varied and significant. This parasellar tumour is divided into internal, medial and external variants, according to its localisation on the sphenoidal rim. The *clinical presentation* of the internal variant is dominated by symptoms of optic nerve compressive lesions, superior orbital fissure syndrome and cavernous sinus with varying degrees of involvement of all three orbital nerves and the 1st branch of the trigeminus, and slowly progressive axial protrusion of the eye. In addition to exophthalmos, the external variant is mainly characterised by a prominent bulging of the temporal fossa. It is caused by a flat meningioma of the outer third of the sphenoid rim, ending in a point called the pterion. The tumour infiltrates the greater wing of the sphenoid bone, and often massive reactive hyperostosis dislocates the temporal fossa, but also reduces the orbital space and dislocates the bulbus. The development varies individually.

1.8 Gliomas—Supratentorial Localization

Neuroepithelial tumours are the most common intra-axial primary brain tumours, divided into three main groups according to differentiation lineage: astrocytic, oligodendroglial (also known collectively as gliomas) and ependymal tumours. From previous classifications, the terms "low grade" and "high grade" tumours established in the clinical community are getting abandoned in favour of the terms "lower/higher grade". WHO grade I borderline gliomas are represented by pilocytic astrocytoma. Diffusely infiltrating gliomas with WHO grades II–IV are represented by diffuse astrocytoma, oligodendroglioma, anaplastic astrocytoma, and glioblastoma (Figs. 11A, B, 12) [33, 43].

Gliomas account for 75% of all malignant brain tumours. Half of these are glioblastomas. Lower grade tumours are neoplasms more typical of younger age groups (mean age 40 years). They are characterised by slow growth and minimal clinical symptoms. Pilocytic astrocytomas (grade I) are minimally invasive and rarely malignant. It is the second most common tumour in childhood. *Ependymomas* account for approximately 5% of all gliomas and 9% of childhood brain tumours. They occur along the entire length of the neural axis, in the ventricular system in about 70% of cases [25].

Risk Factors

- Genetic predisposition syndromes (e.g. NF1 or 2, Li-Fraumenni syndrome)
- Ionising radiation

Clinical Presentation

Symptoms are divided into *focal* (related to a specific localisation in brain tissue) or *general*. General symptoms are mainly due to intracranial hypertension. It is

Neurosurgical Diseases

Fig. 11 A Glial tumour, histologically borderline between low grade (diffuse) astrocytoma (WHO grade II) and anaplastic astrocytoma (WHO grade III) temporomedially on the left, without opacification after contrast agent administration. T2 FLAIR MRI image. *MRI* with contrast remains the gold standard (Figs. 10B, 11A, B). **b** Glial tumour. T1 weighted MRI image after contrast agent administration

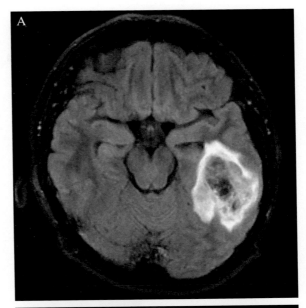

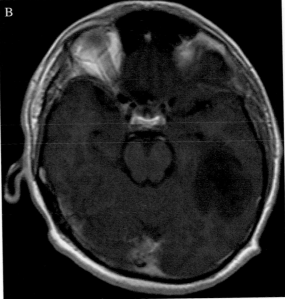

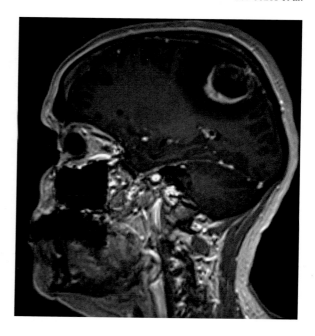

Fig. 12 Multiform glioblastoma (WHO grade IV) parietally on the left. T1 weighted MRI image after contrast agent administration

manifested by headache (30%) and vomiting, mainly in the morning, mental and consciousness disturbances. Localization in some functionally more important areas leads to focal neurological deficits. The first symptoms are most often seizures, sensorimotor deficits and speech disorders [9, 48].

Frontal lobe tumours can cause paresis/plegia, expressive (Broca's) aphasia, dysfunction of the prefrontal cortex (emotional lability, apathy, indifference, incontinence, etc.). *Parietal lobe* involvement can lead to sensory deficits, hemineglect, anosognosia, spatial orientation disorder, apraxia, sensory (Wernicke's) aphasia, acalculia, agraphia, etc. Cortical deafness, personality and mood disorders, short-term memory loss, olfactory hallucinations are typical of *temporal lobe* involvement. Optic radiation damage in the *occipital lobes* may lead to visual hallucinations/illusions with or without prosopagnosia (the affected person does not recognise faces). Damage to the *corpus callosum* will manifest as cognitive dysfunction.

Diagnosis

The method of choice in the diagnosis of gliomas is *MRI* with administration of a contrast agent (gadolinium) (Figs. 11B, 12). Multimodal sequential methods, such as diffusion-weighted imaging (DWI) or diffusion tensor imaging (DTI), functional MRI, MRI perfusion imaging, MRI spectroscopy, and others are used to better characterise cellularity, vascularity, and tumour metabolism. They contribute to differentiate tumours from tumour-like processes. *Computed tomography* contributes to better determination of the relationship of the tumour to bony structures. Contrast administration with the possibility of three-dimensional reconstructions shows the

Neurosurgical Diseases 467

cerebral vasculature (*CT angiography*). Digital subtraction angiography (*DSA*) is performed in highly vascularised tumours, with the possibility of preoperative embolization (skull base tumours), or in lesions with a close relationship to important vascular structures. Positron emission tomography (*PET*) used to determine metabolic changes in the tumour tissue, allows distinguish between tumour recurrence and postradiotherapy changes.

Differential Diagnosis

- Metastases, primary lymphoma of the CNS
- Embryonal tumours, meningiomas, tumour-like lesions

Therapy

The therapeutic strategy for glial processes depends on the size, localization, biological nature of the tumour, age, and general condition of the patient. The main therapeutic options include *surgical resection*, followed by radiotherapy (*RT*) and chemotherapy (*CT*). *Immunotherapy* and *gene therapy* can be also helpful. Another option (for low grade tumours) is *observation* (wait-and-scan). Surgical resections are refined using navigation and ultrasound (*US*). Perioperative monitoring using *electrophysiological techniques* (somatosensory and motor evoked potentials, cortical stimulation) significantly contributes not only to increase the extent of resection, but also to increase the safety of the surgical procedure, especially if it concerns functionally important brain area [25]. The *awake surgery*, where the patient is awakened at a certain stage of the procedure, is performed mainly in tumours located in speech or important motricity regions. For *higher grade gliomas*, surgical cytoreduction followed by RT or concomitant CHT with temozolomide is indicated. In some cases, targeted radiation with stereotactic RT may be considered. In recent years, *biological intratumoural therapies* have also come into use [25].

1.9 Ocular Manifestations of Supratentorial Tumours

Clinical manifestations of supratentorial tumours should be divided according to the brain lobes in which the tumour is located. *Frontal lobe* tumours, due to the absence of vital centres, are often clinically silent for a long time and, from the ophthalmologist's point of view, most often manifest only with symptoms of intracranial hypertension. Rarely, they may manifest with supranuclear gaze palsy and conjugate deviation of the eyes laterally.

Lesions of the *parietal* and *temporal lobes* are most often manifested optically by homonymous contralateral quadrantopsia to hemianopsia due to compression of the radiatio optica. Parietal lobe lesions may have associated tracking movement disorders and asymmetry of optokinetic nystagmus gain.

Occipital lobe tumours typically manifest with congruent homonymous hemianoptic discharges of varying magnitude; when the tumour is located near the midline, these discharges may be bilateral. Further subdivision of supratentorial tumours listed below is on histological and anatomical bases.

Neuroepithelial Tumours

Neuroepithelial tumours arise from the supporting brain cells of the glia. These tumours include mainly *astrocytic* tumours, as well as *oligodendroglial* and *ependymal* tumours. This is a broad group of tumours with different predilection localisation and biological nature. Astrocytic tumours are the most common, with four histological forms, ranging from grade I pilocytic astrocytoma to grade IV glioblastoma multiforme. The clinical manifestation depends on the localisation of the tumour, its growth rate and its biological nature. Therapy is mainly surgical, but adjuvant chemo- or radiotherapy is also possible. High-grade gliomas have a poor prognosis and most patients die within months to years.

Choroid Plexus Tumours

Choroid plexus tumours are rare, intraventricularly localised masses arising from the tissue of the choroid plexus, where cerebrospinal fluid is formed under physiological circumstances. These tumours are more frequent in childhood. Histologically, papilloma is the most common variant, carcinoma is rarer. Clinically, they usually manifest symptoms of intracranial hypertension in hydrocephalus. Direct obstruction of the liquor pathways of the tumour tissues, increased production of cerebrospinal fluid or its impaired absorption due to intraventricular haemorrhages may be involved in the development of hydrocephalus. Therapy is surgical, with a good prognosis with complete excision, especially for papillomas.

Embryonal Tumours

These are tumours typical of childhood arising from poorly differentiated cells. The highest incidence is in children under 5 years of age. The most common are medulloblastoma and ependymoblastoma. Depending on the localisation, they manifest with symptoms of intracranial hypertension or focal neurological symptoms. Due to their high malignancy, the prognosis is often poor, despite combined surgical treatment with chemo- or radiotherapy.

1.10 Gliomas of the Optic Nerve and Chiasma

Optic pathway gliomas include gliomas of the optic tract and hypothalamus. They are usually of lower histological grade, predominantly occur in the paediatric population and affect the precortical segment of the optic pathway. They may be sporadic or associated with NF1 in up to one-third of cases [14]. Optic nerve gliomas are the most common primary tumours of the optic nerve, accounting for 2–3% of orbital tumours. The peak incidence is in the first decade of life. 15–20% of patients with NF1 have an optic nerve glioma demonstrated on MRI, but only 1–5% are symptomatic. The presence of NF1 is a favourable prognostic feature,these patients usually have a less aggressive disease course. The majority of these are pilocytic and diffuse astrocytomas (Fig. 13A, B). Tumours of the chiasmatic-hypothalamic region have an increased risk of dissemination [10].

Risk Factors

- NF1
- Child age, female gender

Clinical Presentation

Bulky tumours, growing mainly from the chiasm and the beginning of the optic tract, cause hypothalamic and pituitary dysfunctions. The literature refers is as the diencephalic Russell syndrome (progressive weight loss with vomiting, precocious puberty with hydrocephalus) [17].

Diagnosis

Optic gliomas can be diagnosed above all mostly by *MRI* (Fig. 13A–C). When the optic nerve is affected, solid enlargement of the nerve predominates. In contrast, more centripetally located tumours often contain a cystic component. Bioptic verification is not required in cases with a typical clinical and graphic picture of optic pathway involvement [10].

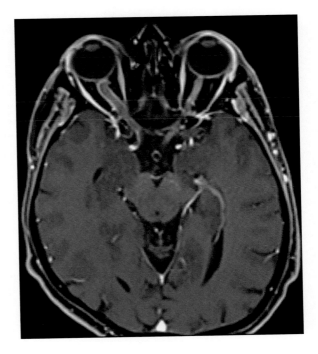

Fig. 13 Optic nerve glioma on the right in a patient with neurofibromatosis type 1. T1-weighted MRI image after contrast agent administration

Differential Diagnosis

- Haemangioma, lymphoma
- Fibrous dysplasia (pseudotumours)
- Pituitary adenoma, craniopharyngioma, meningioma, germinoma

Therapy

Observation is a common practice. Indication for *radical resection* is in a unilateral lesion with progressive exophthalmos, untreatable pain with complete visual loss or severe visual deterioration. Chiasmatic tumours are surgically treated only in exceptional cases. In *young children* with disease progression, first-line treatment is usually long-term chemotherapy. Local *RT* is indicated after failure of chemotherapy [14]. More recently, temozolomide and anti-angiogenic therapy (bevacizumab) are also administrated. In patients with NF1, oncological treatment is indicated only in case of clinical and radiological progression. Overall survival in children with NF1 ranges from 80–90%, in the group without NF1 from 70–80% [10].

1.11 Ocular Manifestations of Optic Nerve and Chiasma Gliomas

Optic glioma, a benign non-metastatic tumour (hamartoma) arises from neuroglia, i.e. astrocytes, oligodendrocytes and their mother cells—spongioblasts, and also contains all of them in varying proportions. The clinical presentation is mainly one-sided, slowly progressive, initially always axial protrusion of the eye without impaired mobility, oedema and redness. Other ocular signs include relative afferent pupillary defect, decreased vision, oedema or atrophy of the optic disc, or strabismus.

Gliomas of the chiasm are divided into two morphologically and clinically distinct types, the anterior optic chiasmatic and the posterior hypothalamochiasmatic. The anterior type is similar in many ways to the optic chiasm glioma. A certain percentage of posterior chiasmatic gliomas have completely different biological characteristics. They represent primary gliomas of the hypothalamus, which infiltrate the chiasm only secondarily. These tumours are usually malignant and their aggressive growth may be lethal. *Clinically*, they present with progressive bilateral visual disturbances and visual field loss is very heterogeneous (central scotomas, laterally asymmetric bitemporal or tract homonymous hemianopsia). On the fundus, there is usually bilateral optic disc oedema, rapidly progressing to atrophy. Internal hydrocephalus with n.VI. palsy and diencephalic or trunk symptomatology is frequent, especially in rapidly growing posterior types of lesions.

Neurosurgical Diseases

1.12 Pineal Region Tumours

The histopathological diversity of the lesions is due to the wide range of different tissues of this region. Non-tumour pineal cysts are a relatively common finding (approximately 10% of all MRI brain scans). In contrast, pineal region tumours are relatively rare. They represent 3–8% of all brain tumours in childhood and less than 1% in adulthood [17]. Histologically, pineal region tumours can be divided into three groups: germ cell, pineal parenchymal (Fig. 14) and others [47]. The most common one is *germinoma* [4].

Risk Factors

- Young age
- Remnants of ectoderm or tissues of other CNS tumours

Clinical Presentation

The most common sign of a *hormonal disorder* in children is precocious puberty. More rarely, diabetes insipidus or hypogonadism may occur due to compression of the hypothalamic-pituitary axis. *Headaches, epileptic seizures and hydrocephalus* are also relatively common [4]. Possible mobility and sensory disturbances result from distant *implantation metastases* in the spinal canal.

Diagnosis

Of the imaging modalities, *MRI* with contrast medium is the first choice (Fig. 14). Tissues with bone-like density or calcifications are revealed by *CT*. Detection

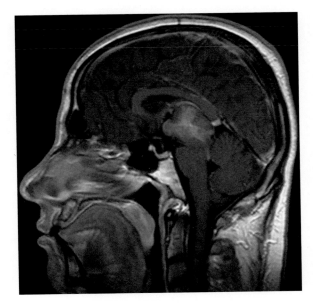

Fig. 14 Tumour of the pineal region (histologically transition between pinealocytoma and pinealoblastoma). T1-weighted MRI image after contrast agent administration

of elevated levels of some *tumour markers* (beta subunit of human chorionic gonadotropin, alpha-fetoprotein, placental alkaline phosphatase) may be helpful to establish the diagnosis.

Differential Diagnosis

- Glial tumours, meningiomas, dermoid/epidermoid cysts, metastases
- Arachnoid cyst
- Vascular lesions (dilatation or malformation of the vein of Galen/basilar artery)

Therapy

There is controversy surrounding the surgical removal. Some authors even suggest that only about 25% are suitable for resection. *RT* is recommended for germinomas. In the case of implantation metastases, irradiation of the entire craniospinal axis is resorted to. Treatment of *pinealocytoma* consists of radical resection [4]. *Radiosurgery* can be effective as a stand-alone treatment modality.

1.13 Ocular Manifestations of Pineal Tumours

Symptomatology of pineal tumours is important from the ocular point of view and can help to diagnose these lesions early. *Parinaud's syndrome* consists of supranuclear visual palsy in the vertical direction (most often upward) and impaired convergence. In addition, various forms of nystagmus may be present when attempting vertical eye movements or convergence. These symptoms are caused by the proximity of the lesion to the mesencephalon, where the gaze centre for vertical eye movement and the centre for convergence are located.

1.14 Intracranial Metastases

They are the most common type of brain tumour (approximately 50%) and its incidence is increasing. It occurs in 20–40% of patients diagnosed with cancer. The most common primary source of brain metastases is lung tumour (45%), followed by breast (10%), kidney (7%), gastrointestinal tract (6%) and melanoma (3%). Most metastases are *supratentorial* and *multiple* (up to 85%) (Fig. 15) [9].

T1-weighted MRI image after contrast agent administration.

Risk Factors

- Risk factors of the origin of metastases (i.e., of primary tumour)
- Adult age, male sex

Neurosurgical Diseases

Fig. 15 Multiple breast cancer metastases supratentorially

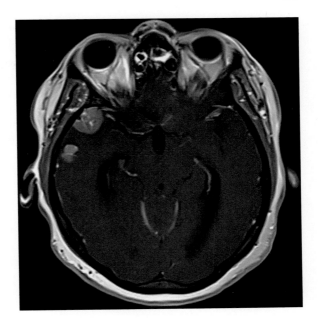

Clinical Presentation

The most common initial symptoms are headache, motor and cognitive impairment, and epileptic seizures.

Diagnosis

CT or MRI with contrast medium administration is used for diagnosis (Fig. 15A, B), with MRI being more sensitive [34]. When metastatic CNS disease is suspected, oncological screening should be performed to facilitate diagnosis and often to detect untreated underlying disease.

Differential Diagnosis

Abscess, glial tumour, lymphoma, meningioma, embryonal tumour, pseudotumour.

Therapy

Due to improvements in cancer therapy, the 5-year survival rate for brain metastases has increased to approximately 70%. *Surgery* for brain metastases is not indicated in patients in poor clinical conditions, having advanced underlying disease, presenting multiple metastases (3 or more) or with lesions in unfavourable anatomical localization [46]. Radiosurgery is more likely to be chosen for smaller or multiple lesions.

1.15 Ocular Manifestations of Intracranial Metastases

The ocular symptoms vary according to the location and size of the CNS lesion; often the metastases may be multiple and may be the first manifestation of the underlying disease. Surgical therapy is a therapeutic option when the tumour is appropriately localised, especially in the case of solitary metastases in patients with a good prognosis for survival. Other therapeutic options include radiotherapy, chemotherapy, and targeted biological therapy, often in combination. Symptomatic therapy (anticonvulsants, analgesics, corticosteroids to reduce oedema and functional problems) is also important to improve the quality of life of patients.

1.16 CNS Lymphomas

CNS lymphomas, either *primary* or *secondary*, represent a rare subset of non-Hodgkin lymphomas (NHL). According to the WHO definition, the incidence of primary CNS lymphoma is limited to the CNS parenchyma, dura mater, cerebral nerves, spinal cord, or intraocular compartment in immunocompromised patients. On the other hand, secondary CNS lymphoma refers to systemic NHL that has spread to the CNS. The most common sites are the frontal and temporal lobes (Fig. 16). Up to 25% develop intraocular lymphoma, which spreads to the CNS in up to 80% of cases [16].

Risk Factors

- Immunodeficiency
- Epstein-Barr virus, lupus erythematosus, Sjogren's syndrome

Clinical Presentation

Similar to glial tumours.

Diagnosis

In patients with suspected CNS lymphoma, MRI is indicated in the first instance (Fig. 16). It gives an indistinct impression with a vaguely demarcated border. The sequence of DWI on MR demonstrates their characteristic restriction of diffusion [22].

Differential Diagnosis

- Neuroepithelial tumour, metastasis
- Embryonal tumour, meningioma, pseudotumour

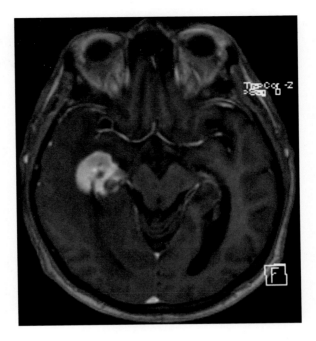

Fig. 16 Primary CNS lymphoma temporally on the right. T1-weighted MRI image after contrast agent administration

Therapy

CNS lymphomas typically regress after *corticosteroid* administration. *RT* is the main treatment modality due to its high radiosensitivity [16].

1.17 Ocular Manifestations of CNS Lymphomas

Primary CNS lymphomas are a relatively rare finding but should be considered when intracranial lesions with rapid progression are found, especially in patients over 65 years of age. The clinical ocular manifestation varies according to the localisation and size of the lesion. Intraorbital and intraocular lymphoma infiltration is also possible. Histological examination is necessary to establish the diagnosis, recommended to be followed by radiological examination. However, due to frequent recurrences, the prognosis is always uncertain.

1.18 Brainstem Tumours

A typical representative of intrinsic brainstem lesions is the group of *brainstem gliomas*. It includes multiple histological entities with variable prognosis (Fig. 17).

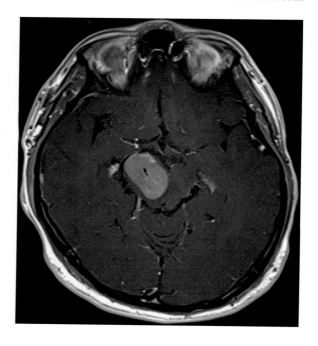

Fig. 17 Multiform glioblastoma (WHO grade IV) in the mesencephalic region on the right. T1 weighted MRI image after contrast agent administration

They can be divided according to localization into *diffuse* (mostly malignant), *local* (in the medulla oblongata), *dorsal exophytic* (in the 4th ventricle), and *cervicomedullary*. Tectal gliomas are mostly called lower grade astrocytomas [19]. Other, rarer, neoplasms of the trunk include atypical *teratoid/rhabdoid tumour* [30].

Risk Factors

See glial tumours—supratentorial.

Clinical Presentation

Brainstem gliomas, due to their infiltrative nature, tend to present with a slow, gradual increase in subtle symptoms that are often disproportionate to the larger volume of the lesion. Lesions localized in the rostral parts of the trunk usually manifest with *cerebellar* and *hydrocephalus symptoms*. Pathologies from the caudal half led to dysfunction of the cranial nerves and neural pathways of the trunk.

Diagnosis

The gold standard is the *MRI* (Fig. 17). Biopsy, to verify the diagnosis, is indicated only in rare cases.

Differential Diagnosis

- Metastases, hemangioblastoma, dermoid, epidermoid
- Postinfectious cysts, vascular malformations, cysticercosis

Neurosurgical Diseases

Therapy

Treatment of the lesion itself is *mostly nonsurgical* [19]. Dorsal exophytic tumours prominent in the IV ventricle are exceptions, as they are usually astrocytomas of low differentiation. Hydrocephalus with clinical manifestations is almost always resolved surgically by shunt surgery. Surgically unfavourable foci are usually only *monitored*. For inoperable gliomas, irradiation in different *radiotherapy regimens* is also an option.

1.19 Ocular Manifestations of Brainstem Tumours

The most common clinical manifestation is nuclear or peripheral oculomotor disorders, often in combination with visual palsy in the horizontal direction. Associated disorders of other cranial nerves may also be present, which may manifest clinically, for example, as corneal reflex disorder, paresis of the facial nerve, dysphagia, and dysarthria. Unlike other posterior fossa tumours, the development of intracranial hypertension is a rarer and late symptom. The prognosis is serious in a large proportion of patients and a significant proportion of patients die within months or years.

1.20 Cerebellar Tumours

The cerebellum is the most common site of CNS tumours in children. Lower grade gliomas (e.g., pilocytic astrocytoma of the cerebellum) are considered as benign lesions. *Embryonal tumours* (especially medulloblastoma) are highly aggressive, and their treatment involves intensive postoperative RT and CHT. In adults, cerebellar *metastases* are the most common lesion (Fig. 15A, B). *Ependymoma* and *hemangioblastoma* complete the list of other less common pathologies in children and adults [18].

The prototype of the embryonal CNS tumour group is *medulloblastoma* (Fig. 18), the most common paediatric CNS malignancy. It accounts for 25% of all intracranial childhood brain tumours [30].

Risk factors (applies to embryonal tumours).

- Age, male sex
- Gorlin, Turcot, Li-Fraumeni syndrome

Clinical Presentation

Common clinical manifestations are the result of increased intracranial pressure (headache, nausea, vomiting, etc.). Cerebellar ataxia, dysdiadochokinesia, cranial nerve palsy may also occur.

Fig. 18 Medulloblastoma (WHO grade IV) in the region of the posterior fossa of the skull and triple chamber hydrocephalus. T1-weighted MRI image after contrast agent administration

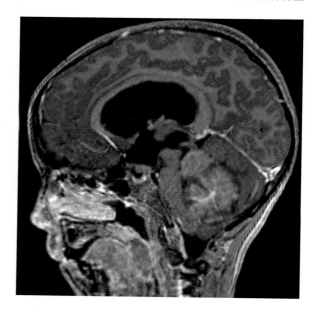

Diagnosis

MRI is the standard method for imaging cerebellar tumours (Fig. 18).

Differential Diagnosis

- Ependymoma, choroid plexus papilloma, dermoid cyst (in children)
- Metastasis, hemangioblastoma, dermoid, epidermoid, lymphoma (in adults)

Therapy

Pilocytic astrocytoma is treated surgically in the first instance. Radical resection does not require further therapy [18]. Surgery is also the first choice for medulloblastomas. They are radiosensitive and RT is often indicated for the entire craniospinal axis.

1.21 Ocular Manifestations of Cerebellar Tumours

The leading clinical manifestation in cerebellar tumours is usually early-onset intracranial hypertension. Cerebellar symptoms usually develop in later stages, due to the good adaptability of the cerebellar tissue, as do symptoms caused by brainstem compression. The prognosis is also largely influenced by the biological nature of the tumour and its extent.

Neurosurgical Diseases

1.22 Tumours of the Cerebellopontine Angle

The cerebellopontine angle (CPA) is the most common site of posterior cranial fossa tumours in adults. Vestibular schwannoma (acoustic neuroma) is the most common tumour in this location, representing 75% of all pathological lesions of the CPA. Meningiomas are the second most common expansion, followed by epidermoid. *Vestibular schwannoma* (Fig. 19) accounts for 8–10% of all primary brain tumours in the adult population.

It occurs sporadically or as part of NF2. Trigeminal neurinomas are the second most common type of cranial nerve schwannomas [37]. *Meningiomas* have been discussed above. *Epidermoid* (epidermoid cyst, primary intracranial cholesteatoma, pearl tumour) accounts for 1% of all intracranial tumour lesions. It is most localised in the CPA, 4th and 3rd ventricles of the brain, in the diploe or parasellar region [9].

Risk Factors

NF2 (for vestibular schwannoma).

Clinical Presentation

Ipsilateral *hearing loss*, *vertigo* and *tinnitus* form a typical triad. Tumour's volume progression often leads to signs of compression of other cranial nerves (n. VII, V, IX, X), brainstem or cerebellum (ataxia, gait disturbances, etc.) [37]. Obstructive hydrocephalus, followed by signs of *intracranial hypertension*, is presented because of blockage of cerebrospinal fluid flow.

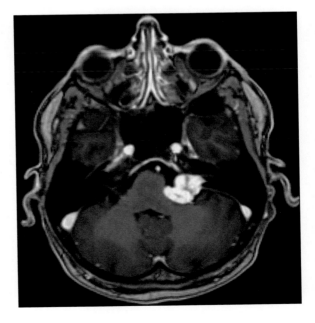

Fig. 19 Vestibular schwannoma on the left with extrameatal promotion. T1-weighted MRI image after contrast agent administration

Diagnosis

Otorhinolaryngological examinations (auditory evoked potentials and PTA—pure tone audiogram) are helpful not only in diagnosis but also in therapy planning. Of the graphic modalities, *MRI* (3D CISS sequence) is the first choice (Fig. 19).

Differential Diagnosis

- Metastasis, arachnoid cyst, lipoma
- Aneurysm, vertebrobasilar dolichoectasia

Therapy

Possible therapies for patients with vestibular schwannoma are as follows: observation, microsurgery and radiosurgery. For patients with small neurinoma and preserved hearing, all three modalities can be offered [37]. Microsurgery is the only radical method of treatment. Radiosurgical therapy (Leksell Gamma Knife and CyberKnife) is well tolerated, however, it is only able to slow, or at best stop, the growth of the tumour mass. Tumour volume reduction is often attributed to natural regressive changes, rather than radiation. Therapy of intracranial epidermoid tumours consists of radical microsurgical extirpation.

1.23 Ocular Manifestations of Cerebellopontine Angle Tumours

The clinical manifestation is subtle, usually due to the compression of n. VIII, there is a gradual unilateral deterioration of hearing. The ocular symptoms may be accompanied by progressive paresis of n. VII with lagophthalmos or decreased corneal sensitivity in n. V lesions.

2 Intracranial Hypertension

Intracranial hypertension is defined as an increase of intracranial pressure (ICP) above 15 mm Hg (1 mm Hg = 1.36 cm H2O). In an adult, the normal mean ICP value is around 15 mm Hg, with a wider range of 2–20 mm Hg [38]. Intracerebral hypertension is a major mechanism of *secondary cerebral damage*. The *underlying causes* of intracranial hypertension include cerebral contusion and bleeding in the context of craniocerebral injuries, hydrocephalus, brain tumours, non-traumatic intra-axial haemorrhage, cerebral oedema, infectious CNS diseases, idiopathic intracranial hypertension, and others.

Neurosurgical Diseases

2.1 *Hydrocephalus*

The term hydrocephalus describes an abnormal accumulation of cerebrospinal fluid (CSF) in the intracranial space (most often in the cerebral ventricles), resulting from a disorder of its production, circulation, or absorption. This condition is associated with an increase in ICP and compression of brain tissue. The basic classification is according to cause: *obstructive* hydrocephalus—arising from blockage of CSF circulation in the ventricular system and/or subarachnoid space (Fig. 18), hydrocephalus due to CSF *hyporesorption/over production*—arising from impaired absorption/excessive CSF production (Fig. 20A, B).

According to the rate of its onset, it can be divided into *acute* and *chronic*. In terms of the site of obstruction, it can then be divided into *non-communicating*—the obstruction is in the ventricular system—and *communicating*—the obstruction is in the subarachnoid spaces or venous system. The communicating hydrocephalus may be due mainly to functional impairment of the arachnoidal granulations. Etiologically, hydrocephalus can be divided into *congenital* or *acquired*. *Complex hydrocephalus* is characterised by the presence obstruction and hyporesorption. An example of a specific type of hydrocephalus is *normotensive hydrocephalus* (form of communicating hydrocephalus). In addition to a dilated ventricular system, it is characterised by the classic clinical Hakim triad (see below), with normal cerebrospinal fluid pressure on lumbar puncture at supine position.

In the *neonatal* age or during *childhood*, hydrocephalus arises due to congenital and acquired causes. The worldwide prevalence of congenital hydrocephalus is 0.5–3 cases/1,000 live births [45]. The most common congenital cause is stenosis of the Sylvian aqueduct (Fig. 21) [45].

Acquired causes include intraventricular haemorrhage, mainly affecting immature neonates, as well as CNS infections, craniocerebral injuries, and intracranial tumours blocking the ventricular system in later life.

Post-haemorrhagic hydrocephalus is the most common form of this disease in adults. It is mainly associated with subarachnoid haemorrhage (SAH). Its incidence in this category varies in a wide range of 6–67%. Another cause may be a disorder of resorption of fluid at the level of arachnoid granulations in *post-traumatic hydrocephalus*, whose incidence also varies in a wide range (0.7–72%) [45]. *Post-infectious hydrocephalus* is encountered in bacterial meningitis, brain abscesses or rarely as a complication after neurosurgical procedures.

Risk Factors

In Children

- Intrauterine infections in pregnancy
- Diabetes, chronic hypertensive disease in the mother
- Neglect of prenatal care; alcohol in pregnancy
- Associations with CNS malformations (e.g. Chiari malformation)

In Adults

Fig. 20 A Mild active hyporesorptive hydrocephalus. T2 FLAIR MRI image. **B** Advanced hypersecretory hydrocephalus in chorioid plexus carcinoma (WHO grade III). T1-weighted MRI image after contrast agent administration

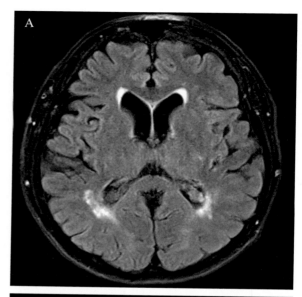

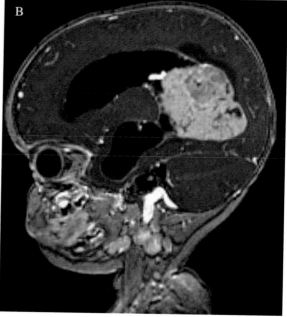

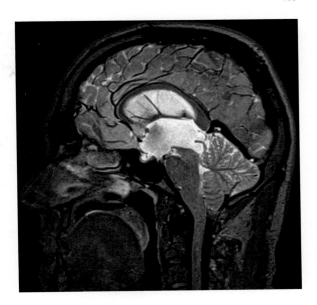

Fig. 21 T2-weighted MRI image of three-chamber obstructive hydrocephalus with stenosis of the mesencephalic aqueduct

- SAH or intraventricular haemorrhage
- Older age, clinical condition

Clinical Presentation

Symptoms of hydrocephalus show interindividual variability. In children whose cranial bones are not fused (up to 12–24 months of age), a *progressive increase in head circumference* is evident. There is inappetence, irritability, thinning of the scalp skin with accentuated venous pattern. The greater fontanelle is tense and diastasis of the sutures is noted. The child thrives poorly. In older children, the symptoms are the same as in adults. Acute hydrocephalus is manifested by syndrome of *intracranial hypertension*. In chronic hydrocephalus, symptoms are creeping. Morning headache, psychomotor slowing, nausea, vomiting, behavioural changes and somnolence are common symptoms. The classic *Hakim triad* consists of cognitive impairment, apraxic gait and urinary incontinence [41].

Diagnosis

In the prenatal period and in children with an open anterior fontanelle, ultrasound is used. In children with no fontanelle and adults, a CT scan of the brain is essential. MRI is the sovereign method to clarify the aetiology of hydrocephalus, as well as to monitor paediatric patients (Figs. 22A–C and 23A–C).

In addition to imaging methods, dynamic testing of CSF is used, which is particularly applicable in the diagnosis of normotensive hydrocephalus. In obstructive hydrocephalus, lumbar puncture is contraindicated, because of concerns about the possible iatrogenic complication of occipital con.

Fig. 22 **A** A picture of empty sella. T1-weighted MRI image. **B** A picture of empty sella. T2-weighted MRI image. **C** A picture of empty sella, accompanied by prominence of the subarachnoid spaces (liquor shrinkage) around the optic nerves. STIR MRI sequence

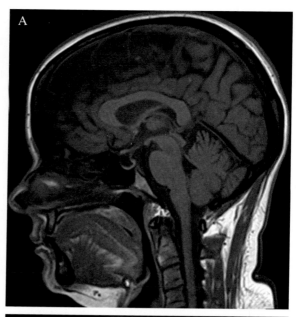

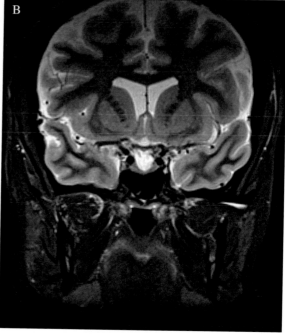

Fig. 22 (continued)

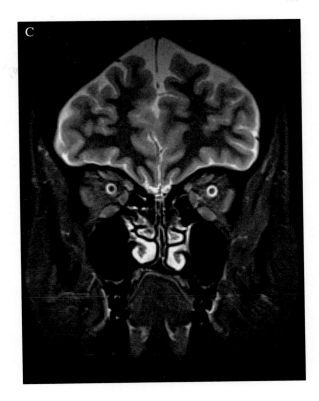

Differential Diagnosis

- Brain atrophy, dementia, headache, brain tumours

Therapy

Conservative treatment of hydrocephalus in children has the role of a temporary therapy before implantation of a drainage system. Pharmacological treatment acts by the mechanism of reducing the production of liquor (acetazolamide and furosemide), on the other hand, affects its increased absorption (hyaluronidase). Osmotically active solutions (mannitol, saline solution) lead only to a temporary decrease in intracranial pressure.

Surgical therapy is dominant in the treatment of hydrocephalus. Shunt insertion, ventriculoperitoneal or ventriculoatrial shunt are a reliable surgical solution for this clinical entity. In today's form, the valves of the drainage sets are equipped with a sophisticated mechanism, allowing non-invasive correction of the liquor pressure according to the current graphic or clinical situation. Endoscopic techniques are mainly indicated in obstructive hydrocephalus. In addition to removing intraventricular tumours, cysts, or other obstructions, they allow restoration of the natural CSF flow. An example is the endoscopic ventriculostomy of the 3rd ventricle (EVT),

Fig. 23 **A** Aneurysm of the anterior communicating artery. Digital subtraction angiography (DSA) in anteroposterior projection. **B** Aneurysm of the anterior communicating artery. 3D reconstruction of the DSA image

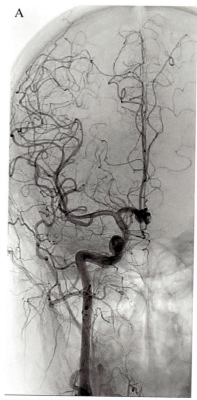

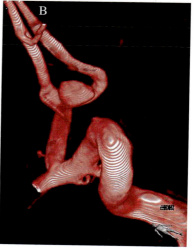

Neurosurgical Diseases

which allows communication of the internal and external liquor compartments and often spares the patient from permanent implantation of a drainage system [26]. Tumour and non-tumour lesions causing obstructive hydrocephalus are also treated by open microsurgery.

2.2 Ocular Manifestations of Hydrocephalus

The clinical manifestations of hydrocephalus depend on the age of the patient and the rate of hydrocephalus onset. Their recognition is important not only for the primary diagnosis but also for early recognition of surgical treatment failure, which may occur several years after the procedure.

In infants and children under two years of age, in the case of acute progression, we observe a tense large fontanelle with spacing of the cranial sutures, paresis of the 6th cranial nerve, vomiting and deviation of the bulbs caudally. In addition, impaired consciousness, bradycardia, hypertension, and respiratory disturbances may occur. The condition requires urgent investigation and surgical intervention. Manifestations of chronic hydrocephalus in older children include papilloedema with signs of congestion and haemorrhages on the eye fundus.

In adults, headaches are at the forefront of symptoms. On the fundus, the papilledema dominates. Sometimes there may be compression in the dorsal mesencephalon, manifested by what is called the *Parinaud syndrome*: the pupils are usually moderately wide with absent photoreaction, but pupil retraction in near vision is preserved, and there is associated vertical gaze palsy, convergence-retraction nystagmus, and eyelid retraction.

2.3 Idiopathic Intracranial Hypertension

Idiopathic intracranial hypertension is a rare clinical entity, characterised by elevated intracranial pressure with normal CSF composition and by absence of graphically demonstrable intracranial pathology. Its incidence is in the range of 1–2 cases/100,000 people per year, with a marked predominance in women [3]. When a group of obese women aged 15–44 years is evaluated, the incidence rises to 19–21 cases/100,000 person-years. Men account for 8–10% of patients [3]. The cause of this disease is still unknown. However, it is well established that weight gain, even in patients who are not obese, is a significant risk factor for its development. Higher BMI is correlated with visual status. For every 10 units of BMI, the risk of severe visual impairment is reported to increase 1.4 times. The literature offers several theories to explain the pathogenesis of elevated ICP. The most cited is the effect of central obesity on central venous pressure, which leads to a subsequent increase in ICP [3, 40]. However, this theory does not explain the gender differences. Intracranial pressure may increase when venous outflow is impaired (dural venous hypertension, stenosis of dural sinuses). On the other hand, stenosis may also result from idiopathic intracranial hypertension due to remodelling, fibrosis and subsequent stenosis of the transverse sinus.

Risk Factors

- Female sex, obesity
- Hypervitaminosis A, use of retinoids
- Exogenous growth hormones, tetracyclines, fluoroquinolones
- Addison's disease, hypoparathyroidism, severe anaemia
- Sleep apnoea syndrome, polycystic ovary syndrome

Clinical Presentation

Typical of idiopathic hypertension, headache (93% of patients) varies with body position (more intense lying down and in the morning) [3]. In practice, it is also possible to encounter patients who seek medical care because of visual disturbances, back pain, spontaneous nasal CSF leak or symptoms of meningitis.

Diagnosis

Due to the nature of the disease, it is a diagnosis per exclusionem [3].

If increased intracranial pressure is suspected, a CT scan is first performed, followed by an MRI, including magnetic resonance cisternography, to rule out stenosis of dural sinuses. Pathognomonic intracranial graphic findings include bilateral or unilateral stenosis of the dural sinus, empty sella, narrower ventricles, multiple anterior and middle cranial fossa defects with or without meningo/meningoencephaloceles, dehiscence of the superior semicircular canal, and thinning of the posterior sclera and distension of the optic nerve sheaths in the orbital compartment (Fig. 22A–C). If imaging does not reveal a structural cause for the elevated ICP, the next step is a lumbar puncture in supine position with measurement of the intracranial pressure ("opening pressure") and evacuation of the liquor (30–40 ml). Values of opening pressure below 200 mm H_2O are normal, above 250 mm H_2O are already evaluated as pathological. Values between 200–250 mm H_2O are borderline and not conclusive for the diagnosis [3, 40]. Modified Dandy criteria are also used in the diagnosis.

Differential Diagnosis

- CNS tumours, venous sinus thrombosis
- Hydrocephalus, malignant systemic hypertension

Therapy

Therapy of idiopathic intracranial hypertension may be conservative or surgical. The simplest therapeutic measure in indicated cases is discontinuation of risky drugs (vit. A, exogenous growth hormones, tetracyclines, fluoroquinolones, etc.) and weight reduction. Among oral drugs, the carbonic anhydrase inhibitor acetazolamide is used. Patients' refractory to conservative treatment, repeated lumbar punctures

Neurosurgical Diseases

are performed initially to reduce the liquor tension, or external lumbar drainage is installed. Surgical management in the sense of permanent drainage (ventriculoperitoneal, lumboperitoneal shunt) is followed if the effect of transient fluid drainage is insufficient. Surgical fenestration of the optic nerve sheaths associated with orbital decompression is an underused method in practice.

2.4 Ocular Manifestations of Idiopathic Intracranial Hypertension

The first cases of patients with idiopathic intracranial hypertension (IIH) were described by Quincke, who mentioned the higher lymphatic pressure shortly after the first lumbar puncture in 1897 [35]. For many years, this condition was also referred to as *pseudotumour cerebri* in medical terminology, but this name is now considered obsolete. In 1955, Foley named increased liquor pressure of unclear aetiology as *benign intracranial hypertension* [12]. However, this term is now completely abandoned in view of published cases of patients with severe visual impairment. IIH may be closely associated with hormonal disorders, nutritional disorders, obstructions in venous outflow, post-meningitis conditions in subarachnoid haemorrhage, hypercoagulable states, and others.

Neuro-ophthalmological symptomatology includes mainly subjectively reported obnubilations, photopsia, blurred vision, diplopia, and pain around the eyes, most often bilateral retrobulbar. Visual field defects with normal visual acuity are found in most patients. The most common type of scotoma is enlargement of the blind spot (Marriott's point). Some patients have horizontal diplopia and 10–20% are diagnosed with 6th cranial nerve paresis. On ophthalmoscopy, bilateral papilledema of varying degrees is found. Conservative *treatment* involves administration of acetazolamide at a dose of up to 1 g/day divided throughout the day. The dose can be increased up to 4 g/day. If the patient does not respond to conservative therapy, interventional methods of treatment are chosen.

3 Selected Vascular Diseases of the CNS

Vascular diseases of the brain are one of the leading causes of morbidity and mortality worldwide. In industrialised countries, they are the third most common cause of death after cardiovascular disease and cancer. The overall incidence rate of cerebrovascular events was 4.9 per 100 person-years worldwide [42]. Stroke is a heterogeneous group of diseases. They include cerebral ischemia (80%), intraparenchymal haemorrhage (15%), subarachnoid haemorrhage (SAH, 5%) and cerebral venous thrombosis (5%).

Cerebral aneurysms represent the most common (95%) source of SAH. Arteriovenous (AV) and cavernous malformations are the sources of intraparenchymal haemorrhages in 5% [24, 48]. Depending on the location of the vascular malformation with hematoma, specific ophthalmological manifestations may be expected.

3.1 Cerebral Aneurysms

A cerebral aneurysm is a circumscribed enlargement of an artery (aneurysm) caused by structural changes in its wall. In the general population, 1–2% of arterial cerebral aneurysms occur, with more than 90% located in the region of the circle of Willis [24]. In terms of clinical manifestation, they are divided into *unruptured* and *ruptured* aneurysms. The annual risk of rupture is estimated to be 1–2% [6]. The size of the most common type (*saccular aneurysm*) ranges from small ("baby" up to 2 mm), medium (6–12 mm) to gigantic size (over 35 mm). Aneurysms located around the entire circumference of the vessel, giving the impression of diffuse enlargement of the vessel, are called *fusiform* (spindle-shaped). A *true* aneurysm is made up of the entire wall of the artery (excluding the inner elastic layer), whereas a *false* aneurysm has a more fragile wall (e.g., post-traumatic aneurysm). More than 80% of aneurysms are located on the vessels of the anterior half of the circle of Willis (including the posterior communicating artery) [6]. The most frequent location of aneurysms (Fig. 23A, B) is the anterior communicating artery then the posterior communicating artery branch from the internal carotid artery, the bifurcation of the middle cerebral artery, and the apex of the basilar artery. From an ophthalmological perspective, the important location in the ophthalmic artery outflow from the internal carotid artery below the optic nerve is where the growth of the aneurysm causes a compressive ophthalmopathy with sectoral visual field loss.

Risk Factors (for Aneurysms)

- Arterial hypertension, smoking, obesity
- Age (50–60 years), female sex
- Population (Japanese and Finnish have higher risk)
- Diabetes, hyperlipidaemia
- Lack of physical activity, stress, excessive alcohol use
- Family anamnesis of aneurysms
- Aortic coarctation, polycystic kidney disease, systemic connective tissue defects—Marfan syndrome

Clinical Presentation

A large proportion of aneurysms are asymptomatic. The most serious manifestations occur after their rupture. *Subarachnoid haemorrhage* is characterised by sudden onset, severe headache, vomiting and often impaired consciousness. Approximately 50% result in rapid death before the patient is taken to hospital [24]. Surviving patients

Neurosurgical Diseases

go on to develop meningeal syndrome and other focal manifestations (limb paresis, speech disorders, brainstem symptoms). Two main classification systems assessing clinical status contribute to better interdisciplinary communication: the Hunt and Hess scale (grades I–V) and the World Federation of Neurological Surgeons scale (WFNS, grades 0–5), which makes use of the Glasgow Coma Score.

Diagnosis

In situations of typical clinical signs with negative CT findings, a diagnostic lumbar puncture should be performed. This may show an admixture of fresh blood in the CSF and thus reveal a slight aneurysm leak. A typical finding suggestive of an older haemorrhage is the presence of haemoglobin degradation products—oxyhaemoglobin/bilirubin on spectrophotometric examination. The gold standard in the diagnosis of aneurysms remains brain angiography (digital subtraction angiography, DSA), despite high-quality CTA imaging (Fig. 23A, B). MRA is used in follow-up after aneurysm repair or for simple observation of findings not indicated for treatment.

Differential Diagnosis

- Ischemic and haemorrhagic stroke, meningitis
- Cerebral venous thrombosis
- Thrombosis of the basilar artery, arterial wall dissection
- Moyamoya disease, malformation of the vein of Galen
- Venous malformations, vasculitis, radiation-induced vasculopathy
- Tumours (especially in the region of the sella turcica), arachnoid cysts

Therapy

Rupture of an aneurysm with SAH is a serious acute situation that requires urgent diagnosis and early management aimed at obliteration of the aneurysm. The eventual recurrence of bleeding usually has a more severe clinical course. The decisive factors considered in the treatment of ruptured aneurysms are the initial neurological status (Hunt-Hess), the size of the aneurysm neck and sac, its orientation, as well as the age and internal comorbidity of the patient. The algorithm for aneurysm treatment is a highly individual process [6, 24]. A detailed description is beyond the scope of this text. However, in principle, treatment consists of direct surgical treatment of the aneurysm, with placement of a titanium clamp on the neck of the aneurysm. The second, currently more widely used technique is endovascular treatment with placement of coils in the aneurysm sac causing the obliteration. The use of one or the other treatment technique is considered from several points of view. It is chosen on a strictly individual basis and requires an interdisciplinary approach involving an interventional radiologist. Observation of unruptured aneurysms may be indicated especially in small, incident, clinically silent aneurysms without growth progression.

3.2 Ocular Manifestations of Cerebral Aneurysms

Clinical Presentation and Objective Findings

Aneurysms Presenting with Compression

These are mainly aneurysms of large size (often more than 3 cm in diameter), which irritate or oppress the surrounding structures by their volume. The most common manifestation of this group is compression of the cranial nerves, especially the oculomotor nerve. When the oculomotor nerve is affected, its inner branch sensitive to compression is typically affected first, and the most common first ocular manifestation of the aneurysm is thus the development of *homolateral mydriasis*, which is often accompanied by sudden and sharp pain localised behind the eyeball or hemicrania. This picture is typical for aneurysms of the posterior communicating artery. In the case of sudden onset of mydriasis accompanied by pain and/or involvement of the orbital part of the 3rd nerve with paralytic ptosis and divergence of the eyeball, it is always necessary to exclude an aneurysm in the incriminated area. In the rarer localisation of the aneurysm on the internal carotid artery in its course through the sinus cavernosus, the clinical presentation may be accompanied by paresis of all nerves running in this area (n. III, n. IV, n. V, n. VI). Very rarely, arterial aneurysms in the region of the anterior circulation of the Circle of Willis and the ophthalmic artery may oppress the same-sided optic nerve or chiasma, presenting with progressive visual field and visual acuity impairment.

Rupture of the Aneurysm

Rupture of an intracranial aneurysm is usually a dramatic event that develops spontaneously from full health or in association with physical exertion of varying intensity. The ophthalmological examination usually follows a time gap and consists mainly of a fundus examination in mydriasis to exclude Terson syndrome. *Terson syndrome* refers to intraocular haemorrhage (IOH) associated with SAH, most commonly with rupture of an intracranial aneurysm. It is described in approximately one-quarter to one-half of these patients. The pathogenesis of IOH has not yet been clearly elucidated. However, the most likely theory currently postulates rupture of the peripapillary retinal vessels due to a sudden increase in intracranial pressure that is transmitted intraocularly through the intervaginal spaces of the optic nerve. This mechanism is suggested by the fact that, rarely, Terson syndrome can arise due to an increase in intracranial pressure for a reason other than SAH, i.e. without the presence of blood in the cerebrospinal fluid. This fact essentially rules out the previously postulated theory of direct propagation of blood from the liquor pathways intraocularly. Patients with SAK with Terson syndrome have a significantly higher mortality rate than patients with SAK without the presence of IOH, which may be explained by the sudden and marked elevation of intracranial pressure required for the development of IOH. Haemorrhages in the eye may be localised subretinally, intraretinally, preretinally, and intravitreally, and with more massive findings may completely obscure the posterior pole region of the eye. Other possible ocular manifestations of intracranial

Neurosurgical Diseases

aneurysm rupture include homolateral mydriasis, possibly associated with an oculomotor disorder and ptosis caused by compression of the 3rd nerve with a significant increase in intracranial pressure.

Therapy

Pars plana vitrectomy is an option in the treatment of Terson syndrome. This procedure is especially approached in younger patients and patients with bilateral findings, where the procedure shortens the duration of visual deterioration and thus improves the possibility of rehabilitation. Of course, the overall prognosis of the patient must be considered when the procedure is indicated. In some cases, it is possible to choose a conservative procedure and wait for possible spontaneous absorption of intraocular haemorrhage.

3.3 Arteriovenous and Cavernous Malformations

Cerebral vascular malformations represent aberrant persistence of embryonic vascular connections between arteries and veins. Their incidence in the population is estimated to be about 4.5% [39]. They are usually divided into four groups: *arteriovenous malformations* (AVMs), cerebral *cavernomas* (cavernous haemangiomas), *venous angiomas* (developmental venous anomalies) and *capillary telangiectasias*.

Arteriovenous malformations forming a pathological convoluted dilated vasculature with abnormal communication between arteries and veins that lacks its own embedded pre-capillary and capillary network. The central cluster of coiled and dysplastic vessels is called a nidus (Fig. 24).

A classification system (Spetzler-Martin, grades I–V) assesses and subdivides malformations according to their size, character of drainage, and eloquent localization. They are more frequent at the supratentorial level, in the frontal or parietal lobe. Clinical manifestation, associated mainly to the presence of haemorrhage, occurs most often between 20–50 years of age. However, they may also manifest with ischemic episodes followed by epileptic equivalents [39].

Brain cavernomas are benign lesions, usually ovoid in shape, consisting of sinusoidal structures with a single layer of endothelial lining (Fig. 25).

They occur in both sporadic and familial forms. Cavernomas comprise 5–3% of all CNS vascular malformations, with an incidence of up to 4% in the population. Up to 85% of cavernomas occur supratentorially and an equal percentage may be multiple [11].

Risk Factors

- Male sex in AVMs
- Some are part of hereditary syndromes (Osler-Weber-Rendu)

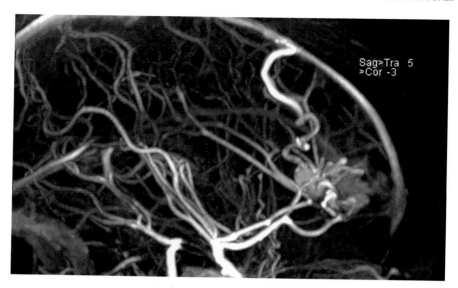

Fig. 24 Arteriovenous malformation frontal left. Maximum intensity projection (MIP) MRI angiography

Fig. 25 Cavernoma at the base of the fourth cerebral ventricle. T2-weighted MRI image

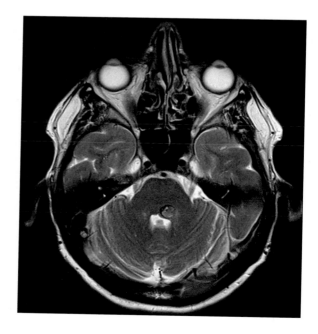

Neurosurgical Diseases

Clinical Presentation

Symptoms of *intracerebral haemorrhage* are the most common manifestation of AVM (50–61%) and *epilepsy* in cavernomas (up to 44%). The second most frequent symptom in AVMs is epilepsy, and symptomatic haemorrhage in cavernomas (15%) [11].

Diagnosis

Native CT will help to detect bleeding from the malformation, CTA will then show the basic characteristics. MRA contributes to the unequivocal diagnosis of a malformation (Fig. 24). However, AVMs will only appear in the necessary detail on DSA. Cavernomas prone to recurrent bleeding, especially those that are multiple and deep-seated, can be diagnosed by CT and MRI (Fig. 25).

Differential Diagnosis

- Haemorrhagic metastases, brain tumours, haemangioma
- Venous malformations, vasculitis, radiation-induced vasculopathy
- Infectious CNS diseases

Therapy

In lower grade AVMs (I–II), surgical resection is the method of choice. Grade III AVM is a matter of literary debate and is judged strictly on an individual basis. Endovascular treatment (embolization) has specific indications. It is usually indicated for preoperative reduction of AVM vascularity to facilitate surgery. It may also be used to treat the most dangerous part of the AVM in otherwise inoperable lesions, e.g., intranidal aneurysm. Primary radiosurgical treatment of AVMs is usually indicated when safe and radical microsurgical extirpation (stages IV and V) cannot be performed, or when it is the patient's choice [39]. Another legitimate modality when dealing with AVMs is observation, especially in situations where the risk of treating exceeds the risk of rupture.

Treatment of cavernomas consists of their surgical removal. Observation is recommended for multiple, asymptomatic and unfavourably located lesions (brainstem, deep brain structures). Radiosurgery is not effective in the treatment of cavernomas. It does not statistically reduce the risk of haemorrhage and is therefore not recommended in the treatment of this clinical entity [13].

3.4 Ocular Manifestations of Arteriovenous and Cavernous Malformations

Epidemiology

The number of incidentally detected AVMs has been increasing in recent years, reflecting the increased availability of imaging methods in clinical practice and the higher number of incidental asymptomatic findings. In the absence of large-scale studies, epidemiological data vary considerably, but the prevalence of AVMs is estimated to be approximately 20/100,000 population, and approximately 90% of AVMs remain asymptomatic throughout life.

Approximately one-half of cavernomas are reported to be familial with autosomal dominant inheritance, the other half occur sporadically. The overall prevalence in the population is reported to be between 400–800/100,000 inhabitants.

Clinical Presentation and Objective Findings

The *ocular manifestation* is relatively rare. Intracranial AVM, when localised near the retrochiasmatic part of the visual pathway, may cause compression of the latter with the finding of homonymous hemianopsia of varying extent. In the case of AVM rupture and SAH, intraocular haemorrhages may be found in the context of Terson syndrome during the examination of the fundus, as well as in SAH in the case of intracranial aneurysm rupture. The presence of a retinal arteriovenous malformation is also rare, which is called *Wyburn-Mason syndrome* when an intracranial AVM is present. Isolated cases of ocular manifestations of AVM caused by impaired venous outflow from the orbit by increased resistance in the superior ophthalmic vein are also described in the literature. This condition is explained by an alteration of intracranial blood flow caused by the presence of a vascular malformation. In such a case, on ocular examination, there is a widening of episcleral and conjunctival vessels of different extent; elevation of intraocular pressure may be present without significant effect of antiglaucoma therapy; possible protrusion of the bulb with eyelid oedema and other symptoms mimicking the image of carotid-cavernous fistula.

The *ocular symptomatology* of *cavernomas* may be due to visual impairment or visual field depression anywhere along the visual pathway, or possibly oculomotor disorders when the optic nerves or their nuclei are affected. When the cavernous malformation is located intraorbitally, the patient may be referred to the physician for eyeball protrusion, ptosis or impaired ocular motility.

References

1. Berman D, Miller NR. New concepts in the management of optic nerve sheath meningiomas. Ann Acad Med Singapore. 2006;35(3):168–74.
2. Boetto J, Birzu C, Kalamarides M, et al. Meningiomas: update on current knowledge. Rev Med Internal. 2022;43(2):98–105.
3. Boyter E. Idiopathic intracranial hypertension. JAAPA. 2019;32(5):30–5.
4. Buchvald P, Suchomel P, Benes V, et al. Expansion of the pineal gland. Cesk Slov Neurol N. 2013;76/109(6):667–8.
5. Cesak T, Nahlovsky J, Latr I, et al. Neoplastic diseases of the pituitary gland. In: Nahlovsky J, editor., et al., Neurochosurgery. Prague: Galen; 2006. p. 155–74.
6. Darsaut TE, Desal H, Cognard C, et al. Comprehensive aneurysm management (CAM): an all-inclusive care trial for unruptured intracranial aneurysms. World Neurosurg. 2020;141:770–7.
7. de Robles P, Fiest KM, Frolkis AD, et al. The worldwide incidence and prevalence of primary brain tumors: a systematic review and meta-analysis. Neuro Oncol. 2015;17(6):776–83.

Neurosurgical Diseases

8. Efenterre R, Boch A. Craniopharyngiomas. In: Tonn JC, Westphal M, Rutka JT, editors. Oncology of CNS tumors. 2nd ed. London: Springer Verlag; 2010. p. 297–307.
9. Fadrus P, Lakomy R, Hubnerova P, et al. Intracranial tumors—diagnosis and therapy. Internal Med, 2010;12(7,8):376–81.
10. Farazdaghi MK, Katowitz WR, Avery RA. Current treatment of optic nerve gliomas. Curr Opin Ophthalmol. 2019;30(5):356–63.
11. Flemming KD. Incidence, prevalence, and clinical presentation of cerebral cavernous malformations. Methods Mol Biol. 2020;2152:27–33.
12. Foley J. Benign forms of intracranial hypertension—"toxic" and "otitic" hydrocephalus. Brain. 1955;78:1–41.
13. Fontanella MM, Zanin L, Fiorindi A, et al. Surgical management of brain cavernous malformations. Methods Mol Biol. 2020;2152:109–28.
14. Fried I, Tabori U, Tihan T, et al. Optic pathway gliomas: a review. CNS Oncol. 2013;2(2):143–59.
15. Gabalec F, Cap J. Pharmacological treatment of pituitary tumors. Practical Pharmacy. 2014;10(5):1746.
16. Ghozy S, Dibas M, Afifi AM, et al. Primary cerebral lymphoma' characteristics, incidence, survival, and causes of death in the United States. J Neurol Sci. 2020;415: 116890.
17. Greenberg MS. Primary tumors of the nervous and related systems. In: Greenberg MS, editor. Handbook of Neurosurgery. New York: Thieme; 2016. p. 584–774.
18. Grossman R, Ram Z. Posterior Fossa intra-axial tumors in adults. World Neurosurg. 2016;88:140–5.
19. Hu J, Western S, Kesari S. Brainstem Glioma in adults. Front. Oncol. 2016;6:180.
20. Huisman TA. Tumor-like lesions of the brain. Cancer Imaging. 2009;9:10–3.
21. Jiraskova N. Neuroophthalmology—minimum for practice. Prague: Triton; 2001.
22. Ko CC, Tai MH, Li CF, et al. Differentiation between Glioblastoma multiforme and primary cerebral lymphoma: additional benefits of quantitative diffusion-weighted MR imaging. PLoS ONE. 2016;11(9): e0162565.
23. Komori T. Updating the grading criteria for adult diffuse gliomas: beyond the WHO2016CNS classification. Brain Tumor Pathol. 2020;37(1):1–4.
24. Krajina A, Lojik M, Cesak T, et al. Endovascular treatment of intracranial aneurysms—methodology, indications, complications. Cesk Slov Neurol. 2012;75/108(5):552–60.
25. Lapointe S, Perry A, Butowski NA. Primary brain tumours in adults. Lancet. 2018;392(10145):432–46.
26. Lipina R, Palecek T. Surgical treatment of hydrocephalus in childhood. Pediatrician Practice. 2004;3:133–6.
27. Mombaerts I, Ramberg I, Coupland SE, et al. Diagnosis of orbital mass lesions: clinical, radiological, and pathological recommendations. Surv Ophthalmol. 2019;64(6):741–56.
28. Netuka D, Masopust V, Benes V. Treatment of pituitary adenomas. Czech Slov Neurol. 2011;74(107):240–3.
29. Otradovec J. Clinical neuroophthalmology. Prague: Grada; 2003.
30. Pavelka Z, Zitterbart K. Tumors of the central nervous system in children. Neurol for practice. 2011;12(1):52–8.
31. Penn DL, Burke WT, Laws ER. Management of non-functioning pituitary adenomas: surgery. Pituitary. 2018;21(2):145–53.
32. Poczos P, Kremlacek J, Cesak T, et al. Use of optical coherence tomography in patients with optic chiasm compression. Cesk Slov Oftalmol. 2019;75(3):120–7.
33. Polivka J, Repik T, Holubec L, et al. Classification of tumors of the central nervous system—WHO 2016 Update. Czech Words Neurol N. 2017;80/113(3):353–6.
34. Pope WB. Brain metastases: neuroimaging. Handb Clin Neurol. 2018;149:89–112.
35. Quincke H. Ueber meningitis serosa und verwandte zustande. Dtsch Z Nervenheilk. 1897;9:149–68.
36. Rindi G, Mete O, Uccella S, et al. Overview of the 2022 WHO classification of neuroendocrine neoplasms. Endocr Pathol. 2022;33(1):115–54.

37. Sames M, Vachata P, Zolal A, et al. Cranial base surgery. Cesk Slov Neurol N. 2013;76/109(4):402–24.
38. Schizodimos T, Soulountsi V, Iasonidou C, et al. An overview of management of intracranial hypertension in the intensive care unit. J Anesth. 2020;34(5):741–57.
39. Simons M, Morgan MK, Davidson AS. Cohort studies, trials, and tribulations: systematic review and an evidence-based approach to arteriovenous malformation treatment. J Neurosurg Sci. 2018;62(4):444–53.
40. Sklenka P, Kuthan P. Idiopathic intracranial hypertension—pseudotumor cerebri from the ophthalmologist's point of view. Neurol Practice. 2011;12(3):167–9.
41. Sonkova Z. Causes and Clinical presentation of intracranial hypertension. Neurol Practice. 2009;10(1):9–12.
42. Sozio SM, Armstrong PA, Coresh J, et al. Cerebrovascular disease incidence, characteristics, and outcomes in patients initiating dialysis: the choices for healthy outcomes in caring for ESRD (CHOICE) study. Am J Kidney Dis. 2009;54(3):468–77.
43. Svajdler M, Rychly B, Zamecnik J, et al. News in the WHO classification of tumors of the central nervous system 2016. Part 1: Diffuse infiltrating gliomas. Czech Pathol. 2017;53(1):12–21.
44. Vachata P, Zikmund L, Kozak J, et al. Tumors of the eye. Czech Words Neurol N. 2015;78/111(6):617–38.
45. Vybihal V, Smrcka M, Roskova I, et al. Surgical treatment of brain metastases. Czech Words Neurol N. 2020;83(2):156–65.
46. Vybihal V. Surgical treatment of hydrocephalus. Cesk Slov Neurol N. 2014;77/110(1):7–22.
47. Zamecnik J, Rychly B, Svajdler M. News in the WHO classification of tumors of the central nervous system 2016. Part 2: Embryonic tumors of the CNS and other groups of tumors (except diffuse gliomas). Czech Pathol. 2017;53(1):22–8.
48. Zeman M. et al. Special surgery. Prague: Galen; 2004.

Infectious Diseases

Alexandr Stepanov◉, Michal Holub, Milan Zlamal, Ondrej Beran, Zofia Bartovska, and Michal Ptacek

1 Lyme Disease

Lyme borreliosis (LB) is caused by *Borrelia burgdorferi*, a spirochete, gram-negative motile bacterium, mainly its species *B. Burgdorferi* sensu stricto, *B. garinii, B. afzelii* and, more recently known, *B. bavariensis.* LB is a tick-borne zoonosis. Reservoirs of Borrelia are mainly mammals, but also birds and reptiles. The disease is endemic mainly in Central Europe, some areas of the USA and in North-East Asia. The adherence of Borrelia to nerve cells, fibroblasts, endothelium, and epithelia is important for the pathogenesis of the disease, hence the typical manifestation on the skin, joints, nervous system, and heart, but any organ can be affected. Some manifestations are based on immunological mechanisms.

A. Stepanov (✉)
Ophthalmology Department, Klaudian's Hospital, Vaclava Klementa 147, 293 01 Mlada Boleslav, Czech Republic
e-mail: stepanov.doctor@gmail.com

Third Faculty of Medicine in Prague, Charles University, Ruska 2411, 100 00 Prague, Czech Republic

Department of Ophthalmology, University Hospital and Faculty of Medicine of Charles University in Hradec Kralove, Sokolska 581, 500 05 Hradec Kralove, Czech Republic

M. Holub · M. Zlamal · O. Beran · Z. Bartovska
Department of Infectious diseases, Central Military Hospital in Prague, U Vojenske nemocnice 1200, 169 02 Prague, Czech Republic
e-mail: Michal.Holub@lf1.cuni.cz

M. Zlamal
e-mail: milan.zlamal@lf1.cuni.cz

O. Beran
e-mail: ondrej.beran@lf1.cuni.cz

© The Author(s), under exclusive license to Springer Nature Switzerland AG 2024
A. Stepanov and J. Studnicka (eds.), *Ocular Manifestations of Systemic Diseases*,
https://doi.org/10.1007/978-3-031-58592-0_12

Clinical Presentation

Clinical manifestation occurs in only 4% of cases, with most cases being cutaneous forms, followed by 10–15% of nervous forms and 5% of articular/musculoskeletal manifestations; other forms include cardiac and ocular involvement or orchitis [19]. The disease is predominantly acute, with only 2% of chronic forms. The different stages of the disease with clinical forms are shown in Table 1.

The *skin manifestations* are characterised especially by erythema migrans, a reddening of at least 3 cm in diameter, which may be accompanied by flu-like symptoms in the days to weeks following the tick bite. In addition, an early stage borrelial lymphocytoma with an acral localisation (on the auricle, nipple, nasal wing, or scrotum) resembling a tumour may be present and is typical in childhood. The late stage represents acrodermatitis chronica atroficans (ACA) of the upper limbs, where early livid oedema and nodules in the subcutaneous tissue are followed by a late atrophic phase that can lead to destruction of peripheral nerves and joints. LB can affect the *peripheral and central nervous system* at all stages. Most cases of neuroborreliosis (95%) are early forms, where symptoms last less than 6 months, have a sudden onset and usually resolve spontaneously [19]. This is called Banwarth's syndrome, characterised by aseptic meningitis, cranial neuropathy—most often palsy of *the facial nerve*, but also of other cranial nerves (*n. oculomotorius* and *n. abducens, n. vestibulocochlearis*) and radiculoneuritis with root pain and motor-sensory impairment. Late neuroborreliosis accounts for only 5% of cases; the chronic course is

Table 1 Stages and clinical manifestations of Lyme disease

Stage	Affected
Early localized (up to two weeks)	Erythema migrans
Early disseminated (weeks to months)	Multiple erythema migrans Borrelial lymphocytoma Acute neuroborreliosis—cranial neuritis, Aseptic meningitis, Bannwarth's syndrome Lyme arthritis Lyme carditis
Late disseminated (months to years)	Acrodermatitis chronica atroficans Late neuroborreliosis—chronic progressive Encephalomyelitis, chronic polyneuritis Late Lyme arthritis

Z. Bartovska
e-mail: zofia.bartovska@lf1.cuni.cz

First Faculty of Medicine in Prague, Charles University, Katerinska 1660/32, 121 08 Prague, Czech Republic

M. Ptacek
Department of Infectious Disease, Silesian Hospital, Olomoucka 470/86, 746 01 Opava, Czech Republic
e-mail: radar115@seznam.cz

Infectious Diseases

prolonged and is sometimes associated with ACA. It mainly involves asymmetric paraesthesias, pain and paresis in the root regions on the distal parts of the limbs. The post-LB syndrome, reported by 10–50% of patients with neuroborreliosis, should be distinguished from the neurological forms [19]. It includes subjective nonspecific polymorphic complaints (fatigue, paraesthesias, sleep disordes, cognitive impairment, headache, arthralgia, and myalgia) that persist for more than 6 months after adequate treatment, with poor clinical and laboratory correlates. Repeated therapy or prolonged antibiotic regimens are not indicated. Another manifestation of LB is *lyme arthritis*, which is divided into early and late form. Early arthritis is characterized by migratory arthralgias to arthritis of small joints or, more rarely, musculoskeletal involvement (e.g. bursitis, tendovaginitis, fasciitis, and myositis) that usually resolves. In contrast, late arthritis is mono- or oligoarticular in nature with asymmetric, intermittent to persistent involvement of large joints, especially the knees. Immune and genetic mechanisms play an important role, which is why up to 10% of arthritis is refractory to antibiotic treatment. *Cardiac involvement* is present in about 1% of clinical manifestation of LB and is mainly atrioventricular block, myocarditis, pericarditis, and cardiomyopathy [19].

Diagnosis

Diagnosis is based on two-step serology. The first is performed by ELISA IgG and IgM immunoassay, which if positive is confirmed by Western blot. Serology carries several pitfalls (late production and short duration of IgM presence, simultaneous IgM false positivity, cross-reactivity, persistence of antibodies, and others). Therefore, it is always necessary to assess the results in the context of the clinical presentation and medical history [21]. In some cases, the detection of Borrelia DNA by PCR, especially in synovial fluid or skin biopsies, may help in establishing a diagnosis. For the diagnosis of neuroborreliosis, the proof of intrathecal synthesis of borrelial antibodies—the antibody index—is essential, in combination with the corresponding clinical presentation and serous cerebrospinal fluid formula.

Therapy

Therapy of LB consists of antibiotics. In cutaneous, articular and musculoskeletal forms, the first-choice antibiotic is doxycycline (with contraindications in pregnant or breast-feeding women and children under 8 years of age), and amoxicillin, cefuroxime or macrolide antibiotics may also be used. In neurological and cardiac forms, or in refractory articular forms, 3rd- generation cephalosporins or penicillin are given intravenously. The duration of therapy is usually 2 weeks for acute forms and 3–4 weeks for chronic forms. Lyme arthritis is the only indication for repeat antibiotic therapy.

2 Ocular Manifestations of Lyme Disease

The ocular manifestations of LB vary, depending on the stage of the disease, and patients may be asymptomatic at all stages. The ocular form of LB is very similar to the clinical presentation of ocular complications of syphilis. Most descriptions of ocular findings of LB in the literature are from single case reports or a series of case reports [27].

Clinical Presentation

Clinical manifestations of LB include eye pain, decreased visual acuity, photophobia, floating dots in the visual field, diplopia and impaired accommodation.

Objective Findings

Orbit

Orbital involvement is manifested by myositis or posterior scleritis.

Conjunctiva

Follicular conjunctivitis is present in approximately 10% of patients [27]. Since the ocular signs and symptoms are generally mild, the patient often delays a visit to the ophthalmologist.

Keratitis

Keratitis occurs months to years after primo infection. Patients complain of a slight decrease in visual acuity and photophobia. Objective findings include subepithelial and stromal infiltration, mostly bilateral. The infiltrates have indistinct margins, may be peripheral or diffuse, and may involve both superficial and deep stroma [57]. Corneal neovascularisation is minimal or absent. Episcleritis may accompany keratitis or occur in isolation as a late manifestation. Because LB-based keratitis responds only to topical steroids, it is presumed to be an autoimmune process.

Neuro-ophthalmological Complications

In the disseminated phase of the disease, neuro-ophthalmological complications predominate. The most common are cranial neuropathy and optic nerve involvement [27]. Optic nerve complications include optic neuritis, optic nerve swelling and papillitis. Isolated optic nerve involvement is not uncommon. Swelling of the optic nerve occurs because of meningitis and increased intracranial pressure and may manifest as transient blurring of vision. Optic neuritis can lead to subsequent atrophy of the optic nerve. Papillitis often occurs in association with Lyme uveitis [21].

Neuropathy of the cranial nerves is the result of a direct infection of the nerve or secondary to meningitis, an autoimmune process or increased intracranial pressure. Facial nerve palsy (Bell's palsy) is the most common neurological manifestation of LB, occurring in up to 10% of patients [27]. Bilateral involvement occurs in up to one-third of affected patients. Cranial nerve palsy can also be both unilateral and

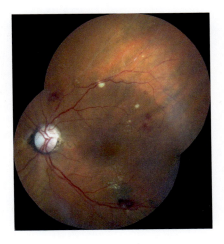

Fig. 1 Focal neuroretinitis and occlusive retinal vasculitis in Lyme disease

bilateral. Neuropathies of the 3rd, 4th and 5th cranial nerves are less common [57]. Multiple cranial nerves may be affected in one patient. Neuropathies often resolve without sequelae within weeks to months, but the condition may recur after treatment.

Posterior Eye Segment

Anterior and intermediate uveitis, neuroretinitis, retinal vasculitis, choroiditis and panuveitis have been described (Fig. 1).

The most common manifestation is intermediate uveitis, with often severe vitritis accompanied by a granulomatous reaction in the anterior chamber [27, 57]. Long-term choroidal involvement leads gradually to atrophy of the RPE.

Diagnosis

It includes examination of the anterior segment of the eye using biomicroscopy, and documentation of the findings on the posterior segment using digital fundus photography. Fluorescence angiography (FAG) shows delayed or patchy choriocapillary filling with areas of choroidal hyperfluorescence and blockage of filling by pigment changes. Late filling of retinal vessels is noted because of vasculitis or occlusive vascular changes.

Differential Diagnosis

- Vogt-Koyanagi-Harada syndrome
- Clinical presentation of any uveitis

Therapy

For treatment, the following regimen of treatment with systemic antibiotics is used.

3 Bartonellosis

Infection is caused by bartonellae, which are gram-negative bacteria adapted to mammalian hosts. The affinity of bartonellae for the endothelium and the ability to induce angiogenesis play a major role in the pathogenesis [31]. Bartonellae adapted to humans include *Bartonella quintana* and *B. bacilliformis*, which are transmitted by insects. Other bartonellae have other mammalian hosts but can occasionally cause disease in humans following contact with an infected animal, notably *B. henselae* (cat) and *B. elizabethae* (rat).

3.1 Cat Scratch Disease

One of the most common zoonoses worldwide is Cat Scratch Disease (also felinosis) caused by *B. henselae*. The most common source of infection for humans is the cat (more rarely, also the dog, squirrel, or goat). Infection occurs after being scratched or bitten by the animal, but also by ocular inoculation and, rarely, transmission by vectors—lice or ticks [22]. Felinosis is particularly common in children. After an incubation period of 1–3 weeks, lymphadenopathy occurs, localized according to the the site of entry of infection, often accompanied by skin vesicle/ulcer and systemic symptoms [5]. Occasionally, in immunosuppressed individuals, generalisation of the disease by haematogenous spread occurs. When the gateway to infection is conjunctiva, granulomatous conjunctivitis with preauricular lymphadenitis called Perinaud's syndrome develops.

The diagnosis of felinosis is based on the clinical manifestation, epidemiological history, and an increase of inflammatory parameters. The aetiological diagnosis is confirmed serologically.

Therapy consists of administration of doxycycline, quinolones, or macrolides for 14 days. In more severe courses, these antibiotics can be combined with rifampicin. In ocular forms, supportive corticoid therapy is sometimes administrated.

3.2 Volhynia Fever

Among the bartonellae adapted to humans B. quintana is the causative agent of Volhynia fever (also trench fever, five-day fever) the vector is a louse, and the aetiological agent is introduced into the skin by scratching. This disease occurred during World War I and World War II due to poor hygienic conditions [31]. After a 2-week incubation period, symptoms lasted for about 5 days and included fever, lower limb pain, and sometimes gastrointestinal symptoms and meningeal irritation. Symptoms returned several times and gradually diminished over several weeks. At present, diseases caused by *B. quintana* are mainly encountered in homeless people in

Infectious Diseases

Europe and the United States and include febrile bacteriaemia, infective endocarditis or bacillary angiomatosis. Bacillary angiomatosis with cutaneous and subcutaneous manifestations and bone lesions was also described in HIV + patients in the 1990s [31].

Diagnosis is based on serology in the case of a positive epidemiological history; it is possible to use prolonged blood culture incubation, or PCR examination.

The therapy consists of the administration of antibiotics—doxycycline, macrolides are used; in more severe courses, they are recommended in combination with gentamicin or rifampicin, or the 3rd-generation cephalosporins intravenously.

3.3 Oroya Fever and Verruga Peruana

Another of the bartonellae, *B. bacilliformis*, is associated with Oroya Fever and Verruga Peruanaperuana (also Carrión's disease). It is endemic in the mountainous regions of South America, the reservoir being humans and the vector of transmission being mosquitoes of *Lutzomyia*. After an incubation period of 2–12 weeks, Oroya Fever with influenza-like symptoms may develop, gastroenterological or neurological symptoms, haemorrhagic manifestations and severe anaemia may occur, with a lethality of tens of percent in untreated patients [31]. The course is biphasic, with an eruptive phase of infection, called Verruga Peruana, after several weeks to months of asymptomatic bacteraemia, skin manifestations resembling haemangiomas, mainly on the upper limbs and face, and more rarely haemorrhagic nodules forming on mucous membranes.

Diagnosis differs from other bartonellae—microscopic examination or culture, or histology and PCR tests are essential.

Therapy consists of administration of quinolone or macrolide antibiotics or 3rd-generation cephalosporins in more severe cases.

4 Ocular Manifestations of Bartonellosis

The incidence of ocular involvement in bartonellosis (specifically cat scratch disease) is not known with certainty, because current knowledge of the disease is based on small patient groups, case series and case reports. It is estimated that approximately 5–10% of patients develop conjunctivitis and 0.15% of cases may develop neuroretinitis [29].

Clinical Presentation and Objective Findings

Anterior Eye Segment

Systemic signs and symptoms usually precede ocular manifestations and are essential for diagnosis. Three to ten days after the scratch, a small erythematous papule forms on the skin. Seven to fourteen days later, superficial injection and conjunctival chemosis with serous secretion may follow. Follicular conjunctivitis affects both the bulbar and palpebral conjunctiva, and if the conjunctiva is the site of inoculation, a conjunctival granuloma may be present at this site. Two to three weeks after infection, regional lymphadenopathy occurs and is often accompanied by myalgias, malaise, fatigue, and fever [29]. The finding of conjunctivitis accompanied by regional lymphadenopathy is called Parinaud's oculoglandular syndrome. Other forms of ocular manifestations of cat scratch disease include anterior uveitis and orbital abscess.

Posterior Eye Segment

The clinical presentation of the posterior segment of the eye is dominated by focal or multifocal neuroretinitis, choroiditis, intermediate uveitis, and vaso-occlusive conditions. The first clinical manifestation of ocular involvement usually occurs within one month after infection with *B. henselae*, with a decrease in visual acuity with gradual progression over the following 2–3 weeks. Visual acuity usually ranges from 20/25 to 20/200, in some cases even worse [29]. Unilateral involvement is more common, only in immunocompromised patients is the disease bilateral [29]. A relative afferent pupillary defect is often present. Clinical findings in the posterior segment of the eye are dominated by optic disc oedema and star-shaped hard exudates in the macula. The macular star may be complete or partial. In the case of incomplete macular star, the deposition of exudates occurs mostly in the nasal part of the macula and is absorbed within 8–12 weeks. Other findings include local or multifocal neuroretinitis and chorioretinitis. In the case of inner retinal barrier involvement, intraretinal haemorrhages and soft exudates on the fundus are found. Branch arteriolar or venous occlusions associated with areas of focal neuroretinitis can be noted quite rarely. Quite rarely, cat scratch disease manifests as a large, highly vascularised inflammatory deposit on the fundus. In an immunocompetent person, the prognosis is favourable, and in most patients with neuroretinitis, visual acuity improves to physiological values.

Diagnosis

On FAG, gradual hyperfluorescence can be observed around the papilla of the optic nerve and perivascularly. On the perimeter, a cecocentral or paracentral scotoma is seen, as well as enlargement of the blind spot. Visual evoked potentials (VEP) are reduced in the affected eye compared to the healthy eye, but electroretinography (ERG) remains normal. For diagnostic purposes, a PCR test is used to determine the presence of a given bacterium from the intraocular fluid by detecting or amplifying a small fragment of the bacterial 16S rRNA gene [29].

Differential Diagnosis

- Tuberculosis
- Toxoplasmosis
- Toxocariasis
- Syphilis

Infectious Diseases

- Lyme disease
- Leptospirosis
- Varicella zoster and herpes simplex neuroretinitis
- Macular star findings—systemic vascular disease (e.g. acute arterial hypertension, increased intracranial pressure (pseudotumour cerebri), diabetic papillopathy, and also anterior ischaemic optic neuropathy)
- Multifocal neuroretinitis—non-infectious diseases with white focal lesions (e.g. white dot syndrome, acute posterior multifocal placoid pigment epitheliopathy and Vogt-Koyanagi-Harad disease)

Therapy

Common oral antibiotics (doxycycline, erythromycin) are used in usual doses.

5 Leptospirosis

It is an infection caused by leptospires, gram-negative bacteria that belong to the spirochetes. The most important human pathogens are the species *Leptospira interrogans* (serovars Icterohaemorrhagiae, Pomona and others), *L. noguchii* and *L. Kirschnerii* (serovar Grippotyphosa). The reservoir are mainly rodents, which excrete leptospires in the urine and contaminate mainly water sources. Infection occurs through direct contact with rodents and their urine, or contaminated water and food. Drinking and bathing in unverified water sources is particularly risky, and professional infection may also occur. The disease is endemic especially in the tropics [51]. Pathogenetically, vasculitis occurs and the target organ is the kidney. The incubation period is 5–14 days and the course of the disease varies in severity from asymptomatic to lethal. The disease usually has a biphasic course—an acute septic phase is followed by a phase with signs of organ involvement (immune phase).

Clinical Presentation

The most frequent form is *Harvest (Swamp) Fever* caused by the serovar Grippotyphosa, which in the first phase manifests like influenza, sometimes with dyspeptic symptoms, and, in some patients, passes to the second phase with manifestations of aseptic meningitis, myalgias, splenomegaly and exanthema [51]. Hepatic and renal parameters may be elevated. The prognosis of the disease is favourable. In contrast, *Weil's disease* caused by serovar Icterohaemorrhagiae has a more severe course. The dramatic septic phase is immediately followed by organ damage, especially cholestatic icterus, renal failure, haemorrhagic manifestations are common, conjunctival suffusion, and the lungs, myocardium and CNS may be affected. In these cases, death of the patient is not infrequent, due mainly to hepatic or renal failure and disseminated intravascular coagulopathy.

Diagnosis

Diagnosis is based on the clinical presentation associated with elevation of liver and renal parameters, or the presence of serous meningitis and haemorrhagic skin manifestations. For aetiological diagnosis, PCR detection of leptospira in blood or cerebrospinal fluid early in the disease and later in urine is used [28]. Serological diagnosis is also used, despite some pitfalls (positivity after 1–3 weeks, cross-reactivity with other spirochetes).

Therapy

Antibiotic therapy is therefore usually initiated empirically—for milder forms, weekly oral antibiotic therapy with doxycycline, amoxicillin or azithromycin. For more severe forms, penicillin, ceftriaxone, or ampicillin is used intravenously for two weeks. In the most severe cases, hospitalisation in an Intensive Care Unit with haemodialysis, support of vital functions and haemocoagulation factor replacement is necessary.

6 Ocular Manifestations of Leptospirosis

The ocular complications of systemic leptospirosis were first described by Adolf Weilem [52]. The incidence of ocular symptoms during the acute systemic phase ranges from 2 to 90% [42]. In some cases, however, ocular manifestations may be subclinical or mild. The prolonged asymptomatic period between systemic and ocular manifestations makes it difficult for the ophthalmologist to link uveitis to leptospirosis. The lack of laboratory testing further impairs the accuracy of diagnosis.

Risk Factors

- Age, uveitis usually affects young and middle-aged patients
- Gender—more often affects men

Clinical Presentation and Objective Findings

Anterior Eye Segment

The earliest and most common manifestation of ocular leptospirosis is conjunctival hyperaemia or subconjunctival suffusion. Other typical manifestations of anterior segment involvement include nongranulomatous anterior uveitis (92%), the occurrence of posterior synechiae (24%) and hypopyon (13%) [42].

Leptospirosis is generally rather underdiagnosed, therefore leptospiral uveitis often occurs many months after the manifestation of systemic disease. There are two distinct forms of leptospiral uveitis. In patients with the first type, anterior uveitis with photophobia, blurred vision and pain are found.

Infectious Diseases

Posterior Eye Segment

The second type includes posterior uveitis, including vitritis, choroiditis, papillitis or even panuveitis [42]. Vitritis is very often severe, with formation of vitreous opacities or inflammatory membranes associated with optic nerve papillae. Occasionally, a feature known as "snowballs" occurs. Another finding may be non-occlusive vasculitis.

Diagnosis

For diagnostic purposes, testing to detect the presence of antibodies to Leptospira interrogans by ELISA or PCR in a sample of intraocular fluid is used.

Differential Diagnosis

- HLA-B27 uveitis
- Idiopathic pars planitis
- Occlusive vasculitis in Behçet's disease
- Eales disease
- Ocular complications of TB

Therapy

In the case of signs of anterior uveitis, corticosteroids topically and mydriatic agents are applied.

7 Brucellosis

The infection is caused by Brucella, gram-negative coccobacilli, intracellular pathogens surviving in macrophages and infecting mainly lymphoid tissues with subsequent granulomatous inflammation [3]. Cellular immunity is crucial. Brucellae include several species, endemic mainly in the Mediterranean and Arabian Peninsula, sub-Saharan Africa, South and Central America [3]. Hosts of brucellae are domestic animals that excrete them into the birth canal—*Brucella abortus* (cattle, camel), *B. suis* (pig, reindeer, camel), *B. canis* (dog), *B. melitensis* (goat, sheep). It is the most common zoonosis with a severe impact in endemic areas worldwide. Infection transmits either by ingestion of unpasteurised milk and dairy products or by direct inoculation of infected tissue or body fluids into a wound or conjunctiva, or more rarely by inhalation of contaminated aerosol [4]. The incubation period is 2–4 weeks, after which a progressive systemic disease develops with involvement of various organs. The severity of the course varies and the disease may mimic specific tuberculous processes or systemic diseases.

Clinical Presentation

Brucellosis may begin acutely or gradually with non-specific symptoms—undulant fever, general weakness, night sweats, lumbago and arthralgia, hepatosplenomegaly, lymphadenopathy, dyspeptic and musculoskeletal impairment, pulmonary manifestations, and more rarely neurobrucellosis or abortion in pregnant women. Recovery is long lasting, sometimes with permanent sequelae, and the disease often progresses to chronicity or relapses. Chronic musculoskeletal impairment, especially of the sacroiliac joint with low lethality, caused by *B. abortus* is referred to as *Bang's disease*. Higher lethality with fevers and organ complications is seen in *Malta fever*—the causative agent is *B. melitensis*. The most severe courses are caused by *B. suis* (febris undulans Traum) with sepsis, liver abscesses and a mortality rate approaching 50% [3].

Diagnosis

Diagnosis is difficult due to nonspecific clinical manifestations. Epidemiological anamnesis, elevation of liver function tests and changes in blood count can lead to the correct diagnosis. The aetiological diagnosis of brucellosis is confirmed by culture of blood, bone marrow and body fluids. Serology and PCR detection of brucellae are also reliable.

Therapy

Antibiotic therapy of brucellosis takes a long time (6–24 weeks), with the most common combination being doxycycline with gentamicin or rifampicin. Cotrimoxazole is given instead of doxycycline in children under 8 years of age, and 3rd-generation cephalosporins are appropriate for treatment of neurobrucellosis.

8 Ocular Manifestations of Brucellosis

Brucellosis is one of the world's most widespread, highly contagious zoonotic bacterial diseases in animals and humans. Ocular complications of systemic brucellosis are estimated to occur in 2–3% of cases, with a very wide range of manifestations [49]. Uveitis is the most common ocular manifestation of brucellosis, occurring in up to 83% of patients with ocular complications of the disease [49]. Although bilateral involvement is not uncommon, in most cases, only one eye is affected.

Clinical presentations include photophobia, eye pain and, in the case of uveitis, a decrease in central visual acuity, metamorphopsia and a decrease in contrast sensitivity. In the case of cystoid macular oedema, positive scotoma in the visual field, retrobulbar neuritis and serous retinal detachment.

Objective Findings

Anterior Eye Segment

Anterior uveitis can be either granulomatous or non-granulomatous, ranging in severity from mild inflammation with typical keratic "scopulose" precipitates to severe inflammation with development of hypopyon, metastatic endophthalmitis and phthisis of the eye. Chronic iridocyclitis can cause formation of Koeppe's

Infectious Diseases

nodules, posterior synechiae, lens opacities and secondary glaucoma. Unusual ocular manifestations of brucellosis include conjunctivitis, nummular subepithelial corneal infiltrates, corneal ulceration with accompanying iritis and focal or diffuse scleritis [49].

Posterior Eye Segment

The typical picture of posterior uveitis includes vitritis, panuveitis, multifocal choroiditis, retinitis, vasculitis, cystoid macular oedema, serous retinal detachment and retrobulbar optic neuritis [1].

Diagnosis

It includes examination of the anterior segment of the eye using biomicroscopy, and the posterior segment using digital fundus photography. Other methods used in patients with complications of brucellosis include OCT to demonstrate macular oedema, FAG to show vasculitis and retinitis, and ultrasound to rule out serous retinal detachment.

Differential Diagnosis

The differential diagnosis of ocular brucellosis is broad and requires systematic exclusion of other infectious and non-infectious causes of uveitis, especially those with findings of multifocal choroiditis [2].

- Infectious diseases: TB and syphilis, Lyme disease, toxoplasmosis, diffuse unilateral subacute neuroretinitis, septic choroiditis, viral retinitis (CMV, HSV, HZV) and presumed ocular histoplasmosis syndrome
- Non-infectious diseases: sarcoidosis, Vogt-Koyanagi-Harad disease, acute posterior multifocal placoid pigment epitheliopathy, multiple white dot syndrome, internal choroidopathy, sympathetic ophthalmia, etc.

Therapy

It requires early and effective treatment of the underlying disease. In severe cases, antibiotic therapy is given in combination with local or total steroids.

9 Herpetic Infections

Human infections are caused by 8 herpes viruses, which are divided into three groups as listed in Table 2.

Human herpes viruses share many common characteristics: their genome consists of linear double-stranded DNA, they replicate within the cell nucleus, and cells infected with them usually die. Human herpes viruses usually persist asymptomatically in their host throughout its lifetime (going into latency), but from time to time they reactivate (especially when immunity is compromised), which may be accompanied by various clinical manifestations.

Table 2 Taxonomy of human herpes viruses

Group	Virus
Alphaherpesvirinae	Herpes simplex virus type 1 (HSV-1)
	Herpes simplex virus type 2 (HSV-2)
	Varicella-zoster virus (VZV)
Betaherpesvirinae	Cytomegalovirus (CMV)
	Human herpesvirus type 6 (HHV-6)
	Human herpesvirus type 7 (HHV-7)
Gammaherpesvirinae	Epstein-Barr virus (EBV)
	Human herpesvirus type 8 (HHV-8)

9.1 Herpes Simplex Viruses

Infections caused by the herpes simplex viruses HSV-1 and HSV-2 occur from early childhood into adulthood. HSV-1 virus is mostly transmitted through saliva. In contrast, HSV-2 infection is typically transmitted through sexual contact and therefore only occurs in young adults (the exception is neonatal infections, where the infected mother is the source). Infection with HSV (primary infection) is usually asymptomatic but may have nonspecific symptoms (e.g. flu-like) or be fully clinically expressed [55].

Clinical Presentation

Clinical manifestations of HSV primary infection include gingivostomatitis, tonsillopharyngitis, keratoconjunctivitis, genital herpes, necrotising encephalitis and myelitis, various neuritis, and possibly cystitis. The most common clinical manifestations of reactivation of latent HSV infection are labial herpes, aphthae, conjunctivitis, and genital herpes [55]. Reinfection, in which HSV is introduced into damaged skin areas, is also possible. An example is what is called Kaposi's varicella dermatitis in the predilection sites of atopic eczema.

Diagnosis

Diagnosis of HSV infection is mostly clinical; in unclear cases, direct detection of viral DNA in material collected from the affected area (vesicles), or in cerebrospinal fluid, blood, amniotic fluid, or urine can be used.

Therapy

Therapy consists of administering aciclovir (orally or parenterally, depending on the severity of the condition). Valacyclovir can also be used for oral treatment, and famciclovir is an available alternative in the case of allergy to aciclovir.

Infectious Diseases

9.2 Varicella-Zoster Virus

Primary infection caused by varicella-zoster virus (VZV) is almost always clinically manifested and manifests as chickenpox (varicella), a highly contagious infectious disease most commonly affecting children, with a few cases occurring in adults.

Clinical Presentation

The clinical manifestation is characterised by high fever and skin rash, which has a maximum on the trunk. The skin efflorescences most often start as macules and within hours change to papules, vesicles, and pustules, which dry up after a few days and turn into crusts. All these types of skin efflorescence are usually visible on the body of the affected person, as the rash occurs in waves during the first 3–4 days of the disease [15]. The rash is almost always also present in the hairy part of the head and not infrequently affects the mucous membranes, including the conjunctiva. Varicella has numerous complications, either caused directly by VZV (cerebellitis in children and primary interstitial pneumonia in adults being the most common), or due to secondary staphylococcal or streptococcal skin infections.

Diagnosis and Therapy

Diagnosis is in most cases clinical; in case of doubt, DNA detection of VZV by PCR can be used. Therapy consists of administration of aciclovir for more severe disease or in the case of virus-induced complications.

9.3 Shingles

Reactivation of latent VZV infection is most often manifested as shingles (herpes zoster), which is characterised by localised vesicular rash, most often in the thoracic or lumbar region. In some patients, the eruption manifests in the face, often in the area innervated by *n. ophthalmicus*. Herpes zoster has numerous complications—the most important is postherpetic neuralgia, which affects up to 20% of patients [39].

Therapy of herpes zoster and complicated varicella courses consists of administration of aciclovir, which is administered orally or parenterally, depending on the severity of the disease, localisation of exanthema and immune status.

9.4 Epstein-Barr Virus, Cytomegalovirus, Human Herpesviruses 6–8

Clinical Presentation

Clinically manifested primary infections caused by Epstein and Barr virus (EBV), cytomegalovirus (CMV), human herpesviruses 6 and 7 (HHV-6 and HHV-7) most commonly present as sore throat, fever, and lymphadenopathy. On clinical examination, there is often pseudomembranous tonsillitis with marked enlargement of the cervical nodes, generalised lymphadenopathy, and splenomegaly with hepatomegaly in almost one-half of patients. If EBV is the cause of these findings, it is infectious mononucleosis. If CMV, HHV-6 or HHV-7 infection is responsible for the clinical presentation, it is infectious mononucleosis syndrome. The most common complication of both these diagnoses is bacterial superinfection of the tonsils.

Diagnosis

The diagnosis of infectious mononucleosis is based on the detection of specific antibodies in the blood. It should be emphasised that serious malignancies such as Burkitt's lymphoma, primary cerebral lymphoma, Hodgkin's lymphoma, and nasopharyngeal carcinoma are also associated with EBV. Primoinfections or reactivations of these latent herpetic infections in immunodeficient patients with impaired cellular immunity are very serious.

Therapy

Therapy is significantly limited, because there is no effective antiviral drug available, and the disease is treated symptomatically. Antibiotics are given for bacterial superinfection (aminopenicillins are contraindicated) and corticosteroids for upper airway obstruction.

CMV Infection

CMV infection can present as retinitis, encephalitis and pneumonitis in AIDS, congenital infection, or as systemic infection after transplantation. **Diagnosis** consists of the detection of low-avidity antibodies in the blood during primary infection; detection of viral DNA by PCR in blood, cerebrospinal fluid, amniotic fluid, respiratory aspirate, and urine is used to detect reactivation of latent infection or primary infection in immunosuppressed patients. Patients with inflammatory bowel disease (especially those on biologic therapy) and AIDS patients may also develop CMV colitis. **Therapy** is fully indicated in immunosuppressed patients and ganciclovir, valganciclovir, foscarnet, or cidofovir may be indicated.

HHV-6, HHV-7 and HHV-8 Infections

Primary infection with HHV-6 and HHV-7 can occur as the Sixth childhood disease (exanthema subitum) in addition to infectious mononucleosis syndrome. Reactivation of latent HHV-6 infection can cause fatal encephalitis in immunosuppressed patients, which is difficult to treat in the absence of effective antiviral therapy. Primary HHV-8 infection is asymptomatic. Reactivation of latent HHV-8 infection in patients with severe immunodeficiency affecting cellular immunity (e.g. in AIDS) can lead to serious cancers, such as Kaposi's sarcoma, angiosarcoma or primary effusion lymphoma, which are difficult to treat.

Infectious Diseases

9.5 Ocular Manifestations of Herpesviruses

Herpesviruses (family Herpesviridae) are among the largest known viral agents. They are widespread in populations worldwide. Their characteristic feature is that they remain latent in the body after primary infection (opportunistic infection). The main human herpes viruses causing ocular infections include: two types of herpes simplex virus, HSV-1 and HSV-2, herpes zoster virus—HZV, Epstein-Barr virus—EBV, cytomegalovirus—CMV. Ocular herpetic diseases associated with primary or recurrent infection can range from anterior to posterior segment inflammation. Inflammations may combine or accompany each other.

Risk Factors

- Promiscuous lifestyle
- Female gender
- Immunosuppressive state
- Co-infection with sexually transmitted diseases

Clinical Presentation and Objective Findings

Anterior Eye Segment

Typical clinical presentations on the anterior segment of the eye caused by alpha herpesviruses (HSV and VZV) include endotheliitis, trabeculitis and iridocyclitis.

Iritis or trabeculitis due to HSV may present with or without signs of corneal involvement. According to recommendations, iritis with a known history of herpetic keratitis should be considered herpetic until clinical findings or laboratory tests prove otherwise. Patients report redness of the eye, photophobia, pain, and decreased visual acuity. Anterior uveitis is manifested by the finding of fine or mutton-fat precipitates and varying degrees of cellular reaction in the anterior chamber. In general, herpetic iritis can be focal or diffuse. In the case of focal iritis, circumscribed iris hyperaemia, posterior synechiae, and iris pigment epithelial defects may be noted. The diffuse form of HSV iritis is much more widespread. It presents with severe cellular reaction in the anterior chamber and is often complicated by fulminant fibrin deposition, hypopyon, pupillary seclusion or secondary glaucoma. Inflammation may involve the trabecular meshwork, called "trabeculitis". Clinically, trabeculitis is characterised by a sudden increase in intraocular pressure and is associated with decompensation of the corneal endothelium. Glaucomatous crises may be temporary, but in some individuals glaucomatous damage to the optic nerve follows.

VZV-based iridocyclitis is the most common finding after herpes zoster ophthalmicus and usually occurs during the first week of acute illness. However, exacerbations have been observed even months after acute illness [12]. Cutaneous vesicles on the tip of the nose (Hutchinson's sign) suggest involvement of the nasociliary nerve and an increased likelihood of involvement of the eye. The diagnosis of VZV uveitis can be particularly difficult in cases without a previous skin eruption or zoster dermatitis ("zoster sine herpete"). The course of iridocyclitis may be mild or severe. Other typical findings are iris atrophy and damage to the m. sphincter pupillae. Hypopyon, hyphema, hypotony of the eyeball and very rarely phthisis of the eye occur. Secondary glaucoma is present in 10% of patients [12].

Posterior Eye Segment

9.6 Acute Retinal Necrosis

The clinical presentation was first described by Urayama in 1971, and 7 years later the term "acute retinal necrosis" (ARN) was officially introduced [50]. In 1982, Culbertson examined the enucleated eye histopathologically for the first time and the aetiology of ARN was suspected to be herpesviruses [10]. This is an infectious retinitis caused by herpesviruses, which is part of the spectrum of necrotising herpetic retinopathies. Recent studies based on PCR testing have shown that VZV is the most common cause of ARN, followed by HSV and, in rare cases, CMV [32]. HSV-1 and VZV infection are more commonly encountered in patients of older age, whereas patients with ARN caused by HSV-2 are younger than 25 years of age. Ocular involvement occurs in approximately 36% of cases, usually within 6 weeks of the onset of symptoms, although it may be delayed for several years after infection [32]. Retinitis may occur without systemic prodrome after primary infection or after cutaneous or systemic herpetic infection, such as herpes zoster of the skin, smallpox, or herpetic encephalitis. The incidence hardly differs between the two sexes. The disease has two peaks, with the first at age 20 and the second at about age 50. Genetic predisposition increases the relative risk of ARN in patients with specific HLA haplotypes.

Clinical Presentation and Objective Findings

The disease usually begins with anterior uveitis, with acute unilateral decrease in visual acuity, photophobia, floaters in the visual field and eye pain. In the following two weeks, the classic triad involving occlusive retinal vasculitis, vitritis, and multifocal yellow-white peripheral retinitis develops in the posterior segment of the eye. In the following 3–21 days, the peripheral retinal lesions coalesce into a picture of confluent creamy retinitis that progresses to necrosis with intraretinal haemorrhages (Fig. 2).

During the disease, several quadrants of the retina to the vascular arcades or the entire retinal surface may be affected [32]. The macular zone often remains unaffected. In some cases, retinal neovascularisation arises in the periphery underlying zones of vascular nonperfusion. Regression of ARN is first evident in the outer periphery, with the affected area having a pattern similar to Swiss Emmental cheese. The creamy retinal staining recedes and a "salt and pepper" appearance pigmentation follows, with sharp borders between normal and affected retina. At the same time, cellular infiltration of the vitreous progresses significantly with subsequent development of proliferative vitreoretinopathy (PVR). 75% of patients develop retinal

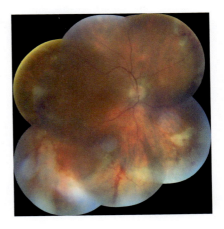

Fig. 2 Acute retinal necrosis due to VZV. Predominantly peripheral necrotizing retinitis, occlusive vasculitis with numerous haemorrhages

necrosis, multiple retinal tears and PVR to retinal detachment [32]. In patients with afferent pupillary defect and severe visual loss, optic nerve involvement should be suspected. Optic nerve oedema is a common finding at the onset of the disease. Optic neuropathy due to vasculitis, optic nerve ischaemia, and direct invasion of the optic nerve by herpesvirus is quite common in these patients.

In addition to ARN, three other types of posterior segment involvement in herpetic infection have been described: (1) the slow type with ARN-like necrotic lesions located in the periphery of the retina, characterised by slow progression, (2) vasculitis or papillitis with absence of retinal necrotic lesions, and (3) panuveitis without overt vasculitis or papillitis [32].

Diagnosis

The diagnosis of ARN is based on the typical clinical presentation and confirmed by the detection of specific antibodies or the presence of viral DNA. Antibody production can be assessed using the Goldmann-Witmer (GW) coefficient: the ratio of specific antibody/total IgG (from anterior chamber fluid or vitreous fluid) to specific antibody (serum)/total IgG (serum), measured by ELISA analysis. A ratio greater than 3.0 is considered diagnostic of local antibody production. Combining the GW ratio with PCR may increase the diagnostic benefit, especially for viral infections. PCR is probably the most sensitive, specific, and rapid diagnostic method for the detection of infectious posterior uveitis in general and ARN specifically, largely replacing viral culture and intraocular antibody titres. Quantitative PCR can add additional information regarding viral load, disease activity and response to therapy.

In rare cases where PCR is negative but clinical suspicion of ARN is high, endoretinal biopsy may be indicated [32]. FAG findings in the acute stage of ARN demonstrate leakage of fluorescein from retinal veins, arterioles, capillaries and often from the papilla of the optic nerve. Occlusions of vessels, especially arterioles and capillaries, can be noted in the affected peripheral parts of the retina.

Differential Diagnosis

- Progressive outer retinal necrosis (PORN)
- CMV retinitis
- Toxoplasma retinochoroiditis
- Syphilis
- Lymphoma
- Autoimmune retinal vasculitis

9.7 Progressive Outer Retinal Necrosis

In 1990, Forster described the condition now known as PORN [14]. It is a severe form of necrotising herpetic retinopathy, occurring most commonly in patients with advanced HIV/AIDS infection (CD4 + T cells < 50 cells/mm^3) or in severely immunocompromised patients [12]. VZV infection is the most common cause of PORN.

Clinical Presentation and Objective Findings

At the onset of this disease, multifocal flat creamy areas of retinal necrosis are seen, which rapidly coalesce. However, unlike ARN, there is no inflammatory reaction in the vitreous or accompanying retinal vasculitis. Approximately 71% of cases involve both eyes, and in 67% skin involvement can be found [12].

Therapy

Treatment with antiviral therapy alone is associated with an unsatisfactory prognosis for visual acuity. Better results are achieved by combining more than one antiviral agent (e.g. acyclovir with ganciclovir or ganciclovir with foscarnet) and by combining systemic and intravitreal antiviral therapy with foscarnet and ganciclovir.

9.8 Epstein-Barr Virus

Clinical Presentation and Objective Findings

Ocular complications of EBV are either due to congenital infection or, more commonly, to primary infection in the form of infectious mononucleosis. The typical finding is unilateral long-standing multifocal choroiditis without signs of anterior uveitis.

Differential Diagnosis

- Sarcoidosis
- Tuberculosis
- Syphilis
- Toxoplasmosis
- Histoplasmosis

Infectious Diseases

- White dot syndrome

9.9 Ocular Manifestations of Cytomegalovirus

Ocular complications of CMV were first described in a new-born in 1947 [24] and in an adult after chemotherapy in 1964 [45]. The most common ocular manifestation is CMV retinitis, which, in the pre-AIDS era, was a rare disease that occurred only in immunocompromised persons. With the advent of HAART (highly active antiretroviral therapy) in AIDS patients, the incidence of CMV retinitis has decreased significantly, yet it is the most common cause of blindness in AIDS patients [47].

Clinical Presentation and Objective Findings

Cytomegalovirus Anterior Uveitis

In rare cases, unilateral, chronic, or recurrent anterior uveitis associated with CMV with or without iris atrophy may occur in immunocompetent individuals.

Cytomegalovirus Retinitis

Congenital CMV retinitis is associated with other systemic manifestations of disseminated infection, including fever, thrombocytopenia, anaemia, pneumonia, and hepatosplenomegaly. Children with proven congenital CMV may not develop pathologic ocular complications, yet regular follow-up is needed for possible ocular involvement later in life. Symptoms of early disease may be quite minimal, such as blurred vision and floaters, especially when the involvement is in the periphery of the retina. Only in the case of macular involvement does a positive scotoma develop. In patients with CD4 + lymphocyte counts < 50 cells/mm^3 or if there is evidence of involvement of other organs, ophthalmological screening in artificial mydriasis is recommended every 3–4 months [47].

Three different variants of the clinical presentation of CMV retinitis have been described [47]:

1. Classic or fulminant haemorrhagic necrotising retinitis spreading mainly along the main vascular arcades (Fig. 3).
2. Granular indolent form, occurring more often on the periphery of the retina, is characterised by fewer haemorrhages, mild retinal oedema and retinal atrophy with active retinitis progressing from the lesion borders.
3. Perivascular form with a clinical presentation reminiscent of the syndrome of "frosted branch angiiti". The affected area is irregularly bordered and surrounded by satellite infiltrates. The optic disc may be infiltrated during the progression of retinitis towards the posterior pole.

The clinical course depends on the overall immune status of the patient. The progression of retinal necrosis is usually slow without treatment, approximately 0.2 mm/week, thus the entire retina is affected in approximately 3–6 months [47].

Fig. 3 Cytomegalovirus retinitis. Haemorrhagic necrotizing retinitis in the nasal periphery

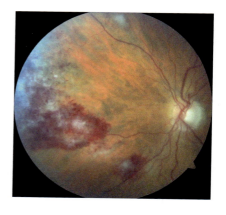

With anti-CMV treatment, the infiltration at the margins becomes transparent and the active lesion progresses to atrophy.

Diagnosis

Continuous photodocumentation appears to be much more sensitive for monitoring the progress of CMV retinitis than biomicroscopic examination. Follow-up at monthly intervals is recommended for inactive lesions. The diagnosis of CMV retinitis is usually based on the clinical presentation in an immunosuppressed individual. In distinguishing between active and inactive stages of the disease, the clinical presentation alone is more important than laboratory tests. Serum antibodies are often positive, even in most healthy persons and thus have no significant diagnostic value. Antibody levels from vitreous and anterior chamber fluid compared with serum levels (using the Goldmann-Witmer coefficient) may support the diagnosis in complicated cases. Because CMV can persist in tissue in an inactive state, these laboratory tests are useful only in conjunction with the clinical presentation.

Differential Diagnosis

- ARN
- PORN
- Syphilitic retinitis
- Fungal infections
- Toxoplasma involvement of the retina and choroid
- Intraocular lymphoma

Therapy

In the case of progression of retinitis despite systemic treatment, the first choice is intravitreal administration of anti-CMV drug. However, this treatment does not prevent extraocular spread of CMV or eventual involvement of the other eye. Local therapy should therefore be combined with systemic therapy. Intravitreal injections of ganciclovir (200–2,000 μg in 0.1 mL) or foscarnet (2.4 mg in 0.1 mL) can be given

Infectious Diseases 521

2–3 times a week at the start of treatment and once a week thereafter. The clinical response to treatment is very good in most cases. In cases of fulminant disease, the first choice is an intraocular implant with ganciclovir, which has a sustained release and provides a consistently high level of drug. In this case, progression of retinitis occurs after 221 days post-implantation, whereas after conventional intravitreal injection of ganciclovir, after 71 days.

9.10 Measles

The measles virus disease (lat. *morbilli*) has been repeatedly described in Europe since antiquity. The aetiological agent is an enveloped RNA virus of the *paramyxovirus* family. Measles is transmitted directly by droplets through the mucous membranes of the respiratory tract or conjunctivae. The only source of infection is the sick person, from the first symptoms of the prodromal stage until the 4th day after the onset of the rash. The incubation period is 10 days to catarrhal stage and 14 days to exanthem seeding; transmission by vaccinia virus has not been demonstrated. Measles is one of the most infectious viral diseases ever, and in developing countries where it is not vaccinated even today, it is still a common cause of childhood deaths [40].

Measles affects susceptible people at any age, and the disease can also be life-threatening at any age, especially if complications occur. In Europe, the annual incidence is described as about 2/100,000 persons, while the mortality rate in developed countries is described as about 1/1,000 measles cases, although data vary [40]. Once the virus has entered the body, there is a transient and severe decline in cellular immunity: this may be clinically manifested, e.g. by development of severe sessile bacterial infections of the respiratory tract (bronchitis, bronchopneumonia, sinusitis, bronchiolitis in young children—the cause of death in the youngest patients is respiratory failure), otitis media, conjunctivitis, exacerbation of the tuberculous process due to weakening of the organism may also occur.

Clinical Presentation

Clinically, after the incubation period, the disease is divided into two stages, *catarrhal* and *exanthemic*. In the first stage—catarrhal (prodromal)—which lasts about 3 to 5 days, patients are weak, have conjunctivitis, sweating, fever, runny nose, and dry, tracheal cough. Even before the exanthema is sown, grey-white macules with a red margin, called Koplik spots, appear on the buccal mucosa at the level of the molars in some cases. These may resemble sores; the Koplik spots disappear with the onset of exanthema. The second—exanthematous—stage appears on about Day 4 after the onset of the troubles. The fever is accompanied by the appearance of a confluent deep red to reddish-purple maculopapular exanthema: typically starting behind the ears and on the back of the neck, it spreads gradually over about 4 days to the face, neck, trunk, and extremities (including the palms and hands). After about 5 days, the exanthema disappears in the same order, and the conjunctivitis and persistent high fever subside, responding only very reluctantly to antipyretics. Sometimes hyperpigmentation may remain transiently, or the skin may peel. In severe cases, the exanthema may be haemorrhagic. Similar exanthema—but with a different clinical appearance and different time course—is also seen as pollen, toxoallergic, in some viruses including coronaviruses, and in scarlet fever or rubella [56].

Throughout the disease period, patients are limp, weak, and sleepy, children are restless and irritable. A less severe or incompletely expressed course in under-immunised (e.g. unvaccinated, etc.) persons is called mitigated measles.

In addition to the seeding bacterial complications of weakened cellular immunity in measles, complications of measles caused directly by the measles virus can occur rarely: viral interstitial pneumonia, encephalitis, meningitis, very rarely laryngitis and appendicitis. Very rarely, rather in young patients, a late complication of measles or even measles vaccination—subacute sclerosing panencephalitis—is also described [40].

Diagnosis

The diagnosis of measles clinically in a typical course is not difficult if it is thought of (at least 3 days of prodromes and at least 3 days of exanthema). Epidemiological anamnesis—travel history or measles in the vicinity can be very helpful. Parents of unvaccinated children do not always readily admit this fact (whether they are vaccine refusers or families who, for example, have lived abroad for a long time and their children have willingly or unwillingly avoided vaccination) [40]. Direct laboratory confirmation is done by PCR testing of nasopharyngeal swabs, possibly saliva or urine, ideally by Day 3 of the problem. Another option used is serological—determination of antibody titres (IgG—passed or vaccinated, IgM—ongoing infection).

Therapy

The treatment is only supportive and symptomatic—analgesics and antipyretics, sufficient fluids, or adjustment of the mineralogram in the case of heavy sweating. Antibiotics are indicated when a seeding bacterial superinfection is proven. There is no effective antiviral agent. The patient expels viruses through the respiratory tract about 6 days before the onset of the prodromal stage and by Day 6 of the rash. The disease is notifiable, and patients should be isolated and hospitalised for a mandatory period of infectiousness. Pregnant women do not develop congenital foetal malformations, but there is a risk of spontaneous abortion. Patients with measles and a history of tuberculosis should have a follow-up chest X-ray approximately 6 weeks apart. Vitamin A levels decline with the disease and there is a risk (especially in poorly nourished children) of corneal involvement; vitamin A replacement is recommended in malnourished patients (in the developing world, measles is still described in about 30 million children per year).

Prevention

Proper vaccination is an option for prevention. It is a live vaccine administered subcutaneously or intramuscularly. Up to one-third of vaccinated persons develop a

Infectious Diseases   523

physiological post-vaccination reaction (subfebrile, conjunctivitis, upper respiratory tract catarrh) in the second week after vaccination, but this is not contagious and resolves spontaneously [40]. Immunity after vaccination can be extinguished in a small proportion of the population: the effective antibody level status can be determined by testing serum IgG antibody levels. In the case of insufficient immunity, re-vaccination with 1 dose of the regular vaccine is then indicated. In contrast, after measles infection, permanent, lifelong immunity is established.

9.11   Ocular Manifestations of Measles

Measles is one of the leading causes of childhood blindness worldwide. According to some estimates, measles causes up to 60,000 cases of blindness worldwide each year [44]. Poor access to measles vaccination and malnutrition are often linked to higher rates of eye disability.

Clinical Presentation and Objective Findings

Anterior Eye Segment

Conjunctivitis has a mild course with a papillary reaction on the conjunctiva. Pseudomembranes may occur and a severe course of the disease cannot be excluded in immunocompromised patients. Associated epithelial keratitis is the most common ocular manifestation of measles. In most cases, it begins at the limbus and progresses centrally; it does not usually affect Bowman's membrane. It is usually bilateral and has a mild course. The incidence is relatively high, reaching up to 76% [44]. Keratitis develops in the prodromal phase or at the onset of the rash and resolves a few days later. However, in some patients it may persist for up to 4 months. Corneal sensitivity is not affected, and the corneal lesions resolve without signs of scarring.

Other less common ocular findings include Koplik spots, which can occur on the caruncle and conjunctiva, where they are also called Hirschberg spots. Blepharitis and gangrene of the eyelids are rare.

Posterior Eye Segment

Patients with posterior segment involvement due to measles have a sudden bilateral decrease in visual acuity approximately 6–12 days after the onset of skin manifestations of the disease [44]. In the acute stage of measles retinitis, can be seen diffuse star-shaped macular oedema with hard exudates, optic disc oedema, arteriolar narrowing, and multiple intraretinal haemorrhages. In the remission stage, the clinical presentation of the disease includes a pale optic disc, peripapillary vasoconstriction and secondary RPE changes in the shape of "bone cells" or a "salt and pepper" image. Several years after acute infection, retinochoroidal atrophy develops along the veins with pathological perimeter and ERG.

Diagnosis

The diagnosis of measles retinopathy is made based on a positive anamnesis of measles infection and the typical finding of "bone cell" or "salt and pepper" RPE changes on the fundus.

Therapy

Treatment of the general disease and, in the case of signs of anterior uveitis, corticosteroids are administered topically.

9.12 Histoplasmosis

Histoplasmosis is an infectious disease caused by *Histoplasma capsulatum* (an American histoplasmosis found in the interior of North and Central America) or *Histoplasma duboisi* (an African histoplasmosis endemic to tropical Africa). The fungus is found in soil contaminated with bird or bat excrement and humans become infected by inhaling the spores of the fungus.

Clinical Presentation

The clinical course is usually asymptomatic, or the infection may be manifested as upper respiratory tract involvement. More severe forms, of which *pneumonia* is most common, may occur with massive inhalation of spores (e.g. in cavers) or in immunocompromised persons. This is characterised by inhomogeneous infiltrates, calcifications, and hilar lymphadenopathy, which may falsely raise suspicion of pulmonary tuberculosis. Another manifestation of acute histoplasmosis is *pericarditis*, which affects approximately 5% of infected persons [9]. In patients with a defect in cellular immunity or in elderly patients, an *acute progressive disseminated form* with multiple organ involvement may occur. This form, for example, affects HIV-positive patients with CD4 + lymphocyte counts below 200 cells/mm^3 in blood [9]. Disseminated histoplasmosis may also be subacute, with clinical manifestations including bloodstream or brain infections (most commonly meningitis).

Diagnosis

Diagnosis of histoplasmosis is based on indirect diagnostic methods, the most common being the detection of antibodies to *H. capsulatum* or *H. duboisi* antigens in blood, using the complement fixation reaction. Another option is direct diagnostic methods where fungal antigen is typically detected in blood, urine, or cerebrospinal fluid. Histological diagnosis is also possible by means of silver staining of the specimen.

Therapy

Therapy consists of the administration of antifungal agents. Treatment is initiated with liposomal amphotericin B is administered intravenously for 1–2 weeks as part of the attack phase of therapy, followed by long-term oral itraconazole therapy for 12 months.

9.13 Ocular Manifestations of Presumed Ocular Histoplasmosis Syndrome

According to the latest findings, the disease results from the interaction of the fungal pathogen Histoplasma capsulatum and the immune response of the infected person. Typically, chorioretinal scars in the macula and in the periphery of the retina ("histo spots") are found, without an accompanying inflammatory reaction in the vitreous [53].

Clinical symptoms are a manifestation of macular involvement, and the main sign is a decrease in central visual acuity.

Objective Findings

The findings in classic presumed ocular histoplasmosis syndrome (POHS) include the presence of multiple small chorioretinal lesions ("histo spots"). These are small depigmented atrophic chorioretinal scars approximately 0.2–0.7 PD in diameter, which may have a cluster of pigment in their centre (Fig. 4).

They commonly occur in numbers of 4 to 8, but there are reports in the literature of numbers ranging from 1 to 70 [25, 53]. In two-thirds of cases, this finding occurs bilaterally and the deposits tend to be randomly distributed throughout the retinal periphery [46]. The greatest number of foci are typically in areas of the highest blood supply, so the possibility of haematogenous spread of the fungus is assumed.

In 5% of patients with POHS, parallel to the ora serrata, stripes are found, consisting of hypo- and hyperpigmented peripheral chorioretinal scars, which are formed by linearly arranged clusters of "histo spots" [25, 53]. These stripes are

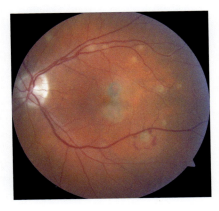

Fig. 4 Presumed ocular histoplasmosis syndrome. Numerous "histo spots" on the fundus

also seen in idiopathic multifocal choroiditis and panuveitis syndromes, which may mimic POHS and pathological myopia in some respects.

Another finding in classic POHS is maculopathy with chorioretinal scar, as well as peripapillary chorioretinal degenerative changes (atrophic and pigmentary) with or without secondary choroidal neovascularisation (CNV) in the macula.

POHS is not accompanied by an inflammatory reaction in the vitreous, therefore its signs include the finding of "clear vitreous".

Diagnosis

For diagnostic purposes, serological detection of antibodies against histoplasma and HLA-B7, HLA-DR2 positivity are important.

Differential Diagnosis

- Foster-Fuchs spots
- White dot syndrome
- Peripapillary choroidal coloboma
- Drusen of the optic disc
- Angioid streaks of the retina
- Choroidal rupture

Therapy

Inactive and atrophic lesions do not need any treatment. In the case of reactivation, administration of systemic or periocular corticosteroids is recommended, either overall or periocularly.

9.14 Candidiasis

Diseases caused by yeasts of the *Candida* genus can occur as benign, localised forms, but also as severe, systemic infections. The main representatives include *Candida albicans, C. krusei, C. guilliermondii, C. parapsilosis, C. tropicalis, C. pseudotropicalis, C. lusitaniae, C. dubliniensis* and *C. glabrata.* Newer yeast species such as *C. inconspicua, C. orthopsilosis* and *C. metapsilosis* are resistant to azole preparations. Severe disease caused by these yeasts occurs mainly in patients with secondary immunodeficiency, or in diabetics. Candida is found in soil, food, animals, and humans. In humans, they colonise mucous membranes, the gastrointestinal tract, the respiratory and urogenital systems. Most infections are caused endogenously but interpersonal transmission can also occur, for example in balanitis in men or colpitis in women [41]. Risk factors for the development of candidiasis are diabetes mellitus, chemotherapy, neutropenia, AIDS, corticosteroid treatment, antibiotic treatment associated with dysmicrobia, and the presence of invasive inputs

Infectious Diseases 527

[41]. Combination of factors increases the risk of developing infection. Manifestations of candida infections can be distinguished by the location of involvement into cutaneous, mucosal, and systemic forms.

Clinical Presentation

Cutaneous forms are typically manifested as wet patches. Cutaneous forms of candidiasis include dermatitis (intertrigo), balanitis, onychomycosis, and interdigital mycosis. The usual symptom is reddening of the skin with the formation of macerated foci with whitish plaques. A special form in the gluteal region is the formation of hyperplastic foci (granuloma inguinale infantum).

Mucosal forms are manifested in the oral cavity (oral thrush) as whitish coatings on the vivid red mucosa. The mucous membrane bleeds profusely when the plaques come off. With progressing oral thrush, the oesophagus may become affected (candida oesophagitis), which affects severely immunocompromised persons. The disease is usually accompanied by marked dysphagia. The mucosal manifestations in women are vaginitis and colpitis. The disease is manifested by itching, genital pain, and discharge. A typical risk factor leading to development of mucosal candidiasis is antibiotic treatment and subsequent vaginal dysmicrobia, which leads to yeast overgrowth in a naturally moist environment. Cystitis caused by candida is a less common disease. Urinary tract obstruction and the presence of lithiasis in risk patients enhance its development. Chronic mucocutaneous candidiasis is a disease that does not respond to appropriate antifungal therapy. In this disease, disorders of cellular immunity should be sought, and it is rarely associated with endocrine disorders in APECED (autoimmune polyendocrinopathy candidosis ectodermal dystrophy) syndrome [41].

Systemic and organ forms of candidiasis are severe diseases. Candida can affect any organ in a severely immunosuppressed person. Manifestations tend to be general—fever, chills, dyspepsia, myalgia, and arthralgia. Generalised cutaneous candidiasis is manifested in the hepatobiliary system, abscesses in the kidneys and skin lesions of up to 1 cm in size. This form with a protracted course typically occurs in patients with haematological malignancies. Candidiasis of the gastrointestinal tract (GIT) may manifest itself in the upper part as oesophagitis, gastritis, or a combination of both [41]. When the lower GIT is affected, inflammation of the small and large intestine may occur, with the formation of abscesses that may perforate. When perforated, candida can cause peritonitis. The respiratory system in systemic candidiasis is most often affected by endobronchial inoculation. Rarely, candida can cause laryngitis, bronchitis, pneumonia, and chest empyema. In haematogenous dissemination, the lungs, any site of the urogenital system and ocular involvement in the form of endophthalmitis may rarely be affected [8]. Exogenous, traumatic, or iatrogenic candida infection in risk patients is rare.

Disseminated candidiasis and sepsis is usually caused by embolisation of mycotic masses from venous inlets, or more rarely in candida endocarditis. Intravenous nutrition is a risk factor. With haematogenous spread, organ forms of candidiasis may then arise. Differential diagnostic, invasive forms of candidiasis should be thought of in atypical courses of febrile illness in patients with risk factors. Localised mucosal forms may be thought of as bacterial infection, tumour, or autoimmune mucosal manifestations.

Diagnosis

Diagnosis of candida infections consists of a comprehensive evaluation of clinical status, physical examination, and risk factors. Basic laboratory parameters are not specified. In invasive forms, mannan detection from blood or aspirate can be used. Aetiological diagnosis is based on culture of samples—swabbing is performed when mucous membranes are affected, haemoculture when the infection is disseminated into the bloodstream, as well as culture of urine, tissues obtained by biopsy or puncture [41]. Due to the difficulty of yeast growth, culture is performed on special mycotic media. It is also necessary to consider the importance of the pre-analytical phase of the examination and to send the material via a transport medium quickly and in suitable thermal conditions. The advantage of culture examination is the possibility of determining the sensitivity to antifungal preparations. Microscopic examination of the specimen is also useful in diagnosis. Another option is PCR testing that is rapid and accurate but not conclusive about the sensitivity of the agent to antifungal agents.

Therapy

Therapy of candida infections depends on the location and type of disease. Mild mucosal and skin infections can be treated with topical administration of antifungal agents, nystatin or clotrimazole is used. Severe mucosal infections and disseminated forms require systemic antifungal therapy. The drug of first choice is fluconazole to which, for example, *C. krusei* is primarily resistant. In risk patients in whom resistant candida can be presumed, echinocandin therapy (anidulafungin, caspofungin) is recommended. Antifungal therapy is guided by culture results and determination of susceptibility to antifungal agents. In immunodeficient patients, antifungal agents can be given prophylactically as primary or secondary prophylaxis.

9.15 Ocular Manifestations of Candidiasis

Candidemia is often associated with significant mortality. The incidence of endophthalmitis due to Candida ranges from 0% to 1.6% and the rate of total ocular involvement ranges from 2.7% to 37% [37].

Clinical Presentation and Objective Findings

Endogenous Candida Endophthalmitis

The clinical presentation of patients with candida endophthalmitis includes floaters, a gradual decrease in visual acuity, red eyes and general ocular discomfort. In the typical picture of candida chorioretinitis, we find predominantly numerous white chorioretinal lesions (often 10 or more in number) occurring bilaterally [37]. In

Infectious Diseases

addition, nerve fibre infarcts, intraretinal haemorrhages, and Roth's spots are usually present and represent an early nonspecific indicator of candida infection. The opacities in the vitreous form a pearl-necklace-shaped chain, and the finding of optic nerve papillitis is no exception.

Exogenous Candida Endophthalmitis

Exogenous mycotic endophthalmitis is a rare finding but is a devastating complication of penetrating eye injury. Foreign material, especially wood or other plant matter, is a source of mycotic infection based on contamination of the wound by septal filamentous fungi (e.g. Fusarium solani and Aspergillus species) [38]. Due to the often-considerable tissue damage caused by the trauma itself, the symptoms of fungal infection tend to be underestimated, correct diagnosis is delayed and with it the subsequent treatment. All these factors thus contribute to the overall poor prognosis of post-traumatic fungal endophthalmitis.

Postoperative candida endophthalmitis is a rare sight-threatening complication of intraocular surgery. Due to the morphology of the self-limiting postoperative corneal wound, mycotic infection manifests primarily as scleritis or keratitis [38]. The picture of mycotic endophthalmitis includes precipitates on the corneal endothelium, intracapsular fibrin fibres, whitish infiltrates in the anterior vitreous, and mild diffuse vitritis. The early symptoms of fungal endophthalmitis closely mimic bacterial endophthalmitis, so in some cases it is misdiagnosed and mismanaged as a postoperative reaction or surgically induced necrotising scleritis [37].

Diagnosis

To reliably confirm candida endophthalmitis, the only option is to obtain a vitreous sample by vitrectomy. The aim of vitrectomy is to confirm the diagnosis, remove the contaminated vitreous and subsequent intravitreal administration of antifungal agents. Detection of candida DNA in intraocular fluids can be performed using a PCR assay to detect the 28S rRNA gene [38]. This method has been shown to be sensitive and rapid, does not require viable organisms and a small sample volume is sufficient.

Differential Diagnosis

- Necrotising retinitis caused by herpes viruses such as CMV, HSV, VZV, ARN
- Toxoplasma retinochoroiditis or nematode infection (e.g. Toxocara canis)
- Bacterial endophthalmitis
- Choroidal granulomas (e.g. in ocular sarcoidosis)
- Retinoblastoma and large cell lymphoma

Therapy

Although a standard therapeutic strategy for mycotic endophthalmitis has not yet been established, early aggressive treatment is needed because of the potentially devastating consequences. Systemic administration of antifungal agents is important, not only in the treatment of endophthalmitis but also in the therapy of systemic manifestations of the infection. The empirical treatment for candida endophthalmitis is a combination of systemic and intravitreally administered amphotericin B, possibly supplemented by pars plana vitrectomy.

9.16 Cryptococcosis

The causative agents of cryptococcosis are the mycotic agents *Cryptococcus neoformans* or, more rarely, *C. gattii*, which cause disease in immunosuppressed patients with diabetes, advanced HIV infection, lymphoproliferation, or monoclonal antibody therapy [7]. Cryptococci are found in the external environment, typically in the excreta of birds and mammals. Humans can become infected by inhaling contaminated air. In immunocompetent persons, the cryptococcus is eliminated by macrophages in the pulmonary alveoli; however, persons with impaired cellular immunity may develop pulmonary or disseminated cryptococcosis [7]. In dissemination, infection of the CNS may occur with the development of meningitis, and other organs that may be affected are the prostate, eye and skin. Risk factors include diabetes mellitus, chemotherapy, monoclonal antibody therapy, AIDS, lupus erythematosus, sarcoidosis, liver cirrhosis, peritoneal dialysis, and corticosteroid therapy [33].

Clinical Presentation

Pulmonary infection manifests as protracted, subacute cryptococcal pneumonia. Patients tend to have nonspecific symptoms with fever, and cough may not be present. Cryptococcal meningitis develops gradually and presents with fever, significant cephalea and varying degrees of impaired consciousness. Disseminated disease may be accompanied by cutaneous manifestations, which typically occur in patients in profound immunodeficiency (e.g. AIDS) [7, 33]. A papular exanthema with a central incision may be present on the skin, which may resemble molluscum contagiosum. Localisation of *C. neoformans* in the prostate is often asymptomatic and may be a source of relapse. Involvement of other organs is possible but rare [48]. Differential diagnosis of cryptococcosis should be considered in at-risk patients with atypical pneumonia, meningitis, skin manifestations and rarely with involvement of other organs.

Diagnosis

Diagnosis is based on the detection of cryptococcal antigen, which is a wall polysaccharide [7]. Culture and PCR can also be used to establish an aetiological diagnosis. Cryptococci can be observed microscopically on ink-stained slides. Imaging in pulmonary involvement (lung X-ray) is not specific. In CNS disease, a purulent liquor formula is usually present in the lumbar puncture.

Infectious Diseases

Therapy

Therapy of milder forms consists in administration of fluconazole, for severe cases (pneumonia, meningitis) intravenous amphotericin B for 14–21 days is recommended in the initial phase and then a maintenance treatment with fluconazole.

9.17 Ocular Manifestations of Cryptococcosis

Cryptococcosis is a common cause of infectious choroiditis in immunodeficient patients, especially those with HIV. Choroidal lesions are the initial manifestation of disseminated disease or secondary meningitis.

Clinical Presentation and Objective Findings

The most common symptom is blurred or reduced vision, followed by eye redness, pain, floaters and photophobia. The most common intraocular complication of cryptococcosis is multifocal chorioretinitis with the finding of focal or multifocal subretinal lesions of yellowish to white colour. This is followed by retinitis, vitritis, anterior uveitis, then keratitis, scleral abscesses, periorbital necrotising fasciitis as well as endogenous and exogenous endophthalmitis. Endogenous cryptococcal endophthalmitis was first described in 1948 [54]. An immune reconstitution ocular inflammatory syndrome manifested by fulminant chorioretinitis, and optic disc swelling has been described in association with the initiation of HAART.

Differential Diagnosis

- Toxoplasmosis
- Syphilis
- Tuberculosis
- Sarcoidosis
- Cytomegalovirus and herpetic retinochoroiditis

Therapy

Both cryptococcal chorioretinitis and endophthalmitis respond best to a combination of systemic antifungal therapy and intravitreally administered amphotericin B (5–10 μg) during pars plana vitrectomy. Intravitreal injections can be given twice weekly and repeated until clinical improvement is achieved.

9.18 Toxoplasmosis

Toxoplasmosis is an infectious disease caused by the parasitic protozoan *Toxoplasma gondii*. Humans become infected by ingesting or possibly inhaling infectious cysts (called oocysts) from an environment contaminated with cat faeces (the cat is the definitive host of *T. gondii*). Acute (primary) infection is asymptomatic in most infected patients, and only about 20% of patients become infected [34]. After infection, *T. gondii* survives in the host for life, and reactivation of latent infection can occur in severe deficiencies of cellular immunity.

Clinical Presentation

Acute toxoplasmosis can manifest as infectious mononucleosis syndrome with pharyngitis, cervical and sometimes generalised lymphadenopathy, and hepatosplenomegaly. Another manifestation of acute *T. gondii* infection is unilateral cervical lymphadenopathy, or the eye may be affected and manifest as chorioretinitis. The eye may also be affected in acute foetal infection in *congenital toxoplasmosis*. The highest risk to the foetus is posed by infection of the woman with *T. gondii* just before conception (within 2–3 months) or during the first trimester. Although foetal lesions are not common during the first trimester (risk is approximately 15%), they can be very severe and lead to miscarriage or severe malformations [34]. The confluence of the three most common manifestations in the affected neonate is referred to as the Sabin triad and includes hydrocephalus, chorioretinitis and the presence of intracranial calcifications. Foetal infection during the second and third trimesters is very common compared to the first trimester (risk is 30–60%), but its manifestations are less severe and most often manifest as chorioretinitis in children or young adults [34]. Persons with severe defects in cellular immunity (e.g. AIDS or bone marrow transplantation) have *reactivation of latent toxoplasma infection.* In HIV + persons, this occurs when CD4 + lymphocytes fall below 200 cells/mm^3 and reactivation most often manifests as a focal encephalitis that resembles a brain abscess on computed tomography or magnetic resonance imaging [34].

Diagnosis

Diagnosis in most cases is based on the detection of specific IgA, IgE and IgM antibodies in the blood. Specific antibody avidity testing can also be used to diagnose acute toxoplasmosis, with low avidity indicating recent infection. Other body fluids, such as cerebrospinal fluid or posterior chamber fluid, can also be tested for specific antibodies or possibly *T. gondii* DNA. However, due to their limited specificity, these investigations are little used, and preference is given to therapeutic detection of the cerebral or ocular form of toxoplasmosis, with significant improvement in clinical findings after 7–10 days of antimicrobial therapy.

Therapy

Therapy of toxoplasmosis consists of the administration of chemotherapeutic drugs, which are recommended only for more severe forms of infection. The mainstay of antimicrobial therapy is pyrimethamine in combination with sulfadiazine (folic acid is administered during treatment with these chemotherapeutic agents); alternatives include cotrimoxazole, spiramycin (especially in pregnant women) and clindamycin. In persons with a known severe defect in cellular immunity (e.g. AIDS), long-term primary prophylaxis of toxoplasmosis is given with cotrimoxazole, which

Infectious Diseases 533

can also be used for secondary prophylaxis after toxoplasmosis in immunocompromised patients or, for example, in the case of recurrent toxoplasmic chorioretinitis in immunocompetent patients [34].

9.19 Ocular Manifestations of Toxoplasmosis

Toxoplasmosis is considered the leading cause of infectious posterior uveitis worldwide, causing more than 80% of cases in some regions [18]. If the macula and optic disc are affected, toxoplasma retinochoroiditis can permanently damage vision in immunocompetent subjects. In developed countries, ocular complications of toxoplasmosis occur in approximately 2–3% of postnatally infected individuals, whereas in some highly endemic areas (e.g. Brazil), up to 20% of the population may be affected [18]. Ocular toxoplasmosis is a recurrent disease in up to 75% of cases. There are three main theories to explain the cause of recurrent toxoplasmic retinochoroiditis. The first theory postulates recurrent rupture of cysts with subsequent release of *T. gondii*, which actively attacks the retina. Another is that the cysts produce antigens that trigger a focal inflammatory reaction. The second theory leans toward an autoimmune response to retinal antigens such as retinal S-antigen with accompanying retinochoroidal inflammation. A third theory proposes that relapses are the result of reinfection.

Clinical Presentation and Objective Findings

Congenital Toxoplasmosis

The most common manifestation of congenital toxoplasmosis is retinochoroiditis, which occurs in 10–80% of infected new-borns soon after birth [18]. It is not uncommon for the new-born to develop a variable combination of systemic involvement such as anaemia, skin rash, thrombocytopenia, hepatitis, hepatosplenomegaly, pneumonitis, encephalitis and myocarditis. The classic Sabin tetrad of congenital toxoplasmosis consists of hydrocephalus or microcephaly, intracranial calcification, mental retardation, and retinochoroiditis. However, most cases are asymptomatic. The most common sequelae of ocular involvement include chorioretinal scar (Fig. 5), complicated cataract, microphthalmia, optic nerve atrophy, strabismus, nystagmus, and even eyeball phthisis.

Early detection of subclinical infection is essential to initiate intensive treatment to improve prognosis.

Postnatally Acquired Toxoplasmosis

The disease has a subclinical and nonspecific course which often leads to misdiagnosis. Up to 70% of immunocompromised patients are completely asymptomatic [18]. If the disease manifests, it is mainly a lymphadenopathy of one or more lymph nodes.

Fig. 5 Congenital toxoplasmosis. Hyperpigmented macular scar

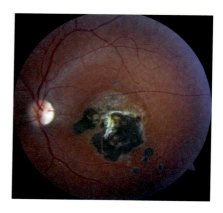

Ocular Toxoplasmosis

Anterior Eye Segment

The anterior segment of the eye may be affected by granulomatous or nongranulomatous inflammation. This process is considered reactive, because the finding of live *T. gondii* has never been demonstrated in the anterior chamber of an immunocompetent patient. Clinical findings include precipitates on the corneal endothelium of the "mutton fat" image, posterior synechiae, fibrin, and Koeppe and Busacca nodules [18]. Corneal oedema may also be present in eyes with normal intraocular pressure, due to endothelial dysfunction. Iridocyclitis is usually transient, yet early initiation of treatment is necessary to prevent complications such as secondary glaucoma and complicated cataract.

Posterior Eye Segment

Recurrent lesions occur singly and typically at the edges of old chorioretinal scars as what are called "satellite lesions". Unilateral, solitary, active lesions without evidence of previous involvement are found in recently acquired postnatal disease. Primary lesions form first in the superficial layers of the neuroretina. As the inflammation progresses, they affect the full thickness of the retina, choroid and sclera.

On ophthalmoscopic examination, focal grey exudate is visible, which has poorly demarcated edges due to surrounding retinal oedema. The size of the lesions ranges from 1/10 PD to two quadrants of the retina. In almost all cases, vitritis is present. In severe vitritis, active retinal lesions have a "reflector in the haze" appearance; the vitreous contracts, and tractional retinal detachment may occur along with posterior hyaloid membrane detachment [18]. With time, the margins of the lesion become circumscribed, exudation and vitritis diminish. Subsequently, the lesions, especially at the margins, become pigmented. The healed scar usually has well-defined borders with central chorioretinal atrophy and peripheral RPE hyperplasia. Either choroidal vessels or sclera are observed in the centre of the atrophied area. Traction bands may also be present, connecting the old scar to the optic disc (Franceschetti's sign) or to

Infectious Diseases

Fig. 6 Postnatal disseminated toxoplasmic retinochoroiditis. Traction bands connecting the scar in the upper periphery with the adjacent scar and with the optic disc (Franceschetti's sign)

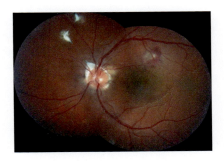

an adjacent scar (Fig. 6). Vitreous opacities are slowly absorbed but may persist for years after complete healing of the lesions.

Diagnosis

The diagnosis of ocular toxoplasmosis is usually based on clinical findings. Laboratory tests are mainly used in case of atypical course of the disease. Diagnosis should not be based on laboratory examination alone, as active lesions on the fundus may not induce elevated systemic antibody titres. However, in an immunocompetent individual, the absence of autoantibodies to *T. gondii* in the serum virtually excludes this diagnosis.

Differential Diagnosis

Congenital toxoplasmosis of new-borns.

- Other diseases of the TORCHS group (toxoplasmosis, rubella, CMV, herpes simplex virus, HIV, syphilis)
- Infection with lymphocytic choriomeningitis virus
- Chorioretinal coloboma
- Persistent hyperplastic primary vitreous
- Retinoblastoma
- Necrotising retinitis caused by herpes viruses (CMV, herpes simplex, herpes zoster)
- Septic retinitis
- Ocular toxocariasis
- Sarcoidosis, syphilis and TB
- Serpiginous choroiditis
- White dot syndrome
- Diffuse unilateral subacute neuroretinitis

Therapy

Due to the incompletely understood pathogenesis of this disease, there are no standard treatments yet. Administration of pyrimethamine (75–100 mg on the first day, then 25–50 mg once a day) + sulfadiazine (0.5–1.0 g every 6 h), or pyrimethamine +

clindamycin (300–900 mg every 6 to 8 h), in combination with folic acid (10–15 mg once daily, about 6–8 h apart from pyrimethamine) and corticosteroid (prednisone 0.5–1.0 mg/kg/day) is still considered the classic treatment with the highest efficacy.

9.20 Pneumocystosis

The main representative of pneumocysts is *Pneumocystis jiroveci*. It is an atypical fungal microorganism that can cause protracted lung infection in immunocompromised persons, abbreviated as PJP (Pneumocystis jiroveci pneumonia) [30]. Rarely, pneumocystis affects other organs. Infection occurs by inhalation of pneumocysts from the environment, the source being birds, rodents, and their droppings. Primoinfection usually occurs asymptomatically or as a mild respiratory disease. In neonates, especially premature infants, the infection may be severe. Development of the disease in adulthood may occur when cellular immunity is reduced and CD4 + lymphocyte counts fall below 200 cells/mm^3 [30].

Clinical Presentation

The clinical manifestation is often progressively increasing and worsening dyspnoea, dry cough, subfebrile or febrile state accompanied by malaise. The disease has a subacute course. The bone marrow, nodules, spleen, and retina may be affected. The risk factor is a decrease in cellular immunity due to biological therapy, AIDS, corticosteroid therapy, cyclophosphamide, but also in persons with primary immunodeficiency [30]. On X-ray lung imaging, a diffuse reticulonodular pattern with a maximum in the middle fields is seen, and on high-resolution computed tomography (HR CT), a typical picture of interstitial pneumonitis with milk glass opacities can be observed.

Diagnosis

Diagnosis is based on direct detection of pneumocysts in sputum, bronchoalveolar lavage fluid or other material by PCR. Microscopic diagnosis in Grocott-Gomori staining is possible. Nonspecific inflammatory markers may not be significantly elevated. Serum LDH (lactate dehydrogenase) levels tend to be elevated and their dynamics reflect the efficacy of therapy. Indirect evidence (serology) is not used in practice. Differential diagnostic consideration is given to viral and atypical bacterial pneumonia.

Therapy

Therapy is based on the administration of high dose cotrimoxazole in combination with corticosteroids. In the case of allergy to cotrimoxazole, pentacarinate can be administered. Clindamycin, in combination with primaquine, is also an alternative. After the initial treatment phase, secondary prophylaxis is usually given with cotrimoxazole or inhaled pentacarinate, which are also used for primary prophylaxis in at-risk patients with profound immunodeficiency [30].

Infectious Diseases

9.21 Ocular Manifestations of Pneumocystosis

In 1987, Macher et al. described the first case of histologically proven choroidopathy due to Pneumocystis carinii infection in a patient with AIDS [30]. The initiation of HAART subsequently led to a sharp decline in the incidence of all AIDS-related opportunistic infections, particularly pneumocystosis.

Clinical Presentation and Objective Findings

Choroidopathy due to Pneumocystis carinii infection is usually an incidental finding during routine examination. The finding is bilateral in up to 76% of cases [20]. One or several yellow-white, plaque-like, slightly striated, spherical lesions with a diameter of 0.5 PD are found on the fundus. The lesions are located mainly at the posterior pole and extend to the equator, but never anterior to it. Without treatment, the margins of the lesions enlarge by an average of 0.5 PD per month [20]. These lesions usually do not lead to a decrease in visual acuity. As a rule, inflammatory manifestations in the anterior chamber and vitreous are absent, in part because cellular immunity is greatly suppressed.

Diagnosis

Diagnosis is based on the clinical presentation and FAG examination, which shows hypofluorescence in early stages and homogeneous staining, with indistinct lesion borders in later stages. Choroidal biopsy is not recommended because of the high risk of retinal complications.

Differential Diagnosis

- Tuberculous choroiditis
- Toxoplasmosis
- Candidiasis
- Cryptococcosis
- Intraocular lymphoma
- Histoplasmosis
- Vogt-Koyanagi-Harada syndrome
- Sympathetic ophthalmia

Therapy

Systemic therapy includes administration of trimethoprim (15 mg/kg/day) and sulfamethoxazole (75 mg/kg/day) or pentamidine (4 mg/kg/day) for at least three weeks.

9.22 Larval Toxocariasis

Larval toxocariasis is a parasitic infection most caused by the larvae of the canine or feline roundworm—*Toxocara canis* and *T. cati*. It is a common infectious disease affecting humans, with an estimated population prevalence of 20% [6]. Humans are most infected by ingesting food contaminated with parasite eggs, and infections of young children from sandboxes are also common. Once ingested, the eggs hatch into larvae in the small intestine, which migrate through the intestinal wall into the blood and organs.

Clinical Presentation

Clinical manifestations depend on the size of the infectious dose. Most cases are asymptomatic, or present with uncharacteristic symptoms such as nausea, lack of appetite and abdominal pain. Rarely, in massive infestations (i.e. ingestion of large numbers of larvae), general symptoms with fever, cough with pulmonary infiltrates on lung X-ray, or hepatosplenomegaly or urticarial skin rash may be present. In dissemination of the infection, cardiac, CNS or ocular involvement may occur.

Diagnosis

Diagnosis is based on the correct assessment of clinical symptoms—for example, in children, the eye may be affected by strabismus or in adults by visual disturbances. Rarely, a migrating larva may be observed on eye examination. The basis of laboratory investigations is the differential blood count, in which significant eosinophilia is found, ranging from 10–90% [6]. Biochemical examination may show a slight increase in transaminases. The aetiological diagnosis is based on the detection of total serum antibodies by immunoassay, and their total concentration is assessed. Since these antibodies persist for a long time, they cannot be used to distinguish acute from past infection. It should be emphasised that both eosinophils and specific antibodies may be absent in the ocular form of larval toxocariasis. In this case, the examination of specific antibodies in the fluid from the eye chamber can be used.

Therapy

Therapy varies according to the severity—lighter forms of larval toxocariasis are not treated, while for more severe forms the anthelmintics thiabendazole and diethylcarbamazine are recommended. Since this therapy is associated with an inflammatory reaction caused by breakdown of dead larvae, the treatment is supplemented with corticosteroids.

9.23 Ocular Manifestations of Toxocariasis

Ocular toxocariasis is a common infectious disease with a worldwide incidence. The main risk factor is contact with dogs, especially puppies. The disease affects

Infectious Diseases

both children and adults. Although human toxocariasis is one of the most common zoonotic infections worldwide, there are few studies estimating the prevalence of ocular involvement. For example, the number of reported cases of ocular toxocariasis in Alabama during a half-year follow-up was 11 cases per 1,000 toxocariasis patients [6]. Infection of the eye by larvae of Toxocara occurs through the bloodstream. The retina is most affected, but they can occur in various tissues of the eye.

Clinical Presentation and Objective Findings

Secondary scleritis can be noted on the anterior segment of the eye after penetration of Toxocara larvae. Less common manifestations, such as keratitis and optic neuritis, are part of the wide spectrum of clinical manifestations seen in this entity. In the most severe course, Toxocara infection can be fatal.

In approximately 44% of eyes, the most common finding is peripheral granuloma, with neuroretinal striae throughout the posterior pole [6]. The lesions are spherical in shape with a diameter of 1 to 2 PD. They are white or grey in colour and occasionally a dark crescent-shaped area representing the larva may be noted. Localisation may be anywhere in the posterior pole including the juxtapapillary and subfoveolar zones [43]. Depending on the number of larvae and their localisations, vitritis of varying degrees may be present.

Diagnosis

Currently, ELISA is the most accurate serological test available. It is important to determine the titre levels of antibodies, leukocytes, eosinophils, and enzyme-linked immunosorbent assays.

Differential Diagnosis

- Retinoblastoma
- Infectious endophthalmitis
- Retinopathy of prematurity
- Toxoplasmosis
- Coats disease and familial exudative vitreoretinopathy

Therapy

The first choice of treatment is topical or general corticosteroids, sometimes in combination with anthelmintics. Surgical procedures such as pars plana vitrectomy, cryoretinopexy and laser photocoagulation are also used. Treatment is primarily concerned with targeting the inflammatory response and thus preventing structural damage with subsequent visual decline.

9.24 Onchocerciasis

Onchocerciasis (River Blindness) is a chronic disease caused by the parasite *Onchocerca volvulus*, a helminth belonging to the nematode family. Humans are the only natural hosts and the stinging flies of the genus *Simulium*, which live mainly around rivers, act as vectors. Given the high incidence of this disease in the form of dermatitis, visual impairment, and blindness, it is a major health problem in endemic areas. More than 99% of onchocerciasis cases occur in sub-Saharan Africa, with smaller outbreaks in Latin America [23]. When a person is bitten by a fly, the larvae are transmitted through the bloodstream and form subcutaneous nodules 0.5–3.0 cm in size. Here the adult females again produce larvae (microfilariae) 300 × 8 μm in size. Adults can survive under the skin for 10–15 years. In addition to the skin, microfilariae can also be trapped in blood or urine and spread directly to the eye from the surrounding skin. Microfilariae from the skin can be ingested by sucking moths and the life cycle repeats. Adult worms have a reproductive period of about 10 years and microfilariae survive for 1–2 years. Clinically severe manifestations of infection are usually due to an inflammatory response to the microfilariae present in the skin or eyes [23]. *Onchocerca volvulus* actively inhibits the specific defence response and thus limits tissue damage. Clinical manifestations appear long after exposure and their severity is related to the infectious dose and host immunity [35].

Diagnosis

Diagnosis is mainly clinical, considering the epidemiological anamnesis of stay in endemic areas, while other possible causes of dermatitis or subcutaneous nodules must be distinguished. Definitive diagnosis is based on microscopic evidence from skin biopsy. Serological or PCR testing in specialised laboratories may also be used.

Therapy

Therapy consists of the administration of antiparasitic agents; the drug of choice for onchocerciasis is ivermectin, which effectively destroys only microfilariae, and therefore the treatment must be repeated several times at 3- to 6-month intervals. In prevention, protection from fly bites is applied; there is no vaccine.

9.25 Ocular Manifestations of Onchocerciasis

Onchocerciasis is the second-most common infectious cause of blindness worldwide after trachoma. Worldwide, approximately 17.7 million individuals are affected by the disease—270,000 of whom are blind and another 500,000 who have severe visual impairment [11]. Almost 99% of all affected individuals (and those blind due to the disease) live in Africa and their life expectancy is reduced by approximately 10–13 years [11].

Infectious Diseases

Clinical Presentation

Ocular signs and symptoms result from the presence of dead microfilariae. Only 30% of cases show the presence of live intraretinal microfilariae [13]. Typical subjective complaints of patients with onchocerciasis include photophobia, foreign body sensation, pain and decreased visual acuity.

Objective Findings

Anterior Eye Segment

Keratitis punctata is an early manifestation of corneal involvement in younger patients, with an average age of 24.6 years [13]. Corneal changes on biomicroscopy include the finding of 0.5–1.5 mm "snowflakes" around dead microfilariae, especially in the anterior stroma. Sclerotic keratitis is associated with long-standing massive onchocerca infection. The mean age of patients with sclerosing keratitis is 41.2 years [13]. The highest density of microfilariae and opacities is at the periphery of the cornea. Chronic keratitis causes scarring with neovascularisation. Corneal opacification usually begins nasally and temporally from the limbus, progresses slowly and merges in the optical axis of the cornea with an accompanying marked decrease in visual acuity. Small round nodules 0.5–2.0 mm in diameter may be present in the conjunctiva.

Anterior uveitis may present clinically as mild chronic non-granulomatous inflammation to severe granulomatous uveitis with iris atrophy, anterior and posterior synechiae and pupillary seclusion.

Posterior Eye Segment

Chorioretinal manifestations of onchocerciasis are usually bilateral and symmetrical. Ocular infection manifests as diffuse or geographic atrophy of the RPE, sometimes accompanied by atrophy of the choriocapillaris [13]. More advanced changes include intraretinal pigment deposition, haemorrhage, and soft exudates. Active retinitis or choroiditis are not typical of the disease.

Diagnosis

The finding of microfilariae in the cornea can be captured using high magnification biomicroscopy or retroillumination. Dead filariae are easy to visualise because they are flat and opaque in the cornea. Live microfilariae can be found in the anterior chamber in 25% of patients with onchocerciasis. Intraretinal microfilariae can be observed by direct ophthalmoscopy when they appear as small reflective opacities with a green tint. For diagnostic purposes, examination of tear or urine samples by ELISA is important.

Differential Diagnosis

- Mansonella streptocerca infection
- Insect bites
- Contact dermatitis

- Sycosis cruris
- Post-traumatic and post-inflammatory depigmentation and mycosis
- Toxoplasmosis
- Syphilis
- Tuberculosis

Therapy

There are two main treatment strategies: (1) chemotherapy treatment and (2) insect movement control. Treatment is primarily concerned with preventing pathological changes in the eyes and skin and stopping the life cycle of the parasite.

9.26 Schistosomiasis

Schistosomiasis is a parasitic disease caused by a species of flukes of the genus *Schistosoma* (previously, this helminthosis was also called bilharziasis after a German pathologist working in Cairo in the nineteenth century) [16]. It is a human disease that is endemic in the tropics and subtropics (especially in sub-Saharan Africa, including Lakes Malawi and Victoria) and is one of the most important parasitic diseases. Infection often occurs in standing water (lakes, rivers), with various species of gastropods as intermediate hosts. The most important representatives are *S. mansoni* causing intestinal schistosomiasis, *S. haematobium* (urinary form) and *S. japonicum* (oriental form). Adult schistosomes are 6–20 mm long, invade the venous plexus and feed on red blood cells. On average, they live for 3–7 years, but can live up to 30 years. The females produce thousands of eggs that invade the tissues of the intestine and bladder. They are then excreted in the faeces or urine and enter freshwater, where the larvae attack the relevant gastropods. The infective larvae, called cercariae, leave the intermediate host and invade the skin of humans. They migrate through the bloodstream to the lungs and liver, where they develop into adult worms. Eggs that do not penetrate the intestines or bladder accumulate in the tissues and trigger an inflammatory response with the formation of granulomas. They can also be introduced into more distant tissues, such as the CNS or lungs. Dermatitis may occur a few days after cercariae penetrate the skin; the incubation period of acute schistosomiasis is 3–8 weeks. The next stage is chronic schistosomiasis, which develops over several months to years.

Diagnosis

Diagnosis consists of microscopic detection of eggs in stool or urine; serological detection of antibodies can also be used. In the acute and chronic stages, eosinophilia and later anaemia are present [16].

Infectious Diseases

Therapy

In therapy, the drug of choice is praziquantel at a minimum dose of 40 mg/kg, which kills adult flukes. Sometimes it is advisable to use anti-inflammatory corticosteroid therapy. Treatment should be repeated in one month. In 2 months, a control parasitological examination for the presence of eggs in the urine and faeces should be performed [16].

9.27 Ocular Manifestations of Schistosomiasis

Although it is primarily an intestinal or urogenital disease, if it enters the eye, it can cause devastating damage.

Clinical signs are associated with the presence of parasite eggs, but the finding of an adult worm in the patient's eye is no exception. Subjective complaints of patients include photophobia and a decrease in visual acuity.

Objective Findings

Although the ocular form of schistosomiasis is rare, involvement of the lacrimal gland, sclera, uveal tissue, RPE and optic nerve has been described. Approximately 10% of patients with the hepatosplenic form of the disease are found to have choroidal granulomas when the choroid is affected [36]. These have the appearance of multiple yellow-whitish foci of varying size. Histologically, they are a granulomatous reaction of epithelioid histiocytes, lymphocytes, plasma cells and eosinophils surrounding the parasite eggs.

Diagnosis

Biomicroscopy of the anterior segment of the eye and ophthalmoscopy or fundus photography of the posterior segment.

Therapy

In the presence of a worm in the conjunctiva, anterior chamber, vitreous or in the orbit near the optic nerve, surgical treatment is recommended.

9.28 Ocular Myiasis

Ocular myiasis is a disease in which humans or other vertebrates are infested with the larvae of flies of the order of the two-winged fly. The incidence of myiasis is higher in rural areas of the tropics and subtropics in Africa and the Americas [26]. Exceptionally, infestation with the fly *Lucilia sericata* may occur in persons with low hygiene standards. Myiasis can be classified as obligate or facultative according to the relationship between the host and the parasite, and, according to the site of infestation, cutaneous, ocular, ear, nasopharyngeal, intestinal, or urogenital forms are distinguished. For example, the following species are important for humans: *Wohlfartia magnifica*, *Chrysomia bezziana*, *Cochliomyia anthropophaga* and *Dermatobia hominis*. *Dermatobia hominis* may be among the souvenirs imported from Mexico and other countries in Central and South America, and mosquitoes may play a role as egg carriers [26]. The skin lesion usually begins as a painful red papule that gradually enlarges and may form a furuncle with a central opening. Here the posterior part through which the larva breathes can be seen. Lesions tend to be localised on the arms, around the waist or on the lower back and buttocks. Cutaneous myiasis is usually a benign disease, the larva leaves the skin at some stage. In some cases, the process can be accelerated by rubbing with cream and squeezing or by minor surgical incision after prior disinfection. Ocular myiasis arises from infestation of the eye or tissues around the orbit and accounts for about 5% of human cases, and, depending on the invasiveness of the larvae, an external or more severe internal form develops [17, 26]. Other forms are rare in humans.

9.29 Ocular Manifestations of Myiasis

Ocular myiasis is a condition in which fly larvae (Diptera) penetrate the orbit and surrounding tissues. Infection occurs by attachment of the immature airborne larvae to the mucous membrane or conjunctiva of a person. Infection occurs randomly throughout the world, especially in sheep-farming areas [17]. If the superficial structures of the eye are affected, this is external ocular myiasis; if the intraocular structures are affected, internal ocular myiasis occurs.

Clinical Presentation and Objective Findings

External ocular myiasis is typically unilateral, internal myiasis can be unilateral or bilateral [26]. Patients with internal ocular myiasis are characterised by a long asymptomatic period, a gradual unilateral decrease in visual acuity and redness of the eye [17]. In the later stages of the disease, the parasite dies, causing secondary intraocular inflammation complicated by pain and photophobia. During biomicroscopy of the anterior and posterior segments of the eye, a white to translucent larva can be seen (Fig. 7).

At both ends, the body of the parasite is segmented and constricted, and, in some cases, movement can be noted. The larvae are found in the anterior chamber, lens, vitreous and subretinal space. They can migrate from the anterior chamber to the vitreous and leave the eye completely. If the larva is located below the neuroretinas, its migration leaves characteristic linear "railroad track" scars at the level of the RPE. In cases of intraocular myiasis, chorioretinitis, endophthalmitis, vitreous haemorrhage and retinal detachment have been reported after larval death.

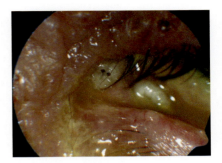

Fig. 7 Diptera larva on the anterior eye segment. Note: used with permission of Adam Kopecky, MD, PhD, FEBO

Diagnosis

Biomicroscopy of the anterior segment of the eye and ophthalmoscopy or fundus photography of the posterior segment.

Differential Diagnosis

- Histoplasmosis
- Other helminth infestations
- Traumatic tears of the choroid

Therapy

Treatment of external ocular myiasis consists of removing the larva from the ocular surface. In patients with a dead larva inside the eye without accompanying signs of uveitis, only monitoring of the condition can be continued. Argon laser photocoagulation was successfully used to kill the live larva, the laser settings were as follows: trace size 200 μm, energy 400 mW, time 0.1 s. Photocoagulation denatures the larval antigens and prevents the development of a secondary inflammatory reaction. Local and systemic corticosteroids can be used in the treatment of uveitis associated with larval death. Vitrectomy and subretinal surgical techniques can be used to remove intraocular parasites.

References

1. Abd EM. Brucella optic neuritis. Arch Intern Med. 1991;151:776–8.
2. Akduman L, Or M, Hasanreisoglu B, et al. A case of ocular brucellosis: importance of vitreous specimen. Acta Ophthalmol (Copenh). 1993;71:130–2.
3. Benes J. Infectious diseases. 1st ed. Prague: Galen; 2009.
4. Bennett JE, Dolin R, Blaser MJ. Mandell, Douglas, and Bennett's principles and practice of infectious diseases. 9th ed. Elsevier; 2020.
5. Boulouis HJ, Chang CC, Henn JB, et al. Factors associated with the rapid emergence of Bartonella infections. Vet Res. 2005;36:383–410.
6. Brown DH. Ocular Toxocara canis: Part II. Clinical review Pediatr Ophthalmol. 1970;7:182.
7. Chayakulkeeree M, Perfect JR. Cryptococcosis. Infect Dis Clin North Am. 2006;20:507–44.

8. Chen JY. Neonatal candidiasis associated with meningitis and endophthalmitis. Acta Paediatr Jap. 1994;36:261–5.
9. Cohen PR, Grossman ME, Silvers DN. Disseminated histoplasmosis and human immunodeficiency virus. Int J Dermatol. 1991;30:614–22.
10. Culbertson WW, Blumenkranz, Haines H, et al. The acute retinal necrosis syndrome. Part 2: Histopathology and etiology. Ophthalmology. 1982;89:1317–25.
11. Dent AE, Kazura JW. Other tissue nematodes. Nelson Textbook of Pediatrics. 2011;1225–7.
12. Devilliers MJ, Ben Hadj Salah W, Barreau E, et al. Ocular manifestations of viral diseases. Rev Med Interne. 2021;42(6):401–10.
13. Diemert DJ. Tissue nematode infections. Goldman's Cecil Medicine. 2011;193–200.
14. Forster DJ, Dugel PU, Frangieh GT, et al. Rapidly progressive outer retinal necrosis in the acquired immunodeficiency syndrome. Am J Ophthalmol. 1990;110(4):341–8.
15. Freer G, Pistello M. Varicella-zoster virus infection: natural history, clinical manifestations, immunity and current and future vaccination strategies. New Microbiol. 2018;41(2):95–105.
16. Gray DJ, Ross AG, Li YS, et al. Diagnosis and management of Schistosomiasis. BMJ. 2011;342: d2651.
17. Hoffman BL, Goldsmid JM. Ophthalmomyiasis caused by Oestrus ovis L. (Diptera: Oestridae) in Rhodesia. S Afr Med J. 1970;44:644–5.
18. Holland GN. Ocular toxoplasmosis: a global reassessment. Part I: epidemiology and course of disease. Am J Ophthalmol. 2003;136(6):973–88.
19. Hu LT. Lyme disease. Ann Intern Med. 2016;164(9):ITC65-ITC80.
20. Jabs DA. Ocular manifestations of HIV infection. Trans Am Ophthalmol Soc. 1995;93:623–83.
21. Jacobson DM, Marx JJ, Dlesk A. Frequency and clinical signicance of Lyme seropositivity in patients with isolated optic neuritis. Neurology. 1991;41(5):706–11.
22. Jerris RC, Regnery RL. Will the real agent of cat scratch disease please stand up? Ann Rev Microbiol. 1996;50:707–25.
23. Kaiser C, Asaba G, Leichsenring M, et al. High incidence of epilepsy related to onchocerciasis in West Uganda. Epilepsy Res. 1998;30:247–51.
24. Kalfayan B. Inclusion disease of infancy. Arch Pathol (Chic). 1947;44(5):467–76.
25. Katz BJ, Scott WE, Folk JC. Acute histoplasmosis choroiditis in 2 immunocompetent brothers. Arch Ophthalmol. 1997;115:1470–2.
26. Kersten RC, Shoukrey NM, Tabbara KF. Orbital myiasis. Ophthalmology. 1986;93:1228–32.
27. Lesser RL. Ocular manifestations of Lyme disease. Am J Med. 1995;98(4):60–2.
28. Letocart M, Baranton G, Perolat P. Rapid identification of pathogenic Leptospira species (Leptospira interrogans, L. borgpetersenii and L. kirsneri) with species-specific DNA probes produced by arbitrarily primed PCR. J. Clin Microbiol. 1997;35(1):248–53.
29. Mabra D, Yeh S, Shantha JG. Ocular manifestations of bartonellosis. Curr Opin Ophthalmol. 2018;29(6):582–7.
30. Macher AM, Bardenstein DS, Zimmerman LE, et al. Pneumocystis carinii choroiditis in a male homosexual with AIDS and disseminated pulmonary and extrapulmonary P. carinii infection. N Engl J Med. 1987;316:1092.
31. Maurin M, Birtles R, Raoult D. Current knowledge of Bartonella species. Eur J Clin Microbiol Infect Dis. 1997;16:487–506.
32. Meghpara B, Sulkowski G, Kesen MR, et al. Long-term follow-up of acute retinal necrosis. Retina. 2010;30:795–800.
33. Mitchell TG, Perfect JR. Cryptococcosis in the era of AIDS—100 years after the discovery of Cryptococcus neoformans. Clin Microbiol Rev. 1995;8(4):515–48.
34. Montoya JG, Liesenfeld O. Toxoplasmosis Lancet. 2004;363(9425):1965–76.
35. Newell ED, Vyungimana F, Bradley JE. Epilepsy, retarded growth and onchocerciasis, in two areas of different endemicity of onchocerciasis in Burundi. Trans R Soc Trop Med Hyg. 1997;91:525–7.
36. Newton JC, Kanchanaranya C, Previte LR. Intraocular Schistosoma mansoni. Am J Ophthalmol. 1968;65(5):774–8.

Infectious Diseases

37. Oude Lashof AM, Rothova A, Sobel JD, et al. Ocular manifestations of candidemia. Clin Infect Dis. 2011;53(3):262–8.
38. Park SS, To KW, Fried AH, et al. Infectious causes of posterior uveitis. In: Albert DM, Jakobiec FA (Eds). Principles and practice of ophthalmology. W.B. Saunders; 1994. p. 450–64.
39. Patil A, Goldust M, Wollina U. Herpes zoster: A Review of Clinical Manifestations and Management. Viruses. 2022;14(2):192.
40. Paules CI, Marston HD, Fauci AS. Measles in 2019—going backward. N Engl J Med. 2019;380(23):2185–7.
41. Pfaller MA. Nosocomial candidiasis: emerging species, reservoirs, and modes of transmission. Clin Infect Dis. 1996;22:89–94.
42. Rathinam SR. Ocular leptospirosis. Curr Opin Ophthalmol. 2002;13(6):381–6.
43. Schimek RA, Perez WA, Carrera GM. Ophthalmic manifestations of visceral larva migrans. Ann Ophthalmol. 1979;11:1387–90.
44. Semba RD, Bloem MW. Measles blindness. Surv Ophthalmol. 2004;49(2):243–55.
45. Smith ME. Retinal involvement in adult cytomegalic inclusion disease. Arch Ophthalmol. 1964;72:44–9.
46. Specht CS, Mitchell KT, Bauman AE, et al. Ocular histoplasmosis with retinitis in a patient with acquired immune deficiency syndrome. Ophthalmology. 1991;98:1356–9.
47. Stewart MW, Bolling JP, Mendez JC. Cytomegalovirus retinitis in an immunocompetent patient. Arch Ophthalmol. 2005;123:572–4.
48. Subramanian S, Mathai D. Clinical manifestations and management of cryptococcal infection. J Postgrad Med. 2005;51:21–6.
49. Tabbara KF. Al-Kassimi H. Ocular brucellosis Br J Ophthalmol. 1990;74:249–50.
50. Urayama A, Yamada N, Sasaki T, et al. Unilateral acute uveitis with retinal periarteritis and detachment. Jpn J Clin Ophthalmol. 1971;25:607–19.
51. Vijayachari P, Sugunan AP, Shriram AN. Leptospirosis an emerging global public health problem. J Biosci. 2008;33(4):557–69.
52. Weil A. Ueber eine eigentümliche, mit Milztumor, Icterus und Nephritis einhergehende akute Infektionskrankheit. Dtsche Arch Klin Med. 1886;39:209–32.
53. Weingeist TA, Watzke RC. Ocular involvement by Histoplasma capsulatum. Int Ophthalmol Clin. 1983;23:33–47.
54. Weiss C, Perry IH, Shevky MC. Infection of the human eye with cryptococcus neoformans; torula histolytica; cryptococcus hominis; a clinical and experimental study with a new diagnostic method. Arch Ophthal. 1948;39(6):739–51.
55. Whitley RJ, Kimberlin DW, Roizman B. Herpes simplex viruses. Clin Infect Dis. 1998;26(3):541–53.
56. Yanoff M, Schaefer DB, Scheie HG. Rubella ocular syndrome: clinical significance of viral and pathological studies. Trans Am Acad Ophthalmol Otol. 1968;72(6):896–902.
57. Zaidman GW. The ocular manifestations of Lyme disease. Int Ophthalmol Clin. 1997;37:13–28.

Printed in the United States
by Baker & Taylor Publisher Services

Global Agricultural Production: Resilience to Climate Change

Mukhtar Ahmed
Editor

Global Agricultural Production: Resilience to Climate Change

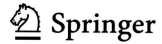

Editor
Mukhtar Ahmed
Department of Agronomy
PMAS Arid Agriculture University
Rawalpindi, Pakistan

ISBN 978-3-031-14972-6 ISBN 978-3-031-14973-3 (eBook)
https://doi.org/10.1007/978-3-031-14973-3

© The Editor(s) (if applicable) and The Author(s), under exclusive license to Springer Nature Switzerland AG 2022

This work is subject to copyright. All rights are solely and exclusively licensed by the Publisher, whether the whole or part of the material is concerned, specifically the rights of translation, reprinting, reuse of illustrations, recitation, broadcasting, reproduction on microfilms or in any other physical way, and transmission or information storage and retrieval, electronic adaptation, computer software, or by similar or dissimilar methodology now known or hereafter developed.

The use of general descriptive names, registered names, trademarks, service marks, etc. in this publication does not imply, even in the absence of a specific statement, that such names are exempt from the relevant protective laws and regulations and therefore free for general use.

The publisher, the authors, and the editors are safe to assume that the advice and information in this book are believed to be true and accurate at the date of publication. Neither the publisher nor the authors or the editors give a warranty, expressed or implied, with respect to the material contained herein or for any errors or omissions that may have been made. The publisher remains neutral with regard to jurisdictional claims in published maps and institutional affiliations.

This Springer imprint is published by the registered company Springer Nature Switzerland AG
The registered company address is: Gewerbestrasse 11, 6330 Cham, Switzerland

Contents

1 Climate Change: An Overview 1
Mukhtar Ahmed, Shakeel Ahmad, and Ahmed M. S. Kheir

2 Climate Change, Agricultural Productivity, and Food Security 31
Mukhtar Ahmed, Muhammad Asim, Shakeel Ahmad,
and Muhammad Aslam

3 Climate Change and Process-Based Soil Modeling 73
Mukhtar Ahmed, Sajid Ali, Adnan Zahid, Shakeel Ahmad,
Nasim Ahmad Yasin, and Rifat Hayat

4 Soil Microbes and Climate-Smart Agriculture 107
Muhammad Nadeem, Rabia Khalid, Sabiha Kanwal,
Ghulam Mujtaba, Ghulam Qadir, Mukhtar Ahmed, and Rifat Hayat

**5 Climate Change Impacts on Legume Crop Production
and Adaptation Strategies** 149
Mukhtar Ahmed, Aashir Sameen, Hajra Parveen,
Muhammad Inaam Ullah, Shah Fahad, and Rifat Hayat

6 Cereal Crop Modeling for Food and Nutrition Security 183
Ahmed M. S. Kheir, Khalil A. Ammar, Ahmed Attia,
Abdelrazek Elnashar, Shakeel Ahmad, Sherif F. El-Gioushy,
and Mukhtar Ahmed

**7 Changing Climate Scenario: Perspectives of *Camelina sativa*
as Low-Input Biofuel and Oilseed Crop** 197
Muhammad Ahmad, Ejaz Ahmad Waraich, Muhammad Bilal Hafeez,
Usman Zulfiqar, Zahoor Ahmad, Muhammad Aamir Iqbal, Ali Raza,
M. Sohidul Slam, Abdul Rehman, Uzma Younis,
Muhammad Kamran, Muhammad Ammar Raza, Javeed Ahmad Lone,
and Ayman El Sabagh

v

8 Greenhouse Gas Emissions and Mitigation Strategies in Rice Production Systems 237
Zeeshan Ahmed, Dongwei Gui, Zhiming Qi, Junhe Liu, Abid Ali, Ghulam Murtaza, Rana Nauman Shabbir, Muhammad Tariq, Muhammad Shareef, Sadia Zafar, Muhammad Saadullah Khan, and Shakeel Ahmad

9 Fiber Crops in Changing Climate 267
Muhammad Tariq, Muhammad Ayaz Khan, Wali Muhammad, and Shakeel Ahmad

10 Estimation of Crop Genetic Coefficients to Simulate Growth and Yield Under Changing Climate 283
P. K. Jha, P. V. V. Prasad, A. Araya, and I. A. Ciampitti

11 Climate Change Impacts on Animal Production 311
Raman Jasrotia, Menakshi Dhar, and Seema Langer

12 Climate Change and Global Insect Dynamics 335
Raman Jasrotia, Menakshi Dhar, Neha Jamwal, and Seema Langer

13 Sustainable Solutions to Food Insecurity in Nigeria: Perspectives on Irrigation, Crop-Water Productivity, and Antecedents 353
Abdulazeez Hudu Wudil, Asghar Ali, Hafiz Ali Raza, Muhammad Usman Hameed, Nugun P. Jellason, Chukwuma C. Ogbaga, Kulvir Singh, Fatih Çiğ, Murat Erman, and Ayman El Sabagh

14 Functions of Soil Microbes Under Stress Environment 373
Sana Zahra, Rifat Hayat, and Mukhtar Ahmed

15 Modeling Impacts of Climate Change and Adaptation Strategies for Cereal Crops in Ethiopia 383
A. Araya, P. V. V. Prasad, P. K. Jha, H. Singh, I. A. Ciampitti, and D. Min

16 Strategies for Mitigating Greenhouse Gas Emissions from Agricultural Ecosystems 409
H. Singh, P. V. V. Prasad, B. K. Northup, I. A. Ciampitti, and C. W. Rice

17 Environmental and Economic Benefits of Sustainable Sugarcane Initiative and Production Constraints in Pakistan: A Review 441
Hafiz Ali Raza, Muhammad Usman Hameed, Mohammad Sohidul Islam, Naveed Ahmad Lone, Muhammad Ammar Raza, and Ayman E. L. Sabagh

Contents

18 Modeling Photoperiod Response of Canola Under Changing Climate Conditions 469
Ameer Hamza, Fayyaz-ul-Hassan, Mukhtar Ahmed, Emaan Yaqub, Muhammad Iftikhar Hussain, and Ghulam Shabbir

19 Modelling and Field-Based Evaluation of Vernalisation Requirement of Canola for Higher Yield Potential 517
Emaan Yaqub, Mukhtar Ahmed, Ameer Hamza, Ghulam Shabbir, Muhammad Iftikhar Hussain, and Fayyaz-ul-Hassan

20 Integrated Crop–Livestock System Case Study: Prospectus for Jordan's Climate Change Adaptation 565
Muhammad Iftikhar Hussain, Abdullah J. Al-Dakheel, and Mukhtar Ahmed

21 Effect of Salinity Intrusion on Sediments in Paddy Fields and Farmers' Adaptation Initiative: A Case Study 587
Prabal Barua, Anisa Mitra, and Mazharul Islam

22 Climatic Challenge for Global Viticulture and Adaptation Strategies 611
Rizwan Rafique, Touqeer Ahmad, Tahira Kalsoom, Muhammad Azam Khan, and Mukhtar Ahmed

Chapter 1
Climate Change: An Overview

Mukhtar Ahmed, Shakeel Ahmad, and Ahmed M. S. Kheir

Abstract Climate variability and change is the main concern for scientific communities since the past decades. This chapter gives an overview about the basics of climate change. It firstly provides detail information about climate change and its responsible factors. Techniques that have been used to quantify climate change were discussed. It includes the application of general circulation or global climate models (GCMs) and use of borehole temperature, cores from deep accumulations of ice, flora and fauna records, sea records and sediment layer analysis. Furthermore, a historical milestone in the science of climate change was given. The Coupled Model Intercomparison Project (CMIP) and its application were discussed in detail. Similarly, the relationship between radiative forcing (RF) and climate change showed that the earth's radiative balance is changed. This was mainly because of the climate change drivers that resulted to the change in air temperature. True picture about climate change was further confirmed by using different climate change drivers coming from different sources. Data showed that climate change is a real phenomenon causing real threat to the human race on planet earth. Meanwhile, the applications of strategic management tools that include RCP (representative concentration pathway), SSP (shared socio-economic pathways) and SPA (shared climate policy assumptions) were presented as they give clear directions in the field of climate change research. Furthermore, they give directions to do climate impact assessments and design climate and socio-economic adaptation and mitigation options. Finally,

M. Ahmed (✉)
Department of Agronomy, PMAS Arid Agriculture University, Rawalpindi, Pakistan
e-mail: ahmadmukhtar@uaar.edu.pk

S. Ahmad
Department of Agronomy, Bahauddin Zakariya University, Multan, Pakistan

A. M. S. Kheir
International Center for Biosaline Agriculture, Directorate of Programs, Dubai, United Arab Emirates

Soils, Water and Environment Research Institute, Agricultural Research Center, Giza, Egypt

© The Author(s), under exclusive license to Springer Nature Switzerland AG 2022
M. Ahmed (ed.), *Global Agricultural Production: Resilience to Climate Change*,
https://doi.org/10.1007/978-3-031-14973-3_1

the responses of the different systems to climatic variables were given as indicators of climate change.

Keywords Climate change · Radiative forcing · Scenario analysis · Climate change drivers · Indicators

1.1 What Is Climate Change?

Climate variability and change is the centre of work in most of the research activities across the globe in the recent decade. Climate variability is the fluctuations in the climatic parameters from its long-term mean. Climate change is the significant variation in weather conditions for the longer period. It is the change in the climatic variables on decadal timescale, i.e. conditions becoming wetter, drier or warmer over several decades. It is different from the natural weather variability as it deals with only shorter time or seasonal climate variability. Climate change is affecting every living being, and it is displaying itself in myriad ways. It can be seen across the globe in the form of extreme events of raging storms, record floods and deadly heat. Different natural and anthropogenic factors are responsible for climate variability and change.

Several techniques have been used to collect data that can be applied to understand the past and future climate. These include borehole temperature, cores from deep accumulations of ice, records of flora and fauna, sediment layer analysis and sea records. GCMs are used extensively to confirm past data and make future projections. GCMs are mathematical models that can model the response of global climate to the increasing greenhouse gas (GHG) emission (IPCC 2013). These models can represent the earth in a few latitudinal bands and can be divided into atmospheric GCMs (AGCMs), the ocean GCMs (OGCMs) and both atmospheric and ocean GCMs (AOGCMs). The basic structure of GCM is shown in Fig. 1.1. The history of these models is closely connected with computing power. Thus, these models are in continuous state of development and evolution so that they can give accurate prediction. Details of the commonly used GCMs have been given in Table 1.1, which are in the process of improvement since their origin as they have shortcomings in computing power due to incompetence to solve crucial climate mechanisms. Similarly, low-resolution models are not capable to portray phenomena at local and smaller scales while its downscaling to higher-resolution propagate error (Lupo et al. 2013). One example of application of GCM has been shown in Fig. 1.2. It shows simulation of global average annual surface temperature changes (°C) from 1860 to 2005 by the geophysical fluid dynamics laboratory coupled model (GFDL-CM3) under four 'representative concentration pathway' (RCP) scenarios. Another category of models includes earth system model (ESM). It can predict CO_2 in atmosphere by using carbon cycle approach. It also has also biological and chemical models that can simulate aerosols, trace gases and cloud condensation nuclei (Hartmann 2016). In most of the earlier GCM simulations, atmosphere and ocean data was generated by fixing different climate drivers. These drivers include

1 Climate Change: An Overview

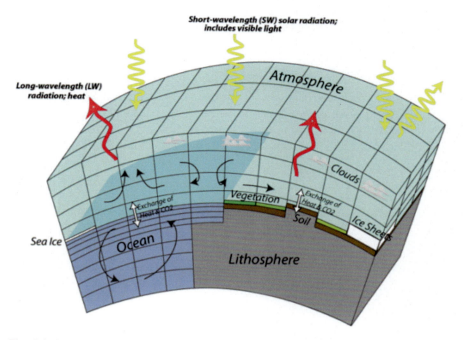

Fig. 1.1 Schematic representation of general circulation model (GCM). (Source: Penn State University)

wind stress, air temperature, sea surface temperature (SST), precipitation and radiative forcing. They all determined the fluxes of heat, exchange of moisture and momentum between the ocean and the atmosphere. However, coupled atmosphere-ocean climate models have shown deficiencies that could be solved by including ESM that consider land surface processes. The components of ESM are shown in Fig. 1.3. It includes physical climate system, biosphere and human influences. ESM can predict vegetation changes, atmospheric composition, biogeochemical cycling, elevated CO_2 effect on leaf stomata, transpiration losses, soil moisture and temperature. Diagrammatic representation of the physical components of GCM has been shown in Fig. 1.4. It has three physical components of the climate system (atmosphere, ocean and land). The frozen places of planet earth are called cryosphere, and it has a significant impact on climate as it has high albedo/reflectivity, acts as insulator, requires latent heat of fusion and absorbs GHG (e.g. permafrost contains 1400–1600 billion tonnes of carbon). Under 1.5 °C–2.0 °C climate warming scenario, it has been reported that the melting of permafrost will produce 150–200 and 220–300 Gt CO_2-eq emissions, respectively (Pörtner et al. 2019). The atmosphere component of GCMs mainly involved weather forecasting through numerical weather prediction systems that can forecast weather in advance for short intervals. However, for longer forecasts, different climatology-based models have been used. In numerical modelling the components of systems (atmosphere or ocean) are

Table 1.1 List of the commonly used GCMs with resolution

S. No.	GCMs	Resolution	
		Latitude	Longitude
1.	ACCESS-CM (Australian Community Climate and Earth System Simulator Coupled Model) (ACCESS1.0 & 1.3)	1.25	1.875
2.	BCC_CSM1.1 (Beijing Climate Centre Climate System Model)	2.7906	2.8125
3.	BNU-ESM (Beijing Normal University Earth System Model)	2.7906	2.8125
4.	CCSM (Community Climate System Model)	0.9424	1.25
5.	CESM (Community Earth System Model)	0.9424	1.25
6.	CESM1(BGC) (Community Earth System Model (CESM1) carbon cycle)	0.9424	1.25
7.	CESM1(CAM5) (Community Earth System Model version 1 (Community Atmospheric Model; CAM))	0.9424	1.25
8.	CESM1(FASTCHEM) (Community Earth System Model version 1 (CAM and Chemistry Model))	0.9424	1.25
9.	CESM1(WACCM) (NCAR Community Earth System Model (Whole Atmosphere Community Climate Model))	1.8848	2.5
10.	CFSv2–2011(National Centers for Environmental Prediction (NCEP) Climate Forecast System Version 2)	1	1
11.	CMCC-CESM (Centro Euro-Mediterraneo per I Cambiamenti Climatici-Earth System Model)	3.4431	3.75
12.	CMCC-CM (Centro Euro-Mediterraneo per I Cambiamenti Climatici-Climate Model)	0.7484	0.75
13.	CMCC-CMS (Centro Euro-Mediterraneo per I Cambiamenti Climatici-Climate Model with a resolved stratosphere)	3.7111	3.75
14.	CNRM-CM5 (Centre National de Recherches Météorologiques-Coupled Model Intercomparison Project)	1.4008	1.40625
15.	CSIRO-Mk3.6.0 (Centre of Excellence and Commonwealth Scientific and Industrial Research Organization)	1.8653	1.875
16.	CSIRO Mk3L (a computationally efficient coupled atmosphere-sea ice-ocean general circulation model)	3.1857	5.625
17.	CanAM4 (Canadian Fourth Generation Atmospheric Global Climate Model)	2.7906	2.8125
18.	CanCM4 (Canadian Fourth Generation Coupled Global Climate Model)	2.7906	2.8125
19.	CanESM2 (Canadian Second Generation Earth System Model)	2.7906	2.8125
20.	EC-EARTH (European Earth System Model)	1.1215	1.125
21.	FGOALS-g2 (Flexible Global Ocean-Atmosphere-Land System Model: Grid-point Version 2)	2.7906	2.8125
22.	FGOALS-gl (Flexible Global Ocean-Atmosphere-Land-Sea-ice)	4.1026	5
23.	GFDL-CM3 (Geophysical Fluid Dynamics Laboratory-Coupled Model 3)	2	2.5
24.	GISS-E2_R (Goddard Institute for Space Studies, USA)	2	2.5
25.	HadGEM2 (Hadley Centre Global Environment Model version 2/UK)	1.25	1.875
26.	MIROC5 (Model for Interdisciplinary Research On Climate/ Japan)	2.7906	2.8125
27.	MPI-ESM-MR (The Max Planck Institute for Meteorology-Earth System Model)	1.8653	1.875
28.	MRI-CGCM3 (Meteorological Research Institute Coupled Global Climate Model Version Three, Japan)	1.12148	1.125

1 Climate Change: An Overview

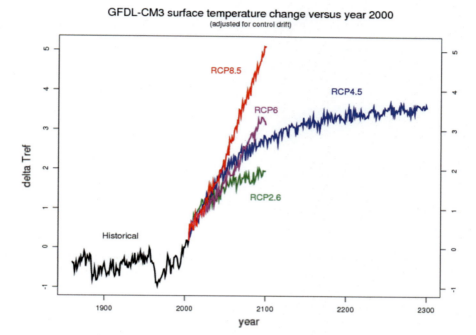

Fig. 1.2 Simulation of changes in surface temperature by GFDL-CM3

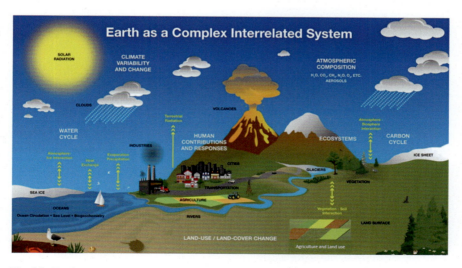

Fig. 1.3 Earth as a complex interrelated system. (Source: NASA)

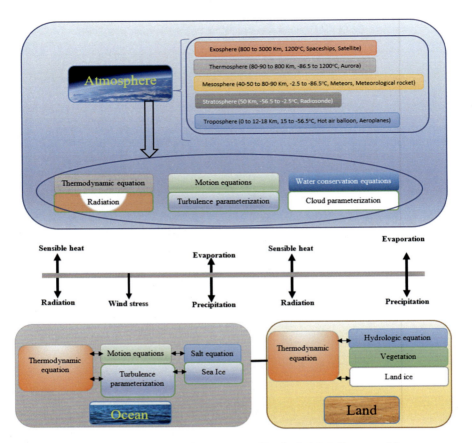

Fig. 1.4 Physical components (atmosphere, ocean and land) of global climate model

divided into spatial grid work with further application of physics equations. The land component of GCM considers surface heat balance and moisture equation as well as model for snow cover. In the case of the ocean component of GCM, the motion equations explaining the general circulation of the ocean were considered. Recent accelerated work in climate change science resulted to the improvement of GCMs. This includes incorporation of physical processes in GCMs that can accurately simulate different phenomena at ocean-atmosphere and land scale (Fig. 1.5). Hence, GCMs could be used to accurately detect climate change causes, future predictions and matching of past climate data (Bhattacharya 2019). Different causes or drivers of climate are called climate forcings. These include alterations in solar radiation, changes in the earth's orbits and albedo/reflectivity of the continents and changes in GHG concentrations.

The Intergovernmental Panel on Climate Change (IPCC) published its first assessment report (FAR) in 1990, and nobody accepted at that time that climate change will be a real issue in the future. The IPCC is the leading body that provides

1 Climate Change: An Overview   7

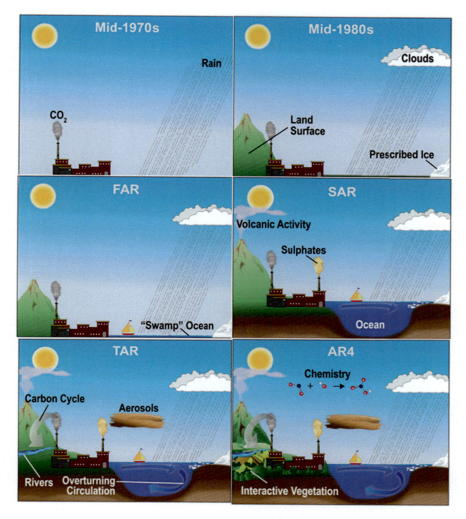

Fig. 1.5 Pictorial description in the climate model complexity over the last few decades. (Source: Le Treut 2007)

true scientific picture about climate change. It also illustrates the potential socio-economic and environmental consequences across the globe. In the 2007 IPCC report, it has been elaborated that significant climate changes are going to happen, which will be mainly due to higher GHGs (Solomon 2007). Higher build-up of GHGs in the environment leads to global warming. Thus, climate change is a broader term that could be due to global warming resulting to the changes in rainfall and ocean acidification. The different important terms that the reader should know to understand the phenomenon of climate change include the following: abatement (decreased greenhouse gas emission); adaptation (adjustment/shifting); adaptability (adjustment ability); adaptive capacity (system ability to adjust to climate change); aerosols; afforestation; agriculture, forestry and other land use (AFOLU); albedo; black carbon; biogeochemical cycle; CO_2 equivalent (scale to compare the emissions from GHGs based upon their GWP (global warming potential)); CO_2 fertilization; carbon footprint; carbon sequestration; Conference of the Parties (COP); chlorofluorocarbons; El Niño-Southern Oscillation (ENSO); enteric fermentation; greenhouse gases; global warming; GWP (total energy a GHG can absorb per 100 years); greenhouse effect; nitrogen oxides (NOX); mitigation; parameterization; risk; risk assessment; uncertainty; validation; and vulnerability.

Climate change importance was already pointed by the Swedish scientist Svante Arrhenius in 1896. He has given the relationship between fossil fuels and increased amount of CO_2 in the air. Detailed historical milestones in the field of climate science had been given in Table 1.2.

Table 1.2 History of milestones in the field of climate change

Years	Milestones
1820	Fourier description about atmosphere contribution to planetary temperature
1850	Foote observed heat-trapping variability in H_2O and CO_2
1859	Tyndall described CO_2 blocking of infrared and elaborated radiative properties of gases
1896	Warming due to doubling of CO_2 by Arrhenius (father of climate change science)
1928	Rate of lunar heat loss was measured
1932	Calculation of 4 °C warming due to doubling of CO_2 by Hulburt
1938	Callendar confirms that warming is occurring
1950–60	CO_2 sources were identified, and models described the earth systems, carbon cycle and climate
1960	Charles keeling started Mauna Loa observatory
1965	Water vapour feedback was described
1965	Warnings by climate scientist to policymakers
1967	Syukuro Manabe and Richard Wetherald (CO_2 and temperature rise have perfect relationship)
1967–68	The first climate models by Syukuro Manabe and Richard Wetherald showing that global temperatures would increase by 2.0 °C (3.6 °F) if the CO_2 content of the atmosphere doubled
1979	Charney report (carbon dioxide and climate: A scientific assessment) doubling of CO_2 leads to 3 °C change in temperature with probable error of 1.5 °C
1988	Hansen predictions about warming
1988	Birth of the IPCC
1992	Establishment of the United Nations framework convention on climate change (UNFCCC) with the aim to combat climate change
1995	Conference of the parties 1 (COP1): The first conference of the parties to the UNFCCC (COP-1) met in Berlin
1996	COP2 in Geneva
1997	COP3, Kyoto protocol; GHG reduction treaty
1998	COP4-Buenos Aires-Argentina

(continued)

1 Climate Change: An Overview

Table 1.2 (continued)

Years	Milestones
1999	COP5-Bonn-Germany
2000	COP6-The Hague-Netherlands
2001	COP7-Marrakech-Morocco
2002	COP8-New Delhi-India-Technology transfer
2003	COP9-Milan-Italy-Adaptation Fund
2004	COP10, Buenos Aires, Argentina, climate change mitigation and adaptation
2005	COP11-Montreal-Canada (biggest intergovernmental conferences on climate change)
2006	COP12-Nairobi-Kenya
2007	COP13-Bali-Indonesia
2008	COP14-Poznań-Poland-Funding to poorest nations
2009	COP15-Copenhagen-Denmark (the Copenhagen accord)
2010	COP16-Cancún-Mexico (Green climate fund and climate technology centre/network)
2011	COP17-Durban-South Africa (Green Climate Fund (GCF))
2012	COP18, Doha, Qatar, the Doha climate gateway
2013	COP19-Warsaw-Poland
2014	COP20-Lima-Peru
2015	COP21-Paris-France (Paris agreement)
2016	COP22-Marrakech-Morocco (water-related sustainability, reduction in GHG emissions and utilization of low-carbon energy sources)
2017	COP23-Bonn-Germany
2018	COP24-Katowice-Poland
2020	COP25-Madrid-Spain
2021	COP26-Glasgow-Scotland (Glasgow climate pact to keep 1.5oC alive and finalize the outstanding elements of the Paris agreement)

1.2 Climate Change and Coupled Model Intercomparison Project (CMIP)

The CMIP (Coupled Model Intercomparison Project) was started by the Working Group on Coupled Modelling (WGCM) of the World Climate Research Programme (WCRP) in 1995 to better recognize the past, present and future climate changes that arise from different natural, unforced variability or due to changes in the radiative forcing. This includes historical assessments of model performance and quantifications of the causes of the spread in future climate projections. The results from CMIP have been used in the IPCC assessment reports. CMIP is the foundational element of climate science, and it includes coupled models of the earth's climate (Fig. 1.6). The CMIP's first two phases were simple. In CMIP1, 18 GCMs were involved in data collection. In CMIP2, simulation was conducted with assumptions of no inter-annual changes in radiative forcing (RF) and doubling of CO_2 concentration at a rate of 1% per year (Stouffer et al. 2017). CMIP3 resulted to the paradigm shift in the field of climate science. It has given the state-of-the-art climate change simulations that have

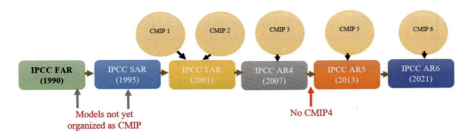

Fig. 1.6 Historical description of Coupled Model Intercomparison Projects (CMIPs) and their contributions to IPCC assessment reports (ARS)

been used on larger scale (Meehl et al. 2007). However, there was no CMIP4, so CMIP5 was developed upon CMIP3. CMIP5 can help to understand the climate system accurately. It generated 2 petabits (PB) of output from different experiments completed through climate models. The salient features of CMIP5 include climate responses to perturbed atmospheric CO_2, impact of atmospheric chemistry on climate, carbon-climate interactions, troposphere-stratosphere interactions, feedbacks and idealized model configurations. The idea of near- and long-term time horizons was implemented in CMIP5. Furthermore, to address the range of advanced scientific questions that come from different scientific communities, CMIP6 was implemented. It has three major components: (i) the DECK (Diagnostic, Evaluation and Characterization of Klima) and CMIP historical simulations (1850–near present); (ii) characterization of the model ensemble and dissemination of model outputs through common standards, coordination, infrastructure and documentation (SCID); and (iii) filling of scientific gaps through the ensemble of CMIP-Endorsed Model Intercomparison Projects (MIPs) that will build on the DECK and CMIP historical simulations. The following three broad questions will be addressed in CMIP6: (i) how does the earth system respond to forcing?; (ii) what are the origins/consequences of model biases?; and (iii) how can future climate change be assessed under the scenarios of uncertainties, predictability and internal climate variability? (Eyring et al. 2016). Further description about CMIP6 has been shown in Fig. 1.7.

1.2.1 Application of CMIP

CMIP/CMIP6 have been widely used in different studies across the globe to quantify the effect of climate change. This includes the climate change effect on soil organic carbon (Wang et al. 2022a); agronomic managements to boost crop yield (Ali et al. 2022); simulation of air-sea CO_2 fluxes (FCO_2) (Jing et al. 2022); anthropogenic aerosol emission inventory (Wang et al. 2022b); heatwave simulation (Hirsch et al. 2021); prediction of future precipitation and hydrological hazard (Nashwan and Shahid 2022); drought prediction (Mondal et al. 2021; Supharatid and Nafung

1 Climate Change: An Overview

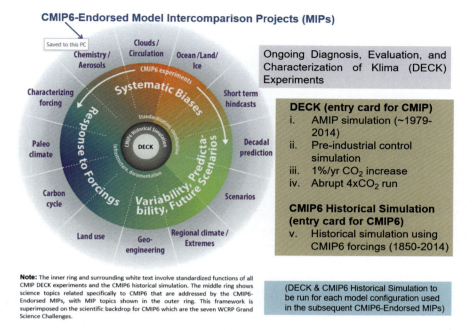

Fig. 1.7 Schematic representation of CMIP6 experiment design. (Source with permission: Eyring et al. 2016)

2021); evaluation of spatio-temporal variability in drought/rainfall in Bangladesh (Kamal et al. 2021); global assessment of meteorological, hydrological and agricultural drought (Zeng et al. 2021); prediction of crop yield and water footprint (Arunrat et al. 2022); temperature simulations over Thailand (Kamworapan et al. 2021); climate projections for Canada (Sobie et al. 2021); ENSO evaluation (Lee et al. 2021); and simulation of ENSO phase-locking (Chen and Jin 2021).

1.3 Radiative Forcing (RF) and Climate Change

Total (downward minus upward) radiative flux (expressed in W m^{-2}) at the top of the atmosphere due to changes in the external drivers of climate change (mainly GHGs) is called radiative forcing (RF). Mathematically, it can be expressed as follows:

$$Radiative\ forcing = Incoming\ energy\ (short\ wavelength)\\ - Outgoing\ energy (both\ short\ \&\ long\ wavelength)$$

Radiative forcing determines the energy budget of the earth (Fig. 1.8). It can be positive or negative. If radiative forcing is positive, it means the earth is getting higher energy from the sun than it is returning to space. This net gain causes warming. However, if the earth loses more energy to space, then what it gets from the sun it produces cooling. Hence, the temperature of the earth is determined by the RF. Around one-third (29.4%) of radiation that comes from the sun is reflected, while the rest is absorbed by the earth system. Calculation about the earth's energy budget has been presented in Table 1.3. Factors that determine the sunlight reflection back into space include land surfaces and the reflectivity (albedo) of clouds, oceans and particles in the atmosphere. However, the strong determinants are cloud albedo, snow and ice cover as they have much higher albedos. Furthermore, important factors that regulate the earth's temperature are incoming sunlight, absorbed/reflected sunlight, emitted infrared radiation and absorbed and re-emitted infrared radiation (mainly by GHGs). The earth's radiative balance has been changed due to changes in these factors, which resulted to the change in air temperature. Anthropogenic activities have changed radiative balance of the earth (Table 1.4), which resulted to the changes in the rainfall pattern, temperature extremes and other climatic variables through a complicated set of coupled physical processes. Radiative forcing caused by human activities since 1750 has been shown in Fig. 1.9.

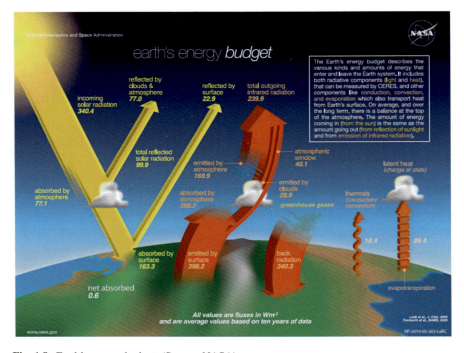

Fig. 1.8 Earth's energy budget. (Source: NASA)

1 Climate Change: An Overview

Table 1.3 Calculation about the earth's energy budget

Incoming solar radiation at the top of the atmosphere (TOA)	Outgoing radiation at TOA	Downwelling (back radiation at the surface from GHGs in the atmosphere)	Solar radiation reflected into space
$= 340.4$ Wm^{-2}. (1/4th of 1361.6 Wm^{-2} solar constant, i.e. total solar irradiance at the top of the atmosphere) Solar constant average varies from 1360 to 1370 Wm^{-2}	$= 239.9$ Wm^{-2} IR $+ 77.0 + 22.9 = 339.8$ W/m^2, which is 0.6 W/m^2 less than the incoming solar radiation	$= 340.3$ Wm^{-2} (same as the solar irradiance at TOA)	$= 22.6\%$ (77 W/m^2)

Source: Kramer et al. (2021)

Table 1.4 The earth's radiative forcing relative to 1750

Year	Radiative forcing relative to 1750 (Wm^{-2})
1750	0.0
1950	0.57
1980	11.25
2011	2.29

Source: IPCC AR5 WG1

1.4 Drivers of Climate Change

Most of the climate change drivers are mainly associated with anthropogenic activity and, to a lesser extent, with natural origin. Well-known natural climate drivers are solar irradiance, volcanic eruptions and ENSO. Drivers of climate change can be categorized into two types: (i) natural and (ii) man induced. Natural climate drivers consist of radiative forcing, variations in the earth's orbital cycle, ocean cycles and volcanic and geologic activity. Human-induced drivers of climate change are burning fossil fuels, cutting down forests and farming livestock. These human activities resulted to global warming due to increased accumulation of GHGs and changes in the reflectivity or absorption of the sun's energy. Details about the drivers of climate change have been further elaborated below.

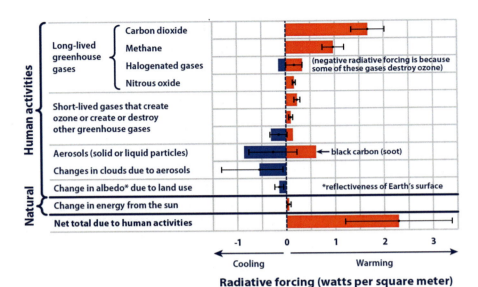

Fig. 1.9 Radiative forcing caused by human activities since 1750. (Source: IPCC 2013)

1.4.1 Anthropogenic Drivers

1.4.1.1 Greenhouse Gases

Greenhouse gases (GHGs) are the main drivers of global climate change. The principal GHGs are carbon dioxide (CO_2), methane (CH_4) and nitrous oxide (N_2O). Concentrations of these GHGs have increased significantly since from the industrial revolution, which resulted to the increased greenhouse effect. On annual scale over 30 billion tonnes of CO_2 have been released into atmosphere due to human activities. The levels of CO_2 have been increased by more than 40% since pre-industrial times. It has been increased from 280 ppm to 417 ppm in 2022. The trend of CO_2 based on C. David Keeling (Keeling Curve) has been shown in Fig. 1.10. CO_2 has global sources and sinks. The major sources of the rise in the concentration of CO_2 are fossil fuel burning, cement industry and changes in land use (e.g. housing sector and deforestation). Sink of CO_2 includes absorption by the oceans, carbonation of finished cement products and its use by the plants in the process of photosynthesis. The data depicted that CO_2 atmospheric growth rate has been increased exponentially, and it has shown the largest RF as compared to other GHGs (Fig. 1.11). Global distribution of GHGs in percentage with their emissions from different economic sector and countries has been shown in Fig. 1.12. CO_2 has been used as reference to define the global warming potential (GWP) of other GHGs. The GWP of CO_2 is 1 as it is used as reference, while for CH_4 (methane)

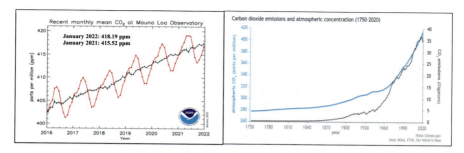

Fig. 1.10 Trend of CO_2 measured at Mauna Loa Observatory, Hawaii. (Source: NOAA)

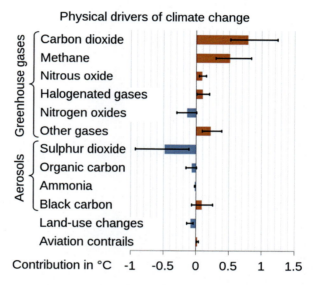

Fig. 1.11 Radiative forcing of physical drivers of climate change. (IPCC 2013)

it is 28–36 per 100 year and N_2O has a GWP of 265–298 times that of CO_2 for a 100-year timescale. Halogen's derivatives (CFCs (chlorofluorocarbons), HFCs (hydrofluorocarbons), HCFCs (hydrochlorofluorocarbons), PFCs (perfluorocarbons)) and SF_6 (sulphur hexafluoride) are called high-ranking GWP gases as they can trap more heat than CO_2 (Fig. 1.13) (Vallero 2019). Most of our daily activities are responsible for GHG emissions, and it can be calculated by using apps like carbon footprint calculator and greenhouse gas equivalencies calculator. The methane concentration and RF have also been increased since the industrial era. Unlike CO_2, CH_4 is increasing at faster rate (Saunois et al. 2016). The major sources of CH_4 include decaying of organic material, seepage from underground deposits, digestion of food by cattle, rice farming and waste management (IPCC 2013; Liu et al. 2021; Matthews and Wassmann 2003). N_2O has a variety of natural and human-caused sources that include use of artificial nitrogenous fertilizers, animal waste, biological N_2 fixation, crop residue, animal husbandry, burning of waste,

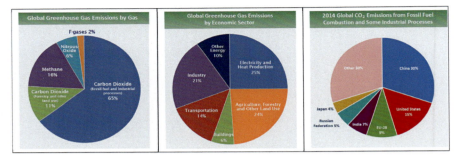

Fig. 1.12 Percentage distribution of GHG emissions by gas, economic sector and CO_2 emissions from fossil fuels. (Source: NOAA)

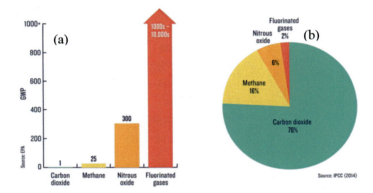

Fig. 1.13 The global warming potential (GWP) of human-generated GHGs (**a**) and per person share to GHG emissions (**b**). (Source: USA, Environment Protection Agency (EPA); IPCC 2014)

combustion of fuel in automobiles and wastewater treatment. Another issue related to N_2O is its destruction in the stratosphere due to photochemical reactions, which form nitrogen oxides (NOX) that destroy ozone (O_3) (Skiba and Rees 2014). Projection of future climate using different climate change scenarios has been well elaborated by the IPCC and presented in Fig. 1.14.

1.4.1.2 Water Vapours

Water vapours account for 60% of the earth's greenhouse warming effect. Water vapours are the most abundant GHG. Researchers from the NASA using novel data from AIRS (Atmospheric Infrared Sounder) on NASA's Aqua satellite have estimated that water also has heat-trapping effect in the air. Furthermore, powerful heat-amplifying effect of water has been confirmed, which can double the climate warming effect caused by higher concentrations of CO_2 (Matthews 2018). The

1 Climate Change: An Overview

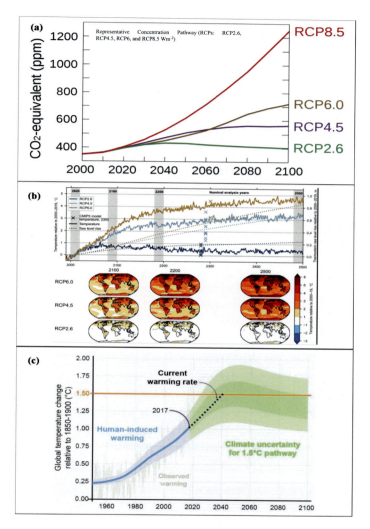

Fig. 1.14 Diagrammatic representation of future climate using (**a**) RCPs, (**b**) global temperature and (**c**) global temperature trend if the current emissions continue. (Source: IPCC 2014)

strength of water vapour feedback has been estimated by climate models and experts that have found that if the earth warms by 1.8 °F, then the increase in water vapour will trap an extra 2 watts m^{-2}. The energy-trapping potential of water vapour at different latitudes has been shown in Fig. 1.15. Water vapours are significantly increasing the earth's temperature. Abundance of water vapours in the troposphere is controlled by two factors: (i) transport from troposphere (the lower atmosphere layer) and (ii) oxidation of CH_4. Since the level of CH_4 is increasing because of anthropogenic activities, it will, hence, increase stratosphere water vapour that will

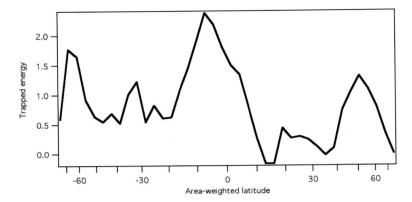

Fig. 1.15 Water vapour trapped energy (southern to northern latitudes). (Source: NASA, Credit: Andrew Dessler)

lead to positive RF (Solomon et al. 2010; Hegglin et al. 2014). Other less important sources of water vapours include hydrogen oxidation, volcanic eruptions and aircraft exhaust. The relationship between increased stratospheric water vapour and ozone and climate change has been reported in earlier work (Shindell 2001). However, water vapour in the troposphere is controlled by temperature. Circulation in the atmosphere limits the build-up of water vapours. Direct changes in water vapours are negligible as compared to indirect changes due to temperature variability that comes from RF. Hence, water vapours are considered as feedback in the climate system as increase in GHG concentration warms the atmosphere that leads to increase in water vapour concentrations, thus amplifying the warming effect.

1.4.1.3 Ozone

Ozone (O_3) is a naturally occurring GHG. It is mainly present in the stratosphere (ozone layer), but a small amount, which is harmful, also generates in the troposphere. O_3 is produced and destroyed due to anthropogenic and natural emissions. CH_4, NOX, carbon monoxide and volatile organic compounds (VOC) are producing O_3 photochemically. This increase in O_3 production results to positive RF (Dentener et al. 2005). However, in polar regions, O_3 has been destroyed due to halocarbons, which leads to negative RF. O_3 is harmful for plants, animals and humans. In plants higher concentration of O_3 causes closure of stomata, decrease in photosynthesis and reduced plant growth. Similarly, O_3 could cause oxidative damage to the plant cells (McAdam et al. 2017; Vainonen and Kangasjärvi 2015; Li et al. 2021; Jimenez-Montenegro et al. 2021).

1 Climate Change: An Overview

1.4.1.4 Aerosols

Aerosols are suspended particles from the surface of planet earth to the edge of space. Aerosols are dispersion of solid/liquid particles in a gas (Hidy 2003). Smoke, particulate air pollutants, dust, soot and sea salt are primary aerosols that come from the anthropogenic activities. Open burning is a major cause of aerosols in the atmosphere (Kumar et al. 2022). Natural aerosols are forest exudates, geyser steam, dust and fog/mist. Aerosols have a significant impact on climate as higher concentrations of aerosols lead to the rise in the temperature. Aerosols have shown an impact on climate change through its two-way interactions: (i) aerosol-radiation interactions (direct effect) and (ii) aerosol-cloud interactions/cloud albedo (indirect effect). The RF for both of this interaction is negative; however, it changes with the types of aerosols. The aerosol, such as black carbon, absorbs light, so they produces positive RF and warms the atmosphere (Flanner et al. 2009).

1.4.1.5 Land Use Change (LUC)

Changes and variability in land use resulted to the alterations in surface features, and it is a major driver of climate change but given less preference (Vose et al. 2004). LUC leads to higher aerosols, CH_4 and CO_2 in the atmosphere. Similarly, it modifies the surface albedo, which alters the climate variables (e.g. temperature, precipitation, etc.). Spatio-temporal variability in the pattern of thunderstorms and ENSO are well-known examples of LUC (Pielke 2005). LUC influences the mass-energy fluxes, which alter the climate of the surroundings. LUC resulted to the change in the albedo, particularly due to deforestation and afforestation. This leads to alteration in RF and carbon and hydrologic cycles.

1.4.1.6 Contrails

Clouds that are line (linear) shaped are produced by the aircraft engine exhaust in the mid to upper troposphere under elevated ambient humidity. Contrail's production resulted to the change in the earth's radiative balance by absorbing outgoing long-wave radiation. Contrails have intensified the effect of global warming, and it can account for more than half of the entire climate impact of aviation. It can interact with solar and thermal radiation, thus producing global net positive RF. Tweaking flight altitude could minimize the impact of contrails (Caldeira and McKay 2021).

1.4.2 Natural Drivers

1.4.2.1 Solar Irradiance

Solar irradiance is the number of solar radiation that reaches the surface of the earth without being absorbed or dispersed. It is a promising source of energy. It also affects different processes such as evaporation, hydrological cycle, ice melting, photosynthesis and carbon uptake and diurnal and seasonal changes in the surface temperatures (Wild 2012). The relationship between climate, solar cycles and trends in solar irradiance has been discussed earlier (Lean 2010). The connection between solar irradiance and climate indicators (global temperature, sea level, sea ice content and precipitation) has been reported in the work of Bhargawa and Singh (2019).

1.4.2.2 Volcanoes

Volcanic eruptions are minor events that lead to significant change in the climate. Active volcanoes inject significant amount of sulphur dioxide (SO_2) in the air. On oxidation SO_2 changes to sulphuric acid (H_2SO_4), which resulted to increase in the earth albedo and negative RF. Furthermore, volcanic eruptions also result to O_3 depletion and changes in the heating and circulation. It also emits CO_2 and water vapour, which then change the climate of surrounding. Volcanic activity has triggered El Niño events due to volcanic radiative forcing. Similarly, decrease in global temperature of 0.5 °C was recorded due to Mount Pinatubo eruption (Cole-Dai 2010).

1.5 Scenario Analysis (RCP, SSP and SPA)

A scenario analysis that includes RCP (representative concentration pathway), shared socio-economic pathways (SSP) and shared climate policy assumptions (SPA) is a strategic management tool that has been used to explore future changes across the globe. They can also be used to design adaptation options under the changing climate (Kebede et al. 2018). Furthermore, they can investigate the consequences of long-term climatic-environmental-anthropogenic futures to design robust policies (Harrison et al. 2015). In initial scenarios most of the focus was on climate change (Hulme et al. 1999) that was addressed by the IPCC through SRES (Special Report on Emission Scenarios), which includes both socio-economic and climate change (Arnell et al. 2004). In the IPCC AR5 three-dimensional aspects (climate/socio-economic/policy dimensions of change) were presented using RCP-SSP-SPA scenarios (van Vuuren et al. 2011; O'Neill et al. 2014; Kriegler et al. 2014). These three dimensional frameworks provide basis for the climate change impact assessment, adaptation and mitigation under a wide range of climate and socio-economic scenarios (Fig. 1.16).

1 Climate Change: An Overview

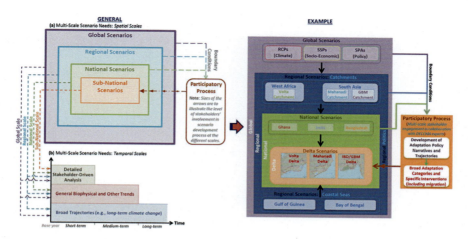

Fig. 1.16 Application of integrated scenario frameworks. (Source: Kebede et al. 2018)

Table 1.5 Temperature and mean sea level change under different RCPs in the mid- and late-twenty-first century

RCP Scenarios	2046–2065 Temperature mean (range)	2081–2100 Temperature mean (range)	2046–2065 Mean sea level (m) increase (range)	2081–2100 Mean sea level (m) increase (range)
RCP2.6	1.0 (0.4 to 1.6)	1.0 (0.3 to 1.7)	0.24 (0.17 to 0.32)	0.40 (0.26 to 0.55)
RCP4.5	1.4 (0.9 to 2.0)	1.8 (1.1 to 2.6)	0.26 (0.19 to 0.33)	0.47 (0.32 to 0.63)
RCP6	1.3 (0.8 to 1.8)	2.2 (1.4 to 3.1)	0.25 (0.18 to 0.32)	0.48 (0.33 to 0.63)
RCP8.5	2.0 (1.4 to 2.6)	3.7 (2.6 to 4.8)	0.30 (0.22 to 0.38)	0.63 (0.45 to 0.82)

Source: IPCC (2013)

A representative concentration pathway (RCP) is a GHG trajectory provided by the IPCC. It has been used in climate modelling and impact assessments for the IPCC AR5 and includes four pathways (RCP2.6 (2.6 Wm^{-2} RF), RCP4.5 (4.5 Wm^{-2} RF), RCP6 (6.0 Wm^{-2} RF) and RCP8.5 (8.5 Wm^{-2} RF)). RCP can be further divided into RCP1.9 (limit global warming <1.5 °C as per the Paris Agreement), RCP2.6, RCP3.4, RCP4.5, RCP6, RCP7 and RCP8.5. RCP2.6 is a very strict pathway, and it requires that CO_2 emissions should be declined by 2020 and should go to zero by 2100. Similarly, CH_4 should be dropped to half by 2020, and SO_2 emissions need to be declined by 10%. RCP2.6 requires that global temperature should be kept below 2 °C through absorption of CO_2. The most possible pathway is RCP3.4, which forces to keep temperature between 2.0 and 2.4 °C till 2100. RCP4.5 is an intermediate scenario that suggests dropping CO_2 and other GHGs by 2045. However, most of the plant and animal species will not be able to adapt because of RCP4.5. Further details about RCP scenarios are given in Table 1.5. The scenarios that are used to project socio-economic changes across the globe are called SSPs. It deals with socio-economic development by working on the aspects of impact assessments of climate change, adaptation and mitigation. Further detail about SSP is given in Fig. 1.17.

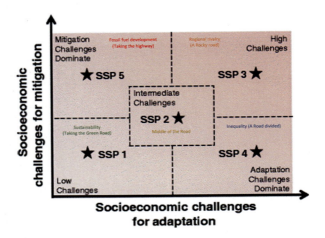

Fig. 1.17 Concept of SSP (shared socio-economic pathways). (Source: O'Neill et al. 2014)

1.6 Indicators of Climate Change

Different indicators could be utilized as early warning signals to identify the impact of climate change. The gathered information can help to design adaptation and mitigation option to the climate change. The major indicators of climate change have been shown in Fig. 1.18. Temperature is the topmost indicator that showed that climate change is a real phenomenon affecting global environment. The average temperature of planet earth has been risen to 1.18 °C since the nineteenth century. Higher concentration of CO_2 and human activities are the main drivers of this rise in temperature. However, this temperature rise is not uniform across the globe (Fig. 1.19). The higher temperature will be more on the land particularly in the tropics as compared to the sea. At 1.5 °C rise in temperature, extreme heatwaves will be more common and widespread across the globe. Deadly heatwave due to 2 °C warming was seen in 2015 in India and Pakistan. Cold extremes will be visible in the Arctic land regions. Temperature extremes will lead to drought in some part of the world while extreme precipitation on the other part. The connection between ENSO (El Niño/Southern Oscillation) phenomenon and extreme temperature in Southeast Asia have been seen in April 2016. Results indicated that 49% of the 2016 anomaly was caused by El Niño while 29% due to warming (Thirumalai et al. 2017). Intensification of hydrological cycle (extreme precipitation and flood) due to global warming has been reported over all climatic regions (Tabari 2020). Furthermore, the intensity of drought under the changing climate was studied using different indices (Bouabdelli et al. 2022). The indices include (i) precipitation only and (ii) overall climate (precipitation plus temperature). Results showed that drought events in plains will be more and long-lasting in hot season that will threaten the agricultural production as well as food security under RCP4.5. Temperature extremes will modify crop life cycle and productivity. Since crop vegetative development requires higher optimum temperature than reproductive phase, rise in temperature will,

1 Climate Change: An Overview

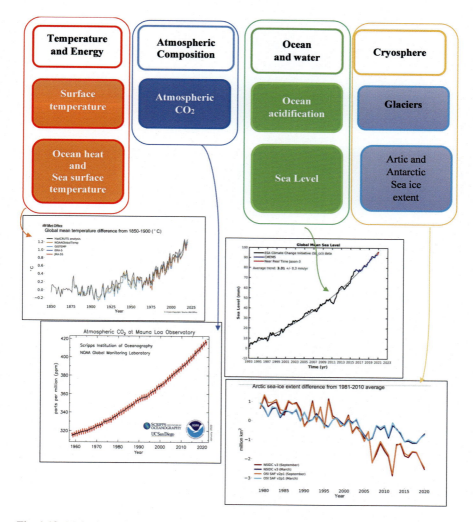

Fig. 1.18 Major indicators of climate change

hence, severely affect pollen viability, grain development and grain weight. The impact is visible on photoperiod sensitive crops (e.g. soybean). Meanwhile, in crops, pollen viability will be decreased due to its exposure to temperature greater than 35 °C. Similarly, in rice, pollen capability and production decreases when daytime temperature goes above 33 °C and stops when it exceeds 40 °C (Hatfield et al. 2011, 2020; Hatfield and Prueger 2015). Other indirect indicators of climate change include plant pathogens (Hatfield et al. 2020; Garrett et al. 2016), crops and livestock systems (Hatfield et al. 2020), biodiversity (Mashwani 2020; Habibullah et al. 2022), loss of species and extinction (Caro et al. 2022), shift in herbicide paradigm (Ziska 2020) and human health (Carlson 2022). Further details about the responses of different systems to different climatic variables have been given in Table 1.6.

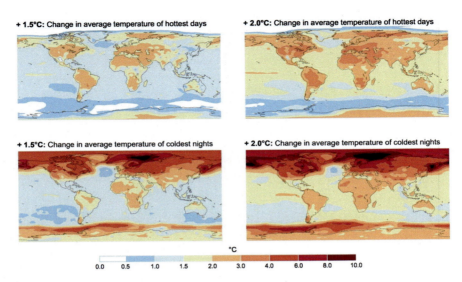

Fig. 1.19 Projection of global warming of 1.5 and 2 °C with hottest and cold days. (Source: NASA)

1.7 Humidity as a Driver of Climate Change

A recent study published in the Proceedings of the National Academy of Sciences (PNAS) by climate scientists reported that temperature is not the only best way to measure climate change (Song et al. 2022). Instead, humidity should also be used as an indicator to measure global warming. They showed that surface equivalent potential temperature (temperature and humidity) is a comprehensive metric to monitor global warming. Similarly, this also has an impact on climate and weather extremes.

1.8 Solar Dimming

The earth is dimming due to climate change as shown in Fig. 1.20. The light reflected from the earth, called the earth's reflectance or albedo, is decreasing. It is now ½ a watt less light per m^2 than what was received 20 years ago, which is equal to 0.5% reduction in the earth's reflectance. About 30% of the sunlight is reflected by the earth, since the earth's albedo has been dropped due to air pollution, which will reduce the intensity of photosynthetically active radiation (PAR) and agricultural production (Yadav et al. 2022). However, on the other hand, researchers are planning to spray sunlight-reflecting particles (the sun dimmers) into the stratosphere to lower the planet temperature (Tollefson 2018).

1 Climate Change: An Overview

Table 1.6 Responses of different systems to climatic variables

Systems	Climatic variables	Impact on system	Indicators
Plants	Temperature	Plant phenology	Phenological changes
		Chilling hours	Flowering timing
		Growing degree days	Crop zoning
	Elevated CO_2	Stimulate photosynthesis, plant productivity, fertilization effect, modified water and nutrient cycles	Crop quality
	Elevated CO_2 and soil nutrients	Nutrient's availability	Beneficial to legumes, N-dilution
	Temperature, precipitation and elevated CO_2	Plant productivity, water use efficiency (WUE), N-deposition, yield, biomass	Variable response in plant productivity, more beneficial for C3
Soil	Extreme rainfall	Nutrient run-off/soil erosion/loss of topsoil	Rainfall intensity
	GHG exchange and carbon sequestration	Soil health	Changes in organic carbon
	Precipitation	Soil nutrients, soil water content and infiltration	Water availability for plant production
	Temperature	Soil health	Loss in organic carbon and microbial biomass
Weeds	Temperature	Plant phenology	Changes in onset of phenological development, e.g. bud break, first flower
		Good biomass and establishment	Higher stand
			Crop zoning
	Elevated CO_2	Stimulate photosynthesis, modified water, nutrient cycles	Higher weed abundance
	Temperature, precipitation and CO_2	Plant productivity, yield, biomass	Variable response in plant productivity
Livestock	Extreme events (hot and cold)	Animal productivity	Temperature humidity index, climate index
Pests	CO_2-temperature interactions	Plant productivity	More attacks
	Temperature/ humidity	Insect or disease pressures	Pressures of insects/ diseases
	Temperature/ precipitation	Weed pressures	More weed distribution
Disease	Climate extremes	System productivity	Promote plantdisease and pest outbreaks
Economics	Extreme events	Declined productivity	Insurance

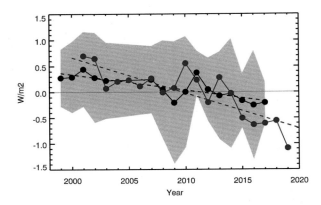

Fig. 1.20 Earth dimming due to climate change. (Source: Goode et al. 2021)

1.9 Conclusion

Climate change is a major environmental concern for the people in all fields of life starting from researchers to policymakers. It is a real phenomenon happening, and its rising impacts cannot be denied. Natural (solar variability, volcanic activity and plate tectonics) and anthropogenic drivers (greenhouse gas emissions, water vapours, ozone, aerosols, land use change and contrails) are the major reasons of accelerated climate change. Another factor includes urbanization, which is the main cause of urban climate change. Since IPCC in AR5 reported that global average surface temperature has increased by 0.85 °C (1880–2012), 0.3–0.7 °C (2016–2036 in comparison with 1986–2005) and 0.3–4.8 °C (end of century in comparison with 1986–2005). Thus, it is essential to use climate change information and adopt measures to control the drivers responsible for this increased climate change. If swift measures will not be taken, these climatic drivers will be responsible for higher possibilities of extreme events, issues of food security, increased weed pressures and occurrence of pest and disease attacks. Climate models are good tools that can give accurate prediction to design adaptation and mitigation strategies for different systems. For example, consider agriculture systems which provides food fuel and fibre to human being is strongly affected by climate change could be managed by using different climate models. The data obtained from these models could be used to understand the relationship between agriculture and climate. The information generated could be used afterwards to improve agricultural systems by adopting different adaptation measures, which can reduce GHG emissions, enhance soil organic carbon and bring sustainability in the system.

References

Ali MGM, Ahmed M, Ibrahim MM, El Baroudy AA, Ali EF, Shokr MS, Aldosari AA, Majrashi A, Kheir AMS (2022) Optimizing sowing window, cultivar choice, and plant density to boost maize yield under RCP8.5 climate scenario of CMIP5. Int J Biometeorol. https://doi.org/10.1007/s00484-022-02253-x

1 Climate Change: An Overview

Arnell NW, Livermore MJL, Kovats S, Levy PE, Nicholls R, Parry ML, Gaffin SR (2004) Climate and socio-economic scenarios for global-scale climate change impacts assessments: characterising the SRES storylines. Glob Environ Chang 14(1):3–20. https://doi.org/10.1016/j.gloenvcha.2003.10.004

Arunrat N, Sereenonchai S, Chaowiwat W, Wang C (2022) Climate change impact on major crop yield and water footprint under CMIP6 climate projections in repeated drought and flood areas in Thailand. Sci Total Environ 807:150741. https://doi.org/10.1016/j.scitotenv.2021.150741

Bhargawa A, Singh AK (2019) Solar irradiance, climatic indicators and climate change – an empirical analysis. Adv Space Res 64(1):271–277. https://doi.org/10.1016/j.asr.2019.03.018

Bhattacharya A (2019) Chapter 1 - global climate change and its impact on agriculture. In: Bhattacharya A (ed) Changing climate and resource use efficiency in plants. Academic Press, pp 1–50. https://doi.org/10.1016/B978-0-12-816209-5.00001-5

Bouabdelli S, Zeroual A, Meddi M, Assani A (2022) Impact of temperature on agricultural drought occurrence under the effects of climate change. Theor Appl Climatol. https://doi.org/10.1007/s00704-022-03935-7

Caldeira K, McKay I (2021) Contrails: tweaking flight altitude could be a climate win. Nature 593(7859):341–341

Carlson G (2022) Human health and the climate crisis. Jones & Bartlett Learning

Caro T, Rowe Z, Berger J, Wholey P, Dobson A (2022) An inconvenient misconception: climate change is not the principal driver of biodiversity loss. Conservation Letters 15:e12868. https://doi.org/10.1111/conl.12868

Chen H-C, Jin F-F (2021) Simulations of ENSO phase-locking in CMIP5 and CMIP6. J Clim 34(12):5135–5149. https://doi.org/10.1175/jcli-d-20-0874.1

Cole-Dai J (2010) Volcanoes and climate. WIREs Climate Change 1(6):824–839. https://doi.org/10.1002/wcc.76

Dentener F, Stevenson D, Cofala J, Mechler R, Amann M, Bergamaschi P, Raes F, Derwent R (2005) The impact of air pollutant and methane emission controls on tropospheric ozone and radiative forcing: CTM calculations for the period 1990-2030. Atmos Chem Phys 5(7):1731–1755. https://doi.org/10.5194/acp-5-1731-2005

Eyring V, Bony S, Meehl GA, Senior CA, Stevens B, Stouffer RJ, Taylor KE (2016) Overview of the coupled model intercomparison project phase 6 (CMIP6) experimental design and organization. Geosci Model Dev 9(5):1937–1958. https://doi.org/10.5194/gmd-9-1937-2016

Flanner MG, Zender CS, Hess PG, Mahowald NM, Painter TH, Ramanathan V, Rasch PJ (2009) Springtime warming and reduced snow cover from carbonaceous particles. Atmos Chem Phys 9(7):2481–2497. https://doi.org/10.5194/acp-9-2481-2009

Garrett KA, Nita M, De Wolf ED, Esker PD, Gomez-Montano L, Sparks AH (2016) Chapter 21 – plant pathogens as indicators of climate change. In: Letcher TM (ed) Climate change, 2nd edn. Elsevier, Boston, pp 325–338. https://doi.org/10.1016/B978-0-444-63524-2.00021-X

Goode PR, Pallé E, Shoumko A, Shoumko S, Montañes-Rodriguez P, Koonin SE (2021) Earth's Albedo 1998–2017 as measured from earthshine. Geophysical Research Letters 48(17):e2021GL094888. https://doi.org/10.1029/2021GL094888

Habibullah MS, Din BH, Tan S-H, Zahid H (2022) Impact of climate change on biodiversity loss: global evidence. Environ Sci Pollut Res 29(1):1073–1086. https://doi.org/10.1007/s11356-021-15702-8

Harrison PA, Holman IP, Berry PM (2015) Assessing cross-sectoral climate change impacts, vulnerability and adaptation: an introduction to the CLIMSAVE project. Clim Chang 128(3):153–167. https://doi.org/10.1007/s10584-015-1324-3

Hartmann DL (2016) Chapter 11 – global climate models. In: Hartmann DL (ed) Global physical climatology, 2nd edn. Elsevier, Boston, pp 325–360. https://doi.org/10.1016/B978-0-12-328531-7.00011-6

Hatfield JL, Prueger JH (2015) Temperature extremes: effect on plant growth and development. Weather and Climate Extremes 10:4–10. https://doi.org/10.1016/j.wace.2015.08.001

Hatfield JL, Boote KJ, Kimball BA, Ziska LH, Izaurralde RC, Ort D, Thomson AM, Wolfe D (2011) Climate impacts on agriculture: implications for crop production. Agron J 103(2): 351–370. https://doi.org/10.2134/agronj2010.0303

Hatfield JL, Antle J, Garrett KA, Izaurralde RC, Mader T, Marshall E, Nearing M, Philip Robertson G, Ziska L (2020) Indicators of climate change in agricultural systems. Clim Chang 163(4):1719–1732. https://doi.org/10.1007/s10584-018-2222-2

Hegglin MI, Plummer DA, Shepherd TG, Scinocca JF, Anderson J, Froidevaux L, Funke B, Hurst D, Rozanov A, Urban J, von Clarmann T, Walker KA, Wang HJ, Tegtmeier S, Weigel K (2014) Vertical structure of stratospheric water vapour trends derived from merged satellite data. Nat Geosci 7(10):768–776. https://doi.org/10.1038/ngeo2236

Hidy GM (2003) Aerosols. In: Meyers RA (ed) Encyclopedia of physical science and technology, 3rd edn. Academic Press, New York, pp 273–299. https://doi.org/10.1016/B0-12-227410-5/00014-4

Hirsch AL, Ridder NN, Perkins-Kirkpatrick SE, Ukkola A (2021) CMIP6 MultiModel Evaluation of Present-Day Heatwave Attributes. Geophysical Research Letters 48(22):e2021GL095161. https://doi.org/10.1029/2021GL095161

Hulme M, Mitchell J, Ingram W, Lowe J, Johns T, New M, Viner D (1999) Climate change scenarios for global impacts studies. Glob Environ Chang 9:S3–S19. https://doi.org/10.1016/S0959-3780(99)00015-1

IPCC (2013) In: Stocker TF, Qin D, Plattner G-K, Tignor M, Allen SK, Boschung J, Nauels A, Xia Y, Bex V, Midgley PM (eds) Climate change 2013: the physical science basis. Contribution of working group I to the fifth assessment report of the intergovernmental panel on climate change. Cambridge University Press, Cambridge/New York

IPCC (2014) In: Field CB, Barros VR, Dokken DJ, Mach KJ, Mastrandrea MD, Bilir TE, Chatterjee M, Ebi KL, Estrada YO, Genova RC, Girma B, Kissel ES, Levy AN, MacCracken S, Mastrandrea PR, White LL (eds) Climate change 2014: impacts, adaptation, and vulnerability. Part A: global and sectoral aspects. Contribution of working group II to the fifth assessment report of the intergovernmental panel on climate change. Cambridge University Press, Cambridge/New York

Jimenez-Montenegro L, Lopez-Fernandez M, Gimenez E (2021) Worldwide research on the ozone influence in plants. Agronomy 11(8):1504

Jing Y, Li Y, Xu Y (2022) An assessment of the North Atlantic (25–75°N) air-sea CO2 flux in 12 CMIP6 models. Deep-Sea Res I Oceanogr Res Pap 180:103682. https://doi.org/10.1016/j.dsr.2021.103682

Kamal ASMM, Hossain F, Shahid S (2021) Spatiotemporal changes in rainfall and droughts of Bangladesh for 1.5 and 2 °C temperature rise scenarios of CMIP6 models. Theor Appl Climatol 146(1):527–542. https://doi.org/10.1007/s00704-021-03735-5

Kamworapan S, Bich Thao PT, Gheewala SH, Pimonsree S, Prueksakorn K (2021) Evaluation of CMIP6 GCMs for simulations of temperature over Thailand and nearby areas in the early 21st century. Heliyon 7(11):e08263. https://doi.org/10.1016/j.heliyon.2021.e08263

Kebede AS, Nicholls RJ, Allan A, Arto I, Cazcarro I, Fernandes JA, Hill CT, Hutton CW, Kay S, Lázár AN, Macadam I, Palmer M, Suckall N, Tompkins EL, Vincent K, Whitehead PW (2018) Applying the global RCP–SSP–SPA scenario framework at sub-national scale: a multi-scale and participatory scenario approach. Sci Total Environ 635:659–672. https://doi.org/10.1016/j.scitotenv.2018.03.368

Kramer RJ, He H, Soden BJ, Oreopoulos L, Myhre G, Forster PM, Smith CJ (2021) Observational evidence of increasing global radiative forcing. Geophysical Research Letters 48(7): e2020GL091585. https://doi.org/10.1029/2020GL091585

Kriegler E, Edmonds J, Hallegatte S, Ebi KL, Kram T, Riahi K, Winkler H, van Vuuren DP (2014) A new scenario framework for climate change research: the concept of shared climate policy assumptions. Clim Chang 122(3):401–414. https://doi.org/10.1007/s10584-013-0971-5

Kumar M, Ojha N, Singh N (2022) Chapter 4 – atmospheric aerosols from open burning in South and Southeast Asia. In: Singh RP (ed) Asian atmospheric pollution. Elsevier, pp 75–96. https://doi.org/10.1016/B978-0-12-816693-2.00001-9

Le Treut H (2007) Historical overview of climate change. Climate Change 2007: The Physical Science Basis Contribution of Working Group I to the Fourth Assessment Report of the Intergovernmental Panel on Climate Change

Lean JL (2010) Cycles and trends in solar irradiance and climate. WIREs Climate Change 1(1):111–122. https://doi.org/10.1002/wcc.18

Lee J, Planton YY, Gleckler PJ, Sperber KR, Guilyardi E, Wittenberg AT, McPhaden MJ, Pallotta G (2021) Robust evaluation of ENSO in climate models: how many ensemble members are needed? Geophysical Research Letters 48(20):e2021GL095041. https://doi.org/10.1029/2021GL095041

Li C, Gu X, Wu Z, Qin T, Guo L, Wang T, Zhang L, Jiang G (2021) Assessing the effects of elevated ozone on physiology, growth, yield and quality of soybean in the past 40 years: a meta-analysis. Ecotoxicol Environ Saf 208:111644. https://doi.org/10.1016/j.ecoenv.2020.111644

Liu S, Proudman J, Mitloehner FM (2021) Rethinking methane from animal agriculture. CABI Agriculture and Bioscience 2(1):22. https://doi.org/10.1186/s43170-021-00041-y

Lupo A, Kininmonth W, Armstrong J, Green K (2013) Global climate models and their limitations. Climate change reconsidered II: Physical science 9:148

Mashwani Z-u-R (2020) Environment, climate change and biodiversity. In: Fahad S, Hasanuzzaman M, Alam M et al (eds) Environment, climate, plant and vegetation growth. Springer International Publishing, Cham, pp 473–501. https://doi.org/10.1007/978-3-030-49732-3_19

Matthews T (2018) Humid heat and climate change. Progress in Physical Geography: Earth and Environment 42(3):391–405. https://doi.org/10.1177/0309133318776490

Matthews R, Wassmann R (2003) Modelling the impacts of climate change and methane emission reductions on rice production: a review. Eur J Agron 19(4):573–598. https://doi.org/10.1016/S1161-0301(03)00005-4

McAdam EL, Brodribb TJ, McAdam SAM (2017) Does ozone increase ABA levels by non-enzymatic synthesis causing stomata to close? Plant. Cell & Environment 40(5):741–747. https://doi.org/10.1111/pce.12893

Meehl GA, Taylor KE, Delworth T, Stouffer RJ, Latif M, McAvaney B, Mitchell JFB (2007) The WCRP CMIP3 multimodel dataset: a new era in climate change research. Bull Amer Meteor Soc 88:1383–1394. https://doi.org/10.1175/bams-88-9-1383

Mondal SK, Huang J, Wang Y, Su B, Zhai J, Tao H, Wang G, Fischer T, Wen S, Jiang T (2021) Doubling of the population exposed to drought over South Asia: CMIP6 multi-model-based analysis. Sci Total Environ 771:145186. https://doi.org/10.1016/j.scitotenv.2021.145186

Nashwan MS, Shahid S (2022) Future precipitation changes in Egypt under the 1.5 and 2.0 °C global warming goals using CMIP6 multimodel ensemble. Atmos Res 265:105908. https://doi.org/10.1016/j.atmosres.2021.105908

O'Neill BC, Kriegler E, Riahi K, Ebi KL, Hallegatte S, Carter TR, Mathur R, van Vuuren DP (2014) A new scenario framework for climate change research: the concept of shared socio-economic pathways. Clim Chang 122(3):387–400. https://doi.org/10.1007/s10584-013-0905-2

Pielke RA (2005) Land use and climate change. Science 310(5754):1625–1626. https://doi.org/10.1126/science.1120529

Pörtner H-O, Roberts DC, Masson-Delmotte V, Zhai P, Tignor M, Poloczanska E, Weyer N (2019) The ocean and cryosphere in a changing climate. IPCC Special Report on the Ocean and Cryosphere in a Changing Climate

Saunois M, Jackson R, Bousquet P, Poulter B, Canadell J (2016) The growing role of methane in anthropogenic climate change. Environ Res Lett 11(12):120207

Shindell DT (2001) Climate and ozone response to increased stratospheric water vapor. Geophys Res Lett 28(8):1551–1554. https://doi.org/10.1029/1999GL011197

Skiba U, Rees B (2014) Nitrous oxide, climate change and agriculture. CAB Rev 9(010):1–7

Sobie SR, Zwiers FW, Curry CL (2021) Climate model projections for Canada: a comparison of CMIP5 and CMIP6. Atmosphere-Ocean 59(4–5):269–284. https://doi.org/10.1080/07055900.2021.2011103

Solomon S (2007) Climate change 2007-the physical science basis: working group I contribution to the fourth assessment report of the IPCC, vol 4. Cambridge University Press

Solomon S, Rosenlof KH, Portmann RW, Daniel JS, Davis SM, Sanford TJ, Plattner G-K (2010) Contributions of stratospheric water vapor to decadal changes in the rate of global warming. Science 327(5970):1219–1223. https://doi.org/10.1126/science.1182488

Song F, Zhang GJ, Ramanathan V, Leung LR (2022) Trends in surface equivalent potential temperature: a more comprehensive metric for global warming and weather extremes. Proc Natl Acad Sci 119(6):e2117832119. https://doi.org/10.1073/pnas.2117832119

Stouffer RJ, Eyring V, Meehl GA, Bony S, Senior C, Stevens B, Taylor K (2017) CMIP5 scientific gaps and recommendations for CMIP6. Bull Am Meteorol Soc 98(1):95–105

Supharatid S, Nafung J (2021) Projected drought conditions by CMIP6 multimodel ensemble over Southeast Asia. Journal of Water and Climate Change 12(7):3330–3354. https://doi.org/10.2166/wcc.2021.308

Tabari H (2020) Climate change impact on flood and extreme precipitation increases with water availability. Sci Rep 10(1):13768. https://doi.org/10.1038/s41598-020-70816-2

Thirumalai K, DiNezio PN, Okumura Y, Deser C (2017) Extreme temperatures in Southeast Asia caused by El Niño and worsened by global warming. Nat Commun 8(1):15531. https://doi.org/10.1038/ncomms15531

Tollefson J (2018) The sun dimmers. Nature 563(7733):613–615

Vainonen UP, Kangasjärvi J (2015) Plant signalling in acute ozone exposure. Plant Cell Environ 38(2):240–252. https://doi.org/10.1111/pce.12273

Vallero DA (2019) Chapter 8 – Air pollution biogeochemistry. In: Vallero DA (ed) Air pollution calculations. Elsevier, pp 175–206. https://doi.org/10.1016/B978-0-12-814934-8.00008-9

van Vuuren DP, Edmonds J, Kainuma M, Riahi K, Thomson A, Hibbard K, Hurtt GC, Kram T, Krey V, Lamarque J-F, Masui T, Meinshausen M, Nakicenovic N, Smith SJ, Rose SK (2011) The representative concentration pathways: an overview. Clim Chang 109(1):5. https://doi.org/10.1007/s10584-011-0148-z

Vose RS, Karl TR, Easterling DR, Williams CN, Menne MJ (2004) Impact of land-use change on climate. Nature 427(6971):213–214. https://doi.org/10.1038/427213b

Wang B, Gray JM, Waters CM, Rajin Anwar M, Orgill SE, Cowie AL, Feng P, Li Liu D (2022a) Modelling and mapping soil organic carbon stocks under future climate change in South-Eastern Australia. Geoderma 405:115442. https://doi.org/10.1016/j.geoderma.2021.115442

Wang Z, Wang C, Yang S, Lei Y, Che H, Zhang X, Wang Q (2022b) Evaluation of surface solar radiation trends over China since the 1960s in the CMIP6 models and potential impact of aerosol emissions. Atmos Res 268:105991. https://doi.org/10.1016/j.atmosres.2021.105991

Wild M (2012) Solar radiation surface solar radiation versus climate change solar radiation versus climate change. In: Meyers RA (ed) Encyclopedia of sustainability science and technology. Springer, New York, pp 9731–9740. https://doi.org/10.1007/978-1-4419-0851-3_448

Yadav P, Usha K, Singh B (2022) Chapter 10 – air pollution mitigation and global dimming: a challenge to agriculture under changing climate. In: Shanker AK, Shanker C, Anand A, Maheswari M (eds) Climate change and crop stress. Academic Press, pp 271–298. https://doi.org/10.1016/B978-0-12-816091-6.00015-8

Zeng J, Li J, Lu X, Wei Z, Shangguan W, Zhang S, Dai Y, Zhang S (2021) Assessment of global meteorological, hydrological and agricultural drought under future warming based on CMIP6. Atmospheric and Oceanic Science Letters:100143. https://doi.org/10.1016/j.aosl.2021.100143

Ziska LH (2020) Climate change and the herbicide paradigm: visiting the future. Agronomy 10(12):1953

Chapter 2
Climate Change, Agricultural Productivity, and Food Security

Mukhtar Ahmed, Muhammad Asim, Shakeel Ahmad, and Muhammad Aslam

Abstract Food security and agricultural-based livelihoods of smallholder farmers are under threat due to climate change and political conflicts. However, quality firm data is needed to assess the damages on food security to suggest appropriate adaptive measures. This chapter gives an overview about the climate change, agricultural productivity, and food security. It firstly provides detailed information about agricultural sector contributions to the climate change with information about water and agriculture footprint. Similarly, the reasons for the declined agricultural productivity and loss of biodiversity were discussed with possible solutions. Results depicted that without adaptations, genetic improvement, and CO_2 fertilization, every 1 °C rise in temperature could reduce yields of wheat (6.0%), rice (3.2%), maize (7.4%), and soybean (3.1%). Afterward, linkage with sustainable agriculture and food security was elaborated. Furthermore, detail about global food security was presented followed by the scenario of food security in Pakistan. The impact of climate change on food security was established through different climatic drivers, e.g., ENSO (El Niño–Southern Oscillation) and SOI (Southern Oscillation Index). These drivers are responsible for the climatic extreme events; hence, earlier prediction of these drivers could help to design appropriate adoptive measures for the agriculture sector, and they could be considered as early warning tool for the risk managements. Afterward, simulation analysis between climate change and rainfed wheat yield was presented, which confirms that climate change is affecting crop production and food security. Hence, adaptive measures, such as improved impact assessments

M. Ahmed (✉)
Department of Agronomy, PMAS Arid Agriculture University, Rawalpindi, Pakistan
e-mail: ahmadmukhtar@uaar.edu.pk

M. Asim
Plant Sciences Division, Pakistan Agricultural Research Council, Islamabad, Pakistan

S. Ahmad
Department of Agronomy, Bahauddin Zakariya University, Multan, Pakistan

M. Aslam
Ministry of National Food Security and Research, Islamabad, Pakistan

© The Author(s), under exclusive license to Springer Nature Switzerland AG 2022
M. Ahmed (ed.), *Global Agricultural Production: Resilience to Climate Change*,
https://doi.org/10.1007/978-3-031-14973-3_2

through modeling, efficient production technologies, changes in sowing windows, precision and smart farming, modernization of water supply and irrigation systems, conservation tillage, inputs and management adjustments, and improved short- and long-term climate prediction, cluster-based agriculture transformation with connections with policy makers could be good adaptation options to ensure food security.

Keywords Food security · Agricultural productivity · Climatic drivers · Adaptation options

2.1 Introduction

Climate change and variability are major causes of declined agricultural productivity across the globe. Agriculture in future will face multiple challenges that include the production of more food and fiber for billions of populations and higher production of feedstocks for bioenergy production. Generally, we think that the major threats to the environment are greenhouse gases (GHGs) coming from different anthropogenic activities, not food needed for our breakfast, lunch, and dinner. But the truth is food will be the biggest dangers to the planet Earth. Agriculture is contributing a lot to GHG emissions as compared to buses, cars, trucks, trains, and airplanes (Fig. 2.1). Methane (CH_4) mainly comes from cattle and rice farms, while oxides of nitrogen are coming from fertilized fields. Higher emissions of carbon dioxide (CO_2) are due to cutting of rain forest to clear land that can be further used to raise animal and grow crops (Crippa et al. 2021; Poore and Nemecek 2018; Lynch et al. 2021). Similarly, farming is using a lot of water, and it pollutes nearby water bodies and underground water via runoff from manure and fertilizers. Water footprint of agriculture is increasing day by day, and it is using 70% of existing freshwater as shown in Fig. 2.2. Water footprint is further divided into blue (consumption of ground and surface water), green (use of rainwater), and gray (water use in the dilution of pollutants). In future, climate change will result to the further increase in water footprint from north to south as irrigation demands will rise from 6% to 16% (Elbeltagi et al. 2020). Decrease in green water footprint was estimated due to change in precipitation (Yeşilköy and Şaylan 2021). Among crops, rice is the crop, which have a higher water footprint, and simulated outcome of study reported that blue water footprint in rice will increase as compared to green water footprint (Zheng et al. 2020). Gray and green water footprint in Amazon for soybean have been increased by 268% and 304%, respectively, in 2050, if current soybean expansion and intensification will remained as such (Miguel Ayala et al. 2016). Thus, in future, efficient water resource management (e.g., reduction of evapotranspiration and crop water use, and optimal fertilizer application) is necessary to ensure food security under changing climate.

Agriculture is also the main cause of accelerated loss of biodiversity (Dudley and Alexander 2017). In future, agriculture will pose more threat to the environment, as we must feed two billion more mouth (>9 billion) to feed by mid-century (Fig. 2.3). The countries with the highest population will need more meat, eggs, and dairy,

2 Climate Change, Agricultural Productivity, and Food Security   33

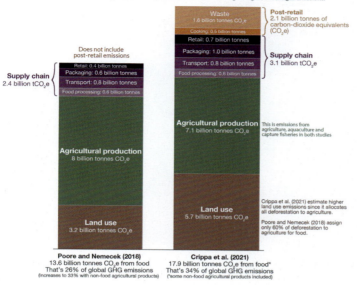

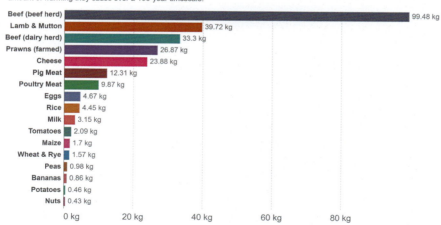

Fig. 2.1 Global greenhouse gas emissions from food system

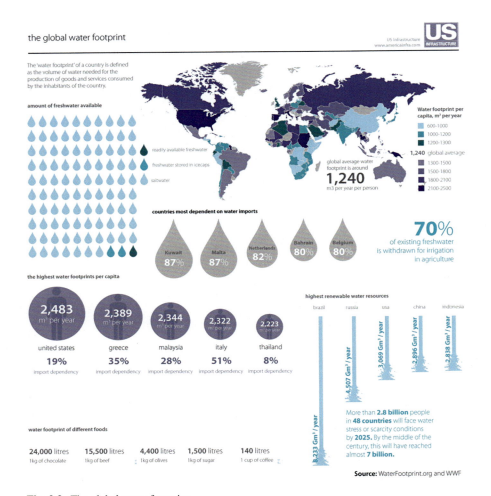

Fig. 2.2 The global water footprint

which will boost pressure to grow more crops like corn and soybean to feed animals. Hence, with this population growth and diet habits, we must double the amounts of crops production by mid-century. Furthermore, debates among conventional agriculture/global commerce and local food systems/organic farms to address the global food challenge have been polarized. Both are right in their point of views, as conventional agriculture talks more about higher food production through the applications of modern tools while organic farming produces quality food with higher benefits to the small-scale farmers and ecosystems. Jonathan Foley asked a question from team of experts, and it has been published in National Geographic magazine. The question was how world can double food availability by minimizing the environmental harm (https://www.nationalgeographic.com/foodfeatures/

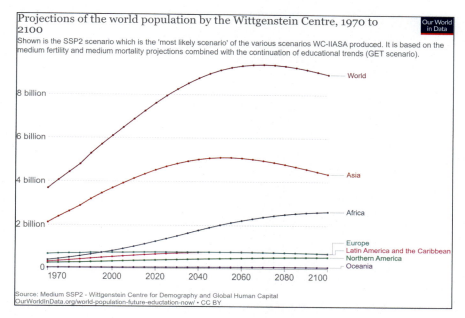

Fig. 2.3 Trend of world population

feeding-9-billion/). Jonathan Foley and team of scientist proposed a five-step mechanism to solve the world's food dilemma, which they got after analyzing a huge amount of data on agriculture and environment. It includes the following: (i) Freeze agriculture footprint (stop deforestation for crop production). (ii) Grow more on farms we have got. (iii) Use resources more efficiently. (iv) Shift diets. (v) And reduce waste. Agriculture footprint has caused the loss of whole ecosystems across the globe, e.g., prairies of North America and the Atlantic Forest of Brazil and tropical forests (Fig. 2.4) (Litskas et al. 2020). Converting tropical forest to agriculture was one of the most damaging acts to the environment by human beings, although it does not contribute a lot to global food security (Fig. 2.5). Reducing yield gaps and increasing yield on less productive areas could bring global food security and that needs to be opted by all researchers across the globe. Yield gap could be minimized by identifying yield-limiting factors, designing crop ideotypes, opting high-tech precision farming systems, as well as approaches from organic farming (Rong et al. 2021; Senapati and Semenov 2019). Similarly, using resources more efficiently through commercial and organic farming can improve soil health, conserve water, and build up nutrients. Shift in diets from livestock to crops could help to feed 9 billion population by 2050 as well as it can minimize agriculture footprint. Waste minimization is another very good option suggested by Jonathan Foley to ensure food security, as 50% of total food weights and 25% of global food calories have been lost before it should be consumed. These proposed five steps could help to double the world's food supply, cut the environmental impact of global agriculture, and ensure food security. Furthermore, the next sections in this chapter

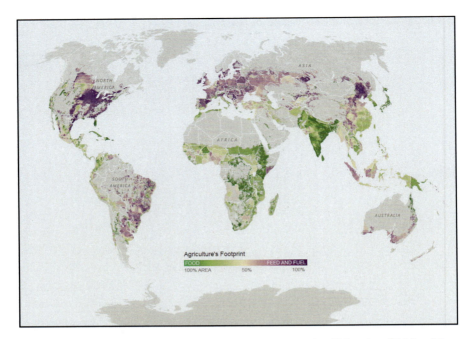

Fig. 2.4 Global agriculture footprint. (Source: Roger LeB. Hooke, University of Maine. Maps, source: Global Landscapes Initiative, Institute on the Environment, University of Minnesota)

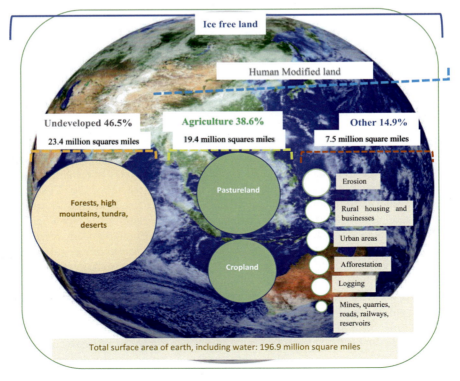

Fig. 2.5 Ratio of human modified land with total surface area of Earth

will be about agricultural productivity, food security, and its linkage with climate change.

2.2 Agricultural Productivity

Output per unit of inputs is called productivity. It is one of closely watched economic performance indicator as it contributes to a healthy economy. Agriculture is an important economic sector for most of the countries, but its output growth as compared to other sectors of economy is not same. This is because of differential response to the inputs used in agriculture sector and their interactions with climatic variables. Similarly, productivity in agriculture is also linked with investments in research and development, extension, education, and infrastructure. Dharmasiri (2012) defined agricultural productivity (AP) as the output per unit of input, and it has two measures: (i) partial measure of productivity (output per unit of a single input) and (ii) total measure of productivity (output in response to all inputs). Partial measure of productivity is generally easy to use because of the availability of data. Agricultural productivity is a good indicator to see the gap in output, e.g., yield gap. The global yield of major crops has been presented in Fig. 2.6, which shows a big gap in the crop yield among countries due to a number of different reasons. It includes land degradation (soil fertility, soil erosion, soil salinity, and waterlogging), climatic extremes (extreme temperature, drought, Flood), poor irrigation water management, agronomic, technological, socioeconomic, and institutional constraints. In Pakistan, the major factors, which contribute a lot to AP, include fertilizer consumption, seed, and credit distribution as concluded by Rehman et al. (2019). Increase in AP is a good option to solve the issue of food crisis, but it has been stalled. The growth rate of major grain crops is about 1% per year, which is lower than the population growth. Since increase in cultivated area is not a possibility to fulfill the future needs of growing population; thus, the only option is increase in AP. However, there are no silver bullet solutions, but AP could be increased by opting options like (i) water availability, (ii) education for farmers, (iii) credit availability, (iv) land reforms, (v) transport and marketing, (vi) policies, (vii) markets and agribusiness, and (viii) outreach programs to disseminate new research findings. Furthermore, new approaches to facilitate small-scale farmers in developing countries are instruments to guarantee food security. AP and yield gaps for the major crops in Pakistan have been presented in Table 2.1.

2.3 Food Security

Food security exists when "all people, at all times, have physical and economic access to sufficient, safe, and nutritious food that meets their dietary needs and food preferences for an active and healthy life" (Shaw 2007). This definition gives rise to the four

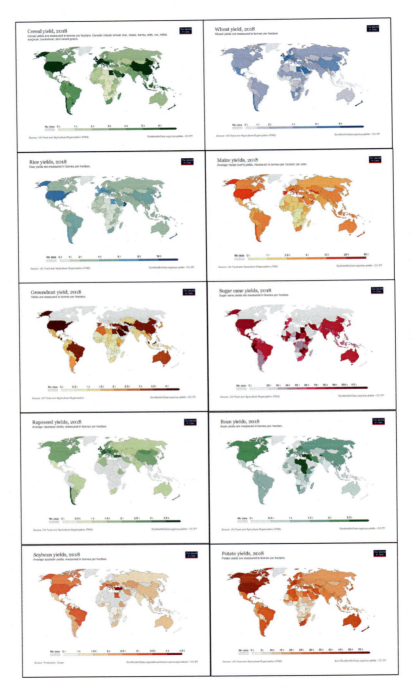

Fig. 2.6 Yield of major crops across the world

2 Climate Change, Agricultural Productivity, and Food Security

Table 2.1 Yield gap for major crops in Pakistan

Crops	World average (t ha^{-1}) (Source: FAOSTAT)	Pakistan average (t ha^{-1}) (Source: Pakistan Economic Survey, Ministry of Finance)	Yield gap
Wheat	8	2.84	5.16
Rice	6.5	2.51	3.99
Maize	10	4.75	5.25
Cotton	3	0.68	2.32
Sugarcane	112	64	48

dimensions of food security: availability of food, accessibility (economically and physically), utilization (the way it is used and assimilated by the human body), and stability of these three dimensions. According to the United Nations, food security can be defined as physical, social, and economic access to food by all people at all times to sufficient, safe, and nutritious food to meet their dietary needs according to their food preferences for an active and healthy life. Under current international scenario, food security is becoming a formidable challenge. In a developed world, most attention is given to biofuel production, and it is using huge quantities of grain, e.g., 50 million tons of maize is used to produce biofuel products (Veljković et al. 2018; Schwietzke et al. 2009). Similarly, increased used of corn grain to produce ethanol is altering the landscape and ecosystem services (Landis et al. 2008). Food security is also on stake due to climate change, increased prices of food grain, and livestock product which has been further aggravated by continuous rise in fuel prices. The cascading effects of climate change on food security have been shown in Fig. 2.7. The earlier world was striving hard to meet the Millennium Development Goals (MDGs) to reduce hunger and poverty to half by 2015 but unable to achieve the UN target. There were eight MDGs with less attention to environmental sustainability (Lomazzi et al. 2014). In Rio +20 conference, MDGs were replaced with the Sustainable Development Goals (SDGs) (Fig. 2.8) with the objectives to end poverty and protect the planet with peace and prosperity for all till 2030 (Fukuda-Parr 2016). Zero hunger (SDG2) was the top priority of the SDGs to ensure food security by 2030. SDG2 was further divided into SDG2.1 (end hunger and access to food), SDG2.2 (end malnutrition), and SDG2.3 (doubling of agricultural productivity and income of small-scale farmers) (UN 2018). Laborde et al. (2016) reported 11 billion USD per year will be required to end hunger by 2030, while Schmidhuber et al. (2011) and the FAO and UNICEF (2014) estimated 50.2 billion USD by 2025. Different interventions were recommended by previous studies to uplift agriculture and small-scale farmers to achieve SDG2 and ensure food security (Gil et al. 2019). These include investment in rural infrastructure and value chains, easy access to market, credit transfer programs, farm insurance, good governance, gender equality, and connection with research, development, and extension services (Ton et al. 2013; Atukunda et al. 2021). Furthermore, Bizikova et al. (2020) identified five different types of interventions (three single and two multiples) that can have significant impacts on food security. Single intervention was input subsidy, extension, and value chains, while multiple interventions include input subsidy-food voucher and input subsidy-extension.

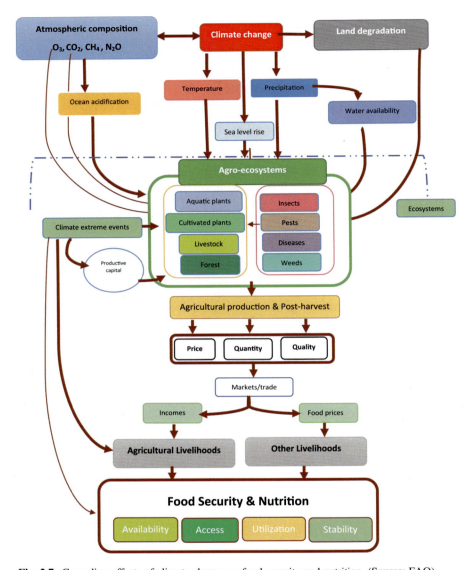

Fig. 2.7 Cascading effects of climate change on food security and nutrition. (Source: FAO)

2.3.1 Sustainable Agriculture and Food Security

Agriculture can be the cause and solution for the climate change, but sustainable agriculture (SA) has the potential to mitigate climate change and ensure food security. SA includes ecological and sustainable intensification, organic farming, integrated farming, climate smart and precision agriculture, vertical farming, and

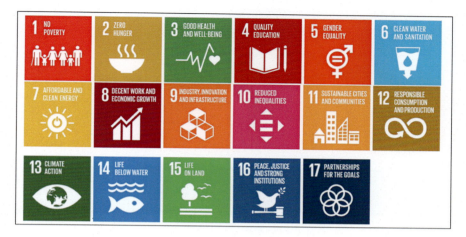

Fig. 2.8 The 17 Sustainable Development Goals (SDGs). (Source: UNDP)

permaculture. Arora (2018) suggested integration of innovative biotechnology and bioengineering techniques with traditional biological methods to achieve goals of food security and sustainability. Similarly, mycorrhizal fungi and beneficial microbes could help to enhance food production by countering biotic and abiotic stresses. They also play vital roles in efficient utilization of resources, mineral solubilization, production of growth regulators, nitrogen fixation, recycling of organic matter, and restoration of degraded soil (Salwan and Sharma 2022). Spiertz (2009) reviewed about nitrogen and SA and concluded that for SA and food security, nitrogen supply should be matched with N demand in spatiotemporal scale, not only for single crops but also for all crops in rotation to have higher agronomic nitrogen use efficiency. Similarly, the role of biofertilizers in SA was discussed by Rehman et al. (2022), while Hussain et al. (2022) reported biochar a critical input and game changer for SA. Furthermore, nuclear techniques as proposed by the IAEA (International Atomic Energy Agency) and FAO could help to improve the food production from farm to fork and bring sustainability in agriculture.

2.3.2 Global Food Security

The world is at a critical juncture as reported in the FAO report of the State of Food Security and Nutrition in the World 2021 (FAO 2021). At present, the world is in chaos as it is committed earlier to end hunger, food insecurity, and malnutrition by 2030. This is mainly because of climate variability and extreme climate events, COVID-19 pandemic, and economic slowdown. Hence, the pathway toward SDG2 became steeper. Hunger level in the world is on rise, and it has been climbing to 9.9% in 2020 as around 720–811 million people faced hunger in 2020 (Fig. 2.9). Bold actions are needed to address the major drivers of food insecurity and

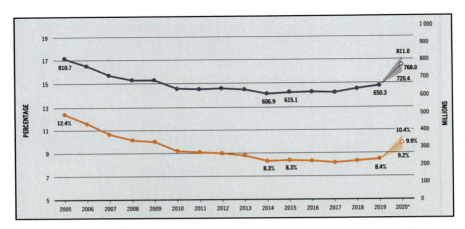

Fig. 2.9 The prevalence and number of undernourished people in the world. (Source: FAO 2021)

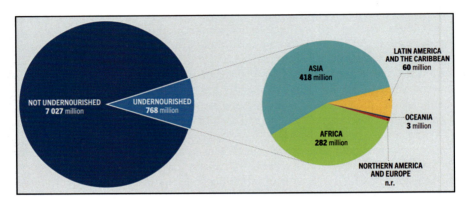

Fig. 2.10 Hunger prevalence among continents. (Source: FAO 2021)

malnutrition. More than half of the world population who are affected due to hunger lives in Asia as shown in Fig. 2.10. More than 30% of the world population has been affected due to moderate or severe food insecurity since the past 6 years (Fig. 2.11) and healthy diets are out of reach for billions of people. The COVID-19 pandemic has shown severe impact on the world economy (Afesorgbor et al. 2022). To end hunger and malnutrition, the way forward is transformation in the food system with greater resilience to major drivers, e.g., climate variability and extremes, conflicts, and economic slowdown. Six pathways were suggested for food system transformation to ensure food security and nutritive food for all. It includes (i) promotion of integrated policies (Humanitarian-Development-Peacekeeping) in affected areas, (ii) augmenting climate resilience across food systems, (iii) increasing resilience of most affected to economic hardship, (iv) lowering the cost of nutrition foods by improving food supply chains, (v) reducing poverty and inequalities, and

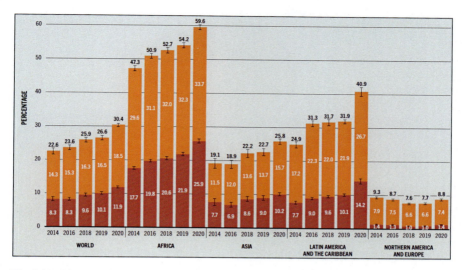

Fig. 2.11 Global food insecurity (moderate or severe) in the past 6 years. (Source: FAO 2021)

(vi) improving food environments and change in dietary habits to have more positive impacts to health and environment. Furthermore, van Dijk and Meijerink (2014) presented different drivers of food and nutrition security, which include climate change, population growth, income growth, food demand, dietary habits, and technical change. These drivers could be used to design integrated approach for the global food security (Fig. 2.12). However, these drivers may vary from country to country as elaborated in Fig. 2.13. High level of panel of experts (HLPE) on world food security have given new dimensions to ensure food security (HLPE 2019, 2020). Furthermore, relationship between different drivers, food systems, and food security have been presented in Fig. 2.14, which shows that these drivers have impacts on diet attributes (e.g., quantity, quality, diversity, safety, and adequacy) as well as on nutrition and health. The drivers, which have a major contribution to recent hunger and slowdown in progress, are given in dark blue boxes. Similarly, Fig. 2.14 elaborates circular feedback loops (e.g., increase in the consumption of unhealthy food due to economic crisis resulted toward higher emissions of GHGs) that can generate higher impacts with time. Hence, food environments have a negative relationship with food security and nutrition. Similarly, the recent COVID-19 pandemic has given a devastating blow to global food security and nutrition with multiple impacts on food systems (Fig. 2.15).

2.3.3 Food Security in Pakistan

Pakistan is committed to divert all possible efforts and resources for increasing food production and ensuring that people at large have access to food at affordable prices.

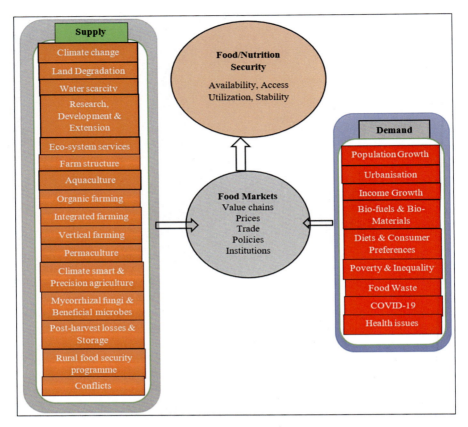

Fig. 2.12 Drivers of food/nutrition security across globe. (Modified from van Dijk and Meijerink 2014)

Pakistan agriculture sector contributes 19.2% to GDP with an employment share of 38.5%. Over 65–70% of Pakistan population depends upon agriculture sector for its livelihood. It is the engine of national economic growth and poverty reduction. However, the growth rate in this sector is on declining trend. This is mainly because of shrinkage of arable land, climate variability and climate change, water scarcity, and higher population shift from rural to urban areas. Government have implemented different agricultural policies to improve farm productivity through untapped productivity potential of crop and livestock subsectors. It includes introduction of agri-input regime and agriculture transformation plan. However, Pakistan is still a net food-importing country with high level of food insecurity that includes lack of food availability and high population growth. The other reason includes small land holdings (32% less than 1 hectare and 24% less than 2 hectare) that is not permitting to enhance farm productivity or incomes beyond a certain limit (Bashir et al. 2013; Abdullah et al. 2019). Data from different sources depicted that daily

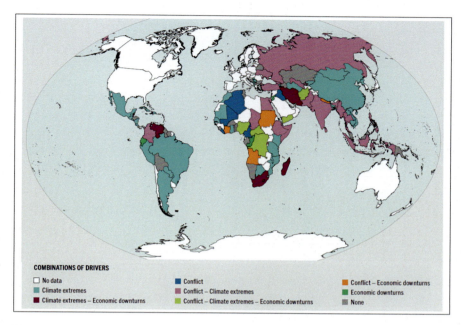

Fig. 2.13 Food security drivers across the globe

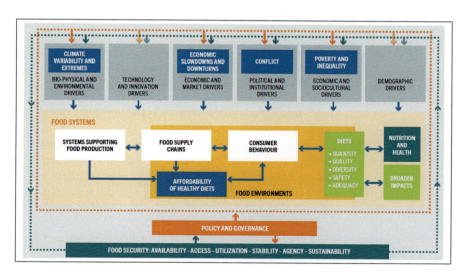

Fig. 2.14 Relationship between different drivers, food systems, and food security. (Source: FAO 2021)

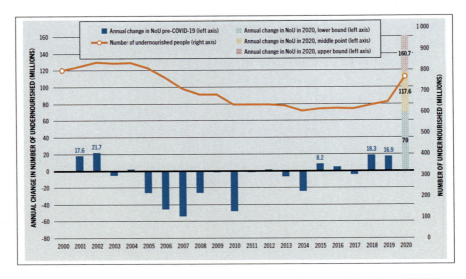

Fig. 2.15 Time series analysis of annual change in number of undernourished due to COVID

average availability of calories per person in Pakistan is lower by 10% and 26% relative to the average in developing and developed counties, respectively (Hameed et al. 2021). Pakistan has been trying to maintain the 2350 calories per person per day since the early 1990s from a level of 1754 calories per person per day in 1961. The average per capita availability of calories during 2015–2016 was 2473 kcal day^{-1}, which exceeds the minimum energy requirements (Shabnam et al. 2021). However, a higher rate of malnutrition was observed due to low nutritional intake (IFPRI 2016). In Pakistan, around half of the caloric needs are met through cereals only. Wheat and rice are the staple food crops, and shortfalls in production adversely affect both food security and national economy. Wheat production (2020–2021) was 27.3 million tons, which was 8.1% higher than the last year. However, still Pakistan has to import 3 million tons to build strategic reserves, a euphemistic indicator of local shortage. Factors which are responsible for the food insecurity in Pakistan are (i) small land holdings, (ii) technological constraints to achieve productivity potential in farming system and climate change perspective, (iii) land and soil health degradation, (iv) deteriorating irrigation and drainage system, (v) poorly regulated markets, (vi) lack of mechanization and skilled farm labor, and (vii) ineffective research-extension linkages. Per capita availability of food items in Pakistan from 2002 to 2007 have been shown in Table 2.2, while food security and related indicators for some years have also been given (Table 2.3), which shows that proper measures are needed to end hunger and malnutrition in Pakistan. Crop productivity scenario to ensure food security in Pakistan is presented in Table 2.4.

2 Climate Change, Agricultural Productivity, and Food Security

Table 2.2 Per capita availability of food items

Items	Unit	2002	2003	2004	2005	2006	2007
Wheat	Kg	114.7	112.0	116.3	115.8	123.2	127.0
Rice	Kg	13.9	17.2	16.8	17.6	10.0	16.6
Other grains	Kg	11.1	11.1	11.6	11.5	17.0	16.0
Pulses	Kg	7.02	5.8	8.00	6.8	7.9	7.2
Edible oils	Kg	11.5	11.9	11.5	11.7	12.9	13.1
Fruits and veg.	Kg	80.5	83.3	87.5	82.9	77.9	77.6
Sugar	Kg	30.3	30.8	30.5	30.7	34.8	32.2
Milk	Lit.	83.1	83.8	85.9	85.9	90.3	94.2
Meat	Kg	21.3	21.3	21.5	21.0	21.8	23.3
Eggs	Doz.	4.5	4.5	4.6	4.6	4.8	5.0

Table 2.3 Food security and related indicators

Indicators	1996	2001	2005	2008
Average per person dietary energy supply (Kcal)	2522	2706	2381	2529
Food production index	–	100	92	111
Cereal supply per person (all food grains) (Kg)	180	203	174	191
Animal protein supply per person (gram) per day	67.3	71.7	–	46.3
Value of gross investment in agriculture (mil US $)	51.5	45.1	22.8	33.3
Food price index (2000–2001 = 100)	82.9	100	111.7	169.5
Index of variability of food production (1999–2000 = 100)	–	91	95	111
Consumer price index	72.5	100	106.7	155.7

Table 2.4 Crop productivity scenario to ensure food security in Pakistan

Scenarios	Average (tons/hectare)				
	Wheat	Cotton	Rice	Maize	Sugarcane
Productivity at research stations	6.5	14.6	8.0	12.5	189.0
Productivity at progressive farmers	5.5	3.5	4.8	7.5	106.7
National average productivity	2.6	2.0	2.1	3.5	48.9
% gap between progressive farmer and national average	52.5	41.3	58.9	53.6	54.2
% gap between potential and national average	59.8	55.3	73.5	72.1	74.1

2.4 Climate Change and Food Security: Impacts

Food security is the topmost challenge of the twenty-first century, but it has been threatened by the climate change. However, ensuring food security is an important task to feed billions in future by sustaining stressed environmental resources (Lal 2005). Magadza (2000) reported more severe impacts of climate change on food security, water, and human health for African countries. Kang et al. (2009) reviewed that uncertainty in food production has been increased due to climate change. Climate change is increasing the intensity and frequency of extreme events across

Table 2.5 Crop productivity variation and climate change

Variation	Causes
Variation from field to field on the same farm under the same management	Soil and microenvironment
	Agro-management
Variation from farm to farm even on similar soil and area	Weather and climate variability
Variation from year to year on the same site, soil, and similar management	

the globe, which resulted to the disasters in livestock, crops, and food production and supply sectors (Hallegatte et al. 2007; Dastagir 2015). Climate change and variability resulted to the depletion in water resources and declined agricultural productivity (Fatima et al. 2022; Arunrat et al. 2022; Yeşilköy and Şaylan 2021). Similarly, it has been well-documented that global temperature at the end of the twenty-first century may increase by 1.4–5.8 °C, which will reduce freshwater and agricultural crop yield and ultimately leads toward the issue of food security (Misra 2014). Furthermore, variation in crop productivity due to climate change have been listed in Table 2.5. Climate change impacts are now visible in the form of growing deserts, more occurrence of floods, heat waves and droughts. These climate extremes cause reduction in crop yields, food shortages, and increase in food inflation. Hence, to protect different crops and production systems from the damaging effect of climate change, most of the recent studies are focused on the climate impacts and adaptation strategies (Naz et al. 2022; Ahmad et al. 2019; Hoogenboom et al. 2017; Li et al. 2015; Asseng et al. 2015; Araya et al. 2015; White et al. 2011). Crop growth models have been significantly used to study the impacts of climate change and furthermore in the designing of adaptation strategies (Tui et al. 2021; Kapur et al. 2019; Dubey and Sharma 2018; Hussain et al. 2018; Mohanty et al. 2012; Akponikpè et al. 2010; Pearson et al. 2008). Simulation models are good tools to study climate impacts and addressed them in a risk management context (both food security and climate change). Similarly, assessing both impacts and adaptations through modeling will help to increase our understanding of climate processes and food production. Thus, understanding the link between food requirements and climate variability is important to design appropriate future sustainable food production options.

2.4.1 Climate Factors Affecting Food Security

Different direct and indirect climate factors are affecting food security. Direct factor changes crop biodynamism, and it includes carbon dioxide (CO_2), temperature, rainfall, solar radiation, frost, fog, and smog. Elevated CO_2 has shown positive effect (fertilization effect) on crop production and water use efficiency but affected negatively the produce quality (Varga et al. 2015; Sulieman et al. 2015; Fitzgerald et al. 2016; O'Leary et al. 2015; Erbs et al. 2015; Manderscheid et al. 2015). The nutritional quality of produce is at stake under elevated CO_2, as in C3 plants higher CO_2 concentrations resulted to the production of more carbohydrates and less

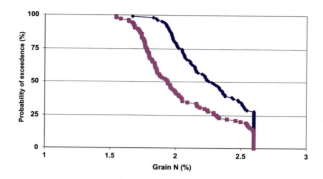

Fig. 2.16 Grain nitrogen in response to elevated CO_2

minerals (zinc and iron) (Ebi and Loladze 2019). Higher CO_2 is directly affecting crops' nutritional quality by decreasing protein and mineral concentration by 5–15% and B vitamins by 30% (Loladze 2014; Myers et al. 2014; Zhu et al. 2018). Reduction in grain nitrogen due to elevated CO_2 is shown in Fig. 2.16. Loladze (2002) reported declined essential element to carbon ratio, which could intensify the problem of micronutrient malnutrition in future. Furthermore, micronutrient deficiencies will cause higher disease burden than food insecurity. However, legume plants have shown more positive response to elevated CO_2 due to increased nitrogen fixation (Hikosaka et al. 2011). C4 crops, although get less benefits from elevated CO_2 as carbon uptake in these plants, is saturated at ambient CO_2 levels, so no carbon dilution occurs with no effect on protein and micronutrients levels (von Caemmerer and Furbank 2003). Hence, C4 crops have great potential to fulfill nutritional needs of human beings under changing climate as they have good adaptability to warm and dry climates. But to have full potential of C4 crops under future changing climate, complete understanding and linkage between mineral nutrition and C4 photosynthesis is needed (Jobe et al. 2020). Rise in temperature is another important limiting factor, which is affecting food security at global scale. Recent temperature anomalies generated by the NASA (the National Aeronautics and Space Administration) have clearly shown that global surface temperature have increased by +1 °C in almost every month (Fig. 2.17). The climate spiral (designed by climate scientist Ed Hawkins from NASA) has been widely distributed during Rio de Janeiro Olympics to show clearly how important it is to address the issue of climate change (https://svs.gsfc.nasa.gov/4975). Increased temperature is the major reason of reduced crop yield and poor quality, as higher temperature decreases water use efficiency, crop growth period, photosynthesis, and yield (Ahmad et al. 2019; Urban et al. 2018; Mäkinen et al. 2018; Lizaso et al. 2018; Prasad and Jagadish 2015). Zhao et al. (2017) investigated the impacts of temperature on yields of four crops, i.e., wheat, rice, maize, and soybean, using published work, where they have used different analytical techniques (e.g., field warming experiments, regression, and global grid-based and local point-based models). Results depicted that without adaptations, genetic improvement, and CO_2 fertilization, every 1 °C rise in temperature could reduce yields of wheat (6.0%), rice (3.2%), maize (7.4%), and soybean (3.1%). Iizumi et al. (2017) studied the responses of crop yield growth to

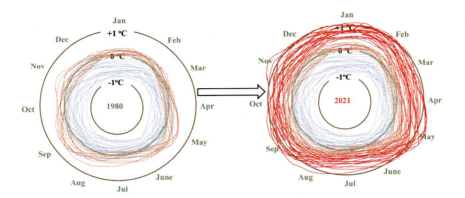

Fig. 2.17 Monthly global surface temperatures from 1980 to 2021. (Modified from NASA)

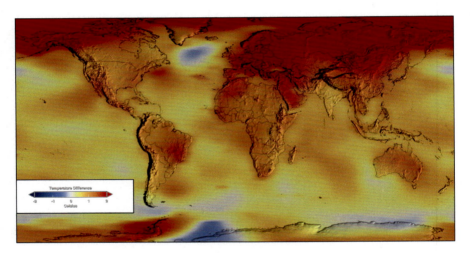

Fig. 2.18 Global temperature anomalies (°C) from 1880 to 2020 (higher than normal temperature = red and lower than normal temperature = blue and normal temperature = average over thirty years baseline period 1951–1980). (Source: NASA's Scientific Visualization Studio)

temperature and concluded that intensive mitigation is needed in low-income countries to improve food security and prevents damage to major crops. The map of global temperature changes for the year 2020 in comparison to baseline period (1951–1980) showed that across the globe there is significant increase in temperature (Fig. 2.18). The dramatic increase is more in far northern latitudes. CO_2 concentration, temperature, rainfall, and solar radiation changes will interactively effect crop productivity and ultimately food security. However, indirect factors of climate change which affect crop existence and food security include water resources, floods, soil degradation, drought spells, pest, and diseases.

2.4.2 Climate Change Extreme Events

Climate change is visible in the form of different extreme events happening across the globe in recent decades. Intensification of weather extremes is important facets of climate change (Jentsch et al. 2007). It includes extreme heat wave (>49.6 °C temperature in Canada on June 29), Hurricane Ida, European summer flood, and flooding in China, July 2021: Earth's warmest month in recorded history and melting of glaciers. These extreme events are causing disasters in vulnerable communities and ecosystems (Mal et al. 2017, 2018). Changes in global precipitation is one of the clear indicators because of global warming. Some parts of the world (mainly northern latitudes) are experiencing increased precipitation, whereas other regions will experience decreased precipitation (Fig. 2.19). Hence, understanding of climate extremes is important to design disaster risk reduction mechanism.

2.4.3 Understanding Climate Change Extreme Events to Ensure Food Security

Understating of climate change is important to ensure food security. Climate change has already threatened agriculture, food production, and food security. Hence, understanding of climate extreme is the first step to design adaptation strategies. Different climatic drivers could be used to understand the future climatic changes. ENSO (El Niño–Southern Oscillation) is the topmost driver which has been used to predict future climatic changes before time (Lee et al. 2021; Thirumalai et al. 2017; Tack and Ubilava 2015; Woli et al. 2015). ENSO changes the global atmospheric

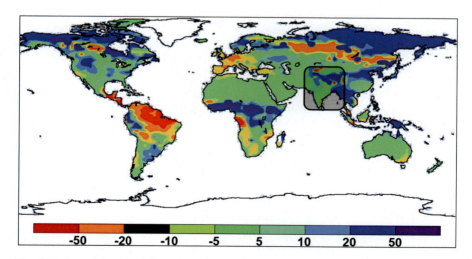

Fig. 2.19 Potential worldwide precipitation changes

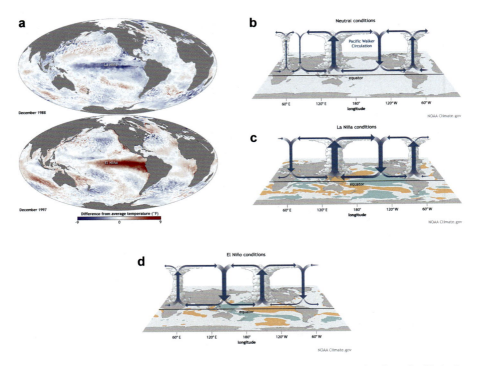

Fig. 2.20 Neutral, La Niña, and El Niño three phases of ENSO (El Niño–Southern Oscillation). (Source: NOAA)

circulation, which results to the change in precipitation and temperature across the globe. Prediction of ENSO arrival in advance is helpful to understand future weather and climate. ENSO has three states or phases, i.e., (i) El Niño (warming of ocean surface or above-average sea-surface temperatures (SST)), (ii) La Niña (cooling of ocean surface or below average SST), and (iii) neutral (neither El Niño or La Niña) (Fig. 2.20). Hence, process-based seasonal forecasting using ENSO could be the most practical way of designing risk management options for dealing with both climate variability and climate change (Davey et al. 2014; Singh et al. 2022). Similarly, prediction of regional heat waves over the South Asian region, particularly over Pakistan, could help to design adaptation options for agriculture sector (Rashid et al. 2022). Wangchen and Dorji (2022) examined the potential impact of agrometeorology initiative for climate change adaptation and food security in Bhutan. Study reported that food security challenges will be further aggravated due to the changing climate. Hence, adaptation is necessary to enhance food security. They suggested the use of agromet decision support system to generate and disseminate information to the stakeholders so that they can plan accordingly. Similarly, information can also be used to manage smart irrigation system and development of pest forecasting system. Thus, the overall enhancement of food security is possible through the establishment of early warning system using climatological information.

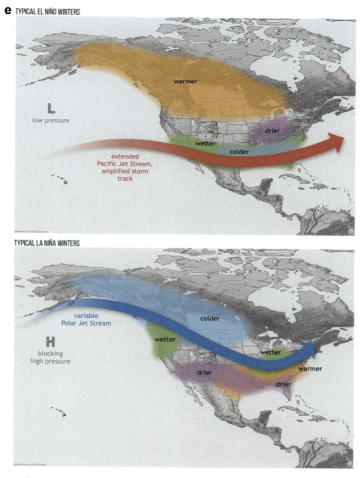

Fig. 2.20 (continued)

van Ogtrop et al. (2014) developed a time-lagged relationship between SSTs and rainfall periods and provided forecast system for the rainfed agriculture. The impact of climate change events (El Niño and La Niña) on rainfed wheat production has been presented in Table 2.6. Variability in yield data during different cropping year was due to variability in rainfall, which has strong connections with ENSO and SOI phases. Therefore, ENSO can be used as an early warning tool for the risk managements in different sectors of life (e.g., agriculture sector) as reported in previously published work (Ludescher et al. 2014; Rashid et al. 2022; Lee et al. 2021; Thirumalai et al. 2017; Tack and Ubilava 2015; Woli et al. 2015). Similarly, rainwater dynamics for rainfed agriculture could be accurately modeled by making teleconnections with climatic drivers like SST and pressure (Ahmed et al. 2014). Long-term rainfall data for rainfed area of Pakistan, i.e., Islamabad, shows a slight

54   M. Ahmed et al.

Table 2.6 Effects of climate events on rainfed wheat production

Cropping Year	Yield (Kg/ha)	% change	Climate events	SOI Phase (July)
1999-00	1319	-25	Drought Year (Weak La Niña)	4
2000-01	534	-70	Drought +Terminal heat stress (Non El Niño drought)	5
2001-02	717	-59	Drought +Terminal heat stress (Non El Niño drought)	5
2002-03	1310	-25	Drought Year (Moderate El Niño)	5
2003-04	1321	-25	Terminal heat stress (Non El Niño drought)	4
2004-05	1730	-1	(Weak El Niño)	1
2005-06	1354	-23	Terminal heat stress (Non El Niño drought)	5
2006-07	1755	=	Bumper Year as Benchmark (Moderate El Niño)	5
2007-08	1205	-31	Frost +Terminal heat stress (Moderate La Niña)	3
2008-09	1290	-31	Drought Year (Weak La Niña)	5
2009-10	1276	-26	Drought & Moderate El Niño	4
2010-11	1375	-27	Strong La Niña	4
2011-12	1357	-22	Moderate La Niña	4
2012-13	1398	-23	Heat stress without El Niño	2
2013-14	1412	-20	-	5
2014-15	1363	-20	Weak El Niño	1
2015-16	1376	-22	Very Strong El Niño	5
2016-17	1486	-22	Weak Lanina	4
2017-18	1425	-15	Weak Lanina	4
2018-19	1403	-19	Weak El Niño	1
2019-20	1433	-20	-	4
2020-21	1487	-18	Moderate La Niña	4

decreasing trend in winter rainfall while increasing trends in the occurrence of summer rainfall (Fig. 2.21). Similarly, rainfall intensity in the month of July has increased overtime (Fig. 2.22), which shows the importance of monsoon rainfall. Hence, simulation models provide the way to focus on risks and responses of food system in relation to climate.

2 Climate Change, Agricultural Productivity, and Food Security

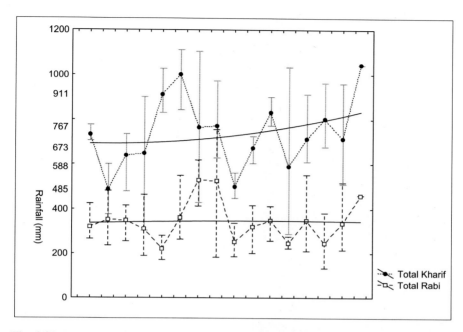

Fig. 2.21 Long-term rainfall pattern in Islamabad during summer (*kharif*) and winter (*rabi*) seasons

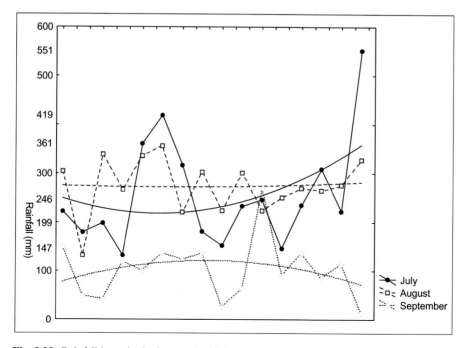

Fig. 2.22 Rainfall intensity in the month of July, August, and September

The strength of El Niño and La Niña events can be further gauged by using the Southern Oscillation Index (SOI), which is the measure of the strength of the Walker circulation (ENSO's atmospheric buddy) (Fig. 2.23). The SOI measures the difference in air pressure between Tahiti and Darwin. The phases of the SOI were defined by Stone et al. (1996), who used cluster analysis to group 2-month pairs of the SOI from 1882 to 1991 into five clusters as phases. The phases are as follows: Phase 1, consistently negative; Phase 2, consistently positive; Phase 3, falling; Phase

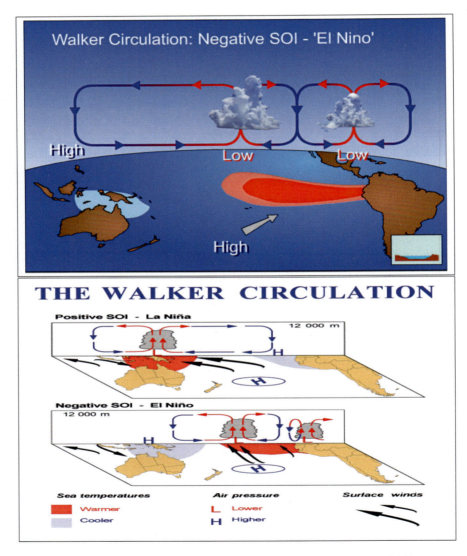

Fig. 2.23 The Walker circulation showing negative and positive SOI. (Source: NOAA)

2 Climate Change, Agricultural Productivity, and Food Security   57

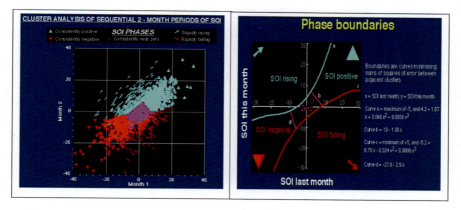

Fig. 2.24 Five clusters of SOI. (Source: Stone et al. 1996)

4, rising; and Phase 5, consistently near zero (Fig. 2.24). Stone et al. (1996) reported that accurate prediction of ENSO is helpful to accurately predict the global rainfall variations, which can be further used to manage agricultural production, reduce risks, and maximize profits. Furthermore, the SOI provides a good basis for rainfall forecasting with accuracy of 2 months which is helpful for key management decisions (Cobon and Toombs 2013).

2.4.4 Climate Change and Rainfed Wheat Production: Simulation Study

The Agricultural Production Systems Simulator (APSIM) was calibrated and evaluated for wheat genotypes in rainfed region of Pakistan (Table 2.7), which shows close association with the field observed yield data. Furthermore, simulation study was conducted to study the impact of rise in temperature and elevated CO_2 on rainfed wheat. Results showed that rise in temperature resulted to the reduction in the days to maturity, but this effect was compensated by the elevated CO_2, which resulted to the higher grain yield (Table 2.8). Guoju et al. (2005) studied the interactive effect of rise in temperature and elevated CO_2 on wheat yield and reported similar outcome. However, when temperature increase was 1.8 °C, then wheat yield was reduced. They suggested supplemental irrigation as an adaptation strategy to minimize the loss of yield. Similarly, variability in temperature during wheat growing season is shown in Fig. 2.25, which confirms that climate is changing, and adaptation options are need of time. Growing degree day or heat unit is the best indicator to monitor temperature response on crop phenology. Temperature requirement of wheat (thermal times/degree days) under normal conditions have been given in Table 2.9. However, with the rise in temperature, availability of heat unit during different phenological stages will be changed (Fatima et al. 2020; Ahmad

Table 2.7 Simulation of different wheat genotypes yield (kg ha^{-1})

Genotypes	Measured		Simulated		Bias	t	Regression equation	r^2
	Mean	SD	Mean	SD				
Wafaq-2001	3245	485	3177	444	−68	−0.36	S = 0.88M + 324.3	0.92
Chakwal-97	3056	542	3017	464	−39	−0.19	S = 0.83M + 473.5	0.94
NR-55	2729	466	2729	483	0.2	0.001	S = 1.02M − 61.73	0.98
NR-232	3062	524	3067	462	5	0.02	S = 0.83M + 528.5	0.88
R-234	3184	485	3180	417	−3	−0.02	S = 0.60M + 1273	0.49
Margalla-99	2938	559	3067	455	129	0.54	S = 0.69M + 1028	0.73

Table 2.8 Simulation of impact of climate change on wheat crop parameters

Variables	Baseline	2020	2050
	1990	0.9 °C	1.8 °C
CO_2 concentration	360 ppm		
Maturity days	183	180	175
Grain yield (Kg ha^{-1})	4090	4425	4397
Grain (number/spike)	28	30	30
Grain weight (mg)	34	37	39
CO_2 concentration	500 ppm		
Maturity days	183	180	175
Grain yield (Kg ha^{-1})	4090	4781	4781
Grain (number/spike)	28	30	29
Grain weight (mg)	34	38	30

et al. 2019). Relationship between wheat critical growth stages and degree days utilized and rainfall received has been elaborated in Fig. 2.26. Kapur et al. (2019) reviewed the impact of climate change and CO_2 on wheat yield. They reported around 25% increase in wheat yield with a twofold increase in CO_2 concentration. However, this increase due to elevated CO_2 was offset by the temperature rise of 3 °C. Hence, they suggested application of proper irrigation management techniques to coup the future water stress. Hernandez-Ochoa et al. (2018) quantified the impact of future climate change on wheat production and reported reduction in yield.

2.4.5 Changing Planting Window: Adaptation Option for Enhancing Food Security

Change in planting window can be a good option to adapt to climate change for enhanced crop productivity and improved food security. Different crops and varieties can give variable yield for different combinations with ENSO phenomenon of climate. The response of wheat crop under different plating windows has been shown in Fig. 2.27. It is clearly visible that delayed sowing resulted to the earlier anthesis and maturity with reduction in grain yield (Fig. 2.28). Furthermore, the

2 Climate Change, Agricultural Productivity, and Food Security

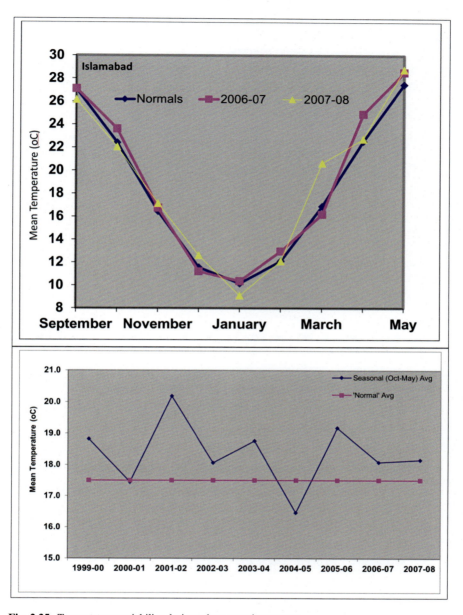

Fig. 2.25 Temperature variability during wheat growing season

impact of SOI phases on wheat yield was simulated, which showed that planting after mid-November (PW3 and PW4) was vulnerable to climatic fluctuation governed by SOI phase in July (Figs. 2.29 and 2.30). Moreover, different wheat

Table 2.9 Temperature requirement of wheat (thermal times/degree days)

At normal seeding depth, thermal time required for germination 65 °Cd
After emergence, the crop takes up to 450 °Cd to reach anthesis
The duration of grain filling is cultivar specific and varies between 500 and 800 °Cd
From sowing to maturity, wheat crop generally requires thermal time between 1350 and 1450 °Cd

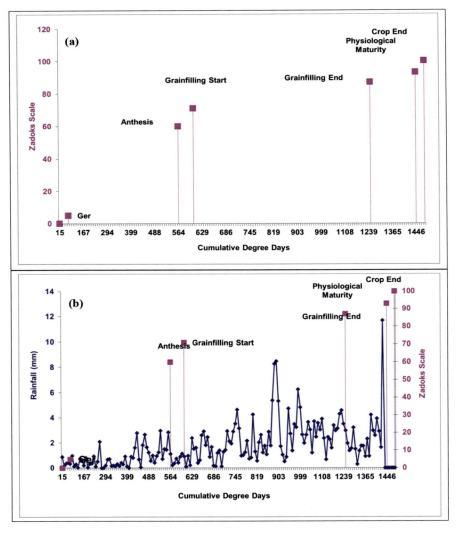

Fig. 2.26 Wheat critical growth stages and degree days utilized (a) and rainfall received (b)

varieties responded differently to SOI phase (Fig. 2.31). Similar to our recommendations, Ali et al. (2022) suggested change in planting date as suitable adaptation

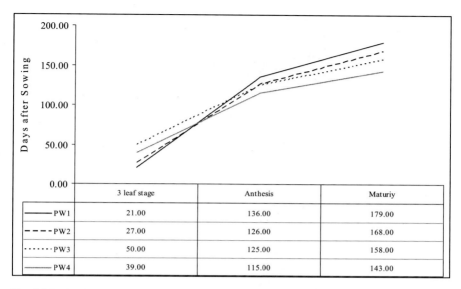

Fig. 2.27 Planting windows (PW) and duration of wheat phenological stages (PW1 = sowing between 15 and 25 October, PW2 = sowing between 10 and 17 November, PW3 = sowing between 27 November and 02 December, PW4 = Sowing between 10 and 24 December)

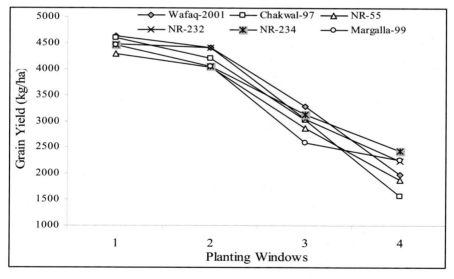

Fig. 2.28 Planting windows and wheat yield (PW1 = sowing between 15 and 25 October, PW2 = sowing between 10 and 17 November, PW3 = sowing between 27 November and 02 December, PW4 = sowing between 10 and 24 December)

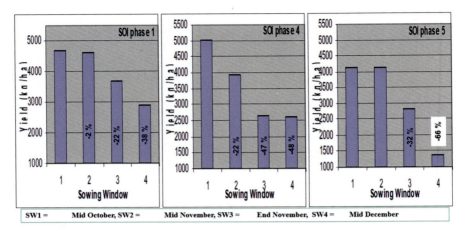

Fig. 2.29 Simulated yield variations in relation to sowing time partitioned against the prevailing SOI phase in July

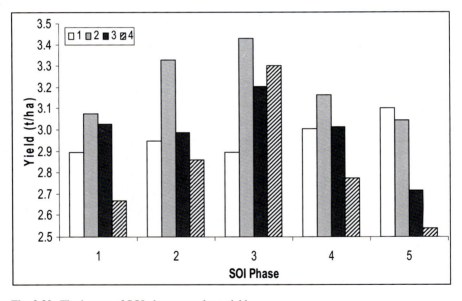

Fig. 2.30 The impact of SOI phases on wheat yield

option to minimize the potential impact of climate change. Similarly, the productivity of rainfed crops could be improved by opting an optimal timing for sowing (Tsegay et al. 2015). Sadras et al. (2015) reported sowing date trials as an effective, practical, inexpensive, and reliable screening method for crop adaptation to high temperature stress. Additionally, He et al. (2015) indicated that later sowing dates and new cultivars with longer thermal time could be helpful to have sustainable crop

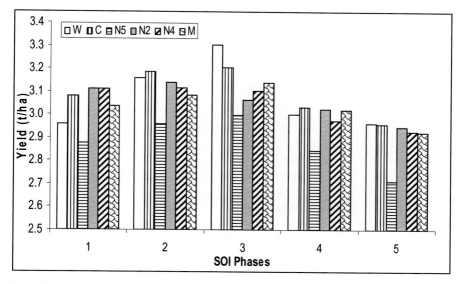

Fig. 2.31 Simulated wheat yield partitioned against July SOI phases (*W* Wafaq-2001, *C* Chakwal-97, *N5* NR-55, *N2* NR-232, *N4* NR-234, *M* Margalla-99)

yield under future rise in temperature. Sowing date as an adaptation to climate warming was studied by different researchers, and they reported sowing date as an important management tool to ensure food security by minimizing yield losses (Naz et al. 2022; Ding et al. 2015; Ahmad et al. 2019; Fletcher et al. 2019; Matthews et al. 1997).

2.5 Potential Options to Manage Food Security and Climate Change

Different measures can be used to manage the issue of food security and climate change. It includes bringing new areas under crops, using improved crop variety or species, and adoption of improved production technologies (e.g., changes in sowing windows, precision and smart farming, modernization of water supply and irrigation systems, inputs and management adjustments, and tillage). Similarly, improved short- and long-term climate prediction can help to identify vulnerabilities of present agricultural systems to climate extremes, which can be used to minimize risk. Furthermore, robustness of new farming strategies to meet the challenges of food security and climate change could be modeled for policy makers. Hence, advanced strategies to ensure food security could be tested accurately through models. Moreover, networking among different research groups and stations is very crucial to design national adaptation plan to mitigate climate change. Similarly, interactive communication can bring research results to different stakeholders (e.g., policy makers and farmers) that could solve the issue of food insecurity. Furthermore, the yield gap in the agricultural commodities could be minimized by cluster development initiative started by the planning commission of Pakistan with the name Cluster Development-Based Agriculture Transformation (CDBAT)-Vision 2025. Different food security programs already going on in Pakistan are listed below:

- Agriculture transformation plan, which includes first- and second-generation interventions. The focus of first-generation interventions is bridging the yield.
- Crop Maximization Programme (costing Rs 8 billions) covering 1,020 villages in four provinces, AJK and FATA/NA, with the objectives to (i) enhance crop productivity of small farmers; (ii) support them to start income-generating activities of livestock, fisheries, on sustainable basis; and (iii) create required systems for value addition of crop and livestock produce coupled with improved market linkages.
- The National Oilseed Development and Commercial Production Program to increase the production of oilseeds in the country to reduce the import bill.
- Two projects of 3.0 billion rupees for livestock farming to enhance community-driven milk and dairy production and increase red meat production.
- The Prime Minister's special initiatives to enhance productivity of livestock through the provision of extension services at farmers' doorsteps.
- For the promotion of commercialization in the livestock sector, two private sector-led companies, namely, "Livestock and Dairy Development Board (LDDB)" and "Pakistan Dairy Company (PDC)" have been established.
- To boost the overall production of crops and improve water use efficiency a mega On-Farm Water Management program has been started, with a cost of Rs. 66.0 billion to renovate 87,000 watercourses.
- Program for the promotion of high efficiency irrigation system, including drip and sprinkler.
- High-value crop production especially horticulture sector.
- The Wheat Maximization Program being launched at a cost of Rs.1.5 billion to increase the production of wheat.
- The Prime Minister's Special Initiative for White Revolution is being launched with an allocation of Rs. 500.0 million for increasing the milk production in the country.
- In line with the Prime Minister's 100-day program National Commercial Seed Production Program.
- Social safety nets are being strengthened, and the government has launched a new Bachat Card Scheme and Income Support Program for the poorest.

2.6 Conclusion

Ensuring food security is very important to feed billions in future, and it is only possible by understanding the impacts of different drivers on food system through different innovative techniques. After impact assessments, different adaptation options, e.g., early warning systems, water management, changes in sowing dates, choice of cultivar, and diversification of agricultural systems could be opted to minimize the devastating effects of climate change. However, the implementation of these adaptive measures in third world countries is a big concern, which is mainly due to lack of coordination between researchers, policy makers, and farmers. Hence, policy and institutional reforms are necessary to implement appropriate adaptive measures. Similarly, policy makers should understand the complex war of hunger, which has been increased due to climate change shocks. Thus, it should be handled carefully so that solution to the food insecurity could be implemented on a ground scale with true pace. Integration of climate predictions with policies could help to adapt food systems to climate change impacts, thus minimizing vulnerability and food insecurity.

References

Abdullah ZD, Shah T, Ali S, Ahmad W, Din IU, Ilyas A (2019) Factors affecting household food security in rural northern hinterland of Pakistan. J Saudi Soc Agric Sci 18(2):201–210. https://doi.org/10.1016/j.jssas.2017.05.003

Afesorgbor SK, van Bergeijk PAG, Demena BA (2022) COVID-19 and the threat to globalization: an optimistic note. In: Papyrakis E (ed) COVID-19 and international development. Springer, Cham, pp 29–44. https://doi.org/10.1007/978-3-030-82339-9_3

Ahmad S, Abbas G, Ahmed M, Fatima Z, Anjum MA, Rasul G, Khan MA, Hoogenboom G (2019) Climate warming and management impact on the change of phenology of the rice-wheat cropping system in Punjab, Pakistan. Field Crop Res 230:46–61. https://doi.org/10.1016/j.fcr.2018.10.008

Ahmed M, Fayyaz Ul H, Van Ogtrop FF (2014) Can models help to forecast rainwater dynamics for rainfed ecosystem? Weather Clim Extremes 5–6:48–55. https://doi.org/10.1016/j.wace.2014.07.001

Akponikpè PBI, Gérard B, Michels K, Bielders C (2010) Use of the APSIM model in long term simulation to support decision making regarding nitrogen management for pearl millet in the Sahel. Eur J Agron 32(2):144–154. https://doi.org/10.1016/j.eja.2009.09.005

Ali MGM, Ahmed M, Ibrahim MM, El Baroudy AA, Ali EF, Shokr MS, Aldosari AA, Majrashi A, Kheir AMS (2022) Optimizing sowing window, cultivar choice, and plant density to boost maize yield under RCP8.5 climate scenario of CMIP5. Int J Biometeorol. https://doi.org/10.1007/s00484-022-02253-x

Araya A, Hoogenboom G, Luedeling E, Hadgu KM, Kisekka I, Martorano LG (2015) Assessment of maize growth and yield using crop models under present and future climate in southwestern Ethiopia. Agric For Meteorol 214–215:252–265. https://doi.org/10.1016/j.agrformet.2015.08.259

Arora NK (2018) Agricultural sustainability and food security. Environ Sustain 1(3):217–219. https://doi.org/10.1007/s42398-018-00032-2

Arunrat N, Sereenonchai S, Chaowiwat W, Wang C (2022) Climate change impact on major crop yield and water footprint under CMIP6 climate projections in repeated drought and flood areas in Thailand. Sci Total Environ 807:150741. https://doi.org/10.1016/j.scitotenv.2021.150741

Asseng S, Ewert F, Martre P, Rotter RP, Lobell DB, Cammarano D, Kimball BA, Ottman MJ, Wall GW, White JW, Reynolds MP, Alderman PD, Prasad PVV, Aggarwal PK, Anothai J, Basso B, Biernath C, Challinor AJ, De Sanctis G, Doltra J, Fereres E, Garcia-Vila M, Gayler S, Hoogenboom G, Hunt LA, Izaurralde RC, Jabloun M, Jones CD, Kersebaum KC, Koehler AK, Muller C, Naresh Kumar S, Nendel C, O'Leary G, Olesen JE, Palosuo T, Priesack E, Eyshi Rezaei E, Ruane AC, Semenov MA, Shcherbak I, Stockle C, Stratonovitch P, Streck T, Supit I, Tao F, Thorburn PJ, Waha K, Wang E, Wallach D, Wolf J, Zhao Z, Zhu Y (2015) Rising temperatures reduce global wheat production. Nature Clim Change 5(2):143–147. https://doi.org/10.1038/nclimate2470. http://www.nature.com/nclimate/journal/v5/n2/abs/nclimate2470.html#supplementary-information

Atukunda P, Eide WB, Kardel KR, Iversen PO, Westerberg AC (2021) Unlocking the potential for achievement of the UN Sustainable Development Goal 2 – 'Zero Hunger' – in Africa: targets, strategies, synergies and challenges. Food. Nutr Res 65. https://doi.org/10.29219/fnr.v65.7686

Bashir M, Schilizzi S, Pandit R (2013) Impact of socio-economic characteristics of rural households on food security: the case of the Punjab, Pakistan. JAPS 23(2):611–618

Bizikova L, Jungcurt S, McDougal K, Tyler S (2020) How can agricultural interventions enhance contribution to food security and SDG 2.1? Global. Food Secur 26:100450. https://doi.org/10.1016/j.gfs.2020.100450

Cobon DH, Toombs NR (2013) Forecasting rainfall based on the Southern Oscillation Index phases at longer lead-times in Australia. Rangeland J 35(4):373–383. https://doi.org/10.1071/RJ12105

Crippa M, Solazzo E, Guizzardi D, Monforti-Ferrario F, Tubiello FN, Leip A (2021) Food systems are responsible for a third of global anthropogenic GHG emissions. Nature Food 2(3):198–209. https://doi.org/10.1038/s43016-021-00225-9

Dastagir MR (2015) Modeling recent climate change induced extreme events in Bangladesh: a review. Weather Clim Extremes 7:49–60. https://doi.org/10.1016/j.wace.2014.10.003

Davey MK, Brookshaw A, Ineson S (2014) The probability of the impact of ENSO on precipitation and near-surface temperature. Clim Risk Manag 1:5–24. https://doi.org/10.1016/j.crm.2013.12.002

Decision Support System for Agrotechnology Transfer (DSSAT) Version 4.7 (2017). https://DSSAT.net

Dharmasiri LM (2012) Measuring agricultural productivity using the average productivity index (API). Sri Lanka J Adv Soc Stud 1(2):25–44

Ding DY, Feng H, Zhao Y, He JQ, Zou YF, Jin JM (2015) Modifying winter wheat sowing date as an adaptation to climate change on the Loess plateau. Agron J. https://doi.org/10.2134/agronj15.0262

Dubey SK, Sharma D (2018) Assessment of climate change impact on yield of major crops in the Banas River Basin, India. Sci Total Environ 635:10–19. https://doi.org/10.1016/j.scitotenv.2018.03.343

Dudley N, Alexander S (2017) Agriculture and biodiversity: a review. Biodiversity 18(2-3):45–49

Ebi KL, Loladze I (2019) Elevated atmospheric CO_2 concentrations and climate change will affect our food's quality and quantity. Lancet Planet Health 3(7):e283–e284. https://doi.org/10.1016/S2542-5196(19)30108-1

Elbeltagi A, Aslam MR, Malik A, Mehdinejadiani B, Srivastava A, Bhatia AS, Deng J (2020) The impact of climate changes on the water footprint of wheat and maize production in the Nile Delta, Egypt. Sci Total Environ 743:140770. https://doi.org/10.1016/j.scitotenv.2020.140770

Erbs M, Manderscheid R, Jansen G, Seddig S, Wroblewitz S, Hüther L, Schenderlein A, Wieser H, Dänicke S, Weigel H-J (2015) Elevated CO_2 (FACE) affects food and feed quality of cereals (Wheat, Barley, Maize): interactions with N and water supply. Procedia Environ Sci 29:57–58. https://doi.org/10.1016/j.proenv.2015.07.155

FAO I, UNICEF (2014) WFP, and WHO 2018. The State of Food Security and Nutrition in the World 2018. Building climate resilience for food security and nutrition. Rome

FAO I, UNICEF, WFP and WHO (2021) The State of Food Security and Nutrition in the World 2021. Transforming food systems for food security, improved nutrition and affordable healthy diets for all. FAO, Rome. https://doi.org/10.4060/cb4474en

Fatima Z, Ahmed M, Hussain M, Abbas G, Ul-Allah S, Ahmad S, Ahmed N, Ali MA, Sarwar G, Haque E, Iqbal P, Hussain S (2020) The fingerprints of climate warming on cereal crops phenology and adaptation options. Sci Rep 10(1):18013. https://doi.org/10.1038/s41598-020-74740-3

Fatima Z, Naz S, Iqbal P, Khan A, Ullah H, Abbas G, Ahmed M, Mubeen M, Ahmad S (2022) Field crops and climate change. In: Jatoi WN, Mubeen M, Ahmad A, Cheema MA, Lin Z, Hashmi MZ (eds) Building climate resilience in agriculture: theory, practice and future perspective. Springer, Cham, pp 83–94. https://doi.org/10.1007/978-3-030-79408-8_6

Fitzgerald GJ, Tausz M, O'Leary G, Mollah MR, Tausz-Posch S, Seneweera S, Mock I, Löw M, Partington DL, McNeil D, Norton RM (2016) Elevated atmospheric [CO₂] can dramatically increase wheat yields in semi-arid environments and buffer against heat waves. Glob Chang Biol 22(6):2269–2284. https://doi.org/10.1111/gcb.13263

Fletcher A, Ogden G, Sharma D (2019) Mixing it up – wheat cultivar mixtures can increase yield and buffer the risk of flowering too early or too late. Eur J Agron 103:90–97. https://doi.org/10.1016/j.eja.2018.12.001

Fukuda-Parr S (2016) From the Millennium Development Goals to the Sustainable Development Goals: shifts in purpose, concept, and politics of global goal setting for development. Gend Dev 24(1):43–52. https://doi.org/10.1080/13552074.2016.1145895

Gil JDB, Reidsma P, Giller K, Todman L, Whitmore A, van Ittersum M (2019) Sustainable development goal 2: improved targets and indicators for agriculture and food security. Ambio 48(7):685–698. https://doi.org/10.1007/s13280-018-1101-4

Guoju X, Weixiang L, Qiang X, Zhaojun S, Jing W (2005) Effects of temperature increase and elevated CO₂ concentration, with supplemental irrigation, on the yield of rain-fed spring wheat in a semiarid region of China. Agric Water Manag 74(3):243–255. https://doi.org/10.1016/j.agwat.2004.11.006

Hallegatte S, Hourcade J-C, Dumas P (2007) Why economic dynamics matter in assessing climate change damages: Illustration on extreme events. Ecol Econ 62(2):330–340. https://doi.org/10.1016/j.ecolecon.2006.06.006

Hameed A, Padda IUH, Salam A (2021) Analysis of food and nutrition security in Pakistan: a contribution to zero hunger policies. Sarhad J Agric 37(3)

He L, Asseng S, Zhao G, Wu D, Yang X, Zhuang W, Jin N, Yu Q (2015) Impacts of recent climate warming, cultivar changes, and crop management on winter wheat phenology across the Loess Plateau of China. Agric For Meteorol 200:135–143. https://doi.org/10.1016/j.agrformet.2014.09.011

Hernandez-Ochoa IM, Asseng S, Kassie BT, Xiong W, Robertson R, Luz Pequeno DN, Sonder K, Reynolds M, Babar MA, Molero Milan A, Hoogenboom G (2018) Climate change impact on Mexico wheat production. Agric For Meteorol 263:373–387. https://doi.org/10.1016/j.agrformet.2018.09.008

Hikosaka K, Kinugasa T, Oikawa S, Onoda Y, Hirose T (2011) Effects of elevated CO₂ concentration on seed production in C3 annual plants. J Exp Bot 62(4):1523–1530. https://doi.org/10.1093/jxb/erq401

HLPE (2019) Agroecological and other innovative approaches for sustainable agriculture and food systems that enhance food security and nutrition. High Level Panel of Experts on Food Security and Nutrition of the Committee on World Food Security, Rome

HLPE HLPoEoFSaN (2020) Food security and nutrition: building a global narrative towards 2030. Rome. Available at www.fao.org/3/ca9731en/ca9731en.pdf

Hoogenboom G, Porter CH, Shelia V, Boote KJ, Singh U, White JW, Hunt LA, Ogoshi R, Lizaso JL, Koo J, Asseng S, Singels A, Moreno LP, Jones JW (2017) Decision support system for agrotechnology transfer (DSSAT) version 4.7. DSSAT Foundation, Gainesville, Florida, USA

Hussain J, Khaliq T, Ahmad A, Akhtar J (2018) Performance of four crop model for simulations of wheat phenology, leaf growth, biomass and yield across planting dates. PLoS One 13(6): e0197546. https://doi.org/10.1371/journal.pone.0197546

Hussain MM, Mohy-Ud-Din W, Younas F, Niazi NK, Bibi I, Yang X, Rasheed F, Farooqi ZUR (2022) Biochar: a game changer for sustainable agriculture. In: Bandh SA (ed) Sustainable agriculture: technical progressions and transitions. Springer, Cham, pp 143–157. https://doi.org/10.1007/978-3-030-83066-3_8

IFPRI (2016) Global nutrition report 2016: from promise to impact: ending malnutrition by 2030. International Food Policy Research Institute, Washington, DC

Iizumi T, Furuya J, Shen Z, Kim W, Okada M, Fujimori S, Hasegawa T, Nishimori M (2017) Responses of crop yield growth to global temperature and socioeconomic changes. Sci Rep 7(1): 7800. https://doi.org/10.1038/s41598-017-08214-4

Jentsch A, Kreyling J, Beierkuhnlein C (2007) A new generation of climate-change experiments: events, not trends. Front Ecol Environ 5(7):365–374. https://doi.org/10.1890/1540-9295(2007) 5[365:ANGOCE]2.0.CO;2

Jobe TO, Rahimzadeh Karvansara P, Zenzen I, Kopriva S (2020) Ensuring nutritious food under elevated CO_2 conditions: a case for improved C4 crops. Front Plant Sci 11. https://doi.org/10.3389/fpls.2020.01267

Kang Y, Khan S, Ma X (2009) Climate change impacts on crop yield, crop water productivity and food security – a review. Prog Nat Sci 19(12):1665–1674. https://doi.org/10.1016/j.pnsc.2009.08.001

Kapur B, Aydın M, Yano T, Koç M, Barutçular C (2019) Interactive effects of elevated CO_2 and climate change on wheat production in the Mediterranean region. In: Watanabe T, Kapur S, Aydın M, Kanber R, Akça E (eds) Climate change impacts on basin agro-ecosystems. Springer, Cham, pp 245–268. https://doi.org/10.1007/978-3-030-01036-2_12

Laborde D, Bizikova L, Lallemant T, Smaller C (2016) Ending hunger: what would it cost? IISD and IFPRI, Winnipeg

Lal R (2005) Climate change, soil carbon dynamics, and global food security. Climate change and global food security. CRC Press, Boca Raton

Landis DA, Gardiner MM, van der Werf W, Swinton SM (2008) Increasing corn for biofuel production reduces biocontrol services in agricultural landscapes. Proc Natl Acad Sci 105(51):20552–20557. https://doi.org/10.1073/pnas.0804951106

Lee J, Planton YY, Gleckler PJ, Sperber KR, Guilyardi E, Wittenberg AT, McPhaden MJ, Pallotta G (2021) Robust evaluation of ENSO in climate models: how many ensemble members are needed? Geophys Res Lett 48(20):e2021GL095041. https://doi.org/10.1029/2021GL095041

Li ZT, Yang JY, Drury CF, Hoogenboom G (2015) Evaluation of the DSSAT-CSM for simulating yield and soil organic C and N of a long-term maize and wheat rotation experiment in the Loess Plateau of Northwestern China. Agric Syst 135:90–104. https://doi.org/10.1016/j.agsy.2014.12.006

Litskas VD, Platis DP, Anagnostopoulos CD, Tsaboula AC, Menexes GC, Kalburtji KL, Stavrinides MC, Mamolos AP (2020) Chapter 3 – climate change and agriculture: carbon footprint estimation for agricultural products and labeling for emissions mitigation. In: Betoret N, Betoret E (eds) Sustainability of the food system. Academic, Amsterdam, pp 33–49. https://doi.org/10.1016/B978-0-12-818293-2.00003-3

Lizaso JI, Ruiz-Ramos M, Rodríguez L, Gabaldon-Leal C, Oliveira JA, Lorite IJ, Sánchez D, García E, Rodríguez A (2018) Impact of high temperatures in maize: phenology and yield components. Field Crop Res 216:129–140. https://doi.org/10.1016/j.fcr.2017.11.013

Loladze I (2002) Rising atmospheric CO_2 and human nutrition: toward globally imbalanced plant stoichiometry? Trends Ecol Evol 17(10):457–461. https://doi.org/10.1016/S0169-5347(02)02587-9

Loladze I (2014) Hidden shift of the ionome of plants exposed to elevated CO_2 depletes minerals at the base of human nutrition. elife 3:e02245

Lomazzi M, Borisch B, Laaser U (2014) The Millennium Development Goals: experiences, achievements and what's next. Glob Health Action 7(1):23695. https://doi.org/10.3402/gha.v7.23695

Ludescher J, Gozolchiani A, Bogachev MI, Bunde A, Havlin S, Schellnhuber HJ (2014) Very early warning of next El Niño. Proc Natl Acad Sci 111(6):2064–2066. https://doi.org/10.1073/pnas.1323058111

Lynch J, Cain M, Frame D, Pierrehumbert R (2021) Agriculture's contribution to climate change and role in mitigation is distinct from predominantly fossil CO_2-emitting sectors. Front Sustain Food Syst 4. https://doi.org/10.3389/fsufs.2020.518039

Magadza CH (2000) Climate change impacts and human settlements in Africa: prospects for adaptation. Environ Monit Assess 61(1):193–205

Mäkinen H, Kaseva J, Trnka M, Balek J, Kersebaum KC, Nendel C, Gobin A, Olesen JE, Bindi M, Ferrise R, Moriondo M, Rodríguez A, Ruiz-Ramos M, Takáč J, Bezák P, Ventrella D, Ruget F, Capellades G, Kahiluoto H (2018) Sensitivity of European wheat to extreme weather. Field Crop Res 222:209–217. https://doi.org/10.1016/j.fcr.2017.11.008

Mal S, Singh RB, Huggel C (2017) Climate change, extreme events and disaster risk reduction: towards sustainable development goals. Springer, Cham

Mal S, Singh RB, Huggel C, Grover A (2018) Introducing linkages between climate change, extreme events, and disaster risk reduction. In: Mal S, Singh RB, Huggel C (eds) Climate change, extreme events and disaster risk reduction: towards sustainable development goals. Springer, Cham, pp 1–14. https://doi.org/10.1007/978-3-319-56469-2_1

Manderscheid R, Sickora J, Dier M, Erbs M, Weigel H-J (2015) Interactive effects of CO_2 enrichment and N fertilization on N-acquisition, -remobilization and grain protein concentration in wheat. Procedia Environ Sci 29:88. https://doi.org/10.1016/j.proenv.2015.07.173

Matthews RB, Kropff MJ, Horie T, Bachelet D (1997) Simulating the impact of climate change on rice production in Asia and evaluating options for adaptation. Agric Syst 54(3):399–425. https://doi.org/10.1016/S0308-521X(95)00060-I

Miguel Ayala L, van Eupen M, Zhang G, Pérez-Soba M, Martorano LG, Lisboa LS, Beltrao NE (2016) Impact of agricultural expansion on water footprint in the Amazon under climate change scenarios. Sci Total Environ 569-570:1159–1173. https://doi.org/10.1016/j.scitotenv.2016.06.191

Misra AK (2014) Climate change and challenges of water and food security. Int J Sustain Built Environ 3(1):153–165. https://doi.org/10.1016/j.ijsbe.2014.04.006

Mohanty M, Probert ME, Reddy KS, Dalal RC, Mishra AK, Subba Rao A, Singh M, Menzies NW (2012) Simulating soybean–wheat cropping system: APSIM model parameterization and validation. Agric Ecosyst Environ 152:68–78. https://doi.org/10.1016/j.agee.2012.02.013

Myers SS, Zanobetti A, Kloog I, Huybers P, Leakey AD, Bloom AJ, Carlisle E, Dietterich LH, Fitzgerald G, Hasegawa T, Holbrook NM, Nelson RL, Ottman MJ, Raboy V, Sakai H, Sartor KA, Schwartz J, Seneweera S, Tausz M, Usui Y (2014) Increasing CO_2 threatens human nutrition. Nature 510(7503):139–142. https://doi.org/10.1038/nature13179

Naz S, Ahmad S, Abbas G, Fatima Z, Hussain S, Ahmed M, Khan MA, Khan A, Fahad S, Nasim W, Ercisli S, Wilkerson CJ, Hoogenboom G (2022) Modeling the impact of climate warming on potato phenology. Eur J Agron 132:126404. https://doi.org/10.1016/j.eja.2021.126404

O'Leary GJ, Christy B, Nuttall J, Huth N, Cammarano D, Stöckle C, Basso B, Shcherbak I, Fitzgerald G, Luo Q, Farre-Codina I, Palta J, Asseng S (2015) Response of wheat growth, grain yield and water use to elevated CO_2 under a Free-Air CO_2 Enrichment (FACE) experiment and modelling in a semi-arid environment. Glob Chang Biol 21(7):2670–2686. https://doi.org/10.1111/gcb.12830

Pearson CJ, Bucknell D, Laughlin GP (2008) Modelling crop productivity and variability for policy and impacts of climate change in eastern Canada. Environ Model Softw 23(12):1345–1355. https://doi.org/10.1016/j.envsoft.2008.02.008

Poore J, Nemecek T (2018) Reducing food's environmental impacts through producers and consumers. Science 360(6392):987–992. https://doi.org/10.1126/science.aaq0216

Prasad PVV, Jagadish SVK (2015) Field crops and the fear of heat stress – opportunities, challenges and future directions. Procedia Environ Sci 29:36–37. https://doi.org/10.1016/j.proenv.2015.07.144

Rashid IU, Abid MA, Almazroui M, Kucharski F, Hanif M, Ali S, Ismail M (2022) Early summer surface air temperature variability over Pakistan and the role of El Niño–Southern Oscillation teleconnections. Int J Climatol. https://doi.org/10.1002/joc.7560

Rehman A, Chandio AA, Hussain I, Jingdong L (2019) Fertilizer consumption, water availability and credit distribution: major factors affecting agricultural productivity in Pakistan. J Saudi Soc Agric Sci 18(3):269–274. https://doi.org/10.1016/j.jssas.2017.08.002

Rehman IU, Islam T, Wani AH, Rashid I, Sheergojri IA, Bandh MM, Rehman S (2022) Biofertilizers: the role in sustainable agriculture. In: Bandh SA (ed) Sustainable agriculture: technical progressions and transitions. Springer, Cham, pp 25–38. https://doi.org/10.1007/978-3-030-83066-3_2

Rong L-b, Gong K-y, Duan F-y, Li S-k, Zhao M, He J, Zhou W-b, Yu Q (2021) Yield gap and resource utilization efficiency of three major food crops in the world – a review. J Integr Agric 20(2):349–362. https://doi.org/10.1016/S2095-3119(20)63555-9

Sadras VO, Vadez V, Purushothaman R, Lake L, Marrou H (2015) Unscrambling confounded effects of sowing date trials to screen for crop adaptation to high temperature. Field Crop Res 177:1–8. https://doi.org/10.1016/j.fcr.2015.02.024

Salwan R, Sharma V (2022) Chapter 19 – plant beneficial microbes in mitigating the nutrient cycling for sustainable agriculture and food security. In: Kumar V, Srivastava AK, Suprasanna P (eds) Plant nutrition and food security in the era of climate change. Academic, London, pp 483–512. https://doi.org/10.1016/B978-0-12-822916-3.00010-X

Schmidhuber J, Bruinsma J, Prakash A (2011) Investing towards a world free of hunger: lowering vulnerability and enhancing resilience. In: Safeguarding food security in volatile global markets. FAO, Rome, pp 543–569

Schwietzke S, Kim Y, Ximenes E, Mosier N, Ladisch M (2009) Ethanol production from maize. In: Kriz AL, Larkins BA (eds) Molecular genetic approaches to maize improvement. Springer, Berlin/Heidelberg, pp 347–364. https://doi.org/10.1007/978-3-540-68922-5_23

Senapati N, Semenov MA (2019) Assessing yield gap in high productive countries by designing wheat ideotypes. Sci Rep 9(1):5516. https://doi.org/10.1038/s41598-019-40981-0

Shabnam N, Ashraf MA, Laar RA, Ashraf R (2021) Increased household income improves nutrient consumption in Pakistan: a cross-sectional study. Front Nutr 8:672754. https://doi.org/10.3389/fnut.2021.672754

Shaw DJ (2007) World Food Summit, 1996. In: World food security: Springer, pp 347–360

Singh J, Ashfaq M, Skinner CB, Anderson WB, Mishra V, Singh D (2022) Enhanced risk of concurrent regional droughts with increased ENSO variability and warming. Nat Clim Chang 12(2):163–170. https://doi.org/10.1038/s41558-021-01276-3

Spiertz JHJ (2009) Nitrogen, sustainable agriculture and food security: a review. In: Lichtfouse E, Navarrete M, Debaeke P, Véronique S, Alberola C (eds) Sustainable agriculture. Springer, Dordrecht, pp 635–651. https://doi.org/10.1007/978-90-481-2666-8_39

Stone RC, Hammer GL, Marcussen T (1996) Prediction of global rainfall probabilities using phases of the Southern Oscillation Index. Nature 384(6606):252–255. https://doi.org/10.1038/384252a0

Sulieman S, Thao N, Tran L-S (2015) Does elevated CO_2 provide real benefits for N2-fixing leguminous symbioses? In: Sulieman S, Tran L-SP (eds) Legume nitrogen fixation in a changing environment. Springer, New York, pp 89–112. https://doi.org/10.1007/978-3-319-06212-9_5

Tack JB, Ubilava D (2015) Climate and agricultural risk: measuring the effect of ENSO on U.S. crop insurance. Agric Econ. https://doi.org/10.1111/agec.12154

Thirumalai K, DiNezio PN, Okumura Y, Deser C (2017) Extreme temperatures in Southeast Asia caused by El Niño and worsened by global warming. Nat Commun 8(1):15531. https://doi.org/10.1038/ncomms15531

Ton G, de Grip K, Klerkx L, Rau M, Douma M, Friis-Hansen E, Triomphe B, Waters-Bayer A, Wongtschowski M (2013) Effectiveness of innovation grants to smallholder agricultural producers: an explorative systematic review. EPPI-Centre, Social Science Research Unit, Institute of Education

Tsegay A, Vanuytrecht E, Abrha B, Deckers J, Gebrehiwot K, Raes D (2015) Sowing and irrigation strategies for improving rainfed tef (Eragrostis tef (Zucc.) Trotter) production in the water scarce Tigray region, Ethiopia. Agric Water Manag 150:81–91. https://doi.org/10.1016/j.agwat.2014.11.014

Tui SH-K, Descheemaeker K, Valdivia RO, Masikati P, Sisito G, Moyo EN, Crespo O, Ruane AC, Rosenzweig C (2021) Climate change impacts and adaptation for dryland farming systems in Zimbabwe: a stakeholder-driven integrated multi-model assessment. Clim Chang 168(1):10. https://doi.org/10.1007/s10584-021-03151-8

UN (2018) Sustainable Development Goal 2. Sustainable Development Knowledge Platform. United Nations. https://sdgs.un.org/goals/goal2. Accessed 27 Feb 2022

Urban O, Hlaváčová M, Klem K, Novotná K, Rapantová B, Smutná P, Horáková V, Hlavinka P, Škarpa P, Trnka M (2018) Combined effects of drought and high temperature on photosynthetic characteristics in four winter wheat genotypes. Field Crop Res 223:137–149. https://doi.org/10.1016/j.fcr.2018.02.029

van Dijk M, Meijerink GW (2014) A review of global food security scenario and assessment studies: results, gaps and research priorities. Glob Food Secur 3(3):227–238. https://doi.org/10.1016/j.gfs.2014.09.004

van Ogtrop F, Ahmad M, Moeller C (2014) Principal components of sea surface temperatures as predictors of seasonal rainfall in rainfed wheat growing areas of Pakistan. Meteorol Appl 21(2):431–443. https://doi.org/10.1002/met.1429

Varga B, Bencze S, Balla K, Veisz O (2015) Effects of the elevated atmospheric CO_2 concentration on the water use efficiency of winter wheat. Procedia Environ Sci 29:180–181. https://doi.org/10.1016/j.proenv.2015.07.249

Veljković VB, Biberdžić MO, Banković-Ilić IB, Djalović IG, Tasić MB, Nježić ZB, Stamenković OS (2018) Biodiesel production from corn oil: a review. Renew Sust Energ Rev 91:531–548. https://doi.org/10.1016/j.rser.2018.04.024

von Caemmerer S, Furbank RT (2003) The C_4 pathway: an efficient CO_2 pump. Photosynth Res 77(2–3):191–207. https://doi.org/10.1023/a:1025830019591

Wangchen T, Dorji T (2022) Examining the potential impacts of agro-meteorology initiatives for climate change adaptation and food security in Bhutan. In: Poshiwa X, Ravindra Chary G (eds) Climate change adaptations in dryland agriculture in semi-arid areas. Springer, Singapore, pp 19–32. https://doi.org/10.1007/978-981-16-7861-5_2

White JW, Hoogenboom G, Kimball BA, Wall GW (2011) Methodologies for simulating impacts of climate change on crop production. Field Crop Res 124(3):357–368. https://doi.org/10.1016/j.fcr.2011.07.001

Woli P, Ortiz BV, Johnson J, Hoogenboom G (2015) El Niño–Southern oscillation effects on winter wheat in the southeastern United States. Agron J. https://doi.org/10.2134/agronj14.0651

Yeşilköy S, Şaylan L (2021) Yields and water footprints of sunflower and winter wheat under different climate projections. J Clean Prod 298:126780. https://doi.org/10.1016/j.jclepro.2021.126780

Zhao C, Liu B, Piao S, Wang X, Lobell DB, Huang Y, Huang M, Yao Y, Bassu S, Ciais P, Durand J-L, Elliott J, Ewert F, Janssens IA, Li T, Lin E, Liu Q, Martre P, Müller C, Peng S, Peñuelas J, Ruane AC, Wallach D, Wang T, Wu D, Liu Z, Zhu Y, Zhu Z, Asseng S (2017) Temperature increase reduces global yields of major crops in four independent estimates. Proc Natl Acad Sci 114(35):9326–9331. https://doi.org/10.1073/pnas.1701762114

Zheng J, Wang W, Ding Y, Liu G, Xing W, Cao X, Chen D (2020) Assessment of climate change impact on the water footprint in rice production: historical simulation and future projections at two representative rice cropping sites of China. Sci Total Environ 709:136190. https://doi.org/10.1016/j.scitotenv.2019.136190

Zhu C, Kobayashi K, Loladze I, Zhu J, Jiang Q, Xu X, Liu G, Seneweera S, Ebi KL, Drewnowski A, Fukagawa NK, Ziska LH (2018) Carbon dioxide (CO_2) levels this century will alter the protein, micronutrients, and vitamin content of rice grains with potential health consequences for the poorest rice-dependent countries. Sci Adv 4(5):eaaq1012. https://doi.org/10.1126/sciadv.aaq1012

Chapter 3
Climate Change and Process-Based Soil Modeling

Mukhtar Ahmed, Sajid Ali, Adnan Zahid, Shakeel Ahmad, Nasim Ahmad Yasin, and Rifat Hayat

Abstract Soil is under pressure due to climate change. Higher temperature is increasing decomposition and mineralization of the soil organic matter (SOM), thus reducing soil organic carbon, which is the blood of the soil. Furthermore, rise in temperature is causing changes in soil moisture. In addition, elevated concentration of carbon dioxide (CO_2) could cause higher activity of soil microbes, thus breaking SOM at a faster rate and releasing more CO_2. Similarly, the production of methane (CH_4) will be more in future if current traditional agricultural practices would be carried out at the same pace. Thus, it is clear that warming is a responsible factor of higher greenhouse gas (GHGs) emissions from soil. Hence, in this chapter, we are proposing different techniques, which could be used to keep the carbon underground, thus making soil as sink, not the source. Carbon (C) sequestration is low-hanging fruit nowadays, being used to improve SOM. However, understanding or quantification of soil health is important to design adaptation and mitigation strategies to climate change. Modern day tools, such as remote sensing and modeling, can be used to quantify the health status of soil, as mentioned in this chapter. Similarly, knowledge of soil physical processes (e.g., hydrologic dynamics, energy dynamics, and overwinter dynamics) is utmost important to get good returns from the soil. Thus, the Green-Ampt approach, Darcy law, and moving multifront (MMF)

M. Ahmed (✉)
Department of Agronomy, PMAS Arid Agriculture University, Rawalpindi, Pakistan
e-mail: ahmadmukhtar@uaar.edu.pk

S. Ali · A. Zahid
Department of Agronomy, Faculty of Agricultural Sciences, Quaid-e-Azam Campus, University of the Punjab, Lahore, Pakistan

S. Ahmad
Department of Agronomy, Bahauddin Zakariya University, Multan, Pakistan

N. A. Yasin
SSG, RO-II Department, University of the Punjab, Lahore, Pakistan

R. Hayat
Institute of Soil and Environmental Sciences, Pir Mehr Ali Shah Arid Agriculture University, Rawalpindi, Pakistan

© The Author(s), under exclusive license to Springer Nature Switzerland AG 2022
M. Ahmed (ed.), *Global Agricultural Production: Resilience to Climate Change*,
https://doi.org/10.1007/978-3-031-14973-3_3

were discussed in this chapter. Similarly, the approaches used by the different process-based models in their soil modules were elaborated. At the end of this chapter, the practical application of remote sensing and modeling was given at different spatiotemporal scale. Finally, it can be concluded that multiple adaptation and mitigation strategies should be used to improve SOM, which can further help to achieve sustainable development goals (SDGs), the blueprint to achieve a sustainable future for all.

Keywords SoilClimate change · Soil organic matter · Greenhouse gasses · Adaptation and mitigation · Remote sensing · Modeling

3.1 Soils and Climate Change

Soil is the loose surface material that covers the land, and it is the basic resource needed for the survival of living organisms. It contains organic and inorganic material. It is a living treasurer under our feet. Soil is a mixture of mineral matter, water, air, and organic matter as shown in Fig. 3.1. It is the natural medium which nourishes and supports plants. Soil is the end product of decomposition of the parent material. This weathering of the parent material is dependent upon climate, topography, and organisms like flora, fauna, and human. Hence, soil differs in texture, structure, color, physical, chemical, and biological properties. Soil is an important component of land and ecosystems, and it also determines the social and economic conditions of the region. Soil is the second largest store or sink of carbon after ocean, and to mitigate climate change, it is essential to improve soil organic matter (SOM) through different land management's techniques. The relationship between soil and climate change has been well described by the European Environmental Agency (Fig. 3.2). Similarly, soil management can play an important role in climate change adaptation and mitigation (Fig. 3.3). Improving carbon (C) in soil will help to protect

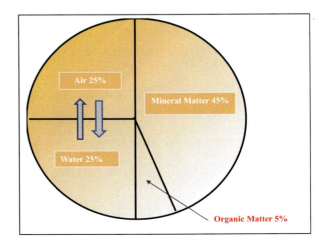

Fig. 3.1 Composition by volume of soil

3 Climate Change and Process-Based Soil Modeling 75

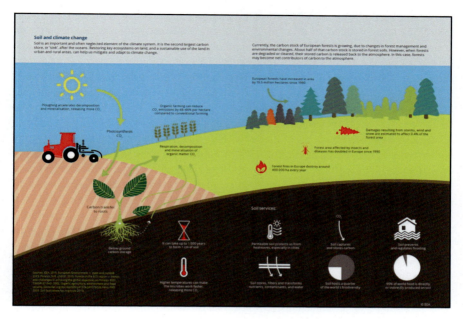

Fig. 3.2 Soil and climate change. (Source: European Environmental Agency (EEA))

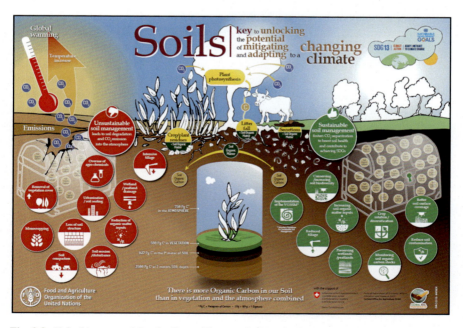

Fig. 3.3 Unlocking potentials of soil to mitigate and adapt to climate change. (Source: FAO)

soil from degradation, increases water holding capacity (WHC) of the soil, promotes microbial growth, and ensures food security. C-sequestration is the transfer of atmospheric CO_2 into different global pools (e.g., oceanic/pedologic/biotic and geological strata) to reduce the increase of CO_2 in the atmosphere. It is a very important technique which can help to maintain the concentration of carbon dioxide (CO_2) in the atmosphere, as concentration of CO_2 is increasing at a rapid pace. It has been increased from 280 ppm (1850) to 417 ppm (2022). This higher CO_2 concentration resulted to the increased surface temperature (1.5–5.8 °C) (IPCC 2001, 2014). C-sequestration have two basic methods, i.e., (i) direct (immediate binding at the source) and (ii) indirect (fixation of CO_2 by photosynthesis or its binding in a soil environment). Agriculture can play a significant role in C-sequestration. It is possible through agroforestry, soil mulching, residue incorporation, application of biochar, proper fertilization, intercropping, crop rotation, and growing of cover crops, which can further improve soil health by preventing soil degradation. Mattila et al. (2022) conducted a farmer participatory research to explore how farmers consider carbon (C) sequestration (low-hanging fruit). Farmers were given training about the basics of C-farming and C-farming plans to improve C-stocks in the field. The study suggested the use of remote sensing, modeling, and soil sampling as an integrated approach to verify the C storage in the field (Diaz-Gonzalez et al. 2022). C-sequestration is an important climate change mitigation approach. Therefore, C-farming was promoted to reduce climate change impact (Paustian et al. 2019). Lal (2008) suggested that reduction in atmospheric CO_2 loading is possible through biological, chemical, and technological options. Biological pumping, a C-sequestration technique in which CO_2 is injected below the ground surface to form carbonates, has so many benefits, which can enhance ecosystem services (e.g., improving soil quality and health, enhancing biodiversity, improving ground water quality, and increasing use efficiency of agronomic inputs), and ensures food security. Furthermore, C-sequestration reduces greenhouse effect (Kowalska et al. 2020; Lal 2005, 2008). Amundson and Biardeau (2018) reported that annual increase in atmospheric CO_2 can be halted if soil carbon could be increased by 0.4% on a yearly basis. Hence, soil C- sequestration is an important mitigation tool. Paustian et al. (2019) reported C-sequestration as an effective CO_2 removal strategy. Different management practices as elaborated in Table 3.1 could be opted to minimize the impact of climate change from soil.

3.2 Understanding Soil

Understanding of soil is very important to design adaptation and mitigation strategies to climate change as mentioned above. Knowledge of soil physical processes is utmost important to get good returns from soil. Soil physical processes include (i) hydrologic dynamics (infiltration, runoff, macropore flow, chemical transport, water table and tile flow, redistribution), (ii) energy dynamics (potential evapotranspiration, soil heat transport and temperatures, energy balance), and (iii) overwinter

3 Climate Change and Process-Based Soil Modeling 77

Table 3.1 Management practices to increase soil C-sequestration and CO_2 removals

S. No	Management practices	Benefits	References
1.	Crop rotations and cover cropping	Higher C-sequester and economic returns Mitigating climate change Improvement in the soil quality Decrease CO_2 emission Improvement in soil temperature, moisture, and total aboveground biomass Reduces erosion and nitrogen leaching, fix atmospheric nitrogen and improves soil health Mitigation of CO_2 emissions	Chahal et al. (2020), Smith et al. (2008), Abdollahi and Munkholm (2014), Nguyen and Kravchenko (2021), Kaye and Quemada (2017) and Rigon and Calonego (2020)
2.	Composting	Reduces emissions of greenhouse gases (GHGs)	Favoino and Hogg (2008)
3.	Manuring	Reduction in GHGs emissions	Dalgaard et al. (2011)
4.	No tillage, zero tillage	Mitigate GHG emissions Viable greenhouse gas mitigation strategy Lower GHGs fluxes Application of DAYCENT model in the estimation of GHGs Minimizing emissions of GHGs Preservation of soil organic carbon	Ogle et al. (2019), Krauss et al. (2017), Forte et al. (2017), Rafique et al. (2014), Mangalassery et al. (2014) and Haddaway et al. (2017)
5.	Cultivation of perennial grasses and legumes	Higher soil C storage Reduced N_2O emissions Suppress weed invasion Reduced use of inorganic fertilizer Lowering of C-footprint	Yang et al. (2019), Liu et al. (2016) and Gan et al. (2014)
6.	Plantation of deep-rooted crops	Improved soil carbon budget Reduced emissions of CO_2 Improves soil structure Improves water and nutrient retention	Jansson et al. (2021) and Kell (2011)
7.	Rewetting organic soils	Lowering CO_2 and N_2O emissions	Wilson et al. (2016) and Paustian et al. (2016)
8.	Grazing land management	Lowers atmospheric CO_2 emissions and surface temperature Improvement of soil carbon stocks	Mayer et al. (2018) and Conant et al. (2017)
9.	Biochar application	Reduced N_2O emissions Improved soil water holding capacity Suppression of soil CO_2 emissions Variable response in CO_2 production Soil greenhouse gas (GHG) fluxes remained variable in response to different biochar application	Martin et al. (2015), Conant et al. (2017), Spokas and Reicosky (2009) and He et al. (2017)
10.	Plant-soil interactions	Restoration of degraded soil	Maiti and Ghosh (2020)

dynamics (simplistic snow accumulation and melt process). Infiltration of water into a layered soil could be monitored by the Green-Ampt approach, which requires saturated hydraulic conductivity K_S and wetting-front suction S_{WF} of each soil layer (Green and Ampt 1911). It is a mechanistic model for infiltration under ponded conditions with well-defined wetting front. The following equation elaborates parameters in the Green-Ampt infiltration model:

$$V = \overline{K}_S \frac{(S_{wf} + H_O + Z_{WF})}{Z_{WF}}$$

where S_{WF} = integral of relative unsaturated hydraulic conductivity $K(h)/K_s$, known or derived from soil-water retention curve, $\theta(h)$ and θ = volumetric soil water content, and h = soil-water pressure head (−ive soil-water suction). Due to air entrapment, field-saturated θ_s is about 0.90 and effective K_s is approximately $K_s/2$. Further description about Green-Ampt infiltration model has been shown in Fig. 3.4.

Water penetration from the ground into the soil is governed by the soil surface condition, vegetation cover, soil properties, hydraulic conductivity, and antecedent

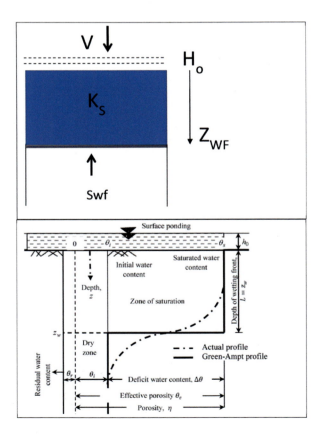

Fig. 3.4 Green-Ampt infiltration model. (Source: Kale and Sahoo 2011)

Fig. 3.5 Green-Ampt piston flow. (Source with permission via Rightslink: Alastal and Ababou 2019)

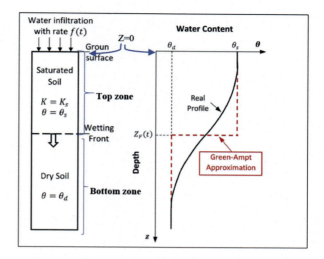

soil moisture. Generally, it has four zones (i) saturated, (ii) transmission, (iii) wetting, and (iv) wetting front. The rate at which water enters the soil is called infiltration rate, represented as f(t), while cumulative infiltration (F(t)) is the accumulated depth of water infiltrating during given time period. The Green-Ampt infiltration model (GAIM) assumes saturated piston-type flow into the dry soil (flow is modeled as the displacement of a single sharp wetting front into a dry soil). The front sharply separates in two regions, i.e., (i) fully saturated region (above) and (ii) very dry region (Below). The wetting front move downward due to gravity and capillary suction (Fig. 3.5). The GAIM is a single front model as it is based on the movement of a single front (Zf(t)) as shown in Fig. 3.5. The GAIM divides the soil into two zones as shown in Fig. 3.5.

Darcy law could be used to describes water flux (q). For example, in case of two-layered soil as shown in Fig. 3.6, water flux for the first layer (q_1) and second layer could be monitored by the following equations:

Water flux for the 1st layer(q_1) (Volume per unit area per unit time)

$$= \text{Hydraulic conductivity of 1st layer } (K_1) \times \frac{\text{Hydraulic gradient}(\Delta H_1)}{L_1 \text{ (Thickness of 1st layer)}}$$

$$= K_1 \frac{H_A - H_B}{L_1}$$

$$\therefore \frac{q_1 L_1}{K_1} - H_A = -H_B$$

$$\therefore -\frac{q_1 L_1}{K_1} + H_A = H_B$$

Fig. 3.6 Darcy law for layered soils

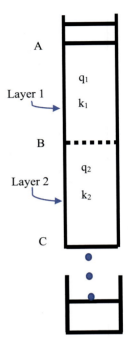

$$H_B = H_A - \frac{q_1 L_1}{K_1}$$

Water flux for the 2nd layer (q_2) (Volume per unit area per unit time)

$$= \text{Hydraulic conductivity of 1st layer } (K_2) \times \frac{\text{Hydraulic gradient}(\Delta H_2)}{L_2 \text{ (Thickness of 2nd layer)}}$$

$$= K_2 \frac{H_B - H_C}{L_2}$$

$$\therefore q_2 = \frac{K_2}{L_2}(H_B - H_c)$$

Putting the value of H_B from the first layer into second-layered equation generates the following equation:

$$q_2 = \frac{K_2}{L_2}\left(H_A - \frac{q_1 L_1}{K_1} - H_c\right)$$

For a steady state system, flux will be:

$$q_1 = q_2 = q$$

Hence,

3 Climate Change and Process-Based Soil Modeling

$$q = \frac{K_2}{L_2}\left(H_A - \frac{qL_1}{K_1} - H_c\right)$$

After rearrangement, equation will be:

$$\frac{qL_2}{K_2} + \frac{qL_1}{K_1} = H_A - H_C$$

$$q\left(\frac{L_2}{K_2} + \frac{L_1}{K_1}\right) = H_A - H_C$$

Hence, Dracy's law for layered soil will be:

$$q = \frac{H_A - H_C}{\frac{L_2}{K_2} + \frac{L_1}{K_1}}$$

Let $\dfrac{L \text{ (lenght of the given soil layer)}}{K \text{ (Hysraulic conductivity of the soil layer)}} = \text{Hydraulic resistance} = R_h$

Then

$$q = \frac{H_A - H_C}{R_{h_1} + R_{h_2}} = \frac{\Delta H}{R_{h_1} + R_{h_2}} =$$

Alastal and Ababou (2019) developed and tested moving multifront (MMF) to solve the Richards equation (Fig. 3.7). The root uptake part of the sink term $W(z,t)$ could be evaluated by using the approach of Nimah and Hanks (1973). Evapotranspiration is generally monitored by using the Penman-Montieth or Shuttleworth and Wallace methods.

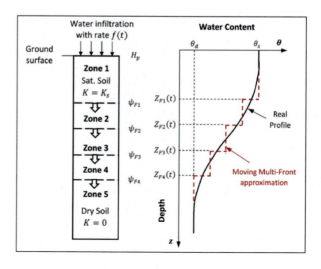

Fig. 3.7 Moving multifront (MMF) model. (Source with permission via Rightslink: Alastal and Ababou 2019)

3.3 Soil Modules in Different Models

3.3.1 AquaCrop

AquaCrop is a FAO model, and it uses soil water balance, soil water movement, and soil profile characteristic modules. The functioning of soil water module in AquaCrop is elaborated in Fig. 3.8. AquaCrop derives soil texture, organic matter, soil compaction, and stoniness by using hydraulic properties calculator developed by the USDA and Washington State University (https://hrsl.ba.ars.usda.gov/soilwater/Index.htm).

3.3.2 Agricultural Production Systems sIMulator (APSIM)_Soil Module

The APSIM is an internationally well-known model (https://www.apsim.info/). The APSIM soil module has multiple components, i.e., (i) erosion, (ii) fertilizer, (iii)

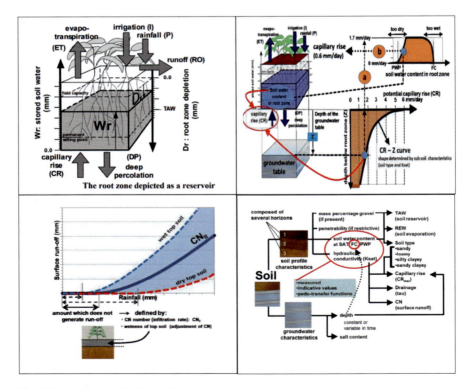

Fig. 3.8 Description of soil module in AquaCrop

3 Climate Change and Process-Based Soil Modeling   83

irrigation, (iv) map, (v) SoilN, (vi) SoilP, (vii) SoilTemp, (viii), SoilWat (ix), solute, (x) surface, (xi) SurfaceOM, (xii) SWIM, (xiii) SWIM3, and (xiv) WaterSuppl. The APSIM soil module is diagrammatically presented in Fig. 3.9. Both C and N dynamics has been described by SoilN module as elaborated in Fig. 3.10, where

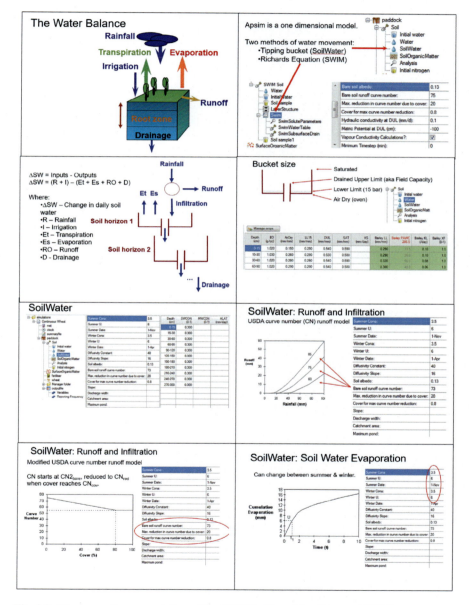

Fig. 3.9 Diagrammatic representation of the APSIM soil module. (Source: APSIM)

Fig. 3.10 Transformation in the APSIM_soilN module. (Source: APSIM)

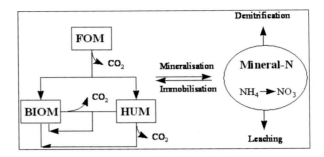

SOM is divided into two pools (Hum and Biom). Labile, soil microbial biomass, and microbial products are represented by "biom" pool, while the rest of the SOM comprises "hum." The flow between different pools is quantified in terms of C, while N flows depend upon C:N ratio of receiving pool. The "ini file" is used to specified C:N for "biom," while for "hum" it comes from the soil as an input. Decomposition in these two pools were calculated as first-order processes with a rate constant being modified by soil moisture and temperature in the layer. The CERES_Maize approach was used to represent fresh organic matter pool (fom), while C:N factor determines "fom" rate of decomposition (Jones 1986). Mineral N is determined though balance between decomposition and immobilization. At initialization, "hum" and "biom" C amount is calculated using soil inputs. The following equations will represent total, organic C, inert C, biom_C, and hum_C at initialization:

$$\text{Total C} = \text{Fresh organic matter (FOM) C} + \text{Orgnaic carbon (OC)}$$

$$\text{Organic Carbon} \left(\text{Kg ha}^{-1}\right) = \text{biom\_C} + \text{hum\_C}$$

$$\text{inert\_C} = F_{\text{inert}} \times \text{OC}(\text{Kg ha}^{-1})$$

$$\text{biom\_C} = F_{\text{biom}} \times (\text{hum\_C} - \text{inert\_C})$$

since

$$\text{hum\_C} = \text{OC} - \text{biom\_C}$$

Thus, biom_C equation will be:

$$\text{biom\_C} = \frac{(F_{\text{biom}} \times (\text{OC} - \text{inert\_C}))}{(1 - F_{\text{biom}})}$$

$$\text{hum\_C} = \text{OC} - \text{biom\_C}$$

3 Climate Change and Process-Based Soil Modeling

Soil temperature in the APSIM_Soil module is calculated using the Williams (1984) approach as applied in the EPIC (erosion-productivity impact calculator) model. The following equations were used in the EPIC model:

$$T(Z, t) = \overline{T} + \frac{AM}{2} \exp\left(\frac{-Z}{DD}\right) \cos\left(\frac{2\pi}{365}(t - 200) - \frac{Z}{DD}\right)$$

where Z = depth from the soil surface (mm), t = time (days), T = average annual air temperature (°C), AM = annual amplitude in daily average temperature (°C), and DD = damping depth for the soil (mm). However, this equation provides the same value for soil temperature as is for air temperature. Hence, to use air temperature as a driver for the soil temperature, the new equation developed was:

$$TG_{IDA} = (1 - AB)\left(\frac{T_{max} + T_{min}}{2}\right)\left(1 - \frac{RA}{800}\right) + T_{max}\frac{RA}{800} + (AB)$$
$$\times (TG_{IDA-1}) \ldots \ldots$$

where TG = soil surface temperature (oC), AB = surface albedo, T_{max} = maximum daily air temperature, T_{min} = minimum daily air temperature, and RA = daily solar radiation.

The final equation for calculating soil temperature at any depth is:

$$T(Z, t) = \overline{T} + \left(\frac{AM}{2}\cos\left(\frac{2\pi}{365}(t - 200) + TG - T(O, t)\right)\right)e^{-Z/DD}$$

Decomposition of SOM pools in the APSIM_Soil module was calculated using the following equations:

$$\begin{aligned}
\text{fom decomposition} = {}& F_{pool}(\text{Carbohydate, cellulose or lignin fraction}) \\
& \times \text{decay rate (rd)for a give fraction}(rd_{carb}, rd_{cell}, rd_{lign}) \\
& \times \text{Soil water factor} \times \text{Soil tempearture factor} \times C \\
& : \text{N factor}
\end{aligned}$$

$$\begin{aligned}
\text{biom decomposition} = {}& \text{biom} \times rd_{biom} \times \text{Soil water factor} \\
& \times \text{Soil temperature factor}
\end{aligned}$$

$$\begin{aligned}
\text{hum decomposition} = {}& (\text{hum} - \text{inert\_C}) \times rd_{hum} \times \text{Soil water factor} \\
& \times \text{Soil temperature factor}
\end{aligned}$$

The factors affecting individual decay rates are shown in Fig. 3.11. Nitrification is an APSIM_Soil module which is calculated using the Michaelis-Menton kinetics. The following equations have been used to determine the nitrification rate:

$$\text{Potential rate} = \frac{\text{Nitrification}_{pot}(\text{mg N/kg soil/day}) \times NH_{4(ppm)}}{\left(NH_{4(ppm)} + NH_{4 \text{ at half pot (ppm)}}\right)}$$

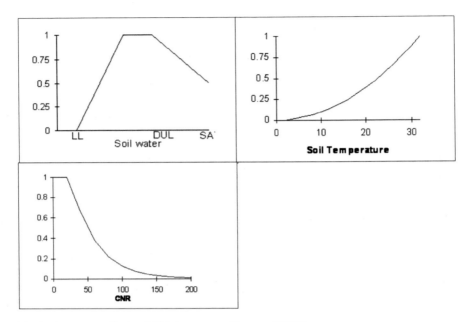

Fig. 3.11 Factors affecting SOM decay rates. (Source: APSIM)

$$\text{Nitrification rate} = \text{Potential rate} \times \min(\text{water factor, temperature factor, pH factor})$$

Factors, i.e., soil water, temperature, and pH, affecting the nitrification rate of ammonium, are shown in Fig. 3.12. Nitrous oxide (N_2O) emission from nitrification is calculated using the following equation:

$$N_2O = K2 \times R_{nit}$$

where R_{nit} = rate of nitrification ((kg N ha^{-1} day^{-1}) and range of values as were used for $K2$ (Li 2000). Denitrification in APSIM_Soil module was taken from CERES-Maize V1, which uses the following equations:

$$\text{Denitrification rate} = 0.0006 \times NO_3 \times \text{Active } C_{ppm} \times \text{water factor} \times \text{temperature factor}$$

where

$$\text{Active } C_{ppm} = 0.0031 \times \left(\text{hum\_C}_{ppm} + \text{FOM\_C}_{ppm}\right) + 24.5$$

Factors affecting denitrification of nitrate is shown in Fig. 3.13. Further details of all other components in APSIM_Soil module are available on https://www.apsim.info/documentation/model-documentation/soil-modules-documentation/

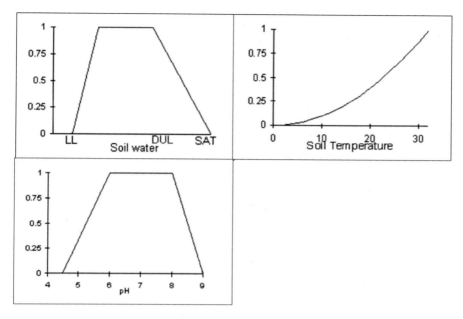

Fig. 3.12 Factors affecting *nitrification rate of ammonium.* (Source: APSIM)

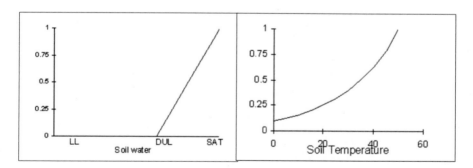

Fig. 3.13 Factors affecting *denitrification.* (Source: APSIM)

3.3.3 Decision Support System for Agrotechnology Transfer (DSSAT)_Soil Module

The simulation of the dynamics of soil in DSSAT is possible through different soil modules. These include soil water, inorganic soil N, soil P, and soil K modules. DSSAT also has soil organic matter modules with two options: (i) CERES-Godwin soil organic matter module and (ii) CENTURY (Parton) soil organic matter module. Furthermore, DSSAT has GHG emission modules, i.e., CERES denitrification, DayCent denitrification, N-gas emissions, and methane emissions. The DSSAT_soil module can also simulate dynamic soil properties as well as flood N dynamics. Further detail is available at https://dssat.net/models-overview/components/soil-module/

3.3.4 CropSyst_Soil

CropSyst simulates soil water budgets (precipitation, irrigation, runoff, interception, water infiltration, water redistribution in the soil profile), nutrients budgets (N and P), and C cycling on daily as well as hourly time step. Soil water fluxes in CropSyst is determined by a simple cascading approach or by a finite difference approach. Evapotranspiration in CropSyst can be calculated by three approaches, i.e., (i) Penman-Monteith model (ii) Priestley-Taylor model, and (iii) simpler implementation of the Priestley-Taylor, which considers only air temperature (Stöckle et al. 2003).

3.3.4.1 CropSyst Carbon/Nitrogen Model

This portion of the carbon/nitrogen model only includes the description of decay and mineralization of organic residues (crop, manure, etc.) incorporated into soil layers and dead roots. Surface residues are treated in a separate module using a slightly different approach. The pools included in the model are given in Table 3.2, all of them with units of kg m^{-2} ground area and with specified carbon/nitrogen ratios, except for residues whose ratio depends on their specific nitrogen content. The separate set of pools are defined for each soil layer. Figure 3.1 depicts the relations and exchanges of carbon (and nitrogen indirectly) among pools. Decomposition of organic residues and organic matter follows first-order kinetics with the following decomposition constants (day^{-1}).

A significant fraction of the carbon resulting from the decomposition of the different pools is lost as CO_2, and the rest is transferred to other pools (Fig. 3.14) according to the following carbon distribution fractions, where $F_{X->Y}$ represents the fraction of carbon transferred from pool X to pool Y (Badini et al. 2007).

$$F_{R \to CO_2} = 0.55$$

$$F_{R \to MB} = 1 - F_{R \to CO_2}$$

$$F_{MB \to CO_2} = \text{Minimum} \left[(0.55), \left(0.85 - 0.68 \left(F_{Silt} + F_{clay} \right) \right) \right]$$

where F_{Silt} and F_{Clay} are the soil silt and clay fractions, respectively.

$$F_{MB \to P} = 0.003 + 0.032 \, F_{Clay}$$

Table 3.2 Description of different pools in the CropSyst carbon/nitrogen model

Acronym	Description	Carbon/nitrogen ratio
R	Organic residue	Variable
MB	Microbial biomass	10
LA	Labile active soil organic matter	10
MA	Metastable active soil organic matter	10
P	Passive soil organic matter	10
Pool	**Notation**	**Value**
R	K_R	0.02
MB	K_{MB}	0.02 [1–0.75($F_{Silt}+F_{Clay}$)]
LA	K_{LA}	0.01
MA	K_{MA}	0.00055
P	K_P	0.000019

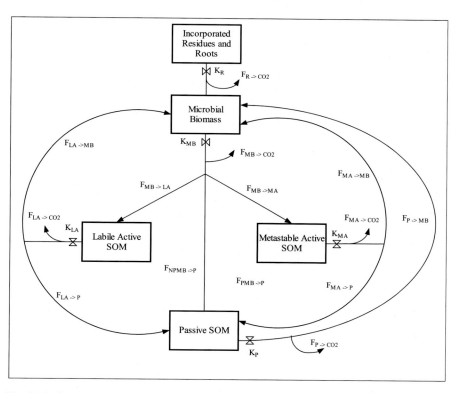

Fig. 3.14 CropSyst conceptual carbon flow model. (Source with permission: Badini et al. 2007)

$$F_{MB \to LA} = (1 - F_{MB \to CO_2} - F_{MB \to P})\text{FNPSV}$$

$$F_{MB \to MA} = (1 - F_{MB \to CO_2} - F_{MB \to P})(1 - \text{FNPSV})$$

where FNPSV is the fraction of non-protected soil volume, which is zero or low for consolidated and undisturbed soil layers and higher for layers recently disturbed by tillage.

$$F_{\text{LA}\to\text{CO}_2} = F_{\text{MA}\to\text{CO}_2} = F_{P\to\text{CO}_2} = 0.55$$

$$F_{\text{LA}\to P} = F_{\text{MA}\to P} = \text{Maximum}\left[(0.0), (0.003 - 0.009 F_{\text{Clay}})\right]$$

$$F_{\text{LA}\to\text{MB}} = 1 - F_{\text{LA}\to\text{CO}_2} - F_{\text{LA}\to P}$$

$$F_{\text{MA}\to\text{MB}} = 1 - F_{\text{MA}\to\text{CO}_2} - F_{\text{MA}\to P}$$

$$F_{P\to\text{MB}} = (1 - F_{P\to\text{CO}_2})$$

The carbon transferred among pools also determines the nitrogen transfer, which is equal to the amount of nitrogen required to preserve the carbon/nitrogen ratio of the receiving pools. In this process, if the amount of nitrogen released by the decomposing pool is greater than the amount of nitrogen required by the receiving pools, mineral nitrogen in the form of ammonium is released to the soil layer (mineralization). If the opposite is true, ammonium (first source) and nitrate (secondary source) from the soil layer is taken up for microbial consumption (immobilization). If no sufficient mineral nitrogen is available in the soil to supply the microbial demand, the decomposition is reduced in all pools requiring immobilization proportionally to the fraction of immobilization demand not satisfied. The initial amount of carbon allocated to each soil organic matter (SOM) pool in Fig. 3.14 depends on the organic matter content of the soil layer, expressed in kg carbon per square meter ground area. The total amount of carbon initially present in the soil layer is apportioned to each pool as mentioned in Table 3.3.

3.3.5 STTCS (Simulateur mulTIdisciplinaire Pour les Cultures Standard)

STICS is a model developed by INRA (France), now called as INRAE (Brisson et al. 2003). Soil surface can modify the water and heat balances in STICS, and it is linked

Table 3.3 Total amount of carbon in different pools

Pool	Fraction
Microbial biomass	0.02
Labile active SOM	(1 – Microbial biomass fraction – passive SOM fraction) physically non-protected soil volume
Metastable active SOM	(1 – Microbial biomass fraction – passive SOM fraction) physically protected soil volume
Passive SOM	Minimum (0.5, 0.3 + 0.4 F_{Clay}) for grasslands Minimum (0.5, 0.4 + 0.2 F_{Clay}) for croplands

Source: Badini et al. (2007)

Fig. 3.15 C and N fluxes in STICS. (Source with permission: Brisson et al. 2003)

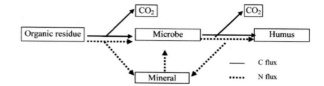

with the albedo of soil in dry state. Runoff coefficients determines the runoff proportion above a threshold in the presence of plants or mulch. Water balance in STICS is computed by using precipitation, irrigation, and reference evapotranspiration. Bulk density, field capacity, and wilting point was assumed constant in each soil horizon. The whole soil profile in STICS was characterized by five horizons of different depth. Beer's law is applied to calculate potential evaporation. N balance in STICS is calculated through N mineralization that originates from the three pools of organic matter (OM), i.e., (i) humified OM, (ii) microbial biomass (BIOM), and (iii) crop residues (RES) (Fig. 3.15). Denitrification (the gaseous loss) was calculated by using the NEMIS model (Hénault and Germon 2000). Nitrogen absorption is linked to crop requirements and supply from soil root system. Crop requirements was connected with the upper envelop of N dilution curves as reported by Lemaire and Gastal (1997). Soil N supply is equal to two fluxes, i.e. (i) transport flux (NO_3^{-1} transport via convection and diffusion from soil to closet root) and (ii) sink flux (active absorption by the root). In case of legumes, symbiotic fixation option is available that maintains N nutrition at the critical N level, and it depends on nodule activity, NO_3^{-1} presence, water stress, anoxia, and temperature. Soil temperature in STICS is calculated by using the model of McCann et al. (1991), which considers daily crop temperature and its amplitude (Brisson et al. 1998, 2003).

3.3.6 Erosion Productivity Impact Calculator (EPIC)

The EPIC model was developed by Williams (1984) to quantify the relationship between erosion and productivity. It is one of the comprehensive cropping system models developed initially (Williams et al. 1989; Williams 1990, 1995; Rosenberg et al. 1992; Stockle et al. 1992). The extended version of EPIC is APEX (Agricultural Policy/Environmental eXtender) developed by Texas A&M University (Jones et al. 2021; Gassman et al. 2009). Izaurralde et al. (2012) elaborated the development and application of EPIC in C-cycle, GHG mitigation. The EPIC model can simulate more than 100 crops, and it uses the Seligman and Keulen (1980) approach to calculate N transformations and dynamics. Afterward, soil organic carbon was calculated using a fixed fraction of soil organic N and C:N ratio of 10. This gives realistic picture of soil C dynamics and fluxes of C. However, EPIC performance to simulate long-term C dynamics was not up to mark as compared to other models, i.e., CENTURY, DNDC (DeNitrification DeComposition), ecosys, RothC, SOCRATES (Soil Organic Carbon Reserves And Transformations in agro-EcoSystems) used in

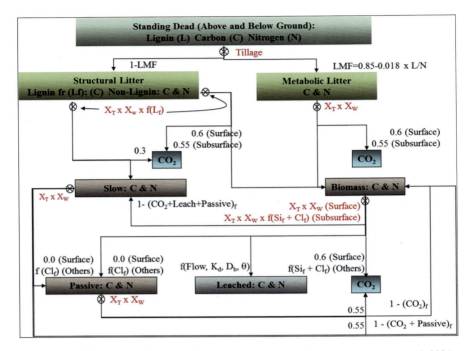

Fig. 3.16 EPIC soil C and N pools with their flows. (Source with permission: Jones et al. 2021)

the study conducted in Canada (Izaurralde et al. 2001). Hence, for improvement in EPIC, C-dynamics was needed, as elaborated by Jones et al. (2021). The C and N in SOM are distributed among the three pools as shown in Fig. 3.16 Furthermore, C balance in ecosystem prospective is given in Fig. 3.17, as EPIC generally gives C only in plant material, but with this modification, EPIC can describe C cycling at an ecosystem scale (Jones et al. 2021).

3.3.7 *WOrld FOod Studies Crop Simulation Model (WOFOST)*

WOFOST is a mechanistic, dynamic simulation model, which can simulate the production of annual crops (van Diepen et al. 1989; de Wit et al. 2019) in response to different managements and climate change. The WOFOST_Soil module includes soil water balance using tipping bucket and SWAP (soil-water-atmosphere-plant) approach. SWAP uses the Richards equation to simulate the flow of water and solutes among different layers (Kroes et al. 2009). WOFOST has also been connected through the BioMA framework to simulate soil water balance (Donatelli et al. 2010). WOFOST has the potential to be used in precision agriculture and smart farming.

3 Climate Change and Process-Based Soil Modeling 93

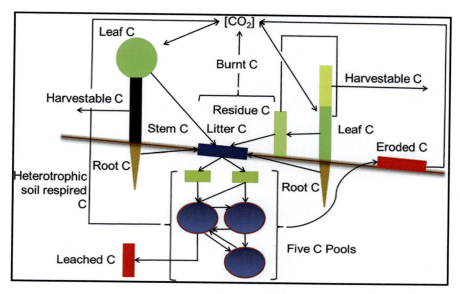

Fig. 3.17 EPIC ecosystem C balance. (Source with permission: Jones et al. 2021)

3.3.8 DNDC (DeNitrification DeComposition)

DNDC is a mathematical model that has been used in the study of management and climate change impacts on agriculture. DNDC has the potential to simulate dynamics (production, consumption, and transport) of nitrous oxide from different sources in agricultural systems (Gilhespy et al. 2014). Initially, DNDC (1–7) has three submodels, i.e., (i) denitrification (ii), decomposition (three soil organic carbon pools), and (iii) Soil_Climate_thermal hydraulic flux (Li et al. 1992). However, in DNDC_7.1, an additional empirical plant growth submodel was added; thus, it has four submodels. DNDC has so many further versions (e.g., PnET-N-DNDC, DNDC v. 8.0, Crop-DNDC, DNDC v. 8.2, Wetland-DNDC, UK-DNDC, DNDC v. 8.5, Forest-DNDC, NZ-DNDC, Forest-DNDC-Tropica, EFEM-DNDC, BE-DNDC, DNDC v. 9.0, DNDC-Europe, DNDC-Rice, and Mobile-DNDC), which was built to answer multiple questions of different scenarios. Smith et al. (2010) suggested improvement in the DNDCv9.3. estimation of soil evaporation. Manure-DNDC can quantify the manure life cycle on farms, and DNDCv.9.5 is the latest updated version, which can quantify hydrological features and GHGs estimation (Zhang and Niu 2016). Fluxes of GHGs among soil, plant, and atmosphere that elaborate DNDC mechanisms are shown in Fig. 3.18. Li et al. (2019) conducted a study to suggest improvement in the DNDC simulation of ammonia (NH_3) volatilization. They suggested major modifications in the source code. These include pedo-transfer functions in soil hydraulic parameters to simulate soil moisture, temperature effect on ammonium bicarbonate decomposition, and soil texture effect on NH_3 volatilization (Fig. 3.19).

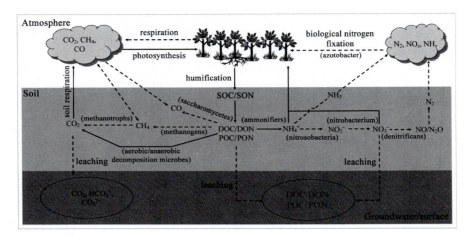

Fig. 3.18 Diagrammatic representation of DNDC showing carbon dioxide (CO_2), nitrous oxide (N_2O), and methane (CH_4) fluxes in forest/arable soil. (Source with permission: Zhang and Niu 2016)

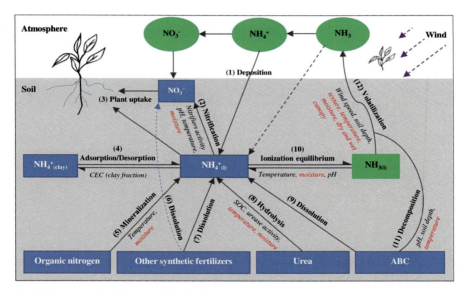

Fig. 3.19 Ammonia (NH_3) volatilization in DNDC. (Source with permission: Li et al. 2019)

3.4 Monitoring Soil Through Remote Sensing

Soil quality has been deteriorated due to intensive agriculture, and it poses big challenge to ensure food security. Traditional and modern soil quality assessment tools for data collection and processing can offer good opportunities to improve soil

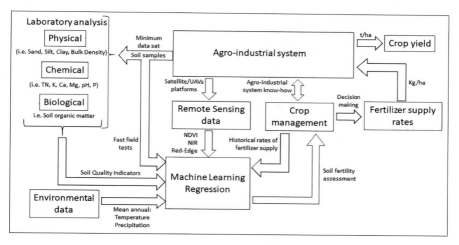

Fig. 3.20 Application of remote sensing and machine learning in soil quality assessments. (Source with permission: Diaz-Gonzalez et al. 2022)

health through different managements (Jung et al. 2021; Ge et al. 2011; Campbell et al. 2022; Bretreger et al. 2022; Angelopoulou et al. 2019). Artificial intelligence techniques provide useful information to farmers to decide treatments as per need. Generally, soil is assessed before the sowing of crop to select accurate management practices. But soil quality cannot be determined directly, and it can only be estimated by a wide range of quality indicators/indices. Traditional indicators to assess soil quality are (i) physical, (ii) chemical, and (iii) biological. Remote sensing is a powerful tool, which can be used to build different types of soil quality indicators based on soil nutrients and SOC contents (Fig. 3.20). However, to process data from remote sensing systems, different machine learning techniques are used. It includes supervised learning methods, i.e., random forest, support vector regression, artificial neural network, bagging decision tree, Bayesian models, boosted regression trees, cubist model, regression tree, regression kriging, random forest regression, partial least squares, k-nearest neighbor, generalized linear model, and deep learning (Diaz-Gonzalez et al. 2022; Harrington 2012; Loureiro et al. 2019; Bhatnagar and Gohain 2020).

3.5 Models Applications

Climate change is negatively affecting the crop productivity and food security due to its direct or indirect effect on different soil processes. Thus, adaptation options are needed to address the issue of climate change. The AquaCrop model was used by Alvar-Beltrán et al. (2021) to study the impact of climate change on the major crops (What and Sugarcane) of Pakistan, which is fifth in number due to the occurrence of extreme weather events. The study suggested that policy makers should act swiftly with solid adaptation options to cope with the changing environmental conditions in Pakistan. Bird et al. (2016) studied the relationship of future yield (2040–2070) variability with soil texture and climate models using AquaCrop to develop possible adaptation strategies. Results showed that yield was reduced by 64% on clay loams while it was increased by 8% on sandy loams and 26% on sandy clay loams soils. They suggested change in plant date and mulching as sustainable adaptation options to reduce crop losses. AquaCrop and DRAINMOD-S were used in a paddy field to simulate salt concentration. Both models were able to simulate soil salinity with good accuracy; thus, they can be used to manage salinity at field scale (Pourgholam-Amiji et al. 2021). Water and fertilizer management is important to get good crop yield and higher nitrogen use efficiency. Hence, Wu et al. (2022) developed a framework to simulate evapotranspiration under water and N stress in modified version of AquaCrop. The accurate performance of AquaCrop has shown that it can be used as a robust tool to develop precise managements for arid areas. Optimization of irrigation scheduling requires knowledge of crop and soil, which is possible through a decision support system. The AquaCrop and MOPECO models were used by Martínez-Romero et al. (2021) to optimize irrigation for barley crop. The results showed that both models were complementary to simulate gross irrigation water depths to attain the potential crop yield (e.g., 310 mm is required by barley to give potential yield). Rahimikhoob et al. (2021) applied AquaCrop a semiquantitative approach to simulate crop response to N stress using the critical N-concentration idea. Results depicted that direct simulation by using crop N status is a good option to improve soil fertility management. Biochar is a climate-friendly practice that can ensure food security by preventing water stress and fertilizer overuse. The AquaCrop model was used by Huang et al. (2022) to optimize the integrated strategies that involves irrigation, N, and biochar regimes. Results showed that AquaCrop simulated treatments impacts on crop yield with good accuracy. Hence, it can be used as a reliable tool for the optimization of field management, e.g., addition of fertilizer, biochar, and irrigation. Adeboye et al. (2019) evaluated AquaCrop to simulate soil water storage and water productivity of soybean. The model has shown low performance in simulating evapotranspiration and water productivity that needs to be fixed for dryland agriculture. AquaCrop-OSPy was proposed as an open source to be used to bridge the gap between research and practice (Kelly and Foster 2021). Groundnut is crop of dryland regions; hence, its simulation is tricky. Chibarabada et al. (2020) tested AquaCrop to simulate evapotranspiration, crop canopy cover, biomass, and yield under water stress conditions. Overall, the model shown good performance under water stress conditions, but it should be further tested under different soils and climates. Han et al. (2020) suggested that performance of crop models could be improved by upscaling the approach through remote sensing, as it can generate spatial distribution of crop parameters.

Soil organic carbon (SOC) is an important C pool, which can minimize atmospheric CO_2 concentration if managed properly. Wan et al. (2011) used the RothC model to study the impact of climate change on SOC stock. Results depicted that

SOC will decrease at higher rate in future if adaptation options, such as adding organic matter in soil through residues management and manure applications, will not be opted quickly. Furthermore, SOC could be increased by applying conservation agriculture practices, intercropping, cover cropping, and mixed farming. Lychuk et al. (2021) used the EPIC model to assess the losses of NO_3-N and labile P under changing climate, three levels of agricultural inputs (organic, reduced, and high), and three levels of cropping diversity (low, diversified annual crops, mixture of annual and perennial crops). Results showed that climate change resulted to the increase losses of NO_3-N, which can be mitigated by increasing cropping diversity as suggested in this work. LPJ-GUESS (Lund-Potsdam-Jena General Ecosystem Simulator) was used by Ma et al. (2022) to assess the impacts of agricultural managements on soil C stocks, nitrogen loss, and crop production. Conservation agriculture practices, i.e., no tillage, cover crop, residue, and manure application, have shown positive effect on SOC, while loss of N was also minimum under these practices. A hydro-biogeochemical model (SWAT-DayCent) was used to investigate the effect of climate warming and root zone soil water contents on SOC. Three Representative Concentration Pathways (RCP2.6, 4.5, and 8.5) and five global climate models were used in this study. The results showed that SOC will decrease in future due to higher warming but higher soil water content could depress SOC losses (Zhao et al. 2021).

Climate change will negatively affect SOM dynamics, soil organisms, and soil properties, but warmer conditions could lead to the higher availability of soil N due to higher mineralization rate. Hence, soil management particularly N application will be governed by future climate change (Jat et al. 2018). SOC dynamics is the core of interlinked environmental problems. However, its management is a mystery due to its complex relationship with N availability, moisture, and temperature. Srivastava et al. (2017) reviewed soil C dynamics under changing climate and suggested that soil may act as a potential C sink if managed properly (e.g., management of soil inorganic N pools and its proper linkage with microbial processes). Climate change mitigation is the implementation of efforts to halt or reverse climate change through behavior, technological, and management strategies (Fig. 3.21). With practical on ground mitigation practices, soil can play a role to reduce CO_2 emissions. It can be a carbon sink instead of the source (Lal 2004; Paustian et al. 2016). On the other hand, the adaptation is to achieve higher resilience toward extreme climatic events. It is possible through different managements as shown in Figure 3.21, which can improve SOC. This higher SOC will help to retain more water and could produce crops even under drought. Sustainable development goals (SDGs), which are the blueprint to achieve a sustainable future for all, could be achieved through improving SOC. The benefit of improvement of SOC to achieve SDGs is elaborated in Fig. 3.22. Mitigation and adaptation both offer solutions to climate change, and they are directly and indirectly related to SDGs. However, they are not always complementary as sometimes they can be independent from each other. Balanced fertilization is the key adaptation strategy, which can sustain SOC on long term basis. Mohanty et al. (2020) simulated C-sequestration potential of balanced fertilization (N and farmyard manure) in soybean-wheat cropping system using the

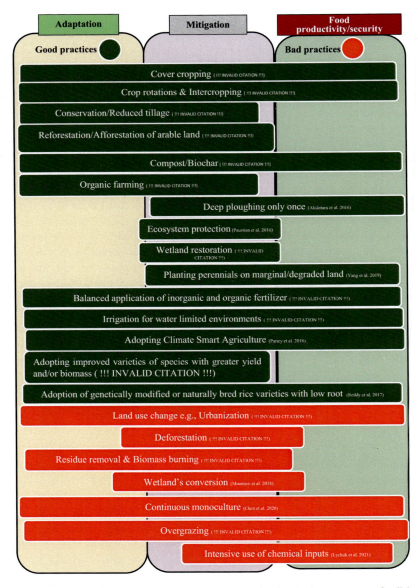

Fig. 3.21 Management strategies (Suggested and dissuaded) for the improvement of soil health and their impacts on climate change adaptation, mitigation, and food productivity/security

43-year long-term experimental dataset. The APSIM results showed that improved N and FYM management had the potential to increase SOC. Chaki et al. (2022) evaluated the APSIM potential to simulate conservation and conventional tillage practices in rice-wheat system. Results showed that the model was able to capture the

3 Climate Change and Process-Based Soil Modeling

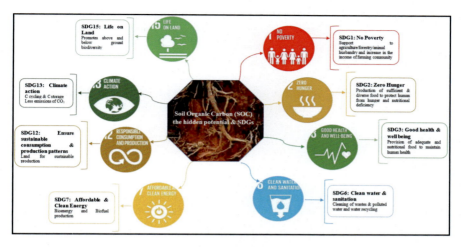

Fig. 3.22 Relationship between SOC and SDGs

effect of tillage, residue, N application, and cropping system; thus, it can be a good tool for designing the adaptation and mitigation options to climate change. Furthermore, the APSIM model was used evaluate the potential of conservation agriculture to mitigate climate change in water-scarce region Tunisia. Results depicted that mulching (residue retention) is more effective than conservation tillage under semi-arid and subhumid conditions. It can increase crop yield, WUE, and SOC as well as would help in the prevention of erosion (Bahri et al. 2019). Singh et al. (2022) compared the simulated potential of DRAINMOD-DSSAT and RZWQM2 to simulate the effects of management practices (N application rates and timings) on NO_3-N losses and crop yield. Results showed that both models provided the same conclusion for the N management strategy. Similarly, DSSAT was used as a valuable tool to suggest conservation agriculture as a potential way to adapt to climate change (Ngwira et al. 2014). Since process-based models are a good tool to design adaptation practices to climate change and, hence, to use them in real sense and to have true field picture, these models should be properly calibrated using different upscaling strategies (Chen et al. 2021).

3.6 Conclusion

Climate change is posing a major threat to food security through soil degradation. Since soil is the largest source of C, then it is necessary to conserve and improve SOM through its judicious use and management. Soil heath improvement will help to combat soil degradation, address food security, and mitigate climate change. Understanding and quantification of soil health through modern tools (e.g., remote sensing and modeling) are utmost important to design adaptation and mitigation strategies. Different adaptation and mitigation strategies are already available, which should be used to improve SOM. These includes reforestation, use of conservation tillage, intercropping, residue management, cover cropping, application of compost and biochar, balanced use of inorganic and organic fertilizer, and adoption of climate smart agriculture. However, these interventions need to be implemented properly through their dissemination to the real stakeholders, i.e., policy makers and farmers.

References

Abdollahi L, Munkholm LJ (2014) Tillage system and cover crop effects on soil quality: I. Chemical, mechanical, and biological properties. Soil Sci Soc Am J 78(1):262–270

Adeboye OB, Schultz B, Adekalu KO, Prasad KC (2019) Performance evaluation of AquaCrop in simulating soil water storage, yield, and water productivity of rainfed soybeans (Glycine max L. merr) in Ile-Ife, Nigeria. Agric Water Manag 213:1130–1146. https://doi.org/10.1016/j.agwat.2018.11.006

Alastal K, Ababou R (2019) Moving Multi-Front (MMF): a generalized Green-Ampt approach for vertical unsaturated flows. J Hydrol 579:124184. https://doi.org/10.1016/j.jhydrol.2019.124184

Alvar-Beltrán J, Heureux A, Soldan R, Manzanas R, Khan B, Dalla Marta A (2021) Assessing the impact of climate change on wheat and sugarcane with the AquaCrop model along the Indus River Basin. Pakis Agric Water Manag 253:106909. https://doi.org/10.1016/j.agwat.2021.106909

Amundson R, Biardeau L (2018) Soil carbon sequestration is an elusive climate mitigation tool. Proc Natl Acad Sci 115(46):11652–11656. https://doi.org/10.1073/pnas.1815901115

Angelopoulou T, Tziolas N, Balafoutis A, Zalidis G, Bochtis D (2019) Remote sensing techniques for soil organic carbon estimation: a review. Remote Sens 11(6):676

Badini O, Stöckle CO, Jones JW, Nelson R, Kodio A, Keita M (2007) A simulation-based analysis of productivity and soil carbon in response to time-controlled rotational grazing in the West African Sahel region. Agric Syst 94(1):87–96. https://doi.org/10.1016/j.agsy.2005.09.010

Bahri H, Annabi M, Cheikh M'Hamed H, Frija A (2019) Assessing the long-term impact of conservation agriculture on wheat-based systems in Tunisia using APSIM simulations under a climate change context. Sci Total Environ 692:1223–1233. https://doi.org/10.1016/j.scitotenv.2019.07.307

Bhatnagar R, Gohain GB (2020) Crop yield estimation using decision trees and random forest machine learning algorithms on data from terra (EOS AM-1) & Aqua (EOS PM-1) satellite data. In: Machine learning and data mining in aerospace technology. Springer, pp 107–124

Bird DN, Benabdallah S, Gouda N, Hummel F, Koeberl J, La Jeunesse I, Meyer S, Prettenthaler F, Soddu A, Woess-Gallasch S (2016) Modelling climate change impacts on and adaptation strategies for agriculture in Sardinia and Tunisia using AquaCrop and value-at-risk. Sci Total Environ 543:1019–1027. https://doi.org/10.1016/j.scitotenv.2015.07.035

Bretreger D, Yeo I-Y, Hancock G (2022) Quantifying irrigation water use with remote sensing: soil water deficit modelling with uncertain soil parameters. Agric Water Manag 260:107299. https://doi.org/10.1016/j.agwat.2021.107299

Brisson N, Mary B, Ripoche D, Jeuffroy MH, Ruget F, Nicoullaud B, Gate P, Devienne-Barret F, Antonioletti R, Durr C, Richard G, Beaudoin N, Recous S, Tayot X, Plenet D, Cellier P, Machet J-M, Meynard JM, Delécolle R (1998) STICS: a generic model for the simulation of crops and their water and nitrogen balances. I. Theory and parameterization applied to wheat and corn. Agronomie 18(5–6):311–346

3 Climate Change and Process-Based Soil Modeling

Brisson N, Gary C, Justes E, Roche R, Mary B, Ripoche D, Zimmer D, Sierra J, Bertuzzi P, Burger P, Bussière F, Cabidoche YM, Cellier P, Debaeke P, Gaudillère JP, Hénault C, Maraux F, Seguin B, Sinoquet H (2003) An overview of the crop model stics. Eur J Agron 18(3–4):309–332. https://doi.org/10.1016/S1161-0301(02)00110-7

Campbell AD, Fatoyinbo T, Charles SP, Bourgeau-Chavez LL, Goes J, Gomes H, Halabisky M, Holmquist J, Lohrenz S, Mitchell C, Moskal LM, Poulter B, Qiu H, Resende De Sousa CH, Sayers M, Simard M, Stewart AJ, Singh D, Trettin C, Wu J, Zhang X, Lagomasino D (2022) A review of carbon monitoring in wet carbon systems using remote sensing. Environ Res Lett 17(2):025009. https://doi.org/10.1088/1748-9326/ac4d4d

Chahal I, Vyn RJ, Mayers D, Van Eerd LL (2020) Cumulative impact of cover crops on soil carbon sequestration and profitability in a temperate humid climate. Sci Rep 10(1):13381. https://doi.org/10.1038/s41598-020-70224-6

Chaki AK, Gaydon DS, Dalal RC, Bellotti WD, Gathala MK, Hossain A, Menzies NW (2022) How we used APSIM to simulate conservation agriculture practices in the rice-wheat system of the Eastern Gangetic Plains. Field Crop Res 275:108344. https://doi.org/10.1016/j.fcr.2021.108344

Chen S, He L, Cao Y, Wang R, Wu L, Wang Z, Zou Y, Siddique KHM, Xiong W, Liu M, Feng H, Yu Q, Wang X, He J (2021) Comparisons among four different upscaling strategies for cultivar genetic parameters in rainfed spring wheat phenology simulations with the DSSAT-CERES-wheat model. Agric Water Manag 258:107181. https://doi.org/10.1016/j.agwat.2021.107181

Chibarabada TP, Modi AT, Mabhaudhi T (2020) Calibration and evaluation of aquacrop for groundnut (Arachis hypogaea) under water deficit conditions. Agric For Meteorol 281:107850. https://doi.org/10.1016/j.agrformet.2019.107850

Conant RT, Cerri CE, Osborne BB, Paustian K (2017) Grassland management impacts on soil carbon stocks: a new synthesis. Ecol Appl 27(2):662–668. https://doi.org/10.1002/eap.1473

Dalgaard T, Olesen JE, Petersen SO, Petersen BM, Jørgensen U, Kristensen T, Hutchings NJ, Gyldenkærne S, Hermansen JE (2011) Developments in greenhouse gas emissions and net energy use in Danish agriculture – how to achieve substantial CO_2 reductions? Environ Pollut 159(11):3193–3203. https://doi.org/10.1016/j.envpol.2011.02.024

de Wit A, Boogaard H, Fumagalli D, Janssen S, Knapen R, van Kraalingen D, Supit I, van der Wijngaart R, van Diepen K (2019) 25 years of the WOFOST cropping systems model. Agric Syst 168:154–167. https://doi.org/10.1016/j.agsy.2018.06.018

Diaz-Gonzalez FA, Vuelvas J, Correa CA, Vallejo VE, Patino D (2022) Machine learning and remote sensing techniques applied to estimate soil indicators – review. Ecol Indic 135:108517. https://doi.org/10.1016/j.ecolind.2021.108517

Donatelli M, Russell G, Rizzoli A, Acutis M, Adam M, Athanasiadis I, Balderacchi M, Bechini L, Belhouchette H, Bellocchi G, Bergez J-E, Botta M, Braudeau E, Bregaglio S, Carlini L, Casellas E, Celette F, Ceotto E, Charron-Moirez M, Confalonieri R, Corbeels M, Criscuolo L, Cruz P, di Guardo A, Ditto D, Dupraz C, Duru M, Fiorani D, Gentile A, Ewert F, Gary C, Habyarimana E, Jouany C, Kansou K, Knapen R, Filippi G, Leffelaar P, Manici L, Martin G, Martin P, Meuter E, Mugueta N, Mulia R, van Noordwijk M, Oomen R, Rosenmund A, Rossi V, Salinari F, Serrano A, Sorce A, Vincent G, Theau J-P, Thérond O, Trevisan M, Trevisiol P, van Evert F, Wallach D, Wery J, Zerourou A (2010) A component-based framework for simulating agricultural production and externalities. In: Brouwer FM, Ittersum MK (eds) Environmental and agricultural modelling. Springer Netherlands, pp 63–108. https://doi.org/10.1007/978-90-481-3619-3_4

Favoino E, Hogg D (2008) The potential role of compost in reducing greenhouse gases. Waste Manag Res 26(1):61–69. https://doi.org/10.1177/0734242x08088584

Forte A, Fiorentino N, Fagnano M, Fierro A (2017) Mitigation impact of minimum tillage on CO_2 and N_2O emissions from a Mediterranean maize cropped soil under low-water input management. Soil Tillage Res 166:167–178. https://doi.org/10.1016/j.still.2016.09.014

Gan Y, Liang C, Chai Q, Lemke RL, Campbell CA, Zentner RP (2014) Improving farming practices reduces the carbon footprint of spring wheat production. Nat Commun 5(1):5012. https://doi.org/10.1038/ncomms6012

Gassman PW, Williams JR, Wang X, Saleh A, Osei E, Hauck LM, Izaurralde RC, Flowers JD (2009) The agricultural policy environmental extender (APEX) model: an emerging tool for landscape and watershed environmental analyses. Trans ASABE 53:09-tr49

Ge Y, Thomasson JA, Sui R (2011) Remote sensing of soil properties in precision agriculture: a review. Front Earth Sci 5(3):229–238. https://doi.org/10.1007/s11707-011-0175-0

Gilhespy SL, Anthony S, Cardenas L, Chadwick D, del Prado A, Li C, Misselbrook T, Rees RM, Salas W, Sanz-Cobena A, Smith P, Tilston EL, Topp CFE, Vetter S, Yeluripati JB (2014) First 20 years of DNDC (DeNitrification DeComposition): model evolution. Ecol Model 292:51–62. https://doi.org/10.1016/j.ecolmodel.2014.09.004

Green W, Ampt G (1911) The flow of air and water through soils. J Agric Sci 4:1–24

Haddaway NR, Hedlund K, Jackson LE, Kätterer T, Lugato E, Thomsen IK, Jørgensen HB, Isberg P-E (2017) How does tillage intensity affect soil organic carbon? A systematic review. Environ Evid 6(1):30. https://doi.org/10.1186/s13750-017-0108-9

Han C, Zhang B, Chen H, Liu Y, Wei Z (2020) Novel approach of upscaling the FAO AquaCrop model into regional scale by using distributed crop parameters derived from remote sensing data. Agric Water Manag 240:106288. https://doi.org/10.1016/j.agwat.2020.106288

Harrington P (2012) Machine learning in action. Simon and Schuster

He Y, Zhou X, Jiang L, Li M, Du Z, Zhou G, Shao J, Wang X, Xu Z, Hosseini Bai S, Wallace H, Xu C (2017) Effects of biochar application on soil greenhouse gas fluxes: a meta-analysis. GCB Bioenergy 9(4):743–755. https://doi.org/10.1111/gcbb.12376

Hénault C, Germon JC (2000) NEMIS, a predictive model of denitrification on the field scale. Eur J Soil Sci 51(2):257–270. https://doi.org/10.1046/j.1365-2389.2000.00314.x

Huang M, Wang C, Qi W, Zhang Z, Xu H (2022) Modelling the integrated strategies of deficit irrigation, nitrogen fertilization, and biochar addition for winter wheat by AquaCrop based on a two-year field study. Field Crop Res 282:108510. https://doi.org/10.1016/j.fcr.2022.108510

IPCC (2001) Climate change 2001: the scientific basis. Contribution of Working Group I to the Third Assessment Report of the Intergovernmental Panel on Climate Change. Cambridge University Press, Cambridge

IPCC (2014) Climate change 2014: impacts, adaptation, and vulnerability. In: Field CB, Barros VR, Dokken DJ, Mach KJ, Mastrandrea MD, Bilir TE, Chatterjee M, Ebi KL, Estrada YO, Genova RC, Girma B, Kissel ES, Levy AN, MacCracken S, Mastrandrea PR, White LL (eds) Part A: global and sectoral aspects. Contribution of Working Group II to the Fifth Assessment Report of the Intergovernmental Panel on Climate Change. Cambridge University Press, Cambridge/ New York

Izaurralde RC, Haugen-Kozyra K, Jans D, Mcgill WB, Grant R, Hiley J (2001) Soil C dynamics: measurement, simulation and site-to-region scale-up. Pacific Northwest National Lab (PNNL), Richland

Izaurralde RC, McGill WB, Williams JR (2012) Chapter 17 – development and application of the EPIC model for carbon cycle, greenhouse gas mitigation, and biofuel studies. In: Liebig MA, Franzluebbers AJ, Follett RF (eds) Managing agricultural greenhouse gases. Academic, San Diego, pp 293–308. https://doi.org/10.1016/B978-0-12-386897-8.00017-6

Jansson C, Faiola C, Wingler A, Zhu X-G, Kravchenko A, de Graaff M-A, Ogden AJ, Handakumbura PP, Werner C, Beckles DM (2021) Crops for carbon farming. Front Plant Sci 12. https://doi.org/10.3389/fpls.2021.636709

Jat ML, Bijay S, Stirling CM, Jat HS, Tetarwal JP, Jat RK, Singh R, Lopez-Ridaura S, Shirsath PB (2018) Chapter four – soil processes and wheat cropping under emerging climate change scenarios in South Asia. In: Sparks DL (ed) Advances in agronomy, vol 148. Academic Press, pp 111–171. https://doi.org/10.1016/bs.agron.2017.11.006

Jones CA (1986) CERES-Maize; a simulation model of maize growth and development. vol 04; SB91. M2, J6

Jones CD, Reddy AD, Jeong J, Williams JR, Hamilton SK, Hussain MZ, Bandaru V, Izaurralde RC (2021) Improved hydrological modeling with APEX and EPIC: model description, testing, and assessment of bioenergy producing landscape scenarios. Environ Model Softw 143:105111. https://doi.org/10.1016/j.envsoft.2021.105111

3 Climate Change and Process-Based Soil Modeling

Jung J, Maeda M, Chang A, Bhandari M, Ashapure A, Landivar-Bowles J (2021) The potential of remote sensing and artificial intelligence as tools to improve the resilience of agriculture production systems. Curr Opin Biotechnol 70:15–22

Kale RV, Sahoo B (2011) Green-Ampt infiltration models for varied field conditions: a revisit. Water Resour Manag 25(14):3505. https://doi.org/10.1007/s11269-011-9868-0

Kaye JP, Quemada M (2017) Using cover crops to mitigate and adapt to climate change. A review. Agron Sustain Dev 37(1):4. https://doi.org/10.1007/s13593-016-0410-x

Kell DB (2011) Breeding crop plants with deep roots: their role in sustainable carbon, nutrient and water sequestration. Ann Bot 108(3):407–418. https://doi.org/10.1093/aob/mcr175

Kelly TD, Foster T (2021) AquaCrop-OSPy: bridging the gap between research and practice in crop-water modeling. Agric Water Manag 254:106976. https://doi.org/10.1016/j.agwat.2021.106976

Kowalska A, Pawlewicz A, Dusza M, Jaskulak M, Grobelak A (2020) Chapter 23 – plant–soil interactions in soil organic carbon sequestration as a restoration tool. In: Prasad MNV, Pietrzykowski M (eds) Climate change and soil interactions. Elsevier, pp 663–688. https://doi.org/10.1016/B978-0-12-818032-7.00023-0

Krauss M, Ruser R, Müller T, Hansen S, Mäder P, Gattinger A (2017) Impact of reduced tillage on greenhouse gas emissions and soil carbon stocks in an organic grass-clover ley – winter wheat cropping sequence. Agric Ecosyst Environ 239:324–333. https://doi.org/10.1016/j.agee.2017.01.029

Kroes J, Van Dam J, Groenendijk P, Hendriks R, Jacobs C (2009) SWAP version 3.2. Theory description and user manual. Alterra

Lal R (2004) Soil carbon sequestration impacts on global climate change and food security. Science 304(5677):1623–1627. https://doi.org/10.1126/science.1097396

Lal R (2005) Climate change, soil carbon dynamics, and global food security. Climate change and global food security. CRC Press, Boca Raton

Lal R (2008) Sequestration of atmospheric CO_2 in global carbon pools. Energy Environ Sci 1(1):86–100. https://doi.org/10.1039/B809492F

Lemaire G, Gastal F (1997) N uptake and distribution in plant canopies. In: Lemaire G (ed) Diagnosis of the nitrogen status in crops. Springer Berlin Heidelberg, Berlin/Heidelberg, pp 3–43. https://doi.org/10.1007/978-3-642-60684-7_1

Li CS (2000) Modeling trace gas emissions from agricultural ecosystems. Nutr Cycl Agroecosyst 58(1):259–276. https://doi.org/10.1023/A:1009859006242

Li C, Frolking S, Frolking TA (1992) A model of nitrous oxide evolution from soil driven by rainfall events: 1. Model structure and sensitivity. J Geophys Res Atmos 97(D9):9759–9776

Li S, Zheng X, Zhang W, Han S, Deng J, Wang K, Wang R, Yao Z, Liu C (2019) Modeling ammonia volatilization following the application of synthetic fertilizers to cultivated uplands with calcareous soils using an improved DNDC biogeochemistry model. Sci Total Environ 660:931–946. https://doi.org/10.1016/j.scitotenv.2018.12.379

Liu C, Cutforth H, Chai Q, Gan Y (2016) Farming tactics to reduce the carbon footprint of crop cultivation in semiarid areas. A review. Agron Sustain Dev 36(4):69. https://doi.org/10.1007/s13593-016-0404-8

Loureiro R, Prado FFD, Riggio G (2019) OMNICROP – an integrated systems alternative to ideal crop site localization and cultivation chamber self-management utilizing machine learning. J Crop Improv 33(1):110–124

Lychuk TE, Moulin AP, Lemke RL, Izaurralde RC, Johnson EN, Olfert OO, Brandt SA (2021) Modelling the effects of climate change, agricultural inputs, cropping diversity, and environment on soil nitrogen and phosphorus: a case study in Saskatchewan, Canada. Agric Water Manag 252:106850. https://doi.org/10.1016/j.agwat.2021.106850

Ma J, Rabin SS, Anthoni P, Bayer AD, Nyawira SS, Olin S, Xia L, Arneth A (2022) Assessing the impacts of agricultural managements on soil carbon stocks, nitrogen loss and crop production – a modelling study in Eastern Africa. Biogeosci Discuss 2022:1–31. https://doi.org/10.5194/bg-2021-352

Maiti SK, Ghosh D (2020) Chapter 24 – plant–soil interactions as a restoration tool. In: Prasad MNV, Pietrzykowski M (eds) Climate change and soil interactions. Elsevier, pp 689–730. https://doi.org/10.1016/B978-0-12-818032-7.00024-2

Mangalassery S, Sjögersten S, Sparkes DL, Sturrock CJ, Craigon J, Mooney SJ (2014) To what extent can zero tillage lead to a reduction in greenhouse gas emissions from temperate soils? Sci Rep 4(1):4586. https://doi.org/10.1038/srep04586

Martin SL, Clarke ML, Othman M, Ramsden SJ, West HM (2015) Biochar-mediated reductions in greenhouse gas emissions from soil amended with anaerobic digestates. Biomass Bioenergy 79: 39–49. https://doi.org/10.1016/j.biombioe.2015.04.030

Martínez-Romero A, López-Urrea R, Montoya F, Pardo JJ, Domínguez A (2021) Optimization of irrigation scheduling for barley crop, combining AquaCrop and MOPECO models to simulate various water-deficit regimes. Agric Water Manag 258:107219. https://doi.org/10.1016/j.agwat.2021.107219

Mattila TJ, Hagelberg E, Söderlund S, Joona J (2022) How farmers approach soil carbon sequestration? Lessons learned from 105 carbon-farming plans. Soil Tillage Res 215:105204. https://doi.org/10.1016/j.still.2021.105204

Mayer A, Hausfather Z, Jones AD, Silver WL (2018) The potential of agricultural land management to contribute to lower global surface temperatures. Sci Adv 4(8):eaaq0932. https://doi.org/10.1126/sciadv.aaq0932

McCann RJ, McFarland MA, Witz J (1991) Near-surface bare soil temperature model for biophysical models. Trans ASAE 34(3):748–0755. https://doi.org/10.13031/2013.31726

Mohanty M, Sinha NK, Somasundaram J, McDermid SS, Patra AK, Singh M, Dwivedi AK, Reddy KS, Rao CS, Prabhakar M, Hati KM, Jha P, Singh RK, Chaudhary RS, Kumar SN, Tripathi P, Dalal RC, Gaydon DS, Chaudhari SK (2020) Soil carbon sequestration potential in a Vertisol in Central India – results from a 43-year long-term experiment and APSIM modeling. Agric Syst 184:102906. https://doi.org/10.1016/j.agsy.2020.102906

Nguyen LTT, Kravchenko AN (2021) Effects of cover crops on soil CO_2 and N_2O emissions across topographically diverse agricultural landscapes in corn-soybean-wheat organic transition. Eur J Agron 122:126189. https://doi.org/10.1016/j.eja.2020.126189

Ngwira AR, Aune JB, Thierfelder C (2014) DSSAT modelling of conservation agriculture maize response to climate change in Malawi. Soil Tillage Res 143:85–94. https://doi.org/10.1016/j.still.2014.05.003

Nimah MN, Hanks RJ (1973) Model for estimating soil water, plant, and atmospheric interrelations: II. Field test of model. Soil Sci Soc Am J 37(4):528–532. https://doi.org/10.2136/sssaj1973.03615995003700040019x

Ogle SM, Alsaker C, Baldock J, Bernoux M, Breidt FJ, McConkey B, Regina K, Vazquez-Amabile GG (2019) Climate and soil characteristics determine where no-till management can store carbon in soils and mitigate greenhouse gas emissions. Sci Rep 9(1):11665. https://doi.org/10.1038/s41598-019-47861-7

Paustian K, Lehmann J, Ogle S, Reay D, Robertson GP, Smith P (2016) Climate-smart soils. Nature 532(7597):49–57

Paustian K, Larson E, Kent J, Marx E, Swan A (2019) Soil C sequestration as a biological negative emission strategy. Front Climate 1. https://doi.org/10.3389/fclim.2019.00008

Pourgholam-Amiji M, Liaghat A, Ghameshlou AN, Khoshravesh M (2021) The evaluation of DRAINMOD-S and AquaCrop models for simulating the salt concentration in soil profiles in areas with a saline and shallow water table. J Hydrol 598:126259. https://doi.org/10.1016/j.jhydrol.2021.126259

Rafique R, Kumar S, Luo Y, Xu X, Li D, Zhang W, Asam Z-u-Z (2014) Estimation of greenhouse gases (N2O, CH4 and CO2) from no-till cropland under increased temperature and altered precipitation regime: a DAYCENT model approach. Glob Planet Chang 118:106–114. https://doi.org/10.1016/j.gloplacha.2014.05.001

Rahimikhoob H, Sohrabi T, Delshad M (2021) Simulating crop response to nitrogen-deficiency stress using the critical nitrogen concentration concept and the AquaCrop semi-quantitative approach. Sci Hortic 285:110194. https://doi.org/10.1016/j.scienta.2021.110194

Rigon JPG, Calonego JC (2020) Soil carbon fluxes and balances of crop rotations under long-term no-till. Carbon Balance Manag 15(1):19. https://doi.org/10.1186/s13021-020-00154-3

Rosenberg NJ, McKenney MS, Easterling WE, Lemon KM (1992) Validation of EPIC model simulations of crop responses to current climate and CO_2 conditions: comparisons with census, expert judgment and experimental plot data. Agric For Meteorol 59(1–2):35–51. https://doi.org/10.1016/0168-1923(92)90085-I

Seligman N, Keulen H (1980) PAPRAN: a simulation model of annual pasture production limited by rainfall and nitrogen. In: Simulation of nitrogen behaviour of soil-plant systems. Pudoc, Wageningen, pp 192–221

Singh S, Negm L, Jeong H, Cooke R, Bhattarai R (2022) Comparison of simulated nitrogen management strategies using DRAINMOD-DSSAT and RZWQM2. Agric Water Manag 266:107597. https://doi.org/10.1016/j.agwat.2022.107597

Smith P, Martino D, Cai Z, Gwary D, Janzen H, Kumar P, McCarl B, Ogle S, O'Mara F, Rice C (2008) Greenhouse gas mitigation in agriculture. Philos Trans R Soc Lond Ser B Biol Sci 363(1492):789–813

Smith W, Grant B, Desjardins R, Worth D, Li C, Boles S, Huffman E (2010) A tool to link agricultural activity data with the DNDC model to estimate GHG emission factors in Canada. Agric Ecosyst Environ 136(3–4):301–309

Spokas KA, Reicosky DC (2009) Impacts of sixteen different biochars on soil greenhouse gas production. Ann Environ Sci 3:4

Srivastava P, Singh R, Tripathi S, Singh P, Singh S, Singh H, Raghubanshi AS, Mishra PK (2017) Soil carbon dynamics under changing climate – a research transition from absolute to relative roles of inorganic nitrogen pools and associated microbial processes: a review. Pedosphere 27(5):792–806. https://doi.org/10.1016/S1002-0160(17)60488-0

Stockle CO, Williams JR, Rosenberg NJ, Jones CA (1992) A method for estimating the direct and climatic effects of rising atmospheric carbon dioxide on growth and yield of crops: part I – modification of the EPIC model for climate change analysis. Agric Syst 38(3):225–238. https://doi.org/10.1016/0308-521X(92)90067-X

Stöckle CO, Donatelli M, Nelson R (2003) CropSyst, a cropping systems simulation model. Eur J Agron 18(3–4):289–307. https://doi.org/10.1016/S1161-0301(02)00109-0

van Diepen CA, Wolf J, van Keulen H, Rappoldt C (1989) WOFOST: a simulation model of crop production. Soil Use Manag 5(1):16–24. https://doi.org/10.1111/j.1475-2743.1989.tb00755.x

Wan Y, Lin E, Xiong W, Ye L, Guo L (2011) Modeling the impact of climate change on soil organic carbon stock in upland soils in the 21st century in China. Agric Ecosyst Environ 141(1):23–31. https://doi.org/10.1016/j.agee.2011.02.004

Williams JR (1990) The erosion-productivity impact calculator (EPIC) model: a case history. Philos Trans Biol Sci 329(1255):421–428. https://doi.org/10.2307/76847

Williams JR (1995) The EPIC model. In: Singh VP (ed) Computer models of watershed hydrology. Water Resources Publications, Colorado, pp 909–1000

Williams JR, Jones CA, Dyke PT (1984) A modeling approach to determining the relationship between erosion and soil productivity. Trans ASAE 27(1):129–144. https://doi.org/10.13031/2013.32748

Williams JR, Jones CA, Kiniry JR, Spanel DA (1989) The EPIC crop growth model. Trans ASAE 32(2):497–511. https://doi.org/10.13031/2013.31032

Wilson D, Blain D, Couwenberg J, Evans C, Murdiyarso D, Page S, Renou-Wilson F, Rieley J, Sirin A, Strack M (2016) Greenhouse gas emission factors associated with rewetting of organic soils. Mires Peat 17:222

Wu H, Yue Q, Guo P, Xu X, Huang X (2022) Improving the AquaCrop model to achieve direct simulation of evapotranspiration under nitrogen stress and joint simulation-optimization of irrigation and fertilizer schedules. Agric Water Manag 266:107599. https://doi.org/10.1016/j.agwat.2022.107599

Yang Y, Reilly EC, Jungers JM, Chen J, Smith TM (2019) Climate benefits of increasing plant diversity in perennial bioenergy crops. One Earth 1(4):434–445. https://doi.org/10.1016/j.oneear.2019.11.011

Zhang Y, Niu H (2016) The development of the DNDC plant growth sub-model and the application of DNDC in agriculture: a review. Agric Ecosyst Environ 230:271–282. https://doi.org/10.1016/j.agee.2016.06.017

Zhao F, Wu Y, Hui J, Sivakumar B, Meng X, Liu S (2021) Projected soil organic carbon loss in response to climate warming and soil water content in a loess watershed. Carbon Balance Manag 16(1):24. https://doi.org/10.1186/s13021-021-00187-2

Chapter 4
Soil Microbes and Climate-Smart Agriculture

Muhammad Nadeem, Rabia Khalid, Sabiha Kanwal, Ghulam Mujtaba, Ghulam Qadir, Mukhtar Ahmed, and Rifat Hayat

Abstract Climate-smart agriculture (CSA) includes approaches that help in reducing climatic extremities and agricultural greenhouse gas (GHG) responsible to global warming. CSA also focuses to balanced and reasonable transformations for agricultural practices. Soil is very diversified due to variations in physical and chemical properties, depending upon the quality and quantity of organic matter, redox potential, and pH status of soil, which also significantly impact the population, growth, and activity of microbes. The microorganism as an arbitrate ensures the sustainable farming by designing effective nutrient cycling strategies and pest control process and minimizing the negative impact of abiotic stress. Therefore, proper managing and development of beneficial microbes can help to achieve sustainable goals and reduce negative effects on the environment. The microbial biofertilizers, biopesticides, and plant growth-promoting rhizosphere bacteria (PGPR) will replace or at least supplement agrochemicals. Soil microbes also provide carbon sinks and help sequester carbon through various processes like the formation of recalcitrant vegetative tissues, bio-products, and different metabolic and biochemical mechanisms that capture CO_2 from the atmosphere; capacity of carbonate sedimentation; and formation of stable soil aggregates, which holds up carbon. Microbes contribute to carbon sequestration by the interactions between the amount of microbial biomass, microbial by-products, its community structure, and soil properties, like clay mineralogy, texture, pore-size distribution, and aggregate dynamics. Soil microbes play a role in climate change through decomposition of organic matter in soil. The diversity and population of soil microorganisms are indirectly influenced by changes in microclimate due to its effects on growth of plant and alignment of vegetation. Soil microbes endorse the sustainability of agriculture and effective operation of agroecosystem through precision agriculture under climate-smart agriculture.

M. Nadeem · R. Khalid · S. Kanwal · G. Mujtaba · R. Hayat (✉)
Institute of Soil and Environmental Sciences, Pir Mehr Ali Shah Arid Agriculture University, Rawalpindi, Pakistan
e-mail: hayat@uaar.edu.pk

G. Qadir · M. Ahmed
Department of Agronomy, PMAS Arid Agriculture University, Rawalpindi, Pakistan

© The Author(s), under exclusive license to Springer Nature Switzerland AG 2022
M. Ahmed (ed.), *Global Agricultural Production: Resilience to Climate Change*,
https://doi.org/10.1007/978-3-031-14973-3_4

Keywords Soil microbes · CAS · Climate change · Precision agriculture · Sustainability

4.1 Introduction

Agriculture is the backbone of Pakistan economy like many other nations around globe. The world population is expecting to be more than 9 billion in 2050, and to feed this growing population, agricultural production system needs to be transformed based on sustainable land management technologies. The basic objective of this transformation would be to increase food production without depleting soil and water resources under changing climate scenarios (Branca et al. 2011). Sustainable agricultural practices lead to reduce gaseous emission and increased carbon sequestration necessary for mitigating climate change. Continuous vulnerabilities in climate, especially changes in temperature, wind, and precipitation pattern, is the cause of uncertainty, risk, and real threat to food security. The modern approach like climate-smart agriculture (CSA) can help to improve the sustainability in the production system by increasing resilience and resource use efficiency (Lipper et al. 2014). Soils are integral to the function of all terrestrial ecosystems and to food and fiber production. Soil microbes are main drivers of different ecosystem processes, and their population and functions determine the sustainable soil productivity, water resources, and gaseous emissions (Wagg et al. 2014). The change in climate, such as elevated atmospheric CO_2 concentration (eCO_2), temperature, and drought, adversely affects the soil microbial activities. The removal of nutrient-rich topsoil through dusty winds also threatens food security. Soil microbes are farmers' allies and can help in dealing the climate challenges faced by agriculture. Soil microbes play a role in fighting against this climate change challenge very effectively and can restore depleted or degraded soil. Soil microbes improve soil health, crop growth, water holding capacity, and carbon sequestration and allow for increased agricultural productivity on existing land. Soil microbes can help crops to tolerate elevated temperature and svere moisture shortage. Crops inoculated with soil microbes have a deeper root system helping to withstand drought and, consequently, accept more water effectively from drying soil. Soil microbes also minimize insect pest deleterious crop diseases and improve the overall crop growth and yield. Soil holds three times more carbon as exists in the atmosphere, and more carbon storage in the soils minimizes greenhouse gas concentrations between 50% and 80% (Paustian et al. 2016).

The terminology climate-smart agriculture (CSA) has established to portray an array of approaches that could facilitate these obstacles by enhancing toughness to climatic extremities, acclimatizing to varying climate, and reducing agricultural greenhouse gas (GHG) that causes global warming. CSA also focuses to augment balanced and reasonable transformations for agricultural practices and employments across balances, varying from small-hold owners to transnational alliances, making an essential fragment of the wider green development plan for agriculture (Braimoh 2013; Palombi and Sessa 2013). Soil is very diversified in the world due to variations in physical and chemical properties (Quesada et al. 2010). The chemical and physical properties of soil depend upon the quality and quantity of organic matter, redox potential, and pH status of soil, which also significantly impact the population, growth, and activity of microbes along with soil productivity (Lombard et al. 2011). Production of food, feed, fiber, and shelter depends upon the agricultural land (Toor and Adnan 2020). In many developing countries, agriculture offers self-employment and is vital for their economic development (Gindling and Newhouse 2014). To meet the need of food, feed, fiber, fuel, and raw material, burden on agricultural soils is increased in recent years due to the heavy increment in the human population. Although the synthetic fertilizers and pesticides are applied to increase the crop growth, they worsen the soil and environment and deteriorate soil organisms (Jacobsen and Hjelmsø 2014). Climate-smart agriculture (CSA) is an approach and addressed to mitigate the issues endeavoring to elevate agriculture production, increase adaptation, and facilitate GHG discharge drops. CSA focuses on emerging agricultural approaches not just to safeguard food security in varying climatic conditions but also to diminish GHG liberations and to ameliorate soil C sequestration (Lipper et al. 2014). Biochar (the C abundant solid produced via biomass pyrolysis) improvement in agriculture lands has been recommended as a tactic to subside climate modification by sequestering C and lessening GHG (specifically N_2O) whereas concurrently enhancing the crop productivity (Woolf et al. 2010; Jiang et al. 2020).

4.2 Soil Microbes and Sustainable Agriculture

Sustainable farming is known as a part of agriculture, which aims on the production of lasting crops and domestic animal despite causing the minimum effect on the environment. In the environment, this type of farming creates a suitable balance between food production demand and protection of ecosystem. The main standard, which ensures the sustainable farming, is the property of soil, in which the role of microorganism is very vital. The key achievements for maintaining sustainability are designing effective nutrient cycling strategies and pest control process and minimizing the negative impact of abiotic stress. Microbial services are acting as an arbitrate in such type of activities; therefore, proper managing and development of beneficial microbes can help to achieve sustainable goals and reduce negative effects on the environment. On the sustainable agriculture, the main impact of agriculture microbiology will be the replacement and addition of the fertilizers and pesticides (agrochemicals) with the microbial preparation. Some of the most common explanations for the use of microorganisms in sustainable farming are biofertilizers, biopesticides, and plant growth-promoting rhizosphere bacteria (PGPR) (Mohanty and Swain 2018).

Biofertilizers are the best tools for sustainable agriculture and considered as a gift from the latest agriculture. Moreover, biofertilizers, being used in agricultural sector, are more efficient and the best substitute to organic fertilizers and manures. Organic fertilizers consist of household wastes, compost, farmyard manure, and green manure, which can help to uphold the quality and sustainability of soil for longer period but not able to cover the instant requirements of crop. Meanwhile, manufactured chemical fertilizers influence the environment like burning of fossil fuels and emission of greenhouse gases (GHGs), which lead to the pollution of soil, air, and water. Furthermore, the constant use of chemical fertilizer for a longer period leads to nutrient imbalance in soil, which also impacts its sustainability. Microbes are also present in biofertilizers, which endorse the adequate availability of primary and secondary nutrients to their host plants and make sure to improve their physiological regulation and structural growth efficiently. In the production of biofertilizers, living microorganisms with specific functions are used to improve plant growth and reproduction. Biofertilizers are an essential element of organic agriculture and perform a key role to maintain the fertility and resilience of plants for long term. Specific microbes are identified and reproduced in vitro that have the ability to absorb nitrogen (N2) directly through the atmosphere, which can be applied in the rhizosphere to make nitrogen available to plants. Such plants or microorganisms containing such materials are knowns as biofertilizers. *Rhizobium*, *Azolla*, *Azospirillum*, *Azotobacter*, and blue-green algae are the frequently used biofertilizers in organic farming (Mohanty and Swain 2018).

Biological pesticides are made of organic components, like bacteria and plants, comprising of minerals that are commonly utilized to fight against disease-causing insects and pathogens. They are classified into microbial pesticides, crop protection agents, and biochemical pesticides. Biopesticides are made up of natural substances that fight with pests through harmless mechanisms. Microbial insecticides, such as *Bacillus thuringiensis*, release toxin A, which paralyzes the insect's midgut and prevents further food intake. Similarly, the spores of *Metarhizium anisopliae* and *Beauveria bassiana* enter the skin/cuticle of the host and releases lethal metabolites, known as destruxin and bovericin, respectively, that lead to insect death. Hence, biological pesticides are intrinsically low in toxicity, only target the relevant host pest, can easily be biodegraded, and have low exposure, because they are effective in lesser amounts. Moreover, they can solve the problem of environmental pollution (Mohanty and Swain 2018). Plant growth-promoting rhizosphere bacteria (PGPR) are found naturally in soil, which improve the productivity and immunity of plant; but these PGPRs are present in the rhizosphere, that is, a soil influenced by the roots of plant and their secretions and exudates. Because of their plant collaboration and interaction, these beneficial rhizobacteria are divided into mutually symbiotic rhizobacteria (living inside the host plant and directly exchanging nutrients and metabolites) and nonsymbiotic bacteria that live freely outside the plant roots (Gray and Smith 2005). In addition, some genera of symbiotic bacteria can physiologically incorporate with plants to make specific root structures. Depending on their working principle, beneficial bacteria are categorized as a biofertilizer, biopesticide, and plant stimulant, and certain bacteria have an overlapping application such as the adhesion of the ACC (1-aminocyclopropane 1-carboxylate) deaminase gene and the availability of phytohormones such as IAA (indoleacetic acid), siderophores on the side, intertorkinin, gibberellin, etc. In this way, they can improve the yield and

4.3 Soil Microbes and Carbon Sequestration

growth of the plant as well as the availability and uptake of nutrients from the several types of crop plants in diverse agroecosystems. Due to multiple uses of growth-promoting bacteria, they become a pivotal part for managing sustainable agricultural systems (Mohanty and Swain 2018).

4.3 Soil Microbes and Carbon Sequestration

In broad terms, carbon sequestration is defined as the elimination, removal, or sequestration carbon dioxide from the atmosphere to moderate or reverse atmospheric CO_2 contamination and to mitigate or reverse climate change. Carbon dioxide (CO_2) is naturally captured from the atmosphere through physical, chemical, and biological processes. While in the agriculture sector, carbon sequestration is defined as the capability of forests and agriculture lands to minimize CO_2 concentration from atmosphere. The removal of CO_2 from the environment is done by its absorbance by means of photosynthesis by crops, plants, and trees and deposition of carbon in foliage, branches, roots, tree trunks, and soil (Schahczenski and Hill 2009).

In general, there are a number of technologies for sequestering carbon from the atmosphere. The main three categories are (i) ocean sequestration, (ii) geologic sequestration, and (iii) terrestrial sequestration. The world's oceans are the primary long-term sink for CO_2 emissions by the anthropogenic activities. Naturally, oceans absorb 2 giga tons of carbon annually through the chemical reactions between seawater and CO_2 in the atmosphere. As a result of these reactions, oceans become more acidic. Numerous marine bodies and ecosystems depend on the formation of sediments and carbonate skeletons, which are vulnerable to dissolution in acidic H_2O. Near the surface, most of the carbon is fixed by photosynthesis of phytoplankton, which are then eaten by sea animals (Sundquist et al. 2008). In geological sequestration, CO_2 is captured from the exhaust of fossil fuel power plants and other major sources, and then, it is supplied through pipes from 1–4 km beneath the Earth's crust layer and incorporated into the formations of porous rock. This type of sequestration is currently utilized for stocking a very lesser amounts of C per year. Many sequestrations are visualized to take advantage of the durability and capacity of geologic storage. Terrestrial sequestration/bio-sequestration is conducted by means of conserving techniques to sequester C in soil and forest that also intensify and enhance its storage (like establishing and restoring forests, wetlands, and grasslands) or reduce CO_2 emissions (like suppressing wildfires and reducing agricultural tillage). These practices are used to meet a variety of land management objectives. Carbon is released in the form of carbon dioxide into the atmosphere by different anthropogenic activities, like the burning of fossil fuels that releases carbon from its long-term geologic storage (such as coal, petroleum, and natural gas). Naturally, CO_2 is emitted through the respiration of living organisms and decomposition of plants and animals. Since the beginning of the industrial era, the amount of carbon dioxide in the atmosphere has increased due to the extensive burning of fossil fuels. CO_2, being a high potential greenhouse gas (GHG), has led to increase the normal temperature of Earth's atmosphere (Klafehn 2019). Carbon sinks are the reservoirs that store carbon and keep it from entering the Earth's atmosphere. For example, afforestation helps in sequestration and capturing of carbon from the atmosphere while C is released into atmosphere through deforestation. Naturally, carbon dioxide present in the atmosphere is sequestered through photosynthesis to the carbon sinks on Earth like plant biomass above soil or inside soils. Other than the plant's natural growth, some terrestrial mechanisms, like cropland management practices, also take part in the atmospheric carbon sequestration. It should be kept in mind that, depending upon the land use, the sequestered carbon in the above-ground vegetation and in soils can be emitted again into the atmosphere.

Microbes also provide carbon sinks and help sequester carbon through various processes like formation of recalcitrant vegetative tissues and bio-products, different metabolic and biochemical mechanisms that capture CO_2 from the atmosphere, capacity of carbonates sedimentation, and formation of stable soil aggregates, which holds up carbon. Microbes contribute to carbon sequestration by the interactions between the amount of microbial biomass, microbial by-products, its community structure, and soil properties, like clay mineralogy, texture, pore-size distribution, and aggregate dynamics. Accumulation of derived organic matter by microbes depends on the balance between decomposition and production of microbial products in the soil. Microbial growth efficiency (the efficiency with which substrates are incorporated into microbial biomass and by-products) is dependent on the (i) degree of protection of microbial biomass in soil structure and (ii) rate of decomposition of by-products by other microorganisms (Six et al. 2006). Microbes adopted different strategies for carbon sequestration like fungal and bacterial dominance (Strickland and Rousk 2010), mycorrhizal association for carbon sequestration (Wright and Upadhyaya 1998), microalgae for CO_2 capture (Buragohain 2019), etc. The bacterial and fungal soils are linked with carbon sequestration potential. If there is a greater number of fungi, then there is a greater C storage (Strickland and Rousk 2010). In the soil, where the microbial community is composed of fungi, the production of microbial biomass and by-products will be larger, because they have higher growth efficiency rates than other microbes like bacteria. Therefore, these communities will retain more carbon in biomass per unit substrate consumed and release less as carbon dioxide. Degradation of microbial-derived organic matter is slower in soils having greater proportion of fungi, as fungal products are chemically resistant to decompose, because of their interactions with clay minerals and soil aggregates (Simpson et al. 2004). The total carbon assimilation increases significantly by mycorrhizal-plant symbiosis. In this association, arbuscular mycorrhiza fungi capture carbon in soil and translocate photosynthetic metabolites present inside the associative plants to the intra-radical of arbuscular mycorrhiza fungi and succeeding extra-radical hyphae, which are then released to the soil medium (Leake et al. 2004). This mycorrhizal association could drain 4–20% of C present in the symbiotic plant to their hyphae and indirectly impact soil carbon sequestration (Graham 2000). The increasing growth and development of fungal extra-radical hyphae within the rhizospheric soil directly enhances the soil carbon sequestration. Soil carbon sequestration by arbuscular mycorrhiza relies upon the turnover time of

4 Soil Microbes and Climate-Smart Agriculture

accumulated biomass of fungal hyphae, the volume of hyphal biomass produced, and the role of fungi to stabilize the formation of soil aggregates (Zhu and Miller 2003). Hyphae produce glomalin protein, which increases the stability of aggregates; this increase in stability leads to larger amounts of protected organic carbon and thereby larger carbon sequestration (Wright and Upadhyaya 1998). Carbon dioxide fixation through microalgae is a favorable and potential technique to sequester CO_2 (Zhao and Su 2014). Microalgae fix and store carbon dioxide through photosynthesis in carbon dioxide and water are transformed into organic assimilates without consuming additional energy having no secondary pollutants. Comparing with the other C capturing and storing methods, fixation of carbon dioxide through microalgae has many benefits, like a rapid growth rate, a high photosynthesis rate (Suali and Sarbatly 2012), efficient adaptability to the environment, and less operational cost. The rate of carbon dioxide fixation through biomass and microalgae production is dependent upon the species of microalgae, soil environment (e.g., pH, light, temperature, and availability and amount of nutrients), and concentration of CO_2. In short, microbes contribute to ecosystem carbon budgets through their roles as pathogens, plant symbionts, or detritivores, thereby influencing the C turnover and modifying the nutrient availability and retention in soil. On decomposition of biomass, carbon losses from the soil due to microbial respiration, while a small proportion of the carbon is retained in the soil by the formation of stable organic matter. Carbon sequestration occurs when SOC levels increase over time as carbon inputs from photosynthesis exceed C losses through soil respiration. Terrestrial ecosystems can be manipulated through land management practices and land use for the development of distinct microbial communities that enhance C sequestration.

4.4 Agricultural Practices and Carbon Sequestration

Vegetative and root systems of grass species and forest trees can store a huge amount of carbon for an extended period; therefore, they are known as sinks for carbon. Agricultural lands can also hold an accountable amount of sequestered carbon; however, their ability to store or sequester carbon depends on climatic conditions, soil and crop or vegetation types, as well as management systems of the cropping land. The total carbon stored in the soil is also affected by the addition of dead plant and animal materials, respiration, and decomposition losses of carbon. However, the carbon losses could be reserved through farming practices through minimal soil disturbance and encouraging carbon sequestration. Overall, there are two distinct trends of the effect of nitrogen fertilization on soil organic carbon fertilizer. On the one hand, nitrogen fertilizer stimulates primary production, resulting in increased above- and below-ground biomass, which can enrich SOC reserves (Chaudhary et al. 2017). Nitrogen fertilization, on the other hand, can promote litter and soil organic matter's biodegradation (Recous et al. 1995). This results in the reduction of SOC stocks (Ladha et al. 2011). Thus, a sufficient supply may be critical for soil carbon sequestration (Van Groenigen et al. 2017). By affecting arbuscular mycorrhizal fungi, phosphorus fertilizers can influence soil carbon sequestration. In contrast to simple nitrogen fertilizers, NPK application inhibits arbuscular mycorrhizal fungi colonization, therefore limiting fungal-mediated nutrient plant absorption, which has a detrimental impact on soil carbon sequestration (Joner 2000; Liu et al. 2020).

Organic additives have numerous effects on SOC pool. Organic fertilization stimulates net primary production, allowing atmospheric carbon to be fixed through photosynthesis (Jacobs et al. 2020; Mathew et al. 2020; Sykes et al. 2020). Source of SOC provide an additional organic alterations for the prevailing pool (Maillard and Angers 2014), and organic fertilization may stimulate SOC biodegradation in the same way that mineral fertilization does (Chenu et al. 2019). When organic fertilizers are used, the outcome is predominantly translation with higher organic carbon intensities at certain sites and lower concentrations at contributing sites (Wiesmeier et al. 2020). Overall, the alternative uses of organic materials are critical, and net appropriation will happen when manures and organic fertilizers are made for a specific farmland field and when C in contemporary fertilizer will then be distributed into the atmosphere (Sykes et al. 2020). Integrating crop wastes into agronomic soils modifies soil structure, decreases bulk density, shrinks erosion, diminishes evaporation, and magnifies the infiltration ratio in soils and in supplement to cumulative SOC stocks (Bronick and Lal 2005; Lehtinen et al. 2014; Spiegel et al. 2018; Trajanov et al. 2019). Straw and hay are exploited for animal suckling or the production of thermal energy in agricultural organization systems. SOC stocks were amended by using deposits (Lehtinen et al. 2014). The carbon impounding influences a fresh equipoise, that is a constant soil organic carbon (SOC) reservoirs in top layer of soil a span after straw is unified (Wang et al. 2018). Numerous crop species and crop alternation are an important module of the natural C cycle, since plants absorb over 10% of atmospheric C production's complete photosynthesis (Raich and Potter 1995). Carbon is consumed via plants, which may be united as biomass, satisfied like root exudes or exhaled back into the atmosphere as CO_2 (Ostle et al. 2003). Maize integrates the atmospheric C more competently than C3 crops like barley, due to its C4 photosynthetic pathway and higher leaf area (Wang et al. 2012). SOC storing is prejudiced by the vegetative cover of agricultural soils and how it is accomplished. Plant biomass delivers the mainstream of organic matter contribution in the topsoil, which reductions as soil depth upsurges (Kaiser and Kalbitz 2012). Varied agricultural spins with several primary crops, cover crops, perennial crops, and forages provide suggestively greater soil organic stocks (SOC) than single cropping systems of monoculture with cereals or maize (Jarecki and Lal 2003; Poeplau and Don 2015). Crop rotational assortment, organic fertilizer/alteration use, and/or perennial farming patterns, all of these can be possible to accrue higher soil organic carbon (SOC) than traditional mono-cropping systems (Don et al. 2018; Minasny et al. 2017).

Root exudations (e.g., organic acids, amino acids, and sugars) from deep delving species and cultivars of crop can transport C into the soil subsurface, where there is a high carbon impounding potential (Sokol et al. 2019), particularly if organic compounds are endangered in organo-mineral aggregates (Paustian et al. 2016). Sunflower (*Helianthus annuus*), alfalfa (*Medicago sativa*), or perennial crops like grass clover, grass, legume, and alfalfa grass amalgamations have deep rooting systems. After the primary crops (e.g., cereals) have been harvested, catch crops are grown or they are undersown in/with the main crops. This consequences in a perpetual vegetative cover on arable land as well as a supplementary period of carbon fascination (Chahal et al. 2020). Traditional tillage practices like plowing eliminate soil aggregates from topsoil, revealing previously endangered SOM to microbial deprivation (Dignac et al. 2017). It also stimulates soil erosion and in lowering SOC stages (De Clercq et al. 2015; Six et al. 2000; Veloso et al. 2019). SOC satisfied in the topsoil (0–10 cm) was originated to be higher in fields refined with no- or reduced-tillage performs than in fields refined with conservative tillage, such as moldboard plowing (Beniston et al. 2015; Francaviglia et al. 2019; Mazzoncini et al. 2016). However, no consequence of tillage practices on SOC accretion was seen as soil depth (>10 cm) increased (Mazzoncini et al. 2016). Soil erosion was allied to the SOC sufferers caused by tillage (Beniston et al. 2015). Besides, lowering mechanical instabilities improves soil health by increasing combined constancy, which decreases erosion (Abid and Lal 2009; Mikha and Rice 2004). By evaluating the complete soil profile (from 0 cm to 60 cm), the impacts of minimal and no-tillage practices on C sequestration are imperfect and inconsequential (Haddaway et al. 2017; Luo et al. 2010; Minasny et al. 2017; Powlson et al. 2014; Sanderman et al. 2009; Spiegel 2012). Biochar is completed by a thermal process of burning organic materials (animal or plant-based) at high temperatures prodigious 350 °C and with a low oxygen source called pyrolysis (Meena et al. 2020). Biochar delivers a long-term carbon sink in soils due to its strong resistance. Biochar treatment is said to boost SOC stocks in agricultural areas (Liu et al. 2016a, b; Maestrini et al. 2015) by cumulative primary output, (Lorenz and Lal 2014) rebellious fractions of SOC, and subsurface SOC pools (Lorenz and Lal 2014; Mao et al. 2012; Rumpel and Kögel-Knabner 2011; Solomon et al. 2012). Moreover, it also can advance soil water retaining, collective stability, soil erosion discount, and soil biota action (Liang et al. 2014; Palansooriya et al. 2019; Schmidt et al. 2014). Agroforestry is the combination of woody perennials like shrubs and trees with grasslands or an agricultural crop. Agroforestry, in all-purpose, assists various roles at the same time, comprising environmental (like better soil fertility and maximized SOC pools) and socioeconomic aids (e.g., increased crop efficiency and to deliver fodder, crops, or timber) (Shi et al. 2018; Sun et al. 2018; Wiesmeier et al. 2020). Deforestation is the loss of forest land for other purposes, such as agricultural crops, growth, or mining processes around the world. Deforestation has impaired the natural ecosystems, the biodiversity, and the climate and has been amplified by human activity since 1960 (Allen and Barnes 1985). Substantial amounts of carbon are stored in forests. As trees and other plants grow, they take carbon dioxide from the atmosphere. This is altered to carbon, which the plant stores in its leaves, trunks, branches, roots, and soil (Gorte and Sheikh 2010). When forests are expurgated or scorched, the carbon that has been deposited is released into the atmosphere, mostly as carbon dioxide. Because trees absorb and store CO_2 throughout their life, deforestation has an important impact on climate change. According to the World Wildlife Fund, tropical forests store more than 210 gigatons of carbon. What's more regarding is that the exclusion of these trees has two major negative consequences (Shukla et al. 1990). To begin with, chopping down trees results in CO_2 emissions into the atmosphere. Additionally, with a smaller number of trees, the general aptitude of planet to capture and sequester CO_2 is abridged. These both processes aggravate the greenhouse gas emission, which contribute to global warming and climate change (Moutinho and Schwartzman 2005).

4.5 Climate Change and Soil Health Indicators

Soil quality consists of active and inherent constituents. Inherent soil qualities, e.g., types of clay, depth to bedrock, and consistency, are difficult to change and take over thousands of years to form as a result of climate changes, such as topography, time, biota, and parent material (Wienhold and Awada 2013). On the other side, dynamic properties of soil quality are established due to human activities and human management practices and can be changed over a brief period. Soil quality comprises physical, chemical, and biological features required to nurture agricultural sustainability and environmental health (Cardoso et al. 2013). Soil is more complex than air and water because it is module part of solid, liquid, and gaseous phases and used in substantial number of variety of determinations assessed for natural ecosystems and efficiency having major focus is on the management biodiversity and environmental quality includes human activities, cultural and geographic heritance. Reaction of soil in comeback to the management practices is slow; thus, it is complex to understand the changes caused in the soil before nonreversible changes. The most significant part for evaluating soil health is the credit of diplomatic soil features that proves the job of soil to work and can be measured as the indicator of soil quality (Nortcliff 2002). The chemical indicators for soil quality evaluation are pH, available phosphorous, and available potassium. The physical indicators include aggregate stability and available water capacity. Biological indicators are represented by organic matter content and active carbon content. Indicators can be restrained from the composite sample of patent sites (Rashidi et al. 2010).

In recent views, soil health assessment is progressively integrated with land evaluation, because its policies are using multiple aspects and for a variety of designs involving sustainable land management. Common management are dependent on long lived land potential conditional on climate, topography and inherent soil properties and can be altered with respect to weather conditions and dynamic soil properties (Herrick et al. 2016). There are three soil indicators, and these are (i) soil physical indicators, (ii) soil chemical indicators, and (iii) soil biological indicators. Physical soil indicators include aggregate stability, porosity, bulk density and texture, and matchup with hydrological processes counting erosion, aeration, runoff, infiltration rate, and water holding capacity. Physical indicators of soil health overall comprise easy, quick, and low budget methods. A soil is reviewed poor in physical aspects when appears having low rates of root density, low aeration, water infiltration, difficulty of mechanization, enhanced surface runoff, and poor cohesion

4 Soil Microbes and Climate-Smart Agriculture

(Dexter 2004). Soil particles with a size of less than 0.2 micron meter are assembled to make aggregates of 20–250 micron meter that are considered as microaggregates, and when these microaggregates cling together, they form macroaggregates. A substantial portion of soil organic matter is composed of carbohydrates that contribute up to 5–25% and is responsible for the stabilization of soil aggregates. Microaggregates have a low organic matter content and are very less disturbed by the microorganisms and more Fe and Al content responsible for the encouragement of microaggregation and, due to micro mass quality, are less disturbed by management practices (Cardoso et al. 2013) Plus, soil organic carbon in microaggregates is less responsive to changes (Zhou et al. 2020) than macro aggregates, which are more vulnerable to management practices and land use and specifically linked to the of the soil organic matter variations. Microbial activity in soil is understood indication toward more organic matter content also dispersion of soil aggregates following land use management practices is low intensive in soils. However, as the organic matter decreased, the accompanying aggregate dispersion lowers soil oxygenation and macroporosity and reduces the interpretation of microbiota causing decomposition and approach to the organic material. Air and water exist in the macro- and micropores of soil particles (Easton and Bock 2016), and soil texture plays a vital role in balancing between water and gases, which become substantial with time and management practices. However, the total porosity and bulk density can demonstrate the consequences of land management and usage on air and water relationships in a better way. Low bulk density of the soil particles are thought to be responsible for boosting up the structure of soil under low anthropogenic assumptions like local forests (Bini et al. 2013). The good amount of the SOM (soil organic matter) is also allowed to play a key role in boosting up the soil structure. In return, it improves soil macroporosity for plant roots, air, and water. The total soil porosity have relationship with texture (proportion of soil particles), and structure (biopores and macrostructure). The structure can easily get damaged by maximum use of land and plowing techniques, due to which distinctive soil water retention curve based on structural pores may change. Cropping methods and intensive management practice alert the structure, which is described as the arrangement of main soil particles (sand, silt, and clay) (Dexter 2004). Organic matter in soil imposes beneficial impact on soil structure in contrast to physical properties, including water infiltration, water retention, bulk density, porosity, and aeration; these are less responsive toward organic matter content. Soil aggregates regulate nutrient cycling, controls aeration and permeability, and acts as a home for soil microbes; as a result, the soil microbes, including microorganisms (bacteria, fungi, and virus), plants, and fauna, affect the soil aggregates. Organic matter (OM) and biological phase are the basic source of water and nutrient supply in soil; as a result, these factors allocate the physical structure of soil and hydrological processes (i.e., erosion, drainage, runoff, and infiltration). As a result, losses of soil function such as synthesis and mineralization of the soil organic matter, as well as consequences on biochemical cycles, may result from the reduction of the soil microbial activity owing to water limits (Bini et al. 2013). Different soil microbes act different on the restriction of water in soil. In the dry soil, water film is more strongly connected with the soil particles due to the restricted movement of bacteria, but, on the other side, in the dry soil, hyphae of fungi can travel in soil pores, which are filled with the air. Availability of the water depends on biological, chemical, and physical characteristics, but these characteristics are influenced by organic matter.

Chemical indicators of soil strength are coordinated with measurement of supplying the nutrients to plants and keeping of chemical elements that cause damages to the ecosystem. The chemical indicators pertaining toward soil strength evaluations are soil CEC, soil OM, soil pH, and nutrients availability (Kelly et al. 2009). Electrical conductivity (EC) and available nutrients in turn favor good crop production, nutrients availability, and microbial activity. Electrical conductivity is defined as the measurement of salt concentration; one of the chemical indicators for measuring soil health can easily be measured due to its very delicate and one-step conductivity measuring instrument. While soil pH is used to detect impact on soil by land use and plowing techniques and eventually climate change will impact on nutrient cycling, organic matter content, carbon cycling, water availability and plant productivity. Although a high amount of OM content also shows adverse impact on the health of soil by reducing the efficiency of pesticides. Electrical conductivity (EC) lets us know the current scenario in biological activity, crop performance, nutrient cycling, and salinity/sodicity in the soil (Arnold et al. 2005). CEC and sorption abilities of soil are important regarding assessment of soil chemical quality the retention of major nutrient cations calcium, magnesium, potassium, and immobilization of potentially toxic cations aluminum, and manganese. These characteristics reveal important signs of soil health, such as the soil ability to absorb nutrients and the presence of pesticides and pollutants (Ross et al. 2008). Due to the hot temperature, decomposition and loss of the soil organic matter will be increased, as a result, the CEC loss of coarse textured/sandy and clay soils with low biological activity, which results in low cation exchange capacity, and soils with low CEC causes poor holding of nutrients and leads to the leaching of nutrients in high rainfall and heavy irrigation applying areas. Nitrogen cycling closely associated with soil organic carbon cycling, consequently operators of change in climate, e.g., hot temperatures, irregular precipitation, and decomposition of atmospheric N cause effect on N cycling and changes the cycling of other plant-available nutrients like phosphorus and sulfur, from direction and exact magnitude of change in plant-available nutrients must be examined in detail. Heavy metals are collected in the soil through chemical and metallurgical industries (Pantelica et al. 2008), and that type of soil will eventually affect plant growth and human health, including adverse effect on soil ecology and agricultural existence of heavy metals in production quality and ground water quality. Concentrations of free metal ions in soil solution are significant to govern because these impact on bio availability to plants which in outcome are achieved by the metal ion speciation in the soil. The free metal ion concentration depends on the total metal content and metal species present in the soil. Irrigation with wastewater increases the amount of heavy metal adulteration in soil, and as there are large amount of heavy metal contaminants in the soil, plants will uptake more heavy metals, depending on the soil types. Other sources of heavy metal gathering are industrial production, mining, transportation, chemical industries, iron, steel industries, agriculture, and domestic activities responsible for the addition of excessive amounts of heavy metals into the water, including both surface and ground water; soils; and the atmosphere. Heavy metal growth in plants is of considerable responsibility because of the chances of food pollution through the soil-root interface. Some heavy metals, like Ni, Cd, and Pb, are not important for plant growth, and they are taken up and accumulated by plants in toxic forms. Soil chemical indicators are directly correlated with the crop production and soil health for higher plants production and sustainability and are quickly interpreted and improved by using fertilizers (Bini et al. 2013). The soil organic carbon is the basic chemical gauge for soil health and yield, as it affects the major functional operations in the soil like the storage of nutrients nitrogen, water holding capacity, stability of aggregates, and microbial activity. The applications of organic alterations in the soil are helpful even in the chemical maintenance of mine soil and the impact of microbial populations present in the adjustments on soil native microbial communities. Sheep and paper supplements are effective at raising the soil pH and decreasing the metal bioavailability and phytotoxicity, whereas poultry and cow dung resulted in greater soil microbial property values, including respiration and functional diversity. Beneficial effects reported under poultry at the start of the research because of the existence of easily degradable organic matter (microbial and chemical) and phytotoxicity to definitively diagnose bottlenecks during amendment selection for chemical stabilization in combination with low metal bioavailability and improved soil health (Galende et al. 2014). N is a required essential in the soil so that plants can accept to fulfill their required needs and is available in different chemical forms like mineral N (especially nitrate) and organic N stored in the soil organic matter. The use of nitrogen for the soil health indicating parameter put through the factors including climatic conditions, turning insufficient the analysis of the real availability for plants, based on soil chemical analysis. After N, phosphorus (P) is also a chief nutrient for crop growth and is essential in defining soil quality that limits the agricultural yields in tropical soils, particularly in highly weathered, oxidic soils, where the main part of the total soil P is fixed in clay minerals and oxides. The available P in the soil solution is found as orthophosphates, but the microbial P and organic P are also stocks that can rapidly become available (Bini et al. 2013).

Soil health pointers concerning biological indicators all needs sufficiently of soil bacteria, fungi and actinomycetes, earthworms, nematodes, protozoa, soil biomass carbon and N and biomass nitrogen. Soil biological indicators call attention to some actions and performances of microorganisms in the soil (Russo et al. 2012). Favorable activities of microorganisms present in the soil include the following: plant nutrients are unconfined from inexplicable inorganic substances; organic residues are decomposed and nutrients are released; beneficial soil humus is composed by breaking down residues that are organic in nature and application of fresh compounds; compounds that increase plant growth are produced; and nutrition of plant is enhanced symbiotically, which leads to the convert nitrogen from atmosphere into the form available to plants. Increasing surface area of roots for absorption of phosphorous; improving soil accumulation by the obligatory agent's production like glomalin and polysaccharides from mycorrhizal fungi and bacteria, respectively;

refining aeration of soil and infiltration of water; having toxic effect against pests and insects and against pathogens of plants weeds; and supporting degradation of pesticides and bioremediation. Soil organic matter indicators turned out to be used in long-time soil conduct experiment for the evaluation of change in climate; however, the reaction of soil organic matter toward elevated temperature is scientifically debatable. It is understood that the increasing temperature improves the decomposition rate of OM, increases the productivity of plant and supply of soil organic matter, as well as improves warmth and precipitation. Carbon dioxide fertilization and deposition of atmospheric nitrogen may promote productivity of plant and supply of organic matter to soil and hence enrich the soil organic matter. According to Kuzyakov and Gavrichkova (2010), the reason for soil organic matter loss is the availability of SOM to microorganisms, despite the rate modification in climate influence like temperature. The microbial biomass of soil is produced by the living portion of the SOM made by the living organisms, including bacteria, algae, fungi, and protozoa, which are the vital source of micronutrients and can be certainly cycled to fulfill the plants' demand. Soil microbial variety performs essential purposes in the sustainability for soil health, considering nutrient and carbon cycles. Microbial indicators are more responsive toward adjustments imposed to the land use and management (Masto et al. 2009). Not only microbial biomass but also soil exhalation has been used on a large scale in agricultural soils as bioindicator of soil health. Modifications in vegetation, including deforestation, reduces the microbial respiration for a long time, because of the low level of organic carbon inputs into the soil through land outer layer or rhizosphere. The less influencing management methods causes higher microbial activity (Babujia et al. 2010). The OM regulates the activity of microorganisms for the source of carbon, nutrients, and energy, which lead to the availability of CO_2 and mineralization, and the rate of mineralization relies on the quantity and quality of SOM. Balance between demands of farmer and needs of community can be fulfilled by healthy soils. Due to the deterioration in soil qualities, soil health is comprised of the complex network functioning as biological, chemical, and physical indicators. Soil organic matter supports to stimulate the soil health, maintain inactivate compounds that are toxic, and destroy pathogens and its implicit interactions between the internal and external soil elements to sustain agriculture. The soil has an ample variety of microbes. Concerning the global expertise of soil microbial dynamics, its function is enhancing rapidly, and the knowledge of rhizosphere complex is constrained to a limit, excluding its value in regulation soil plant systems (Sahu et al. 2017). Soil enzymes including dehydrogenase, urease, protease, phosphatase, and β-glycosidase (Mohammadi 2011) and enzymatic activity work as an indicator to variations occur in the soil plant system as it is nearly mention to the nutrients cycling and biology of soil, can be measured, combine information on the physicochemical status of soil and microbial level and show quick reaction to changes in management of soil (García-Ruiz et al. 2009). By modifying the quality and quantity of underground C input by plants, microbial enzyme activities may be stimulated by elevated CO_2, C change, and plenty of microbial enzymes affecting the function of microbial community in soil on a level. Plus, possibly soil aggregate size has the long-term effect on stimulation of microbial enzyme activities (Dorodnikov et al. 2009). Atmospheric N deposition causes impact on enzymes (extracellular), which are concerned in the processes of soil organic carbon decomposition and nutrient cycling. Soil faunae include the invertebrate community that may live their whole life or half of their life cycle in the soil, as soil fauna has become an important soil health indicator since recent years. Important in processes related to structure of terrestrial ecosystem, disintegration of residues of plants and creating relationships at different degrees with microorganisms. So, their active participation in processes causes effects on the soil properties, considered as great indicators of changes in the soil. OM is decomposed and transformed into various available forms of nutrients, which are conducted by the microorganism and microbial activities. Microbes will work more effectively as the organic matter quantity available to them at large and soil organic matter will be more shattered and spread out along the soil profile. Also, increasing the surface area of contact, earthworms enhance the distribution of organic material in the soil layers vertically or horizontally (Kostina et al. 2011). Higher permanence of soil accumulation has been seen in soil with elevated biomasses of microbes and earthworm. Further, the fauna actions combine particles of soil and generate blocks, tunnels, pores, and other biological chambers that make the movement of water and air, promote the microbial activity, and hence make the soil more accessible for agricultural creations and enhance plant harvests. On the other hand, soils having less activity of fauna reveals more compaction in soil fragments which makes complicated for plant roots for saturation have low accessible water content and less air in the soil triggers poor agricultural construction and have low variety of microbes. Soil fauna can be categorized by the food which they choose to eat, by flexibility, by diversity in their functions, and primarily by size. The most distinctive organisms examined as soil health indicators are members of mesofauna in soil that are present in places between soil macropores and in the soil, litter maintain feeding on organic matter and fungal hyphae and thus take part in process of nutrient cycling and soil accumulation. Some of the experiments have revealed that some species of springtail are good gauges of soil health. The macrofauna comprise bigger soil organisms, consisting of nematodes, proturans, and sauropods feeding on soil microorganisms, decaying plants, and animal materials, which intermittently are active in the soil ecosystem.. Differences in the environment may have different impacts on family, species, or functional group arrangement of the soil faunae. Practical groups as bioindicators have been preferred to use even though of the variety of total species because of the role which they are producing in biological performs. As some species of earthworm are distinct, the organic material accrued on the soil outside, and for that purpose, the activity of the species (individually) was deemed considered restrictive. In fact, in the presence of other functional groups of organisms, they are incompetent to change the role earlier performed by the earthworm species. But the existence or deficiency of some species may be constraining for an ecosystem operating directly influence on the vitality index is considered in evaluations of soil condition.

4.6 Soil Microbe Mitigating Climate Variability

The activity and growth of microorganisms is highly dependent upon the environmental factors, like moisture, temperature, and substrate disposal, and therefore the microbial responses and processes are influenced by climate change. The interests and growth of soil microorganisms may be directly and indirectly influenced by change in climate. The direct effects include change in precipitation pattern, temperature effects, and harsh climatic results, whereas ancillary effects comprise variants due to climate that amends the plant productivity and physicochemical estates of soil. Soil microbes play a key role in climate change through decomposition of organic matter in soil, and ratios of heterotrophic microscopic action stimulate the CO_2 effluence to the atmosphere that will improve global warming. The variety or diversity and population of soil microorganisms are indirectly influenced by changes in microclimate due to its effects on growth of plant and alignment of vegetation. On the first hand, the soil microorganisms are affected indirectly by increasing concentrations of CO_2 in the atmosphere, and in the second phase, there is enhanced photosynthesis and transport of carbon (photosynthate) to mycorrhizal fungi roots (Bardgett et al. 2008; Zak et al. 1993) and microbes that are heterotrophic in nature (Högberg and Read 2006). Because of excess concentration of CO_2, photosynthesis process in plant rises and plant growth may be doubled (Curtis and Wang 1998) that in return encourages the carbon flux in plant roots and microorganisms that are heterotrophic in nature through root exudation of sugars, which degrades it easily (Diaz et al. 1993; Zak et al. 1993). Soil microorganisms may be applied to support adaptation to change in climate by development and growth promotion and improving resistance against various abiotic and biotic stresses. Soil microorganisms take part in the formation of soil; maintain its properties; regulate its fertility, breakdown, and remediation of toxic contaminants; increase sustainable production; and eventually enhance ecosystem sustainability and resilience. Microbes are applied for management of soil health and resilience of ecosystem to lower the demand for production and transportation of synthetic fertilizers. Novel microbes and organic regulating agents can be applied to diminish the damaging influences of novel and advancing pests and pathogens in climate change setting. Frequently found natural managing agents comprise rust fungus *Maravalia cryptostegiae*, applied in country Australia for managing the weed rubber vine and *Neozygites fresenii* (parasitoid) applied for controlling the pest of cotton *Aphis gossypii*. The bacterium *Bacillus thuringiensis* is cast off at field condition, because it produces crystalline toxins, which demolish the *Diptera* and *Lepidoptera larvae*. Beneficial microorganism plant relations can efficiently enhance the growth of plant and increase their resistance to abiotic stresses and deteriorating diseases. Bacteria that are beneficial for plants help in the acquisition of nutrient, secrete PGP (plant growth promoting) hormones, and modify biochemical and physiological characters of the host plant and, so in this way, protect the plant roots from soil-borne deleterious pathogens. Bacterial genera like *Serratia*, *Bacillus*, *Azospirillum*, *Streptomyces*, *Rhizobium*, and *Pseudomonas* reduction in this class. These plant-growth

4 Soil Microbes and Climate-Smart Agriculture

indorsing useful bacteria can be applied for increased growth of plant and improved resistance against disease in altering conditions of climate. According to researches, right strains of mycorrhizal fungi, when inoculated with C4 plant, help against raised levels of CO_2 (Tang et al. 2009). Novel species of *Rhizobia* affiliated with *Medicago sativa* holds the potential to work under several circumstances (abiotic) like high or low pH or temperature, or low concentrations of SOM. The vast unmapped reservoirs of genetic and metabolic diversity of microorganisms offer a marvelous opportunity for the identification of novel genes to control the pest, biodegradation, and N_2-fixation with the help of the latest improved tools like metagenomics.

Soil microorganisms and their metabolism can impact the atmosphere-land carbon exchange cycles in several ways, which can be categorized into diverse groups like those which influence the ecosystem by CO_2 and methane uptake and which also affect the loss of carbon from the soil by respiration. Methane-oxidizing bacteria (MOB) or methanotrophs found in aerobic soils can function as effective biological sink to minimize emissions of methane to the atmosphere. They depend upon CH_4 for energy and carbon. About 15% of the total worldwide CH_4 is contributed by MOBs. They are sensitive to environmental calamities and hard to isolate because of their fixed attachment to soil particles and slow growth rate. A bacterial specie *Methylokorus infernorum*, which is present in geothermal zones in hot and acidic locations, exploits methane CH_4 gas. These bacteria have the ability to use a high amount of methane, which is up to 11 kg year^{-1} and can also be used to reduce emissions of methane from CH_4-producing areas and factories. Moreover, *Methylobacillus* utilize carbon-containing compounds, like methanol, methylated amines, and methane. Additionally, there exist some natural microorganisms, which transform CO_2 into calcium carbonate ($CaCO_3$). Some species of microbes (denitrifying) are accountable to transform nitrous oxide (NO) into nitrogen (N_2) gas. The microorganisms have the propensity to reduce and mitigate emissions of GHGs. The microbial nutrients, gasses, and climate change pathway are explained in Fig. 4.1.

Soil microorganisms improved productivity, influencing the greenhouse gas budget in sense of discharges of greenhouse gas per part food fabrication. The advantage acquired by using the beneficial microorganisms in case of productivity can be thought as a role of microorganism to mitigate the change in climate. The world of microorganisms is very large, and only a very little portion <10% is characterized and identified so far (Bhattacharyya and Jha 2012). Soil microbes sense the biochemical created stimuli and releases the chemicals from their body, which can trigger complex mechanisms of plant defenses (Glick 2012). They effectively contribute in utilizing the greenhouse gases like N_2O, CH_4, CO_2, and nitric oxide (Bardgett et al. 2008). Microbes are essential for crop protection by promoting the capacity of disease resistance in plants opposed to the damaging pathogens and exposing destructive structures or auxiliary as biological elicitors against several biological and ecological influences. The fungi among microorganisms have the ability to colonize the external parts of plants and offer protection from several living and nonliving agents like pathogens, pests and insects attack, heat, and drought (Singh et al. 2011). Usage of microbial biofertilizer in agriculture system is

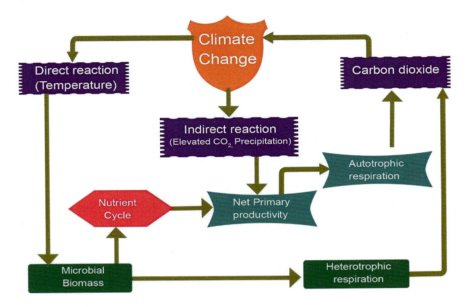

Fig. 4.1 The microbial nutrients, gasses, and climate change pathway. (Dutta and Dutta 2016)

not yet so common because of the problems of identification and tracking of inoculated strains and uncertainty of results. Nowadays, the application of microbial biotechnology is very important in sustainable agricultural development. Conserving the microorganism diversity is vital to maintain the species variety of higher living organisms and strategies for nutrient management and disease of plants (Colwell and Munneke 1997). Changes in climate encourage modification processes in the microorganisms and plants (Grover et al. 2011) and therefore alter the efficiency of microbe-plant linkages. The concept of microclimate difference-microbe response and potential negative and encouraging position of microorganisms in worldwide environment difference is important to use them for changes in climate improvement and variation.

The three main factors affecting climate modification consist of natural, human, and atmospheric influence. The sun radiates solar energy that affects the planet and raises temperature; and rising temperatures cause global warming (Lean 1991). Improved amounts of human-generated glasshouse gases reason much more warming than current fluctuations in solar action. Satellites have been observing the sun's energy harvest for more than 40 years, and it has oscillated by less than 0.1%. The life on Earth exists due to the sun, which keeps its temperature warm and makes the conditions favorable for the survival of humans. It also influences Earth's atmosphere. However, the contemporary warming has been far too swift to be credited to the changes in Earth's orbit and far too huge to be caused by the solar endeavor (Assessment 2018). In a single solar cycle, which is of 11 years, the sun

4 Soil Microbes and Climate-Smart Agriculture

never brightens the same way it brightens and dims slightly. The sun undergoes various changes in activity and looks over each cycle. The level of the radiations coming from the sun changes, as does the quantity of material discharged into space by the sun, as well as the volume or size and number of solar flares and sunspots. Long- and short-term disparities in solar activity play only a minor effect on Earth's climate. Warming caused by the rising amounts of human-produced greenhouse gases is many times more commanding than any effects caused by the recent vagaries in solar activity. Satellites have been tracing the sun's energy output for more than 40 years, and it has been altered by less than 0.1% over that time. Since 1750, the warming produced by greenhouse gases unconfined by human use of fossil fuels has been more than 50 times more than the small extra warming caused by the sun (Birat 2021). Global climate change has been linked to huge volcanic explosions (Altman et al. 2021). Volcanic explosions have two major effects on the climate. First, they radiate the greenhouse gas carbon dioxide, which promotes global warming. However, the influence is negligible. Volcanic emissions have been projected to be at least 100 times lower than those from fossil fuel incineration since 1750 (Wilson 2021). Climate change is influenced by volcanoes. Massive quantity of volcanic gas, drips of aerosol, and ash are inserted into the stratosphere layer during a huge explosive outbreak. Although volcanic gases such as SO_2 can provide a cooling effect globally, on the other hand, volcanic gas like carbon dioxide, which is a greenhouse gas, has the ability to raise the temperature of the globe (Sigurdsson et al. 2015).

Climate alteration and air pollution have an intricate relationship. Pollutants, such as ozone O_3 and black carbon, raise the Earth temperature by entrapping the heat in the atmosphere, while others like SO_2 that form light-indicating elements cool the temperature (Stern 1977). Sustained decrease in air pollution and GHG emissions are dangerous because they cause significant health and ecological hazards around the world. Air property and climate lineups can be an advantage to one another: change in climate vindication enterprises can help decrease pollution of air, while policies related to clean air can help reduce greenhouse gas emissions, resulting in lower global warming. If decrease in a specific emission of pollutant results in increased atmospheric temperature rather than cooling, there may be trade-offs (Seinfeld and Pandis 2016). All through complex interactions in the environment, difference in climate, and pollution in air influence each other. raising levels of greenhouse gases interrupt the balance of energy between the atmosphere and the surface of Earth, which results in temperature changes that alter the atmosphere's chemical makeup. This balance of energy can also be influenced by direct emissions of air pollutants, for example, black carbon or those pollutants formed from emissions like sulfate and ozone. As a result, climate change and air pollution organizations have common impacts (Paoletti et al. 2007). The less gasoline we burn up, the better we are at decreasing air pollution and the dangerous effects of climate change. Make wise shipping verdicts. Walk, ride a bike, or operate public transportation wherever possible. Buying food in the vicinity decreases the quantity of fossil fuels need to transport or fly food across the country and possibly most prominently, "Support leaders who promoter for clean air and water, as well as accountable climate change action" (Mackenzie 2016). Water vaporization is the most plentiful GHG, but it also functions as a climate response. As the temperature of Earth increases, degree of water vapors increases, but, as a result, chances of clouds and rainfall also increase, making these two response mechanisms important to the greenhouse effect. CO_2 levels in the atmosphere raised from 280 ppm to 414 ppm in the last 150 years, due to the industries that underlie our modern society. Generated greenhouse gases, such as carbon dioxide, methane, and nitrous oxide, are produced by humans, likely to be responsible for much of the rise in Earth's temperature during the past 50 years (Oreskes 2004; Karl et al. 2009). Increase temperatures result in higher evaporation costs, since the amount of energy required for evaporation decreases as the temperature rises. In a sunny, warm weather, water loss is increased due the high evaporation as compared to depressing and cool weather. As a result, when the weather is bright, hot, dry, and windy, evaporation rates are higher. Due to the water vapor functioning as a greenhouse gas in the atmosphere, evaporation might have a warm effect on the global climate. Increases in the evaporation intensity tend to induce clouds to develop low in the atmosphere, which function as a signal that the sun's warming rays are being reflected back into the space (Spracklen et al. 2018).

The emissions of greenhouse gas have a wide range of environmental and physical condition inferences. They contribute to respirational ailments due to air pollution and smog, along with triggering environmental difference through confining the heat up. Other consequences of climate change produced by greenhouse gases include extreme weather, food supply shortages, and more wildfires (Nunez 2019). Carbon dioxide is a minor but vital component of the environment. Ecological practices like respiration and volcano explosions emit carbon dioxide, as do human endeavors like deforestation, land use changes, and fossil fuels burning are only a few examples. Human has raised CO_2 level in the atmosphere by 47% since the beginning of the industrial revolution, which is the most significant long-term "forcing" of climate change (Fig. 4.2).

4.7   Climate-Smart Agriculture

Soil health is indispensable for creating more climate flexible agricultural systems, and it may be enhanced through an assortment of climate-smart agriculture (CSA) advances. Climate-smart agriculture (CSA) has been suggested as a general attempt to establishing agricultural practices to ensure long-term food insurance in the face of climate alteration (Palombi and Sessa 2013). One of CSA's pivotal goals is to minimize the emission of greenhouse gases while also enhancing the soil carbon appropriation and soil physical condition (Campbell et al. 2014; Lipper et al. 2014). Increasing the carbon consequences while lowering the carbon outputs is the key to distinguish more carbon in soils. Adding cover crops to the crop rotation, utilizing biochar to soils, and decreasing soil tillage are all often recommended ways for SOC

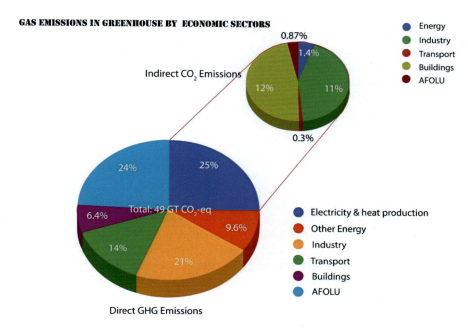

Fig. 4.2 The greenhouse gasses that affect climate change. (FAOSTAT 2022)

sequestration (i.e., conservation tillage). These administration tactics have been used in important agricultural zones around the world in the latest decades, developing in an enormous number of examinations and statistics (Chen et al. 2009; Clark et al. 2017). Encouraging effects of CSA regulating methods on SOC appropriation have been described by several processes. Conservation tillage, for instance, minimizes the organic matter rate in the soil and also minimizes the soil disturbance (Salinas-Garcia et al. 1997) and stimulates earthworm and mycological biomass (Fragoso et al. 1999; Briones and Schmidt 2017), thereby advancing SOC stability (Wang et al. 2021). Cover crop boosts carbon and nitrogen inputs, improving the agroecosystem biodiversity, and offers extra biomass inputs from above- and below-ground (Blanco-Canqui et al. 2011) (Lal 2004). Furthermore, cover crop can increase soil aggregation and structure (Sainju et al. 2003), reducing carbon loss from soil erosion indirectly (De Baets et al. 2011). Biochar alterations prejudiced the soil organic carbon diminuendos 2 ways: (1) enhancing soil combination and physical protection of aggregate related with soil organic matter from microorganisms attack; and (2) increasing the pool of intractable organic material, resultant in a low soil organic matter putrefaction amount and significant adverse priming (Du et al. 2017; Weng et al. 2017; Zhang et al. 2012). Even though these climate-smart agriculture governing techniques have been commonly utilized to improve the soil physical condition (Denef et al. 2007; Fungo et al. 2017; Thomsen and Christensen 2004; Weng et al. 2017), their effects on CO_2 sequestration change over time and are highly dependent on experiment design and site-specific factors, including climate and soil condition (Abdalla et al. 2016; Liu et al. 2016a, b; Paustian et al. 2016; Vickers 2017). The aptitude of CSA methods to sequester soil carbon differs widely. Some research has also claimed that CSA management techniques have a negative impact on SOC (Liang et al. 2007) (Tian et al. 2005). Most mathematical exploration intensive on the impacts of a single climate-smart agriculture practice on soil organic carbon (Abdalla et al. 2016; Liu et al. 2016a, b; Vickers 2017) and very few studies estimated the joint effects of varied CSA and conventional management practices. A combination of cover harvest and preharvest tillage, according to several recent research, may dramatically improve SOC when compared to a single management strategy. When no-tillage and cover crop practice were combined, soil carbon sequestration increased by 0.267 Mg C ha^{-1} year^{-1}, with the latter being a varied culture of hairy vetch (*Vicia villoma*) and rye (*Secale cereale*); when only no tillage was used, soil carbon sequestration decreased by 0.967 Mg C ha^{-1} year^{-1} (Ashworth et al. 2014; Blanco-Canqui et al. 2013; Duval et al. 2016; Sheehy et al. 2015). When biochar was added to conservation tillage, Agegnehu et al. (2016) found that 1.58% and 0.25% more of SOC were sequestered in the midway and end season, respectively, under conservation tillage.

Climate-smart agriculture (CSA) is emerging progressively more popular as a solution in many nations. CSA is a comprehensive approach to landscape organization that improves productivity, improves flexibility, and lowers greenhouse gas emissions. The World Bank, as one of the major agricultural financiers, assists countries in their attempts to scale-up climate-smart agriculture. Climate-smart agriculture (CSA) is a management strategy for farmers in the face of climate change. The CSA wants to advance internationally relevant agriculture management practices for food security. The concept was initially introduced in 2009, and it has since grown based on feedback and interactions from a variety of stakeholders. The CSA strategy was established in response to arguments and disputes in environmental change and agricultural policies for long-term development (Lipper et al. 2017). Enhancement in mitigation by decreasing GHGs is an important CSA goal and a key to long-term efficient climate change adaptation; therefore, it comprises inventions and implementation of cultural techniques, varieties of crop, managing techniques, and organizations that will speed up improvement. Transitioning to no- or small tillage methods has already been recognized as a significant resource of carbon sequestration, and implementing more varieties of yields and conservation practices that decrease agriculture's land, ecological, and nonrenewable fuel resources is an additional significant reduction policy (Lal 2011; McCarthy et al. 2012). Climate-smart agriculture may work as an agent for developing resistance, better modification, and adaptation approaches within sociobiological structure (Steenwerth et al. 2014) (Fig. 4.3).

Precision agriculture is one such implement that is useful in making an agriculture more "climate savvy" by minimizing its environmental influence. Thus, precision agriculture is an intensive system that entails the usage of a world aligning system, several instruments for observing soil moisture content, nutrients availability, and geo reference map for various soil characteristics, but when implemented on a huge scale, it can support to increase productivity, reduce resource ingesting, and reduce ecological impact. Precision agriculture is a contemporary day climate-smart

4 Soil Microbes and Climate-Smart Agriculture

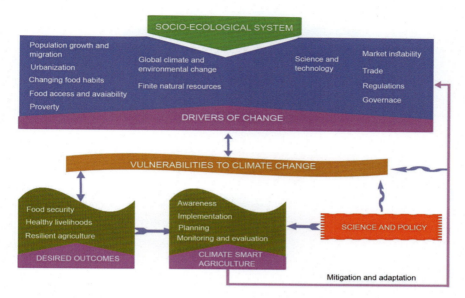

Fig. 4.3 Climate-smart agriculture for improving resilience, better mitigation, and adaptation. (Steenwerth et al. 2014)

agricultural technique that has the potential to address the food problems insecurity in poor nations and combine as a strong instrument and solution to the agriculture sector's numerous challenges (Roy 2020). The practice of "no-till farming," which avoids soil manipulation for crop production, is one approach to sequester carbon. No-till farming has numerous potential benefits for gardeners, farmers, and the environment when combined with cover cropping. The combination of no-till farming and cover cropping is always found suitable for increasing organic matter. Through this way, a shield is created over the soil to protect it during the driest times as well as a sponge in the soil to protect it during heavy rains. So, while the two activities combined generate organic matter and store carbon in the soil, they also offer additional advantages. Because all that organic waste is now decomposing, they give nutrients to the food. There are numerous environmental advantages to no-till farming. It increases carbon sequestration in the soil and reduces fossil fuel use in farm activities. The quantity of nutrients that the soil can contain increases as soil organic carbon levels rise, implying less petroleum-based fertilizers and runoff into nearby water bodies. Farmers would benefit from the method in the event of harsh weather, such as drought, because soil rich in soil organic matter absorbs water better than tilled ground. Agricultural practices in poor nations frequently result in poor soil quality. Climate change-related extreme weather may exacerbate the problem, unless better agronomic techniques are implemented. The goal of soil and land management must be to enhance yield while preserving soil and water resources. It also intends to sequester carbon. Organic fertilization, least soil disruption, residue absorption, terraces, water gathering, preservation, and agroforestry are all illustrations of this administration (Branca et al. 2013), but there are several

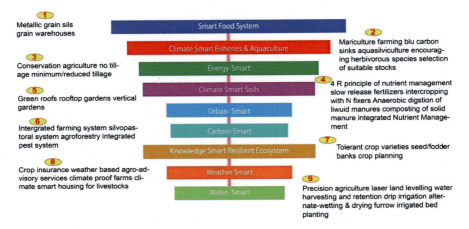

Fig. 4.4 Climate-smart agriculture technologies. (Adopted from Source: Khatri-Chhetri et al. 2017)

prospects for improving new management methods and improving existing ones to adjust spatial and climatic erraticism.

All agroecosystems require climate-smart agriculture (CSA) equipment, methods, and help. These approaches can help to improve agriculture, protect it from climate change, and ensure food security. The biophysical environment, farmer socioeconomic traits, and the benefits of CSA technology all play a role in CSA adoption (Khatri-Chhetri et al. 2017) (Fig. 4.4).

For countries that rely on agriculture for subsistence, CSA technologies provide at least two benefits in terms of production, resilience, and mitigation, with productivity being the most important. Metrics nested under these broad CSA categories can be used to track progress against a realistic baseline. For example, improved productivity could be assessed in terms of yields, income, or internal rate of return. CSA aspires to maximize synergies and minimize trade-offs across all of its pillars (Rosenstock et al. 2016). While boosting food security, CSA technologies manage climate- or weather-related risk. Extreme occurrences (such as floods) as well as slow-onset threats may be considered (such as delayed onset of seasonal rains). CSA technology should assist in mitigating the effects of these risks in the short term (by increasing the amount of production per farm, hectare, season, etc.) as well as in the long run (by increasing the amount of production per farm, hectare, season, and so on and decreasing the variability in production over time, despite climate change).

4.8 Soil Microbes and Global Agriculture

Food security becomes a major challenge in the twenty-first century in response to the increase in demand of sufficient food with respect to population rate. Nowadays, the other main factor influencing food security is climate change (Alamgir et al.

2020; Borrill et al. 2019). The alteration in environment, such as extreme temperatures and fluctuation in rainfall intensity, becomes a global aspect that concerns agricultural production (Abberton et al. 2016; Milus et al. 2009). These alterations have high impact on soil, microbiota, agricultural output, and global food security (Adger et al. 2009; Hill et al. 2009; Nelson et al. 2009; Campbell et al. 2016; Durán et al. 2016). As per contemplates, the normal world temperature has risen, and freshwater supplies will be fundamentally decreased before the end of the twenty-first century. Varieties in snowfall and territorial precipitation have additionally been noticed, and these variations are required to deteriorate in the coming days (Misra 2014; Reidsma and Ewert 2008; Reidsma et al. 2010; Stocker et al. 2013). Climate is fundamentally affected by farming. Farming emanates enormous volume of ozone-harming substances, i.e., GHGs like CO_2, CH_4, N_2O, and corona carbons into the environment, where they assume a critical part in ingest sun-powered energy (Valizadeh et al. 2014). Farming is responsible for an expected 17–32% of all worldwide greenhouse gas emanations (Cotter and Tirado 2008). Agribusiness can lessen GHG discharges and ease environmental change. While certain harvests may profit with environmental change in certain areas, expanding temperatures may in the long run lower rural yields on a worldwide scale, especially in dry and hot areas (Smith and Gregory 2013; Valizadeh et al. 2014). Moreover, extreme temperatures have increased weed and creepy crawly attacks, bringing about lower farming yields (Nelson et al. 2009; Reidsma and Ewert 2008). Without a debate, the combined impacts of environmental change on agribusiness are negative, representing a risk to worldwide horticultural creation and, thus, imperiling sanitation (Glenn et al. 2013; Malhotra 2017).

Farming usefulness is associated with conditions both straightforwardly and by implication, through giving and related cycles; environmental change will put a strain on this fragile equilibrium (Altieri et al. 2015; Smith and Gregory 2013). In spite of the fact that environmental change will impact our overall ability to get food, it is plausible that underestimated individuals in nonindustrial countries would be the most exceedingly awful hit (Sanchez and Stern 2016). It is clear that future requirements for food and environment administrations will require more extreme changes underway, utilizations, and strategies (Davidson 2016). CO_2 and other fellow gases are growing, and these additions will in the end affect the world's environment (Ortiz-Bobea 2021). Plant constructions and thus crop productions are prejudiced by various organic parts, and these components similar to suddenness and temperature may act either synergistically or ridiculously with various variable quantities in selecting yields (Yevessé 2021). Controlled field preludes can make information on how the yield of a specific gather arrangement responds to a given lift, like water or fertilizer. Nevertheless, by their disposition, such controlled tests consider only a confined extent of biological factors (Jiang et al. 2021). An elective method to manage and check out crop yield (changes) is the use of gather biophysical diversion models that introduce limits drawn from crop tests (Gurgel et al. 2021). Since natural change is likely to cut across a huge gathering of living components, such collect proliferation models give the most quantitative examinations of changes in ecology impacts on crop yields (Manzoor et al. 2021). However, the usage of gather reenactment models makes the examination of climate impacts over an area of yields logical; these kinds of models furthermore have limits, counting the separation from the grouping of components and state that impact creation in the field (Lal 2021). feasible ecological circumstances that changes, consolidate increased temperatures, variations in rainfall or snowfall, and increased air CO_2 obsessions. Regardless of the way that temperature additions can have both positive and antagonistic outcomes on crop yields, with everything taken into account, temperature increases have been found to diminish yields and nature of various harvests (Avagyan 2021).

A climate with greater CO_2 intensity would achieve higher net photosynthetic values (Horton et al. 2021). Higher centers may equally reduce arising (water disaster) as plants decline their stomata holes, the little cavities in the leaves through which CO_2 and water seethe are replaced with the air (Ortiz et al. 2021). The net change in crop yields is limited by the affability between these negative and positive direct ramifications for plant improvement and progress and by deceitful effects that can impact creation. These inadvertent effects have been usually disregarded in the examination of ecological change impacts (Zougmoré et al. 2021). Typical effects may rise up out of changes in the event and course of vermin and microorganisms, extended speeds of soil crashing down and defilement, and increased troposphere ozone levels in view of rising temperatures (Kehler et al. 2021). Extra deceitful effects may rise up out of changes in overflow and groundwater re-invigorate rates, which impact water supplies, and changes in capital or mechanical supplies, for instance, surface water accumulating and water support practices (Koutsoyiannis 2021) (Fig. 4.5).

Fig. 4.5 Soil microbial response to climate change. (Jansson and Hofmockel 2020)

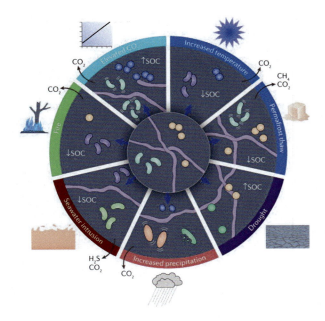

Naturally, more than 90 billion bacteria are preset in one-gram soil that promotes the plat growth by making the unavailable nutrients in the available form for plant uptake. Nowadays, the biotic stress is a big challenge for agriculture due to day-by-day increase in the world population, which causes increase in food demands. The use of chemical means of nutrients increases the crop production, but it also deteriorates the environment causing a reduction in soil fertility and plan growth (Armstrong and Taylor 2014). For agricultural production, the health of soil is very important, which depends on different reactions, such as chemical, biological, and physical, collaborated by microorganisms. The beneficial microorganisms are group of naturally occurring microorganisms, like plant growth-promoting rhizobacteria, fermenting fungi, actinomycetes, yeast, lactic acid bacteria, etc. These microorganisms play a very important role in improving the soil structure and soil fertility, suppressing soil-borne pathogen, fixing nitrogen, increasing the decomposition of organic matter, and enhancing the level of nutrients and of plant strength and ultimately crop yield (Joshi et al. 2019).

Soil microorganism is involved in different biogeochemical cycling of all major (N, P, K, S, etc.) and minor nutrients (Fe, Mn, Co, B, Zn, etc.) required for crop growth and other life (Jansson and Hofmockel 2020). The impact of climate change on soil microbes in different climate-sensitive soil ecosystem is illustrated in Fig. 4.1 (Dutaa and Dutta 2016). Mycorrhizal fungi and bacteria that live near the roots offer numerous advantages to the host plant, including faster growth, enhanced nutrition, better drought resistance, and defense against pathogens. Mycorrhizal fungi are broadly characterized into two groups. The first one is vesicular arbuscular mycorrhizas (VAM or AM) and the second is eco-mycorrhizas (EM), which differ extensively in structure and function. The structures produce by VAM within the roots of plants are known as arbuscules and vesicles, which participate in the transfer process of nutrients. This symbiotic relation benefits the host plants directly, through the solubilization of phosphate and other mineral nutrients from the soil by the fungus, while the fungus obtains a carbon source from the host plants. The symbiosis also improves the resistance of plants to biotic and abiotic stresses. Ectomycorrhizas (EM) frequently produce large aboveground fruiting bodies like that of a mushroom and toadstool as well as a hyphal net around the root of plant. Vesicles and arbuscules are absent, and the hyphal penetration of the root is incomplete. EM fungi are amenable to axenic culture. Potential inoculum can also be produced in the field from mycelium (Harrier 2001; Thomson et al. 1994). The soil microorganisms play a vital role in soil health and sustainability. The density and diversity of microorganisms' population indirectly depend on the level of organic matter, because it provides energy for soil microorganisms and improves the structure, stability, and moisture of the soil and plant nutrient availability and stops the occurrence of soil-borne disease (Zhang et al. 2007).

4.9 Microbial Contribution in Climate-Smart Agriculture

Worldwide, agriculture participate in and is an agriculture both promotes to and is endangered by climate change over. Corresponding to the account of IPCC, agriculture brings part in 58% and 47% of the total anthropogenetic constructions of N_2O and CH_4, respectively. Agriculture is previously facing the severe impacts of climate adjustment (Lobell et al. 2011), and consequently, the food production is also being affected directly and indirectly by it. Fluctuations in rainfall pattern, upsurge in mean temperature, and intensification in occurrence of intense climatic effects, like scarcity, floods, and cyclones, will highly affect the agriculture (Lee 2007). The growth of population in the world is forecasted up to one third by 2050, and most of the people (about 2 billion). The world's residents are expected to improve by one third by 2050, and most of the added two billion people will survive in improving states (Boettcher et al. 2015). With the aim to fulfill the constraints of food and feeding, agricultural production is predicted to grow by 60%. It is a big challenge for the upcoming food security, as the resources required to maintain the present agricultural growth are already being endangered. Furthermore, worldwide agriculture is already being harmfully impacted by global climate change, and climatic hazards to livestock, fisheries, and cropping are predicted to rise in the coming years. In the period of such rapid change in climate, alteration and redirection of agricultural production led to the strategy of climate-smart agriculture (CSA). Microorganisms are vital members of the soil-plant ecosystem, and simply no food production is possible without them. Microorganisms perform a vital role in the cycling of plant nutrients in the system of microbe plant soil and atmosphere. Microbes are crucial to nitrogen and carbon cycles and take part in the consumption and production of greenhouse gases (GHGs), like nitrous oxide, methane, and carbon dioxide. A vast diversity of microorganisms offers an unexploited way to improve the quality and quantity of agricultural products, leading to adaptation and mitigation of changing climate outcomes, thus helping to attain the target of climate-smart agriculture. The microbes that cause diseases to insect pest and weeds are utilized as biopesticides. There are many microbes in the soil, which promote plant growth through various biocontrol mechanisms. The free-living soil microbes help to maintain the soil structure, carbon sequestration, and nutrient storage and availability (Das et al. 2019).

Microbe variety in soil enhances the numerous mechanisms that are a vital part of biogeochemical cycles and henceforward promotes and maintains a lot of agroecosystem's biochemical reactions, such as decomposition of organic matter, nutrient availability to plants, and overall productivity of plant and soil. Many times, the microorganisms make associations, and many limiting resources are made available to plants by them. Furthermore, the host-specific microorganisms like mycorrhiza and N_2 fixers also make available limited and fixed plant nutrients to enhance plant growth. Consequently, microbes endorse the sustainability of agriculture and effective operation of agroecosystem (Das et al. 2019) (Fig. 4.6).

4 Soil Microbes and Climate-Smart Agriculture

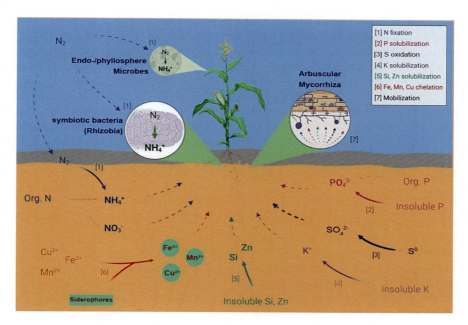

Fig. 4.6 Microbial-mediated nutrient transformation pathway. (Mitter et al. 2021)

The process in which complex organic biopolymers present in the dead remains, and residues of animals and plants are broken down into simpler inorganic and organic monomers through various biochemical reactions, referred to as organic matter decomposition (Juma 1998). During this microbial process of organic matter decomposition, nutrients and energy are recycled, and the surplus plant nutrients, like N, S, and P, are added to the soil in the plant-available form; this transformation is known as mineralization. Hence, in this way, microbes are crucial for the availability of essential plant nutrients and necessary inorganic compounds in the soil through the processes of nutrient recycling, by decomposing the plant residues and dead bodies of animals (Das et al. 2019). Fixation of atmospheric elemental nitrogen (N_2) into plant-available forms is one of the most important biochemical reactions that is highly essential and beneficial for global agricultural sustainability and efficient ecosystem functioning. Worldwide, the annual incorporation of the fixed nitrogen through symbiosis between rhizobia and legume is assessed to be 18.5 million tones and 2.95 million tones for oilseed legumes and pulses, respectively (Howieson et al. 2005). However, the symbiotic bacteria nodulating the legume crops belong to the genera *Brady rhizobium*, *Ensifer*, *Rhizobium*, and *Mesorhizobium* that are conscientious of about 80% N accumulation in grains, causing high nutrition and profit. The bacteria, which live freely and do not form a symbiotic relation with the host crop, are known as free-living N_2-fixing bacteria. Some of them are *Azospirillum*, present in temperate region cereal-growing soils; Beijerinckia, associated with sugarcane in tropical areas; and *Azotobacter*, prominent for N2 fixation in rice growing soil and also used as a biofertilizer for tobacco, tea, coffee, coconuts beetroot, sunflowers, oat, barley, maize, and wheat crops. Moreover, the species that belongs to the genera *Herbaspirillum*, *Gluconacetobacter*, and *Azospirillum* are endophytes of sugarcane and provide nitrogen to the crop. *Azorhizobium* strains that fix the N2 are isolated from the rhizosphere of wheat crop, while *Bradyrhizobium* and *Rhizobium* are from the roots of paddy. Additionally, there are specific diazotrophic bacteria that form a true beneficial mutualism (symbiosis) with some host plants by forming the nodules with its roots (García-Fraile et al. 2015). Phosphorus solubilizing microorganisms (PSMs) release the plant unavailable inorganic and organic soil phosphorus through mechanisms like solubilization and mineralization and make P available to crop plants, thus playing a vital role in soil fertility (Sharma et al. 2013; Walpola and Yoon 2012). In the P-deficient soils, a diversified variety of PSMs like fungi (*Penicillium* and *Aspergillus*) and bacteria (*Bacillus*, *Pseudomonas*, and *Actinomycetes*) can be inoculated in the soil to increase the P availability, through their mineralizing and solubilizing capability (Gyaneshwar et al. 2002). P solubilization by bacteria is more efficient than fungi (Sharma et al. 2013). *Penicillium bilaii* is also a beneficial P-solubilizing bacterium that effectively takes part in the phosphate solubilization in native soils. Secretion of organic acid by fungi solubilizes the phosphate reservoirs in soil, making P easily available to plant roots. Potential phosphate-solubilizing bacterial genera in the soil include *Pseudomonas*, *Rhizobium*, endosymbiotic rhizobia, and ectorhizospheric strains of *Enterobacter* and *Bacilli* (Khan et al. 2009). A mutual exchange of nutrients and carbon occurs between mycorrhizal symbiosis of arbuscular mycorrhizal fungi (AMF) and host plant. The host plant acquires nutrients, e.g., phosphate and nitrogen, from fungus, which promotes plant's resistance against abiotic and biotic stress, and, in response, fungi get 4–20% C fixed by photosynthesis. Mycorrhizal symbiosis is quite common, and its symbiotic functions depends upon the variations between the soil properties, host plants, and AMF species. Generally, the AMF symbiotic linkages are thought to be nonspecific and diffused due to their several linkages by many species to different plants (Selosse et al. 2006). AMF symbiosis is an important biological mechanism to remediate polluted soils and mining spots (S. E. Smith and Read 2010). The microbes that benefit the health when consumed are known as probiotics. The concept of probiotics was given by the Nobel Scientist Élie Metchnikoff, who recommended that food requirement by intestinal microorganisms helps to exchange the detrimental microorganisms by beneficial microbes and to follow measures to adapt the microbial flora in our bodies. Soil probiotics are normally thought as soil-based organisms (SBOs), since they are advantageous bacteria which live in the soil. As the plants do not genetically acclimatize in the rapidly changing environment, i.e., drought, limited nutrients, and toxins, therefore, they may utilize the microorganisms to build the capacity for fast growth in the fluctuating environmental conditions for shorter life period. Hence, in this way, plants show the same mechanism as humans using probiotics to progress their health. Stimulation of plant-specific microbial species in their rhizosphere region tells us that plants can support and stimulate tactically to certain microbes, which have the ability to produce antibiotics that defend the plants against diseases causing soil pathogenic organisms (Weller et al. 2002). The bacterial species of the genus *Pseudomonas* are universal in many soils and participate in a lot of reactions, like bioremediation, nitrogen (N2) fixation, nutrient cycling, control, and inhibition of diseases, therefore promoting the plant growth. Pseudomonads work as a potential biocontrol agent against oomycete and fungi pathogens over the last two decades (de Souza 2002). Their most frequent property is antibiosis that is responsible for their reactions against the disease-causing plant pathogens, and a variety of antipathogenic compounds are also recognized, e.g., biosurfactant, hydrogen cyanide (HCN), pyoluteorin, pyrrolnitrin, phenazines, and 2,4-diacetylphloroglucinol (2,4-DAPG) (Picard and Bosco 2008). Their quick response capability to variations in nutritional, carbon, chemical, and physical conditions in the soil is very highly beneficial in agriculture, environment, and ecosystem functioning.

References

Abberton M, Batley J, Bentley A, Bryant J, Cai H, Cockram J et al (2016) Global agricultural intensification during climate change: a role for genomics. Plant Biotechnol J 14(4):1095–1098. https://doi.org/10.1111/pbi.12467

Abdalla K, Chivenge P, Ciais P, Chaplot V (2016) No-tillage lessens soil CO 2 emissions the most under arid and sandy soil conditions: results from a meta-analysis. Biogeosciences 13(12): 3619–3633

Abid M, Lal R (2009) Tillage and drainage impact on soil quality: II. Tensile strength of aggregates, moisture retention and water infiltration. Soil Tillage Res 103(2):364–372

Adger WN, Dessai S, Goulden M, Hulme M, Lorenzoni I, Nelson DR et al (2009) Are there social limits to adaptation to climate change? Clim Chang 93(3):335–354. https://doi.org/10.1007/s10584-008-9520-z

Agegnehu G, Bass AM, Nelson PN, Bird MI (2016) Benefits of biochar, compost and biochar–compost for soil quality, maize yield and greenhouse gas emissions in a tropical agricultural soil. Sci Total Environ 543:295–306

Alamgir M, Khan N, Shahid S, Yaseen ZM, Dewan A, Hassan Q, Rasheed B (2020) Evaluating severity–area–frequency (SAF) of seasonal droughts in Bangladesh under climate change scenarios. Stoch Env Res Risk A:1–18. https://doi.org/10.1007/s00477-020-01768-2

Allen JC, Barnes DF (1985) The causes of deforestation in developing countries. Ann Assoc Am Geogr 75(2):163–184

Altieri MA, Nicholls CI, Henao A, Lana MA (2015) Agroecology and the design of climate change-resilient farming systems. Agron Sustain Dev 35(3):869–890. https://doi.org/10.1007/s13593-015-0285-2

Altman J, Saurer M, Dolezal J, Maredova N, Song J-S, Ho C-H, Treydte K (2021) Large volcanic eruptions reduce landfalling tropical cyclone activity: evidence from tree rings. Sci Total Environ 775:145899

Armstrong M, Taylor S (2014) Armstrong's handbook of human resource management practice: Edition 13. Kogan Page

Arnold S, Doran JW, Schepers J, Wienhold B, Ginting D, Amos B, Gomes S (2005) Portable probes to measure electrical conductivity and soil quality in the field. Commun Soil Sci Plant Anal 36(15–16):2271–2287

Ashworth AJ, Allen FL, Wight JP, Saxton AM, Tyler DD (2014) Long-term soil organic carbon changes as affected by crop rotation and bio-covers in no-till crop systems. In: Soil carbon. Springer, pp 271–279

Assessment C (2018) Fourth national climate assessment

Avagyan AB (2021) Theory of bioenergy accumulation and transformation: application to evolution, energy, sustainable development, climate change, manufacturing, agriculture, military activity and pandemic challenges Athens. J Sci 8(1):57–80

Babujia L, Hungria M, Franchini J, Brookes P (2010) Microbial biomass and activity at various soil depths in a Brazilian oxisol after two decades of no-tillage and conventional tillage. Soil Biol Biochem 42(12):2174–2181

Bardgett RD, Freeman C, Ostle NJ (2008) Microbial contributions to climate change through carbon cycle feedbacks. ISME J 2(8):805–814

Beniston JW, Shipitalo MJ, Lal R, Dayton EA, Hopkins DW, Jones F et al (2015) Carbon and macronutrient losses during accelerated erosion under different tillage and residue management. Eur J Soil Sci 66(1):218–225

Bhattacharyya PN, Jha DK (2012) Plant growth-promoting rhizobacteria (PGPR): emergence in agriculture. World J Microbiol Biotechnol 28(4):1327–1350

Bini D, dos Santos CA, do Carmo KB, Kishino N, Andrade G, Zangaro W, Nogueira MA (2013) Effects of land use on soil organic carbon and microbial processes associated with soil health in southern Brazil. Eur J Soil Biol 55:117–123

Birat J-P (2021) Materials, greenhouse gas emissions and climate change. In: Sustainable materials science-environmental metallurgy. EDP Sciences, pp 43–120

Blanco-Canqui H, Mikha MM, Presley DR, Claassen MM (2011) Addition of cover crops enhances no-till potential for improving soil physical properties. Soil Sci Soc Am J 75(4):1471–1482

Blanco-Canqui H, Holman JD, Schlegel AJ, Tatarko J, Shaver TM (2013) Replacing fallow with cover crops in a semiarid soil: effects on soil properties. Soil Sci Soc Am J 77(3):1026–1034

Boettcher PJ, Hoffmann I, Baumung R, Drucker AG, McManus C, Berg P et al (2015) Genetic resources and genomics for adaptation of livestock to climate change. Front Genet 5:461

Borrill P, Harrington SA, Uauy C (2019) Applying the latest advances in genomics and phenomics for trait discovery in polyploid wheat. Plant J 97(1):56–72. https://doi.org/10.1111/tpj.14150

Braimoh AK (2013) Global agriculture needs smart science and policies. BioMed Central

Branca G, McCarthy N, Lipper L, Jolejole MC (2011) Climate-smart agriculture: a synthesis of empirical evidence of food security and mitigation benefits from improved cropland management. Mitigat Clim Change Agric Ser 3:1–42

Branca G, Lipper L, McCarthy N, Jolejole MC (2013) Food security, climate change, and sustainable land management. A review. Agron Sustain Dev 33(4):635–650

Briones MJI, Schmidt O (2017) Conventional tillage decreases the abundance and biomass of earthworms and alters their community structure in a global meta-analysis. Glob Chang Biol 23(10):4396–4419

Bronick CJ, Lal R (2005) Soil structure and management: a review. Geoderma 124(1–2):3–22

Buragohain P (2019) Role of microbes on carbon sequestration. Int J Microbiol Res. ISSN:0975-5276

Campbell BM, Thornton P, Zougmoré R, Van Asten P, Lipper L (2014) Sustainable intensification: what is its role in climate smart agriculture? Curr Opin Environ Sustain 8:39–43

Campbell BM, Vermeulen SJ, Aggarwal PK, Corner-Dolloff C, Girvetz E, Loboguerrero AM et al (2016) Reducing risks to food security from climate change. Glob Food Secur 11:34–43. https://doi.org/10.1016/j.gfs.2016.06.002

Cardoso EJBN, Vasconcellos RLF, Bini D, Miyauchi MYH, Santos CAD, Alves PRL et al (2013) Soil health: looking for suitable indicators. What should be considered to assess the effects of use and management on soil health? Sci Agric 70:274–289

Chahal I, Vyn RJ, Mayers D, Van Eerd LL (2020) Cumulative impact of cover crops on soil carbon sequestration and profitability in a temperate humid climate. Sci Rep 10(1):1–11

4 Soil Microbes and Climate-Smart Agriculture

Chaudhary S, Dheri GS, Brar BS (2017) Long-term effects of NPK fertilizers and organic manures on carbon stabilization and management index under rice-wheat cropping system. Soil Tillage Res 166:59–66

Chen H, Marhan S, Billen N, Stahr K (2009) Soil organic-carbon and total nitrogen stocks as affected by different land uses in Baden-Württemberg (southwest Germany). J Plant Nutr Soil Sci 172(1):32–42

Chenu C, Angers DA, Barré P, Derrien D, Arrouays D, Balesdent J (2019) Increasing organic stocks in agricultural soils: knowledge gaps and potential innovations. Soil Tillage Res 188:41–52

Clark KM, Boardman DL, Staples JS, Easterby S, Reinbott TM, Kremer RJ et al (2017) Crop yield and soil organic carbon in conventional and no-till organic systems on a claypan soil. Agron J 109(2):588–599

Colwell PF, Munneke HJ (1997) The structure of urban land prices. J Urban Econ 41(3):321–336

Cotter J, Tirado R (2008) Food security and climate change: the answer is biodiversity. A review of scientific publications on climate change adaptation in agriculture. Greenpeace, Exeter

Curtis PS, Wang X (1998) A meta-analysis of elevated CO 2 effects on woody plant mass, form, and physiology. Oecologia 113(3):299–313

Das S, Ho A, Kim PJ (2019) Role of microbes in climate smart agriculture. Front Microbiol 10:2756

Davidson D (2016) Gaps in agricultural climate adaptation research. Nat Clim Chang 6(5):433–435

De Baets S, Poesen J, Meersmans J, Serlet L (2011) Cover crops and their erosion-reducing effects during concentrated flow erosion. Catena 85(3):237–244

De Clercq T, Heiling M, Dercon G, Resch C, Aigner M, Mayer L et al (2015) Predicting soil organic matter stability in agricultural fields through carbon and nitrogen stable isotopes. Soil Biol Biochem 88:29–38

de Souza, J. T. (2002). Distribution, diversity, and activity of antibiotic-producing Pseudomonas spp.

Denef K, Zotarelli L, Boddey RM, Six J (2007) Microaggregate-associated carbon as a diagnostic fraction for management-induced changes in soil organic carbon in two Oxisols. Soil Biol Biochem 39(5):1165–1172

Dexter AR (2004) Soil physical quality: Part I. Theory, effects of soil texture, density, and organic matter, and effects on root growth. Geoderma 120(3-4):201–214

Diaz S, Grime J, Harris J, McPherson E (1993) Evidence of a feedback mechanism limiting plant response to elevated carbon dioxide. Nature 364(6438):616–617

Dignac M-F, Derrien D, Barre P, Barot S, Cécillon L, Chenu C et al (2017) Increasing soil carbon storage: mechanisms, effects of agricultural practices and proxies. A review. Agron Sustain Dev 37(2):14

Don A, Flessa H, Marx K, Poeplau C, Tiemeyer B, Osterburg B (2018) Die 4-promille-initiative "Böden für Ernährungssicherung und Klima": Wissenschaftliche Bewertung und Diskussion möglicher Beiträge in Deutschland

Dorodnikov M, Blagodatskaya E, Blagodatsky S, Marhan S, Fangmeier A, Kuzyakov Y (2009) Stimulation of microbial extracellular enzyme activities by elevated CO2 depends on soil aggregate size. Glob Chang Biol 15(6):1603–1614

Du Z-L, Zhao J-K, Wang Y-D, Zhang Q-Z (2017) Biochar addition drives soil aggregation and carbon sequestration in aggregate fractions from an intensive agricultural system. J Soils Sediments 17(3):581–589

Durán J, Morse JL, Groffman PM, Campbell JL, Christenson LM, Driscoll CT et al (2016) Climate change decreases nitrogen pools and mineralization rates in northern hardwood forests. Ecosphere 7(3):e01251. https://doi.org/10.1002/ecs2.1251

Dutta H, Dutta A (2016) The microbial aspect of climate change. Energy Ecol Environ 1(4):209–232. https://doi.org/10.1007/s40974-016-0034-7

FAOSTAT (2022) The state of food security and nutrition in the world 2021. Transforming food systems for food security, improved nutrition and affordable healthy diets for all. FAO, Rome. https://doi.org/10.4060/cb4474en

Duval ME, Galantini JA, Capurro JE, Martinez JM (2016) Winter cover crops in soybean monoculture: effects on soil organic carbon and its fractions. Soil Tillage Res 161:95–105

Easton ZM, Bock E (2016) Soil and soil water relationships

Fragoso C, Kanyonyo J, Moreno A, Senapati BK, Blanchart E, Rodriguez C (1999) A survey of tropical earthworms: taxonomy, biogeography and environmental plasticity. Earthworm Manag Trop Agroecosyst:1–26

Francaviglia R, Di Bene C, Farina R, Salvati L, Vicente-Vicente JL (2019) Assessing "4 per 1000" soil organic carbon storage rates under Mediterranean climate: a comprehensive data analysis. Mitig Adapt Strateg Glob Chang 24(5):795–818

Fungo B, Lehmann J, Kalbitz K, Thiongo M, Okeyo I, Tenywa M, Neufeldt H (2017) Aggregate size distribution in a biochar-amended tropical Ultisol under conventional hand-hoe tillage. Soil Tillage Res 165:190–197

Galende M, Becerril J, Gómez-Sagasti M, Barrutia O, Epelde L, Garbisu C, Hernández A (2014) Chemical stabilization of metal-contaminated mine soil: early short-term soil-amendment interactions and their effects on biological and chemical parameters. Water Air Soil Pollut 225(2): 1–13

García-Fraile P, Menéndez E, Rivas R (2015) Role of bacterial biofertilizers in agriculture and forestry. AIMS Bioeng 2:183–205

García-Ruiz R, Ochoa V, Vinegla B, Hinojosa M, Pena-Santiago R, Liébanas G et al (2009) Soil enzymes, nematode community and selected physico-chemical properties as soil quality indicators in organic and conventional olive oil farming: Influence of seasonality and site features. Appl Soil Ecol 41(3):305–314

Gindling TH, Newhouse D (2014) Self-employment in the developing world. World Dev 56:313–331

Glenn M, Kim S-H, Ramirez-Villegas J, Laderach P (2013) Response of perennial horticultural crops to climate change. Hortic Rev 41:47–130

Glick BR (2012) Plant growth-promoting bacteria: mechanisms and applications. Scientifica 2012

Gorte RW, Sheikh PA (2010) Deforestation and climate change. Congressional Research Service, Washington, DC

Graham JH (2000) Assessing costs of arbuscular mycorrhizal symbiosis in agroecosystems. Curr Adv Mycorrhizae Res:127–140

Gray E, Smith D (2005) Intracellular and extracellular PGPR: commonalities and distinctions in the plant–bacterium signaling processes. Soil Biol Biochem 37(3):395–412

Grover M, Ali SZ, Sandhya V, Rasul A, Venkateswarlu B (2011) Role of microorganisms in adaptation of agriculture crops to abiotic stresses. World J Microbiol Biotechnol 27(5): 1231–1240

Gurgel AC, Reilly J, Blanc E (2021) Challenges in simulating economic effects of climate change on global agricultural markets. Clim Chang 166(3):1–21

Gyaneshwar P, Kumar GN, Parekh L, Poole P (2002) Role of soil microorganisms in improving P nutrition of plants. Plant Soil 245(1):83–93

Haddaway NR, Hedlund K, Jackson LE, Kätterer T, Lugato E, Thomsen IK et al (2017) How does tillage intensity affect soil organic carbon? A systematic review. Environ Evid 6(1):1–48

Harrier L (2001) The arbuscular mycorrhizal symbiosis: a molecular review of the fungal dimension. J Exp Bot 52(suppl_1):469–478

Herrick JE, Beh A, Barrios E, Bouvier I, Coetzee M, Dent D et al (2016) The land-potential knowledge system (LandPKS): mobile apps and collaboration for optimizing climate change investments. Ecosyst Health Sustain 2(3):e01209

Hill J, Polasky S, Nelson E, Tilman D, Huo H, Ludwig L et al (2009) Climate change and health costs of air emissions from biofuels and gasoline. Proc Natl Acad Sci 106(6):2077–2082. https://doi.org/10.1073/pnas.0812835106

Högberg P, Read DJ (2006) Towards a more plant physiological perspective on soil ecology. Trends Ecol Evol 21(10):548–554

4 Soil Microbes and Climate-Smart Agriculture

Horton P, Long SP, Smith P, Banwart SA, Beerling DJ (2021) Technologies to deliver food and climate security through agriculture. Nat Plants 7(3):250–255

Howieson J, Yates R, O'hara G, Ryder M, Real D (2005) The interactions of Rhizobium leguminosarum biovar trifolii in nodulation of annual and perennial Trifolium spp. from diverse centres of origin. Aust J Exp Agric 45(3):199–207

Jacobs A, Poeplau C, Weiser C, Fahrion-Nitschke A, Don A (2020) Exports and inputs of organic carbon on agricultural soils in Germany. Nutr Cycl Agroecosyst 118(3):249–271

Jacobsen CS, Hjelmsø MH (2014) Agricultural soils, pesticides and microbial diversity. Curr Opin Biotechnol 27:15–20

Jansson JK, Hofmockel KS (2020) Soil microbiomes and climate change. Nat Rev Microbiol 18 (1):35–46

Jarecki MK, Lal R (2003) Crop management for soil carbon sequestration. Crit Rev Plant Sci 22(6): 471–502

Jiang Z, Lian F, Wang Z, Xing B (2020) The role of biochars in sustainable crop production and soil resiliency. J Exp Bot 71(2):520–542

Jiang R, He W, He L, Yang JY, Qian B, Zhou W, He P (2021) Modelling adaptation strategies to reduce adverse impacts of climate change on maize cropping system in Northeast China. Sci Rep 11(1):1–13

Joner EJ (2000) The effect of long-term fertilization with organic or inorganic fertilizers on mycorrhiza-mediated phosphorus uptake in subterranean clover. Biol Fertil Soils 32(5): 435–440

Joshi H, Somduttand CP, Mundra S (2019) Role of effective microorganisms (EM) in sustainable agriculture. Int J Curr Microbiol App Sci 8(3):172–181

Juma N (1998) The pedosphere and its dynamics: a systems approach to soil science, vol 1. Quality Color Press, Edmonton

Kaiser K, Kalbitz K (2012) Cycling downwards–dissolved organic matter in soils. Soil Biol Biochem 52:29–32

Karl TR, Melillo JM, Peterson TC (2009) United states global change research program. Global Climate Change Impacts in the United States

Kehler A, Haygarth P, Tamburini F, Blackwell M (2021) Cycling of reduced phosphorus compounds in soil and potential impacts of climate change. Eur J Soil Sci

Kelly B, Allan C, Wilson B (2009) Corrigendum to: soil indicators and their use by farmers in the Billabong Catchment, southern New South Wales. Soil Res 47(3):340–340

Khan AA, Jilani G, Akhtar MS, Naqvi SMS, Rasheed M (2009) Phosphorus solubilizing bacteria: occurrence, mechanisms and their role in crop production. J Agric Biol Sci 1(1):48–58

Khatri-Chhetri A, Aggarwal PK, Joshi PK, Vyas S (2017) Farmers' prioritization of climate-smart agriculture (CSA) technologies. Agric Syst 151:184–191

Klafehn R (2019) Burning down the house: do Brazil's forest management policies violate the no-harm rule under the CBD and customary international law? Am U Intl L Rev 35:941

Kostina N, Bogdanova T, Umarov M (2011) Biological activity of the coprolites of earthworms. Moscow Univ Soil Sci Bull 66(1):18–23

Koutsoyiannis D (2021) Rethinking climate, climate change, and their relationship with water. Water 13(6):849

Kuzyakov Y, Gavrichkova O (2010) Time lag between photosynthesis and carbon dioxide efflux from soil: a review of mechanisms and controls. Glob Chang Biol 16(12):3386–3406

Ladha JK, Reddy CK, Padre AT, van Kessel C (2011) Role of nitrogen fertilization in sustaining organic matter in cultivated soils. J Environ Qual 40(6):1756–1766

Lal R (2004) Soil carbon sequestration to mitigate climate change. Geoderma 123(1-2):1–22

Lal R (2011) Sequestering carbon in soils of agro-ecosystems. Food Policy 36:S33–S39

Lal R (2021) Climate change and agriculture. In: Climate change. Elsevier, pp 661–686

Leake J, Johnson D, Donnelly D, Muckle G, Boddy L, Read D (2004) Networks of power and influence: the role of mycorrhizal mycelium in controlling plant communities and agroecosystem functioning. Can J Bot 82(8):1016–1045

Lean J (1991) Variations in the Sun's radiative output. Rev Geophys 29(4):505–535

Lee H (2007) Intergovernmental Panel on Climate Change

Lehtinen T, Schlatter N, Baumgarten A, Bechini L, Krüger J, Grignani C et al (2014) Effect of crop residue incorporation on soil organic carbon and greenhouse gas emissions in European agricultural soils. Soil Use Manag 30(4):524–538

Liang A-Z, Zhang X-P, Hua-Jun F, Xue-Ming Y, Drury CF (2007) Short-term effects of tillage practices on organic carbon in clay loam soil of northeast China. Pedosphere 17(5):619–623

Liang C, Zhu X, Fu S, Méndez A, Gascó G, Paz-Ferreiro J (2014) Biochar alters the resistance and resilience to drought in a tropical soil. Environ Res Lett 9(6):064013

Lipper L, Thornton P, Campbell BM, Baedeker T, Braimoh A, Bwalya M et al (2014) Climate-smart agriculture for food security. Nat Clim Chang 4(12):1068–1072

Lipper L, McCarthy N, Zilberman D, Asfaw S, Branca G (2017) Climate smart agriculture: building resilience to climate change. Springer

Liu S, Zhang Y, Zong Y, Hu Z, Wu S, Zhou J et al (2016a) Response of soil carbon dioxide fluxes, soil organic carbon and microbial biomass carbon to biochar amendment: a meta-analysis. GCB Bioenergy 8(2):392–406

Liu Z, Dugan B, Masiello CA, Barnes RT, Gallagher ME, Gonnermann H (2016b) Impacts of biochar concentration and particle size on hydraulic conductivity and DOC leaching of biochar–sand mixtures. J Hydrol 533:461–472

Liu J, Zhang J, Li D, Xu C, Xiang X (2020) Differential responses of arbuscular mycorrhizal fungal communities to mineral and organic fertilization. MicrobiologyOpen 9(1):e00920

Lobell DB, Bänziger M, Magorokosho C, Vivek B (2011) Nonlinear heat effects on African maize as evidenced by historical yield trials. Nat Clim Chang 1(1):42–45

Lombard N, Prestat E, van Elsas JD, Simonet P (2011) Soil-specific limitations for access and analysis of soil microbial communities by metagenomics. FEMS Microbiol Ecol 78(1):31–49

Lorenz K, Lal R (2014) Soil organic carbon sequestration in agroforestry systems. A review. Agron Sustain Dev 34(2):443–454

Luo Z, Wang E, Sun OJ (2010) Can no-tillage stimulate carbon sequestration in agricultural soils? A meta-analysis of paired experiments. Agric Ecosyst Environ 139(1-2):224–231

Mackenzie J (2016) Air pollution: everything you need to know. Natural Resources Defense Council

Maestrini B, Nannipieri P, Abiven S (2015) A meta-analysis on pyrogenic organic matter induced priming effect. GCB Bioenergy 7(4):577–590

Maillard É, Angers DA (2014) Animal manure application and soil organic carbon stocks: a meta-analysis. Glob Chang Biol 20(2):666–679

Malhotra SK (2017) Horticultural crops and climate change: a review. Indian J Agric Sci 87(1): 12–22. https://doi.org/10.1002/9781118707418

Manzoor SA, Griffiths G, Lukac M (2021) Land use and climate change interaction triggers contrasting trajectories of biological invasion. Ecol Indic 120:106936

Mao JD, Johnson RL, Lehmann J, Olk DC, Neves EG, Thompson ML, Schmidt-Rohr K (2012) Abundant and stable char residues in soils: implications for soil fertility and carbon sequestration. Environ Sci Technol 46(17):9571–9576

Masto RE, Chhonkar PK, Singh D, Patra AK (2009) Changes in soil quality indicators under long-term sewage irrigation in a sub-tropical environment. Environ Geol 56(6):1237–1243

Mathew I, Shimelis H, Mutema M, Minasny B, Chaplot V (2020) Crops for increasing soil organic carbon stocks – a global meta analysis. Geoderma 367:114230

Mazzoncini M, Antichi D, Di Bene C, Risaliti R, Petri M, Bonari E (2016) Soil carbon and nitrogen changes after 28 years of no-tillage management under Mediterranean conditions. Eur J Agron 77:156–165

McCarthy N, Lipper L, Mann W, Branca G, Capaldo J (2012) Evaluating synergies and trade-offs among food security, development and climate change. Clim Change Mitigat Agric:39–49

Meena RS, Kumar S, Yadav GS (2020) Soil carbon sequestration in crop production. In: Nutrient dynamics for sustainable crop production. Springer, pp 1–39

Mikha MM, Rice CW (2004) Tillage and manure effects on soil and aggregate-associated carbon and nitrogen. Soil Sci Soc Am J 68(3):809–816

Milus EA, Kristensen K, Hovmøller MS (2009) Evidence for increased aggressiveness in a recent widespread strain of Puccinia striiformis f. sp. tritici causing stripe rust of wheat. Phytopathology 99(1):89–94. https://doi.org/10.1094/PHYTO-99-1-0089

Minasny B, Malone BP, McBratney AB, Angers DA, Arrouays D, Chambers A et al (2017) Soil carbon 4 per mille. Geoderma 292:59–86

Misra AK (2014) Climate change and challenges of water and food security. Int J Sustain Built Environ 3(1):153–165. https://doi.org/10.1016/j.ijsbe.2014.04.006

Mitter EK, Tosi M, Obregón D, Dunfield KE, Germida JJ (2021) Rethinking crop nutrition in times of modern microbiology: innovative biofertilizer technologies. Front Sustain Food Syst 5:606815

Mohammadi K (2011) Soil microbial activity and biomass as influenced by tillage and fertilization in wheat production. Am Eur J Agric Environ Sci 10:330–337

Mohanty S, Swain CK (2018) Role of microbes in climate smart agriculture. In: Microorganisms for green revolution. Springer, pp 129–140

Moutinho P, Schwartzman S (2005) Tropical deforestation and climate change

Nelson GC, Rosegrant MW, Koo J, Robertson R, Sulser T, Zhu T et al (2009) Climate change: impact on agriculture and costs of adaptation. Intl Food Policy Res Inst 21

Nortcliff S (2002) Standardisation of soil quality attributes. Agric Ecosyst Environ 88(2):161–168

Nunez C (2019) Carbon dioxide levels are at a record high. Here's what you need to know. National Geographic. https://www.nationalgeographic.com/environment/global-warming/greenhousegases/. Accessed 8 Nov 2019

Oreskes N (2004) The scientific consensus on climate change. Science 306(5702):1686–1686

Ortiz AMD, Outhwaite CL, Dalin C, Newbold T (2021) A review of the interactions between biodiversity, agriculture, climate change, and international trade: research and policy priorities. One Earth 4(1):88–101

Ortiz-Bobea A (2021) Climate, agriculture and food. arXiv preprint arXiv:2105.12044

Ostle N, Whiteley AS, Bailey MJ, Sleep D, Ineson P, Manefield M (2003) Active microbial RNA turnover in a grassland soil estimated using a 13CO2 spike. Soil Biol Biochem 35(7):877–885

Palansooriya KN, Ok YS, Awad YM, Lee SS, Sung J-K, Koutsospyros A, Moon DH (2019) Impacts of biochar application on upland agriculture: a review. J Environ Manag 234:52–64

Palombi L, Sessa R (2013) Climate-smart agriculture: sourcebook. In: Climate-smart agriculture: sourcebook

Pantelica A, Cercasov V, Steinnes E, Bode P, Wolterbeek B (2008) Investigation by INAA, XRF, ICPMS and PIXE of air pollution levels at Galati (Siderurgical Site), Book of abstracts. In: 4th national conference of applied physics (NCAP4), Galati, Romania, September

Paoletti E, Bytnerowicz A, Andersen C, Augustaitis A, Ferretti M, Grulke N et al (2007) Impacts of air pollution and climate change on forest ecosystems – emerging research needs. TheScientificWorldJOURNAL 7:1–8

Paustian K, Lehmann J, Ogle S, Reay D, Robertson GP, Smith P (2016) Climate-smart soils. Nature 532(7597):49–57

Picard C, Bosco M (2008) Genotypic and phenotypic diversity in populations of plant-probiotic Pseudomonas spp. colonizing roots. Naturwissenschaften 95(1):1–16

Poeplau C, Don A (2015) Carbon sequestration in agricultural soils via cultivation of cover crops – a meta-analysis. Agric Ecosyst Environ 200:33–41

Powlson DS, Stirling CM, Jat ML, Gerard BG, Palm CA, Sanchez PA, Cassman KG (2014) Limited potential of no-till agriculture for climate change mitigation. Nat Clim Chang 4(8):678–683

Quesada C, Lloyd J, Schwarz M, Patiño S, Baker T, Czimczik C et al (2010) Variations in chemical and physical properties of Amazon forest soils in relation to their genesis. Biogeosciences 7(5):1515–1541

Raich JW, Potter CS (1995) Global patterns of carbon dioxide emissions from soils. Glob Biogeochem Cycles 9(1):23–36

Rashidi M, Seilsepour M, Ranjbar I, Gholami M, Abbassi S (2010) Evaluation of some soil quality indicators in the Varamin region, Iran. World Appl Sci J 9(1):101–108

Recous S, Robin D, Darwis D, Mary B (1995) Soil inorganic N availability: effect on maize residue decomposition. Soil Biol Biochem 27(12):1529–1538

Reidsma P, Ewert F (2008) Regional farm diversity can reduce vulnerability of food production to climate change. Ecol Soc 13(1)

Reidsma P, Ewert F, Lansink AO, Leemans R (2010) Adaptation to climate change and climate variability in European agriculture: the importance of farm level responses. Eur J Agron 32(1): 91–102. https://doi.org/10.1016/j.eja.2009.06.003

Rosenstock TS, Lamanna C, Chesterman S, Bell P, Arslan A, Richards M, Cheng Z (2016) The scientific basis of climate-smart agriculture: a systematic review protocol

Ross D, Matschonat G, Skyllberg U (2008) Cation exchange in forest soils: the need for a new perspective. Eur J Soil Sci 59(6):1141–1159

Roy T (2020) Precision farming: a step towards sustainable, climate-smart agriculture. In: Global climate change: resilient and smart agriculture. Springer, pp 199–220

Rumpel C, Kögel-Knabner I (2011) Deep soil organic matter – a key but poorly understood component of terrestrial C cycle. Plant Soil 338(1):143–158

Russo A, Carrozza GP, Vettori L, Felici C, Cinelli F, Toffanin A (2012) Plant beneficial microbes and their application in plant biotechnology. Innov Biotechnol:57–72

Sahu N, Vasu D, Sahu A, Lal N, Singh S (2017) Strength of microbes in nutrient cycling: a key to soil health. In: Agriculturally important microbes for sustainable agriculture. Springer, pp 69–86

Sainju UM, Whitehead WF, Singh BP (2003) Cover crops and nitrogen fertilization effects on soil aggregation and carbon and nitrogen pools. Can J Soil Sci 83(2):155–165

Salinas-Garcia JR, Hons FM, Matocha JE (1997) Long-term effects of tillage and fertilization on soil organic matter dynamics. Soil Sci Soc Am J 61(1):152–159

Sanchez LF, Stern DI (2016) Drivers of industrial and non-industrial greenhouse gas emissions. Ecol Econ 124:17–24. https://doi.org/10.1016/j.ecolecon.2016.01.008

Sanderman J, Farquharson R, Baldock J (2009) Soil carbon sequestration potential: a review for Australian agriculture

Schahczenski J, Hill H (2009) Agriculture, climate change and carbon sequestration. ATTRA Melbourne

Schmidt H-P, Kammann C, Niggli C, Evangelou MWH, Mackie KA, Abiven S (2014) Biochar and biochar-compost as soil amendments to a vineyard soil: influences on plant growth, nutrient uptake, plant health and grape quality. Agric Ecosyst Environ 191:117–123

Seinfeld JH, Pandis SN (2016) Atmospheric chemistry and physics: from air pollution to climate change. Wiley

Selosse M-A, Richard F, He X, Simard SW (2006) Mycorrhizal networks: des liaisons dangereuses? Trends Ecol Evol 21(11):621–628

Sharma SB, Sayyed RZ, Trivedi MH, Gobi TA (2013) Phosphate solubilizing microbes: sustainable approach for managing phosphorus deficiency in agricultural soils. Springerplus 2(1):1–14

Sheehy J, Regina K, Alakukku L, Six J (2015) Impact of no-till and reduced tillage on aggregation and aggregate-associated carbon in Northern European agroecosystems. Soil Tillage Res 150: 107–113

Shi L, Feng W, Xu J, Kuzyakov Y (2018) Agroforestry systems: meta-analysis of soil carbon stocks, sequestration processes, and future potentials. Land Degrad Dev 29(11):3886–3897

Shukla J, Nobre C, Sellers P (1990) Amazon deforestation and climate change. Science 247(4948): 1322–1325

Sigurdsson H, Houghton B, McNutt S, Rymer H, Stix J (2015) The encyclopedia of volcanoes. Elsevier

Simpson RT, Frey SD, Six J, Thiet RK (2004) Preferential accumulation of microbial carbon in aggregate structures of no-tillage soils. Soil Sci Soc Am J 68(4):1249–1255

Singh LP, Gill SS, Tuteja N (2011) Unraveling the role of fungal symbionts in plant abiotic stress tolerance. Plant Signal Behav 6(2):175–191

Six J, Elliott ET, Paustian K (2000) Soil macroaggregate turnover and microaggregate formation: a mechanism for C sequestration under no-tillage agriculture. Soil Biol Biochem 32(14): 2099–2103

Six J, Frey SD, Thiet RK, Batten KM (2006) Bacterial and fungal contributions to carbon sequestration in agroecosystems. Soil Sci Soc Am J 70(2):555–569

Smith P, Gregory PJ (2013) Climate change and sustainable food production. Proc Nutr Soc 72(1): 21–28. https://doi.org/10.1017/S0029665112002832

Smith SE, Read DJ (2010) Mycorrhizal symbiosis. Academic

Sokol NW, Kuebbing SE, Karlsen-Ayala E, Bradford MA (2019) Evidence for the primacy of living root inputs, not root or shoot litter, in forming soil organic carbon. New Phytol 221(1): 233–246

Solomon D, Lehmann J, Wang J, Kinyangi J, Heymann K, Lu Y et al (2012) Micro-and nano-environments of C sequestration in soil: a multi-elemental STXM–NEXAFS assessment of black C and organomineral associations. Sci Total Environ 438:372–388

Spiegel H (2012) Impacts of arable management on soil organic carbon and nutritionally relevant elements in the soil-plant system

Spiegel H, Mosleitner T, Sandén T, Zaller JG (2018) Effects of two decades of organic and mineral fertilization of arable crops on earthworms and standardized litter decomposition. Die Bodenkultur J Land Manag Food Environ 69(1):17–28

Spracklen DV, Baker JCA, Garcia-Carreras L, Marsham JH (2018) The effects of tropical vegetation on rainfall. Annu Rev Environ Resour

Steenwerth KL, Hodson AK, Bloom AJ, Carter MR, Cattaneo A, Chartres CJ, Hatfield JL, Henry K, Hopmans JW, Horwath WR (2014) Climate-smart agriculture global research agenda: scientific basis for action. Agric Food Sec 3(1):1–39

Stern AC (1977) Air pollution: the effects of air pollution, vol 2. Elsevier

Stocker BD, Roth R, Joos F, Spahni R, Steinacher M, Zaehle S et al (2013) Multiple greenhouse-gas feedbacks from the land biosphere under future climate change scenarios. Nat Clim Chang 3(7): 666–672. https://doi.org/10.1038/nclimate1864

Strickland MS, Rousk J (2010) Considering fungal: bacterial dominance in soils–methods, controls, and ecosystem implications. Soil Biol Biochem 42(9):1385–1395

Suali E, Sarbatly R (2012) Conversion of microalgae to biofuel. Renew Sust Energ Rev 16(6): 4316–4342

Sun H, Koal P, Gerl G, Schroll R, Gattinger A, Joergensen RG, Munch JC (2018) Microbial communities and residues in robinia-and poplar-based alley-cropping systems under organic and integrated management. Agrofor Syst 92(1):35–46

Sundquist E, Burruss R, Faulkner S, Gleason R, Harden J, Kharaka Y et al (2008) Carbon sequestration to mitigate climate change. US Geol Surv Fact Sheet 3097:2008

Sykes AJ, Macleod M, Eory V, Rees RM, Payen F, Myrgiotis V et al (2020) Characterising the biophysical, economic and social impacts of soil carbon sequestration as a greenhouse gas removal technology. Glob Chang Biol 26(3):1085–1108

Tang J, Xu L, Chen X, Hu S (2009) Interaction between C4 barnyard grass and C3 upland rice under elevated CO2: impact of mycorrhizae. Acta Oecol 35(2):227–235

Thomsen IK, Christensen BT (2004) Yields of wheat and soil carbon and nitrogen contents following long-term incorporation of barley straw and ryegrass catch crops. Soil Use Manag 20(4):432–438

Thomson B, Grove T, Malajczuk N, Hardy GSJ (1994) The effectiveness of ectomycorrhizal fungi in increasing the growth of Eucalyptus globulus Labill. in relation to root colonization and hyphal development in soil. New Phytol 126(3):517–524

Tian G, Kang BT, Kolawole GO, Idinoba P, Salako FK (2005) Long-term effects of fallow systems and lengths on crop production and soil fertility maintenance in West Africa. Nutr Cycl Agroecosyst 71(2):139–150

Toor MD, Adnan M (2020) Role of soil microbes in agriculture: a review. Open Access J Biogeneric Res 10

Trajanov A, Spiegel H, Debeljak M, Sandén T (2019) Using data mining techniques to model primary productivity from international long-term ecological research (ILTER) agricultural experiments in Austria. Reg Environ Chang 19(2):325–337

Valizadeh J, Ziaei SM, Mazloumzadeh SM (2014) Assessing climate change impacts on wheat production (a case study). J Saudi Soc Agric Sci 13(2):107–115. https://doi.org/10.1016/j.jssas.2013.02.002

Van Groenigen JW, Van Kessel C, Hungate BA, Oenema O, Powlson DS, Van Groenigen KJ (2017) Sequestering soil organic carbon: a nitrogen dilemma. ACS Publications

Veloso MG, Cecagno D, Bayer C (2019) Legume cover crops under no-tillage favor organomineral association in microaggregates and soil C accumulation. Soil Tillage Res 190:139–146

Vickers NJ (2017) Animal communication: when i'm calling you, will you answer too? Curr Biol 27(14):R713–R715

Wagg C, Bender SF, Widmer F, Van Der Heijden MG (2014) Soil biodiversity and soil community composition determine ecosystem multifunctionality. Proc Natl Acad Sci 111(14):5266–5270

Walpola BC, Yoon M-H (2012) Prospectus of phosphate solubilizing microorganisms and phosphorus availability in agricultural soils: a review. Afr J Microbiol Res 6(37):6600–6605

Wang C, Guo L, Li Y, Wang Z (2012) Systematic comparison of C3 and C4 plants based on metabolic network analysis

Wang B, Liu C, Chen Y, Dong F, Chen S, Zhang D, Zhu J (2018) Structural characteristics, analytical techniques and interactions with organic contaminants of dissolved organic matter derived from crop straw: a critical review. RSC Adv 8(64):36927–36938

Wang D, Zang S, Wu X, Ma D, Li M, Chen Q, Liu X, Zhang N (2021) Soil organic carbon stabilization in permafrost peatlands. Saudi J Biol Sci 28(12):7037–7045. https://doi.org/10.1016/j.sjbs.2021.07.088

Weller DM, Raaijmakers JM, Gardener BBM, Thomashow LS (2002) Microbial populations responsible for specific soil suppressiveness to plant pathogens. Annu Rev Phytopathol 40(1):309–348

Weng ZH, Van Zwieten L, Singh BP, Tavakkoli E, Joseph S, Macdonald LM et al (2017) Biochar built soil carbon over a decade by stabilizing rhizodeposits. Nat Clim Chang 7(5):371–376

Wienhold BJ, Awada T (2013) Long-term agro-ecosystem research (LTAR) network to establish the platte river–high plains aquifer LTAR

Wiesmeier M, Mayer S, Burmeister J, Hübner R, Kögel-Knabner I (2020) Feasibility of the 4 per 1000 initiative in Bavaria: A reality check of agricultural soil management and carbon sequestration scenarios. Geoderma 369:114333

Wilson B (2021) Past the tipping point, but with hope of return: how creating a geoengineering compulsory licensing scheme can incentivize innovation. Wash Lee J Civ Rights Soc Justice 27(2):791

Woolf D, Street-Perrott FA, Lehmann J, Josheph S (2010) Sustainable biochar to mitigate global climate change. Nat Commun 1(56):1

Wright SF, Upadhyaya A (1998) A survey of soils for aggregate stability and glomalin, a glycoprotein produced by hyphae of arbuscular mycorrhizal fungi. Plant Soil 198(1):97–107

Yevessé D (2021) Effects of temperature and rainfall variability on the net income of cereal crops in togo: semiparametric approach

Zak DR, Pregitzer KS, Curtis PS, Teeri JA, Fogel R, Randlett DL (1993) Elevated atmospheric CO 2 and feedback between carbon and nitrogen cycles. Plant Soil 151(1):105–117

Zhang W, Ricketts TH, Kremen C, Carney K, Swinton SM (2007) Ecosystem services and dis-services to agriculture. Ecol Econ 64(2):253–260

Zhang A, Bian R, Pan G, Cui L, Hussain Q, Li L et al (2012) Effects of biochar amendment on soil quality, crop yield and greenhouse gas emission in a Chinese rice paddy: a field study of 2 consecutive rice growing cycles. Field Crop Res 127:153–160

Zhao B, Su Y (2014) Process effect of microalgal-carbon dioxide fixation and biomass production: a review. Renew Sust Energ Rev 31:121–132

Zhou M, Liu C, Wang J, Meng Q, Yuan Y, Ma X et al (2020) Soil aggregates stability and storage of soil organic carbon respond to cropping systems on Black Soils of Northeast China. Sci Rep 10(1):1–13

Zhu Y-G, Miller RM (2003) Carbon cycling by arbuscular mycorrhizal fungi in soil–plant systems. Trends Plant Sci 8(9):407–409

Zougmoré RB, Läderach P, Campbell BM (2021) Transforming food systems in Africa under climate change pressure: role of climate-smart agriculture. Sustainability 13(8):4305

Chapter 5
Climate Change Impacts on Legume Crop Production and Adaptation Strategies

Mukhtar Ahmed, Aashir Sameen, Hajra Parveen, Muhammad Inaam Ullah, Shah Fahad, and Rifat Hayat

Abstract Climate change is a major constraint limiting legume production across the globe. Legume crops are a good source of food, feed and fodder, and they are grown on large scale in the arid and semi-arid tropics. Grain legumes provide great services to the ecosystem by fixing atmospheric nitrogen (N) through bacteria in root nodules, a process called biological N fixation (N-fixing symbiosis). Hence, legume can help to minimize emissions of greenhouse gases (GHGs), e.g. N_2O, CO_2 and CH_4, reduce fossil fuel energy and boost C sequestration in the soil. Climate models have predicted more occurrence of climate extreme events in the future. These events will impede the legume production by disturbing the growth and development of crop. Hence, in this chapter, we discussed the impact of heat stress, elevated CO_2 concentration eCO_2, drought and rainfall variability on legume crop production so that adaptation options can be suggested for the sustainable crop production. Results showed that legumes having C3 fixation pathway have shown higher rate of photosynthesis, reduction in photorespiration, more biomass production and higher water use efficiency under eCO_2. However, with the rise in temperature, plants show faster development rate, shorter life cycle, shorter grain filling duration and lower yield. Similarly, the positive impact of eCO_2 on nodulation was hampered by rise in temperature. In general, legume could cope eCO_2 even up to 1000 ppm by carbohydrate allocation in the form of sucrose and its storage as starch. Moreover, apart from starch mobilization, protein synthesis in legumes helps them to adapt in the

---

M. Ahmed (✉) · A. Sameen · H. Parveen · M. I. Ullah
Department of Agronomy, PMAS Arid Agriculture University, Rawalpindi, Pakistan
e-mail: ahmadmukhtar@uaar.edu.pk

S. Fahad
Hainan Key Laboratory for Sustainable Utilization of Tropical Bioresource,
College of Tropical Crops, Hainan University, Haikou, China

Department of Agronomy, The University of Haripur, Haripur, Pakistan

R. Hayat
Institute of Soil and Environmental Sciences, Pir Mehr Ali Shah Arid Agriculture University,
Rawalpindi, Pakistan

© The Author(s), under exclusive license to Springer Nature Switzerland AG 2022
M. Ahmed (ed.), *Global Agricultural Production: Resilience to Climate Change*,
https://doi.org/10.1007/978-3-031-14973-3_5

149

150 M. Ahmed et al.

changing climate. Water stress is another climate extreme event that limits the legume crop production at all phenological stages, but its impact is more severe during flowering and grain development phases, called terminal drought. Hence, adaptation options such as development of new climate-resilient legume crop cultivars, ideotype designing through use of process-based crop models, change in sowing dates, availability of short duration cultivars, use of precision agriculture tools for accurate application of irrigation and fertilization, intercropping, switching to better adapted legume cultivars and crop diversification are needed to combat the negative impact of climate extreme.

Keywords Climate change · Legume · Heat stress · Elevated CO_2 concentration eCO$_2$ · Drought and adaptation

5.1 Introduction

Legumes belong to the family Leguminosae or Fabaceae. The new name Fabaceae comes from the extinct genus *Faba* now part of *Vicia* genus (vetches). Faba word came from Latin which mean bean. However, the old name still works as it is related to a fruit name, i.e. legume. It is one of the agriculturally important large family of flowering plants. It includes trees, shrubs and annual/perennial herbaceous plants. Legume family has 765 genera and 20,000 species, and it is the third largest family on land. Legumes have worldwide distribution except Antarctica and the high Arctic. Legumes rank third in crop production after cereals and oilseeds. Legume crops are a good source of food, feed and fodder, and they are grown on large scale in the semi-arid tropics (Sita et al. 2017; Cernay et al. 2016). Legume plants can fix atmospheric nitrogen (N_2) through their symbiotic relationship with bacteria present in their root nodules. This fixation of N_2 is called biological nitrogen fixation (BNF). Legume plants are also called nodulated plants as well as additive or restorative plants as they can provide nutrients to the soil. These plants can be easily identified through compound stipulate leaves and dehiscent fruit, which can open in two sides. Legume seeds are also called pulse when used as dry grain, or pulse is the edible seed of legume. Legume is mainly used as a human diet as well as part of livestock forage and silage. Legumes as forage have two broad types: (i) pasture legume grazed by livestock, including alfalfa, clover, vetch, and arachis, and (ii) woody shrub or tree species, e.g. *Leucaena/Albizia*. Legumes have also been used as green manure crops, and they play a key role in crop rotation. Dominated legume plants across the globe include alfalfa, beans (black beans, guar or cluster bean, soybeans, mung bean, mashbean, kidney beans, faba bean, etc.), carob, clover, chickpeas, lentils, lupins, mesquite, peanuts, peas, tamarind, etc. Legume plants use C3 cycle to fix atmospheric carbon dioxide (CO_2). Legumes can be classified into cool season and warm tropical season legumes. Cool season legumes include lentil, lupin, chickpea, dry pea, grass pea, vetch and broad bean (Andrews and Hodge 2010). The legumes that can be grown in warm seasons and in hot and humid conditions are mung bean, pigeon pea, cowpea, common bean and urd bean (Singh and Singh 2011). Duc et al.

5 Climate Change Impacts on Legume Crop Production and Adaptation Strategies

(2015) reported that grain legumes that have been consumed largely across the globe are lentil, chickpea, field pea, mung bean, common bean, broad bean, kidney bean and pigeon pea. Grain legumes are the biggest source (33%) of plant protein. Different types of legumes have been shown in Figs. 5.1a and 5.1b. Mainly, legumes can be divided into oilseed and non-oilseed legumes (Fig. 5.1b). Soybean and peanuts are the main examples of non-oilseed legumes, while oilseed legumes can be divided into fresh and dried legumes. Dried grain legumes are called pulses, and it can be further subdivided into lentil, dry bean, dry pea, chickpea and cowpea. Lentil's name came from the Latin word "lens" as the seed of these legumes looks like small lens. The list of legumes, which are available at FAOSTAT data set,

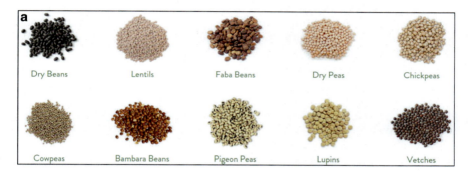

Fig. 5.1a Different types of dry legumes

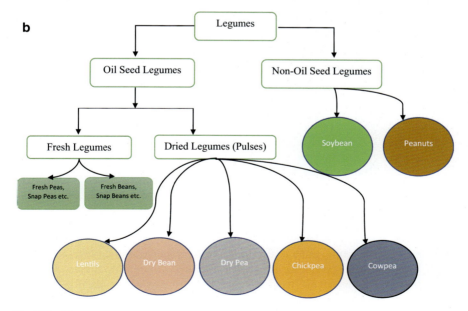

Fig. 5.1b Types of legumes

includes pulses, soybeans, pigeon peas, peas, lupins, lentils, groundnuts with shell, carobs, dry cowpeas, chickpeas, dry beans and Bambara beans. The production trends for these legumes have been shown in Figs. 5.2a and 5.2b. Furthermore, yield map of legumes with yield trend from 1980 to 2020 has been presented in these figures (Figs. 5.3a, 5.3b and 5.3c).

5.2 Nutritional Benefits of Legumes

Grain legumes are a rich source of protein (16–50%), dietary fibre (10–23%), essential elements (Fe, Ca, Mg, Zn and K) and vitamins. They are precious gifts to mankind and often known as the poor man's meat. Wang et al. (2009) reported that grain legumes are a storehouse of multiple nutritional components that include carbohydrates, sugars, vitamins, mono- and polyunsaturated fatty acids as well as more than 15 essential mineral elements. Grain legumes also contain folic acids, lectins, phytate, trypsin inhibitors and polyphenolic non-nutritional bioactive components. Pulse inclusion in a diet plan prevents a person from various health problems (e.g. type 2 diabetes, cardiovascular diseases and some forms of cancer), and it also reduces the risks of obesity. Pulses act as a tonic of the body as they digest slowly and provide slow-burning energy with a good supply of iron, which can help to provide oxygen throughout the body, thus boosting energy production and metabolism. Furthermore, the fibre in the pulses increases stool volume and transit, and it can also bind toxins and cholesterol in the gut so that it can be removed from the body. This helps to improve heart health and lower level of blood cholesterol. Pairing of pulses with grains prepares the ideal balanced diet, as pulses are rich in lysine protein and low in sulphur-containing amino acids, while grains are low in lysine and high in sulphur-containing amino acids. The top ten reasons to recommend pulses in diet plans are as follows: (i) low-fat, (ii) low sodium, (iii) good source of iron, (iv) good source of protein, (v) excellent supplier of fibre, (vi) excellent source of folate, (vii) good supplier of potassium, (viii) low glycaemic index, (ix) cholesterol-free and (x) gluten-free.

5.3 Area, Production and Yield of Grain Legumes

The grain legumes are grown on an area of more than 81 million ha with a global production of greater than 92 million tonnes (FAOSTAT 2022). India is the topmost producer of grain legume production, and it accounts for one-fourth of the global grain legume production. India is also the largest consumer of grain legumes. Other major grain legume-producing countries include China, Myanmar, Canada, Australia, Brazil, Argentina, the USA and Russia. Soybean is the top growing legume with an area of 126.95 million ha, production of 353.46 million tonnes and yield of 27,842 hg ha^{-1}. However, dry bean is the widely grown grain legume

5 Climate Change Impacts on Legume Crop Production and Adaptation Strategies 153

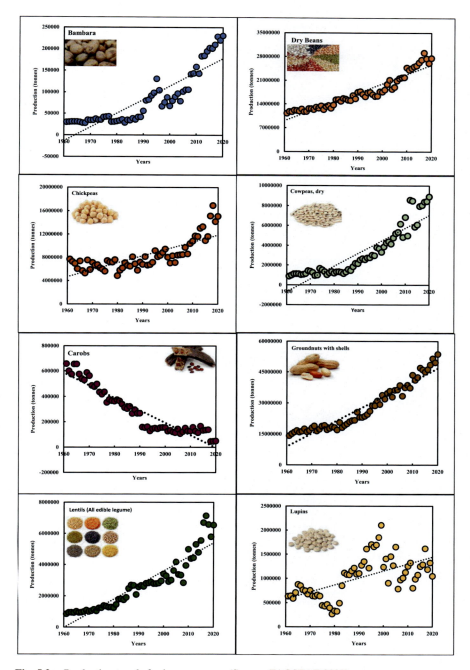

Fig. 5.2a Production trends for legume crops. (Source: FAOSTAT 2022)

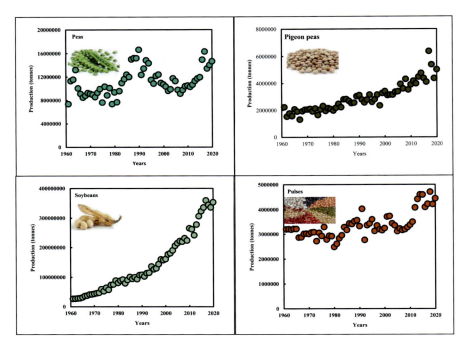

Fig. 5.2b Production trends for legume crops. (Source: FAOSTAT 2022)

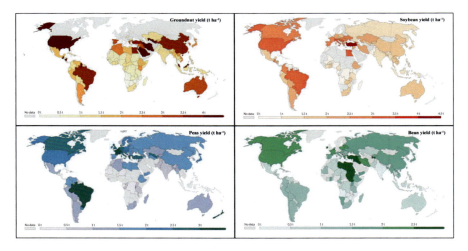

Fig. 5.3a Yield map of some legume crops. (Source: FAOSTAT 2022)

with an area, production and yield of 34.80 million ha, 27.54 million tonnes and 7915 kg ha^{-1}, respectively. Groundnut with shells is grown on an area of 31.56 million ha with production and yield of 53.63 million tonnes and 16,991 kg ha^{-1},

5 Climate Change Impacts on Legume Crop Production and Adaptation Strategies

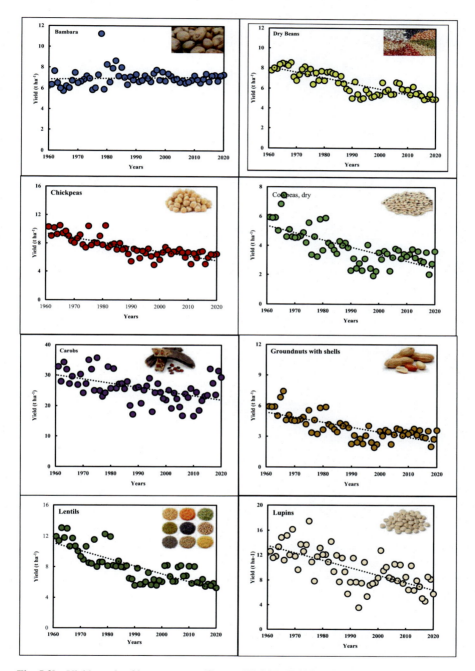

Fig. 5.3b Yield trends of legume crops. (Source: FAOSTAT 2022)

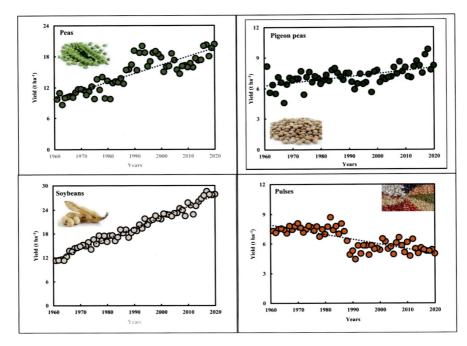

Fig. 5.3c Yield trends of legume crops. (Source: FAOSTAT 2022)

Table 5.1 Area, production and yield of main grain legumes across the globe (FAOSTAT 2022)

Crops	Area (million ha)	Production (million tonnes)	Yield (kg ha^{-1})
Beans, dry	34.80	27.55	7915
Chickpeas	14.84	15.08	10,163
Cowpeas, dry	15.05	8.90	5912
Groundnuts, with shell	31.57	53.64	16,991
Lentils	5.01	6.54	13,049
Peas, dry	7.19	14.64	20,364
Soybeans	126.95	353.46	27,842

respectively. Dry cowpeas occupy an area of 15.05 million ha with production and yield of 8.90 million tonnes and 5912 kg ha^{-1}, respectively (FAOSTAT 2022). Further details about other legumes have been given in Table 5.1.

5.4 Legumes and Ecosystem Services

Grain legumes provide great services to the ecosystem by fixing atmospheric nitrogen (N) through bacteria in root nodules, a process called BNF. This phenomenon can solve the problem of protein malnutrition across the globe as shown in the

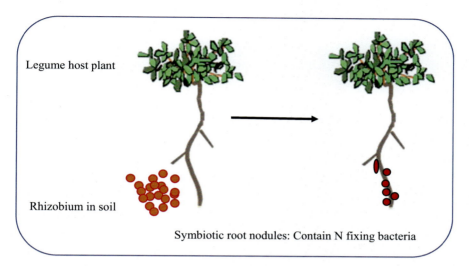

Fig. 5.4 Legume symbiosis with N-fixing bacteria

equation where legume plants in collaboration with *Rhizobium* bacteria can convert molecular nitrogen (N_2) to chemical N. However, these bacteria require energy that comes through plant photosynthesis, and they all are very species specific. Specialized root nodules are formed by legume plants to host N-fixing bacteria (rhizobia). These legume plants can grow without exogenous N fertilizer, and they are high in protein with ability to provide nutrition to the surrounding plants. Legume and bacteria symbiosis has been further elaborated in Figs. 5.4 and 5.5.

Legume plants + Rhizobium bacteria → NH_3 produced inside root → Protein

Biological N fixation could help to minimize the emission of GHGs and groundwater pollution. Yue et al. (2017) reported from China that GHG emission from soybean production is 1% while it was 30%, 8%, 6% and 4% from cereals, vegetables, fruits and cash crops, respectively. Similarly, legumes can curtail global CO_2 emissions (>300 Tg year^{-1}) up to 50% that come from N fertilizer industries. Legume-rich feeds for ruminants can minimize CH_4 emissions as legume-based feeds contain less fibre, condensed tannins and saponins and have faster rate of passage. This leads to reduced cell wall digestion and modified rumen methanogenesis. Jensen et al. (2012) reported lower emissions of nitrous oxide in legumes (1.02 kg N_2O-N ha^{-1} year^{-1}) as compared to cereals (2.71 kg N_2O-N ha^{-1} year^{-1}) where N was applied. Schwenke et al. (2015) documented the positive impact of legume to reduce GHG emission in subtropical Australia. The work was carried out with the objective that introduction of legumes in cereal-based cropping system could help to mitigate nitrous oxide (N_2O) emissions. The results showed that cumulative N_2O emissions (CNE) from N-fertilized canola (624 g N_2O-N ha^{-1}) were much higher than legume crops, i.e. chickpea (127–166 g

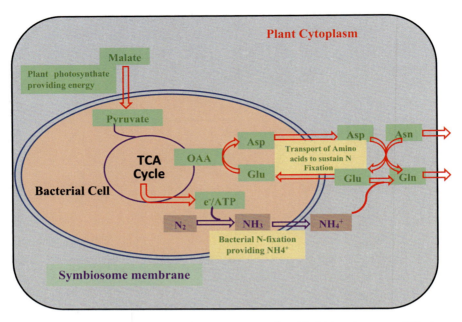

Fig. 5.5 Legume and bacteria symbiosis. *TCA* tricarboxylic acid, *OAA* oxaloacetate, *ATP* adenosine triphosphate, *Asp* aspartic acid, *Glu* glutamic acid, *Asn* asparagine, *Gln* glutamine

N_2O-N ha^{-1}), faba bean (166 g N_2O-N ha^{-1}) and field pea (135 g N_2O-N ha^{-1}). Similarly, N fixation provided higher total plant N biomass in chickpea (37–43%), field pea (54%) and faba bean (64%). Furthermore, the emission factor (EF) (percentage of input N emitted as N_2O) remained highest for canola (0.48–0.78%), while, in the case of legume, it was 0.13–0.31% for chickpea, 0.18% for field pea and 0.04% for faba bean. This study suggests that legumes should be part of all cropping systems as they have low EF. However, in another study conducted by Peyrard et al. (2016), higher N_2O emissions were reported due to legumes, which could be caused by faster decomposition rate of N-rich residues and denitrification. This exception in N_2O emission because of use of legumes could also be due to climatic conditions and management practices (Bayer et al. 2016). Ghosh et al. (2012) described C sequestration potential of legumes as they have deep root system, can fix N and have carbon-rich root exudates. Higher legume crop biomass and moderate rate of C mineralization have resulted to improve soil C retention in reduced tillage as compared to cereal crops (Bayer et al. 2016). Hazra et al. (2018) indicated legume potential to translocate C-photosynthate as root exudates and lignin-rich compounds, thus contributing largely to C sequestration and reducing C footprint. Legumes require less input to grow on marginal land and thus can bring prosperity to farming community living in problem soils. Legume can be a popular choice for farming community as they can withstand abiotic stress. Legumes are critical for the human nutrition as they can help to build resilience in combating system shocks such as COVID-19. It has now been proven that legumes have diverse

5 Climate Change Impacts on Legume Crop Production and Adaptation Strategies

application with unique properties; thus, their use could help in reducing GHG emissions and energy consumption, water conservation, C sequestration and soil health improvement. Furthermore, legume-rich diets provide greater health benefits with lower healthcare costs. Similarly, legumes could play an important role to fulfil the three important challenges in recent times, i.e. (i) population growth, (ii) urbanization and (iii) climate change.

5.5 Pulses: The Dry Edible Legumes

Edible dry grain seeds of legumes are called pulses. According to the Food and Agriculture Organization (FAO) (1994), plants that should be considered as pulses are given in Table 5.2. They grow in pods with variety of shapes, sizes and colours. Eleven types of pulses were recognized by the Food and Agriculture Organization (FAO). These are (i) Bambara beans, (ii) chickpeas, (iii) cowpeas, (iv) dry beans,

Table 5.2 Pulse plants as per FAO (1994) classification

Vernacular name	Scientific name
Common bean	*Phaseolus vulgaris* L
Lima bean	*Phaseolus lunatus* L
Scarlet runner bean	*Phaseolus coccineus* L
Tepary bean	*Phaseolus acutifolius* A Gray
Adzuki bean	*Vigna angularis* (Willd) Ohwi & H. Ohashi
Mung bean	*Vigna radiata* (L) R Wilczek
Mungo bean	*Vigna mungo* (L) Hepper
Rice bean	*Vigna umbellata* (Thunb) Ohwi & H Ohashi
Moth bean	*Vigna aconitifolia* (Jacq) Maréchal
Bambara bean	*Vigna subterranea* (L) Verdc
Broad bean	*Vicia faba* L
Common vetch	*Vicia sativa* L
Pea	*Pisum sativum* L
Chickpea	*Cicer arietinum* L
Cowpea	*Vigna unguiculata* (L) Walp
Pigeon pea	*Cajanus cajan* (L) Huth Lentil
Lentil	*Lens culinaris* Medik
Lupins	Several *Lupinus* L species
Hyacinth beans	*Lablab purpureus* (L) Sweet
Jack beans	*Canavalia ensiformis* (L) DC
Winged beans	*Psophocarpus tetragonolobus* (L) DC
Guar beans	*Cyamopsis tetragonoloba* (L) Taub
Velvet bean	*Mucuna pruriens* (L) DC
African yam beans	*Sphenostylis stenocarpa* (Hochst ex A Rich) Harms

(v) dry broad beans, (vi) dry peas, (vii) lentils, (viii) lupins, (ix) pigeon peas, (x) vetches and (xi) pulses nes (minor pulses). Pulse introduction in the cropping system is very beneficial and sustainable as they can minimize greenhouse gas (GHG) emissions, increase soil heath and use less water. In Pakistan the major grown pulses are chickpea, mung bean, lentil and mashbean, while on minor scale cowpea, faba bean, pigeon pea, common bean and moth bean are also grown.

Pulse production (0.7 Mt) in Pakistan is very low as compared to its requirement (1.5 Mt). Hence, Pakistan needs to import more than 50% of its pulses to fulfil its food requirements. The production and area of the major pulses during the last five decades in Pakistan have been shown in Fig. 5.6 (Ullah et al. 2020). The major reasons for low yield of pulses in Pakistan are as follows: (i) biotic and abiotic stresses; (ii) unavailability of quality seed and farm machinery; (iii) lack of crop improvements; (iv) competition with major crops; (v) soil issues, e.g. high pH, low organic matter and moisture; and (vi) support price and marketing issues. Moreover, climate extreme events, such as drought, heat waves and rainfall variability, are damaging pulse production in Pakistan. According to the Economic Survey of Pakistan, 2021–22 (https://www.finance.gov.pk/survey/chapter_22/PES02-AGRICULTURE.pdf), the area under pulse production is only 5% (1.5 mha), and due to

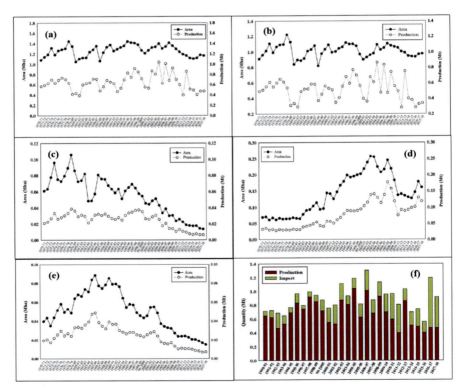

Fig. 5.6 Area and production statistics of (**a**) major pulses, (**b**) chickpea, (**c**) lentil, (**d**) mung bean, (**e**) mashbean and (**f**) import/deficit in Pakistan. (Source with permission: Ullah et al. 2020)

5 Climate Change Impacts on Legume Crop Production and Adaptation Strategies 161

Table 5.3 Pulse area, production and yield during 2020–2021 in Pakistan

Crops	Area (000 ha)	Production (000 t)	Yield (kg/ha)
Chickpea	873	261	299
Lentil	6.5	4.9	754
Mung bean	231	204	833
Mash (black gram)	11	7	636

Source: Agriculture Statistics of Pakistan, 2020–2021

Table 5.4 Pulse area (hectares) in Pothwar region

Crops	Rawalpindi (ha)	Attock (ha)	Chakwal (ha)	Jhelum (ha)	Total (ha)
Chickpea	798	2500	9424	162	12,884
Lentil	1570	193	970	540	3273
Mung bean	618	191	1018	1337	3164
Mash (black gram)	2204	50	691	753	3698
Total	**5190**	**293**	**12,103**	**2792**	**23,019**

above-mentioned reasons, the area and yield declined drastically with the passage of time. The national average yield of pulses in Pakistan is less than one-fourth of the potential average yield of China, India, the USA and Australia. Generally, pulse production in Pakistan is centred in two regions, i.e. (i) Thal desert and (ii) Barani region. The pulse area, production and yield during 2020–2021 in Pakistan are given in Table 5.3. Similarly, pulse area in Pothwar region is given in Table 5.4. Distribution of pulses during kharif and rabi season of Pakistan has been shown in Fig. 5.7, which clearly illustrates that contribution of pulses to the total agricultural production is very low as compared to other kharif and rabi crops. Furthermore, pulse contribution in different cropping systems of Pakistan has been shown in Fig. 5.8. Pulses need attention in Pakistan as they are nature gifted crops, which can ensure food security, uplift human nutrition, improve soil health, bring sustainability in agriculture and help to mitigate climate change impacts. Since pulse production is very low, measures such as availability of quality seed and promotion of short duration pulses intercropped with major cereal crops could, therefore, help to boost pulse production. The Australian Centre for International Agricultural Research (ACIAR) is investing in the region to increase the pulse production in collaboration with the local stakeholders.

5.6 Pulse Benefits to Climate

Crop production, food security and climate change are interlinked with each other. Climate change has shown a profound effect on food production and quality of food. Similarly, climate change is shifting the production areas of food and non-food crops. Hence, urgent sustainable measures are needed to minimize the impact of

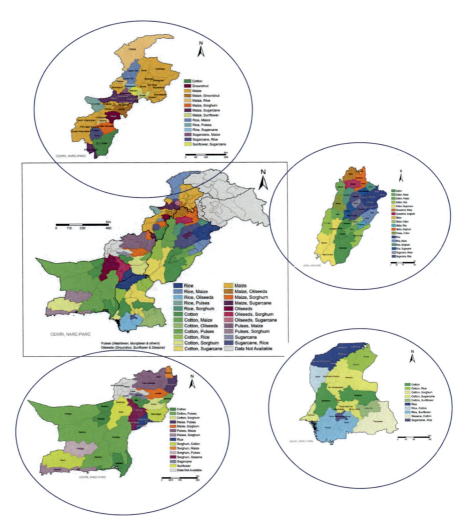

Fig. 5.7 Distribution of pulses in comparison with kharif crops in Pakistan. (Source: CIMMYT-Pakistan)

climate change, and under such circumstances pulses can be a good option. Pulse introduction in the cropping system will increase its resilience to climate change. Furthermore, pulses can increase crop productivity by nourishing the soil. Pulses are climate-smart crops as they can provide 5–7 million tonnes of N in soil, require less fertilizers, reduce the risks of soil depletion/erosion and promote higher C sequestration. However, improved pulse varieties will be required to minimize the impact of heat stress in the future. Pulses are very beneficial to minimize ecological footprint as introduction of pulses in the cropping system results to the fixation of N, which

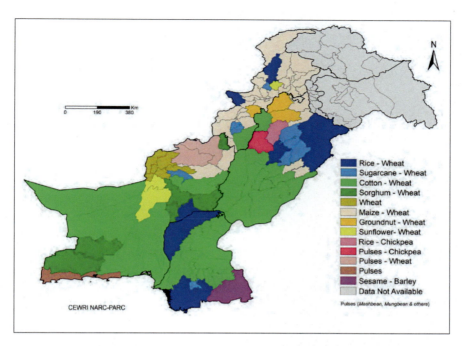

Fig. 5.8 Pulses share in different cropping system of Pakistan. (Source: CIMMYT-Pakistan)

increases grass yield and its feed values. Since grass grown as mixture with pulses resulted to the production of higher protein contents. This feed will further help to reduce GHG emissions from ruminants (Calles 2016) as it has already been well documented that agriculture is the fourth largest source of GHG emissions (Fig. 5.9) (IPCC 2007) and 4% of the global GHG emissions comes from the dairy sector (Gerber et al. 2010). Xu et al. (2021) reported doubled GHG emissions from animal-based foods as compared to the plant-based food. From animal-based foods it was 57% of the global GHG emissions (17,318 ± 1675 Tg CO_2 eq $year^{-1}$), while from plant-based foods it was 29%. The remaining 14% comes from other sources. Furthermore, they reported that farmland management contributes 38% to the total GHG emissions, while the share of GHG emissions from the land use change was 29%. South and Southeast Asia and South America are the largest emitters of the production-based GHG emissions as rice and beef production occurs in these regions. Smith et al. (2014) reported that 11% of the global GHG emissions comes from the agriculture sector and cattle produces 5335 Mt of CO_2 equivalents annually, which is almost 11% of the human-induced GHG emissions. Thus, it is essential to bring down all these GHG emissions, which is possible by adding legumes in the agricultural system as well as in the livestock feed. Furthermore, Rotz (2018) suggested that feeding protein (nitrogen)-rich diet to the cattle could help to reduce the emissions of NH_3, N_2O and nitrates in excreted manure. Data of GHG emissions per kilogram of food product shows that pulses release less GHGs (Fig. 5.10) as

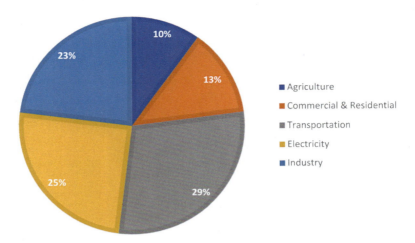

Fig. 5.9 Sector-wise emissions of greenhouse gases (GHGs)

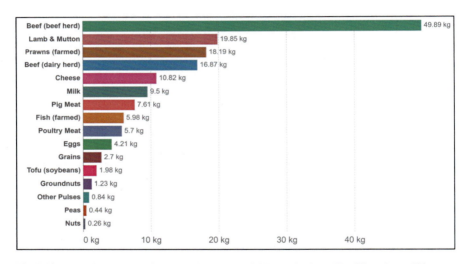

Fig. 5.10 Greenhouse gas emissions in kilograms of CO_2 equivalents (Kg CO_2 eq) per 100 grams of protein. (Source: https://ourworldindata.org/environmental-impacts-of-food)

compared to other sources. Furthermore, pulses can help to build sustainable food systems as they can be good alternatives in the production of bioenergy (Lienhardt et al. 2019). Pulses are environment-friendly crops as they help to reduce the application of synthetic N fertilizer (Jensen et al. 2012). This will help to minimize the emission of CO_2 in the air as synthetic N fertilizer production is also the biggest source of CO_2. Likewise, emissions of N_2O will be lower under pulses than crops and pastures where N will be applied. Leip et al. (2014) reported that the total N requirement to produce one N unit by pulse crop is very low, i.e. 1–2 kg kg^{-1} N product. Pulse acts as break crops in cereal-dominated crop rotations and could reduce insect, pest, disease and weed attacks (Liu et al. 2016).

5.7 Pulses as Food Security Boosters

Pulses have great potential to ensure food security and end hunger, which is a very important Sustainable Development Goal (SDG) of the United Nations, i.e. SDG2-Zero Hunger. Pulses can contribute to food security as it can be grown by small-holder farmers as an affordable source of protein, and due to their longer storability, they have low food wastage footprint (Bessada et al. 2019). Furthermore, pulses are suitable for marginal environments, and they are drought resistant with deep rooting features; thus, they have great potential to provide food and feed to dry environments. Pulses in the cropping system can give economic stability to the farming community. Farmers can get benefits from these crops by using them as feeds as well as storing them for longer period. Pulses also help to diversify the diets in developing countries. Furthermore, pulse incorporation in food systems could help to adapt to climate change.

5.8 Impact of Climate Change on Pulse Production

Climate change is one of the major threats to global pulse crop production. Pulse production from different regions of the world in the last two decades has been shown in Fig. 5.12. Around 25% of pulse production comes from the rainfed areas of the world where climate change is showing a significant impact (Fig. 5.11). India is the topmost producer of pulses followed by China (Fig. 5.12). According to the Intergovernmental Panel on Climate Change (IPCC), irreversible impacts of climate change will be more in the coming decades in the Asian subcontinent. This is already visible in the form of droughts, erratic rainfall and heat waves. Temperature during 2022 in India and Pakistan have reached at highest levels with April temperature (35.9 and 37.78 °C) broken the records of 122 years. This heat wave resulted to significant crop damage. It has been reported by experts that on average 7 °C increase in temperature in the month of April resulted to more than 500 kg ha^{-1} decline in the April wheat yield. Similarly, other crops, which include pulses, e.g. lentil and chickpea, have also been affected due to this rise in temperature. Since most of the pulse crops are heat sensitive, the sudden rise in temperature has, thus, shown significant damage to these crops. Furthermore, terminal heat stress at grain filling stages of rabi-sown pulse crops resulted to the declined yield. Thus, it is essential to develop proper mitigation strategies by considering both agronomic and breeding approaches. Similarly, intervention by the government is also needed to bring policies that can help to stabilize pulse crop yield in the future changing climate (Bera 2021).

Fig. 5.11 Pulse production from different regions of the world in the last two decades

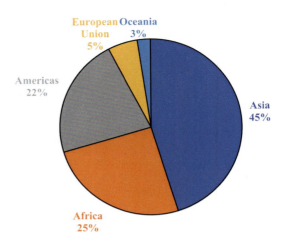

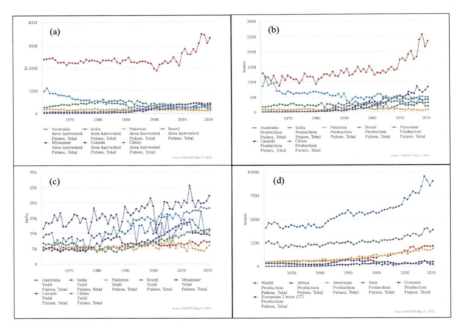

Fig. 5.12 Country-wise scenario of pulse harvested area (**a**), production (**b**), yield (**c**) and regional production in comparison with world production (**d**)

5.9 Institutes Working on Pulse Improvement

The International Center for Agricultural Research in the Dry Areas (ICARDA) is working, since quite a long time, for the promotion of sustainable agriculture in the dry areas of the world. It provides innovative science-based solutions to rural communities. The International Crops Research Institute for the Semi-Arid Tropics (ICRISAT), headquartered in India (Hyderabad), is working on the improvement of pulses. ICRISAT is mainly conducting research for the improvement of dryland farming and agri-food systems. It was established in 1972 by the consortium led by the Ford and Rockefeller Foundations and was supported by the Government of India. ICRISAT provides innovative solutions in collaboration with the international partners to end hunger, poverty, malnutrition and environmental degradation in drylands of sub-Saharan Africa and Asia. ICRISAT has given early-maturing groundnut varieties (drought-escaping groundnut cultivar, ICGV 91114) that can produce higher yields by avoiding mid- and end-season drought. Similarly, high-yielding wilt-resistant chickpea variety was developed through genomics-assisted breeding. The Australian Centre for International Agricultural Research (ACIAR) is funding a lot to improve pulses in different countries. A large ACIAR project (CIM/2015/041) was implemented in Pakistan to increase productivity and profitability of pulses. Similarly, a scientific collaboration was established between ACIAR; National Agriculture Research Centre (NARC), Islamabad; Arid Zone Research Institute (AZRI), Bhakkar; and MNS-University of Agriculture, Multan to improve pulse production in rainfed areas of Pakistan. ACIAR is working hard in collaboration with the local stakeholders in Pakistan to reintroduce legumes in the ongoing cropping systems.

5.10 Quantification of Climate Variability Impacts on Legume Crops

Climate is becoming hostile for food production, particularly in the semi-arid tropics (Cooper et al. 2008; Arunrat et al. 2022; Ahmed et al. 2022; Tui et al. 2021). Climate change in the form of rise in temperature, drought and variability in the rainfall has shown a significant impact on the agricultural production (Aslam et al. 2022; Bouabdelli et al. 2022; Arnell and Freeman 2021; Hernandez-Ochoa et al. 2018). Most of the prediction models had forecasted a 2–4 °C increase in temperature over the next century. Similarly, the concentration of CO_2 has been reached to 421 ppm as compared to pre-industrial time period when it was 278 ppm. CO_2 is now 50% higher than what it was before the industrial revolution. Furthermore, 10–20% increase or decrease in rainfall variability has been predicted. Annual variability in the climatic events is also increasing, and in the future crops will face more extreme events, e.g. heat waves and drought. Hence, it is essential to study the impact of heat stress, elevated CO_2 concentration eCO_2, drought and rainfall variability alone and in interaction on legume crop production so that adaptation options can be suggested for the sustainable crop production. Since legumes are dominantly grown in dryland conditions, drought will, thus, be the main yield-limiting abiotic stress for these crops. Therefore, to keep up the pace of agricultural production, improvement in the tolerance of legume crops to drought is an utmost important task. In the next sections, the response of legume crops to eCO_2, high temperature and water stress has been discussed so that prospects of grain legumes as climate-smart crops could be evaluated.

5.10.1 Impact of Elevated CO_2 Concentration eCO_2 on Legume Crops

Legume as a climate-smart crop sounds exciting, but the adverse effect of climate change on legume crop performance raises questions. eCO_2 has shown direct and indirect impacts on physiology and biochemical characteristics of grain legumes as reported in the past studies (Ainsworth et al. 2002; Mishra and Agrawal 2015; Palit et al. 2020). Legumes having C3 fixation pathway have CO_2 saturation point of 50–150 mg L^{-1} CO_2 as compared to C4 where it is 1–10 mg L^{-1} CO_2. Hence, under eCO_2 legume crops will do higher photosynthesis and maintain growth (Jin et al. 2012). Different studies confirmed the positive response of grain legumes to eCO_2 (Jin et al. 2012, 2013; Dutta et al. 2022; Singer et al. 2020; Sicher and Bunce 2015; Sulieman et al. 2015). Increasing CO_2 concentration from 350 ppm to 550 ppm in open-top chamber (OTC) resulted to 33% and 27% increase in the biomass of black gram and pigeon pea, respectively (Srinivasarao et al. 2016). Similarly, reduction in photorespiration due to eCO_2 was also reported by Srinivasarao et al. (2016). Furthermore, previous studies documented the positive impact of eCO_2 on growth and yield of other grain legumes, e.g. green gram, soybean, lentil, pigeon pea and chickpea (Pandey et al. 2016; Lam et al. 2012; Nasser et al. 2008; Saha et al. 2011; Bhatia et al. 2021). The impact of eCO_2 on biomass and yield of legume crops as reported earlier has been shown in Fig. 5.13.

Grain legume requires optimum supply of nutrients (N, P and K) and soil moisture to perform best as a climate-smart crop. Kimball (2016) reported complex relationship between eCO_2, crop performance and applied inputs through a meta-analysis of FACE (free-air CO_2 enrichment) experiments. Outcomes showed that the availability of N and water in C3 legumes, i.e. soybean and clover, resulted to 25% increase in shoot biomass while increase in C3 cereals (barley, rice and wheat) was 19%. eCO_2 resulted to 10% decrease in evapotranspiration in both C3 and C4 plants. Butterly et al. (2015) reported higher wheat biomass (55%) as compared to field pea (36%) due to eCO_2 and other input application. This higher benefit in wheat was due to dilution of tissue nutrient (Wang and Liu 2021). Furthermore, different past studies reported that in the future plants could be exposed to nutrient imbalance with lower N or higher C:N and C:P ratios due to eCO_2 (Sardans et al. 2012; Cotrufo et al. 1998; Yuan and Chen 2015). Decrease in nutritional quality due to eCO_2 was illustrated by Myers et al. (2014) and Loladze (2014) in their work and depicted Mg (9.2%), Fe (16.0%) and Zn (9.4%) deficiency in wheat, rice, vegetables and other C3 plants. Newton et al. (1996) stated that, in general, legumes (dicots) performed well as compared to cereals (monocots) under eCO_2 but cereals are more prone to water

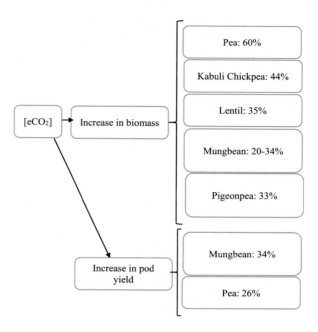

Fig. 5.13 The impact of [eCO$_2$] on biomass and yield of legume crops

stress than legume. Phosphorus (P) is a very important major macronutrient, which plays a critical role in the synthesis of ATP (adenosine triphosphate), the currency of energy as well as other biochemicals. Higher availability of P in the presence of eCO$_2$ resulted in the increase in biomass of field pea and chickpea, but the compensatory impact of eCO$_2$ under lower P was also reported for green gram (Zhang et al. 2014; Pandey et al. 2016). However, there was no consistent correlation observed between P and plant biomass under eCO$_2$ due to a number of reasons. One reason could be duration of exposure to eCO$_2$ as prolonged exposure to eCO$_2$ resulted to photosynthetic downregulation (plants acclimate and show a reduction in photosynthetic activity), which leads to lower crop yield (Sanz-Sáez et al. 2010). Other reasons for the downregulation under eCO$_2$ could be due to poor stomatal conductance and declined activity of rubisco (ribulose-1,5-bisphosphate carboxylase/oxygenase) (Rosenthal et al. 2014). Furthermore, C-sink limitation theory and N limitation hypothesis were given by Rogers et al. (2009) to provide other reasons for this downregulation. According to C-sink limitation theory, additional sinks are needed to translocate the carbon to the linked microbes; otherwise, this excessive carbon will limit the activity of rubisco. However, as per N limitation hypothesis, legumes fulfil additional N requirements by improving nitrogenase activity and nodule mass, which resulted to the overall increase in BNF (Sulieman et al. 2015; Goicoechea et al. 2014). Rogers et al. (2009) illustrated the positive (+), negative (−) and no effect of eCO$_2$ and nutrient supply on legume leaves, nodules and pods per seed parameter as shown in Fig. 5.14. This supports the hypothesis that greater photoassimilate production at eCO$_2$ resulted to higher nodule biomass and N fixation (Rogers et al. 2006; Ross et al. 2004).

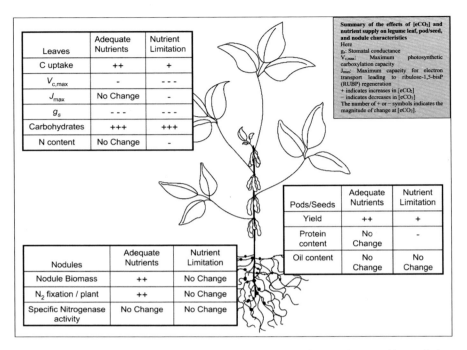

Fig. 5.14 Effect of eCO$_2$ on legume nodules, pods per seed and leaves. (Source with permission: Rogers et al. 2009)

5.10.2 Impact of High Temperature on Legume Crops

Temperature is the determinant factor of plant development, and rise in temperature is happening across the globe due to climate change (Song et al. 2022; Allan et al. 2021). Hence, plant productivity is on decline due to extreme temperature (Aslam et al. 2022; Hatfield and Prueger 2015). Small change in temperature can affect production of those crops, which are already growing close to optimum temperatures (Prasad and Jagadish 2015). Flowering is the most sensitive phenological stage among all crops, and rise in temperature during this crop developmental stage significantly affects crop production. Hatfield et al. (2011) provided cardinal temperature (Tc) values for different annual crops, which showed that vegetative development increases with increase in temperature and has higher optimum temperature. However, with the rise in temperature, plants show faster development rate, shorter life cycle, shorter grain filling duration and lower yield (Hatfield and Prueger 2015; Aslam et al. 2022; Naz et al. 2022; Fatima et al. 2020; Ahmad et al. 2019; Ahmed and Ahmad 2020). Legume crops, e.g. soybean, which is a photoperiod-sensitive crop, have also shown disruption in the phenological development due to rise in temperature. Similarly, extreme high temperature also resulted to a significant effect on pollen viability, fertilization and fruit or grain formation (Hatfield et al.

5 Climate Change Impacts on Legume Crop Production and Adaptation Strategies 171

2011, 2020; Boote 2011). Furthermore, temperature rise (2–4 °C by the end of century) due to the global climate change will also result to the change in the weather parameters, such as solar radiation, wind speed, pan evaporation and vapour pressure deficit (VPD). According to Vadez et al. (2012), VPD and evapotranspiration (ET) are very important climatic variables that determine crop water use efficiency (WUE). Under the changing climate, plants must transpire huge amount of water to sustain biomass accumulation, but it will not be sustainable both environmentally and economically. Hence, drought-tolerant legume cultivars with lower transpiration under higher VPD should be screened to increase WUE under extreme temperatures (Sinclair et al. 2008). The nitrogen fixation potential of rhizobia is very sensitive to temperature, and it performs well at the optimum temperature of 20–25 °C. However, if there is any minor change in soil temperature, it could destroy the symbiotic relationship and BNF (Aranjuelo et al. 2014). Similarly, the positive impact of eCO_2 on nodulation could be hampered by rise in temperature. In general, legume could cope eCO_2 even up to 1000 ppm by carbohydrate allocation in the form of sucrose and its storage as starch. Furthermore, apart from starch mobilization, protein synthesis in legumes helps them to adapt in the changing climate.

5.10.3 Impact of Water Stress on Legume Crops

Water stress limits the legume crop production at all phenological stages, but its impact is more severe during flowering and grain development phases, called terminal drought (Farooq et al. 2017). This kind of drought has shown significant damage to legume crops in the arid and semi-arid tropics (Pushpavalli et al. 2015). Drought reduces biomass, yield and yield components of legume crops as shown in Fig. 5.15. However, the magnitude of reduction depends on the intensity and duration of the drought stress, crop phenological stage and genotypic variability. For example, in chickpea, stress at pod filling stage shows higher yield loss as compared to flower initiation. Terminal drought also leads to leaf senescence, oxidative damage, reduced C fixation, sterility of pollen, inhibition of flowering and reduced pod filling and development (Vadez et al. 2012; Sita et al. 2017; Farooq et al. 2009, 2017).

5.11 Modelling and Simulation

New legume crop varieties are required that can perform well under the changing climate. Plant breeders are targeting specific traits to provide climate-resilient cultivars. However, early assessments of such traits are necessary to get potential benefits to minimize significant investment losses. Process-based crop models can be used to design site-specific crop ideotypes by using crop, soil, environment and management data (Boote et al. 2003). These models have crop coefficients that represent genetic

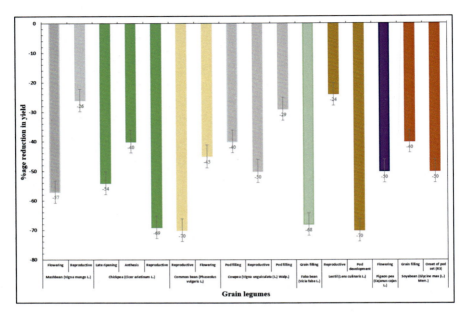

Fig. 5.15 Percentage reduction in the yield of grain legumes due to water stress

traits of cultivars, which can be modified within observed limit of genetic variability to evaluate the potential benefits of incorporating traits singly or in multiple combinations for the target site (Singh et al. 2012). Crop models have already been used by different researchers to suggest genetic improvement of crops under different climate change scenarios (Stöckle and Kemanian 2020; Boote 2011; Boote et al. 1996, 1998, 2001, 2003; Varshney et al. 2020; Hammer et al. 1996, 2002, 2010; Suriharn et al. 2011). Furthermore, the use of omics approaches (e.g. genomics, transcriptomics, epigenomics, proteomics and metabolomics) in combination with modelling and computational analysis could help to understand biological systems accurately (Lavarenne et al. 2018).

CROPGRO-Groundnut model was used by Singh et al. (2014b) with the objectives to develop high-yielding groundnut cultivars under heat and drought stress. Drought and heat tolerance and yield-enhancing traits were incorporated into the commonly grown chickpea cultivars. For drought tolerance enhancement in cultivars, changes were made in the relative root distribution function (WR) and lower limit (LL). Generally, the following equation is used to calculate WR for different soil layers:

$$WR_{(L)} = \exp(-0.02 \times Z(L))$$

where $Z(L)$ is the depth in metres to the midpoint of soil layer L. For the drought-tolerant cultivars, it was assumed that they will have greater rooting density and depth in soil profile; hence, the roots of drought-tolerant cultivars will go deeper to extract soil water. Therefore, the following equation was used to compute greater rooting density:

$$WR_{(L)} = \left[1.0 - Z_{(L)}/5\right]^{P}$$

where P:6 and 5 was used for all soils. This increases WR with depth in soil profile. Furthermore, water in soil layer was also increased by 5% by reducing the LL using the following equation:

$$LL_{(TOL)} = LL - 0.05 \times (DUL - LL)$$

where LL(TOL) is the LL for the drought-tolerant cultivar.

For the incorporation of heat tolerance traits, changes were made in the species file as there is no heat tolerance coefficient in the groundnut model. Thus, temperature tolerance of the three processes, i.e. (i) seed set, (ii) individual seed growth rate and (iii) partitioning of assimilates to reproductive organs, was increased by 2 °C to have heat-tolerant cultivars. The outcome of the study depicted that CROPGRO-Groundnut model could be used to develop heat- and drought-tolerant virtual cultivars, which can be a useful adaptation strategy under the changing climate.

Genetic traits of groundnut were evaluated by Singh et al. (2012) using CROPGRO to suggest adaptation options for the future climate. Modification in crop traits was made by changing crop phenological traits at first. The traits used were emergence to flowering duration (EM-FL) and seed filling to physiological maturity (SD-PM). These traits were increased by 10% alone and in combination. Similarly, SD-PM was increased by 10%, but EM-FL was reduced to keep the maturity the same. Furthermore, crop growth traits, i.e. maximum leaf photosynthesis rate (AMAX), specific leaf area (SLA) and leaf size (SIZLF), were increased by 10%. However, N mobilization from the leaves (NMOB) was reduced by 10%. Among the reproductive traits, pod adding duration (PODUR) was reduced by 10% to make the cultivar more determinant, while seed filling duration (SFDUR) and coefficient for maximum partitioning to pods (XFRT) were increased by 10%. In the case of root traits, the relative distribution of roots in the soil profile (SRGF) was decreased by 10% for 30 cm soil layer, and afterwards below 30 cm layer, it was increased by 10%. Similarly, the rate of rooting depth (RTFAC) was increased by 10%, while assimilate partitioning to the roots were increased by 2% via reducing partitioning to the leaves and stems. Furthermore, the turgor-induced shift of partitioning from shoot to root (ATOP) was reduced from 0.80 to 0.0. The ATOP value of 0 shows no shift, i.e. the root is less adaptive to plant water deficit, while the ATOP value of 1.0 represents maximum adaptive shift. The simulation outcome showed that increasing AMAX, XFRT and SFDUR resulted to higher pod yield in all climates. Similarly, productivity of groundnut under the changing climate could be increased by adjusting the duration of crop life cycle phases, particularly SD-PM. Moreover, under water stress conditions, shorter PODUR is recommended. This study recommended that CROPGRO model should be used to assess the potential of crop traits alone and in combination for multiple environments to design crop ideotypes under multiple stresses. Sennhenn et al. (2015) suggested that well calibrated and evaluated models can be a good tool for ex ante assessment of agricultural management interventions under the changing climate. Furthermore, they recommended that short-season grain legumes can contribute more to climate-resilient and productive farming system in dryland agriculture.

5.12 Adaptation Options for Legumes to Climate Variability

Ideotype to genotype approach can help to adapt crop phenology to climate change (Gouache et al. 2015). Different simulation models can be used to fulfil this task as model parameters could be linked to the markers. The model outcomes showed that earlier phenology can be a good stress-avoidance strategy in the future (Boote 2011; Singh et al. 2012; Boote et al. 1998, 2003, 2011; Suriharn et al. 2011). Similarly, the models themselves can be useful for developing crop adaptation strategies under the changing climate (Singh et al. 2014b). Other adaptation measures that can be useful to cope climate change impacts on legume crops include change in sowing dates, availability of short duration cultivars, application of precision agriculture tools for accurate application of irrigation and fertilization, intercropping, switching to better adapted legume cultivars and crop diversification (Ali et al. 2022; Ejaz et al. 2022; Tsegay et al. 2015; Ge et al. 2011; Thorp et al. 2008; Basso et al. 2001; Weih et al. 2022; Kherif et al. 2022; Wang et al. 2022; Singh et al. 2014a, b; Ahmed et al. 2022; Kollas et al. 2015; Jensen et al. 2012; Ghosh et al. 2012). Boote (2011) suggested use of cultivars with lower leaf area per plant and cultivars with earlier transition ability to reproductive phase in his work about improvement of soybean cultivars for adaptation to climate change and variability. Pulses have potential to outperform others under the changing climate by adopting strategies in which they can allocate more photoassimilates to the roots (Nie et al. 2013). Modification in root architecture under the changing climate is a very good adaptation option by which legumes can explore additional soil volume for water and nutrients. Hence, the investigation of root to shoot ratio in legumes should be considered to develop climate-resilient cultivars (Pritchard 2011). Kumar et al. (2019) emphasized on the use of systematic screening approach for the development of climate-resilient smart pulses.

5.13 Conclusion

Climate change has shown a significant impact on legume production, and risk is likely to increase in the future. The response of future legume crops will not only be dependent on eCO_2, but it will also be having strong association with other abiotic factors. Thus, it is essential to select and develop cultivars that can cope with climate extremes. It might also include cultivars with early vigour, shorter duration and higher root to shoot ratio. Similarly, genotypes with better WUE could help to give sustainable yield under dryland conditions. Furthermore, development of climate-resilient agrotechnologies is needed to adapt legumes to the changing climate and fulfil the food demand of rising population. The agrotechnologies could be adoption of conservation agriculture, use of plastic mulching, screening for heat- and drought-tolerant cultivars, application of precision agriculture, merging modelling with genetics and use of omics techniques in combination with modelling.

References

Ahmad S, Abbas G, Ahmed M, Fatima Z, Anjum MA, Rasul G, Khan MA, Hoogenboom G (2019) Climate warming and management impact on the change of phenology of the rice-wheat cropping system in Punjab, Pakistan. Field Crop Res 230:46–61. https://doi.org/10.1016/j.fcr.2018.10.008

Ahmed M, Ahmad S (2020) Systems modeling. In: Ahmed M (ed) Systems modeling. Springer Singapore, Singapore, pp 1–44. https://doi.org/10.1007/978-981-15-4728-7_1

Ahmed M, Hayat R, Ahmad M, Ul-Hassan M, Kheir AMS, Ul-Hassan F, Ur-Rehman MH, Shaheen FA, Raza MA, Ahmad S (2022) Impact of climate change on dryland agricultural systems: a review of current status, potentials, and further work need. Int J Plant Prod. https://doi.org/10.1007/s42106-022-00197-1

Ainsworth EA, Davey PA, Bernacchi CJ, Dermody OC, Heaton EA, Moore DJ, Morgan PB, Naidu SL, Yoo Ra H-S, Zhu X-G, Curtis PS, Long SP (2002) A meta-analysis of elevated $[CO_2]$ effects on soybean (Glycine max) physiology, growth and yield. Glob Chang Biol 8(8):695–709. https://doi.org/10.1046/j.1365-2486.2002.00498.x

Ali MGM, Ahmed M, Ibrahim MM, El Baroudy AA, Ali EF, Shokr MS, Aldosari AA, Majrashi A, Kheir AMS (2022) Optimizing sowing window, cultivar choice, and plant density to boost maize yield under RCP8.5 climate scenario of CMIP5. Int J Biometeorol. https://doi.org/10.1007/s00484-022-02253-x

Allan RP, Hawkins E, Bellouin N, Collins B (2021) IPCC 2021: summary for policymakers

Andrews M, Hodge S (2010) Climate change, a challenge for cool season grain legume crop production. In: Yadav SS, Redden R (eds) Climate change and management of cool season grain legume crops. Springer Netherlands, Dordrecht, pp 1–9. https://doi.org/10.1007/978-90-481-3709-1_1

Aranjuelo I, Cabrerizo PM, Aparicio-Tejo PM, Arrese-Igor C (2014) Unravelling the mechanisms that improve photosynthetic performance of N_2-fixing pea plants exposed to elevated $[CO_2]$. Environ Exp Bot 99:167–174. https://doi.org/10.1016/j.envexpbot.2013.10.020

Arnell NW, Freeman A (2021) The effect of climate change on agro-climatic indicators in the UK. Clim Chang 165(1):40. https://doi.org/10.1007/s10584-021-03054-8

Arunrat N, Sereenonchai S, Chaowiwat W, Wang C (2022) Climate change impact on major crop yield and water footprint under CMIP6 climate projections in repeated drought and flood areas in Thailand. Sci Total Environ 807:150741. https://doi.org/10.1016/j.scitotenv.2021.150741

Aslam MA, Ahmed M, Hassan F-U, Afzal O, Mehmood MZ, Qadir G, Asif M, Komal S, Hussain T (2022) Impact of temperature fluctuations on plant morphological and physiological traits. In: Jatoi WN, Mubeen M, Ahmad A, Cheema MA, Lin Z, Hashmi MZ (eds) Building climate resilience in agriculture: theory, practice and future perspective. Springer, Cham, pp 25–52. https://doi.org/10.1007/978-3-030-79408-8_3

Basso B, Ritchie JT, Pierce FJ, Braga RP, Jones JW (2001) Spatial validation of crop models for precision agriculture. Agric Syst 68(2):97–112. https://doi.org/10.1016/S0308-521X(00)00063-9

Bayer C, Gomes J, Zanatta JA, Vieira FCB, Dieckow J (2016) Mitigating greenhouse gas emissions from a subtropical Ultisol by using long-term no-tillage in combination with legume cover crops. Soil Tillage Res 161:86–94. https://doi.org/10.1016/j.still.2016.03.011

Bera A (2021) Impact of climate change on pulse production and it's mitigation strategies. Asian J Adv Agric Res:14–28. https://doi.org/10.9734/ajaar/2021/v15i230147

Bessada SMF, Barreira JCM, Oliveira MBPP (2019) Pulses and food security: dietary protein, digestibility, bioactive and functional properties. Trends Food Sci Technol 93:53–68. https://doi.org/10.1016/j.tifs.2019.08.022

Bhatia A, Mina U, Kumar V, Tomer R, Kumar A, Chakrabarti B, Singh RN, Singh B (2021) Effect of elevated ozone and carbon dioxide interaction on growth, yield, nutrient content and wilt disease severity in chickpea grown in Northern India. Heliyon 7(1):e06049. https://doi.org/10.1016/j.heliyon.2021.e06049

Boote KJ (2011) Improving soybean cultivars for adaptation to climate change and climate variability. In: Crop adaptation to climate change. Wiley-Blackwell, pp 370–395. https://doi.org/10.1002/9780470960929.ch26

Boote KJ, Jones JW, Pickering NB (1996) Potential uses and limitations of crop models. Agron J 88(5):704–716. https://doi.org/10.2134/agronj1996.00021962008800050005x

Boote KJ, Jones JW, Hoogenboom G, Pickering NB (1998) The CROPGRO model for grain legumes. In: Tsuji G, Hoogenboom G, Thornton P (eds) Understanding options for agricultural production, vol 7. Systems approaches for sustainable agricultural development. Springer, pp 99–128. https://doi.org/10.1007/978-94-017-3624-4_6

Boote KJ, Kropff MJ, Bindraban PS (2001) Physiology and modelling of traits in crop plants: implications for genetic improvement. Agric Syst 70(2):395–420. https://doi.org/10.1016/S0308-521X(01)00053-1

Boote KJ, Jones JW, Batchelor WD, Nafziger ED, Myers O (2003) Genetic coefficients in the CROPGRO–soybean model. Agron J 95(1):32–51. https://doi.org/10.2134/agronj2003.3200

Boote KJ, Allen LH, Prasad PVV, Jones JW (2011) Testing effects of climate change in crop models. In: Handbook of climate change and agroecosystems. Imperial College Press, pp 109–129. https://doi.org/10.1142/9781848166561_0007

Bouabdelli S, Zeroual A, Meddi M, Assani A (2022) Impact of temperature on agricultural drought occurrence under the effects of climate change. Theor Appl Climatol. https://doi.org/10.1007/s00704-022-03935-7

Butterly C, Armstrong R, Chen D, Tang C (2015) Carbon and nitrogen partitioning of wheat and field pea grown with two nitrogen levels under elevated CO_2. Plant Soil:1–16. https://doi.org/10.1007/s11104-015-2441-5

Calles T (2016) The international year of pulses: what are they and why are they important. Agric Dev 26:40–42

Cernay C, Pelzer E, Makowski D (2016) A global experimental dataset for assessing grain legume production. Sci Data 3(1):160084. https://doi.org/10.1038/sdata.2016.84

Cooper PJM, Dimes J, Rao KPC, Shapiro B, Shiferaw B, Twomlow S (2008) Coping better with current climatic variability in the rain-fed farming systems of sub-Saharan Africa: an essential first step in adapting to future climate change? Agric Ecosyst Environ 126(1–2):24–35. https://doi.org/10.1016/j.agee.2008.01.007

Cotrufo MF, Ineson P, Scott A (1998) Elevated CO_2 reduces the nitrogen concentration of plant tissues. Glob Chang Biol 4(1):43–54. https://doi.org/10.1046/j.1365-2486.1998.00101.x

Duc G, Agrama H, Bao S, Berger J, Bourion V, De Ron AM, Gowda CL, Mikic A, Millot D, Singh KB (2015) Breeding annual grain legumes for sustainable agriculture: new methods to approach complex traits and target new cultivar ideotypes. Crit Rev Plant Sci 34(1–3):381–411

Dutta A, Trivedi A, Nath CP, Gupta DS, Hazra KK (2022) A comprehensive review on grain legumes as climate-smart crops: challenges and prospects. Environ Challenge 7:100479. https://doi.org/10.1016/j.envc.2022.100479

Ejaz M, Abbas G, Fatima Z, Iqbal P, Raza MA, Kheir AMS, Ahmed M, Kakar KM, Ahmad S (2022) Modelling climate uncertainty and adaptations for soybean-based cropping system. Int J Plant Prod. https://doi.org/10.1007/s42106-022-00190-8

FAO (1994) FAO Statistics Division, Food and Agriculture Organization of the United Nations. https://www.fao.org/faostat/en/#data. Accessed 25 Aug 2022

FAOSTAT (2022) Food and Agriculture Organization of the United Nations (FAO). FAOSTAT Database. http://faostat.fao.org/site/291/default.aspx

Farooq M, Wahid A, Kobayashi N, Fujita D, Basra SMA (2009) Plant drought stress: effects, mechanisms and management. Agron Sustain Dev 29(1):185–212. https://doi.org/10.1051/agro:2008021

Farooq M, Gogoi N, Barthakur S, Baroowa B, Bharadwaj N, Alghamdi SS, Siddique KHM (2017) Drought stress in grain legumes during reproduction and grain filling. J Agron Crop Sci 203(2): 81–102. https://doi.org/10.1111/jac.12169

Fatima Z, Ahmed M, Hussain M, Abbas G, Ul-Allah S, Ahmad S, Ahmed N, Ali MA, Sarwar G, Haque EU, Iqbal P, Hussain S (2020) The fingerprints of climate warming on cereal crops phenology and adaptation options. Sci Rep 10(1):18013. https://doi.org/10.1038/s41598-020-74740-3

Ge Y, Thomasson JA, Sui R (2011) Remote sensing of soil properties in precision agriculture: a review. Front Earth Sci 5(3):229–238. https://doi.org/10.1007/s11707-011-0175-0

Gerber P, Vellinga T, Opio C, Henderson B, Steinfeld H (2010) Greenhouse gas emissions from the dairy sector: a life cycle assessment. Food and Agriculture Organization of the United Nations, Rome

Ghosh PK, Venkatesh MS, Hazra KK, Kumar N (2012) Long-term effect of pulses and nutrient management on soil organic carbon dynamics and sustainability on an Inceptisol of Indo-Gangetic Plains of India. Exp Agric 48(4):473–487. https://doi.org/10.1017/S0014479712000130

Goicoechea N, Baslam M, Erice G, Irigoyen JJ (2014) Increased photosynthetic acclimation in alfalfa associated with arbuscular mycorrhizal fungi (AMF) and cultivated in greenhouse under elevated CO_2. J Plant Physiol 171(18):1774–1781. https://doi.org/10.1016/j.jplph.2014.07.027

Gouache D, Bogard M, Thepot S, Pegard M, Le Bris X, Deswarte J-C (2015) From ideotypes to genotypes: approaches to adapt wheat phenology to climate change. Procedia Environ Sci 29: 34–35. https://doi.org/10.1016/j.proenv.2015.07.143

Hammer G, Butler D, Muchow R, Meinke H (1996) Integrating physiological understanding and plant breeding via crop modelling and optimization. In: Plant adaptation and crop improvement. CAB International, pp 419–441

Hammer GL, Kropff MJ, Sinclair TR, Porter JR (2002) Future contributions of crop modelling – from heuristics and supporting decision making to understanding genetic regulation and aiding crop improvement. Eur J Agron 18(1–2):15–31. https://doi.org/10.1016/S1161-0301(02)00093-X

Hammer GL, van Oosterom E, McLean G, Chapman SC, Broad I, Harland P, Muchow RC (2010) Adapting APSIM to model the physiology and genetics of complex adaptive traits in field crops. J Exp Bot 61(8):2185–2202. https://doi.org/10.1093/jxb/erq095

Hatfield JL, Prueger JH (2015) Temperature extremes: effect on plant growth and development. Weather Clim Extremes 10:4–10. https://doi.org/10.1016/j.wace.2015.08.001

Hatfield JL, Boote KJ, Kimball BA, Ziska LH, Izaurralde RC, Ort D, Thomson AM, Wolfe D (2011) Climate impacts on agriculture: implications for crop production. Agron J 103(2): 351–370. https://doi.org/10.2134/agronj2010.0303

Hatfield JL, Antle J, Garrett KA, Izaurralde RC, Mader T, Marshall E, Nearing M, Philip Robertson G, Ziska L (2020) Indicators of climate change in agricultural systems. Clim Chang 163(4):1719–1732. https://doi.org/10.1007/s10584-018-2222-2

Hazra KK, Ghosh PK, Venkatesh MS, Nath CP, Kumar N, Singh M, Singh J, Nadarajan N (2018) Improving soil organic carbon pools through inclusion of summer mungbean in cereal-cereal cropping systems in indo-Gangetic plain. Arch Agron Soil Sci 64(12):1690–1704. https://doi.org/10.1080/03650340.2018.1451638

Hernandez-Ochoa IM, Asseng S, Kassie BT, Xiong W, Robertson R, Luz Pequeno DN, Sonder K, Reynolds M, Babar MA, Molero Milan A, Hoogenboom G (2018) Climate change impact on Mexico wheat production. Agric For Meteorol 263:373–387. https://doi.org/10.1016/j.agrformet.2018.09.008

IPCC (2007) Climate Change 2007: synthesis report. Contribution of working Groups I, II and III to the Fourth Assessment Report of the Intergovernmental Panel on Climate Change (IPCC), Valencia, Spain. IPCC, Geneva

Jensen ES, Peoples MB, Boddey RM, Gresshoff PM, Hauggaard-Nielsen H, Alves BJR, Morrison MJ (2012) Legumes for mitigation of climate change and the provision of feedstock for biofuels and biorefineries. A review. Agron Sustain Dev 32(2):329–364. https://doi.org/10.1007/s13593-011-0056-7

Jin J, Tang C, Armstrong R, Sale P (2012) Phosphorus supply enhances the response of legumes to elevated CO_2 (FACE) in a phosphorus-deficient vertisol. Plant Soil 358(1):91–104. https://doi.org/10.1007/s11104-012-1270-z

Jin J, Tang C, Armstrong R, Butterly C, Sale P (2013) Elevated CO_2 temporally enhances phosphorus immobilization in the rhizosphere of wheat and chickpea. Plant Soil 368(1):315–328. https://doi.org/10.1007/s11104-012-1516-9

Kherif O, Seghouani M, Justes E, Plaza-Bonilla D, Bouhenache A, Zemmouri B, Dokukin P, Latati M (2022) The first calibration and evaluation of the STICS soil-crop model on chickpea-based intercropping system under Mediterranean conditions. Eur J Agron 133:126449. https://doi.org/10.1016/j.eja.2021.126449

Kimball BA (2016) Crop responses to elevated CO_2 and interactions with H_2O, N, and temperature. Curr Opin Plant Biol 31:36–43. https://doi.org/10.1016/j.pbi.2016.03.006

Kollas C, Kersebaum KC, Nendel C, Manevski K, Müller C, Palosuo T, Armas-Herrera CM, Beaudoin N, Bindi M, Charfeddine M, Conradt T, Constantin J, Eitzinger J, Ewert F, Ferrise R, Gaiser T, Cortazar-Atauri IG, Giglio L, Hlavinka P, Hoffmann H, Hoffmann MP, Launay M, Manderscheid R, Mary B, Mirschel W, Moriondo M, Olesen JE, Öztürk I, Pacholski A, Ripoche-Wachter D, Roggero PP, Roncossek S, Rötter RP, Ruget F, Sharif B, Trnka M, Ventrella D, Waha K, Wegehenkel M, Weigel H-J, Wu L (2015) Crop rotation modelling – a European model intercomparison. Eur J Agron 70:98–111. https://doi.org/10.1016/j.eja.2015.06.007

Kumar J, Choudhary AK, Gupta DS, Kumar S (2019) Towards exploitation of adaptive traits for climate-resilient smart pulses. Int J Mol Sci 20(12):2971

Lam SK, Hao X, Lin E, Han X, Norton R, Mosier AR, Seneweera S, Chen D (2012) Effect of elevated carbon dioxide on growth and nitrogen fixation of two soybean cultivars in northern China. Biol Fertil Soils 48(5):603–606. https://doi.org/10.1007/s00374-011-0648-z

Lavarenne J, Guyomarc'h S, Sallaud C, Gantet P, Lucas M (2018) The spring of systems biology-driven breeding. Trends Plant Sci 23(8):706–720. https://doi.org/10.1016/j.tplants.2018.04.005

Leip A, Weiss F, Lesschen J, Westhoek H (2014) The nitrogen footprint of food products in the European Union. J Agric Sci 152(S1):20–33

Lienhardt T, Black K, Saget S, Costa MP, Chadwick D, Rees RM, Williams M, Spillane C, Iannetta PM, Walker G (2019) Just the tonic! Legume biorefining for alcohol has the potential to reduce Europe's protein deficit and mitigate climate change. Environ Int 130:104870

Liu C, Cutforth H, Chai Q, Gan Y (2016) Farming tactics to reduce the carbon footprint of crop cultivation in semiarid areas. A review. Agron Sustain Dev 36(4):69. https://doi.org/10.1007/s13593-016-0404-8

Loladze I (2014) Hidden shift of the ionome of plants exposed to elevated CO_2 depletes minerals at the base of human nutrition. elife 3:e02245

Mishra AK, Agrawal SB (2015) Biochemical and physiological characteristics of tropical mung bean (Vigna radiata L.) cultivars against chronic ozone stress: an insight to cultivar-specific response. Protoplasma 252(3):797–811. https://doi.org/10.1007/s00709-014-0717-x

Myers SS, Zanobetti A, Kloog I, Huybers P, Leakey ADB, Bloom AJ, Carlisle E, Dietterich LH, Fitzgerald G, Hasegawa T, Holbrook NM, Nelson RL, Ottman MJ, Raboy V, Sakai H, Sartor KA, Schwartz J, Seneweera S, Tausz M, Usui Y (2014) Increasing CO_2 threatens human nutrition. Nature 510(7503):139–142. https://doi.org/10.1038/nature13179

Nasser RR, Fuller MP, Jellings AJ (2008) Effect of elevated CO_2 and nitrogen levels on lentil growth and nodulation. Agron Sustain Dev 28(2):175–180. https://doi.org/10.1051/agro:2007056

Naz S, Ahmad S, Abbas G, Fatima Z, Hussain S, Ahmed M, Khan MA, Khan A, Fahad S, Nasim W, Ercisli S, Wilkerson CJ, Hoogenboom G (2022) Modeling the impact of climate warming on potato phenology. Eur J Agron 132:126404. https://doi.org/10.1016/j.eja.2021.126404

Newton PCD, Clark H, Bell CC, Glasgow EM (1996) Interaction of soil moisture and elevated CO_2 on the above-ground growth rate, root length density and gas exchange of turves from temperate pasture. J Exp Bot 47(6):771–779. https://doi.org/10.1093/jxb/47.6.771

Nie M, Lu M, Bell J, Raut S, Pendall E (2013) Altered root traits due to elevated CO_2: a meta-analysis. Glob Ecol Biogeogr 22(10):1095–1105. https://doi.org/10.1111/geb.12062

Palit P, Kudapa H, Zougmore R, Kholova J, Whitbread A, Sharma M, Varshney RK (2020) An integrated research framework combining genomics, systems biology, physiology, modelling and breeding for legume improvement in response to elevated CO_2 under climate change scenario. Curr Plant Biol 22:100149. https://doi.org/10.1016/j.cpb.2020.100149

Pandey R, Meena SK, KrishnapriyaVengavasi SK, Singh MP (2016) Interactive effects of phosphorus nutrition and atmospheric carbon dioxide levels on growth, nitrogen fixation and yield of green gram. Indian J Fertil 12:56

Peyrard C, Mary B, Perrin P, Véricel G, Gréhan E, Justes E, Léonard J (2016) N_2O emissions of low input cropping systems as affected by legume and cover crops use. Agric Ecosyst Environ 224:145–156. https://doi.org/10.1016/j.agee.2016.03.028

Prasad PVV, Jagadish SVK (2015) Field crops and the fear of heat stress – opportunities, challenges and future directions. Procedia Environ Sci 29:36–37. https://doi.org/10.1016/j.proenv.2015.07.144

Pritchard SG (2011) Soil organisms and global climate change. Plant Pathol 60(1):82–99. https://doi.org/10.1111/j.1365-3059.2010.02405.x

Pushpavalli R, Zaman-Allah M, Turner NC, Baddam R, Rao MV, Vadez V (2015) Higher flower and seed number leads to higher yield under water stress conditions imposed during reproduction in chickpea. Funct Plant Biol 42(2):162–174. https://doi.org/10.1071/FP14135

Rogers A, Gibon Y, Stitt M, Morgan PB, Bernacchi CJ, Ort DR, Long SP (2006) Increased C availability at elevated carbon dioxide concentration improves N assimilation in a legume. Plant Cell Environ 29(8):1651–1658. https://doi.org/10.1111/j.1365-3040.2006.01549.x

Rogers A, Ainsworth EA, Leakey ADB (2009) Will elevated carbon dioxide concentration amplify the benefits of nitrogen fixation in legumes? Plant Physiol 151(3):1009–1016. https://doi.org/10.1104/pp.109.144113

Rosenthal DM, Ruiz-Vera UM, Siebers MH, Gray SB, Bernacchi CJ, Ort DR (2014) Biochemical acclimation, stomatal limitation and precipitation patterns underlie decreases in photosynthetic stimulation of soybean (Glycine max) at elevated [CO_2] and temperatures under fully open air field conditions. Plant Sci 226:136–146. https://doi.org/10.1016/j.plantsci.2014.06.013

Ross DJ, Newton PCD, Tate KR (2004) Elevated [CO_2] effects on herbage production and soil carbon and nitrogen pools and mineralization in a species-rich, grazed pasture on a seasonally dry sand. Plant Soil 260(1):183–196. https://doi.org/10.1023/B:PLSO.0000030188.77365.46

Rotz CA (2018) Modeling greenhouse gas emissions from dairy farms. J Dairy Sci 101(7):6675–6690. https://doi.org/10.3168/jds.2017-13272

Saha S, Chakraborty D, Lata PM, Nagarajan S (2011) Impact of elevated CO_2 on utilization of soil moisture and associated soil biophysical parameters in pigeon pea (Cajanus cajan L.). Agric Ecosyst Environ 142(3):213–221. https://doi.org/10.1016/j.agee.2011.05.008

Sanz-Sáez Á, Erice G, Aranjuelo I, Nogués S, Irigoyen JJ, Sánchez-Díaz M (2010) Photosynthetic down-regulation under elevated CO_2 exposure can be prevented by nitrogen supply in nodulated alfalfa. J Plant Physiol 167(18):1558–1565. https://doi.org/10.1016/j.jplph.2010.06.015

Sardans J, Rivas-Ubach A, Peñuelas J (2012) The C:N:P stoichiometry of organisms and ecosystems in a changing world: a review and perspectives. Perspect Plant Ecol Evol Syst 14(1):33–47. https://doi.org/10.1016/j.ppees.2011.08.002

Schwenke GD, Herridge DF, Scheer C, Rowlings DW, Haigh BM, McMullen KG (2015) Soil N_2O emissions under N_2-fixing legumes and N-fertilised canola: a reappraisal of emissions factor calculations. Agric Ecosyst Environ 202:232–242. https://doi.org/10.1016/j.agee.2015.01.017

Sennhenn A, Njarui DMG, Maass BL, Whitbread AM (2015) Can short-season grain legumes contribute to more resilient and productive farming systems in semi-arid Eastern Kenya? Procedia Environ Sci 29:81–82. https://doi.org/10.1016/j.proenv.2015.07.169

Sicher RC, Bunce JA (2015) The impact of enhanced atmospheric CO_2 concentrations on the responses of maize and soybean to elevated growth temperatures. In: Mahalingam R (ed) Combined stresses in plants. Springer, pp 27–48. https://doi.org/10.1007/978-3-319-07899-1_2

Sinclair TR, Zwieniecki MA, Holbrook NM (2008) Low leaf hydraulic conductance associated with drought tolerance in soybean. Physiol Plant 132(4):446–451. https://doi.org/10.1111/j.1399-3054.2007.01028.x

Singer SD, Chatterton S, Soolanayakanahally RY, Subedi U, Chen G, Acharya SN (2020) Potential effects of a high CO_2 future on leguminous species. Plant-Environ Interact 1(2):67–94. https://doi.org/10.1002/pei3.10009

Singh D, Singh B (2011) Breeding for tolerance to abiotic stresses in mungbean. J Food Legum 24(2):83–90

Singh P, Boote KJ, Kumar U, Srinivas K, Nigam SN, Jones JW (2012) Evaluation of genetic traits for improving productivity and adaptation of groundnut to climate change in India. J Agron Crop Sci 198(5):399–413. https://doi.org/10.1111/j.1439-037X.2012.00522.x

Singh P, Nedumaran S, Boote KJ, Gaur PM, Srinivas K, Bantilan MCS (2014a) Climate change impacts and potential benefits of drought and heat tolerance in chickpea in South Asia and East Africa. Eur J Agron 52(Part B):123–137. https://doi.org/10.1016/j.eja.2013.09.018

Singh P, Nedumaran S, Ntare BR, Boote KJ, Singh NP, Srinivas K, Bantilan MCS (2014b) Potential benefits of drought and heat tolerance in groundnut for adaptation to climate change in India and West Africa. Mitig Adapt Strat Glob Change 19(5):509–529. https://doi.org/10.1007/s11027-012-9446-7

Sita K, Sehgal A, HanumanthaRao B, Nair RM, Vara Prasad PV, Kumar S, Gaur PM, Farooq M, Siddique KHM, Varshney RK, Nayyar H (2017) Food legumes and rising temperatures: effects, adaptive functional mechanisms specific to reproductive growth stage and strategies to improve heat tolerance. Front Plant Sci 8. https://doi.org/10.3389/fpls.2017.01658

Smith P, Clark H, Dong H, Elsiddig E, Haberl H, Harper R, House J, Jafari M, Masera O, Mbow C (2014) Agriculture, forestry and other land use (AFOLU). In: Edenhofer O, Pichs-Madruga R, Sokona Y, Farahani E, Kadner S, Seyboth K, Adler A, Baum I, Brunner S, Eickemeier P, Kriemann B, Savolainen J, Schlömer S, von Stechow C, Zwickel T, Minx JC (eds) Climate change 2014: mitigation of climate change. Contribution of working group III to the fifth assessment report of the intergovernmental panel on climate change. Cambridge University Press, Cambridge/New York

Song F, Zhang GJ, Ramanathan V, Leung LR (2022) Trends in surface equivalent potential temperature: a more comprehensive metric for global warming and weather extremes. Proc Natl Acad Sci 119(6):e2117832119. https://doi.org/10.1073/pnas.2117832119

Srinivasarao C, Kundu S, Shanker AK, Naik RP, Vanaja M, Venkanna K, Maruthi Sankar GR, Rao VUM (2016) Continuous cropping under elevated CO_2: differential effects on C4 and C3 crops, soil properties and carbon dynamics in semi-arid alfisols. Agric Ecosyst Environ 218:73–86. https://doi.org/10.1016/j.agee.2015.11.016

5 Climate Change Impacts on Legume Crop Production and Adaptation Strategies

Stöckle CO, Kemanian AR (2020) Can crop models identify critical gaps in genetics, environment, and management interactions? Front Plant Sci 11. https://doi.org/10.3389/fpls.2020.00737

Sulieman S, Thao N, Tran L-S (2015) Does elevated CO_2 provide real benefits for N2-fixing leguminous symbioses? In: Sulieman S, Tran L-SP (eds) Legume nitrogen fixation in a changing environment. Springer, pp 89–112. https://doi.org/10.1007/978-3-319-06212-9_5

Suriharn B, Patanothai A, Boote KJ, Hoogenboom G (2011) Designing a peanut ideotype for a target environment using the CSM-CROPGRO-peanut model. Crop Sci 51(5):1887–1902. https://doi.org/10.2135/cropsci2010.08.0457

Thorp KR, DeJonge KC, Kaleita AL, Batchelor WD, Paz JO (2008) Methodology for the use of DSSAT models for precision agriculture decision support. Comput Electron Agric 64(2): 276–285. https://doi.org/10.1016/j.compag.2008.05.022

Tsegay A, Vanuytrecht E, Abrha B, Deckers J, Gebrehiwot K, Raes D (2015) Sowing and irrigation strategies for improving rainfed tef (Eragrostis tef (Zucc.) Trotter) production in the water scarce Tigray region, Ethiopia. Agric Water Manag 150:81–91. https://doi.org/10.1016/j.agwat.2014.11.014

Tui SH-K, Descheemaeker K, Valdivia RO, Masikati P, Sisito G, Moyo EN, Crespo O, Ruane AC, Rosenzweig C (2021) Climate change impacts and adaptation for dryland farming systems in Zimbabwe: a stakeholder-driven integrated multi-model assessment. Clim Chang 168(1):10. https://doi.org/10.1007/s10584-021-03151-8

Ullah A, Shah TM, Farooq M (2020) Pulses production in Pakistan: status, constraints and opportunities. Int J Plant Prod 14(4):549–569. https://doi.org/10.1007/s42106-020-00108-2

Vadez V, Berger JD, Warkentin T, Asseng S, Ratnakumar P, Rao KPC, Gaur PM, Munier-Jolain N, Larmure A, Voisin A-S, Sharma HC, Pande S, Sharma M, Krishnamurthy L, Zaman MA (2012) Adaptation of grain legumes to climate change: a review. Agron Sustain Dev 32(1):31–44. https://doi.org/10.1007/s13593-011-0020-6

Varshney RK, Sinha P, Singh VK, Kumar A, Zhang Q, Bennetzen JL (2020) 5Gs for crop genetic improvement. Curr Opin Plant Biol 56:190–196. https://doi.org/10.1016/j.pbi.2019.12.004

Wang X, Liu F (2021) Effects of elevated CO_2 and heat on wheat grain quality. Plan Theory 10(5): 1027

Wang N, Hatcher DW, Toews R, Gawalko EJ (2009) Influence of cooking and dehulling on nutritional composition of several varieties of lentils (Lens culinaris). LWT Food Sci Technol 42(4):842–848. https://doi.org/10.1016/j.lwt.2008.10.007

Wang G, Wang D, Zhou X, Shah S, Wang L, Ahmed M, Sayyed RZ, Fahad S (2022) Effects of cotton–peanut intercropping patterns on cotton yield formation and economic benefits. Front Sustain Food Syst 6. https://doi.org/10.3389/fsufs.2022.900230

Weih M, Mínguez MI, Tavoletti S (2022) Intercropping systems for sustainable agriculture. Agriculture 12(2):291

Xu X, Sharma P, Shu S, Lin T-S, Ciais P, Tubiello FN, Smith P, Campbell N, Jain AK (2021) Global greenhouse gas emissions from animal-based foods are twice those of plant-based foods. Nat Food 2(9):724–732. https://doi.org/10.1038/s43016-021-00358-x

Yuan ZY, Chen HYH (2015) Decoupling of nitrogen and phosphorus in terrestrial plants associated with global changes. Nat Clim Chang 5(5):465–469. https://doi.org/10.1038/nclimate2549

Yue Q, Xu X, Hillier J, Cheng K, Pan G (2017) Mitigating greenhouse gas emissions in agriculture: from farm production to food consumption. J Clean Prod 149:1011–1019. https://doi.org/10.1016/j.jclepro.2017.02.172

Zhang Y, Chen X, Zhang C, Pan G, Zhang X (2014) Availability of soil nitrogen and phosphorus under elevated [CO_2] and temperature in the Taihu Lake region, China. J Plant Nutr Soil Sci 177(3):343–348. https://doi.org/10.1002/jpln.201200526

Chapter 6
Cereal Crop Modeling for Food and Nutrition Security

Ahmed M. S. Kheir, Khalil A. Ammar, Ahmed Attia, Abdelrazek Elnashar, Shakeel Ahmad, Sherif F. El-Gioushy, and Mukhtar Ahmed

Abstract Rapid population growth, climate change, and limited natural resources have widened the gap between food production and consumption, contributing to global hunger. Improving cereal crop production is a critical hot spot challenge for closing this gap and ensuring global food security and nutrition. Previous data and findings from published literature demonstrated that cereal crop models have been applied and developed globally over the last 30 years under a wide range of climate, soil, genotype, and management conditions. However, when the models are applied to pests, diseases, phosphorus fertilization, potassium fertilization, iron, and zinc, further improvements are required. Furthermore, the integration of genotypes and phenotypes is critical for food security, necessitating careful consideration in crop models. We examined about 31 cereal crop models for increasing crop production and ensuring food and nutrition security. Furthermore, we discussed the current limitations in crop model application, as well as the critical need to integrate with

---

A. M. S. Kheir (✉)
International Center for Biosaline Agriculture, Directorate of Programs, Dubai, United Arab Emirates

Soils, Water and Environment Research Institute, Agricultural Research Center, Giza, Egypt
e-mail: a.kheir@biosaline.org.ae

K. A. Ammar · A. Attia
International Center for Biosaline Agriculture, Directorate of Programs, Dubai, United Arab Emirates

A. Elnashar
Department of Natural Resources, Faculty of African Postgraduate Studies, Cairo University, Giza, Egypt

S. Ahmad
Department of Agronomy, Bahauddin Zakariya University, Multan, Pakistan

S. F. El-Gioushy
Horticulture Department, Faculty of Agriculture (Moshtohor), Benha University, Moshtohor, Toukh, Egypt

M. Ahmed
Department of Agronomy, PMAS Arid Agriculture University, Rawalpindi, Pakistan

© The Author(s), under exclusive license to Springer Nature Switzerland AG 2022
M. Ahmed (ed.), *Global Agricultural Production: Resilience to Climate Change*,
https://doi.org/10.1007/978-3-031-14973-3_6

183

other cutting-edge sciences, such as remote sensing, machine learning, and deep learning. This will undoubtedly improve crop model accuracy and reduce uncertainty, assisting agronomists and decision makers in ensuring food and nutrition security. In this chapter, we discussed the current and further improvements of cereal crop models in assisting breeders, researchers, agronomists, and policy makers in addressing current and future challenges related to global food security and nutrition.

Keywords Cereal crops · Crop models · Food security · Model limitations and improvements · Uncertainty · Machine learning · Remote sensing · Production

6.1 Introduction

Food security is suffering from many issues worldwide including but not limited to rapid population growth, limited soil and water resources and climate change (Godfray et al. 2010; Kheir et al. 2021), which definitely affected also on nutrition (Godfray et al. 2011). Agriculture provides food security as one of the most significant ecosystem services (Zhang et al. 2007). A sustainable food system (SFS) is a food system that provides food security and nutrition for all while ensuring that the economic, social, and environmental foundations for future generations are not jeopardized (FAO 2018). This means that it is profitable all the time (economic sustainability), has broad-based societal benefits (social sustainability), and has a positive or neutral impact on the natural environment (environmental sustainability). As a result, agricultural intensification and expansion have increased in recent decades to meet global food demand. Given the rising population's demand for food, the agriculture industry has a significant challenge in raising food crop productivity. As the three staple grains of wheat, rice, and maize represent about two-thirds of total daily calorie intake, improving their yields is essential (Cassman 1999). Globally, many attempts worked on enhancing crop production and decreasing the environmental impacts. Such experiments have faced by other encountered factors, such as weather, soil, and genotypes (Basso et al. 2011). Because of the variation in place and time, it's challenging to move crop dataset from region to another for the farming policy makers (Jones et al. 1998). Crop models (CM) are regarded as powerful tools for exploring the complex integration of soil, crop, climate, and management in order to provide valuable recommendations to decision makers that are difficult to provide in trial-and-error experiments (Ali et al. 2020; Asseng et al. 2018, 2019; Ding et al. 2021; Kheir et al. 2019).

During the initial decades, the Crop Environment Resource Synthesis (CERES) models were improved. CERES-Wheat (Otter and Ritchie 1985; Ritchie 1985), CERES-Maize (Jones et al. 1986; Ritchie 1985), and CERES-Rice (Ritchie et al. 1986) were developed first to predict grain yield only and then promoted as decision support tools when Decision Support System for Agrotechnology Transfer (DSSAT) was released (Jones et al. 2003). The CERES models are dynamic crop system models that predict the crop phenology and development on a daily time series (Ahmad et al. 2012, 2013, 2019; Abbas et al. 2017). The main components of water, nitrogen, phenology and soil are important for models to predict yield (Kheir et al. 2022). The most often tested and utilized crops are maize, wheat, and rice, although CERES models also include barley, grain sorghum, and pearl millet (Ritchie 1985). In addition, the crop modeling platforms also include Agricultural Production Systems Simulator (APSIM) (Keating et al. 2003), Environmental Policy Integrated Climate (EPIC) (Kiniry et al. 1995), CropSyst (Stockle et al. 2003), as well as STICS model (Brisson et al. 1998).

Crop models have been developed to investigate the yield gap and highlight potential challenges to food security (Ammar et al. 2022). Applications of the models included quantification of the yield gap (Schils et al. 2018; van Ittersum et al. 2016), gaps between available and consumption of food (Keating et al. 2014), and land reclamation is required to meet the population growth current and in the future (Gerten et al. 2020). However, the use of CM for soil fertility, particularly with potassium and phosphorus, pets, and diseases has received less attention thus far (Donatelli et al. 2017; Kheir et al. 2020). This chapter outlines the global challenges of food security, the role of cereal crop models to address such challenges, and the consequent policy recommendations.

6.2 Global Challenges and Solutions to Ensure Food Security

The United Nations' Sustainable Development Goals (SDGs) outlined the big issues for the coming decades (UN 2015). Based on SDG axes, it was required from the agricultural system to end the hunger and food insecurity and to enhance the nutrition, as well as to protect, restore, and promote the terrestrial ecosystem and alleviate the biodiversity loss (SDG 15) and thus combat climate change (SDG 13). Diverging paradigms about what to produce, where to produce it, and how to produce it will be the fourth major problem for agricultural science in the coming years.

6.3 Food Security and Nutrition

The food wedge analysis highlighted that even if the policy recommendations reduced the food losses and demand via changing the diets, about 46% of food demand in 2050 will be taken from increasing the crop productions (Keating et al. 2014). Understanding the difference between the potential or water-limited yield and the actual yield is required to meet the additional production needed for closing the future food demand (van Ittersum et al. 2013). In the analysis of food systems, health, nutrition, and quality are becoming increasingly important (Brouwer et al. 2020). This is critical in broadening the discourse on food security beyond staple (cereal) crops and evaluating the function of nutritional variety as a crucial component of agricultural systems. It also helps to put health and nutrition into context with other macroeconomic changes such as rising earnings and an expanding middle class.

6.4 Keeping Away from Diversity Loss and Changing Land Use

Land reclamation is important and required to close the food gap by meeting the required food demand (Foley et al. 2011). For the period 2002–2014, global reclamation land grew at a rate of 12.6 million hectares per year, indicating a significant shift that had not occurred previously (Cassman and Grassini 2020). More than half of this increase in farmland was dedicated to cereal crops. Despite the global vast agricultural land resources (Chamberlin et al. 2014), it is critical to conserve land for wildlife and avoid greenhouse gas emissions connected with land removal. This is especially true considering that the majority of biodiversity is situated outside of protected areas in human-managed production landscapes, where agricultural growth poses a substantial danger (Baudron and Giller 2014). Both land sparing and land sharing are viable choices for increasing agricultural productivity while limiting negative impacts on biodiversity, but the best method relies heavily on local conditions.

6.5 Adaptation and Mitigation to Climate Change

Due to its detrimental impact on agricultural yields, climate change is anticipated to place the world's food supply on a knife's edge (Rosenzweig et al. 2014), coupled with decreasing the suitable agricultural land. Increasing CO_2 and other greenhouse gases is the main driver to increase the global temperature, variability of rainfall, and extreme events. Climate change's detrimental effects on cereal wheat output have been assessed using CM (Asseng et al. 2015; Bassu et al. 2014), but this can be offset using appropriate CO_2 fertilization (Long et al. 2006). A considerable number of crop model applications deal with climate change adaptation, but there is an imbalance with other areas that could benefit from crop model insights. Exploratory studies mapping the suitability of a given region to introduce new crops are examples of the latter (Silva and Giller 2021), or regional resource use efficiency. Noticeably, most crop models target the field scale cropping systems (Table 6.1). Extrapolating from field to region is straightforward and appealing, but it ignores explanatory factors at the farm level, which is the most significant decision-making level. To address this constraint, spatially explicit crop models have been integrated with agricultural systems to assess trade-offs in management alternatives while taking farm heterogeneity into account (Antle et al. 2018; Capalbo et al. 2017).

6 Cereal Crop Modeling for Food and Nutrition Security

Table 6.1 What can and cannot crop models do for predicting the yield and cluster levels at which they have been used

Item	Can do	Cannot do	References
Radiation	Yes		Chapman et al. (2020)
Temperature	Yes		Albasha et al. (2020)
Sowing	Yes		Bassu et al. (2020)
Water	Yes		Lopez-Bernal et al. (2020)
Nutrients (largely N)	Yes		Falconnier et al. (2020)
Pests		Yes	Rasche and Taylor (2020)
Diseases		Yes	Bregaglio et al. (2020)
Weeds		Yes	Colbach et al. (2020)
Field scale	Yes		ten Den et al. (2020)
Farm scale		Yes	Ngwira et al. (2020)
Cropping system	Yes		Kersebaum et al. (2020)
Farming system		Yes	None
Food system		Yes	None

Adapted from Silva and Giller (2021)

6.6 The Role of Cereal Crop Models

The CM could be applied to avoid the management problems following appropriate calibration and uncertainty quantification. Dynamic models are fundamentally complex hypotheses, and their testing and development entails identifying and changing the explanatory processes in the model that are responsible for an unsatisfactory representation of reality. The improvement and development is a complexed cycle of simulation experiments to generate and test the hypothesis (Rötter et al. 2018). Different crop models have been created exclusively, and the majority of CM exercises have focused on cereal crops. This is mainly due to the importance of cereals in food security and nutrition in most regions worldwide. Crop models have been applied to support plant breeding and improve cereal crop production and to reduce resource use in various environments (Dingkuhn et al. 2007; Kropff et al. 2013). In the last few decades, there has been evidence of changes in crop cultivar features and their responses to weather in many parts of the world. The creation of new rice varieties, such as semidwarf variants in the 1960s and hybrid rice varieties in the 1970s, has resulted in a rise in rice grain output across Asia. Because of the creation of semidwarf rice varieties, for example, China's rice output potential improved by around 30% (Fang et al. 2004), achieving 20% increase in yield when heteros are used (Virmani et al. 2003). In China, it was found that the vegetative growth in spring wheat decreased by 30% due to warming effect (Tao et al. 2012). Many studies have been conducted to demonstrate the importance of cereal crop models in simulating yield for use in food security strategies and policy recommendations for decision makers (Gautam et al. 2015; Liu et al. 2013; Zhang et al. 2016).

6.7 Principle Disciplines and Integrating Innovations

Most of CM have been used for simulating crop growth and development based on plant physiology and biology. However, combining crop models with other innovations such as remote sensing, machine learning, big data, and deep learning has less attention so far. These innovations frequently necessitate the creation of new sorts of models or the repackaging of current models in new programming languages (i.e., Python, R, C++) that enable their integration with new forms of data and big dataset (de Wit et al. 2019). This integration will undoubtedly improve the accuracy of CM in designing sustainable food systems, especially in light of population growth and large datasets (Basso and Antle 2020). Recently, a big dataset derived from remote sensing images has been generated, which could be used for CM to be applied at a wide range of spatial and temporal resolutions (Dharmawan et al. 2021; Sishodia et al. 2020). For example, spatial satellite image data combined with crop models improved crop yield, water use, N uptake, and resource use efficiency predictions (Huang et al. 2019). Machine learning has also proven useful in calibrating crop models based on big phenotyping data for specific genotypes (Chapman et al. 2020).

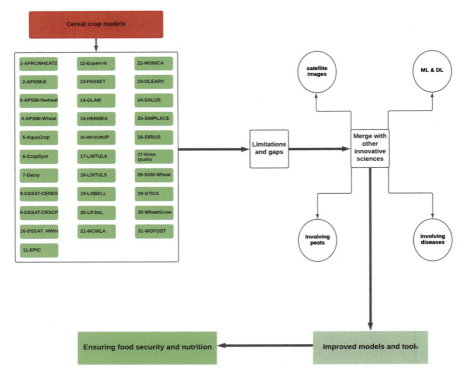

Fig. 6.1 Analytical framework highlighting the cereal crop models in literature and the potential for improvement for ensuring food security. (Own preparation by authors)

Nonetheless, this important field still requires a great deal of attention with multi-machine learning models in various environments. Therefore, we summarized cereal crop models from the literature and developed an analytical framework highlighting the potential for improving such models to ensure food security and nutrition (Fig. 6.1). Furthermore, the relative references for each model were gathered and summarized in Table 6.2.

Table 6.2 Cereal crop models in literatures

No.	Model	References
1	AFRCWHEAT2	Porter (1993)
2	APSIM-E	Keating et al. (2003) and Wang et al. (2002)
3	APSIM-N wheat	Asseng et al. (1998, 2004) and Keating et al. (2003)
4	APSIM-wheat	Keating et al. (2003)
5	AQUACROP	Stedduto et al. (2009) and Vanuytrecht et al. (2014)
6	CropSyst	Stockle et al. (2003)
7	DAISY	(Hansen et al. (1991, 2012)
8	DSSAT-CERES	(Hoogenboom and White (2003), Jones et al. (2003) and Ritchie et al. (1985)
9	DSSAT-CROPSIM	Hunt and Pararajasingham (1995) and Jones et al. (2003)
10	DSSAT-N wheat	Holzworth et al. (2014) and Kassie et al. (2016)
11	EPIC	Kiniry et al. (1995) and Williams et al. (1989)
12	Expert-N	Biernath et al. (2011), Ritchie et al. (1987) and Stenger et al. (1999)
13	FASSET	Berntsen et al. (2003) and Olesen et al. (2002)
14	GLAM	Challinor et al. (2004) and Li et al. (2010)
15	HERMES	Kersebaum (2007, 2011)
16	INFOCROP	Aggarwal et al. (2006)
17	LINTUL4	Shibu et al. (2010) and Spitters and Schapendonk (1990)
18	LOBELL	Gourdji et al. (2013)
19	LPJmL	Beringer et al. (2011) and Gerten et al. (2004)
20	MCWLA-wheat	Tao and Zhang (2013) and Tao et al. (2009)
21	MONICA	Nendel et al. (2011)
22	OLEARY	Latta and O'Leary (2003) and O'Leary et al. (1985)
23	SALUS	Basso et al. (2010) and Senthilkumar et al. (2009)
24	SIMPLACE	Angulo et al. (2013)
25	SIRIUS	Semenov and Shewry (2011)
26	Sirius quality	He et al. (2010)
27	SSM-wheat	Soltani et al. (2013)
28	STICS	Brisson et al. (2003)
29	WHEATGROW	Pan et al. (2007)
30	WOFOST	Boogaard and Kroes (1998)
31	LINTUL5	Shibu et al. (2010) and Spitters and Schapendonk (1990)

Adapted from Kheir et al. (2020)

6.8 Conclusion

The world's food systems face significant challenges, including gaps between food production and consumption caused by land degradation, rapid population growth, climate change, and limited natural resources, such as soil and water. These challenges necessitate the use of unconventional methods to meet the technology trend, large datasets, and the pressing need for food security and nutrition. Cereal crops are the most common and important crops for quantifying and addressing food security but require further improvements in production. The defined cereal crop models can investigate potential future of yield production, and adaptation for stresses. However, with new trials and cultivars, the current crop models will need to be improved and developed further. Furthermore, simulating processes at the cropping system level and contextualizing global model application and food systems should also be considered. Consequently, combining new innovative sciences such as remote sensing, machine learning, and deep learning with crop models will improve prediction accuracy and reduce uncertainty, assisting in the preparation of policy recommendations for decision makers. Integrating cereal crop models with other cutting-edge sciences will improve yield predictions and help policy makers make appropriate adaptation recommendations to ensure food security and nutrition.

References

Abbas G, Ahmad S, Ahmad A, Nasim W, Fatima Z, Hussain S, Habib ur Rehman M, Azam Khan M, Hasanuzzaman M, Fahad S, Boote KJ, Hoogenboom G (2017) Quantification the impacts of climate change and crop management on phenology of maize-based cropping system in Punjab, Pakistan. Agric For Meteorol 247:42–55. https://doi.org/10.1016/j.agrformet.2017.07.012

Aggarwal P et al (2006) InfoCrop: a dynamic simulation model for the assessment of crop yields, losses due to pests, and environmental impact of agro-ecosystems in tropical environments. II. Performance of the model. Agric Syst 89(1):47–67

Ahmad S, Ahmad A, Soler CMT et al (2012) Application of the CSM-CERES-Rice model for evaluation of plant density and nitrogen management of fine transplanted rice for an irrigated semiarid environment. Precis Agric 13:200–218. https://doi.org/10.1007/s11119-011-9238-1

Ahmad S, Ahmad A, Ali H et al (2013) Application of the CSM-CERES-Rice model for evaluation of plant density and irrigation management of transplanted rice for an irrigated semiarid environment. Irrig Sci 31:491–506. https://doi.org/10.1007/s00271-012-0324-6

Ahmad S, Abbas G, Ahmed M, Fatima Z, Anjum MA, Rasul G, Khan MA, Hoogenboom G (2019) Climate warming and management impact on the change of phenology of the rice-wheat cropping system in Punjab, Pakistan. Field Crop Res 230:46–61. https://doi.org/10.1016/j.fcr.2018.10.008

Albasha R, Manceau L, Martre P (2020) When would simulating temperature at the leaf-layer scale improve crop model performance? Conclusions from a wheat model. In: Book of abstracts Second International Crop Modelling Symposium (iCROPM2020): crop modelling for the future

Ali MGM et al (2020) Climate change impact and adaptation on wheat yield, water use and water use efficiency at North Nile Delta. Front Earth Sci 14(3):522–536

Ammar KA, Kheir AMS, Makinas I (2022) Agricultural big data and methods and models for food security analysis—a mini-review. Peer J 10:e13674. https://doi.org/10.7717/peerj.13674

Angulo C et al (2013) Implication of crop model calibration strategies for assessing regional impacts of climate change in Europe. Agric For Meteorol 170:32–46

Antle JM, Homann-KeeTui S, Descheemaeker K, Masikati P, Valdivia RO (2018) Using AgMIP regional integrated assessment methods to evaluate vulnerability, resilience and adaptive capacity for climate smart agricultural systems. In: Lipper L, McCarthy N, Zilberman D, Asfaw S, Branca G (eds) Climate smart agriculture building resilience to climate change. Springer, Cham, p 626

Asseng S et al (1998) Performance of the APSIM-wheat in Western Australia. Field Crop Res 57: 163–179

Asseng S et al (2004) Simulated wheat growth affected by rising temperature, increased water deficit and elevated atmospheric CO_2. Field Crop Res 85:85–102

Asseng S et al (2015) Rising temperatures reduce global wheat production. Nat Clim Chang 5(2): 143–147

Asseng S et al (2018) Can Egypt become self-sufficient in wheat? Environ Res Lett 13(9):094012

Asseng S et al (2019) Climate change impact and adaptation for wheat protein. Glob Chang Biol 25(1):155–173

Basso B, Antle J (2020) Digital agriculture to design sustainable agricultural systems. Nat Sustain 3(4):254–256

Basso B, Cammarano D, Troccoli A, Chen D, Ritchie J (2010) Long-term wheat response to nitrogen in a rainfed Mediterranean environment: field data and simulation analysis. Eur J Agron 33:182–188

Basso B, Ritchie JT, Cammarano D, Sartori L (2011) A strategic and tactical management approach to select optimal N fertilizer rates for wheat in a spatially variable field. Eur J Agron 35:215–222

Bassu S et al (2014) How do various maize crop models vary in their responses to climate change factors? Glob Chang Biol 20(7):2301–2320

Bassu S et al (2020) Potential maize yields in a Mediterranean environment depend on conditions around flowering. In: Book of abstracts Second International Crop Modelling Symposium (iCROPM2020): crop modelling for the future

Baudron F, Giller KE (2014) Agriculture and nature: trouble and strife? Biol Conserv 170:232–245

Beringer T, Lucht W, Schaphoff S (2011) Bioenergy production potential of global biomass plantations under environmental and agricultural constraints. Glob Change Biol Bioenergy 3: 299–312

Berntsen J, Petersen B, Jacobsen B, Olesen J, Hutchings N (2003) Evaluating nitrogen taxation scenarios using the dynamic whole farm simulation model FASSET. Agric Syst 76:817–839

Biernath C et al (2011) Evaluating the ability of four crop models to predict different environmental impacts on spring wheat grown in open-top chambers. Eur J Agron 35:71–82

Boogaard H, Kroes J (1998) Leaching of nitrogen and phosphorus from rural areas to surface waters in the Netherlands. Nutr Cycl Agroecosyst 50:321–324

Bregaglio S et al (2020) Methodological advances to incorporate damage mechanisms from diseases in crop models. In: Book of abstracts Second International Crop Modelling Symposium (iCROPM2020): crop modelling for the future

Brisson N et al (1998) STICS: a generic model for the simulation of crops and their water and nitrogen balances. I. Theory and parameterization applied to wheat and corn. Agronomie 18: 311–346

Brisson N et al (2003) An overview of the crop model STICS. Eur J Agron 18:309–332

Brouwer ID, McDermott J, Ruben R (2020) Food systems everywhere: improving relevance in practice. Glob Food Sec 26:100398

Capalbo SM, Antle JM, Seavert C (2017) Next generation data systems and knowledge products to support agricultural producers and science-based policy decision making. Agric Syst 155:191–199

Cassman KG (1999) Ecological intensification of cereal production systems: yield potential, soil quality, and precision agriculture. Proc Natl Acad Sci U S A 96:5952–5959

Cassman KG, Grassini P (2020) A global perspective on sustainable intensification research. Nat Sustain 3:262–268

Challinor A, Wheeler T, Craufurd P, Slingo J, Grimes D (2004) Design and optimisation of a large area process based model for annual crops. Agric For Meteorol 124:99–120

Chamberlin J, Jayne TS, Headey D (2014) Scarcity amidst abundance? Reassessing the potential for cropland expansion in Africa. Food Policy 48:51–65

Chapman S et al (2020) Extending the phenotype – combining proximal sensing with crop models to characterise radiation use efficiency. In: Book of abstracts Second International Crop Modelling Symposium (iCROPM2020): crop modelling for the future

Colbach N et al (2020) Modelling crop-weed canopies as a tool to optimise crop diversification in agroecological cropping systems. In: Book of abstracts Second International Crop Modelling Symposium (iCROPM2020): crop modelling for the future

de Wit A et al (2019) 25 years of the WOFOST cropping systems model. Agric Syst 168:154–167

Dharmawan IA, Rahadianto MAE, Henry E, Endyana C, Aufaristama M (2021) Application of high-resolution remote-sensing data for land use land cover mapping of university campus. ScientificWorldJournal 2021:5519011–5519011

Ding Z et al (2021) Modeling the combined impacts of deficit irrigation, rising temperature and compost application on wheat yield and water productivity. Agric Water Manag 244:106626

Dingkuhn M et al (2007) Scale and complexity in plant systems research: gene-plant-crop relations. In: Is plant growth driven by sink regulation. Springer, Berlin, pp 157–170

Donatelli M et al (2017) Modelling the impacts of pests and diseases on agricultural systems. Agric Syst 155:213–224

Falconnier GN et al (2020) Modelling climate change impacts on maize yields under low nitrogen input conditions in sub-Saharan Africa. Glob Chang Biol 26(10):5942–5964

Fang F, Zhang X, Wang D, Liao X (2004) Influence of science and technology advancement on development of Chinese rice production and scientific strategy. Res Agric Modern 25:177–181

FAO (2018) Sustainable food systems. Concept and framework. www.fao.org/sustainable-food-value-chain/www.fao.org/about/what-we-do/so4

Foley JA et al (2011) Solutions for a cultivated planet. Nature 478(7369):337–342

Gautam S, Mbonimpa EG, Kumar S, Bonta JV, Lal R (2015) Agricultural policy environmental eXtender model simulation of climate change impacts on runoff from a small no-till watershed. J Soil Water Conserv 70(2):101–109

Gerten D, Schaphoff S, Haberlandt U, Lucht W, Sitch S (2004) Terrestrial vegetation and water balance – hydrological evaluation of a dynamic global vegetation model. J Hydrol 286:249–270

Gerten DV et al (2020) Feeding ten billion people is possible within four terrestrial planetary boundaries. Nat Sustain 3(3):200–208. https://doi.org/10.1038/s41893-019-0465-1

Godfray HCJ et al (2010) Food security: the challenges of feeding 9 billion people. Science 327: 812–818

Godfray HCJ, Pretty J, Thomas SM, Warham JR, Beddington JR (2011) Linking policy on climate and food. Science 331:1013–1014

Gourdji SM, Mathews KL, Reynolds M, Crossa J, Lobell DB (2013) An assessment of wheat yield sensitivity and breeding gains in hot environments. Proc R Soc B Biol Sci 280(1752):20122190

Hansen S, Jensen H, Nielsen N, Svendsen H (1991) Simulation of nitrogen dynamics and biomass production in winter-wheat using the Danish simulation model DAISY. Fertil Res 27:245–259

Hansen S, Abrahamsen P, Petersen CT, Styczen M (2012) DAISY: model use, calibration, and validation. Trans ASABE 55:1317–1335

He J, Stratonovitch P, Allard V, Semenov MA, Martre P (2010) Global sensitivity analysis of the process-based wheat simulation model siriusquality1 identifies key genotypic parameters and unravels parameters interactions. Procedia Soc Behav Sci 2:7676–7677

Holzworth DP et al (2014) APSIM – evolution towards a new generation of agricultural systems simulation. Environ Model Softw 62:327–350

6 Cereal Crop Modeling for Food and Nutrition Security

Hoogenboom G, White JW (2003) Improving physiological assumptions of simulation models by using gene-based approaches. Agron J 95:92–90

Huang J et al (2019) Assimilation of remote sensing into crop growth models: current status and perspectives. Agric For Meteorol 276–277:107609

Hunt LA, Pararajasingham S (1995) CROPSIM-wheat – a model describing the growth and development of wheat. Can J Plant Sci 75:619–632

Jones CA, Kiniry JR, Dyke PT (1986) CERES-maize: a simulation model of maize growth and development. Texas A & M University Press, College Station

Jones JW et al (1998) Decision support system for agrotechnology transfer: DSSAT v3. In: Tsuji G, Hoogenboom G, Thornton P (eds) Understanding options for agricultural production, vol 7. Springer

Jones JW et al (2003) The DSSAT cropping system model. Eur J Agron 18:235–265

Kassie BT, Asseng S, Porter CH, Royce FS (2016) Performance of DSSAT-N wheat across a wide range of current and future growing conditions. Eur J Agron 81:27–36

Keating BA et al (2003) An overview of APSIM, a model designed for farming systems simulation. Eur J Agron 18:267–288

Keating BA, Herrero M, Carberry PS, Gardner J, Cole MB (2014) Food wedges: framing the global food demand and supply challenge towards 2050. Glob Food Sec 3(3):125–132

Kersebaum K (2007) Modelling nitrogen dynamics in soil-crop systems with HERMES. Nutr Cycl Agroecosyst 77:39–52

Kersebaum K (2011) Special features of the HERMES model and additional procedures for parameterization, calibration, validation, and applications. In: Ahuja LR, Ma L (eds) Methods of introducing system models into agricultural research, Advances in agricultural systems modeling series 2. Madison (ASA-CSSA-SSSA), pp 65–94

Kersebaum KC, Wallor E, Schulz S (2020) Effects of climate change on crop rotations and their management across the federal state of Brandenburg/Germany. In: Book of abstracts Second International Crop Modelling Symposium (iCROPM2020): crop modelling for the future

Kheir AMS et al (2019) Impacts of rising temperature, carbon dioxide concentration and sea level on wheat production in North Nile delta. Sci Total Environ 651:3161–3173

Kheir AMS et al (2020) Wheat crop modelling for higher production. In: Ahmed M (ed) Systems modeling. Springer, Singapore. https://doi.org/10.1007/978-981-15-4728-7_6

Kheir AMS et al (2021) Modeling deficit irrigation-based evapotranspiration optimizes wheat yield and water productivity in arid regions. Agric Water Manag 256:107122

Kheir AMS, Hoogenboom G, Ammar KA, Ahmed M, Feike T, Elnashar A, Liu B, Ding Z, Asseng S (2022) Minimizing trade-offs between wheat yield and resource-use efficiency in the Nile Delta – A multimodel analysis. Field Crop Res 287:108638. https://doi.org/10.1016/j.fcr.2022.108638

Kiniry JR et al (1995) EPIC model parameters for cereal, oilseed, and forage crops in the northern great plains region. Can J Plant Sci 75:679–688

Kropff MJ et al (2013) Applications of systems approaches at the field level: volume 2: proceedings of the second international symposium on systems approaches for agricultural development, held at IRRI, Los Baños, Philippines, 6–8 December 1995. Springer, p 6

Latta J, O'Leary G (2003) Long-term comparison of rotation and fallow tillage systems of wheat in Australia. Field Crop Res 83:173–190

Li S et al (2010) Simulating the impacts of global warming on wheat in China using a large area crop model. Acta Meteor Sin 24:123–135

Liu S et al (2013) Modelling crop yield, soil water content and soil temperature for a soybean–maize rotation under conventional and conservation tillage systems in Northeast China. Agric Water Manag 123:32–44

Long SP, Ainsworth EA, Leakey ADB, Nösberger J (2006) Food for thought: lower-than-expected crop yield stimulation with rising CO_2 concentrations. Science 312:1918–1921

Lopez-Bernal A et al (2020) A spatial assessment of climate change impacts on the productivity and irrigation requirements of olive orchards. In: Book of abstracts Second International Crop Modelling Symposium (iCROPM2020): crop modelling for the future

Nendel C et al (2011) The MONICA model: testing predictability for crop growth, soil moisture and nitrogen dynamics. Ecol Model 222:1614–1625

Ngwira A et al (2020) Improving the productivity and resilience of smallholder farmers with maize-legume and legume-legume systems in Malawi. In: Book of abstracts Second International Crop Modelling Symposium (iCROPM2020): crop modelling for the future

O'Leary GJ, Connor DJ, White DH (1985) A simulation-model of the development, growth and yield of the wheat crop. Agric Syst 17:1–26

Olesen J et al (2002) Comparison of methods for simulating effects of nitrogen on green area index and dry matter growth in winter wheat. Field Crop Res 74:131–149

Otter S, Ritchie JT (1985) Validation of the CERES-wheat model in diverse environments. In: Wheat growth and modelling. Springer, Boston, pp 307–310

Pan J, Zhu Y, Cao W (2007) Modeling plant carbon flow and grain starch accumulation in wheat. Field Crop Res 101:276–284

Porter JR (1993) AFRCWHEAT2: a model of the growth and development of wheat incorporating responses to water and nitrogen. Eur J Agron 2:69–82

Rasche L, Taylor R (2020) EPIC-GILSYM: modelling crop-insect interactions and pest management with a novel coupled crop-insect model. In: Book of abstracts Second International Crop Modelling Symposium (iCROPM2020): crop modelling for the future

Ritchie JT (1985) A user-orientated model of the soil water balance in wheat. In: Wheat growth and modelling. Springer, pp 293–305

Ritchie JT, Godwin DC, Otter-Nacke S (1985) CERES-wheat. A simulation model of wheat growth and development. Texas A & M University Press, College Station

Ritchie JT, Alocilja EC, Singh U, Uehara G (1986) IBSNAT and the CERES Rice model. Weather and rice

Ritchie S, Nguyen H, Holaday A (1987) Genetic diversity in photosynthesis and water use efficiency of wheat and wheat relatives. J Cell Biochem 43

Rosenzweig C et al (2014) Assessing agricultural risks of climate change in the 21st century in a global gridded crop model intercomparison. Proc Natl Acad Sci 111(9):3268

Rötter RP et al (2018) Linking modelling and experimentation to better capture crop impacts of agroclimatic extremes – a review. Field Crop Res 221:142–156

Schils R et al (2018) Cereal yield gaps across Europe. Eur J Agron 101:109–120

Semenov MA, Shewry PR (2011) Modelling predicts that heat stress, not drought, will increase vulnerability of wheat in Europe. Sci Rep 1:5

Senthilkumar S, Basso B, Kravchenko AN, Robertson GP (2009) Contemporary evidence of soil carbon loss in the US corn belt. Soil Sci Soc Am J 73:2078–2086

Shibu M, Leffelaar P, van Keulen H, Aggarwal P (2010) LINTUL3, a simulation model for nitrogen-limited situations: application to rice. Eur J Agron 32:255–271

Silva JV, Giller KE (2021) Grand challenges for the 21st century: what crop models can and can't (yet) do. J Agric Sci 158(10):794–805

Sishodia RP, Ray RL, Singh SK (2020) Applications of remote sensing in precision agriculture: a review. Remote Sens 12(19):3136

Soltani A, Maddah V, Sinclair R (2013) SSM-wheat: a simulation model for wheat development, growth and yield. Int J Plant Prod 7:711–740

Spitters CJT, Schapendonk AHCM (1990) Evaluation of breeding strategies for drought tolerance in potato by means of crop growth simulation. Plant Soil 123:193–203

Stedduto P, Hsiao T, Raes D, Fereres E (2009) Aquacrop – the FAO crop model to simulate yield response to water: I. concepts and underlying principles. Agron J 101:426–437

Stenger R, Priesack E, Barkle G, Sperr C (1999) Espert-N A tool for simulating nitrogen and carbon dynamics in the soil-plant-atmosphere system. Land Treatment collective proceedings Technical Session, New Zealand

Stockle C, Donatelli M, Nelso R (2003) CropSyst, a cropping systems simulation model. Eur J Agron 18:289–307

Tao F, Zhang Z (2013) Climate change, wheat productivity and water use in the North China Plain: a new super-ensemble-based probabilistic projection. Agric For Meteorol 170:146–165

Tao F, Zhang Z, Liu J, Yokozawa M (2009) Modelling the impacts of weather and climate variability on crop productivity over a large area: a new super-ensemble-based probabilistic projection. Agric For Meteorol 149:1266–1278

Tao F, Zhang S, Zhang Z (2012) Spatiotemporal changes of wheat phenology in China under the effects of temperature, day length and cultivar thermal characteristics. Eur J Agron 43:201–212

ten Den T et al (2020) The effect of potato cultivar differences on parameters in WOFOST. In: Book of abstracts Second International Crop Modelling Symposium (iCROPM2020): crop modelling for the future

UN (2015) Resolution adopted by the general assembly on 25 September 2015. 70/1 Transforming our world: agenda for sustainable development, Technical report. The 2030 United Nations General Assembly, Washington, DC

van Ittersum MK et al (2013) Yield gap analysis with local to global relevance – a review. Field Crop Res 143:4–17

van Ittersum MK et al (2016) Can sub-Saharan Africa feed itself? Proc Natl Acad Sci 113(52): 14964

Vanuytrecht E et al (2014) AquaCrop: FAO's crop water productivity and yield response model. Environ Model Softw 62:351–360

Virmani SS, Mao CX, Hardy B (2003) Hybrid rice for food security, poverty alleviation, and environmental protection. International Rice Research Institute

Wang E et al (2002) Development of a generic crop model template in the cropping system model APSIM. Eur J Agron 18:121–140

Williams JR, Jones CA, Kiniry JR, Spanel DA (1989) The EPIC crop growth-model. Trans ASABE 32:497–511

Zhang W, Ricketts TH, Kremen C, Carney K, Swinton SM (2007) Ecosystem services and dis-services to agriculture. Ecol Econ 64:253–260

Zhang B et al (2016) Simulating yield potential by irrigation and yield gap of rainfed soybean using APEX model in a humid region. Agric Water Manag 177:440–453

Chapter 7
Changing Climate Scenario: Perspectives of *Camelina sativa* as Low-Input Biofuel and Oilseed Crop

Muhammad Ahmad, Ejaz Ahmad Waraich, Muhammad Bilal Hafeez, Usman Zulfiqar, Zahoor Ahmad, Muhammad Aamir Iqbal, Ali Raza ⓘ, M. Sohidul Slam, Abdul Rehman, Uzma Younis, Muhammad Kamran, Muhammad Ammar Raza, Javeed Ahmad Lone, and Ayman El Sabagh

Abstract High population shifts and climate change are putting thrust on the food industry, especially edible oil production. Monoculture of high-input crops certainly affects the crop yield and soil health. The import of edible oil is increasing in the major part of the world, putting some burden on the national exchequer of the countries. The current oil crops are unable to meet the deficit to address the problems; a crop with distinct features must be incorporated in the cropping system.

M. Ahmad · E. A. Waraich · M. B. Hafeez · U. Zulfiqar
Department of Agronomy, University of Agriculture, Faisalabad, Pakistan

Z. Ahmad
Department of Botany, University of Central Punjab Bahawalpur Campus, Bahawalpur, Pakistan

M. A. Iqbal
Department of Agronomy, Faculty of Agriculture, University of Poonch Rawalakot, Rawalakot, Pakistan

A. Raza
Key Lab of Biology and Genetic Improvement of Oil Crops, Oil Crops Research Institute (OCRI), Chinese Academy of Agricultural Sciences (CAAS), Wuhan, Hubei, China

M. S. Slam
Department of Agronomy, Hajee Mohammad Danesh Science and Technology University, Dinajpur, Bangladesh

A. Rehman
Department of Agronomy, Faculty of Agriculture and Environment, The Islamia University of Bahawalpur, Bahawalpur, Pakistan

U. Younis
Department of Botany, University of Central Punjab, Punjab, Pakistan

M. Kamran
College of Pastoral Agriculture Science and Technology, Lanzhou University, Lanzhou, People's Republic of China

© The Author(s), under exclusive license to Springer Nature Switzerland AG 2022
M. Ahmed (ed.), *Global Agricultural Production: Resilience to Climate Change*,
https://doi.org/10.1007/978-3-031-14973-3_7

[*Camelina sativa* (L.) Crantz], a unique profiled biodiesel crop, is famous as gold of pleasure, and its oil is famous as a golden liquid. Camelina oil is an outstanding feedstock for the bio-based industry since its unique composition allows multiple applications. It is a rich source of oil >43%, which comprises a huge amount of unsaturated fatty acids, which accounts for 90%, containing 30–40% of alpha-linolenic acid and 15–25% of linoleic acid. The revival of this unique oilseed crop was based on (a) numerous inherent promising physiognomies, vigorous agronomic characteristics, eye-catching oil profile, genetic continuity with *Arabidopsis*, and the comfort of genetic remodeling by floral dip; (b) the investment in camelina which is understood as it merits serious considerations as potential biodiesel and oilseed and which shares a big role toward the sustainability along with increasing the diversity and production of plant oils; and (c) a univocal and descriptive portrayal of the different growth stages of camelina which will be used as an important apparatus for agronomy and research. In this review, the extended BBCH (Biologische Bundesanstalt, Bundessortenamt, and Chemische Industrie) scale was used to describe the phenological stages. The best use of camelina in the industrial sector as a drop-in product of packing materials, coatings, and adhesions can be achieved by further research to enlarge the camelina market.

Keywords Agronomic aspects · Industrial products · and biodiesel · BBCH scale · *Camelina sativa* · Diversification · Morpho-phenology · Attainable yield potential

7.1 Introduction

Agriculture productivity has many major challenges including increasing resource depletion, ever-growing cost pressure (Iqbal et al. 2021a), ongoing structural change, and increasingly adverse impacts of climate change (IPPC 2011). Oil crops are high-value agricultural commodities used in refined edible oil products, and with the rising global population, the demand for high-quality seed oils continues to grow (Gupta 2015). Despite numerous efforts to enhance the productivity of oil crops, there is still a huge gap between the demand and supply of oil in the bio-based and edible oil markets extracted from different oilseed crops (Iqbal et al. 2021b). Sustainable oil crops produce high amount of edible oil which could be used in human nutrition and the feedstock could be used in animal feed. Most extensively grown oilseed crops, i.e., rapeseed (*Brassica napus* L.), soybean (*Glycine max* L.), and sunflower (*Helianthus annuus* L.), mainly retrieve the economic values of their oil related to its quality. Having even, or at least predictable, oil quality would

M. A. Raza · J. A. Lone
Department of Field Crops, Faculty of Agriculture, Kezer Campus Siirt University, Siirt, Turkey

A. El Sabagh (✉)
Department of Field Crops, Faculty of Agriculture, Kezer Campus Siirt University, Siirt, Turkey

Department of Agronomy, Faculty of Agriculture, Kafrelsheikh University, Kafrelsheikh, Egypt

characterize an added value for emerging oilseed crops, such as camelina, which has a huge potential in the bio-based market under the eyes of its unique fatty acid profile, as it permits a plethora of numerous applications (Berti et al. 2016). The introduction of a new crop in the existing cropping system to enhance productivity and profitability is directly associated with crop diversification. This is a vital part of the process of structural transformation of the economy of the country. The improvement in the productivity of oilseed crops in the country is the need of the hour. The introduction of the latest technologies brings crop diversification, which results in a positive shift in the area under oilseed crops (Abro 2012). These efforts were fruitful, but still, there is a huge gap between the demand-supply of edible oil in the country. *Camelina sativa* is a golden crop, which is a success story due to its salient features, i.e., environmentally sustainable source of energy (Chaturvedi et al. 2017). The introduction, adoption, and implementation of new technology always need special attention due to certain factors such as economic situation of the farmers. So, it is a challenge to penetrate a new crop into the rural market and agriculture infrastructure. Furthermore, the adoption of the new crop must be superior in a particular section, plus it must have the ability to be a value-added commodity which can give early and handsome returns to the stakeholders. This will also help in resolving the problems associated with monotonous crop rotation and also will enhance the systems health and productivity. To overcome these problems, there should be an alternative solution like another oilseed crop that can compete in the production race and maintains the quality of edible oil and other purposes. In this scenario, *C. sativa* may be used as a commercial, sustainable, and terrestrial source of longer-chain fatty acids and for human food and as aquaculture feedstock (Righini et al. 2019).

C. sativa is a rediscovered oilseed crop that belongs to the family Brassicaceae (Righini et al. 2016); originated from Finland, Northern Europe; and spread around the globe (Schillinger 2019). This crop has gained tremendous attention from stakeholders and re-emerged as an important oilseed crop. It has numerous attributes that give it unique status among other oilseed crops. For instance, it can be grown successfully under suboptimal growth condition and has been reported to perform well under water-deficit environment than major oilseed crop, e.g., rapeseed (*Brassica napus* L.) (Zubr 1997; Gugel and Falk 2006). It requires low inputs compared to other crops (Righini et al. 2019) that makes *C. sativa* the best fit on less fertile and moisture-deficient lands. Its oil has comparatively low glucosinolate content than other members of the Brassicaceae family, making it relatively better option to use its oil in different feed formations (Matthäus and Zubr 2000b).

Biodiesel production from vegetable oils is a great alternative to conventional petroleum-biodiesel due to its remarkable environmentally safe quality. It has a huge market as it can be used in agricultural machinery, automobiles, power generation, and the stationary power sector (Xue et al. 2011). Almost 95% of the world's biodiesel is produced from vegetable oils like canola, sunflower, and soybean (Gui et al. 2008). In recent years, the demand for *C. sativa* has increased due to its ability to grow with few inputs, and its oil can be utilized for a nonfood purpose (Putnam et al. 1993). The fatty acids pattern in *C. sativa* is very particular with the characterization of 30–40% linolenic acid (C18:3), almost 4% of erucic acid, and 15% of eicosenic acid (C20:1) (Budin et al. 1995), making it highly suitable for drying oil, which is used to form environment-friendly paints and coatings (Zaleckas et al. 2012; Kasetaite et al. 2014). Despite its ability to be grown as an alternate oilseed crop for semiarid regions, *C. sativa* remains underexploited due to the limited attention of researchers despite its unique agronomic and industrial potential. The present review describes the agronomic potential of *C. sativa* provided under semiarid conditions as an alternate oilseed crop. It further underscores the industrial potential of *C. sativa* and its nutritive values. Moreover, it also discusses the challenges and projections for future research to ensure the economic feasibility of *C. sativa* production.

7.2 Oilseed and Biofuel Crops Under Changing Climate

The climate change is characterized by various indicators and manifests itself as global warming, CO_2 enrichment of the atmosphere, ozone depletion, melting of glaciers, and permafrosts resulting in rising of sea level and changing of weather patterns (Abbas et al. 2021a; Iqbal et al. 2021a, b; Siddiqui et al. 2019). The net impacts of climate change include erratic rainfalls, emergence of drought spells of varying intensity and duration along with disruption of modern cropping systems with respect to sowing time, and emergence of new insect pest of food and nonfood crops (Iqbal et al. 2020). Besides food and oilseed crops, biofuel crops have also been seriously affected by changing climatic scenario in a direct or an indirect way (Abbas et al. 2021b; Iqbal et al. 2020). The direct influence of climate change and global warming has been significantly adverse for most of C3 crops compared to C4 crops (Iqbal et al. 2020). The indirect impact of changing climate on biofuel crops might be attributed to lesser area available for cultivating nonfood crops owing to uncertain and highly variable productivity of food crops especially wheat, rice, maize, etc. Currently, intensive research is being undertaken to develop strategies for reducing CO_2 emission into the atmosphere, while bioenergy may serve as one of the promising substitutes of the fossil fuels (Somerville et al. 2010). For instance, the USA is using the starch component from 40% of maize for the production of ethanol having consumption in transportation sector. However, optimum amount of fertilizer needs to be applied in addition to field preparation for growing biofuel crops such as maize that ultimately requisite fossil fuel consumption, thus tempering carbon savings strives (Hossain et al. 2020).

Recently, researchers are striving to develop liquid fuel (ethanol) from lignocellulose of crops like camelina that hold potential to mitigate adverse effects of climate change through lesser use of fertilizers and tillage, avoiding numerous disadvantages associated with traditional biofuel crops such as corn which require intensive management and contribute to greenhouse gases emission into the atmosphere. The biofuel term encompasses grown fuels like corn ethanol that might be utilized in transportation sector instead of fossil fuels (like petroleum products). In addition, biofuel term is also used for any fuel synthesized from various types of plant materials belonging to crops such as maize, sorghum, soybean, etc. The biggest advantage of biofuel crops especially camelina is that they greatly suck CO_2 from the air as they grow and thus might be declared as zero net emitter. But considering camelina like biofuel crops as zero emitter crop is not too simplistic as its cultivation requires application of fertilizers, use of fossil fuel-run tractors for performing different operations, transportation of farm inputs to field, and energy for converting the plant material into liquid fuels. Under changing climate, cultivation of camelina can also increase carbon storage in the soil. However, a careful and precise life cycle analysis of camelina encompasses fossil fuel consumption for crop cultivation, harvest, plant material conversion into fuel, transportation of biofuel to distribution facilities, and their combustion effect on environment.

Climate change tends to trigger most of oilseed crop growth and development on the cost of shortening the crop growth duration (Farooq et al. 2022). It has been reported that increased air saturation and vapor pressure owing to higher temperature in the longer run restrict moisture exchange among crop leaves and atmosphere (Faisal et al. 2020). Additionally, high temperature as a result of climate change gives rise to heat stress that is detrimental to crop plants especially at reproductive crop stage which leads to notable reduction in crop yield (Sabagh et al. 2020; Raza et al. 2022). Moreover, warmer climate coupled with CO_2-enriched environment invites significantly higher pests and diseases (both indigenous and exogenous). Oilseed crops have witnessed a sharp decline in their productivity owing to the adverse effects of climate change during the last decade. In particular, heat stress and erratic precipitation have served as the most vital climatic factors determining the seed yield as well as oil concentration of seeds (Ahmad et al. 2021). Therefore, there is a dire need to investigate alternative oilseed crops such as camelina that are either preadapted or hold potential to thrive well under rising temperature and erratic precipitation levels as predicted by numerous climate change models. Despite due recognition of the need to produce biodiesel and cooking oil from alternative crops including camelina, the agroecological requirements of alternative crops and degree of adaptive variation in their seeds and ecophysiological characteristics have remained unclear. Thorough investigations pertaining to determining the ecological requirements for biofuel-cum-oilseed crops like camelina might be used for identification of suitable present as well as future cultivation areas. Moreover, there is need to develop viable analytical tools for appropriate modeling of camelina like crops niches and their potential distributions enabling the projection of changes for their cultivation in climatically suitable areas.

7.3 History

Camelina (*Camelina sativa* L.) originated from Finland to Romania and east to Ural Mountains. The very first cultivation of *C. sativa* was done after the bronze ages (between the stone ages and the iron ages) in Northern Europe (Francis and Warwick 2009; Toncea 2014). It is native to Northern Europe. According to Francis and Warwick (2009), the *Camelina* spp. in the cards originated in southwestern Asia and southeastern Europe, while the exact origin of *C. sativa* is still undefined (Larsson 2013). A number of its species got under the molecular analysis that suggested the center of its origin is Russia and Ukraine (Ghamkhar et al. 2010). According to archaeologists, the origin of *C. sativa* is southern Europe, and its cultivation is started in Neolithic times. Till the iron ages, it was a famous cultivated crop all over Europe (Knörzer 1978). Its introduction to North America is a contaminant in the seed lots of different crops (Francis and Warwick 2009). It was deliberately introduced in Canada in 1863 in Manitoba and then cultivated in the Peace River district during the mid-1990s (Francis and Warwick 2009). In North America, its proper cultivation was started in the late 1990s (Robinson 1987). It belongs to the family Brassicaceae and is famous as "false flax" and "gold of pleasure." It was a well-known oilseed crop before World War II, but after the explosions, the cultivation of *C. sativa* declined and was replaced by other oilseed crops (Ehrensing and Guy 2008; Séguin-Swartz et al. 2013). The very initial trial that was carried out in North America renowned that *C. sativa* bearing a high level of oil content, economic yield, and short duration lifecycle which assets grave consideration as a potential crop (Plessers et al. 1962) and three trials were carried out in Ottawa and Ontario. The second trial was performed at Fort Vermillion, Alberta (Plessers et al. 1962), and found that camellia is performing better than other oilseed crops of the area like rapeseed and flaxseed. These trials were followed, and additional trials were conducted in Denmark, England, and Finland, showing that *C. sativa* has an oil content of 40–44% (Zubr 2003a, b).

7.3.1 Native Range

The native region of *C. sativa* in Asia includes Pakistan, Armenia, Georgia, Azerbaijan, India, Mongolia, Russian Federations, Turkey, Tajikistan, Kazakhstan, and Turkmenistan (USDA 2011), and in Europe, Albania, Macedonia, Austria, Slovakia, Belgium, France (including Corsica), Bosnia and Herzegovina, Montenegro, Bulgaria, Czech Republic, Croatia, Ukraine (Crimea), Denmark, Greece (Crete), Germany, Hungary, Italy, Spain (Sardinia, Sicily), Russian Federation, Moldova, Slovenia, the Netherlands, Switzerland, Sweden, and the UK (USDA 2011).

7.3.2 Range

In Asia, the *C. sativa* was first introduced in China and Japan (USDA 2011), while in Africa, it was introduced in Tunisia (USDA 2011). In Australasia, *C. sativa* was first introduced in Australia (Southern regions of the country, Tasmania, Victoria, and Western regions) and New Zealand (Western Australian Herbarium, 2010, USDA-ARS 2011). In the USA, it was introduced in almost 38 states, including California,

Indiana, Arkansas, Florida, Mississippi, Tennessee, Nevada, Colorado, etc. (USDA 2011). The introduction of *C. sativa* is reported in South America in Uruguay, Chile, Mexico, and Argentina (Francis and Warwick 2009; USDA 2011). In Canada, it was introduced throughout the whole country except Newfoundland province (Govt. of Canada 2011; Francis and Warwick 2009), and in Europe, it was reported as a naturalized crop in Belarus, Ireland, Finland, Estonia, Lithuania, Latvia, Poland, Norway, Romania, and Ukraine (Milbau and Stout 2008; USDA-ARS 2011)

7.4 Classification

7.4.1 Taxonomy and Genetics

The genera Camelina belongs to the tribe Camelineae and family Brassicaceae (mustard family) (Al-Shehbaz et al. 2006). Camelineae tribe also includes the model plant known as *Capsella bursa-pastoris* and *Arabidopsis thaliana*. It is polyploidy in nature, evidenced by the genetic mapping of its genome (Galasso et al. 2011), and the hexaploid genome is also reported (Hutcheon et al. 2010). Chromosome numbers for *C. sativa* are 14 or $n = 6$ or 26 or $2n = 12$, or 40, with $2n = 40$, a common count (Gehringer et al. 2006). USDA-NRCS (2010) stated the taxonomic position of *C. sativa* as it belongs to the kingdom Plantae, subkingdom Tracheobionta, superdivision Spermatophyta, division Magnoliophyta, class Magnoliopsida, subclass Dilleniidae, order Capparales, family Brassicaceae, tribe Camelineae, genus *Camelina* Crantz, and species *Camelina sativa* (L.) Crantz (gold-of-pleasure) (Al-Shehbaz et al. 2006).

7.5 Plant Growth

7.5.1 Morphology

It is assumed that *C. sativa* was originally cultured as a winter oilseed crop (Waraich et al. 2017) that can attain height up to 30–90 cm (Putnam et al. 1993). After germination, the initial growth is conceded on the conical room having axial branches. In the initial growth phase, the plant part above the ground consists of rosettes of leaves. These rosettes then will be turned into an erect stalk having several leaves. Its stem becomes woody when the plant reaches maturity with glabrous or sparse hairs (Klinkenberg 2008). The stem is non-branched most of the time, but sometimes it has branches (Klinkenberg 2008). In the case of hairy stems, the starlike hairs are more in numbers than normal hairs. Leaves are narrow in shape with pointed edges and are 2–8 cm long (Putnam et al. 1993). During the consequent stage of growth, flowering and axial branches having flowers develop from the apex. Its flowers are small and prolific, known as racemes, which are greenish-yellow (Putnam et al. 1993), pale yellow, or white (Klinkenberg 2008) in color. Camelina flowers consist of four petals with 4–5 mm length and sepals with 2–3 mm, style length is 2–2.5 mm, and length of flower stalk is 10–25 mm. Its fruit is known as silique, which is shaped like a pear pod or teardrop-shaped having 5–6 mm width and 7–9 mm in length with a squared-off tip, 0.7–2.5 mm in diameter, brown to orange in color, and results from self-pollination, though they can be cross-pollinated by different pollinator insects. Seed pods resembled the bolls of flax and range 6–14 mm in length, containing 10–25 seeds. The seeds are pale yellow, tiny in size (0.7 mm × 1.5 mm) (Klinkenberg 2008), and oblong with a tough surface (Putnam et al. 1993). Seedling emergence takes around 6 days after sowing, while fluorescence appeared and seed formation initiates 37 and 57 days after sowing and plant takes ~80 days after emergence to reach maturity (Alina and Roman 2009). At harvesting time, the plant reached a height of 51.4 cm, with an average of 87–121 siliques per plant having ~739 seeds/plant and ~6.55 seeds per silique (Alina and Roman 2009; Waraich et al. 2017).

7.5.2 Phenology

C. sativa has got much attention due to its salient features, but the exact depiction of its phenological growth stages is not understood yet. Martinelli and Galasso (2011) planned an experiment to elaborate the phenological growth stages based on the extended BBCH scale (Hack et al. 1992). The knowledge of growth stages is essential and supposed to be fundamental for studying the ability of crops to adopt different environmental conditions, for development of highly suitable and appropriate agronomic techniques, for different breeding programs, and for the setup of application protocols of different fertilizer and herbicide.

7.5.3 Growth of Camelina: Overall Depiction

It can be subdivided into three subspecies on taxonomic bases (*pilosa, foetida*, and *sativa*) (Angelini and Moscheni 1998). So, its cultivation extended from overwintering to spring period. *C. sativa* ssp. *pilosa and sativa* were supposed to be good in an agronomic context. *Pilosa* is known for its character of verbalization requiring the maximum growth of stem and consequent flowering. One of the main characteristics of camelina is its morphological plasticity. This species is characterized as a short-growing seasonal crop that completes its life cycle with 110 days in spring, and it might be shortened under adverse conditions.

7.5.4 BBCH Scale for C. sativa

Table 7.1 shows the ten different growth stages of *C. sativa* based on two- and three-digit BBCH scales. For the overall depiction of development, the two-digit code is

7 Changing Climate Scenario: Perspectives of *Camelina sativa*...

Table 7.1 Depiction of the *C. sativa* phenological growth stages in accordance with the extended BBCH scale (Used with permission of Martinelli and Galasso, 2011)

BBCH codes		
Two digits (00)	Three digits (000)	Explanation
Germination: the principal growth stage 0		
00	000	Dry seed
01	001	Imbibition of seed starts
03	003	Imbibition finished
05	005	Emergence of radicle from seed
07	007	Hypocotyl emergence from seed with cotyledons
08	008	Hypocotyl along with cotyledons mounting toward the soil
09	009	Cotyledons emergence through the soil surface
Leaf enlargement: principal growth stage 1		
10	100	Unfolded Cotyledons (node 0)
11	101	True leaf pair on first node
12	102	Single true leaf on second node
13	103	Single true leaf on third node
14	104	Single true leaf on fourth node
15	105	Single true leaf on fifth node
16	106	Single true leaf on sixth node
17	107	Single true leaf on seventh node
18	108	Single true leaf on eighth node
19	109	Single true leaf on ninth node
	110	Single true leaf on tenth node
	118	Till stage 199 the coding lasts with the same trend
	119	Single true leaf on 19th or succeeding node
Development of side shoots[a]: principal growth stage 2		
21	201	One-sided shoot developed
22	202	Two-sided shoots developed
2.	20.	Coding continues with the same scheme up until stage 29 (209)
29	209	Nine or more side shoots visible
	21.	Till 219 the coding lasts with the same trend
	219	19 or >19 side shoots developed
Elongation of main stem: principal growth stage 3		
31	301	Stem elongated 10% of final extension
32	302	Stem elongated 20% of final extension
3.	30.	Till 39 the coding lasts with the same trend
39	309	Maximum stem elongation
Harvestable vegetative parts development[b]: principal growth stage 4 (mislaid)		
Emergence of inflorescence: principal growth stage 5 (main shoot)		
50	500	Enclosed inflorescence in leaves
51	501	Visible inflorescence
55	505	Enclosed individual flower buds
59	509	First petals visible but still all flowers enclosed

(continued)

Table 7.1 (continued)

BBCH codes		
Two digits (00)	Three digits (000)	Explanation
Flowering: principal growth stage 6 (main shoot)		
60	600	First flower opened
61	601	10% flowers opened
62	602	20% flowers opened
63	603	30% of flowers opened, first petal dried or fallen
64	604	40% flowers opened
65	605	Complete flowering: 50% flowers opened
67	607	Flowering ending: most petals dried or fallen
69	609	Flowering ended: Visibility of fruit
Fruit development: principal growth stage 7 (main shoot)		
71	701	10% siliques touched maximum size
72	702	20% siliques touched maximum size
73	703	30% siliques completed maximum size
7.	70.	Till 79 the coding lasts with the same trend
79	709	All siliques touched maximum size
Ripening: principal growth stage 8		
81	801	Ripened silique 10% (seeds are deep yellow/orange and hard)
82	802	Ripened silique 20%
83	803	Ripened silique 30%
8.	80.	Till 89 the coding lasts with the same trend
89	809	Almost every silique is ripe; the crop is prepared to be reaped
Senescence: principal growth stage 9		
97	907	Plant death and dryness
99	909	Harvested produce[c]

[a]In *C. sativa*, the side shoot development generally happens either concurrently or after inflorescence emergence. Consequently, the second principal growth stage ordinarily mislaid. If formation of side shoot is taken a feature of specific attention, then principal growth stage 2 can be counted in along with principal growth stage 5 by using diagonal stroke
[b]As vegetative part was not harvested, so principal growth stage 4 has been omitted
[c]Storage treatments were applied at this stage

used, but the three-digit code is used in case of more accuracy. The application of three-digit code permits for selecting 19 leaves (Hack et al. 1992), thus allowing the precise depiction of plant growth before the emergence of an inflorescence. This is predominantly essential as in camelina, the scoring of stem enlargement, a phase that generally happens concurrently with the development of leaf, doesn't allow the instant valuation of the existing growth stage stated as a percentage of the final plant height. The accurate knowledge of the growth stage developed before the emergence of fluorescence then goes for the three-digit growth stage. The main-stem elongation can be directly assessed by the scoring of clearly protracted internodes on the main stem, but this is very difficult in the case of *Camelina sativa* as the identification of enlarged internodes is habitually equivocal and mainly operative dependent. To address this problem, main-stem elongation capacity as a percentage of the final stem length was taken as a highly suitable means to measure stem elongation in camelina. As different growth stages in *Camelina sativa* overlapped, like fluorescence emergence and formation of side shoot that take place simultaneously, the operator might skip the advanced stage or consider both the BBCH codes alienated by a diagonal stroke.

7.6 Reproduction

7.6.1 Floral Biology

C. sativa is considered an autogamous, self-compatible species (Mulligan 2002). The selfing process in camelina starts at dusk; stamen turned toward the stigma in the evening and deposited its pollen that lasts for the whole night that results from withering the flower that falls in 2–3 days. The same thing happens next to the stem, which grows longer as a new flower blooms (Schultze-Motel 1986). Out of 10,000 plants, the cross-pollinated were less than 3% (Tedin 1922). Contrastingly results were published by those who erroneously stated that camelina benefited from different pollinators (Goulson 2003).

7.7 Seed Production and Dispersal

7.7.1 Planting Time

Planting date is a key aspect in the satisfactory production of camelina due to favorable and unfavorable environmental conditions, i.e., temperature and soil moisture, which affects seed yield and seed quality. Generally, high-temperature stress might result in plant sterility, seed abortion, reduced number of seeds, and grain filling duration (Hatfield and Prueger 2015). Studies showed that camelina oil content is greater under cool environmental conditions (Obour et al. 2017; Zanetti et al. 2017), as grain weight is affected by seeding date and lower thousand seed weight has been reported in late seeded crop (Liu et al. 2021). Contrastingly, Urbaniak et al. (2008) stated that the seeding date has no effect on the 1000-grain weight and yield in field trials of Canada. Due to climatic variations among different regions globally, it defines the optimum planting time of camelina (Table 7.2).

Table 7.2 Optimum planting times of camelina around the world

Country	Planting time	References
USA/Montana	Late February or early March	McVay and Lamb (2008)
USA/Minnesota	Mid-April to mid-May	Gesch (2014)
USA/Minnesota	Mid-April to mid-May	Sintim et al. (2016a)
USA/Western Nebraska	Late March to end of April	Pavlista et al. (2011)
USA/Kansas State	April	Obeng et al. (2019)
USA/Nevada	Mid-March	Neupane et al. (2019)
Chile	April 30	Berti et al. (2011)
Europe	Mid-March and mid-April	Zanetti et al. (2017)
Canada	Mid-April to mid-May	Gesch (2014)
Pakistan	Mid-November	Waraich et al. (2017)
Poland	September 1	Czarnik et al. (2018)

7.7.2 Seed Rate

Optimization of the seed rate of a crop is a critical aspect for balancing seed cost with proper crop stand establishment to improve yield and, particularly for camelina, to contend with weeds because there are only a few herbicides used for its better performance (Sobiech et al. 2020; Gesch et al. 2018). Urbaniak et al. (2008) demonstrated that 1000-grain weight and yield are significantly affected by seed rate in field trials in Canada. They reported seed yield of 1.34, 1.50, and 1.60 ton ha^{-1}at seed rate of 200, 400, and 600 seed m^{-2}, respectively. They also observed more silique and branches per plant at lower seed rate. In another 3-year trial in Germany, 1.34, 1.16, and 1.80 ton ha^{-1}average yield was recorded each year, respectively, while seed rate of 400 m^{-2} and 120 kg N ha^{-1} application produced the highest yield (2.28 ton ha^{-1}). However, a higher seed rate (800 seed m^{-2}) reduced the total branches plant^{-1}, number of silique plant^{-1}, seeds silique^{-1}, and seed weight plant^{-1}. The positive effect of N application on yield and yield contributing traits was also affirmed by other field studies (Gao et al. 2018).

7.7.3 Seed Banks, Viability, and Germination

C. sativa is not a novel crop in the field, but unfortunately it was being ignored by the researchers despite its unique characters. The literature on seed dormancy and crop volunteers in camelina is very rare. Zhang and Auer (2019) have little information about seed dormancy in camelina as the seeds have shown little dormancy period, and seed emergence was recorded after 2 weeks of harvesting in a 3-year experiment in Ireland by Crowley (1999). Ellis et al. (1989) found that the germination of camelina was related to the dose of white light photon and was subdued by high radiation, which generally hinders emergence, and was significantly stimulated by gibberellic acid (GA$_3$). In Maritime Canada, the rate of germination of camelina was

7 Changing Climate Scenario: Perspectives of *Camelina sativa*...

>95%, although the seedling emergence rate was dependent on the environment (Urbaniak et al. 2008).

7.8 Camelina: Agronomy, Prospects, and Challenges

C. sativa is a short-day plant and completes its life cycle within 100 days (McVay and Lamb 2008). It can't reach the lower soil surfaces in search of water because of the shallow root system (Putnam et al. 1993). It can either be grown as an annual spring or biannual winter crop. It can be successfully grown under various soil and climatic conditions due to its high adaptability.

7.8.1 Sowing Date

The production of *C. sativa* can be optimized by following the basic principle of crop production, starting from the optimum sowing date. Sowing of camelina at an optimum time prevents pod abortion by preventing its exposure to severe heat and drought in early summer. Soil moisture and environmental conditions are the main driving forces behind the optimization of sowing date. Pavlista et al. (2011) did not find any effect of sowing date on the crop yield in western Nebraska. In the summer crop, the sowing after mid-April despite late March or mid-April negatively impacts the yield. The winter sowing in September and October (Gesch and Cermak 2011) bears the chilling conditions of winter and resumes its growth with favorable conditions. Winter-sown camelina has distinctive benefits like proper stand establishment of crop leads to better plant growth which lowers the weed pressure (Gesch and Cermak 2011) and it permits the crop to mature before the start of severe summer leading to early harvesting which helps in soil moisture conservation for the succeeding crop (Gesch and Archer 2009; Gesch and Cermak 2011).

7.8.2 Tillage

This would be best suited in winter-based nonirrigated traditional cropping systems where crop failure could be prevented by moisture availability. Soil preparation must be done carefully. Before the sowing of the crop, multiple harrowing must be done to eliminate the weed infestation. Camelina has the potential to perform under no-till and traditional tillage (Enjalbert and Johnson 2011). However, under no-till/ excessive crop residue, the seed rate needs to be increased as emergence rate can be negatively effected (Enjalbert and Johnson 2011).

7.8.3 Seed Rate

Optimal seed rate is very crucial for proper stand establishment, active plant growth, and high economic yield. There must be 210 plants m^{-2} (20 plants ft^{-2}), which can be achieved with optimal seed rate (6 kg ha^{-1}); seed must be incorporated into the soil. Its seeds must be planted at shallow depths (6–8 mm) due to small seeds for a better crop stand. Primary and secondary tillage, seed rate, sowing method, and sowing depth are the key dynamics that affect the plant population and consequent yield (McVay and Khan 2011). It is known as a drought- and chilling-tolerant crop as compared to canola and can thrive and give satisfactory yield under these conditions (Putnam et al. 1993; McVay and Lamb 2008; Berti et al. 2016). The seedling of camelina can tolerate the freezing temperature up to -2 °C, whereas the seedlings of rapeseed, mustard, and flax cannot survive (Robinson 1987). Schulte et al. (2013) published that the temperature fluctuations do not influence the lipid profile of camelina. However, there is a possibility that the sowing date might affect the lipid profile as late sowing exposes the crop to high summer temperatures.

7.8.4 Herbicide Control

There is no proper post-emergence herbicide of camelina, so pendimethalin and glyphosate could be the better option for pre-emergence control. Camelina is a short-duration biofuel crop having consistent yield without using many weedicides and pesticides (Razeq et al. 2014; Iskandarov et al. 2014). Unlike *Brassica*, camelina is not affected by birds and flea beetle damage (Pavlista et al. 2011). It is also resistant to insect pests (Iskandarov et al. 2014; Kirkhus et al. 2013). Quizalofop is used for post-emergence chemical weed control, while glyphosate is useful for pre-emergence weed control (Jha and Stougaard 2013). Prior researchers had used bonanza and treflan as pre-plant herbicides to restrict weed invasion (Yang et al. 2016). The only labeled herbicide for camelina is sethoxydim, which is ineffective on broad leaves (Obour et al. 2015). *Sclerotinia sclerotiorum* is also documented in *Camelina* fields, reducing its production (Yang et al. 2016). The literature on pre-emergence herbicide (PRE) usage is very limited for weed control in camelina (Schillinger et al. 2012). Consequently, existing substitutes of weed control have to use a labeled pre-emergence broad-spectrum herbicide, while mechanical removal of weeds is a very time-consuming practice (Froment et al. 2006). Sethoxydim is the only registered herbicide for camelina, but it controls narrow-leaf herbs, and quinclorac is suitable for broadleaf herbs (Jha and Stougaard 2013). The lower rates of S-metolachlor, dimethenamid-P, and pendimethalin, keeping in view the toxic level for use, could be approved for camelina (Jha and Stougaard 2013). However, certain residual herbicides from sulfonylurea are reported to affect the crop stand of camelina (Enjalbert and Johnson 2011).

7 Changing Climate Scenario: Perspectives of *Camelina sativa*. . .   211

7.8.5 Fertilizer Applications

Optimum nutrient application is a driving force behind better growth and development, yield quantity, and quality. Depending upon soil type, fertility, and soil moisture, 20–50:10–25:0 kg ha^{-1}of nitrogen (N) and sulfur (S) are required for camelina, respectively (Jiang et al. 2013). Soil organic matter and moisture are the main factors behind the response of *C. sativa* toward N and S (Jankowski et al. 2019). As camelina has shown maximum yield at 45–56 kg N ha^{-1}. *C. sativa* does not need any intercultural practice from the seedling stage till harvesting. The response of camelina toward phosphorus (P) application was not good even in P-deficient soil (Obour et al. 2012), and P at 15–30 kg ha^{-1}might be suitable for the *C. sativa* production.

7.8.6 Harvesting

The plant reached its harvesting maturity when 50–75% of silique got brown, which is the best time to harvest the crop (Sintim et al. 2016b). Harvesting at a proper time decreases the chances of yield loss by shattering, so swathing of the crop must be considered for harvesting at uneven maturity. Regular grain combine harvester can be used to harvest camelina with certain adjustments like the height of header must be fixed at the highest spot to deny the plugging and airflow adjustments to minimize the chances of seed to blow away. However, the cleaning of seed might be needed due to this slow airflow as a seed might be mixed with plant material. The mixing of plant material with seeds could be fixed by installing a 0.35 cm screen before the lower sieves beneath the harvester (Enjalbert and Johnson 2011).

7.8.7 Seed Yield

The nonirrigated areas where the total precipitation recorded was 400–500 mm gave seed yield of 1.68–2.02 ton ha^{-1}and 0.50–1.34 ton ha^{-1} in low rainfall areas (McVay and Lamb 2008). Seed yield of 0.45–1.30 ton ha^{-1} has been recorded in trials in years 2013 and 2014. The trial conducted in Eastern Europe gave 2.88 ton ha^{-1} of seed yield (Vollmann et al. 2008). Camelina seed yield varies in different continents (Table 7.3).

7.9 Potential of *C. sativa* Over Nonirrigated Areas Compared to Other Oilseeds

C. sativa has greater potential in nonirrigated areas due to its lower requirements of water. The intercropping of camelina has been tested in wheat-based cropping systems in dryland regions. The trials under dryland regions resulted that camelina

Table 7.3 The difference in seed yield and oil content of *C. sativa* in experiments conducted in different parts of the world

Location	Oil content range	Yield range (kg ha^{-1})	Major source of variation	References
Iran	33–34.4%	1868–3209	Irrigation levels, sulfur	Amiri-Darban et al. (2020)
Nevada, USA		594–961	Sowing dates, years	Neupane et al. (2019)
Kansas, USA	290 g kg^{-1}	317–483	Sowing dates, years	Obeng et al. (2019)
Germany	32.0–49.0%	1100–2650	Breeding lines	Gehringer et al. (2006) and Berti et al. (2011)
Romania		1761–2892	Cultivars	
Austria	40.5–46.7%	1574–2248	Breeding lines, seed size	Vollmann et al. (2007)
Ireland	43.1–44.7%	1630–3200	Sowing date, N rates	Crowley and Fröhlich (1998) and Berti et al. (2011)
Chili		420–2390	Sowing dates, NPS, Fertilization	
Denmark	40.4–46.7%	1270–2360	Spring/fall sowing	Zubr (1997)
Pakistan		300–400	Drought, selenium	Ahmad et al. (2020)
Germany	34.3–42.4%	1290–3230	Breeding lines	Seehuber et al. (1987)
Germany	32.1–42.3%	500–2620	Genebank accessions	Seehuber (1984) and Katar et al. (2012)
Turkey		572–997	Accessions and breeding lines	
West Canada	37.0–46.3%	1000–3000	N fertilizer rates, environments	Malhi et al. (2014)
Minnesota, USA	37.7–41.0%	800–1900	Cultivars, sowing date	Gesch (2014)
Pacific Northwest USA	29.6–36.8%	127–3302	Cultivars, spring/fall planting	Guy et al. (2014)
East Canada	35.5–37.8%	1400–2050	N, S fertilization	Jiang et al. (2013)
Nebraska, USA	29.8–34.3%	556–1456	Sowing date	Pavlista et al. (2011)
East Canada	35.5–40.1%	426–2568	Cultivars, N rate	Urbaniak et al. (2008)
West Canada	35.8–43.2%	962–3320	Genebank accessions, environments	Gugel and Falk (2006)
Minnesota, USA	34.3–37.5%	1007–1218	Genebank accessions	Putnam et al. (1993) and Rode (2002)
Slovenia		400–800	Cultivars	

yielded more or somewhere the same as other oilseed crops, but the shattering, lodging, disease, and insect factors were minimal compared to others (Putnam et al. 2009; Gao et al. 2018). Likewise, Johnson et al. (2009) stated that the performance of camelina under nonirrigated conditions was way better than rapeseed as camelina produced more seed yield than rapeseed. *C. sativa* can be used as a potential fallow

7 Changing Climate Scenario: Perspectives of *Camelina sativa*. . .

crop in cereal-based crop system, which results in crop diversification, minimizes pest population, and increases the profit of the farmer, log-term crop sustainability, and farm in the region. *C. sativa* proved a potential crop with minimum reduction in yield as it can replace fallow in the wheat-fallow system (McVay and Lamb 2008). Cultivation of *C. sativa* on underutilized fallow wheat-based production systems strips to evade uninterrupted competition for land use.

7.10 Constraints

Several restraints affect the outcome and economic feasibility of *C. sativa* regardless of its capability as a substitute potential bioenergy crop for dryland regions. Information regarding the agronomic practices, production systems, and adapted spring and winter genotype is scarce. *C. sativa* is facing problems regarding the benefit-cost ratio and lack of marketing system that could lose the productivity of the crop. Like other constraints, uneven maturation results in the harvesting problems that might cause shattering, and postharvest losses are another significant constraint in the profitability of camelina (McVay and Khan 2011; Lenssen et al. 2012). Certain fungal infections have been reported in camelina, like downy mildew infestation in Pacific Northwest in the USA (Putnam et al. 2009; Harveson et al. 2011), and the control of downy mildew has not been reported yet for camelina. All these challenges bring much-needed attention of researchers to conduct more research on camelina to optimize its production and profitability.

7.11 Camelina Agronomic Performance, Oil Quality, Properties, and Potential

C. sativa oil has many advantages over other oilseeds. One of them is the presence of unsaturated omega-fatty acid (80%) of total fatty acid and 35–40% of linolenic acid (18: 3n·3) (Belayneh et al. 2015). Camelina oil has many advantages over other oilseeds. Its oil is a rich source of omega-3 fatty acid (80%) of total fatty acid and 35–40% of linolenic acid (18: 3n·3) (Budin et al. 1995; Abramovič and Abram 2005; Abramovič et al. 2007; Schwartz et al. 2008), and it has more than 50% polyunsaturated fatty acids in cold-pressed camelina oil (Budin et al. 1995; Abramovič et al. 2007), and it has tenfold of more oil as compared to other oilseeds (Alice et al. 2007; Tabără et al. 2007). The fatty acids pattern in camelina is very particular with the characterization of 30–40% linolenic acid (C18:3), almost 4% of erucic acid, and 15% of eicosenic acid (C20:1) (Budin et al. 1995). Member of order Brassicales, especially the Brassicaceae family, has a secondary metabolite known as glucosinolates (Clarke 2010). There are almost 120 types of glucosinolates discovered yet which are naturally present in the plants. These secondary metabolites are responsible for the sharp and bitter taste in cruciferous vegetable oil and also release chemicals that act as defensive agents against herbivores and natural pests (Fahey et al. 2003). Glucosinolates can cause damage to plants, and plants compartmentalize this compound to avoid the damage. Camelina also does the same and accumulates the glucosinolates (glucoarabin (9-(methylsulfinyl)nonylglucosinolate – GS9), glucocamelinin (10-(methylsulfinyl)decylglucosinolate – GS10), and 11-(methylsulfinyl)undecylglucosinolate (GS11) in its seeds. Camelina oil is also known as golden liquid, which contains more than 50% of polyunsaturated essential fatty acids primarily linoleic acid and alpha-linoleic acid, and it also contains tenfold more fatty acids than other oilseed crops (Alice et al. 2007; Tabără et al. 2007). It has a significant shelf life due to the presence of Vit-E (tocopherol) that saves it from oxidation (www.simplunatura.ro), and it also plays a vital role in slenderness recovery, the elasticity of skin, and regeneration of cell (Vollmann et al. 1996). The basic properties of camelina make it specifically suitable, which are (1) exceptional aroma and taste, (2) color, (3) chemical and physical composition, and (4) extended conservation duration (up to 2 years). Table 7.4 has shown the fatty acid composition in the camelina oil.

The camelina oil yield and quality has shown variations on different location. Though the modern breeding history of *C. sativa* is relatively little, *C. sativa* trials have shown a satisfactory seed yield and other promising agronomic features than other novel crops that may be due to the long adaptation history of *C. sativa*. A

Table 7.4 Fatty acid profile of *C. sativa* oil (research conducted in the Constanta County, 2009) (Imbrea et al. 2011; El Sabagh et al. 2019; Borzoo et al. 2020; Yuan and Li 2020; Amiri-Darban et al. 2020)

Fatty acids	Bonds ratio	Oil content (%)
Myristic acid	C14:0	0.10
Palmitic acid	C16:0	6.51–8.1
Palmitoleic acid	C16:1	0.18
Stearic acid	C18:0	2.15
Oleic acid	C18:1n–9	16.27–16.38
Linoleic acid	C18:2n–6	20.99–21.52
Linolenic acid	C18:3n–6	32.20–35.58
Conjugated linoleic acid	C18:2	1.06
A-Linolenic acid	C18:3n–3	11.59
Arachidonic acid	C20:4n–6	1.11
Erucic acid	C22:1n–9	1.6
Docosadienoic acid	C22:2n–3	2.24
Gadeolic acid	C20:1	14.4
Eicosadienoic + eicosatrienoic	C20:2	2.64
PUFAs/MUFAs		1.83
Polyunsaturated fatty acid		90.0
Other fatty acids		0.61
Glucosinolate		15.7–28.2

7 Changing Climate Scenario: Perspectives of *Camelina sativa*...
215

detailed number of published research on the difference of camelina seed yield and oil content in European and North American locations are presented (Table 7.4). The use of camelina oil in the human diet has been established in many European countries like the UK, Germany, Finland, Denmark, and Ireland. Camelina is found to be used in the bread of human consumption. It has a specific composition that enriches the bread with essential amino acids (Zubr 2003b), omega-3 fatty acids (Amiri-Darban et al. 2020), fatty acids (Zubr 2003b), dietary fibers (Zubr 2003a), and other minor compounds. It is also rich in oil (Sehgal et al. 2018), fatty acids (Anderson et al. 2019), tocopherols (Zubr 2009; Fernández-Cuesta et al. 2014), bioactive compounds (Matthäus and Zubr 2000b), and amino acids (Zubr 2003b).

7.12 Camelina Response to Insects, Disease, Herbivory, and Higher Plant Parasites

7.12.1 Insects

The insect attack on *C. sativa* is not very extensive because the insect damage has never been enough to warrant control measures (Robinson 1987) for flea beetles (Soroka et al. 2015). It was found that the possible reasons behind the resistance against insects shown by camelina could be due to either the occurrence of repellents or the nonexistence of volatile stimulatory compounds, probably because of the low concentration of glucosinolates (Henderson et al. 2004). The European tainted plant bug is the possible insect species connected with camelina developed as a potential crop (Palagesiu 2000). Further studies have proved that camelina insects susceptibility depends upon the host specificity (Soroka et al. 2015).

7.13 Diseases

7.13.1 Fungal Diseases

Downy mildew, botanically known as *Peronospora parasitica* (Pers. ex Fr.) Fr., was found on camelina in Canada (Conners 1967). *C. sativa* was found resistant to various fungal diseases due to the production of camalexin, methoxycamalexin, and phytoalexins (Browne et al. 1991). The concentration of these compounds can be increased by the inoculation of *A. brassicae* inoculum (Jejelowo et al. 1991), which is the first reported antifungal compound. Pedras et al. (2003) suggested that the resistance in camelina against blackleg could be found by the mixture of phytoalexin production and the destruxin B detoxification pathway. Camelina has also shown massive variability toward different diseases as the variability toward leaf spot was 34% and 10% toward black rot (Westman and Dickson 1998; Westman et al. 1999). The resistance of *Camelina* against several diseases is stated in different

216   M. Ahmad et al.

regions as Camelina was found resistant to blackleg fungus from Australia (Salisbury 1987) and Poland (Karolewski 1999), and no virulence reported yet (Li et al. 2005). *C. sativa* was also found susceptible to *Botrytis* spp. and *Sclerotinia* in Poland (Crowley 1999) and downy mildew in Austria and the USA (Vollmann et al. 2001; Dimmock and Edwards-Jones 2006).

7.13.2 Viral Diseases

C. sativa has shown susceptibility to aster yellows phytoplasma (Zhao et al. 2010), turnip yellow mosaic tymovirus (TYMV) and *erysimum* latent tymovirus (ELV), beet western yellows virus (BWYV) in Germany, and radish mosaic virus (RaMV) in the Czech Republic. TYMV was also transmitted by *C. sativa* seed (Brunt et al. 1996; Špak and Kubelková 2000).

7.13.3 Bacterial Diseases

In Germany, Camelina was reported to be infested by bacterial blight caused by *Pseudomonas syringae* pv. *camelinae* (Mavridis et al. 2002).

7.13.4 Phytoplasmas

C. sativa was reported to be infected by the aster-yellows-phytoplasma disease (Khadhair et al. 2001) from Alberta, Canada.

7.13.5 Invertebrates

In mixed crop with wildflower, *Camelina* seeds have shown big damage by *Arion lusitanicus* Mabille and *Deroceras reticulatum* Muller by destroying more than 50% of seed, but this did not happen in the crop grown in harrowed plots (Kollmann and Bassin 2001).

7.14 Nutritional Values of Camelina Seed

The nutritional values of camelina seed have been shown in Table 7.5. The analysis of water-soluble B series vitamins has found the contents of thiamin (B1), riboflavin (B2), niacin (B3), pantothenic acid (B5), pyridoxine (B6), biotin (B7), and folate

7 Changing Climate Scenario: Perspectives of *Camelina sativa*... 217

Table 7.5 Amount of different compounds, amino acids, sugars, vitamins, and minerals in camelina seed oil (Rode 2002; Bătrîna et al. 2020)

Compounds	Amount (%)	Compounds	Amount	Minerals	Amount
Glucose	0.42	Flavonoid	143 mg/kg of seed	Ca	1%
Fructose	0.04	Polar phenolic	439 mg/kg	Mg	0.51%
Sucrose	5.5	Sitosterol	1884 µg/g of oil	Na	0.06%
Raffinose	0.64	Stigmasterol	103 µg/g of oil	K	1.6%
Stachyose	0.36	Brassicasterol	133 µg/g of oil	Cl	0.04%
Starch	1.21	Campesterol	893 µg/g of oil	P	1.4%
Pectin	0.96	Cholesterol	188 µg/g of oil	S	0.24%
Lignin	7.4	Thiamin	18.8 mg/g	Cu	9.9 mg/g
Crude fiber	12.8	Riboflavin	4.4 mg/g	Mn	40 mg/g
Mucilages	6.7	Niacin	194 mg/g	Ni	1.9 mg/g
		Pantothenic acid	11.3 mg/g	Zn	69 mg/g
		Pyridoxine	1.9 mg/g	Fe	329 mg/g
		Biotin	1.0 mg/g		
		Folate	3.2 mg/g		
Amino acids (%)					
Histidine	4.06	Lysine	4.46	Threonine	2.89
Isoleucine	4.38	Methionine	2.70	Tryptophan	1.21
Leucine	7.04	Phenylalanine	5.06	Valine	6.10
Alanine	6.14	Glutamate	16.03	Proline	5.88
Arginine	8.45	Glycine	5.44	Serine	5.84
Aspartate	8.96	Cysteine	1.84	Tyrosine	3.52

(B9). Camelina oil also possessed phenolics such as polar phenolic compounds (Abramovič et al. 2007; Chaturvedi et al. 2017) and flavonoid (Matthäus and Zubr 2000a). Its oil has a significant amount of sterols as sitosterol, cholesterol, campesterol (Shukla et al. 2002; Szterk et al. 2010), brassicasterol, and stigmasterol (Shukla et al. 2002). Topically applied, a healing effect on bruises, skin scratches, squeezing, and sprains, and skin diseases (e.g., acne) and inflammations, is described in the literature (Rode 2002).

7.15 Agro-industrial Uses

The huge oil content in camelina seeds makes it a special product for industrial use and nutritional application. The seed meal of defatted *C. sativa* has a substantial level of carbohydrates, proteins, and a number of phytochemicals, which can be used in the feed and agriculture sector (Gugel and Falk 2006; Zubr 2009). Its oil has great potential for industrial applications. It is reported that camelina has a unique fatty acid profile that makes it early drier, making it good in making polymers, paints, varnishes, dermatological products, and cosmetics (Kasetaite et al. 2014; Zaleckas et al. 2012). Its epoxidized oil has great industrial uses, like in the making of pressure-sensitive resins, adhesives, and coatings (Kim et al. 2015). Its oil content (106–907 L ha^{-1}) is far more as compared to sunflower (500–750 L ha^{-1}) and soybean (247–562 L ha^{-1}), which make it best fit agriculture industrial growth medium (Moser 2010). Due to the presence of omega-3 fatty acid in such a high percentage, camelina oil is being promoted as a dietary supplement in animals (Ponnampalam et al. 2019) and human diet (Rahman et al. 2018). The composition of hen egg can be changed through alteration in diet. If their feed is rich in long-chain fatty acids like omega-3 fatty acids, their concentration will be increased in the yolk, and flax is the best source of omega-3 fatty acid (Jiang et al. 1992; Pilgeram 2007).

7.16 Camelina and Animal Feed

Oilseed crops can also be used as a source of feed for humans and animals like *C. sativa* (Sawyer 2008), which is a source of protein-rich meal having a unique amino acid profile including cysteine, methionine, glycine, arginine, threonine, and lysine which are more in concentration than soymeal (Pekel et al. 2009). This unique profile of amino acids made the camelina meal a good feed source for poultry. Camelina meal consists of 5–10% lipid content that enhances its nutritive values and provides a high-value meal as compared to soymeal (Zubr 1997). This makes the camelina meal one of the best additions to feeding the livestock and poultry (Frame et al. 2007).The first publication on the use of camelina meal for livestock feed was published in 1962 reported that its meal has more proteins than rapeseed and flaxseed (Plessers et al. 1962). A study has been reported on camelina meal usage as a starter diet in turkey production at 5%, 15%, and 20%, a good source of protein, and 5% is recommended for starter diet (Frame et al. 2007). The replacement of soymeal with *C. sativa* in the ruminant (beef steer) diet resulted in a significant decrease in the stress-responsive hormones (Cappellozza et al. 2012). Its meal contains 23–40 glucosinolates μ moles g^{-1} (Singh et al. 2014), 1–6% phytate (Adhikari et al. 2016), and 100–150 g kg^{-1} crude fiber (Kakani et al. 2012). In addition to this, there was no change noticed in the function of the thyroid. However, camelina meal reduced the acute-phase reduction protein reactions, which are normally enhanced during transportation or when animals are subjected to a feed lot setting (Cappellozza et al. 2012). This research is evidence of the positive role of camelina meal in reducing the stress response in cattle. A fat reduction was observed in the cow milk by using camelina meal (2 kg of DM), but it did not reduce the milk yield (Hurtaud and Peyraud 2007). After oil extraction, the by-products of *C. sativa* seeds can be used as a nutritious feed meal with high levels of crude protein (>45%), omega-3 fatty acids (>35%), fiber (10^{-11}), and vitamin E (Meadus et al. 2014) for livestock.

7 Changing Climate Scenario: Perspectives of *Camelina sativa*...

7.17 Biofuel

Total global fossil reserves are 1707 billion barrels, which is an alarming number because it will only be able to fulfill of global supply for 50.6 years (BP 2017). Due to limited resources, conservation of fossil fuels, and climate change, renewable energy sources such as camelina are under the limelight (Sainger et al. 2017). Oilseed feedstocks counting camelina are estimated to contribute 0.5 billion gallons of the 36 billion gallons of conveyance fuel required by the US economy by 2022 (USDA 2010; Mohammed et al. 2017). The worldwide emphasis on energy security accompanied by the determinations to subordinate the greenhouse gas emissions (GHGs) has pushed many governments to begin with inflexible policies on cleaner-energy production, predominantly biofuels' production goals and utilization, joined with continuous efforts that focused on research and progress of bioenergy crops (e.g., Glithero et al. 2012; Radzi and Droege 2014). Past literature indicated that camelina is apt for aviation fuel and biodiesel production (Keshavarz-Afshar and Chen 2015; Yang et al. 2016). Biodiesel production from vegetable oils is an excellent alternative to conventional petroleum-biodiesel due to its remarkable environmentally safe qualities. It has a huge market as it can be used in agricultural machinery, automobiles, power generation, and stationary power sector (Xue et al. 2011; Tabatabaie and Murthy, 2017). Almost 95% of the world's biodiesel is produced from vegetable oils like canola, sunflower, and soybean (Gui et al. 2008). Besides other advantages and use of oilseed crops, they are projected to play a vital part in alleviating greenhouse gas emissions by their capacity to produce biofuel. USDA report has lightened up the potential of camelina to produce biofuel (USDA 2010). The properties (acid value, the lubricity of the oil, permeability at low temperature, kinematic velocity, and acid value) of biodiesel produced by camelina have the same properties of biodiesel produced by soybean (Moser and Vaughn 2010). This shows the potential of high-quality biodiesel production in camelina. Mineral diesel fuel can produce a power of 38.5 kW, which is less than that of camelina (43.5 kW), which is produced by coldly pressed neat oil of camelina seeds. However, mineral diesel fuel has less consumption efficiency as compared to camelina (Bernardo et al. 2003). In the recent few years, the demand for camelina is increasing due to its ability to grow in fewer input requirement, and its oil can be used for a nonfood purpose (Seehuber 1984; Putnam et al. 1993; Mohammad et al. 2018). The fatty acids pattern in camelina is very particular with the characterization of 30%–40% linolenic acid (C18:3), almost 4% of erucic acid, and 15% of eicosenic acid (C20:1) (Budin et al. 1995); this will make it best for the utilization of drying oil which is used to form environment-friendly paints and coatings same as of linseed oil (Zaleckas et al. 2012; Kasetaite et al. 2014). Camelina oil can be used as biodiesel and can also be an alternative to petroleum due to its huge production ability. Its oil can be utilized in different vehicles as biodiesel (Fröhlich and Rice 2005). As camelina is known for its diverse use in industrial products, that makes it a profitable enterprise (Table 7.6).

Table 7.6 Research has been done in different countries to evaluate the uses of camelina oil in different industries and products

Products	Country	References
Chemicals, paints and coatings, resins, adhesives	Poland, USA	Nosal et al. (2015), Kim et al. (2015) and Li et al. (2015)
Cosmetics and soaps	USA	Obour et al. (2015)
Film, fibers, and thermoplastics	China	Reddy et al. (2012)
Bio-Gum	USA	Li et al. (2016)
Bioplastic	USA	Kim et al. (2015)
Cuticular waxes and suberins	USA	Razeq et al. (2014)
Shelf life enhancer	Ireland	Eidhin et al. (2003)
Phytoremediation	India	Tripathi et al. (2016)
Bio-alkyd resin	Poland	Nosal et al. (2015)
Bioadhesive	USA	Kim et al. (2015) and Obour et al. (2015)
Animal feed	Romania, Turkey, Denmark, India	Ponnampalam et al. (2019), Ciurescu et al. (2016), Pekel et al. (2015) and Singh et al. (2014)
Fish	Canada	Bullerwell et al. (2016) and Booman et al. (2014)
Jet fuel	USA, Canada	Drenth et al. (2015), Li and Mupondwa (2014) and Vollmann and Eynck (2015)
Food and supplements	Egypt	Ibrahim and El Habbasha (2015)
Bio-oils	USA, Ireland, Spain	Mohammad et al. (2018), Drenth et al. (2015) and Gómez-Monedero et al. (2015)
Herbicide, fungicide	USA	Cao et al. (2015) and Ma et al. (2015)
Medical use		
Cancers and tumors	USA	Das et al. (2014)
Ulcers	USA	Cuendet et al. (2006)
Cholesterol reduction	Finland	Karvonen et al. (2002)
Neurological abnormalities	USA	Trumbo et al. (2002)
Coronary heart diseases	Turkey	Gogus and Smith (2010)
Burns and inflammations	USA	Sampath (2009)
Antioxidant	Germany	Terpinc et al. (2012)

7.18 Alternative Uses

The *C. sativa* meal is very nutritious and is used as feed for ewe's milk (Salminen et al. 2006), cattle's, hens, turkey's, rabbits, etc. If we want to expand this industry, we must find new alternative uses of camelina meal. There must be strong collaboration among universities, research wing, and stakeholders to find new ways of camelina meal uses as bio-based products like adhesive, coating, and packing materials (Li et al. 2015; Kalita et al. 2018; Liu et al. 2018). The dearth of a marketing system and less productivity when related to several other oilseeds are currently impeding its adoption. The government policy must be clear about the rates and marketing of *C. sativa* and its products. This will boost camelina production. An extended marketing system will be able to improve the cost-effective feasibility of camelina as a profitable oilseed.

7.19 Camelina in the Fallow Season

This crop can be used as a replacement for the fallow season before sowing wheat in the main winter fallow and can also be sown in the wheat summer fallow system (Obour et al. 2015; Berti et al. 2016; Obour et al. 2018). It will be a big success for agronomic assistance; the crop management is comparatively very easy because the insect pest infestation is very low and no extra mechanization is required which will result in high economic yield. Crops that could replace the wheat-summer crop-fallow phase system must have some unique features, including agronomic assistance, companionable with available technology, comparatively easy to handle, lowest disease and invasion, and increasing the final profitability. In the cereal-based cropping system of dryland area, the incorporation of camelina will diversify the cropping system and increase profitability (Johnston et al. 2002). A yield reduction has been reported in wheat yields following camelina in drier years might be due to sustained fallow period (Hess et al. 2011; Sintim et al. 2014).

7.20 Prospects for Future Research

Unfortunately, price and low seed yield contributed to the decline in camelina production acreage (NASS 2015). Camelina is being grown under contracts in Canada, with about half in the province of Saskatchewan (Li and Mupondwa 2014). Because there is no established market for camelina, many economic studies have used canola prices for economic feasibility evaluations (Gesch et al. 2018). Barriers to wide-scale adoption of this crop as feed or feedstock for biofuels include low seed yield, lack of an open market, low price for the seed, perception as a weed by farmers (Jewett 2015), and anti-nutritional aspects in both the meal and oil.

7.20.1 Agronomic Research

The main concern with camelina is that very little effort is being made in technology development and transformation regarding breeding efforts to updated genotypes, the latest and appropriate production systems, and best agronomic practices. In contrast, many trials have been conducted to produce elite germplasm via conventional breeding efforts to improve the potential of *C. sativa* in field conditions. Several efforts should be made to conduct multi-locational experiments to check its response in water shortage conditions, thermal stress, salinity, or heavy metal stress conditions as were being made for canola by Pavlista et al. (2011). Studies must be made on the optimum fertilizer requirements of *C. sativa* on different soils to enhance its productivity and must try to incorporate it into an existing cropping system. Trials must be conducted to investigate weed and disease control. *C. sativa* is reported to be highly susceptible against residual class two herbicide. Nonetheless, efforts were made to address this problem; they transformed it by *Arabidopsis acetolactate* synthase (ALS) engineered with a number of particular changes/mutations in various combinations in the active site of camelina (Ala122Thr, Pro197Ser, and Trp574Leu). The studies on the camelina issue like shattering, harvesting, and postharvest management must be done to improve its response. Most of the oilseed crops are raised in marginal and submarginal lands which are having poor fertility status. So, it's an agronomist's job to convince the farmers and increase the cultivation area on fertile and productive soils. Agronomic research to recognize the appropriate spring and winter genotypes, seeding dates, and soil fertility requirements are desired to optimize the site-specific production technologies for camelina.

7.20.2 Plant Breeding Efforts

Unlike other oilseed crops, there is a minimum number of breeding efforts being made in *C. sativa*. Most of the cultivars being used in the USA are from their native origin, with minimum improvements that were screened and adjusted to regional conditions. If we want to increase the camelina seed yield, oil content, and oil quality, we need to make plant breeding efforts to develop new high potential varieties. These cultivars must have the ability to cope with environmental stresses effectively. The ability to outcross in *C. sativa* is minimal so efforts must be needed to explore this wing (Julié-Galau et al. 2014). The genotypic research in camelina was very limited because of the self-pollinating nature of camelina that makes it a complex process, so biotechnological techniques could give a breakthrough. However, scientists have forged the utilization of an agrobacterium-mediated transformation by spending ex-plants of camelina and floral dip procedure to incorporate bacterial strains in camelina plant. So, we need to use plant breeding approaches to improve the performance of *C. sativa*.

7.21 Climate Change

A growing global population is driving up the demand for food. This challenge is intensified in agriculture by extreme vulnerability to climate change. Climate change noticeably affects crop productivity and global food security by increasing temperatures, atmospheric carbon dioxide and ground-level ozone concentrations, weather variability, shifting agroecosystem boundaries, invasive crops and pests, and more frequent extreme weather events. However, the changing climate is having far-reaching impacts on agricultural production, which are likely to challenge food security in the future. Therefore, extensive actions will be needed for increasing yield and quality food to meet the future demand.

Agriculture is a foremost part of the climate problem (climate change) and also a major source of greenhouse gases (GHGs) which contribute to the greenhouse effect. Agriculture contributes toward climate change through *anthropogenic* GHG emissions and by the conversion of nonagricultural land such as *forests* into agricultural land (Sarkodie et al. 2019). Blanco et al. (2014) estimated that agriculture, forestry, and land-use change contributes 20–25% of global annual emissions. The food system as a whole contributes 37% of total GHG emissions estimated by *European Union's Scientific Advice Mechanism*, and this figure will increase up to 40% by 2050 due to population growth and dietary change (SAPEA 2020). However, crop insecurity will increase over time and with rising GHG emissions. Therefore, climate change will affect in agriculture, and the potential agrobiodiversity can provide resilient solutions in future agriculture.

7.22 Role of Camelina to Mitigate Climate Change Issues

Camelina can endorse biodiversity, decrease soil erosion, improve water infiltration (Gaba et al. 2015; Meyer et al. 2019), and encourage the sustainable intensification of cropping systems (Sindelar et al. 2017; Struik and Kuyper 2017). Mixed or relay cropping with camelina is valuable and widespread organic farming to overcome weed pressure (Leclère et al. 2019).

The production of plant-based liquid fuels has major implications to improve the environment and to mitigate climate change. Camelina is well known as advanced biofuel producer crop. A biofuel qualifies as an "advanced biofuel" if the fuel reduces GHG emissions by at least 50% compared to baseline petroleum fuel (EISA 2007). In 2013, the US Environmental Protection Agency identified the fuel pathways for biofuels produced from camelina oil and stated that camelina biodiesel could qualify as an advanced biofuel (USEPA 2013). It was estimated that use of camelina biodiesel reduces GHG emissions by 69% compared to 2005 baseline diesel (Dangol et al. 2015). Biofuels have the potential to emit less pollution compared with fossil fuels and, if implemented correctly, could help alleviate the rise of CO_2 levels and climate change (Bernardo et al. 2003). It is often reported that oilseed crops are the most efficient and effective biofuel source (Hill et al. 2006). In another study using camelina in place of mineral-diesel to power trucks showed that emissions of carbon monoxide (CO), carbon dioxide (CO_2), and smoke were significantly less from trucks powered by camelina oil (Bernardo et al. 2003).

7.23 Conclusion and Suggestions

The worldwide alimentary-oil requirement is increasing; thus, despite the development of hybrids and cultivars, improvement in production machinery, and technologies of oil-bearing crops, we need to incorporate the novel species in the cropping system that have the unique fat profile as reserve substances. Camelina as an oilseed holds a promise with the ability as the commercial oilseed, animal feed, and other industrial uses. As camelina has important agronomic characters that must highlight its scope as a new addition in a cropping system. BBCH's two- or three-digit coding system that described the phenological growth stages of a crop provides the phenological information and is complemented by depictions of most descriptive stages. Existing approaches for adjusting endogenous lipid profile and oil yield in camelina have a huge success, and it can also offer industrial products derived from it. The abiotic stress tolerance and low-input requirements are novel characters of this crop that makes it best fit in semiarid and arid conditions like Pakistan. The one biggest harmer of camelina adoption is the lack of a proper marketing system and low productivity in competition with other oilseed crops. The economic yield of camelina needs to improve the challenges relating to seed yield and new lipids. Novel approaches are being instigated to understand the intricate metabolic fluctuations over time and space with synthetic biological apparatuses to fine-tune lipid metabolism for explicit requirements. So, there is a dire need to develop a proper marketing system and a government policy for its production. Research on *Camelina* is limited, and its production systems are not being fully optimized. Agronomic research to identify suitable winter and spring *C. sativa* genotypes, seeding dates, and soil fertility requirements are needed to develop site-specific production recommendations for camelina. A prolonged proper marketing system will improve the financial feasibility of camelina as a salable oilseed. The latter will guarantee the grower's adoption of camelina in the semiarid regions due to its desired agronomic features as a dryland crop.

To attain numerous high-valued lipid foodstuffs, it is vital to reform the enzyme with enhanced activities or precise characteristics. Numerous methods can be employed to alter or produce innovative enzymes essential for the specific lipid amalgamation and accretion, together with focused protein alteration and upright-translation amendments. Lastly, modified metabolic paths for elevating innovative and high-esteemed lipids would be shared with additional breeding plans in camelina, for instance, cumulative harvest and seed oil contents and enlightening resistance to numerous environmental stress circumstances.

Conflict of Interest Authors declare that they have no conflict of interest.

References

Abbas RN, Iqbal A, Iqbal MA, Ali OM, Ahmed R, Ijaz R, Hadifa A, Bethune BJ (2021a) Weed-free durations and fertilization regimes boost nutrient uptake and paddy yield of direct-seeded fine rice (*Oryza sativa* L.). Agronomy 11:2448

Abbas RN, Arshad MA, Iqbal A, Iqbal MA, Imran M, Raza A, Chen JT, Alyemeni MN, Hefft DI (2021b) Weeds spectrum, productivity and land-use efficiency in maize-gram intercropping systems under semi-arid environment. Agronomy 11:1615

Abramovič H, Abram V (2005) Physico-chemical properties, composition and oxidative stability of *Camelina sativa* oil. Food Technol Biotechnol 43(1):63–70

Abramovič H, Butinar B, Nikolič V (2007) Changes occurring in phenolic content, tocopherol composition and oxidative stability of *Camelina sativa* oil during storage. Food Chem 104(3): 903–909. https://doi.org/10.1016/j.foodchem.2006.12.044

Abro AA (2012) Determinants of crop diversification towards high value crops in Pakistan. Int J Bus Manag Econ Res 3(3):536–545

Adhikari PA, Heo JM, Nyachoti CM (2016) Standardized total tract digestibility of phosphorus in Camelina (*Camelina sativa*) meal fed to growing pigs without or phytase supplementation. Anim Feed Sci Technol 214:104–109. https://doi.org/10.1016/j.anifeedsci.2016.02.018

Ahmad Z, Waraich EA, Barutcular C, Alharby H, Bamagoos A, Kizilgeci F, Öztürk F, Hossain A, Bayoumi Y, El Sabagh A (2020) Enhancing drought tolerance in Camelina sativa L. and canola (Brassica napus L.) through application of selenium. Pak J Bot 52(6):1927–1939

Ahmad Z, Anjum S, Skalicky M, Waraich EA, Tariq RMS, Ayub MA, Hossain A, Hassan MM, Brestic M, Sohidul IM, Rahman MH, Allah W, Iqbal MA, Ayman A (2021) Selenium alleviates the adverse effect of drought in oilseed crops Camelina (*Camelina sativa* L.) and canola (*Brassica napus* L.). Molecules 26:1699

Alice P, Sands DC, Boss D, Dale N, Wichmann D, Lamb P, Lu C, Barrows R, Kirkpatrick M, Thompson B, Johnson DL (2007) Camelina sativa, a Montana omega-3 and fuel crop. In: Janick J, Whipkey A (eds) Issues in New Crops and New Uses. ASHS Press, Alexandria, pp 129–131

Alina I, Roman G (2009) Research on morphological and biological peculiarities of Camelina sativa (l.) Crantz species under the conditions of the central part of Roumanian plain. Sci Pap Ser LII:344

Al-Shehbaz IA, Beilstein MA, Kellogg EA (2006) Systematics and phylogeny of the *Brassicaceae* (*Cruciferae*): an overview. Plant Syst Evol 259(2-4):89–120. https://doi.org/10.1007/s00606-006-0415-z

Amiri-Darban N, Nourmohammadi G, Rad AHS, Mirhadi SMJ, Heravan IM (2020) Potassium sulfate and ammonium sulfate affect quality and quantity of Camelina oil grown with different irrigation regimes. Ind Crop Prod 148:112308

Anderson JV, Wittenberg A, Li H, Berti MT (2019) High throughput phenotyping of Camelina sativa seeds for crude protein, total oil, and fatty acids profile by near infrared spectroscopy. Ind Crop Prod 137:501–507

Angelini L, Moscheni E (1998) Camelina (*Camelina sativa* [L.] Crantz). In: Mosca G (ed) Oleaginose non Alimentari. Edagricole, Bologna, pp 82–85

Bǎtrîna ŞL, Jurcoane Ş, Popescu I, Marin F, Crista F, Pop G, Imbrea F (2020) *Camelina sativa*: a study on amino acid content. Biotechnol Lett 25(1):1136–1142

Belayneh HD, Wehling RL, Cahoon E, Ciftci ON (2015) Extraction of omega-3-rich oil from *Camelina sativa* seed using supercritical carbon dioxide. J Supercrit Fluids 104:153–159. https://doi.org/10.1016/j.supflu.2015.06.002

Bernardo A, Howard-Hildige R, O'Connell A, Nichol R, Ryan J, Rice B, Roche E, Leahy JJ (2003) Camelina oil as a fuel for diesel transport engines. Ind Crop Prod 17(3):191–197. https://doi.org/10.1016/S0926-6690(02)00098-5

Berti M, Wilckens R, Fischer S, Solis A, Johnson B (2011) Seeding date influence on Camelina seed yield, yield components, and oil content in Chile. Ind Crop Prod 34(2):1358–1365. https://doi.org/10.1016/j.indcrop.2010.12.008

Berti M, Gesch R, Eynck C, Anderson J, Cermak S (2016) Camelina uses, genetics, genomics, production, and management. Ind Crop Prod 94:690–710. https://doi.org/10.1016/j.indcrop.2016.09.034

Blanco G et al (2014) Agriculture, forestry, other land use: drivers, trends and mitigation (archived 30 December 2014). In: IPCC AR5 WG3 2014, p 383. Emissions aggregated using 100-year global warming potentials from the IPCC Second Assessment Report

Booman M, Xu Q, Rise ML (2014) Evaluation of the impact of Camelina oil-containing diets on the expression of genes involved in the innate anti-viral immune response in Atlantic cod (*Gadus morhua*). Fish Shellfish Immunol 41(1):52–63. https://doi.org/10.1016/j.fsi.2014.05.017

Borzoo S, Mohsenzadeh S, Moradshahi A, Kahrizi D, Zamani H, Zarei M (2020) Characterization of physiological responses and fatty acid compositions of *Camelina sativa* genotypes under water deficit stress and symbiosis with Micrococcus yunnanensis. Symbiosis:1–12

BP (2017) BP statistical review of world energy. British Petroleum, London

Browne LM, Conn KL, Ayert WA, Tewari JP (1991) The camalexins: new phytoalexins produced in the leaves of *Camelina sativa* (*Cruciferae*). Tetrahedron 47(24):3909–3914. https://doi.org/10.1016/S0040-4020(01)86431-0

Brunt A, Crabtree K, Dallwitz MJ, Gibbs AJ, Watson L (1996) Viruses of plants: descriptions and lists from the VIDE database. CAB International, Wallingford, 1504 pp

Budin JT, Breene WM, Putnam DH (1995) Some compositional properties of Camelina (*Camelina sativa* L. Crantz) seeds and oils. J Am Oil Chem Soc 72(3):309–315. https://doi.org/10.1007/BF02541088

Bullerwell CN, Collins SA, Lall SP, Anderson DM (2016) Growth performance, proximate and histological analysis of rainbow trout fed diets containing *Camelina sativa* seeds, meal (high-oil and solvent-extracted) and oil. Aquaculture 452:342–350. https://doi.org/10.1016/j.aquaculture.2015.11.008

Cao Y, Gu Z, Muthukumarappan K, Gibbons W (2015) Separation of glucosinolates from Camelina seed meal via membrane and acidic aluminum oxide column. J Liquid Chromat Relat Technol 38(13):1273–1278. https://doi.org/10.1080/10826076.2015.1037454

Cappellozza BI, Cooke RF, Bohnert DW, Cherian G, Carroll JA (2012) Effects of Camelina meal supplementation on ruminal forage degradability, performance, and physiological responses of beef cattle. J Anim Sci 90(11):4042–4054. https://doi.org/10.2527/jas.2011-4664

Chaturvedi S, Bhattacharya A, Khare SK, Kaushik G (2017) *Camelina sativa*: an emerging biofuel crop. Handb Environ Mater Manag:1–38. https://doi.org/10.1007/978-3-319-58538-3_110-1

Ciurescu G, Ropota M, Toncea I, Habeanu M (2016) Camelina (*Camelina sativa* L. Crantz variety) oil and seeds as n-3 fatty acids rich products in broiler diets and its effects on performance, meat fatty acid composition, immune tissue weights, and plasma metabolic profile. J Agric Sci Technol:315–326

Clarke DB (2010) Glucosinolates, structures and analysis in food. Anal Methods 2(4):310–325. https://doi.org/10.1039/b9ay00280d

Conners IL (1967) An annotated index of plant diseases in Canada and fungi recorded on plants in Alaska, Canada and Greenland. Can Dep Agric Res Branch Ottawa Publ:1251.38

Crowley JG (1999) Evaluation of *Camelina sativa* as an alternative oilseed crop. Teagasc, Dublin

Crowley JG, Fröhlich A (1998) Factors affecting the composition and use of Camelina. Research Report 7, Project 4319, Teagasc, Dublin, Ireland

Cuendet M, Oteham CP, Moon RC, Pezzuto JM (2006) Quinone reductase induction as a biomarker for cancer chemoprevention. J Nat Prod 69(3):460–463

Czarnik M, Jarecki W, Bobrecka-Jamro D (2018) Reaction of winter varieties of false flax (*Camelina sativa* (L.) Crantz) to the varied sowing time. J Cent Eur Agric 19(3):571–586

Dangol N, Shrestha DS, Duffield JA (2015) Am Soc Agric Biol Eng 58(2):465–475. https://doi.org/10.13031/trans.58.10771

Das N, Berhow MA, Angelino D, Jeffery EH (2014) *Camelina sativa* defatted seed meal contains both alkyl sulfinyl glucosinolates and quercetin that synergize bioactivity. J Agric Food Chem 62(33):8385–8391

Dimmock J, Edwards-Jones G (2006) Crop protection in alternative crops. Outlook Pest Manag 17(1):24–27

Drenth AC, Olsen DB, Denef K (2015) Fuel property quantification of triglyceride blends with an emphasis on industrial oilseeds Camelina, Carinata, and pennycress. Fuel 153:19–30. https://doi.org/10.1016/j.fuel.2015.02.090

Ehrensing DT, Guy SO (2008) Camelina. EM 8953-E. Oregon State University Extension Service, Corvallis

Eidhin DN, Burke J, O'Beirne D (2003) Oxidative stability of ω3-rich Camelina oil and Camelina oil-based spread compared with plant and fish oils and sunflower spread. J Food Sci 68(1):345–353

EISA (2007) Energy Independence and Security Act of 2007 (Public Law 110–140). U.-S. Government Printing Office, Washington, DC. Retrieved from www.gpo.gov/fdsys/pkg/PLAW110publ140/pdf/PLAW-110publ140.pdf

El Sabagh A, Hossain A, Barutcular C, Gormus O, Ahmad Z, Hussain S, Akdeniz A (2019) Effects of drought stress on the quality of major oilseed crops: implication and possible mitigation strategies – a review. Appl Ecol Environ Res 17:4019–4043

Ellis RH, Hong TD, Roberts EH (1989) Quantal response of seed germination in seven genera of *Cruciferae* to white light of varying photon flux density and photoperiod. Ann Bot 63(1):145–158

Enjalbert N, Johnson J (2011) Guide for producing dryland Camelina in eastern Colorado. Crop production fact sheet no. 0709. Colorado State University, Fort Collins

Fahey JW, Wade KL, Stephenson KK, Chou FE (2003) Separation and purification of glucosinolates from crude plant homogenates by high-speed counter-current chromatography. J Chromatogr 996(1-2):85–93. https://doi.org/10.1016/S0021-9673(03)00607-1

Faisal F, Iqbal MA, Aydemir SK, Hamid A, Rahim N, El Sabagh A, Khaliq A, Siddiqui MH (2020) Exogenously foliage applied micronutrients efficacious impact on achene yield of sunflower under temperate conditions. Pak J Bot 52(4):1215–1221

Farooq MS, Uzair M, Raza A, Habib M, Xu Y, Yousuf M, Yang SH, Ramzan Khan M (2022) Uncovering the research gaps to alleviate the negative impacts of climate change on food security: a review. Front Plant Sci 13:927535. https://doi.org/10.3389/fpls.2022.927535

Fernández-Cuesta Á, Velasco L, Ruiz-Méndez MV (2014) Novel safflower oil with high γ-tocopherol content has a high oxidative stability. Eur J Lipid Sci Technol 116:832–836

Frame DD, Palmer M, Peterson B (2007) Use of *Camelina sativa* in the diets of young Turkeys. J Appl Poult Res. https://doi.org/10.1093/japr/16.3.381

Francis A, Warwick SI (2009) The biology of Canadian weeds. 142. *Camelina alyssum* (Mill.) Thell.; *C. microcarpa* Andrz. ex DC.; *C. sativa* (L.) Crantz. Can J Plant Sci 89(4):791–810. https://doi.org/10.4141/CJPS08185

Fröhlich A, Rice B (2005) Evaluation of *Camelina sativa* oil as a feedstock for biodiesel production. Ind Crop Prod 21(1):25–31. https://doi.org/10.1016/j.indcrop.2003.12.004

Froment M, Mastebroek D, Van Gorp K (2006) A growers manual for Calendula officinalis L. http://www.defra.gov.uk/farm/crops/industrial/research/reports/Calendula%.20Manual.pdf

Gaba S, Lescourret F, Boudsocq S, Enjalbert J, Hinsinger P, Journet EP, Navas ML, Wery J, Louarn G, Malezieux E, Pelzer E, Prudent M, Ozier-Lafontaine H (2015) Multiple cropping systems as drivers for providing multiple ecosystem services: from concepts to design. Agron Sustain Dev 35:607–623. https://doi.org/10.1007/s13593-014-0272-z

Galasso I, Manca A, Braglia L, Martinelli T, Morello L, Breviario D (2011) h-TBP: An approach based on intron-length polymorphism for the rapid isolation and characterization of the multiple members of the β-tubulin gene family in *Camelina sativa* (L.) Crantz. Mol Breed. https://doi.org/10.1007/s11032-010-9515-0

Gao L, Caldwell CD, Jaing Y (2018) Photosynthesis and growth of Camelina and canola in response to water deficit and applied nitrogen. Crop Sci 58:393–401. https://doi.org/10.2135/cropsci2017.07.0406

Gehringer A, Friedt W, Lühs W, Snowdon RJ (2006) Genetic mapping of agronomic traits in false flax (Camelina sativa subsp. sativa). Genome 49(12):1555–1563. https://doi.org/10.1139/G06-117

Gesch RW (2014) Influence of genotype and sowing date on Camelina growth and yield in the north central U.S. Ind Crop Prod 54:209–215. https://doi.org/10.1016/j.indcrop.2014.01.034

Gesch RW, Archer DW (2009) Camelina: A potential winter annual crop for the northern Corn Belt. (Abstract) (CD-ROM). ASA-CSSASSSA annual meet, Pittsburgh, PA. 1–5 November 2009. ASA, CSSA and SSSA, Madison

Gesch RW, Cermak SC (2011) Sowing date and tillage effects on fall-seeded Camelina in the Northern Corn Belt. Agron J 103(4):980–987. https://doi.org/10.2134/agronj2010.0485

Gesch RW, Matthees HL, Alvarez AL, Gardner RD (2018) Winter Camelina: Crop growth, seed yield, and quality response to cultivar and seeding rate. Crop Sci 58(5):2089–2098

Ghamkhar K, Croser J, Aryamanesh N, Campbell M, Kon'kova N, Francis C (2010) Camelina (Camelina sativa (L.) Crantz) as an alternative oilseed: molecular and ecogeographic analyses. Genome 53(7):558–567. https://doi.org/10.1139/G10-034

Glithero NJ, Ramsden SJ, Wilson P (2012) Farm systems assessment of bioenergy feedstock production: Integrating bioeconomic models and life cycle analysis approaches. Agric Syst 109:53–64. https://doi.org/10.1016/j.agsy.2012.02.005

Gogus U, Smith C (2010) n-3 Omega fatty acids: a review of current knowledge. Int J Food Sci Technol 45(3):417–436

Gómez-Monedero B, Bimbela F, Arauzo J, Faria J, Ruiz MP (2015) Pyrolysis of red eucalyptus, Camelina straw, and wheat straw in an ablative reactor. Energy Fuel. https://doi.org/10.1021/ef5026054

Goulson D (2003) Conserving wild bees for crop pollination. Food Agric Environ 1:142–144

Government of Canada (2011) Plants of Canada database. [Online] Available: https://glfc.cfsnet. nfis.org/mapserver/cfia_taxa/taxa.php?gid=1004663. 9 Mar 2011

Gugel RK, Falk KC (2006) Agronomic and seed quality evaluation of Camelina sativa in Western Canada. Can J Plant Sci 86(4):1047–1058. https://doi.org/10.4141/P04-081

Gui MM, Lee KT, Bhatia S (2008) Feasibility of edible oil vs. non-edible oil vs. waste edible oil as biodiesel feedstock. Energy 33(11):1646–1653. https://doi.org/10.1016/j.energy.2008.06.002

Gupta SK (ed) (2015) Breeding oilseed crops for sustainable production: opportunities and constraints. Academic

Guy SO, Wysocki DJ, Schillinger WF, Chastain TG (2014) Camelina: adaptation and performance of genotypes. Field Crop Res 155:224–232

Hack H, Bleiholder H, Burh L, Meier U, Schnock-Fricke E, Weber E, Witzenberger A (1992) Einheitliche Codierung der phänologischen Entwicklungsstadien mono-und dikotyler Pflanzen—Erweiterte BBCH-Skala Allgemein. Nachrichtenblatt desDeutschen Pflanzenschutzdientes

Harveson RM, Santra DK, Putnam ML, Curtis M, Pavlista AD (2011) A new report for downy mildew [(Hyaloperonospora camelinae Gaum.) Goker, Voglmayr, Riethm., M. Weiss & Oberw. 2003] of camelina [Camelina sativa (L.) Crantz] in the High Plains of the United States. Plant Health Progr. https://doi.org/10.1094/PHP-2011-1014-01-BR

Hatfield JL, Prueger JH (2015) Temperature extremes: Effect on plant growth and development. Weath Cli Ext 10:4–10

Henderson AE, Hallett RH, Soroka JJ (2004) Prefeeding behavior of the crucifer flea beetle, Phyllotreta cruciferae, on host and nonhost crucifers. J Insect Behav 17, 17(1):–39. https://doi.org/10.1023/B:JOIR.0000025130.20327.1a

Hess BW, Chen C, Foulke T, Jacobs J, Johnson D (2011) Evaluation of Camelina sativa as an alternative seed crop and feedstock for biofuel and developing replacement heifers. Project number SW07-049. Sustainable Agriculture Research & Education, University of Maryland

7 Changing Climate Scenario: Perspectives of *Camelina sativa*... 229

Hill J, Nelson E, Tilman D, Polasky S, Tiffany D (2006) Environmental, economic, and energetic costs and benefits of biodiesel and ethanol biofuels. Proc Natl Acad Sci 103:1206–11210

Hossain A, El Sabagh A, Barutcular C, Bhatt R, Çig F, Seydoşoglu S, Turan N, Konuskan O, Iqbal MA, Abdelhamid M, Soler CMT, Laing AM, Saneoka H (2020) Sustainable crop production to ensuring food security under climate change: a Mediterranean perspective. Aust J Crop Sci 14(3):439–446

Hurtaud C, Peyraud JL (2007) Effects of feeding camelina (seeds or meal) on milk fatty acid composition and butter spreadability. J Dairy Sci 90(11):5134–5145

Hutcheon C, Ditt RF, Beilstein M, Comai L, Schroeder J, Goldstein E, Shewmaker CK, Nguyen T, De Rocher J, Kiser J (2010) Polyploid genome of *Camelina sativa* revealed by isolation of fatty acid synthesis genes. BMC Plant Biol 10(1):1–15. https://doi.org/10.1186/1471-2229-10-233

Ibrahim FM, El Habbasha SF (2015) Chemical composition, medicinal impacts and cultivation of Camelina (*Camelina sativa*): review. Int J Pharm Tech Res 8:114–122

Imbrea F, Jurcoane S, Hălmăjan HV, Duda M, Botoş L (2011) *Camelina sativa*: a new source of vegetal oils. Roum Biotechnol Lett 16(3):6263–6270

IPPC (2011) Direct solar energy. Tech Rep. http://www.ipcc-wg3.de/report/IPCC_SRREN_Ch03.pdf

Iqbal MA, Hamid A, Hussain I, Rizwan M, Imran M, Sheikh UAA, Ishaq S (2020) Cactus pear: a weed of drylands for supplementing food security under changing climate. Planta Daninha 38: e020191761

Iqbal MA, Imtiaz H, Abdul H, Bilal A, Saira I, Ayman S, Celaleddin B, Rana DK, Imran M (2021a) Soybean herbage yield, nutritional value and profitability under integrated manures management. An Acad Bras Cienc 93(1):e20181384

Iqbal MA, Iqbal A, Ahmad Z, Raza A, Rahim J, Imran M, Sheikh UAA, Maqsood Q, Soufan W, Sahloul NMA, Sorour S, El Sabagh A (2021b) Cowpea [Vigna unguiculata (L.) Walp] herbage yield and nutritional quality in cowpea-sorghum mixed strip intercropping systems. Revista Mexicana De Ciencias Pecurias 12(2):402–418

Iskandarov U, Kim HJ, Cahoon EB (2014) Camelina: an emerging oilseed platform for advanced biofuels and bio-based materials. In: McCann M, Buckeridge M, Carpita N (eds) Plants and bioenergy. Advances in plant biology, vol 4. Springer, New York

Jankowski KJ, Sokolski M, Kordan B (2019) Camelina: yield and quality response to nitrogen and sulfur fertilization in Poland. Ind Crop Prod 141:111776

Jejelowo OA, Conn KL, Tewari JP (1991) Relationship between conidial concentration, germling growth, and phytoalexin production by *Camelina sativa* leaves inoculated with Alternaria brassicae. Mycol Res 95(8):928–934

Jewett FG (2015) *Camelina sativa*: for biofuels and bioproducts. In: Cruz VMV, Dierig DA (eds) Industrial crops. Springer, pp 157–170

Jha P, Stougaard RN (2013) Camelina (*Camelina sativa*) tolerance to selected preemergence herbicides. Weed Technol 27(4):712–717. https://doi.org/10.1614/wt-d-13-00061.1

Jiang Z, Ahn DU, Ladner L, Sim JS (1992) Influence of feeding full fat flax and sunflower seeds on internal and sensory qualities of eggs. Poult Sci

Jiang Y, Caldwell CD, Falk KC, Lada RR, Macdonald D (2013) Camelina yield and quality response to combined nitrogen and sulfur. Agronomy J105(6):1847–1852. https://doi.org/10.2134/agronj2013.0240

Johnson J, Enjalbert N, Schneekloth J, Helm A, Malhotra R (2009) Development of oilseed crops for biodiesel production under Colorado limited irrigation conditions. Final report no. 211. Colorado Water Institute

Johnston AM, Tanaka DL, Miller PR, Brandt SA, Nielsen DC, Lafond GP, Riveland NR (2002) Oilseed crops for semiarid cropping systems in the northern Great Plains. Agron J 94(2): 231–240. https://doi.org/10.2134/agronj2002.0231

Julié-Galau S, Bellec Y, Faure JD, Tepfer M (2014) Evaluation of the potential for interspecific hybridization between *Camelina sativa* and related wild *Brassicaceae* in anticipation of field trials of GM camelina. Transgenic Res 23(1):67–74. https://doi.org/10.1007/s11248-013-9722-7

Kakani R, Fowler J, Haq AU, Murphy EJ, Rosenberger TA, Berhow M, Bailey CRA (2012) Camelina meal increases egg n-3 fatty acid content without altering quality or production in laying hens. Lipids 47(5):519–526. https://doi.org/10.1007/s11745-012-3656-3

Kalita DJ, Tarnavchyk I, Sibi M, Moser BR, Webster DC, Chisholm BJ (2018) Biobased poly (vinyl ether)s derived from soybean oil, linseed oil, and Camelina oil: synthesis, characterization, and properties of crosslinked networks and surface coatings. Prog Org Coat 125:453–462. https://doi.org/10.1016/j.porgcoat.2018.09.033

Karolewski Z (1999) Characteristics of Leptosphaeria maculans isolates occurring in Wielkopolska region in 1991–1996. Phytopathol Pol:103–111

Karvonen HM, Aro A, Tapola NS, Salminen I, Uusitupa MI, Sarkkinen ES (2002) Effect of [alpha]-linolenic acid-rich *Camelina sativa* oil on serum fatty acid composition and serum lipids in hypercholesterolemic subjects. Metabolism 51(10):1253–1260

Kasetaite S, Ostrauskaite J, Grazuleviciene V, Svediene J, Bridziuviene D (2014) Camelina oil- and linseed oil-based polymers with bisphosphonate crosslinks. J Appl Polym Sci 131(17):10.1002/app.40683

Katar D, Arslan Y, Subasi I (2012) Ankara ekolojik koşullarında farklı ekim zamanlarının ketencik (Camelina sativa (L.) Crantz) bitkisinin yağ oranı ve bileşimi üzerine olan etkisinin belirlenmesi. Tekirdağ Ziraat Fakültesi Dergisi 9(3):84–90

Keshavarz-Afshar R, Chen C (2015) Intensification of dryland cropping systems for bio-feedstock production: energy analysis of Camelina. Bioeng Res 8:1877–1884. https://doi.org/10.1007/s12155-015-9644-8

Khadhair AH, Tewari JP, Howard RJ, Paul VH (2001) Detection of aster yellows phytoplasma in false flax based on PCR and RFLP. Microbiol Res 156(2):179–184. https://doi.org/10.1078/0944-5013-00100

Kim N, Li Y, Sun XS (2015) Epoxidation of *Camelina sativa* oil and peel adhesion properties. Ind Crop Prod 64:1–8. https://doi.org/10.1016/j.indcrop.2014.10.025

Kirkhus B, Lundon AR, Haugen J-E, Vogt G, Borge GIA, Henriksen BI (2013) Effects of environmental factors on edible oil quality of organically grown *Camelina sativa*. J Agric Food Chem 61(13):3179–3185

Klinkenberg B (2008) E-Flora BC: electronic atlas of the plants of British Columbia [www.eflora. bc.ca]. Lab for Advanced Spatial Analysis, Department of Geography, University of British Columbia

Knörzer KH (1978) Entwicklung und Ausbreitung des Leindotters (*Camelina sativa*). Ber Deutsch Bot Ges, Bd

Kollmann J, Bassin S (2001) Effects of management on seed predation in wildflower strips in northern Switzerland. Agric Ecosyst Environ 83(3):285–296. https://doi.org/10.1016/S0167-8809(00)00202-4

Larsson M (2013) Cultivation and processing of *Linum usitatissimum* and *Camelina sativa* in southern Scandinavia during the Roman Iron Age. Veg Hist Archaeobotany 22:509–520

Leclère M, Jeuffroy MH, Butier A, Chatain C, Loyce C (2019) Controlling weeds in Camelina with innovative herbicide-free crop management routes across various environments. Ind Crop Prod 140:111605. https://doi.org/10.1016/j.indcrop.2019.111605

Lenssen AW, Iversen WM, Sainju UM, Caesar-TonThat TC, Blodgett SL, Allen BL, Evans RG (2012) Yield, pests, and water use of durum and selected crucifer oilseeds in two-year rotations. Agronomy J104(5):1295–1304. https://doi.org/10.2134/agronj2012.0057

Li X, Mupondwa E (2014) Life cycle assessment of Camelina oil derived biodiesel and jet fuel in the Canadian Prairies. Sci Total Environ 481:17–26

Li H, Barbetti MJ, Sivasithamparam K (2005) Hazard from reliance on cruciferous hosts as sources of major gene-based resistance for managing blackleg (*Leptosphaeria maculans*) disease. Field Crop Res 91(2-3):185–198. https://doi.org/10.1016/j.fcr.2004.06.006

Li Z, Chakraborty S, Xu G (2016) X-ray crystallographic studies of the extracellular domain of the first plant ATP receptor, DORN1, and the orthologous protein from Camelina sativa. Acta Crystallographica Sect F: Str Biol Comm 72(10):782–787

7 Changing Climate Scenario: Perspectives of *Camelina sativa*...

Li N, Qi G, Sun XS, Xu F, Wang D (2015) Adhesion properties of Camelina protein fractions isolated with different methods. Ind Crop Prod 69:263–272. https://doi.org/10.1016/j.indcrop.2015.02.033

Liu H, Bean S, Sun XS (2018) Camelina protein adhesives enhanced by polyelectrolyte interaction for plywood applications. Ind Crop Prod 124:343–352. https://doi.org/10.1016/j.indcrop.2018.07.068

Liu K, Zhang C, Guan B, Yang R, Liu K, Wang Z, Li X, Xue K, Yin L, Wang X (2021) The effect of different sowing dates on dry matter and nitrogen dynamics for winter wheat: an experimental simulation study. Peer J 9:e11700. https://doi.org/10.7717/peerj.11700. PMID: 35070513; PMCID: PMC8759384

Ma Y, Gentry T, Hu P, Pierson E, Gu M, Yin S (2015) Impact of brassicaceous seed meals on the composition of the soil fungal community and the incidence of Fusarium wilt on chili pepper. Appl Soil Ecol 90:41–48. https://doi.org/10.1016/j.apsoil.2015.01.016

Malhi SS, Johnson EN, Hall LM, May WE, Phelps S, Nybo B (2014) Effect of nitrogen fertilizer application on seed yield, N uptake, and seed quality of *Camelina sativa*. Can J Soil Sci 94(1):35–47. https://doi.org/10.4141/CJSS2012-086

Martinelli T, Galasso I (2011) Phenological growth stages of *Camelina sativa* according to the extended BBCH scale. Ann Appl Biol 158(1):87–94. https://doi.org/10.1111/j.1744-7348.2010.00444.x

Matthäus B, Zubr J (2000a) Bioactive compounds in oil-cakes of *Camelina sativa* (L.) Crantz. Agro Food Industry Hi Tech, September/October

Matthäus B, Zubr J (2000b) Variability of specific components in *Camelina sativa* oilseed cakes. Ind Crop Prod. https://doi.org/10.1016/S0926-6690(99)00040-0

Mavridis A, Paul V, Rudolph K (2002) Bacterial blight of *Camelina sativa* caused by *Pseudomonas syringae* pv. camelinae. Beitr. Zuchtungsf. Bundesanst. Zuchtungsf. Kulturpfl

McVay KA, Khan QA (2011) Camelina yield response to different plant populations under dryland conditions. Agronomy J103(4):1265–1269. https://doi.org/10.2134/agronj2011.0057

Mcvay KA, Lamb PF (2008) Camelina Production in Montana (Report). Bull. MT200701AG

Meadus WJ, Duff P, McDonald T, Caine WR (2014) Pigs fed Camelina meal increase hepatic gene expression of cytochrome 8b1, aldehyde dehydrogenase, and thiosulfate transferase. J Anim Sci Biotechnol. https://doi.org/10.1186/2049-1891-5-1

Meyer JC, Michelutti N, Paterson AM, Cumming BF, Keller WB, Smol JP (2019) The browning and re-browning of lakes: Divergent lake-water organic carbon trends linked to acid deposition and climate change. Sci Rep 9(1):1

Milbau A, Stout JC (2008) Factors associated with alien plants transitioning from casual, to naturalized, to invasive. Conserv Biol 22(2):308–317. https://doi.org/10.1111/j.1523-1739.2007.00877.x

Mohammed YA, Chen C, Lamb P, Afshar RK (2017) Agronomic evaluation of Camelina (*Camelina sativa* L. Crantz) cultivars for biodiesel feedstock. Bioeng Res 10:792–799. https://doi.org/10.1007/s12155-017-9840-9

Mohammad BT, Al-Shannag M, Alnaief M, Singh L, Singsaas E, Alkasrawi M (2018) Production of multiple biofuels from whole Camelina material: a renewable energy crop. BioResources 13(3):4870–4883

Moser BR (2010) Camelina (Camelina sativa L.) oil as a biofuel's feedstock: golden opportunity or false hope. Lipid Tech 22(12):270–273

Moser BR, Vaughn SF (2010) Evaluation of alkyl esters from *Camelina sativa* oil as biodiesel and as blend components in ultra low-sulfur diesel fuel. Bioresour Technol 101(2):646–653. https://doi.org/10.1016/j.biortech.2009.08.054

Mulligan GA (2002) Weedy introduced mustards (*Brassicaceae*) of Canada. Can Field-Naturalist 116(4):623–631

NASS (2015) National agricultural statistical services. USDA. http://www.nass.usda.gov

Neupane D, Solomon JK, Mclennon E, Davison J, Lawry T (2019) Sowing date and sowing method influence on Camelina cultivars grain yield, oil concentration, and biodiesel production. Food Energy Secur 8(3):e00166

Nosal H, Nowicki J, Warzała M, Nowakowska-Bogdan E, Zarębska M (2015) Synthesis and characterization of alkyd resins based on *Camelina sativa* oil and polyglycerol. Prog Org Coat 86:59–70. https://doi.org/10.1016/j.porgcoat.2015.04.009

Obeng E, Obour AK, Nelson NO, Moreno JA, Ciampitti IA, Wang D, Durrett TP (2019) Seed yield and oil quality as affected by Camelina cultivar and planting date. J Crop Improv. https://doi.org/10.1080/15427528.2019.1566186

Obour AK, Krall JM, Nachtman JJ (2012) Influence of nitrogen and phosphorus fertilization on dryland *Camelina sativa* seed yield and oil content. Agricultural Experiment Station 2012 Field Days Bulletin. University of Wyoming, Laramie

Obour AK, Sintim HY, Obeng E, Jeliazkov VD (2015) Oilseed Camelina (*Camelina Sativa* L. Crantz): production systems, prospects and challenges in the USA Great Plains. Adv Plants Agric Res 2:1–9

Obour AK, Obeng E, Mohammed YA, Ciampitti IA, Durrett TP, Aznar-Moreno JA, Chen C (2017) Camelina seed yield and fatty acids as influenced by genotype and environment. Agron J 109(3):947–956

Obour AK, Chen C, Sintim HY, McVay K, Lamb P, Obeng E, Mohammed YA, Khan Q, Afshar RK, Zheljazkov VD (2018) Camelina sativa as a fallow replacement crop in wheat-based crop production systems in the US Great Plains. Ind Crops Prod 111:22–29

Palagesiu I (2000) Contributions to the knowledge of the entomofauna of some prospective oil plants in Romania. Lucrai Stiintifice-Agricultura, Universitatea de Stiinte Agricole si Medicina Veterinara a Banatului Timisoara 32(3):983–992

Pavlista AD, Isbell TA, Baltensperger DD, Hergert GW (2011) Planting date and development of spring-seeded irrigated canola, brown mustard and Camelina. Ind Crop Prod 33(2):451–456. https://doi.org/10.1016/j.indcrop.2010.10.029

Pedras MSC, Montaut S, Zaharia IL, Gai Y, Ward DE (2003) Transformation of the host-selective toxin destruxin B by wild crucifers: Probing a detoxification pathway. Phytochemistry 64(5): 957–963. https://doi.org/10.1016/S0031-9422(03)00444-8

Pekel AY, Patterson PH, Hulet RM, Acar N, Cravener TL, Dowler DB, Hunter JM (2009) Dietary Camelina meal versus flaxseed with and without supplemental copper for broiler chickens: live performance and processing yield. Poult Sci 88(11):2392–2398. https://doi.org/10.3382/ps.2009-00051

Pekel AY, Kim JI, Chapple C, Adeola O (2015) Nutritional characteristics of Camelina meal for 3-week-old broiler chickens. Poult Sci 94(3):371–378. https://doi.org/10.3382/ps/peu066

Pilgeram AL (2007) Camelina sativa, a Montana omega-3 and fuel crop. Terpinc P, Abramovič H (ed). A kinetic approach for evaluation of the antioxidant activity of selected phenolic acids. Food Chem 121(2):366–371

Plessers AG, McGregor WG, Carson RB, Nakoneshny W (1962) Species trials with oilseed plants. II. Camelina. Can J Plant Sci 42(3):452–445

Ponnampalam EN, Kerr MG, Butler KL, Cottrell JJ, Dunshea FR, Jacobs JL (2019) Filling the out of season gaps for lamb and hogget production: diet and genetic influence on carcass yield, carcass composition and retail value of meat. Meat Sci 148:156–163. https://doi.org/10.1016/j.meatsci.2018.08.027

Putnam DH, Budin JT, Field LA, Breene WM (1993) Camelina: a promising low-input oilseed. New Crop. Wiley, New York

Putnam ML, Serdani M, Ehrensing D, Curtis M (2009) Camelina infected by Downy Mildew (*Hyaloperonospora camelinae*) in the Western United States: a first report. Plant Heal Prog 10(1):40. https://doi.org/10.1094/php-2009-0910-01-br

Radzi A, Droege P (2014) Latest perspectives on global renewable energy policies. Curr Sustain Renew Energy Rep 1:85–93. https://doi.org/10.1007/s40518-014-0014-5

Rahman MJ, de Camargo AC, Shahidi F (2018) Phenolic profiles and antioxidant activity of defatted Camelina and sophia seeds. Food Chem 240:917–925. https://doi.org/10.1016/j.foodchem.2017.07.098

Raza A, Charagh S, García-Caparrós P, Rahman MA, Ogwugwa VH, Saeed F, Jin W (2022) Melatonin-mediated temperature stress tolerance in plants. GM Crops Food 13(1):196–217

Razeq FM, Kosma DK, Rowland O, Molina I (2014) Extracellular lipids of *Camelina sativa*: characterization of chloroform-extractable waxes from aerial and subterranean surfaces. Phytochemistry 106:188–196

Reddy N, Jin E, Chen L, Jiang X, Yang Y (2012) Extraction, characterization of components, and potential thermoplastic applications of Camelina meal grafted with vinyl monomers. J Agric Food Chem 60(19):4872–4879

Righini D, Zanetti F, Monti A (2016) The bio-based economy can serve as the springboard for Camelina and crambe to quit the limbo. OCL 23(5):D504

Righini D, Zanetti F, Martínez-Force E, Mandrioli M, Toschi TG, Monti A (2019) Shifting sowing of Camelina from spring to autumn enhances the oil quality for bio-based applications in response to temperature and seed carbon stock. Ind Crop Prod 137:66–73

Robinson R (1987) Camelina: a useful research crop and a potential oilseed crop

Rode J (2002) Study of autochthon *Camelina sativa* (L.) Crantz in Slovenia. Int J Geogr Inf Syst 9(4):313–318. https://doi.org/10.1300/J044v09n04_08

Sabagh AE, Hossain A, Islam MS, Iqbal MA, Raza A, Karademir Ç, Karademir E, Rehman A, Rahman MA, Singhal RK, Llanes A (2020) Elevated CO2 concentration improves heat-tolerant ability in crops. In: Fahad S, Saud S, Chen Y, Wu C, Wang D (eds) Abiotic stress in plants. IntechOpen. https://doi.org/10.5772/intechopen.94128

Sainger M, Jaiwal A, Sainger PA, Chaudhary D, Jaiwal R, Jaiwal PK (2017) Advances in genetic improvement of *Camelina sativa* for biofuel and industrial bio-products. Renew Sustain Energy Rev 68:623–637. https://doi.org/10.1016/j.rser.2016.10.023

Salisbury PA (1987) Blackleg resistance in weedy crucifers. *Eucarpia cruciferae*. Newsletter 12:90

Salminen H, Estévez M, Kivikari R, Heinonen M (2006) Inhibition of protein and lipid oxidation by rapeseed, Camelina and soy meal in cooked pork meat patties. Eur Food Res Technol 223(4): 461. https://doi.org/10.1007/s00217-005-0225-5

Sampath A (2009) Chemical characterization of Camelina seed oil. Rutgers University-Graduate School, New Brunswick

Sarkodie SA, Ntiamoah EB, Dongmei L (2019) Panel heterogeneous distribution analysis of trade and modernized agriculture on CO_2 emissions: the role of renewable and fossil fuel energy consumption. Nat Resour Forum 43(3):135–153. https://doi.org/10.1111/1477-8947.12183

Sawyer K (2008) Is there room for Camelina. Biodiesel Mag 5(7):83–87

Schillinger WF (2019) Camelina: long-term cropping systems research in a dry Mediterranean climate. Field Crop Res 235:87–94

Schillinger WF, Wysocki DJ, Chastain TG, Guy SO, Karow RS (2012) Camelina: planting date and method effects on stand establishment and seed yield. Field Crop Res 130:138–144

Schulte LR, Ballard T, Samarakoon T, Yao L, Vadlani P, Staggenborg S, Rezac M (2013) Increased growing temperature reduces content of polyunsaturated fatty acids in four oilseed crops. Ind Crop Prod 51:212–219. https://doi.org/10.1016/j.indcrop.2013.08.075

Schultze-Motel W (1986) Camelina. In: Hegi G (ed) Illustrierte flora von Mittel-europa, vol 4, 3rd edn. Verlag Paul Parey, Berlin/Hamburg, pp 340–345

Schwartz H, Ollilainen V, Piironen V, Lampi AM (2008) Tocopherol, tocotrienol and plant sterol contents of vegetable oils and industrial fats. J Food Compos Anal 21(2):152–161. https://doi.org/10.1016/j.jfca.2007.07.012

Science Advice for Policy by European Academies (2020) A sustainable food system for the European Union (PDF). SAPEA, Berlin, p 39. https://doi.org/10.26356/sustainablefood. ISBN:978-3-9820301-7-3. Archived from the original (PDF) on 18 April 2020. Retrieved 14 April 2020

Seehuber R (1984) Genotypic variation for yield- and quality-traits in poppy and false flax. Fette-Seifen-Anstrichmittel 86(5):177–180

Seehuber R, Vollmann J, Dambroth M, Anwendung D (1987) Single-seed-descent Methode bei Leindotter (*Camelina sativa* (L.) Crantz) zur Erhöhung des Ertragsniveaus. Landbauforsch. Völken- rode

Séguin-Swartz G, Nettleton JA, Sauder C, Warwick SI, Gugel RK (2013) Hybridization between *Camelina sativa* (L.) Crantz (false flax) and North American Camelina species. Plant Breed 132: 390–396

Sehgal A, Sita K, Siddique KH, Kumar R, Bhogireddy S, Varshney RK, Nayyar H (2018) Drought or/and heatstress effects on seed filling in food crops: impacts on functional biochemistry, seed yields, and nutritional quality. Front Plant Sci 9

Shukla VKS, Dutta PC, Artz WE (2002) Camelina oil and its unusual cholesterol content. JAOCS 79(10):965–969. https://doi.org/10.1007/s11746-002-0588-1

Siddiqui MH, Iqbal MA, Naeem W, Hussain I, Khaliq A (2019) Bio-economic viability of rainfed wheat (Triticum aestivum L.) cultivars under integrated fertilization regimes in Pakistan. Custos e Agronegocio 15(3):81–96

Sindelar AJ, Schmer MR, Gesch RW, Forcella F, Eberle CA, Thom MD, Archer DW (2017) Winter oilseed production for biofuel in the US Corn Belt: opportunities and limitations. GCB Bioenergy 9(3):508–524. https://doi.org/10.1111/gcbb.12297

Singh BK, Bala M, Rai PK (2014) Fatty acid composition and seed meal characteristics of brassica and allied genera. Natl Acad Sci Lett 37(3):219–226. https://doi.org/10.1007/s40009-014-0231-x

Sintim HY, Zheljazkov VD, Obour AK, Garcia-y-Garcia A, Foulke TK (2014) Camelina as a replacement for fallow in wheat-fallow rotation. ASA-CSSA-SSSA International Annual Meeting, Poster No: 323, Long Beach

Sintim HY, Zheljazkov VD, Obour AK, Garcia-y-Garcia A, Foulke TK (2016a) Evaluating agronomic responses of Camelina to seeding date under rain-fed conditions. Agron J 108: 349–357. https://doi.org/10.2134/agronj2015.0153

Sintim HY, Zheljazkov VD, Obour AK, Garcia-y-Garcia A (2016b) Managing harvest time to control pod shattering in oilseed camelina. Agron J 108(2):656–661. https://doi.org/10.2134/agronj2015.0300

Sobiech Ł, Grzanka M, Kurasiak-Popowska D, Radzikowska D (2020) Phytotoxic effect of herbicides on various camelina [Camelina sativa (L.) Crantz] genotypes and plant chlorophyll fluorescence. Agriculture 10(5):185

Somerville C, Youngs H, Taylor C, Davis SC, Long SP (2010) Feedstocks for lignocellulosic biofuels. Science 329(5993):790–792

Soroka J, Olivier C, Grenkow L, Séguin-Swartz G (2015) Interactions between *Camelina sativa* (*Brassicaceae*) and insect pests of canola. Cana Entomol 147(2):193–214

Špak J, Kubelková D (2000) Serological variability among European isolates of radish mosaic virus. Plant Pathol 49(2):295–301. https://doi.org/10.1046/j.1365-3059.2000.00438.x

Struik PC, Kuyper TW (2017) Sustainable intensification in agriculture: the richer shade of green. A review. Agron Sustain Dev 37:39. https://doi.org/10.1007/s13593-017-0445-7

Szterk A, Roszko M, Sosińska E, Derewiaka D, Lewicki PP (2010) Chemical composition and oxidative stability of selected plant oils. JAOCS 87(6):637–645. https://doi.org/10.1007/s11746-009-1539-4

Tabără V, Pop G, Ladislau W, Tabără CG, Mateas I, Prodan M (2007) Plantele, surse deproducție pentru biocombustibil. Buletinul AGIR nr. 3 (iulie-septembrie) in western Canada. Can J Plant Sci 3:17–20

Tabatabaie SMH, Murthy GS (2017) Effect of geographical location and stochastic weather variation on life cycle assessment of biodiesel production from Camelina in the northwestern USA. Int J Life Cycle Assess 22(6):867–882

Tedin O (1922) Zur Blüten- und Befruchtungsbiologie der Leindotter (*Camelina sativa*). Bot Notiser 1922:177–189

7 Changing Climate Scenario: Perspectives of *Camelina sativa*. . . 235

Terpinc P, Čeh B, Ulrih NP, Abramovič H (2012) Studies of the correlation between antioxidant properties and the total phenolic content of different oil cake extracts. Ind Crops Prod 39:210–217

Toncea I (2014) The seed yield potential of Camelia-first Romanian cultivar of Camelina (*Camelina sativa* L. Crantz). Roum Agric Res 31:17–23

Tripathi V, Edrisi SA, Abhilash P (2016) Towards the coupling of phytoremediation with bioenergy production. Renew Sustain Energy Rev 57:1386–1389

Trumbo P, Schlicker S, Yates AA, Poos M (2002) Dietary reference intakes for energy, carbohydrate, fiber, fat, fatty acids, cholesterol, protein and amino acids. J Am Diet Assoc 102(11): 1621–1630

Urbaniak SD, Caldwell CD, Zheljazkov VD, Lada R, Luan L (2008) The effect of seeding rate, seeding date and seeder type on the performance of *Camelina sativa* L. in the Maritime Provinces of Canada. Can J Plant Sci. https://doi.org/10.4141/CJPS07148

USDA (2010) A USDA regional roadmap to meeting the biofuels goals of the renewable fuels standard by 2022. USDA Biofuels Strategic Production Report

USDA (2011) www.ers.usda.gov/Briefing/SoybeansOilcrops/Canola.htm. Accessed Feb 2012

USDA-ARS (2011) National genetic resources program. Germplasm resources information network – (GRIN). National Germplasm Resources Laboratory, Beltsville

USDA-NRCS (2010) Keys to soil taxonomy. Soil Survey Staff, Washington, DC

USEPA (US Environmental Protection Agency) (2013) Regulation of fuels and fuel additives: identification of additional qualifying renewable fuel pathways under the renewable fuel standard program. Fed Regist 78(43):14190–14217

Vollmann J, Eynck C (2015) Camelina as a sustainable oilseed crop: Contributions of plant breeding and genetic engineering. Biotechnol J 10(4):525–535. https://doi.org/10.1002/biot.201400200

Vollmann J, Steinkellner S, Glauninger J (2001) Variation in resistance of Camelina (*Camelina sativa* [L.] Crtz.) to downy mildew (*Peronospora camelinae Gäum.*). J Phytopathol 149(3-4): 129–133. https://doi.org/10.1046/j.1439-0434.2001.00599.x

Vollmann J, Damboeck A, Eckl A, Schrems H, Ruckenbauer P (1996) Improvement of *Camelina sativa*, an underexploited oilseed. In: Janick J (ed) Progress in new crops. ASHS Press, Alexandria, pp 357–362

Vollmann J, Moritz T, Kargl C, Baumgartner S, Wagentristl H (2007) Agronomic evaluation of camelina genotypes selected for seed quality characteristics. Ind Crops and Prod 26(3):270–277

Vollmann K, Qurishi R, Hockemeyer J, Müller CE (2008) Synthesis and properties of a new water-soluble prodrug of the adenosine A2A receptor antagonist MSX-2. Molecule 13(2):348–359

Waraich EA, Ahmed Z, Ahmad R, Shabbir RN (2017) Modulating the phenology and yield of Camelina sativa L. by varying sowing dates under water deficit stress conditions. Soil Environ 36:84–92

Western Australian Herbarium (2010) FloraBase – the Western Australian Flora. Department of Environment and Conservation. [Online] Available: http://florabase.dec.wa.gov.au/. 1 Sept 2010

Westman AL, Dickson MH (1998) Disease reaction to *Alternaria* brassicicola and *Xanthomonas* campestris pv. campestris in *Brassica* nigra and other weedy crucifers. Crucif Newsl

Westman AL, Kresovich S, Dickson MH (1999) Regional variation in *Brassica nigra* and other weedy crucifers for disease reaction to *Alternaria brassicicola* and *Xanthomonas campestris* pv. campestris. Euphytica 106(3):253–259. https://doi.org/10.1023/A:1003544025146

Xue J, Grift TE, Hansen AC (2011) Effect of biodiesel on engine performances and emissions. Renew Sust Energ Rev 15(2):1098–1116. https://doi.org/10.1016/j.rser.2010.11.016

Yang J, Caldwell C, Corscadden K, He QS, Li J (2016) An evaluation of biodiesel production from *Camelina sativa* grown in Nova Scotia. Ind Crop Prod 88:162–168. https://doi.org/10.1016/j.indcrop.2015.11.073

Yuan L, Li R (2020) Metabolic engineering a model oilseed *Camelina sativa* for the sustainable production of high-value designed oils. Front Plant Sci 11:11

Zaleckas E, Makareviciene V, Sendžikiene E (2012) Possibilities of using *Camelina sativa* oil for producing biodiesel fuel. Transport. https://doi.org/10.3846/16484142.2012.664827

Zanetti F, Eynck C, Christou M, Krzyżaniak M, Righini D, Alexopoulou E, Stolarski MJ, Van Loo EN, Puttick D, Monti A (2017) Agronomic performance and seed quality attributes of Camelina (*Camelina sativa* L. Crantz) in multi-environment trials across Europe and Canada. Ind Crop Prod 107:602–608

Zhang CJ, Auer C (2019) Overwintering assessment of Camelina (*Camelina sativa*) cultivars and congeneric species in the northeastern US. Ind Crop Prod 139:111532

Zhao Y, Wei W, Davis RE, Lee IM (2010) Recent advances in 16S rRNA gene-based phytoplasma differentiation, classification and taxonomy. In: Weintraub PG, Jones P (eds) Phytoplasma genomes, plant hosts and vectors. CABI, Cambridge, pp 64–92

Zubr J (1997) Oil-seed crop: *Camelina sativa*. Ind Crop Prod 6(2):113–119

Zubr J (2003a) Dietary fatty acids and amino acids of *Camelina sativa* seed. J Food Qual 26(6): 451–462. https://doi.org/10.1111/j.1745-4557.2003.tb00260.x

Zubr J (2003b) Qualitative variation of *Camelina sativa* seed from different locations. Ind Crop Prod *17*(3):161–169. https://doi.org/10.1016/S0926-6690(02)00091-2

Zubr J (2009) Unique dietary oil from *Camelina sativa* Seed. Agro Food Ind Hi Tech 20(2):42–46

Chapter 8
Greenhouse Gas Emissions and Mitigation Strategies in Rice Production Systems

Zeeshan Ahmed, Dongwei Gui, Zhiming Qi, Junhe Liu, Abid Ali, Ghulam Murtaza, Rana Nauman Shabbir, Muhammad Tariq, Muhammad Shareef, Sadia Zafar, Muhammad Saadullah Khan, and Shakeel Ahmad

Abstract Methane (CH_4) and nitrous oxide (N_2O) are the two critical greenhouse gases (GHGs) that absorb radiation, affect atmospheric chemistry, and contribute to global climate change. Rice being the second largest cultivated food crop around

---

Z. Ahmed · D. Gui · M. Shareef
Xinjiang Institute of Ecology & Geography, Chinese Academy of Sciences, Urumqi, Xinjiang, China

Cele National Station of Observation and Research for Desert-Grassland Ecosystem, Xinjiang Institute of Ecology and Geography, Chinese Academy of Sciences, Xinjiang, China
e-mail: guidwei@ms.xjb.ac.cn

Z. Qi
Department of Bioresource Engineering, McGill University, Saitne-Anne-de-Bellevue, Canada

J. Liu
College of Biological and Food Engineering, Huanghuai University, Zhumadian, Henan, China

A. Ali
College of Life Science, Shenyang Normal University, Shenyang, Liaoning, China

Department of Entomology, University of Agriculture, Faisalabad, Pakistan

G. Murtaza
Faculty of Environmental Science and Engineering, Kunming University of Science and Technology, Kunming, China

R. N. Shabbir · S. Ahmad (✉)
Department of Agronomy, Faculty of Agricultural Science and Technology, Bahauddin Zakariya University, Multan, Pakistan
e-mail: shakeelahmad@bzu.edu.pk

M. Tariq
Agronomy Section, Central Cotton Research Institute, Multan, Pakistan

S. Zafar
Department of Botany, Division of Science and Technology, University of Education, Lahore, Pakistan

M. S. Khan
Department of Agronomy, University of Agriculture, Faisalabad, Pakistan

---

© The Author(s), under exclusive license to Springer Nature Switzerland AG 2022
M. Ahmed (ed.), *Global Agricultural Production: Resilience to Climate Change*,
https://doi.org/10.1007/978-3-031-14973-3_8

237

the world is also a leading anthropogenic source of GHG emissions from agriculture sector. It accounts for 18% CH_4 and 11% N_2O emissions of the total agricultural GHG additions. In the face of rising population, rice production is estimated to be increased by 40% in 2030 along with higher CH_4 and N_2O release to the atmosphere which needs to be reduced on priority basis. We attempted to develop a mechanistic understanding on CH_4 and N_2O production from rice fields and different factors influencing their emission. It has been found that modifications in traditional crop cultivation practices manifested enormous potential to minimize GHG emissions from rice fields. However changes in the existing management practices can simultaneously influence more than one gas, and their effects may be opposite. After assessing the possible mitigation options to abate CH_4 and N_2O emissions, it has been found that modifying irrigation and tillage practices, improving fertilizer management, using low-emitting rice varieties, incorporation of fermented cow dung and leaf manures, addition of nitrification inhibitors, and slow-release fertilizers manifested great potential to abate methane and nitrous oxide emissions. Incorporation of biochar, straw compost, and straw ash could have better results in curtailing GHG emissions compared to direct straw additions. Adoption of these proposed mitigation options singly or in combination is likely to minimize GHG emissions and helpful in sustainable rice production. However successful execution of these practices at farmer's level demands the removal of all social, economic, educational, and political barriers.

Keywords GHG emission · Rice production · CH_4 · N_2O · Climate change · Nitrification · Methanogenesis

Abbreviations

AFOLU	Agriculture, forestry, and other land use
CH_4	Methane
CO_2	Carbon dioxide
FAO	Food and Agriculture Organization
GHG	Greenhouse gas
GWP	Global warming potential
IPCC	Intergovernmental Panel on Climate Change
IRRI	International Rice Research Institute
N_2O	Nitrous oxide
RFESs	Rice field ecosystems

8 Greenhouse Gas Emissions and Mitigation Strategies in Rice Production Systems

8.1 Introduction

Climate change is a major environmental concern of the twenty-first century largely driven by rising greenhouse gas (GHG) emissions (Wang et al. 2017). Rising sea levels, food security, health problems, severe storms, migration, and increasing economic losses are just some of the immediate repercussions of climate change (Yoro and Daramola 2020). This devastating situation advocates the adoption of certain strategies to minimize the GHG emissions and limit the impact of climate change. The three most important GHGs are carbon dioxide (CO_2), methane (CH_4), and nitrous oxide (N_2O), absorb infrared radiation in the atmosphere, retain heat, and warm the surface of the Earth, therefore potentially contributing toward global warming (Synder et al. 2009). Global warming potential (GWP) of these three GHGs differ significantly as GWP of N_2O is 298 times higher than CO_2, while GWP of methane is 265 times greater than CO_2 on a 100-year time span (Shakoor et al. 2020). According to IPCC (2014), power sector (electricity and heat production) accounts for 25%; agriculture, forestry, and other land use (AFOLU) sector 24%; industrial sector 21%; transportation sector 14%; other energy sectors 10%; and building sector 6% contribution in global GHG emissions, respectively (Fig. 8.1).

Agricultural production systems are vital anthropogenic sources of GHGs having share of about 10–14% in global GHG emissions, and agriculture alone contributes about 42% of total CH_4 and 75% of N_2O emissions (FAO 2020). In worldwide agricultural ecosystems, CH_4 emissions are 3.22×10^6 Gg CO_2-eq year^{-1}, while nitrous N_2O emissions amounted 5.99×10^6 Gg CO_2-eq year^{-1} (FAO 2020).

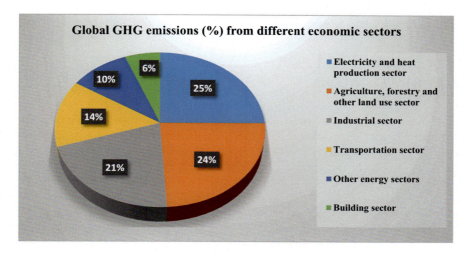

Fig. 8.1 Contribution of different economic sectors in global greenhouse gas emissions. (Source: IPCC 2014)

Rice (*Oryza sativa* L.) is a vital component of agricultural production systems encompassing a harvest area of about 23% of the total area of global cereal farming (FAO 2020). Rice is widely cultivated as a staple food crop globally (Carlson et al. 2017) covering 160 million hectares (ha) of land with 740 million tons of annual production (Pathak et al. 2018). About 92% of the global rice production and consumption occurs in Asia, and it satisfies nearly 35–80% of total calorie consumption of the Asian people (Sarwar et al. 2022). Almost 75% of the global rice supply is dependent on 79 million hectares of irrigated cropland in Asia. Therefore, current and future food security particularly in Asia and around the globe will largely depend on irrigated rice systems (Kumar et al. 2019). Irrigated rice cropping systems significantly contribute toward CH_4 and N_2O emissions into the atmosphere. Global estimates revealed that CH_4 accounts for 18%, while N_2O accounts for 11% emissions of the total agricultural emissions that come from paddy fields (IPCC 2014; FAO 2020). Furthermore, GWP of GHG emissions from rice production systems is approximately four times greater as compared to wheat (*Triticum aestivum* L.) and maize (*Zea mays* L.) (Linquist et al. 2012). According to an estimate, rice production will be increased by 40% at the end of 2030 in response of enormously increasing population (FAO 2009). Hence increase in production will escalate the CH_4 and N_2O emissions to the atmosphere, thereby raising serious concerns regarding climate change and sustainable rice production (Wang et al. 2017). Therefore for sustainable rice production in the future, we have to combine the increase in rice yield with reduced GHG emissions (Faiz-ul Islam et al. 2018). Nonetheless CH_4 and nitrous oxide ejections from rice fields are significantly persuaded by crop production practices such as soil tilling methods, land leveling, plant residue management, irrigation scheduling, drainage system, and organic and inorganic soil modifications. Therefore the appropriate strategy to manage the GHG emissions with gains in rice yields is to modify or improve the traditional crop management practices. It will help to maintain appropriate soil carbon pools and improve nutrient use efficiency with substantial reduction in CH_4 and N_2O productions from paddy fields.

8.2 Rice Ecosystems

Rice crop is widely grown under diverse climatic conditions around the globe. The International Rice Research Institute (IRRI) has classified the rice field ecosystems (RFESs) into four categories: (i) upland, (ii) irrigated, (iii) rain-fed lowland, and (iv) flood-prone rice ecosystems (IRRI 1993) (Fig. 8.2).

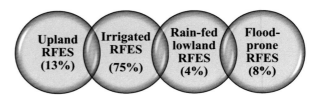

Fig. 8.2 Different types of rice field ecosystems (RFESs) in the world. (Source: IRRI 1993)

8 Greenhouse Gas Emissions and Mitigation Strategies in Rice Production Systems 241

Upland RFES The upland rice field ecosystems comprised of low-lying valleys with undulating steep slopy land having high runoff and sideways water movement. Such kind of system represents less than 13% of the global rice land.

Irrigated RFES Irrigated RFESs have ample quantity of water to support single or more crops annually. Lands under irrigated RFES cover about 50% of world's rice lands controlling nearly 75% of the world's rice production.

Rain-Fed Lowland RFES The rain-fed lowland RFES encounters both drought and flooding problems. Rain-fed low lands cover about 25% (one quarter) of the world's rice fields.

Flood-Prone RFES The rest of the rice fields are categorized as flood-prone RFES holding an area of about 8% of the world rice lands. Uncontrolled flooding is a primary feature of this RFES. The land may remain submerged with water (0.5–4.0 depth) for about 5 months, whereas in some areas get alternate flooding with brackish water caused by tidal fluctuations. These RFESs face multiple problems such as plant nutrition, weeds, and pest problems; therefore they require different rice crop management strategies.

8.3 Paddy Soil Characteristics

Paddy soils represent the second largest manmade wetlands after natural wetlands (Yoon 2009). Primarily paddy soils are characterized by heavy texture with reduced soil horizon indicating continuous or inconsistent signs of waterlogging like splitting of iron and manganese in the soil solution (Kirk 2004). Moreover presence of a hard pan with higher bulk density at a depth of 15–25 cm substantially decreases water percolation and promotes flooding. Utilization of paddy soils through puddling constitutes the artificial submerged conditions accompanying reduced soil conditions hiding the original soil characteristics (Kirk 2004). Management of paddy soils mediates the creation of pedogenetic horizons (Fig. 8.3) a characteristic of paddy soils (FAO 2006).

W: This horizon is characterized by thin layer of standing water containing bacteria, macrophytes, phytoplankton, and small fauna. This horizon is primarily oxic.

Ap: It represents the interface of the soil and standing water with oxic conditions. Thickness of this zone may range from several millimeters to several centimeters.

Arp: It is the top portion of an anthraquic horizon having reduced puddled and flooded layer, indicating a reduced soil matrix with some oxidized root channel. It represents an oxidation reduction site during the period of alternate flooding and drainage of soil. This layer is usually 15 cm thick.

Ardp: It is the lower part of an anthraquic horizon with plough pan. It is compact with high bulk density having platy structure that hinders the water infiltration. Hence stagnant and reduced conditions are retained in this layer.

B or C: A hydragic horizon carrying redoximorphic properties.

Fig. 8.3 Horizon sequence of a typical paddy soil. (Source: FAO 2006)

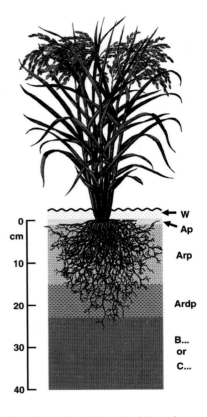

Paddy soil management-induced fluctuations in redox potential control the microbial community structure, function, and therefore short-term biogeochemical processes. Microbial reduction processes after flooding utilize NO_3^-, Mn^{4+}, Fe^{3+}, and SO_4^{2-} as electron acceptors and emit gases including N_2O, N_2, H_2S, and CH_4 and due to reduction-mediated increasing pH-NH_3. This is the main reason of N losses and low N fertilizer use efficiency. Meanwhile, rice roots acquiring atmospheric O_2 via aerenchyma cells modify the rhizosphere environment, causing nitrification and CH_4 oxidation along with precipitation of Mn and Fe oxides. High content and fluxes of dissolved organic matter (DOM) in rice soils from plant remains initiate microbial activity and GHG. DOM confinement by soil minerals and consequent steadiness against microbial decay is highly dependent on the prevailing redox state (e.g., DOM precipitation by Fe^{2+} under anaerobic conditions). Fluctuations in redox conditions may prolong the retention and stabilization of DOM by Fe oxy hydroxides (Kögel-Knabner et al. 2010).

8.4 Methane (CH$_4$) Production and Emissions from Paddy Soils

CH$_4$ is the second crucial GHG after CO$_2$ in terms of GWP and the dominant GHG emitted from rice fields. Its concentration in atmosphere has greatly increased from preindustrial level of 722 ppb to the current level of 1830 ppb (Wang et al. 2017). The cumulative annual CH$_4$ emission from both anthropogenic and natural sources is estimated about 600 CH$_4$ Tg year$^-$1 out of which 20% is added by paddy fields. Globally rice cultivation alone adds up approximately 46 Tg year^{-1} CH$_4$ emissions to atmosphere (James and James 2010).

8.4.1 Methanogenesis and Methanogens

Production of CH$_4$ through bacterial breakdown of complex organic matter under anaerobic conditions in flooded rice is called methanogenesis, whereas the bacteria/archaea accomplishing this process are called methanogens (Penning and Conrad 2007).

Methanogens from Archaea domain are strictly anaerobic obligate in nature (Fazli et al. 2013). Methanogens are also unique as they obtain their energy from CH$_4$ production by utilizing substrates like ethanol, formate, acetate, CO$_2$, and H$_2$ (Conrad 2007). Methanogens are mesophilic in nature, capable of producing CH$_4$ in a temperature range of 20–40 °C (Dubey 2005). Ammonium ion (NH$_4^+$) is the preferred nitrogen source used by all the methanogens, although they can fix molecular nitrogen and also contain nitrogen fixation genes (nif) (Dubey 2005; Serrano-Silva et al. 2014). CH$_4$ formation by methanogens requires some unique enzymes and coenzymes to accomplish this procedure (Nazaries et al. 2013).

Weeds, weed and rice roots, rhizo-deposition by weeds and rice, algal biomass, rice litter, rice stubbles, biomass of microbes, aquatic animals, and organic fertilizers act as organic matter sources. Conversion of this organic matter into preferable food forms (acetate) or alcohols (desired after acetate) for methanogens is executed through following processes (Malyan et al. 2016).

8.4.1.1 Hydrolysis

Both humus and humic components constitute the organic matter in rice soils. The humus consists of specific matter and water-soluble materials. This granular matter comprising of cellulose, hemicellulose, lignin, and proteins is provided by living component, whereas substances such as amino acids, sugars, and nucleotides which are water soluble either contributed by disintegration of the particulate matter through hydrolysis of extracellular enzymes or by rhizo-deposition (Conrad 1999; Brune et al. 2000; Kimura 2000; Liesack et al. 2000; Kimura et al. 2004).

8.4.1.2 Acidogenesis

In acidogenesis the hydrolytic products (monomers) are transformed into volatile fatty acids, ammonia, organic acids, alcohols, hydrogen, and CO_2 (Cairo and Paris 1988). Fermentative bacteria convert monomers of hydrolysis into acids. This kind of fermentative bacteria may be strictly anaerobic or can be facultative aerobic.

8.4.1.3 Acetogenesis

During acetogenesis volatile fatty acids convert themselves into acetic acid, CO_2, and H by acetogens. Acetogen bacteria are primarily obligatory anaerobic bacteria found largely in rice fields (Rosencrantz et al. 1999). Wood–Ljungdahl or reductive acetyl-CoA pathway is used by acetogens to synthesize acetyl-CoA and cell carbon. Formation of acetate from the preformed metabolites (acids) is accomplished by bacteria at a temperature range of 15–50 °C. Globally this range of temperature usually exists in majority of the rice fields across all geographical regions (Malyan et al. 2016).

8.4.1.4 Methanogenesis

Methanogens consume C from formic acid, alcohols, methylated sulfides, methylamines, dimethyl sulfide, acetate, methanethiol, and CO_2/H_2 as substrates producing CH_4 (Nazaries et al. 2013; Dubey 2005). The acetate or CO_2/H_2 acts as an instant methanogenesis precursor. Methanogenesis occurs as a result of decline in non-methanogenic electron-accepting agents (oxygen, nitrate, manganese (IV), iron (III), and sulfate) and transforms thermodynamic conditions (Malyan et al. 2016).

8.4.2 Methane Emission Pathways

CH_4 can be found in rice soils either as dissolved CH_4 or in gas phase (Tokida et al. 2005). An estimation revealed that approximately 33–88% of the total subsurface CH_4 exist in gas form. In contrast dissolved CH_4 content found to be quite low is less soluble (17 mg/l) in water (at 35 °C) and not having any ionic form (Green 2013). Association of methanogens, methanotrophs, and atmospheric-soil CH_4 completely governs the CH_4 cycle in soil. Generally three possible processes facilitate the CH_4 release from soil to the atmosphere.

8.4.2.1 Diffusion

Movement of gas molecules in the most active layer is called diffusion. CH_4 emission through diffusion is relatively slow with less and CH_4 flux from soil because it is less soluble in water. The highest CH_4 diffusion is observed in sandy soil, while in clay soil CH_4 diffusion is negligible mainly due to pore-space differences. In deepwater rice, diffusion operates only in the top portion of water column (Neue 1993), and it also impedes the CH_4 transfer from plants to atmosphere when CH_4 partial pressure in the root zone reaches to its threshold level (Denier van der Gon and Breemen 1993).

8.4.2.2 Ebullition

When CH_4 is transported in the form of bubbles, this process is known as ebullition, and it may be steady or sporadic (Green 2013; Tokida et al. 2005; Strack et al. 2005). Ebullition is much faster compared to diffusion and occurs under high CH_4 production especially during early growth period of rice. Loss of CH_4 during ebullition is common from rice soils, particularly in clay textured soils. It is also noted that ebullition process is largely influenced not only by gaseous pool of CH_4 but also by the plant-derived flux capacity (Tokida et al. 2013). Additionally, CH_4 emission through ebullition is so quick that opportunity of CH_4 oxidation becomes limited.

8.4.2.3 Plant-Mediated Transport

This process of CH_4 emission is assisted by aerenchymatous tissues of rice. Arenchymatous tissues also liberate CH_4 gas (nearly 80–90% of total methane) to air from rhizosphere in paddy fields (Malyan et al. 2016). CH_4 is primarily liberated via micropores present in the leaf sheath on the lower side of the leaf while it is released secondarily through leaf blade stomata (Nouchi et al. 1990). Additionally, Chanton et al. (1997) and Das and Baruah (2008) highlighted the correlation between CH_4 emission rates and stomatal density and further linked this emission with transpiration.

8.4.3 Methane Oxidation

Methane oxidation occurs under both aerobic and anaerobic circumstances (Nazaries et al. 2013). This bacterial oxidation is mediated by methanotrophs (either aerobic or anaerobic). Methanotrophs usually consume CH_4 or methanol to obtain energy for their growth (Malyan et al. 2016). Details about both oxidation processes are presented below.

8.4.3.1 Aerobic Methane Oxidation

In aerobic oxidation CH_4 is changed into CO_2, via stepwise action of enzymes. In the first step, CH_4 is converted into CH_3CHO by methane monooxygenase (MMO) enzyme. Methanol dehydrogenase then oxidizes CH_3CHO to formaldehyde, which is further oxidized to generate formate and lastly to CO_2. The process of CH_4 aerobic oxidation is catalyzed by MMO enzymes. A brief depiction of CH_4 oxidation process to CO_2 is as under:

$$CH_4 \rightarrow CH_3OH \rightarrow HCHO \ (Formaldehyde) \rightarrow HCOOH \rightarrow CO_2$$

8.4.3.2 Anaerobic Methane Oxidation

Anaerobic CH_4 oxidation (AOM) is accomplished through physical combination of anaerobic methanotrophic archaea (ANME) and sulfate-reducing bacteria (SRB) (Nazaries et al. 2013; Chowdhary and Dick 2013). CH_4 oxidation to CO_2 took place via SRB in the presence of sulfate as an electron acceptor agent (Caldwell et al. 2008; Thauer and Shima 2008). Ettwig et al. (2010) described that an anaerobic bacterium *Methylomirabilis oxyfera* that oxidizes CH_4 has been found to reduce nitrite into dinitrogen in pure cultures. Moreover, reduction of nitric oxide to dinitrogen without forming N_2O is mediated by an unknown enzyme (Serrano-Silva et al. 2014). Despite utilization of sulfate and nitrite being electron acceptors, AOM in marine environment largely depends on iron and manganese (Beal et al. 2009).

8.4.4 Factors Affecting Methane Production from Paddy Soils

Methane emission from paddy soils is largely dependent on the production and oxidation rates that are mainly governed by methanogens and methanotroph population dynamics in the system. Interplay of various factors (Fig. 8.4) regulates these processes like SOM content, soil pH and soil texture, redox potential, fertilizers, and soil temperature. These emission processes are also influenced by diurnal and seasonal variation, increasing ozone and carbon dioxide concentration, management practices such as cultivar selection, nutrient application, water management, and pesticide application (Table 8.1) (Malyan et al. 2016).

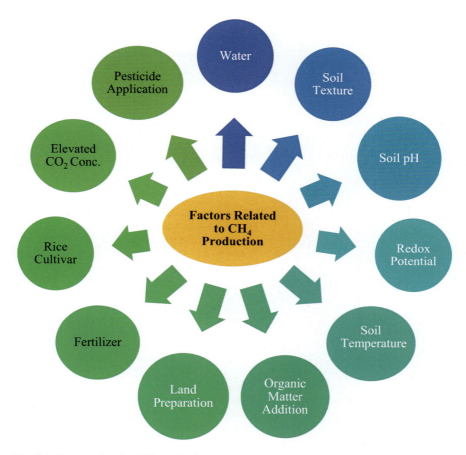

Fig. 8.4 Factors related to CH$_4$ production

8.5 Nitrous Oxide (N$_2$O) Production and Emission from Rice Fields

N$_2$O is a leading anthropogenic GHG and plays a key role in stratospheric ozone depletion. Its share in enhanced global warming effect is approximately 6% (IPCC 2007a, b). Agriculture sector is the largest source of N$_2$O among all the anthropogenic sources (Reay et al. 2012). Rice (*Oryza sativa* L.) farming is an important component of agriculture sector because it fulfills the food needs of nearly half of the global population (Maclean et al. 2013). Paddy fields also contribute toward atmospheric N$_2$O emissions (Maclean et al. 2013; Linquist et al. 2012). Rice fields have a share of about 11% in total global agricultural emissions of N$_2$O (IPCC 2014; FAO 2020). In addition to that on global scale, one-seventh of the nitrogen (N) fertilizer and one-third of irrigation are utilized by paddy globally (Heffer 2009). It creates a

248   Z. Ahmed et al.

Table 8.1 Factors affecting the CH_4 production from rice fields

Factor		Effect on CH_4 production and emission
Water regimes	Submergence	Submerged conditions found to enhance CH_4 production and emission (Ponnamperuma 1972)
	Intermittent drainage	It decreased the CH_4 formation through O_2 influx in soil; consequently CH_4 emission is reduced (Sass et al. 1992; Corton et al. 2000)
Soil	Soil texture	Heavy-textured soils may capture more CH_4 and allow more oxidation, thus releasing less CH_4. Sandy soil manifested high methane emission as compared to clayey soil. CH_4 production also increases with increase in aggregate size of the soil (Neue 1993; Jackel et al. 2000)
	Soil pH	Optimal soil pH range lies between 7.5 and 8.5 for CH_4 production. However soil pH above 8.8 and below 5.8 completely inhibits CH_4 production (Parashar et al. 1991; Pathak et al. 2008)
	Soil redox potential (Eh)	Production of Eh starts at -150 to -160 mV. Production escalates with reduction in Eh maximum production noted at Eh -250 mV (IPCC 2001; Ali et al. 2008)
	Soil temperature	Emission rate doubled when soil temperature ranges between 20 and 25 °C and maximum production takes place at 30 °C of soil. Rising temperature makes gases more soluble in water, thereby increasing the gas emission chances (Holzapfel-Pschorn and Seiler 1986; Lu et al. 2015)
Organic matter application	FYM, straw compost, and green manure	Drastic increase in production and emission occurred with organic matter addition (Yagi et al. 1997; Majumdar et al. 1999; Pandey et al. 2014; Sander et al. 2014; Haque et al. 2013)
	Biochar and cattle manure	Addition of these amendments decreased the CH_4 emission (Feng et al. 2012; Pramanik and Kim 2014)
Land preparation		Intercultural operations can increase emissions, but it is less prevalent in direct-seeded rice because of higher plant density, less weed growth, and mechanical weeding which restrict emissions (Neue 1993)
Fertilizer (type, rate, and mode)		Urea enhances CH_4 emissions, while ammonium sulfate, ammonium thiosulfate, and super single phosphate reduce CH_4 emissions in paddy fields (Wang et al. 1993; Serrano-Silva et al. 2014; Rath et al. 2002; Adhya et al. 1998)
Nitrification inhibitors		Nitrification inhibitors (NI) like dicyandiamide and nitrapyrin inhibit the formation of CH_4 in rice fields. Use of urease inhibitor (hydroquinone), nitrification inhibitor (dicyandiamide), and hydroquinone plus dicyandiamide have been found to decrease CH_4 release by 30, 53, and 58%, respectively (Lindau et al. 1990; Salvas and Taylor 1980; Boeckx et al. 2005)

(continued)

8 Greenhouse Gas Emissions and Mitigation Strategies in Rice Production Systems 249

Table 8.1 (continued)

Factor		Effect on CH_4 production and emission
Rice cultivars		CH_4 flux changes from cultivar to cultivar; increase in production occurs due to root exudate availability; resultantly emission rises by providing conduits (Mitra et al. 1999; Jain et al. 2000)
Diurnal variation		Maximum production noted at 12:00, whereas minimum production was observed at 18:00 (Zhang et al. 2015)
Elevated CO_2 concentration		No significant effect was noted on CH_4 emission (Tokida et al. 2010)
Pesticide effect		15 to 98% decrease in CH_4 emission with butachlor application has been observed compared to control (Mohanty et al. 2004; Jiang et al. 2019)

strong N_2O formation zone, because both N fertilizer application and irrigation management practices promote N_2O emissions (Zhao et al. 2019; Jiang et al. 2019). Hence, chances of rise in global N_2O emissions from paddy in the future are considerably high (Ussiri et al. 2012). Therefore, understanding of N_2O production mechanisms under paddy fields is quite necessary so that promising mitigation strategies should be evolved that could help to curtail rising global warming affect and resultant climate change.

8.5.1 Nitrogen Transformation in Flooded Soils (Volatilization, Leaching)

Some important characteristics of flooded rice soils responsible for N conversion are (i) restricted exchange of atmospheric gases with flooded soils, (ii) rise in pH of acidic soils and decline in calcareous and sodic soil pH, (iii) reduction in soil redox potential, (iv) higher ionic strength and electrical conductivity (EC), and (v) anaerobiosis combined with decomposition of soil organic matter (Savant and De Datta 1982).

Behavior of nitrogen in flooded soils is completely different as compared to dry soils. Flooding in aerobic soils causes rapid depletion of soil O_2, so soil NO_3^- becomes vulnerable to be lost through denitrification and leaching. Soil flooding results in NH_4^+-N accumulation mainly because of inhibited nitrification, unstable NO_3^--N, and less N needed for OM breakdown. Flooding also reduces the utilization efficiency of added nitrogen. In flooded soils conversion of NH_4^+ to NO_3^- is restricted by O_2 deficiency that stops the mineralization at NH_4^+. Therefore, NH_4^+ becomes the leading form of N that gets accumulated. Hence it can be found in three sections: (i) NH_4^+ in exchange sites (ii), NH_4^+ in soil solution, and (iii) non-exchangeable NH_4^+ (De Datta 1995). NH_4^+ present in soil solution and at the exchange sites is easily taken up by rice. The NH_4^+-N may be fixed by clays, lost through volatilization, runoff, leaching, seepage, and nitrification followed by denitrification.

In puddled soils, runoff and leaching losses are less common. Thus, in flooded rice soils, the N_2 and NH_3 gas emissions are the main reason for fertilizer inefficiency. Higher N losses are noted when applied fertilizer yielded ammoniacal N in large amounts under flooded conditions (Simpson et al. 1988), which revealed that NH_3 volatilization is a vital process of N loss. Soil-applied N restricts NH_3 volatilization; however it cannot limit N loss, because after its application, NH_4^+ is transformed to NO_3^-, which is denitrified and lost in the form of N_2 and/or N_2O (Freney et al. 1990). In tropical transplanted rice, NH_3 volatilization losses may range between 10% and 56% of urea nitrogen broadcasted in flooding conditions (Buresh and De datta 1990; Freney et al. 1990). Different factors affecting the pattern of NH_3 loss include fertilizer source, temperature, pH, CEC of the soil, wind speed, and ammoniacal $[NH_4^+ + NH_3]$-N concentration (Freney et al. 1990; De Datta 1995; Cai et al. 2002). During volatilization process, gaseous NH_3 is formed, i.e.,

$$NH_4^+(aq) \rightarrow NH_3 + H^+$$

H^+ ion is liberated in this reaction. Therefore, in both oxidized and reduced soil layers, pH and buffering capacity affect the process of volatilization. In wetland soils, pH dynamics reveal that submerged conditions regulate the pH values in reduced acid and alkali soils within a range of 6.5 and 7.2. Thus volatilized NH_3 may exacerbate indirect N_2O emissions.

Reduced plow layer in flooded soils exists in between thin oxidized surface and somewhat oxidized subsurface soil layers. Reduced soil layer represents a specific pattern with aerobic and anaerobic microsystem in which rice roots get flourished and derive nitrogen. O_2 diffusion from rice roots makes the root rhizosphere somewhat oxidized as compared to the rest of the plow layer soil. Nitrification operating in oxidized soil zones, root rhizosphere, and floodwater transforms ammonical N into NO_3^-, which travels to reduce soil zones and further converted into N_2 and N_2O after denitrification (Reddy and Patrick 1986). Denitrifying bacteria require soil organic matter as an energy source, but the type and quantity of soil organic matter mainly govern the denitrification rate.

Wetland rice soils also experience alternating wet and dry phases, particularly in rain-fed circumstances or in continuous flooding situation. These soils remain saturated during the production period of rice, but become dry and aerated when there is an interval between rice crops. In this interval time, soil is either fallow or under crop cultivation. Under dryland aerobic conditions of soil, NO_3^--N from nitrification of N fertilizer or NH_4^+ after mineralization of soil organic nitrogen may become deposited in the soil or may be utilized by the plants. Although processes of mineralization and immobilization operate at the same time in wetland soils, they are affected by various soil and environmental elements. Near the harvest of rice crop, the amount of soil NO_3^- is minute, whereas soil NH_4^+ also becomes low owing to N taken up by rice plus volatilization losses (Buresh and De Datta 1991).

8.5.2 Processes Enabling Nitrous Oxide Emission from Rice Fields

Intermingling of different biophysical processes of biotic and abiotic origin derives the N_2O production and release from soils (Firestone and Davidson 1989). Flooded rice fields after fertilization facilitate denitrification to produce N_2O and N_2, but the same conditions further promote N_2O reduction to N_2, which is the vital output of denitrification. Soil flooding displaces O_2, and any O_2 in water is used by microbial and root respiration, ultimately depriving the soil from O_2. Rice paddies with anaerobic conditions prevent nitrification and support accumulation of NH_4^+.

8.5.2.1 Nitrification

Nitrification is not a common phenomenon in paddy soils mainly because of unfavorable water environment that favors anaerobic conditions. However, aerobic rice soils or alternatingly flooded soils may facilitate higher nitrification. When rice soils are intermittently flooded, it makes surface soil layer fully or partial aerobic during drainage and for a short time when next irrigation carries dissolved O_2 with water. In this situation with presence of NH_4^+ in the field, substantial amount of N_2O can be produced through nitrification in rice fields.

Nitrification is a microbial process accomplished through ammonium (NH_4^+) oxidation into nitrate (NO_3^-) through nitrite (NO_2^-) (Hayatsu et al. 2008). Nitrification consists of two steps: oxidation of ammonium ($NH_4^+ \rightarrow NO_2^-$) and oxidation of nitrite ($NO_2^- \rightarrow NO_3^-$). Ammonium oxidation can be performed by *Nitrosomonas* spp. and *Nitrosospira* spp. of bacteria and *Nitrosococcus* spp. of *Gammaproteobacteria* called as ammonia-oxidizing bacteria (AOB). Moreover, some archaea known as ammonia-oxidizing archaea (AOA) can also perform ammonia oxidation. Many studies revealed that AOA is more abundant than AOB in the ocean (Francis et al. 2007), while it is assumed that AOB could be more responsible for nitrification than AOA in agricultural soils. In rice paddy soils, a positive relationship has been noticed between nitrification activity and AOB abundance (Li et al. 2007); therefore, AOB might have more important role than AOA in ammonium oxidation in paddy soils. Nitrite oxidation, the second step of nitrification, is completed by nitrite-oxidizing bacteria (NOB) belonging to the genera *Nitrobacter*, *Nitrospina*, *Nitrococcus*, and *Nitrospira* (Hayatsu et al. 2008). Hydroxylamine, an intermediate of ammonia oxidation, and N_2O can be produced as a byproduct of hydroxylamine oxidation (Ishii et al. 2011).

8.5.2.2 Denitrification

Denitrification can occur in significant amount under field during drainage of water at anaerobic microsites containing nitrate and when demand for O_2 surpasses supply (Arah and Smith 1989). This phenomenon takes place either inside the soil mass or in fully saturated areas inside a structureless soil when O_2 diffusion is restricted or when there is unusual O_2 demand. Denitrification process simultaneously serves as both source and sink for N_2O because it forms and uses N_2O in the soil.

Denitrification is a microbial respiratory process, where after stepwise reduction, nitrogen oxides (NO_3^- and NO_2^-) are transformed into gaseous forms (NO, N_2O, and N_2). Nitrogen oxides may work as substitute electron acceptors for oxygen under anaerobic conditions. N_2O can also be consumed as an alternative electron acceptor, but it can be reduced by non-denitrifiers (Zumft and Kroneck 2006). Although N_2O is an intermediate product of denitrification ($NO_3^- \rightarrow NO_2^- \rightarrow NO \rightarrow N_2O \rightarrow N_2$) the final product can be N_2O if a denitrifier is not able to reduce it (Tiedje 1994).

Microorganisms containing assimilatory NO_3^- reduction generate N_2O, whereas respiratory NO_3^- and dissimilatory NO_3^- reduction to NH_4^+ (DNRA). All these metabolic processes normally produce N_2O, and they also produce N_2 without any gain in energy; therefore they are called as non-respiratory N_2O producers (Tiedje 1988). A chemical reaction in which NO_2^- or NH_2OH are decayed in acidic soil can also produce N_2O in small amounts.

8.6 Factors Influencing N_2O Emission from Rice Fields

N_2O emission is a primary outcome of nitrogen source (Eichner 1990). A number of factors can influence the N_2O emission from soils (Table 8.2). Interaction and interplay of these factors actually regulate and determine the N_2O emission rate from paddy soils. However, the main emission curtailing factors are water regimes, fertilizers, plant population, soil texture, management, and cultural practices.

8.7 Strategies to Mitigate CH_4 and N_2O Emissions from Rice Fields

Agriculture is among the largest sectors contributing CH_4 and N_2O gases to atmosphere. For that reason experimentation to develop mitigation strategies of methane and N_2O formation and release from agricultural ecosystems are pretty much in vogue in recent days. It is quite obvious that mitigation of either of these gases from the irrigated rice fields through better management practices may probably give rise to the emission of others. Several studies have reported a negative correlation between the emissions of these two gases (CH_4 and N_2O) from rice soils. A

8 Greenhouse Gas Emissions and Mitigation Strategies in Rice Production Systems

Table 8.2 Factors influencing N_2O formation and release from paddy fields

Factor		Effect on N_2O production in soil	Influence on N_2O liberation to the atmosphere
Water	Submergence	Water controls oxygen amount and diffusion process in soil; it promotes anaerobic conditions and accelerates denitrification process	Controls diffusion process; flooding increases complete denitrification to N_2 and curtails N_2O emission (Granli and Bockman 1994; Majumdar et al. 2000; Hou et al. 2000; Akiyama et al. 2005)
	Intermittent drainage	Switching of aerobic-anaerobic conditions drives switchable processes of nitrification and denitrification. Consequently N_2O production increases	Switching of anaerobic and aerobic processes promotes N_2O emission as compared to constant anaerobic or aerobic conditions (Majumdar et al. 2000)
Fertilizer	Types and application rate	Large amounts of N content scale up the nitrification and denitrification production. Hence N_2O formation is increased due to higher N content	Taken together emissions of N_2O increase in response of higher N application rate rather than type of nitrogen fertilizer applied (Cai et al. 1997)
	Ammonium sulfate vs. urea fertilizers	NH_4^+ facilitates N_2O liberation through nitrification	High amount of N_2O is produced by ammonium sulfate compared to urea with same amount of fertilizer application (Cai et al. 1997; Hua et al. 1997).
	Nitrate fertilizers vs. urea	In flooded soils N_2O formation is favored by NO_3^- via denitrification (Cai et al. 1997)	Nitrate fertilizers increase N_2O emissions compared to ammonium sulfate and urea (Cai et al. 1997)
	Farm yard manure vs. inorganic N fertilizers	FYM is a slow releaser of nitrogen via mineralization compared to inorganic nitrogen fertilizers	It reduces N_2O emissions compared to inorganic nitrogen fertilizers (Pathak et al. 2002, 2003)
Soil texture	Heavy texture	Trapping of high N_2O content leads to slow diffusion	Decline in N_2O emissions occurs because N_2O is completely denitrified to N_2 (Cai et al. 1999; Xu et al. 2000)
	Sandy soils	N_2O diffusion is faster in sandy soils	N_2O emissions are high due to easy movement of N_2O
Nitrification inhibitors		Delay in nitrification minimizes N_2O formation	Controlled nitrification facilitates reduced N_2O emissions (Majumdar et al. 2000)

prominent trade-off effect between CH_4 and N_2O discharges from paddy fields has suggested that it is inevitable to examine the holistic effects of various management practices for minimizing GHG emissions in order to tackle the greenhouse effect backed by rice croplands. Hence the management practices should be adjusted in such a manner that emissions of these greenhouse gases may effectively be mitigated with least atmospheric radiative forcing contribution. Generally farmers give preference to economic crop production over mitigation. However CH_4 and N_2O mitigation controlling factors start from small scale and reach to global scale. Some extensively discussed management strategies may be employed to mitigate CH_4 and N_2O that are exclusively given below.

8.7.1 Water Management

Appropriate management of irrigation practices such as intermittent flood irrigation, midseason drainage (5–20 days) before reaching the maximum tillering stage, controlled irrigation, and multiple short-duration drainages (2–3 days after 3-week interval during the entire growth period) have been found to be effective in minimizing the CH_4 and N_2O emissions (Hussain et al. 2015; Malyan et al. 2016).

CH_4 in puddled soil is produced due to anaerobic decomposition of organic material following the flooding event in rice fields. However, performing field drainage activities completely diminishes the anaerobic condition for a time that not only prohibits the production of CH_4 but also reduces its total quantity to be released into the atmosphere during the entire growing season. On the other hand, N_2O production in rice fields is also regulated by the existence of oxygen. Unlike CH_4, the interchanging aerobic and anaerobic conditions favor bacterial conversion of various nitrogenous compounds to N_2O in the soil and its release to atmosphere. Additionally N_2O production in cropland is synergistically linked with the available nitrogen content in the soil (Hussain et al. 2015).

As far as midseason drainage is concerned, a 43% decrease in CH_4 emission owing to oxygen influx in soil is noted, thus providing conditions suitable for methanotrophic bacteria. Similarly intermittent drainage practice can reduce CH_4 discharge by 47% than flooding. Intermittent irrigation practice consisting of 20- or 40-day period can substantially minimize CH_4 emission compared to continuous flooding. According to an estimate, alternate wetting and drying with 5 cm irrigation depth (3 days and/or 4 days drying in a week) can successfully reduce CH_4 discharge up to 28% compared to continuous flooding with sustainable grain yield (6.71 t/ha). Likewise, midseason drainage has proven to be a good practice to control CH_4 and nitrous oxide emissions from paddy soils (Malyan et al. 2016).

8.7.2 Rice Varietal Selection

Selection of an appropriate variety can successfully regulate the methane emission from paddy croplands. Numerous studies have revealed that cultivated rice varieties having less sterile tillers, short rooting system, high root oxidation capacity, maximum harvest index, and less root excretion tendency and having timely maturing characteristics are best suited for curtailing CH_4 emissions from rice soils (Wang and Adachi 2000; Aulakh et al. 2001). Cultivars differing in CH_4-emitting capacity have differences in their morphological traits and physiological activities, methane gas carriage and root exudation potentials, etc. (Jia et al. 2002; Setyanto et al. 2004). Additionally, qualitative and quantitative transformations in the composition of root exudates among various rice cultivars can significantly influence CH_4 generation rate (Jia et al. 2002). Besides these, it is also narrated that root aerenchyma and root oxidation capacity substantially adjust the methane source strength in the rhizosphere. Conclusively these disparities in rice cultivars could develop significant direct or indirect changes in CH_4 emission rates.

8.7.3 Planting Methods

Adoption of direct-seeded rice (DSR) technique and using system of rice intensification (SRI) planting method are found effective in minimizing GHG emissions. Puddling and seedling transplanting operations are avoided in DSR, and rice seeds are directly sown in plowed or no-tilled soil. The DSR planting significantly reduces CH_4 emissions compared to transplanted rice (TPR) with slight increase in N_2O emission. Cumulative reduction in CH_4 liberation in DSR over transplanted rice has been ranged between 82% and 98% (Gupta et al. 2016; Pathak et al. 2012). Taking into account comparable GWP, higher grain yield and lower GHGI advocate that the DSR substantially lowers the resultant radiative forcing of CH_4 and N_2O releases as compared to TPR cropping system. In SRI planting 15–20-day-old rice seedlings are transplanted per hill in well-puddled soil by avoiding soil flooding but maintaining the soil field capacity level. SRI planting technique showed potential to decrease CH_4 emission by 61% when compared with TPR (Jain et al. 2014). Hence selection of suitable planting techniques can be useful in minimizing the GHG emission rates from rice fields.

8.7.4 Fertilizer Management

CH_4 and N_2O emissions are largely affected by fertilizer management. Type, amount, and fertilizer application method affect CH_4 emission from rice croplands. A recent finding revealed that proper nitrogen management in rice crop can reduce

CH_4 discharge by 30–50% relative to control treatment (Dong et al. 2011). Ammonium-based N fertilizer application as compared to urea showed higher potential to minimize CH_4 emission mainly due to higher CH_4 oxidation rate in the rhizosphere (Bodelier et al. 2000; Ali et al. 2012; Linquist et al. 2012). Sulfate-based fertilizers compel sulfate-reducing bacteria and methanogens to compete for substrate, which results in less CH_4 discharge under anaerobic conditions (Hussain et al. 2015). When ammonium sulfate applied as N source in rice crop, it caused 23% reduction in CH_4 emission (Ali et al. 2012). However in reduced zone, it does not affect CH_4 oxidation, so nitrification and denitrification will be minimum to produce N_2O. Application of potassium fertilizer decreases soil redox potential, reduces CH_4 formation, and stimulates CH_4 oxidation, consequently releasing less CH_4 (Hussain et al. 2015; Babu et al. 2006). Babu et al. (2006) reported a cumulative 49% reduction in CH_4 emissions with 30 kg K ha^{-1} as compared to control in rice crop. Split application of N at critical crop growth stages, especially low N amounts, is recommended because N uptake is low and it will reduce N_2O emission (De Datta and Magnaye 1969; Pillai et al. 1986).

Belowground (8–10 cm deep) application of urea super-granules, urea pellets, and urea briquettes in reduced zone can maximize N recovery and decrease N_2O loss (Pillai et al. 1986). Subsurface application of urea super-granules reduces methane flux over control (Rath et al. 1999).

Bio-fertilizers have capability to improve soil and increase yields on sustainable basis together with CH_4 mitigation in rice crop (Pabby et al. 2003). Bio-fertilizers include *Azolla*, mycorrhizae, cyanobacteria/blue green algae (BGA), and diazotrophs. BGA/*Azolla* with photosynthetic ability provides oxygen to rice soils. Azolla (aquatic pteridophyte) having N_2-fixation ability and symbiotic association with *Anabaena azollae* are widely applied bio-fertilizers in China, India, Bangladesh, and Vietnam in rice field. *Azolla* has curbing effect on CH_4 ejection from flooded soils, as it increases the dissolved oxygen content at the soil-floodwater interface. Lowest CH_4 emission has also been observed, when cyanobacteria applied in combination with *Sesbania* biomass, urea, and silicate fertilizers.

Pre-composted organic matter when added to soil has shown less CH_4 production per unit of carbon as compared to readily mineralizable carbon sources. In contrast, animal dung compost showed more N_2O emission when compared to chemical fertilizers (Chao and Chao 2001). However composts consisting of cow dung and leaves have reduced CH_4 fluxes (Agnihotri et al. 1999). Organic matter-induced aerobic degradation can significantly decrease CH_4 emission, but simultaneously it can increase N_2O emission through nitrification of liberated ammonium. Proper straw management via surface retention/mulching or converting it into biochar or compost rather than burning or incorporation showed potential to curtail GHG discharges from rice soils (Hussain et al. 2015).

8.7.5 Nitrification Inhibitors and Slow-Release Fertilizers

Nitrification inhibitors (NI) or slow-releasing N-based fertilizers have ability to minimize rice field greenhouse gas emissions (Majumdar 2003). NI restricts NH^{+4}-N conversion into NO_3^--N, which directly reduces N_2O emissions via nitrification and availability of NO_3^- for denitrification is also reduced. Aside from artificially prepared materials, some plant-based products have also shown potential to lessen N_2O emissions from rice fields. Dicyandiamide (DCD) and nitrapyrin nitrification inhibitors prevented CH_4 formation and minimized the emissions of CH_4 and nitrous oxide from paddy fields (Lindau et al. 1993; Salvas et al. 1980).

A significant decrease (30, 53, and 58%) in CH_4 emission has been observed with hydroquinone, dicyandiamide, and hydroquinone plus dicyandiamide applications, respectively (Boeckx et al. 2005). Many natural nitrification inhibitors like neem cake and urea coated with neem oil have been found to reduce CH_4 release by 8% and 11%, respectively, than urea fertilizer alone. Application of encapsulated form of calcium carbide (ECC) also reduced CH_4 emission by 13% in rice soils (Malla et al. 2005). Slow-release fertilizers can mitigate N_2O emissions; however slow-release (coated urea) and fast-release (compound fertilizer) N sources did not reveal any significant difference regarding methane emission (Hussain et al. 2015).

8.7.6 Tillage Practices

Soil tillage practices significantly affect the soil physical properties and GHG balance. Looking at GHGs together, soil tilling caused 20% higher net global warming compared to zero tillage indicating climate change mitigation potential of zero tillage system. Compared to conventional tillage system, no or reduced tillage practices significantly lessen (by 6.6%) the overall GWP of methane and N_2O emissions. The possible controlling effect of reduced tillage on CH_4 oxidation may facilitate CH_4 emissions mitigation. Adoption of zero tillage practices on regular basis may promote CH_4 oxidation and conversely minimizes CH_4 emission. In contrast some researchers have the viewpoint that no tillage practices can enhance N_2O emissions from rice soils (Zhang et al. 2011; Nyamadzawo et al. 2013). On the basis of C sequestration and CH_4 mitigation abilities, zero tillage practices have capacity to offset overall GHG emissions. Overall less GWP of zero or reduced tillage compared to conventional tillage practices in rice croplands (Ahmad et al. 2009) suggested that practicing reduced tillage has potential benefits of GHG mitigation and C-smart agriculture, which should be endorsed in rice-based cropping systems. However, the effectiveness of no tillage will largely depend on tillage methods, type of land use, and other management practices. No tillage considerably reduced the overall GWP when the percentage of basal N fertilizer (PBN) was >50% and when tillage duration was >10 years or rain-fed in upland, while when PBN < 50%, tillage duration ranged between 5 and 10 years, or with continuous flooding in paddy fields. Reduced tillage practices also decreased the overall GWP in monoculture system in upland. Therefore, while adopting no tillage or reduced tillage practices to curtail GHG emissions, their interaction with other agronomic practices should also be considered (Feng et al. 2018).

8.8 Conclusion

Rice (*Oryza sativa* L.) is a vital component of agricultural production systems, and its cultivation significantly contributes toward GHG (CH_4 and N_2O) releases and leads to global warming. Increasing population and escalating rice demand in the future raised serious concerns to curtail GHG emissions from rice cultivation without compromising the yield. By understanding the production mechanisms of CH_4 and N_2O from paddy fields, different mitigation strategies have been proposed to decrease methane and N_2O emissions. Site-specific nutrient management, changing irrigation practices like excess water drainage, performing recurrent irrigation, and adoption of DSR are helpful in minimizing the CH_4 and N_2O emissions. Use of fermented cow dung and leaf manures, changing N fertilizer sources (such as urea with ammonium chloride and use of ammonium sulfate in place of prilled urea), application of NI, and slow-release fertilizers are capable to alleviate methane and nitrous oxide releases. Similarly biochar, straw compost, and straw ash incorporation showed more promising results as compared to direct straw incorporation. However, the farmers will accept only those mitigation strategies which will not affect their grain yield.

The abovementioned mitigation possibilities are scientific findings, but to attain full implementation of these options singly or in combination at the farmer level needs a decisive policy and substantial government support. The policy to alleviate or lessen CH_4 and N_2O releases to atmosphere will vary according to a specific region or country, and it will highly be dependent on financial aid given by the government. However for effective and fruitful implementation of such practices to curtail GHG emissions and to sustain rice productivity under changing climate, all social, economic, educational, and political hurdles must be removed.

References

Adhya TK, Patanaik P, Satpathy SN, Kumaraswamy S, Sethunathan N (1998) Influences of phosphorous application on methane emission and production in flooded paddy soils. Soil Biol Biochem 30:177–181

Agnihotri S, Kulshreshtha K, Singh SN (1999) Mitigation strategy to contain methane emissions from rice-fields. Environ Monitor Assess 58:95–104

Ahmad S, Li CF, Dai GZ, Zhan M, Wang JP, Pan SG, Cao CG (2009) Greenhouse gas emission from direct seeding paddy field under different rice tillage systems in Central China. Environ Sci Pollut Res 22:3342–3360

8 Greenhouse Gas Emissions and Mitigation Strategies in Rice Production Systems

Akiyama H, Yagi K, Yan X (2005) Direct N_2O emissions from rice paddy fields: summary of available data. Global Biochem Cycles 19:1005

Ali MA, Oh JH, Kim PJ (2008) Evaluation of silicate iron slag amendment on reducing methane emission from flood water rice farming. Agric Ecosyst Environ 128:21–26

Ali MA, Farouque MG, Haque M, Kabir A (2012) Influence of soil amendments on mitigating methane emissions and sustaining rice productivity in paddy soil ecosystems of Bangladesh. J Environ Sci Nat Resour 5:179–185

Arah JRM, Smith KA (1989) Steady-state denitrification in aggregated soils: a mathematical model. J Soil Sci 40:139–149

Aulakh MS, Wassmann R, Bueno C, Rennenberg H (2001) Impact of root exudates of different cultivars and plant development stages of rice (*Oryza sativa* L.) on methane production in a paddy soil. Plant Soil 230:77–86. https://doi.org/10.1023/A:1004817212321230

Babu YJ, Nayak DR, Adhya TK (2006) Potassium application reduces methane emission from a flooded field planted to rice. Biol Fertil Soils 42:532–541

Beal EJ, House CH, Orphan VJ (2009) Manganese and iron-dependent marine methane oxidation. Science 325:184–187

Bodelier PLE, Roslev P, Henckel T, Frenzel P (2000) Stimulation by ammonium-based fertilizers of methane oxidation in soil around rice roots. Nature 403:421–424

Boeckx P, Xu X, Cleemput OV (2005) Mitigation of N_2O and CH_4 emission from rice and wheat cropping systems using dicyandiamide and hydroquinone. Nutr Cycl Agroecosyst 72:41–49. https://doi.org/10.1007/s10705-004-7352-4

Bouwman AF (1996) Direct emission of nitrous oxide from agricultural soils. Nutr Cycl Agroecosyst 46:53–70

Brune A, Frenzel P, Cypionka H (2000) Life at the oxic–anoxic interface: microbial activities and adaptations. FEMS Microbiol Rev 24:691–710

Buresh RJ, De Datta SK (1991) Nitrogen dynamics and management in rice-legume cropping systems. Adv Agron 45:1–59

Buresh RJ, Dedatta SK (1990) Denitrification losses from puddled rice soils in the tropics. Biol Fertil Soils 9:1–13

Cai ZC, Xing GX, Yan XY, Xu H, Tsuruta H, Yagi K, Minami K (1997) Methane and nitrous oxide emissions from rice paddy fields as affected by nitrogen fertilizers and water management. Plant Soil 196:7–14

Cai ZC, Xing GX, Shen GY, Xu H, Yan XY, Tsuruta H, Yagi K, Minami K (1999) Measurements of CH4 and N20 emissions from rice paddies in Fengqiu, China. Soil Sci Plant Nutr 45(1):1–3

Cai GX, Chen DL, Ding H, Pacholski A, Fan XH, Zhu ZL (2002) Nitrogen losses from fertilizers applied to maize, wheat and rice in the North China plain. Nutr Cycl Agroecosyst 63:187–195

Cairo JJ, Paris JM (1988) Microbiologia de la digestion anaerobia. In: Polanco FF, García PA, Hernándo S (eds) Methanogenesis. 4th Seminario in Depuración Anaerobia de Aguas Residuales. Universidad de Valladolid. ISBN: 8477620547, pp 41–51

Caldwell SL, Laidler JR, Brewer EA, Eberly JO, Sandborgh SC, Colwell FS (2008) Aerobic oxidation of methane mechanisms, bioenergetics and the ecology of associated microorganisms. Environ Sci Technol 7:1127–1138

Carlson KM, Gerber JS, Mueller ND, Herrero M, GK MD, Brauman KA, Havlik P, O'Connell CS, Johnson JA, Saatchi S, West PC (2017) Greenhouse gas emissions intensity of global croplands. Nat Clim Chang 7:63–67

Carriger S, Vallee D (2007) More crop per drop. Rice Today 6:10–13

Chanton JP, Whiting GJ, Blair NE, Lindau CW, Bollich PK (1997) Methane emission from rice: stable isotopes, diurnal variations, and CO2 exchange. Glob Chang Biol 11:15–27

Chao CC, Chao CC (2001) Taiwanese. J Agric Chem Food Sci 39:275–283

Chin KJ, Conrad R (1995) Intermediary metabolism in methanogenic paddy soils and their influences of temperature. FEMS Microbial Ecol 18:85–102

Chowdhary TR, Dick RP (2013) Ecology of aerobic methanotrophs in controlling methane fluxes from wetlands. Appl Soil Ecol 65:8–22

Conrad R (1999) Contribution of hydrogen to methane production and control of hydrogen concentrations in methanogenic soils and sediments. FEMS Microbiol Ecol 28:193–202

Conrad R (2007) Microbial ecology of methanogens and methanotrophs. Adv Agron 96:1–63

Corton TM, Bajita JB, Grospe FS, Pamplona RR, Asis CA Jr, Wassmann R, Lantin RS, Buendia LV (2000) Methane emission from irrigated and intensively managed rice fields in Central Luzon (Philippines). Nutr Cyc Agroecosys 58:37–53

Das K, Baruah KK (2008) Methane emission associated with anatomical and morpho-physiological characteristics of rice (*Oryza sativa* L.) plant. Physiol Plant 134:303–312

De Datta SK (1995) Nitrogen transformations in wetland rice ecosystems. Fertil Res 42:193–203

De Datta SK, Magnaye CP (1969) A survey of the forms and sources of fertilizer nitrogen for flooded rice. Soils Fert 32(2):103–109

Denier van der Gon HAC, Breemen NV (1993) Diffusion-controlled transport of methane from soil to atmosphere as mediated by rice plants. Biogeochemistry 21:177–190

Dong H, Yao Z, Zheng X (2011) Effect of ammonium-based, non-sulfate fertilizers on CH_4 emissions from a paddy field with a typical Chinese water management regime. Atmos Environ 45:1095–1101

Dubey SK (2005) Microbial ecology of methane emission in rice agro-ecosystem: a review. Appl Ecol Environ Res 3:1–27

Eichner MJ (1990) Nitrous oxide emissions from fertilized soils: summary of available data. J Environ Qual 19(2):272–280

Ettwig KF, Butler MK, Le Paslier D, Pelletier E, Mangenot S, Kuypers MMM, Schreiber F, Dutilh BE, Zedelius J, de Beer D, Gloerich J, Wessels JCT, van Alen T, Luesken F, Wu ML, Vande Pas-Schoonen KT, den Camp HJM O, Janssen-Megens EM, Francoijs KJ, Stunnenberg H, Weissenbach J, MSM J, Strous M (2010) Nitrite-driven anaerobic methane oxidation by oxygenic bacteria. Nature 464:543–548

Faiz-ul Islam S, van Groenigen JW, Jensen LS, Sander BO, de Neergaard A (2018) The effective mitigation of greenhouse gas emissions from rice paddies without compromising yield by early-season drainage. Sci Total Environ 612:1329–1339

FAO (2006) Guidelines for soil description, 4th edn. Publishing Management Service, Information Division, FAO, Rome

FAO (2009) Food and agricultural organization of the United Nations. OECD-FAO Agricultural Outlook, Rome, pp 2011–2030

FAO (2020) FAOSTAT Emissions shares, http://www.fao.org/faostat/en/#data/EM

Fazli P, Man HC, Shah UKM, Idris A (2013) Characteristics of methanogens and methanotrophs in rice fields: a review. Pac J Mol Biol Biotechnol 21:3–17

Feng Y, Xu Y, Yu Y, Xie Z, Lin X (2012) Mechanisms of biochar decreasing methane emission from Chinese paddy soils. Soil Biol Biochem 46:80–88

Feng J, Li F, Zhou X, Xu C, Ji L, Chen Z, Fang F (2018) Impact of agronomy practices on the effects of reduced tillage systems on CH_4 and N_2O emissions from agricultural fields: a global meta-analysis. PLoS One 13(5):e0196703

Firestone MK, Davidson EA (1989) Microbiological basis of NO and N_2O production and consumption in soil. Exchange of trace gases between terrestrial ecosystems and the atmosphere 47:7–21

Francis CA, Bemanand JM, Kuypers MMM (2007) New processes and players in the nitrogen cycle: the microbial ecology of anaerobic and archaeal ammonia oxidation. ISME J 1:19–27

Freney JR, Trevitt ACF, De Datta SK, Obcemea WN, Real JG (1990) The interdependence of ammonia volatilization and denitrification as nitrogen loss processes in flooded rice fields in the Philippines. Biol Fertil Soils 9:31–36

Granli T, Bockman OC (1994) Nitrous oxide from agriculture. Norw J Agric Sci 12:7–128

Green SM (2013) Ebullition of methane from rice paddies: the importance of fur the ring understanding. Plant Soil 370:31–34

Gupta DK, Bhatia A, Kumar A, Das TK, Jain N, Tomer R, Malyan SK, Fagodiya RK, Dubey R, Pathak H (2016) Mitigation of greenhouse gas emission from rice–wheat system of the Indo-

8 Greenhouse Gas Emissions and Mitigation Strategies in Rice Production Systems 261

Gangetic plains: through tillage, irrigation and fertilizer management. Agric Ecosyst Environ 230:1–9

Haque MM, Kim SY, Pramanik P, Kim G, Kim PJ (2013) Optimum application level of winter cover crop biomass as green manure under considering methane emission and rice productivity in paddy soil. Biol Fertil Soils 49:487–493

Hayatsu M, Tago K, Saito M (2008) Various players in the nitrogen cycle: diversity and functions of the microorganisms involved in nitrification and denitrification. Soil Sci Plant Nutr 54:33–45

Heffer P (2009) Assessment of fertilizer use by crop at the global level 2006–2007. Paris, France, International Fertilizer Industry Association

Holzapfel-Pschorn A, Conrad R, Seiler W (1986) Effects of vegetation on the emission of methane from submerged paddy soil. Plant Soil 92:223–233

Hou AX, Chen GX, Wang ZP, Van Cleemput O, Patrick WH (2000) Methane and nitrous oxide emissions from a rice field in relation to soil redox and microbiological processes. Soil Sci Soc Am J 64:2180–2186

Hua X, Guangxi X, Cai ZC, Tsuruta H (1997) Nitrous oxide emissions from three rice paddy fields in China. Nutr Cycl Agroecosyst 49:23–28

Hussain S, Peng S, Fahad S, Khaliq A, Huang J, Cui K, Nie L (2015) Rice management interventions to mitigate greenhouse gas emissions: a review. Environ Sci Pollut Res 22(5): 3342–3360

IPCC (1997) In: Houghton JT, Filho LGM, Lim B, Treanton K, Mamaty I, Bonduki Y, Griggs DJ, Callender BA (eds) IPCC Guidelines for National Greenhouse Gas Inventories. UK Meteorological Office, Bracknell

IPCC (2001) In: Houghton JT et al (eds) Climate change: a scientific basis, inter governmental panel on climate change. Cambridge University Press

IPCC (2007a) Climate change 2007: synthesis report. Contribution of Working Groups I, II and III to the Fourth Assessment Report of the Intergovernmental Panel on Climate

IPCC (2007b) Contribution of working group I to the fourth assessment report of the intergovernmental panel on climate change. In: Qin D, Manning M, Marquis M, Averyt K, Marquis M, Tignor MMB (eds) Climate change 2007: the physical science basis; in: Solomon S. Cambridge University Press, Cambridge

IPCC (2014) Climate change 2014: impacts, adaptation, and vulnerability working group II contribution to the fifth assessment report. Cambridge University Press, Cambridge/New York

IRRI (1993) In: Maclean JL, Dawe DC, Hardy B, Hettel GP (eds) Rice Almanac. International Rice Research Institute, Los Banos, p 257

Ishii S, Ikeda S, Minamisawa K, Senoo K (2011) Nitrogen cycling in rice paddy environments: past achievements and future challenges. Microbes Environ 26:282–292

Jackel U, Schnell S, Conard R (2000) Effect of moisture, texture and aggregate size of paddy soil on production and consumption of CH_4. Soil Biol Biochem 33:965–971

Jain MC, Kumar S, Wassmann R, Mitra S, Singh SD, Singh JP, Singh R, Yadav AK, Gupta S (2000) Methane emissions from irrigated rice fields in northern India (New Delhi). Nutr Cycl Agroecosyst 58:75–83. https://doi.org/10.1023/A:1009882216720

Jain N, Dubey R, Dubey DS, Singh J, Khanna M, Pathak H, Bhatia A (2014) Mitigation of greenhouse gas emission with system of rice intensification in the Indo-Gangetic Plains. Paddy Water Environ 12:355–363

James SJ, James C (2010) The food cold-chain and climate change. Food Res Int 43:1944–1956

Jia ZJ, Cai ZC, Xu H, Tsuruta H (2002) Effect of rice cultivars on methane fluxes in a paddy soil. Nutr Cycl Agroecosyst 64:87–94. https://doi.org/10.1023/A:1021102915805

Jiang Y, Carrijo D, Huang S, Chen J, Balaine N, Zhang W, Groenigen KJ, Linquist B (2019) Water management to mitigate the global warming potential of rice systems: a global meta-analysis. Field Crop Res 234:47–54

Kimura M (2000) Anaerobic microbiology in waterlogged rice fields. In: Bollag JM, Stotzky G (eds) Soil biochemistry 10. Marcell Dekker, New York, pp 35–138

Kimura M, Murase J, Lu YH (2004) Carbon cycling in rice field ecosystems in the context of input, decomposition and translocation of organic materials and the fates of their end products (CO_2 and CH_4). Soil Biol Biochem 36:1399–1416

Kirk G (2004) The biogeochemistry of submerged soils. Wiley, Chichester, p 282

Kögel-Knabner I, Amelung W, Cao Z, Fiedler S, Frenzel P, Jahn R, Kalbitz K, Kölbl A, Schloter M (2010) Biogeochemistry of paddy soils. Geoderma 157:1–14

Kumar U, Jain MC, Pathak H, Kumar S, Majumdar D (2000) Nitrous oxide emission from different fertilizers and its mitigation by nitrification inhibitors in irrigated rice. Biol Fertil Soils 32:474–478

Kumar A, Nayak AK, Das BS, Panigrahi N, Dasgupta P, Mohanty S, Kumar U, Panneerselvam P, Pathak H (2019) Effects of water deficit stress on agronomic and physiological responses of rice and greenhouse gas emission from rice soil under elevated atmospheric CO_2. Sci Total Environ 650:2032–2050

Li YL, Zhang YL, Hu J, Shen QR (2007) Contribution of nitrification happened in rhizospheric soil growing with different rice cultivars to N nutrition. Biol Fertil Soils 43:417–425

Liesack W, Schnell S, Revsbech NP (2000) Microbiology of flooded rice paddies. FEMS Microbiol Rev 24:625–645

Lindau CW, Bollich PK, DeLaune RD, Mosier AR, Bronson KF (1993) Methane mitigation in flooded Louisiana rice fields. Bio Fert Soils 15(3):174–178

Lindau CW, Patrick WH, De Laune RD, Reddy KR (1990) Rate of accumulation and emission of N_2, N_2O and CH_4 from a flooded rice soil. Plant Soil 129:269–276

Linquist BA, Adviento-Borbe MA, Pittelkow CM, van Kessel C, van Groenigen KJ (2012) Fertilizer management practices and greenhouse gas emissions from rice systems: a quantitative review and analysis. Field Crop Res 135:10–21

Lu Y, Fu L, Lu Y, Hugenholtz F, Ma K (2015) Effect of temperature on the structure and activity of a methanogenic archaeal community during rice straw decomposition. Soil Biol Biochem 81:17–27

Maclean J, Hardy B, Hettel G (2013) Rice almanac: source book for one of the most important economic activities on earth. IRRI, Manila

Majumdar D (2003) Methane and nitrous oxide emission from irrigated rice fields: proposed mitigation strategies. Curr Sci 84(10):1317–1326

Majumdar D, Kumar S, Jain MC (1999) Methane and nitrous oxide emission from irrigated rice fields: proposed mitigation strategies. Asia Pacific J Environ Dev 6:81–95

Majumdar D, Kumar S, Pathak H, Jain MC, Kumar U (2000) Reducing nitrous oxide emission from an irrigated rice field of North India with nitrification inhibitors. Egric Ecosys Environ 81:163–169

Malla G, Bhatia A, Pathak H, Prasad S, Jain N, Singh J (2005) Mitigating nitrous oxide and methane emissions from soil in rice-wheat system of the Indo-Gangetic plain with nitrification and urease inhibitors. Chemosphere 58:141–147

Malyan SK, Bhatia A, Kumar A, Gupta DK, Singh R, Kumar SS, Tomer R, Kumar O, Jain N (2016) Methane production, oxidation and mitigation: a mechanistic understanding and comprehensive evaluation of influencing factors. Sci Total Environ 572:874–896

Mitra S, Jain MC, Kumar S, Bandyopadhya SK, Kalra N (1999) Effect of rice cultivars on methane emission. Agric Ecosyst Environ 73:177–183

Mohanty SR, Nayak DR, Babu YJ, Adhya TK (2004) Butachlor inhibits production and oxidation of methane in tropical rice soils under flooded condition. Microbio Res 159(3):193–201

Nazaries L, Murrekk JC, Millard P, Baggs L, Singh BK (2013) Methane, microbes and models: fundamental understanding of the soil methane cycle for future predictions. Environ Microbiol 15:2395–2417

Neue H (1993) Methane emission from rice fields: wetland rice fields may make a major contribution to global warming. Bio Sci 43:466–473

Nouchi I, Mariko S, Aoki K (1990) Mechanism of methane transport from the rhizosphere to the atmosphere through rice plants. Plant Physiol 94:59–66

Nyamadzawo G, Wuta M, Chirinda N, Mujuru L, Smith JL (2013) Greenhouse gas emissions from intermittently flooded (Dambo) rice under different tillage practices in chiota smallholder farming area of Zimbabwe. Atmos Clim Sci 3:13–20

Pabby A, Parsanna R, Singh PK (2003) Biological significance of Azolla and its utilization in agriculture. Proc Indian Natl Sci Acad 3:299–333

Palmer RR, Reeve IN (1993) Methanogen genes and the molecular biology of methane biosynthesis. In: Sebald M (ed) Genetics and molecular biology of anaerobic bacteria. Springer, Berlin, pp 13–35

Pandey A, Mai VT, Vu DQ, Bui TPL, Mai TLA, Jensen LS, Neergaaed A (2014) Organic matter and water management strategies to reduce methane and nitrous oxide emissions from rice paddies in Vietnam. Agric Ecosyst Environ 196:137–146

Parashar DC, Rai J, Sharma RC, Singh N (1991) Parameters affecting methane emission from rice paddy fields. Indian J Radio Space Phys 20:12–17

Pathak H (1999) Emissions of nitrous oxide from soil. Curr Sci 77:359–369

Pathak H, Bhatia A, Prasad S, Singh S, Kumar S, Jain MC, Kumar U (2002) Emission of nitrous oxide from rice-wheat systems of indo-Gangetic plains of India. Environ Monit Asses 77:163–178

Pathak H, Arti B, Shiv P, Shalini S, Kumar S, Jain MC, Singh P, Bhatia A, Prasad S, Singh S (2003) Effect of DCD, FYM and moisture regime on nitrous oxide emission from an alluvial soil in rice-wheat cropping system. J Indian Soc Soil Sci 51:139–145

Pathak H, Kumar S, Jain N, Mitra S (2008) Emission of methane from soil. In: Pathak H, Kumar S (eds) Soil and greenhouse effect, monitoring and mitigation, 1st edn. CBS Publishers & Distributors, New Delhi, pp 18–32

Pathak H, Tewari AN, Sankhyan S, Dubey DS, Mina U, Singh VK, Jain N, Bhatia A (2011) Direct-seeded rice: potential, performance and problems – a review. Curr Adv Agric Sci 3:77–88

Pathak H, Chakrabarti B, Bhatia A, Jain N, Aggarwal PK (2012) Potential and cost of low carbon technologies in rice and wheat systems: a case study for the Indo-Gangetic Plains. In: Pathak H, Aggarwal PK (eds) Low carbon technologies for agriculture: a study on rice and wheat systems in the Indo-Gangetic Plains. Indian Agricultural Research Institute, New Delhi, India, pp 12–40

Pathak H, Samal P, Shahid M (2018) Revitalizing rice-systems for enhancing productivity, profitability and climate resilience. In: Pathak H et al (eds) Rice research for enhancing productivity, profitability and climate resilience. ICAR-National Rice Research Institute, Cuttack, Odisha, pp 1–17

Penning H, Conrad R (2007) Quantification of carbon flow from stable isotope fractionation in rice field soils with different organic matter content. Org Geochem 38:2058–2069

Pillai SM, Ravindranathan M, Sivaram S (1986) Dimerization of ethylene and propylene catalyzed by transition-metal complexes. Chem Rev 86(2):353–399

Ponnamperuma FN (1972) The chemistry of submerged soils. Adv in Agron 1(24):29–96

Pramanik P, Kim PJ (2014) Evaluating changes in cellulolytic bacterial population to explain methane emissions from air-dried and composted manure treated rice paddy soils. Sci Total Environ 470:1307–1312

Rath AK, Ramakrishnan B, Sethunathan N (2002) Effect of application of ammonium thiosulphate on production and emission of methane in a tropical rice soil. Agric Ecosyst Environ 90:319–325

Reay DS, Davidson EA, Smith KA, Smith P, Melillo JM, Dentener F, Crutzen PJ (2012) Global agriculture and nitrous oxide emissions. Nat Clim Chang 2:410–416

Reddy KR, Patrick WHJ (1986) Denitrification losses in flooded rice fields. In: De Datta SK, Patrick WHJ (eds) Nitrogen economy of flooded rice soils. Martinus Nijhoff Publishers, Dordrecht, pp 99–116

Rosencrantz D, Rainey FA, Janssen PH (1999) Culturable populations of *Sporomusa spp.* L. and *Desulfovibrio spp.* L. in the anoxic bulk soil of flooded rice microcosms. Appl Environ Microbiol 65:3526–3533

Salvas PL, Taylor BF (1980) Blockage of methanogenesis in marine sediments by the nitrification inhibitor 2-chloro-6- (trichloromethyl) pyridine (nitrapyrin or N-serve)

Sander OB, Samson M, Buresh RJ (2014) Methane and nitrous oxide emissions from flooded rice fields as affected by water and straw management between rice crops. Geoderma 2:235–236

Sarwar N, Atique-ur-Rehman, Ahmad S, Hasanuzzaman, M (2022) Modern Techniques of Rice Crop Production. Springer Nature Singapore Pvt. Ltd., (EBook ISBN (978-981-16-4955-4); Hard Cover ISBN (978-981-16-4954-7); https://doi.org/10.1007/978-981-16-4955-4) (https://www.springer.com/in/book/9789811649547)

Sass RL, Fisher FM, Wang YB, Turner FT, Jund MF (1992) Methane emission from rice fields: the effect of floodwater management. Global Biogeochem Cycle 6:249–262

Savant NK, De Datta SK (1982) Nitrogen transformations in wetland rice soils. Adv Agron 35:241–302

Serrano-Silva N, Sarria-Guzman Y, Dendooven L, Luna-Guido M (2014) Methanogenesis and methanotrophy in soil: a review. Pedosphere 24:291–307

Setyanto P, Rosenani AB, Boer R, Fauziah CI, Khanif MJ (2004) The effect of rice cultivars on methane emission from irrigated rice field. Indones J Agric 5(1):20–31

Shakoor A, Ashraf F, Shakoor S, Mustafa A, Rehman A, Altaf MM (2020) Biogeochemical transformation of greenhouse gas emissions from terrestrial to atmospheric environment and potential feedback to climate forcing. Environ Sci Pollution Res 27:38513–38536. https://doi.org/10.1007/s11356-020-10151-1

Simpson JR, Muirhead WA, Bowmer KH, Cai GX, Freney JR (1988) Control of gaseous nitrogen losses from urea applied to flooded rice soils. Fertil Res 18:31–47

Snyder CS, Bruulsema TW, Jensen T, Fixen PE (2009) Review of greenhouse gas emissions from crop production systems and fertilizer management effects. Agric Ecosys Environ 133:247–266

Strack M, Kellner E, Waddington JM (2005) Dynamics of biogenic gas bubbles in peat and their effects on peatland biogeochemistry. Global Biogeochem Cycles 19:1003

Thauer RK, Shima S (2008) Methane as fuel for anaerobic microorganisms. Ann N Y Acad Sci 1125:158–170

Tiedje JM (1988) Ecology of nitrification and dissimilatory nitrate reduction to ammonium. In: Zehnder AJB (ed) Biology of anaerobic microorganisms. Wiley, New York

Tiedje JM (1994) Denitrifiers. In: Weaver RW, Angle JS, Bottomley PJ (eds) Methods of soil analysis, part 2: microbiological and biochemical properties. Soil Science Society of America, Madison, pp 245–267

Tokida T, Miyazaki T, Mizoguchi M (2005) Ebullition of methane from peat with falling atmospheric pressure. Geophys Res Lett 32:13823

Tokida T, Fumoto T, Cheng W, Matsunami T, Adachi M, Katayanagi N, Mastsushima M, Okawara Y, Nakamura H, Okada M, Sameshima R, Hasegawa T (2010) Effects of free air CO_2 enrichment (FACE) and soil warming on CH_4 emission from a rice paddy field: impact assessment and stoichiometric evaluation. Biogeosciences 7:2639–2653

Tokida T, Cheng W, Adachi M, Matsunami T, Nakamura H, Okada M, Hasegawa T (2013) The contribution of entrapped gas bubbles to the soil methane pool and their role in methane emission from rice paddy soil in free-air (CO_2) enrichment and soil warming experiments. Plant Soil 364:131–143

Ussiri D, Lal R (2012) Soil emission of nitrous oxide and its mitigation. Springer, Dordrecht

Wang B, Adachi K (2000) Differences among rice cultivars in root exudation, methane oxidation, and populations of methanogenic and methanotrophic bacteria in relation to methane emission. Nutr Cycl Agroecosyst 58:349–356. https://doi.org/10.1023/A:1009879610785

Wang ZP, Lindau CW, Delaune RD, Patrick WH (1993) Methane emission and entrapment in flooded rice soils as affected by soil properties. Bio Fert Soils 16(3):163–168

Wang C, Derrick YF, Lai SJ, Wang W, Zeng C, Peñuelas J (2017) Factors related with CH_4 and N_2O emissions from a paddy field: clues for management implications. PLoS One 12(1): e0169254

Xu H, Xing G, Cai Z, Tsuruta H, Xu H, Xing GX, Cai ZC (2000) Effect of soil water regime and soil texture on N2O emission from rice paddy field. Acta Pedol Sin 37:499–505

Yagi K, Tsuruta H, Minami K (1997) Possible options for mitigating methane emission from rice cultivation. Nutr Cycl Agroecosyst 49:213–220

Yoon CG (2009) Wise use of paddy rice fields to partially compensate for the loss of natural wetlands. Paddy Water Environ 7:357

Yoro KO, Daramola MO (2020) CO_2 emission sources, greenhouse gases, and the global warming effect. Adv Carbon Capture 3–28. https://doi.org/10.1016/b978-0-12-819657-1.00001-3

Zhang W, Yu Y, Huang Y, Li T, Wang P (2011) Modelling methane emissions from irrigated rice cultivation in China from 1960 to 2050. Glob Chang Biol 17:3511–3523

Zhang G, Yu H, Fan X, Liu G, Ma J, Xu H (2015) Effect of rice straw application on stable carbon isotopes, methanogenic pathway, and fraction of CH_4 oxidized in a continuously flooded rice field in winter season. Soil Biol Biochem 84:75–82

Zhao X, Pu C, Ma ST, Liu SL, Xue JF, Wang X, Wang YQ, Li SS, Lal R, Chen (2019) Management-induced greenhouse gases emission mitigation in global rice production. Sci Total Environ 649:1299–1306

Zumft WG, Kroneck PMH (2006) Respiratory transformation of nitrous oxide (N_2O) to dinitrogen by bacteria and archaea. Adv Microb Physiol 52:107–227

Chapter 9
Fiber Crops in Changing Climate

Muhammad Tariq, Muhammad Ayaz Khan, Wali Muhammad, and Shakeel Ahmad

Abstract About 2000 plants have been reported in the world as fiber sources; however, only few are being utilized. Cumulatively fiber crops including cotton, jute, flax, agave, sisal, manila fiber, and ramie are being grown on 34.2 million hectares with the annual production of 29.5 million tonnes. The cotton is the leading fiber crop which shares more than 90% area and 80% production across the world. Despite the importance of the other fiber crops, most of the climate change studies were limited to cotton. There is uncertainty in climate of the future as the human actions responsible for greenhouse gas emission are not accurately predicted. The chemicals used for fiber extraction are deteriorating the environment quality, and proper treatments must be performed prior to disposal. Climatic factors are driving force for the crop growth, reproduction, and movement of insect pests. Increase in temperature, concentration of carbon dioxide in air, and rainfall pattern are distinguished climatic factors responsible for change in crop production. The cotton and hemp contributions in greenhouse gas emission are high; however, cotton is more victim of climate change in terms of phenology, yield, and quality. The accelerated development in response to high temperature reduces the duration of various developmental stages, thus reducing the yield as well as quality. Due to weakening of plant protection mechanism in current scenario of climate change, cotton bollworms, mealy bug, mirid bugs, and fall armyworm will be the widely distributing pests of fiber crops in the world. The phenomenon of the climate change is regulated by

---

M. Tariq
Agronomy Section, Central Cotton Research Institute, Multan, Pakistan
e-mail: mtariq131@gmail.com

M. A. Khan
Department of Agronomy, MNS-University of Agriculture, Multan, Pakistan

W. Muhammad
Agriculture Pest Warning & Quality Control of Pesticides, Government of Punjab, Multan, Pakistan

S. Ahmad (✉)
Department of Agronomy, Bahauddin Zakariya University, Multan, Pakistan
e-mail: shakeelahmad@bzu.edu.pk

© The Author(s), under exclusive license to Springer Nature Switzerland AG 2022
M. Ahmed (ed.), *Global Agricultural Production: Resilience to Climate Change*,
https://doi.org/10.1007/978-3-031-14973-3_9

268 M. Tariq et al.

multiple factors, has multiple effects, and requires multiple approaches to strengthen fiber availability.

Keywords Fiber · Greenhouse gas emission · Quality · Pests

9.1 Global Fiber Production

The fibers are important component of the human lives in addition to shelter and food. The fiber crops were primarily grown for raw material of textile industry; however, non-textile applications have been identified since the last few decades back. Some of future uses of fiber crops may be in form of biopolymers, insulation board, particle board, cosmetics, etc. The natural fibers are mainly classified as bast fiber, seed fiber, and leaf fiber. About 2000 species were reported as fiber crops but the number of cultivated species is very few (Pari et al. 2015). The sclerenchyma fibers associated with phloem of the plant are known as bast fiber. The bast fiber accounts 16% in total global production of natural fiber crops. The other categories of fiber crops are seed and leaf fiber. The seed and leaf fibers originated and are extracted from seed and leaves, respectively. The other examples of these fiber categories are listed in Table 9.1.

The latest reports of International Cotton Advisory Committee (ICAC 2021) showed that the global cotton lint production in 2020–2021 was 24,189,000 metric tonnes which was harvested from 32,045,000 ha. The India ranks first in production (6,026,000 metric tonnes) and area (13,477,000 ha); Australia in yield (1905 kg ha^{-1}); China in beginning stock (8,938,000 metric tonnes), consumption (8,400,000 metric tonnes), imports (2,801,000 metric tonnes), and ending stocks (9,219,000 metric tonnes); the USA in exports (3,571,000 metric tonnes); and Hong Kong in ratio of ending stocks (34.08). The cotton is grown in many countries of the world with the prime objective of source of natural fiber along with many other associated uses as raw material in edible oils, bioenergy, and feed industry (Tariq et al. 2018, 2021; Afzal et al. 2018, 2020; Saranga et al. 2001; Mubeen et al. 2021; Abbas et al. 2020).

The fiber of jute is also known as allyott and golden fiber. There are two most common species of jute *Corchorus capsularis* (white jute) and *Corchorus olitorius* (tossa jute). It is believed that the former originated from India and later originated from South Asia. The jute is the major fiber crop followed by cotton. It is mainly grown in Asia (99.7%) particularly India, Bangladesh, and China along with some contribution from South America. Worldwide, 3,375,884 tonnes were harvested in 2019 from an area of 1,437,939 ha. It is a short-season (120–150 days) crop, it is sown in summer season, and irrigation requirements are fulfilled with precipitation. The flax was sown on 259,424 ha with the total production of 1,085,734 tonnes. The Europe (France) is the main producer with share of 74.4% followed by Asia (China and Russian Federation) with global share of 24%. The total agave fiber production was 38,173 tonnes from an area of 64,360 ha. The America contributes about 91.9% in total production and Asia contributes only 8.1%. It is mainly produced from

9 Fiber Crops in Changing Climate

Table 9.1 Description and uses of fiber crops

Fiber crop	Scientific name	Other species	Fiber type	Family	Principal uses
Cotton	*Gossypium hirsutum* L.	*G. arboreum* L., *G. barbadense* L., *G. herbaceum* L.	Seed fiber	Malvaceae	Principal raw material for textile
Flax	*Linum usitatissimum* L.		Bast fiber		Fashionable clothing, raw material for linen, packaging materials, cigarette paper
Sunn hemp	*Crotalaria juncea* L.		Bast fiber	Leguminosae/Fabaceae	Bags, shoes, insulation material, ropes or cords
Kenaf	*Hibiscus cannabinus* L.		Bast fiber	Malvaceae	Composites for automotive cordage, woven
Ramie	*Boehmeria nivea* L.		Bast fiber	Urticaceae	Industrial sewing threads, fishing nets, filter cloth
Jute	*Corchorus capsularis* L. (white jute)	*C. olitorius* L. (black jute)	Bast fiber	Malvaceae	Cloth for wrapping bales, sacks, carpets, curtains
Sisal	*Agave sisalana* L.		Leaf fiber	Asparagaceae	Hats, bags, carpets, rope and twine, geotextile
Manila hemp (abaca)	*Musa textilis* L.		Leaf fiber	Musaceae	Ships' rigging, fishing line, paper making

Columbia, Mexico, and Cuba. The sisal is being grown on 235,670 ha with the production of 602,509 tonnes. Both the area and production of sisal are decreasing since 2011. The Americas share 69.4%, Africa 23.7%, and Asia 6.9% in world total production of sisal. Brazil ranks first in sisal production followed by Mexico and the United Republic of Tanzania. The worldwide Manila fiber (abaca) was grown on 173,206 ha with the global production of 108,582 tonnes. It is mainly produced in Asia (68.9%), America (30.7%), and Africa (0.4%). It is mainly grown in the Philippines followed by Ecuador. Ramie is being grown on 31,587 ha with the production of 60,610 tonnes. Its production and area are continuously decreasing since 2007. It is mainly grown in China and Asia shares about 99.2% global production. The kapok fiber production in the world was 101,300 tonnes in 2013. It is mainly grown in Asia in Indonesia and Thailand (FAO 2019).

9.2 Fiber Crops Contribution in Climate Change

Like other crops, the energy, fertilizer, and pesticide use is an important aspect of fiber crops. Therefore, the greenhouse gas emissions are also linked with production practices of fiber crops. It was concluded that carbon footprint of natural fiber is

Table 9.2 Carbon footprints of fiber crops

Fiber crops	Carbon footprints (CO_2-eq/tonne)
Cotton[a]	2150[c]
Jute[b]	566
Flax[b]	520
Kenaf[b]	445
Sunn hemp[b]	423

[a]Agarwal and Jeffries (2013); [b]Singh et al. (2018b); [c]Average of both Australia and the USA

20–50% lower than those of synthetic fiber. Producing one tonne of jute fiber (carbon footprint) results an emission of 566 kg CO_2-eq (Singh et al. 2018a). The carbon footprints of other fiber crops are given in Table 9.2.

The kenaf plant has ability to absorb very high amount of CO_2, and it was concluded that every tonne of kenaf absorbs 1.5 tonnes of CO_2. The CO_2 requirement of kenaf was regarded much high than other crops (Kimball and Idso 1983). The nitrous oxide (N_2O) from agriculture field is linked with nitrogen fertilization. Since, the nitrogen requirement (50–100 kg N ha^{-1}) of kenaf is very low and very low N_2O emissions are thus reported. The N_2O emissions value for kenaf is 0.7–1.3 kg N ha^{-1} $year^{-1}$ which is very low, and its cultivation did not result in a significant amount of greenhouse gas emissions (Cherubini et al. 2009). It was also further confirmed that 10% of total nitrogen applied to kenaf field is lost through volatilization, loss through runoff/leaching is 5–10 kg ha^{-1} $year^{-1}$, and N_2O emissions are 0.6–1.2 kg ha^{-1} $year^{-1}$, which is only negligible part (IPCC 2006). The hemp has capacity to absorb CO_2 which will reduce the intensity of climate change (Vosper, 2011). It can be successfully grown without irrigation water supply which makes it the future crop of the area which is likely to be affected by drought (Gedik and Avinc 2020).

The study conducted to evaluate the greenhouse gas emissions from various cotton production steps showed that about 400.7 kg CO_2 e/ha. The further fragmentation revealed that harvesting/module building, road cartridge, and primary tillage contribute 141.8, 68.6, and 56.7 kg CO_2 e/ha, respectively. Among the agro-inputs, the nitrogen fertilizers are the main source of greenhouse gas emission followed by insecticides (Maraseni et al. 2010). The pollution during retting process is a common environmental issue of those fiber crops in which retting is essential. It consumes lot of water and pollutes the surface water. The decortication is an essential process of fiber extraction from sisal. Generally wet decortication is used which generates lot of wastewater, i.e., 100 m^3/ton fiber, which require effluent treatment prior to disposal. The pesticide and fertilizer use is very low in Manila hemp; hence, its contribution to greenhouse gas emission is minor. The sodium hydroxide, sodium sulfide, and hydrogen peroxide are used for fiber extraction which is dangerous for environmental quality.

9.3 Impact of Climate Change on Fiber Crop Production

9.3.1 Cotton

Worldwide, cotton is already broadly adapted to growing in temperate, subtropical, and tropical environments, but growth may be challenged by future climate change (Bange et al. 2016). Climate change is likely to affect cotton production both positively and negatively. Temperature influences cotton growth and development by determining rates of fruit production, photosynthesis, and respiration. The high temperature at critical stages during June to September reduced the yield due to flower shedding and less boll setting (Tariq et al. 2017; Ahmad et al. 2017). In addition, high temperature coupled with high humidity boosted whitefly population which is a major cause of yield reduction in 2019. Higher temperatures in cotton-producing areas and regions already suffering from high temperatures could have a negative impact as a result of increased shedding of flower buds. The rise in temperature could have a positive effect on yields, though, in those areas and regions where the effective fruiting period is squeezed between two phases of lower temperatures: one early in the season to start effective flowering and boll formation and one at maturity that results in termination of fruit formation. It has been projected that CO_2 concentration in the atmosphere will rise. Since CO_2 is an important substrate for photosynthesis, there should be increased yield in the future. However, various control environment studies highlighted that crops cannot take the full benefits because of high temperature. The similar findings were confirmed in control experiments in cotton conducted by Reddy et al. (2002).

Another impact of higher atmospheric CO_2 is that weeds will be growing more vigorously as well. When cotton is in the seedling stage, competition with weeds is critical. In spite of the fact that cotton planting and development will start earlier as temperatures rise, the same development will be observed in weeds. The critical period in the development of cotton and weeds will coincide. Unlike cotton (which is a C_3 plant), most weeds are C_4 plants and will show less reaction to CO_2 as C_4 plants let in even more carbon dioxide than C_3 plants, and this reduces, and sometimes eliminates, carbon losses by photorespiration. That is why cotton can compete with weeds more effectively under conditions where there is enough water and nutrition (Kaynak 2007).

There is a global warming phenomenon in the world and same is the case with cotton-growing areas. There are implications of rising temperature on growth and development processes and input requirement. The irrigation requirement is linked with prevailing temperatures and rainfall. The temperature stimulates the evapotranspiration and hence regulates the irrigation requirement, while rainfall serves as supplement to irrigation and support to reduce irrigations. The other impact of warming appears with respect to accelerated crop development, leading to reduce the duration of phenological stages (Ahmad et al. 2017). The earliness of 2.30–5.66 and 4.23 days per decade have been reported for sowing to boll opening and sowing to maturity in Pakistan (Ahmad et al. 2017) (Figs. 9.1, 9.2 and 9.3). The same trend

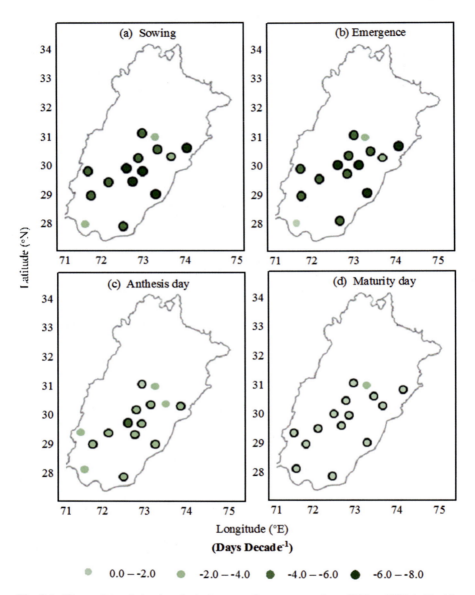

Fig. 9.1 Observed trends in phenological stages of cotton sown from 1980 to 2015 in Punjab, Pakistan: (**a**) sowing, (**b**) emergence, (**c**) anthesis, and (**d**) maturity. Circles with black border indicate statistically significant trends at $p = 0.05$ probability level. (Source: Adapted from Ahmad et al. 2017)

was observed in China where a reduction of 2.16 days from sowing to harvesting was observed. In the future, the temperature in China will increase by 2.3 °C–3.3 °C, and precipitation may change by 5–7% (Arshad et al. 2021). The precipitation during

9 Fiber Crops in Changing Climate

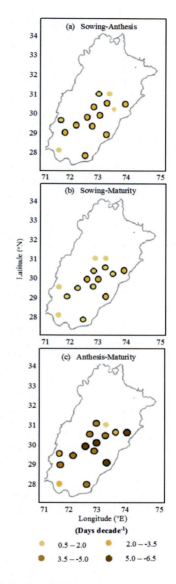

Fig. 9.2 Observed trends in the length of phenological phases for cotton from 1980 to 2015 in Punjab, Pakistan: (**a**) sowing-anthesis, (**b**) anthesis-maturity, and (**c**) sowing-maturity. Circles with black border indicate statistically significant trend at $p = 0.05$ probability level. (Source: Adapted from Ahmad et al. 2017)

the months of September, October, and June will change by 6–20% and 13–44% in Punjab (Pakistan). Temperature will increase in this region by 0.5 °C–1.7 °C in 2025 and 0.5 °C–3.7 °C in 2050 (Amin et al. 2018). The earliness in various stages due to higher temperature have also been confirmed in the Punjab, Pakistan, in the results of study on the impact of quantification of climate warming in cotton (Ahmad et al. 2017).

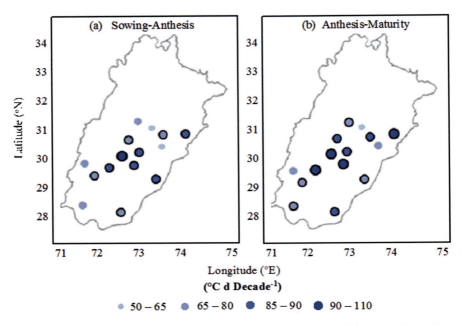

Fig. 9.3 Observed trends in thermal time required for cotton in Punjab, Pakistan, to advance from (**a**) sowing-anthesis and (**b**) anthesis-maturity. Circles with black border indicate statistically significant trend at $p = 0.05$ probability level. (Source: Adapted from Ahmad et al. 2017)

9.3.2 Jute

The temperature and rainfall are two principal factors of climate change which will affect the jute growth performance. Historical weather data of the last 100 years show a noticeable increase in ambient temperature and large variation in monsoon rainfall in the lower Indo-Gangetic Plain (IGP) region where jute is grown. An increase of 1.04 °C in annual average surface air temperature has been recorded (Singh et al. 2017), and by the 2050s, average ambient temperature is expected to rise by another approximately 2 °C (MEF 2004). In recent years, the impact of climatic variability is causing significant fluctuations in jute production and is likely to affect its yields in the long term. The jute is mainly grown under rainfed condition and about 500 mm rainfall is required for its successful growth. The rainfall has been reduced by 40–50% from 12th week to 15th week of the year (Singh 2017). The uneven distribution of rainfall exposes jute to early season drought, a serious abiotic limiting factor inhibiting nutrient acquisition by roots and restricting jute production (Geethalakshmi et al. 2009).

9.3.3 Hemp

Hemp can adapt and grow in different climate circumstances but is also vulnerable to several climate-related events. The early flowering and probable drought stress resulted in decreased stem/fiber yield in the study by Amaducci et al. (2008). The crop does not like wet soils that are prone to soil crusting and soil compaction. In case of high precipitation, these soil conditions increase the chance of waterlogging and full saturation of the soil, which can decrease yield or cause total crop failure. The hemp is a crop of temperate region which may shift to North as a result of climate change in the future (Rubel and Kottek 2010). It showed that farmers should be kept alert for future climate and is most likely that some new areas may be brought under hemp cultivation, while the area in core zone may be reduced. The water requirement of hemp is comparatively high during first 6 weeks of the growth; reducing the precipitation during this period may reduce the growth and yield, particularly in rainfed cultivation.

9.3.4 Flax

Higher accumulated temperatures cause lignin generation within the plant, however, and pose problems during the retting and mechanical separation of fibers. Meanwhile, flower bud differentiation and pollination of flax were influenced by temperature increasing in the reproductive growth phase, which would affect the number of capsules and the seed setting rate per plant and lead to the decrease of flax yield. The annual precipitation also influences the growth of fibers. It has been suggested that during the growing period, the precipitation should be about 110–150 mm (Heller et al. 2015). In climate change scenario, sudden temperature rise, precipitation fluctuations, and floods with windstorms not only affect the crop growth but also have negative impact on flax fiber quality.

9.4 Impact of Climate Change on Fiber Quality

The cotton is a raw material of various textile products in which fiber length determines the yarn quality. There are increasing trends of global warming over the world, and of course it has implications on cotton fiber quality as the crops are already suffering heat stress in arid and semiarid regions. For this controlled environment, experiments were performed for evaluating the impact of increased day and night temperature. The results demonstrated the negative impact of high temperature on fiber length, and the main reason behind these results was identified that high temperature shortened the duration of rapid fiber elongation. The enzymes and genes responsible for fiber elongation had been responsive to high temperature.

It was further investigated that increased night temperature has great influence on reduction of fiber length. Therefore, it was suggested that future projection must be made on the basis of rising trends of night temperature (Dai et al. 2017). In another study, Lokhande and Reddy (2014) concluded on the basis of controlled environment experiment that fiber length linearly increased in response to increased temperature from 18 °C to 22 °C and decreased with further rise in temperature. Similarly, fiber uniformity and micronaire improved with temperature up to 26 °C followed by decline, while fiber strength linearly increased with rising temperature. The immature fiber contents, short fiber contents, and seed coat nips decreased with rising temperature levels up to certain level followed by improvement, whereas maturity ratio improved with rising temperature. Changing temperature has great impact on micronaire followed by fiber strength, length, and uniformity. The decrease in natural water resources during jute harvesting time affects fiber quality, as large volume of clean and slow moving water is required for appropriate retting (Majumdar et al. 2013). In kenaf, the fiber length and core fiber length improved from 2.68 to 3.10 mm and 0.92 to 0.98 mm by increasing concentration of CO_2 from 400 to 800 $\mu mol\ mol^{-1}$. The bast holocellulose, bast α-cellulose, core holocellulose, core α-cellulose, and core lignin had negative association with CO_2 levels (Mahdi et al. 2014). Water stress delays plant growth and fiber maturation in hemp (Abot et al. 2013). Stem height and stem diameter decrease, while fiber layers become thinner in the year with drier conditions.

9.5 Fiber Crop Production Opportunities in Climate Change Scenarios

The concerns about the environmental impacts of various synthetic fibers are growing over time. Therefore, the demand for natural fiber crops is increasing due to ease of biodegradability and recycling. The predicted demand for fiber is likely to increase by 60% (130 million tonnes) in 2050 over 1990 (50 million tons) (https://cordis.europa.eu/).

The flax fiber production though has high pesticides and energy requirement but has minimum global warming impact, eutrophication, and acidification (Yan et al. 2014). The climate change potential of flax fiber production is low as it produces 316 kg CO_2-eq for each tonne of fiber production (Dissanayake et al. 2009). The climate change potential of flax fiber is also low in comparison with hemp because each tonne of hemp fiber production is accompanied with 2600 kg CO_2-eq, while this value is 2000 kg CO_2-eq for flax fiber (van der Werf and Turunen 2008). In another study, the hemp was reported an efficient tool of conversion of CO_2 into biomass as estimated that 1 ha can absorb 2.5 tonnes of CO_2. Moreover, if the crop is grown twice a year, this absorption can be doubled (Kolodziej et al. 2012). The hemp has ability to withstand the waterlogged (Satriani et al. 2021) and drought conditions (Gao et al. 2018); therefore, it may be a potential crop of the future keeping in view the fluctuations in precipitations in changing climate scenarios. The greenhouse gas emission during textile processing does not vary for synthetic and natural fiber. However, synthetic fiber manufacturing from various raw materials resulted in higher emissions than natural fiber. During 120-day growth cycle, the jute plants in 1 ha consume 15 MT CO_2 and release 11 MT of O_2 in the atmosphere (IJSG 2013).

9.6 Climate Change Impacts on Pests

Pest profiles are changing with the change in climate for all the agricultural crops. Fiber crops are also most affected due to climate change. Aphid was a serious pest of cotton crop in Australia, and it was observed to cross Europe, disturbing the cotton crop (Hulle et al. 2010). With early warming of climate, the cotton crop is not much disturbed, and the potato crop in the USA is damaged due to aphids and plant hoppers (Nelson et al. 2013). Temperature has warmer 10 days before in the last 65 years, posing a serious effect on interaction of crops and pests due to interaction of biotic and abiotic factors essential for crop growth and pest population (Baker et al. 2015). Among the fiber crops, cotton is the most sensitive and vulnerable to the climatic factors.

Plant material becomes less nutritive after increase of temperature and decrease of carbon accumulation within the plant tissues. To cope with these changes, insects consume more plant materials for their survival resulting in more damage of crops. Farmers are using more and more insecticides for better pest management. These pesticides are even increasing after the introduction of Bt cotton and pest pressure still increasing specially on genetically engineered cotton verities. In the last 10 years, pink bollworm on cotton crop is remarkably increasing. Similarly, whitefly is also on alarming situation in Pakistan.

9.6.1 Cotton Bollworm

Cotton bollworm (*Helicoverpa armigera* L.) was a common pest of cotton crop in many countries including Australia, Pakistan, and India. This pest goes into the winter diapause into the soil surface depending on the temperature and sunlight availability. After climate change and increasing of mean temperature, adult survival rate of cotton bollworm has decreased, and it is decreasing on cotton crop each year. The increase in carbon dioxide in air causes longer larval stage of *H. armigera* L. (Kriticos et al. 2015). Advanced modeling shows that the coastal areas of southern Australia will receive less attack of this pest in 2090. Similarly, attack will be more in western and northern Australia.

9.6.2 Natural Enemies

The reported changes in phenology of fiber crop pests are also supportive for higher survival of natural enemies of any pest hibernation in winter. Aphid and *H. Armigera* L. survival patterns are totally changed, and the population dynamics of stated pets needs further research to mitigate with climate change adopting the advanced pest management options (Li et al. 2015).

9.6.3 Fall Armyworm

The fall armyworm (*Spodoptera frugiperda* L.) is a moth belonging to the family Noctuidae. It has a host range of hundreds of plant species, inflicting severe damage in grasses – particularly maize and sorghum, which are the preferred hosts – along with other crops, such as rice, cotton, and soybean preferred by different species strains. It is native to tropical and subtropical areas of the Americas, and during summer it migrates into southern and northern temperate American regions (FAO 2021). Still fall armyworm has most choice of maize, but with change of preference, it can be converted to cotton and other fiber crops.

9.6.4 Cotton Mealybug

Mealybugs are severe agricultural pests which reach up to 350 species, but only 158 (about 35 are polyphagous) species are identified as pests worldwide (Franco et al. 2009). Cotton mealybug (*Phenacoccus solenopsis*) has been introduced as serious and alarming pest for cotton crop in Pakistan and India (Noureen et al. 2016). This pest was first time reported in 1991 from the state of Texas and spread throughout the world (Franco et al. 2009). During the initial years of the twenty-first century, cotton mealybug emerged as the most destructive pest of cotton crop, and it was spreading high in high-temperature areas (Arif et al. 2009). With the changing environment of cotton areas, adaptation was carried out from leaves to roots in hottest and dry areas, while it was foliage pest on moderate climate (Hodgson et al. 2008).

9.6.5 Minor Pests

Numbers of mirid bugs (insects of the Miridae family), previously only minor pests in northern China, have increased 12-fold since 1997, they found. Mirids are now a main pest in the region. Mirids can reduce cotton yields just as much as bollworms, up to 50% when not controlled. The insects are also emerging as a threat to crops such as green beans, cereals, vegetables, and various fruits. The rise of mirids has driven Chinese farmers back to pesticides. According to ecologists, genetic modified crops are not a magic bullet for pest control. They have to be part of an integrated pest management system to retain long-term benefits. Whenever a primary pest is targeted, other species are likely to rise in its place. For example, the boll weevil was once the main worldwide threat to cotton. As farmers sprayed pesticides against the weevils, bollworms developed resistance and rose to become the primary pest. Similarly, stink bugs have replaced bollworms as the primary pest in the southeastern USA since *Bt* cotton was introduced (Lu et al. 2010).

9.7 Fiber Crop Diseases

Increased carbon dioxide concentrations and change in mean temperature are also favoring the spread and damage of plant pathogenic bacteria and fungi. Cotton wilt has been increased manyfold in the last 10 years of Pakistan crop history due to which crop gets early matured and farmers can't attain natural maturity of crop.

9.8 Future Recommendations and Conclusion

The detailed studies on the impact of climate change were mainly focused on cotton; however, these studies must be extended to other fiber crops to evaluate the integrated effects of temperature, humidity, CO_2, and water stress on growth, yield, and quality. The development of cultivars tolerant to abiotic stresses including water availability (deficit and waterlogged), heat stress, and capabilities to efficiently utilize the elevated CO_2 to maximize production and minimize losses in variable environments.

References

Abbas G, Fatima Z, Tariq M, Ahmed M, Nasim W, Rasul G, Ahmad S (2020) Applications of crop modeling in cotton production. In: Ahmad S, Hasanuzzaman M (eds) Cotton production and uses. Springer, Singapore, pp 429–445

Abot A, Bonnafous C, Touchard F, Thibault F, Chocinski-Arnault L, Lemoine R, Dedaldechamp F (2013) Effects of cultural conditions on the hemp (Cannabis sativa) phloem fibres: biological development and mechanical properties. J Compos Mater 47(8):1067–1077

Afzal MN, Tariq M, Ahmad M, Mubeen K, Khan MA, Afzal MU, Ahmad S (2018) Dry matter, lint mass and fiber properties of cotton in response to nitrogen application and planting densities. Pak J Agric Res 32(2):229–240

Afzal MN, Tariq M, Ahmed M, Abbas G, Mehmood Z (2020) Managing planting time for cotton production. In: Ahmad S, Hasanuzzaman M (eds) Cotton production and uses. Springer, Singapore, pp 31–44

Agarwal B, Jeffries B (2013) Cutting cotton carbon emissions: findings from Warangal, India. World Wildlife Fund

Ahmad S, Abbas Q, Abbas G, Fatima Z, Naz S, Younis H, Khan RJ, Nasim W, Habib ur Rehman M, Ahmad A, Rasul G, Khan MA, Hasanuzzaman M (2017) Quantification of climate warming and crop management impacts on cotton phenology. Plants 6(1):7. https://doi.org/10.3390/plants6010007

Amaducci S, Zatta A, Raffanini M, Venturi G (2008) Characterisation of hemp (Cannabis sativa L.) roots under different growing conditions. Plant Soil 313(1):227–235

Amin A, Nasim W, Mubeen M, Ahmad A, Nadeem M, Urich P, Hoogenboom G (2018) Simulated CSM-CROPGRO-cotton yield under projected future climate by SimCLIM for southern Punjab, Pakistan. Agric Syst 167:213–222

Arif MI, Rafiq M, Ghaffar A (2009) Host plants of cotton mealybug (Phenacoccus solenopsis): a new menace to cotton agroecosystem of Punjab, Pakistan. Int J Agric Biol 11(2):163–167

Arshad A, Raza MA, Zhang Y, Zhang L, Wang X, Ahmed M, Habib-ur-Rehman M (2021) Impact of climate warming on cotton growth and yields in china and Pakistan: a regional perspective. Agriculture 11(2):97

Baker MB, Venugopal PD, Lamp WO (2015) Climate change and phenology: Empoasca fabae (Hemiptera: Cicadellidae) migration and severity of impact. PLoS One 10(5):e0124915

Bange M, Baker JT, Bauer PJ, Broughton KJ, Constable GA, Luo Q, Oosterhuis DM, Osanai Y, Payton P, Tissue DT, Reddy KR, Singh BK (2016) Climate change and cotton production in modern farming systems, ICAC review articles on cotton production research. CAB International, Boston, 61 pp, Available at: https://books.google.de/books?id=KUJFjwEACAAJ. Last access 12 Apr 2021

Cherubini F, Bird ND, Cowie A, Jungmeier G, Schlamadinger B, Woess-Gallasch S (2009) Energy – and greenhouse gas-based LCA of biofuel and bioenergy systems: key issues, ranges and recommendations. Resour Conserv Recycl 53:434–447

Dai Y, Yang J, Hu W, Zahoor R, Chen B, Zhao W, Zhou Z (2017) Simulative global warming negatively affects cotton fiber length through shortening fiber rapid elongation duration. Sci Rep 7(1):1–13

Dissanayake NP, Summerscales J, Grove SM, Singh MM (2009) Energy use in the production of flax fiber for the reinforcement of composites. J Nat Fibers 6(4):331–346

FAO (2019). http://www.fao.org/faostat/en/#data. Accessed on 21 Sept 2021

FAO (2021) Strategic framework for the International Plant Protection Convention (IPPC) 2020–2030. FAO on Behalf of the IPPC Secretariat, Rome. 40 pp

Franco JC, Zada A, Mendel Z (2009) Novel approaches for the management of mealybug pests. In: Biorational control of arthropod pests. Springer, Dordrecht, pp 233–278

Gao C, Cheng C, Zhao L, Yu Y, Tang Q, Xin P, Zang G (2018) Genome-wide expression profiles of hemp (Cannabis sativa L.) in response to drought stress. Int J Genomics:1–13

Gedik G, Avinc O (2020) Hemp fiber as a sustainable raw material source for textile industry: can we use its potential for more eco-friendly production? In: Muthu SS, Gardetti MA (eds) Sustainability in the textile and apparel industries. Springer, Basel/Cham, pp 87–109

Geethalakshmi V, Palanismy K, Aggarwal PK (2009) Impact of climate change on rice, maize and sorghum productivity in Tamil Nadu. In: Aggarwal PK (ed) Global climate change and Indian agriculture: case studies from the ICAR network project. Indian Council of Agriculture Research (ICAR), New Delhi, pp 13–18

Heller K, Sheng QC, Guan F, Alexopoulou E, Hua LS, Wu GW, Jankauskiene Z, Fu WY (2015) A comparative study between Europe and China in crop management of two types of flax: linseed and fibre flax. Ind Crop Prod 68:24–31

9 Fiber Crops in Changing Climate

Hodgson C, Abbas G, Arif MJ, Saeed S, Karar H (2008) Phenacoccus solenopsis Tinsley (Sternorrhyncha: Coccoidea: Pseudococcidae), an invasive mealybug damaging cotton in Pakistan and India, with a discussion on seasonal morphological variation. Zootaxa 1913(1): 1–35

https://cordis.europa.eu/project/id/311965/reporting

Hulle M, d'Acier AC, Bankhead-Dronnet S, Harrington R (2010) Aphids in the face of global changes. Comptes Rendus Biologies 333(6-7):497–503

ICAC (2021). https://www.icac.org/DataPortal/DataPortal?Units=Area&Year=2020/21. Accessed on 5 Oct 2021

IJSG (2013) Carbon credit of jute and sustainable environment, International Jute Study Group (IJSG). Jute Matter 1(7):1–2

IPCC – Intergovernmental Panel on Climate Change (2006) 2006 IPCC Guidelines for national greenhouse gas inventories. In: Eggleston HS, Buendia L, Miwa K, Ngara T, Tanabe K (eds) Prepared by the National Greenhouse Gas Inventories Programme. IGES

Kaynak MA (2007) Production problems in 2025. In: ICAC (ed) The vision for technology in 2025. International Cotton Advisory Committee (ICAC). United States of America, pp 3–7

Kimball BA, Idso SB (1983) Increasing atmospheric CO_2: effects on crop yield, water use and climate. Agric Water Manag 7(1-3):55–72

Kolodziej J, Wladyka-Przybylak M, Mankowski J, Grabowska L (2012) Heat of combustion of hemp and briquettes made of hemp shives. Renew Energy Energy Effic:163–166

Kriticos DJ, Ota N, Hutchison WD, Beddow J, Walsh T, Tay WT, Zalucki MP (2015) The potential distribution of invading Helicoverpa armigera in North America: is it just a matter of time? PLoS One 10(3):e0119618

Li Z, Zalucki MP, Yonow T, Kriticos DJ, Bao H, Chen H, Hu Z, Feng X, Furlong MJ (2015) Population dynamics and management of diamondback moth (Plutella xylostella) in China: the relative contributions of climate, natural enemies and cropping patterns. Bull Entomol Res:1–18

Lokhande S, Reddy KR (2014) Quantifying temperature effects on cotton reproductive efficiency and fiber quality. Agron J 106(4):1275–1282

Lu Y, Wu K, Jiang Y, Xia B, Li P, Feng H, Guo Y (2010) Mirid bug outbreaks in multiple crops correlated with wide-scale adoption of Bt cotton in China. Science 328(5982):1151–1154

Mahdi KA, Jaafar HZE, Ali Khalatbari A (2014) The impact of CO_2 enrichment on fiber dimension and lignocellulose properties of three varieties of kenaf (Hibiscus cannabinus L.). J Soil Sci Plant Nutr 14(3):676–687

Majumdar B, Suparna D, Saha AR (2013) Improved retting of jute and Mesta with microbial formulation. ICAR-Central Research Institute for Jute and Allied Fibres, Kolkata

Maraseni TN, Cockfield G, Maroulis J (2010) An assessment of greenhouse gas emissions: implications for the Australian cotton industry. J Agric Sci 148(5):501–510

MEF (2004) India's initial national communication to the United Nations Framework Convention on Climate Change. Ministry of Environment and Forests (MEF), New Delhi

Mubeen K, Afzal MN, Tariq M, Ahmad M, Muhammad D, Shehzad M, Yonas MW (2021) Sowing date influences cotton leaf curl disease (CLCuD) incidence and productivity of non-Bt cotton cultivars. Pure Appl Biol 11(1):26–34

Nelson WA, Bjornstad ON, Yamanaka T (2013) Recurrent insect outbreaks caused by temperature-driven changes in system stability. Science 341:796–799

Noureen N, Hussain M, Fatima S, Ghazanfar M (2016) Cotton mealybug management: a review. J Entomol Zool Stud 4(4):657–663

Pari L, Baraniecki P, Kaniewski R, Scarfone A (2015) Harvesting strategies of bast fiber crops in Europe and in China. Ind Crop Prod 68:90–96

Reddy KR, Doma PR, Mearns LO, Boone MY, Hodges HF, Richardson AG, Kakani VG (2002) Simulating the impacts of climate change on cotton production in the Mississippi Delta. Clim Res 22(3):271–281

Rubel F, Kottek M (2010) Observed and projected climate shifts 1901–2100 depicted by world maps of the Köppen-Geiger climate classification. Meteorol Z 19(2):135–141

Saranga Y, Menz M, Jiang CX, Robert JW, Yakir D, Andrew HP (2001) Genomic dissection of genotype x environment interactions conferring adaptation of cotton to arid conditions. Genome Res 11:1988–1995

Satriani A, Loperte A, Pascucci S (2021) The cultivation of industrial hemp as alternative crop in a less-favoured agricultural area in Southern Italy: the Pignola Case Study. Pollutants 1(3): 169–180

Singh AK (2017) The potential of jute crop for mitigation of greenhouse gas emission in the changing climatic scenario. Int J Agric Sci 13(2):419–423

Singh AK, Behera MS, Barman D et al (2018a) Modelling carbon sequestration under jute based agro-ecosystem. Annual report 2017–18. ICAR-Central Research Institute for Jute and Allied Fibres, Kolkata

Singh AK, Kumar M, Mitra S (2018b) Carbon footprint and energy use in jute and allied fibre production

Tariq M, Yasmeen A, Ahmad S, Hussain N, Afzal MN, Hasanuzzaman M (2017) Shedding of fruiting structures in cotton: factors, compensation and prevention. Trop Subtrop Agroecosyst 20(2):251–262

Tariq M, Afzal MN, Muhammad D, Ahmad S, Shahzad AN, Kiran A, Wakeel A (2018) Relationship of tissue potassium content with yield and fiber quality components of Bt cotton as influenced by potassium application methods. Field Crop Res 229:37–43

Tariq M, Fatima Z, Iqbal P, Nahar K, Ahmad S, Hasanuzzaman M (2021) Sowing dates and cultivars mediated changes in phenology and yield traits of cotton-sunflower cropping system in the arid environment. Int J Plant Prod 15(2):291–302

Van der Werf HM, Turunen L (2008) The environmental impacts of the production of hemp and flax textile yarn. Ind Crop Prod 27(1):1–10

Vosper J (2011) The role of industrial hemp in carbon farming, [pdf]. GoodEarth Resources PTY Ltd, Sydney. Available at: https://hemp-copenhagen.com/images/Hemp-cph-Carbon-sink.pdf. Accessed 1 June 2020

Yan L, Chouw N, Jayaraman K (2014) Flax fibre and its composites – a review. Compos Part B 56: 296–317

Chapter 10
Estimation of Crop Genetic Coefficients to Simulate Growth and Yield Under Changing Climate

P. K. Jha, P. V. V. Prasad, A. Araya, and I. A. Ciampitti

Abstract Global climate change has several implications on food security. The task of feeding the growing human population with limited resources is a challenging mission. With modern climate-resilient cultivars and optimized management practices, agronomists are trying to provide solutions to optimize the demand and supply balance in the food system. Crop simulation models play a vital role in assessing cultivar's performances with extrapolated conditions (soil and weather types) and resources (management practices), at varying spatiotemporal scales as large and multilocation field experiments with scarce resources are challenging. New cultivars need to be updated with their genetic coefficients to simulate crop growth and development and hence prediction of phenology and yield under different environments. Most of the modeling studies rely on the calibrated genetic coefficients of crops from different geographical regions and do not calibrate it properly which brings biasness in the model output. Different optimization methods for parameter estimation play a crucial role in meeting these requirements in short period. The selection of methods to estimate genetic coefficients also requires careful cataloguing of input data using standardized and appropriate protocols. With robust estimates of genetic coefficients, the reliability on simulation model will be boosted after proper statistical evaluation on the need of parameterization, testing model symmetry, and improving modeling metrics. Moreover, properly calibrated and validated model can be used to assess crop potential yield analysis, yield gap assessment,

---

P. K. Jha · A. Araya
Sustainable Intensification Innovation Lab, Kansas State University, Manhattan, KS, USA

P. V. V. Prasad (✉)
Sustainable Intensification Innovation Lab, Kansas State University, Manhattan, KS, USA

Department of Agronomy, Kansas State University, Manhattan, KS, USA
e-mail: vara@ksu.edu

I. A. Ciampitti
Department of Agronomy, Kansas State University, Manhattan, KS, USA

© The Author(s), under exclusive license to Springer Nature Switzerland AG 2022
M. Ahmed (ed.), *Global Agricultural Production: Resilience to Climate Change*,
https://doi.org/10.1007/978-3-031-14973-3_10

283

projection of climate and economic, and other decision support analysis which helps growers to enhance profitability and strengthen environmental stewardship. In this chapter, we discuss and describe different method of estimating crop genetic coefficients for simulation models. We also highlight advantages and disadvantages of the individual methods with special emphasis on the need of ensembling methods to minimize bias and inherent uncertainties in the estimation of these coefficients. This chapter will provide crop model developers and users an insight over different optimization methods and ensembling needs.

Keywords Crop modeling · Climate change · Genetic coefficient · Optimization · Calibration · Validation

10.1 Introduction

Global food security has become a growing challenge and will be critical to meet several Sustainable Development Goals (SDGs) (United Nations 2015). The ever-increasing demands for food, water, and energy for growing population are influenced by multiple factors which led to instability in global food production and supply. These factors are compounded by climate change, one of the significant drivers of instability in global food production. The increasing frequency of extreme climate events is of key concern and poses risk to food security (Mehrabi and Ramankutty 2019). To offset the instability in food production, breeders develop climate-resilient crop cultivars, which tend to achieve its potential yield with innovative agronomic interventions including optimal use of inputs such as seeds, nutrients, and water.

Global efforts during the last few decades have shown that yield gain is attributed ~50–60% to improved genetics and ~40–50% to management practices (Sacks and Kucharik 2011). Moreover, the process of developing better crop cultivar with improved tolerance to abiotic (heat and drought) and biotic (pests, diseases, and weeds) stresses along with other consumer-preferred traits demands time and resources. Despite these accomplished traits, cultivars attain lesser yield under field conditions than their potential. Although breeders have leveraged the interaction of genotype and environment (Elias et al. 2016), optimized agronomic management practices help in overcoming the challenges of yield gap (i.e., gap between potential and attainable yields). To realize the interactions of genotype, environment, and management (G × E × M), traditional agronomic experiments are designed for optimizing management practices to minimize the yield gap (Vilayvong et al. 2015). However, these voluminous experiments are constrained by time, spatial scale (heavily focused in a specific site), and resources.

To overcome these constraints, simulations of crop growth and development can facilitate these G × E × M interactions by extrapolating field experiments at spatiotemporal scales having varied location and multiple seasons (Lobell et al. 2009). Dynamic process-based crop simulation models can potentially quantify the physiological behavior and responses of crop cultivars under different G × E × M scenarios. The expression of cultivar to the individual environment is controlled by specific cultivar traits, termed as "genetic coefficients." Crop model algorithm identifies these coefficients to express the interaction among weather, soil characteristics, and management practices for crop growth and development. Moreover, these coefficients define and differentiate crop varieties, and hence estimation of the genetic coefficients is required while introducing new cultivar and when evaluating a known cultivar to a new region within the crop model. Obtaining these coefficients accurately at the field conditions is difficult as it is vulnerable to environmental disturbances within and during seasons and prone to human error while replicating field experiments.

The purpose of this chapter is to describe (a) crop genetic coefficients and their role in simulating crop growth and yield, (b) different methods of estimating the crop genetic coefficients, and (c) statistical evaluation of the performance of genetic coefficients. This chapter also highlights the advantages and disadvantages of different methods of estimating crop genetic coefficients.

10.2 Crop Simulation Models and Genetic Coefficients

The interaction of genetics (G), the biophysical environment (E), and management practices (M) resulting in crop phenological development can be simulated by process-based dynamic ecophysiological models, popularly known as crop models. These models are widely used as a support tool for research and decision-making at a scale, where we need to assess roles of G x E x M scenarios on crop development and yields. The physiological processes are simulated using state- and rate-variable approaches, which are associated and characterize the rate of change in the physiological processes. At the end of crop duration, the total biomass production is determined by the product of the average growth rate and total duration of the crop. And later, economic yield can be quantified as partitioned portion which goes into grain with a certain fraction that depends on environment under which crops are grown. Hence, physiologically, once rate variables are estimated, the state variables are calculated at time interval (Δt) following numerical integration (Forrester 1961) for total crop growth duration. It can be simply represented as Eq. 10.1 and can be depicted as Fig. 10.1:

Fig. 10.1 A relation diagram of dynamic exponential growth

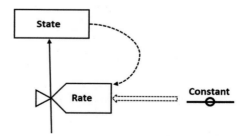

$$\text{Rate} = \text{Constant} \times \text{State} \tag{10.1}$$

These rate variables and constant in models are controlled by the genetic characteristics of the cultivar and are represented as genetic coefficients. These coefficients represent differences among cultivars, and their values are empirically estimated through extensive field experiments (evaluated under varying soil $\times$ weather conditions). To better represent genetic information of cultivar into models, cultivar parameters are estimated as a function of the alleles at different loci. A large set of germplasms are evaluated which vary in loci of interest to quantify their specific effects. In case of limited variation, for pure inbred lines, dominant and recessive alleles are scored 1 and 0, respectively, and their expression under different environments are estimated through linear regression with a physiological rationale. Once cultivar coefficients are determined, the field evaluation data are used to calibrate them conventionally by adjusting and comparing simulated and observed values of crop phenology and yield. This is a tedious task for all specific parameters of a cultivar as many modelers and/or agronomists are not familiar with genetics to evaluate these parameters following these approaches.

10.3 Common Methods of Estimating Genetic Coefficients

10.3.1 Field Experimentation

The development of new cultivars requires a selection of desired traits from screened pool of genotypes. The estimation of desired genotypic characteristics from breeding and field trials usually follows a liner model in the form of

$$Y = X\beta + Z\mu + e \tag{10.2}$$

where y is observed values; β and μ are fixed and random effects of gene under consideration, respectively; X and Z are design matrices for experiment; and e is a random residual error.

As evident from Fig. 10.1, yield is the product of the duration of crop growth and rate of biomass accumulation, both governed by light intercepted over a range of temperatures (Ritchie and Nesmith 1991). Hence temperature and photoperiod response function are critical in determining genetic coefficients. Moreover, for modern cultivars duration of growth is of highest significance than rate of growth, which is of relatively less significance (Evans and Fischer 1999). Temperature is the prime factor for growth duration; however, photoperiod and vernalization also impact growth significantly. Mostly the genes that regulate photoperiod and temperature response are scrutinized for estimating genetic coefficients and are part of fixed effects, β (Eq. 10.2). The randomness, μ (Eq. 10.2) of genotypic values of desired genes, is of major concern for breeders, and hence they look for shrinkage of those values toward desired means and are estimated through best linear unbiased prediction (BLUP) (Henderson 1985).

Photoperiod response function (PRF) is of prime focus for breeders while estimating genetic coefficients. The PRF is a function of basic vegetative phase, maximum optimal photoperiod, and photoperiod sensitivity (Rood and Major 1981). Basic vegetative phase is the time to anthesis under optimum photoperiod. Maximum optimal photoperiod is the longest photoperiod that does not delay flowering time. Photoperiod sensitivity is the delayed anthesis beyond maximum optimal photoperiod. The appearance of leaf, total leaf number, and time to anthesis are influenced by photoperiod. The evaluation under controlled environment is a good source for retrieving this data by determining duration of sensitive phases (Craufurd et al. 2013).

The dynamic nature of photoperiod response and its impact on growth stages and yield attributes have been studied extensively for major crops and their PRF, for example, rice (*Oryza sativa* L.; Yin et al. 1997; Nakagawa et al. 2005; Guo et al. 2020; Clerget et al. 2021; Zong et al. 2021), wheat (*Triticum aestivum* L.; Masle et al. 1989; Miralles and Slafer 1999; Slafer and Rawson 1996; Aslam et al. 2017; Arjona et al. 2020; Hyles et al. 2020), maize (*Zea mays* L.; Kiniry et al. 1983; Warrington and Kanemasu 1983a, b; Kiniry 1991; Birch et al. 1998; Van Bussel et al. 2015; Lin et al. 2021), soybean (*Glycine max* L. Merr.; Hadley et al. 1984; Jones et al. 1991; Sinclair et al. 1991; Mavromatis et al. 2001; Nico et al. 2019; Ohigashi et al. 2019; Bu et al. 2021), and sorghum (*Sorghum bicolor* L. Moench; Alagarswamy and Ritchie 1991; Craufurd et al. 1999; Clerget et al. 2004; Folliard et al. 2004; Dingkuhn et al. 2008; Wolabu and Tadege 2016; Clerget et al. 2021).

Temperature response function (TRF) can be developed by estimating crop phasic development with respect to temperature. Prediction of the crop developmental stages using temperature summation or total heat accumulation which translates into assimilate production leading to growth of plants was first suggested by Reaumur in 1735 (Wang 1960). With that idea, the concept of growing degree days or thermal time has been used extensively by researchers (Gallagher 1979) in the form of

$$t_d = \sum_{i=1}^{n} \left(\overline{T}_a - T_b \right) \tag{10.3}$$

where $\overline{T}_a$ is the daily mean air temperature, T_b is the base temperature at which crop ceases its development, and n is the total number of days used for defining phasic development.

The effects of temperature on crop development have been extensively studied by developing temperature response curve for major crops, for example, rice (Yin et al. 1997; Baker 2004; Prasad et al. 2006; Han et al. 2009; Puteh et al. 2010; Van Oort et al. 2011; Sánchez et al. 2014), wheat (Porter and Gawith 1999; Prasad and Djanaguiraman 2014; Cammarano et al. 2016; Prasad et al. 2017; Maiorano et al. 2017; Wang et al. 2017; Nuttall et al. 2018), maize (Cutforth and Shaykewich 1990;

Ritchie and Nesmith 1991; Stewart et al. 1998; Wang et al. 2018, 2020), soybean (Wilkerson et al. 1983; Hodges and French 1985; Jones et al. 1991; Setiyono et al. 2007; Boote et al. 2018; Alsajri et al. 2020), and sorghum (Hammer et al. 1989; Craufurd et al. 1999; Kumar et al. 2009; Prasad and Djanaguiraman 2011; Boote et al. 2018; Clerget et al. 2021; Liang et al. 2021). Field and controlled environment experiments have been conducted to assess and quantify the effect of temperature and photoperiod or their interactions (Erskine et al. 1990; Jagadish et al. 2007; Prasad et al. 2008; Tao and Zhang 2010). Field experiments measuring key phenological and physiological processes and their interaction primarily generate valuable information on sensitive stages and secondarily the quantification of varietal response which form a basis to estimate genetic coefficients for crop models.

10.3.2 Trial and Error (TE)

The conventional and subjective methodology for parameter estimation is manual trial-and-error (TE) method. In this method the cultivar's genetic coefficients are adjusted by the users until the observed and simulated yield matches or have least root mean square error (RMSE) (Willmott 1981). Although the process is cumbersome and considerably time-consuming, the results are more questionable when parameters of the model are arbitrarily changed to match the observed results – without following more functional approaches of the natural variation for the crop traits. Manual iteration requires expertise and careful calibration. The final estimates vary with the model users, despite with the same dataset and model structure. However, if calibration can be performed carefully, users might get better results in TE than automated optimization as the latter has sometimes been locally optimal and unreliable. An optimization algorithm for estimating genetic coefficients is a complicated process and demands advance programming and computing knowledge; hence the TE method is commonly used and preferred by agronomists. Several modelers have compared different methods of estimation and found the TE method promising and better than others. Mereu et al. (2019) used 10-year datasets to optimize the genetic coefficients and found the TE method performed better in simulating phenology and yield than the objective optimization methods of the generalized likelihood uncertainty estimation (GLUE) (He et al. 2009). The TE method was found to be better than parameter optimization tool PEST (Parameter ESTimation; Doherty et al. 1994) for phenology and yield prediction for wheat and soybean experiments conducted by Ma et al. (2020).

10.3.3 GENotype Coefficient Calculator (GENCALC)

Crop models have been used to simulate growth and development of crops from field scale (Jha et al. 2018; Saravi et al. 2021) to watershed (Eeswaran et al. 2021) and regional scale (Therond et al. 2011). The decision support system for agrotechnology transfer (DSSAT) model is one of the most widely used models (Hoogenboom et al. 2019) which has incorporated the GENotype Coefficient Calculator (GENCALC) method for estimating genetic coefficients based on sequential or gradient search method (Hunt et al. 1993). The basic idea behind a gradient search algorithm is to achieve an optimal solution within a defined search space of set experimental data and initial cultivar. This follows a hill-climbing optimization pattern which consists of moving solution from one point θ_n (phenology coefficients) to θ_{n+1} (growth coefficients) with a gradient of deterministic objective function $J(\theta)$. It is feasible for continuous domain (datasets from cultivar and field experiment), not for multidimensional or nonlinear. The GENCALC estimates cultivar coefficients by iterating them in a preset sequence of coefficients first which controls phenology and then the yield. Iteration involves comparison of outputs based on the simulated and observed variables (phenology and yields) in a sequential manner until it achieves best model fit, i.e., least RMSE between simulated and observed variables.

The GENCALC reads through a set of experimental data using coefficients from a startup cultivar (a closely related cultivar which functions as a reference for desired calibration). With initial startup coefficients, it adjusts and modifies genetic coefficients for best fit, i.e., least RMSE for target variable in each run or search cycle. Several researchers have used GENCALC and compared with other methods to assess its performances. The GENCALC has been used to estimate genetic coefficients of major crops including groundnut (*Arachis hypogea* L.) (Anothai et al. 2008), soybean (Bao et al. 2015), rice (Buddhaboon et al. 2018), wheat (Ibrahim et al. 2016), and maize (Román-Paoli et al. 2000; Hassanien and Medany 2007; Yang et al. 2009; Bao et al. 2017; Adnan et al. 2019). This approach has main limitations of the relatively small sampling area of search space, not optimum for wide ranges of desired targets (Pabico et al. 1999), and the overall inability to estimate uncertainties of the derived parameters, obtaining the crop genetic coefficients as deterministic values (He et al. 2010).

10.3.4 Downhill Simplex Method

Downhill simplex method (Nelder and Mead 1965) is an optimization algorithm which does not use derivatives for optimization and performs optimization quickly. The idea of getting geometric search space in simplex method, with N+1 vertices in N-dimensional space is to get same dimension of simplex and search space. The simplex moves through search space once starting cultivar is defined. Using the initial coefficients, it generates initial simplex, and the target or objective function (phenology and yield) is evaluated for each vertex of simplex (here vertices represent combination of genetic coefficients) by computing RMSE between simulated and observed values. The simplex movement ceases once it achieves lowest RMSE for one of the vertices as compared to others. With a goal of quick optimization, it sometimes captured into local minimum of the target of objective function (phenology and yield) which is determined by genetic coefficients. It is advisable to repeat the process with different initial cultivar to avoid local minima. To overcome this limitation, several evolutions have been practiced in this method; however, it makes this method more complex for crop models (Matsumoto et al. 2002). Researchers have used this method to estimate genetic coefficients for different crops, for example, soybean (Grimm et al. 1993; Piper et al. 1996), maize (Wei et al. 2009), rice (Gilardelli et al. 2019), and sunn hemp (*Crotalaria juncea* L.; Parenti et al. 2021). Correndo et al. (2000) investigated the pros and cons of choosing model to estimate errors and highlighted about the paradox of choices of model users.

10.3.5 Simulated Annealing Method

As the name annealing connotes, optimization is performed akin to annealing in thermodynamics, as first by melting at high temperatures and then slowly lowering the system until it freezes and at each temperature simulation search space runs at its maximum capacity to get best solutions with the lowest RMSE for target function (Brooks and Morgan 1995). Researchers have used this method to estimate genetic coefficients for different crops, for example, soybean (Mavromatis et al. 2002), maize (Ferreyra 2004), and rice (Zha et al. 2021), and soil root parameters (Calmon et al. 1999).

10.3.6 Generalized Likelihood Uncertainty Estimation (GLUE)

The uncertainty in data input and model parameters give biased model output. Likewise, associated uncertainty in cultivar datasets, field experimental datasets, and the derived parameters are difficult to be accounted during optimization. A Bayesian framework that assesses uncertainty of parameters using Monte Carlo technique, called generalized likelihood uncertainty estimation (GLUE), overcomes the limitation of associated uncertainties (Mertens et al. 2004; Candela et al. 2005; He et al. 2010). This method employed the genetic coefficients database of the DSSAT (Hoogenboom et al. 2019) to generate prior parameter distributions (He et al. 2010) and then can be used to develop the posterior distribution based on Bayes' theorem (Makowski et al. 2006). The prior parameter distributions are developed by fitting them to a multivariate normal distribution and then estimate the posterior distributions of each parameter using Bayes' theorem (Eq. 10.4):

$$P(\theta|O) = \frac{P(O|\theta)P(\theta)}{P(O)}, \qquad (10.4)$$

10 Estimation of Crop Genetic Coefficients to Simulate Growth and Yield... 291

where θ and O represent the parameter set and observations, respectively. $P(\theta|O)$ is the posterior distribution. $P(O|\theta)$ is the likelihood, $P(\theta)$ is the prior probability, and $P(O)$ is a normalizing constant.

To calculate likelihood values, random parameter sets θ_i are generated from the prior distributions. A likelihood value $L[\theta_i|O]$ for each observation (anthesis date, maturity date, and yield) is estimated based on Gaussian likelihood function (Eq. 10.5) (He et al. 2010):

$$L[\theta_i|O] = \prod_{j=1}^{M} \frac{1}{\sqrt{(2\pi\sigma_o^2)}} \exp\left\{-\frac{[O_j - Y(\theta_i)]^2}{2\sigma_o^2}\right\} \tag{10.5}$$

where θ_i is the ith parameter set, M is the number of observations, O_j is the jth observation, σ_o^2 is the variance of model error, and $Y(\theta_i)$ is the output of the model. In addition, Eq. 10.6 calculates the probability of the parameter set:

$$p(\theta_i) = \frac{L(\theta_i|O)}{\sum_{j=1}^{N} L(\theta_i|O)} \tag{10.6}$$

where $p(\theta_i)$ is the probability or likelihood weight of the ith parameter's set θ_i and $L(\theta_i|O)$ is the likelihood value of parameter set θ_i, given observations O (He et al. 2010).

The empirical posterior distributions were constructed from the pairs of parameter's set and probabilities $(\theta_i, p(\theta_i), i = 1...,N)$. The means and variances of those chosen parameters were calculated as in Eqs. 10.7 and 10.8 (He et al. 2010):

$$\mu_{post}(\theta) = \sum_{i=1}^{N} p(\theta_i) * \theta_i \tag{10.7}$$

$$\sigma_{post}^2(\theta) = \sum_{i=1}^{N} p(\theta_i) * (\theta_i - \mu_{post}(\theta))^2 \tag{10.8}$$

where $\mu_{post}(\theta)$ and $\sigma_{post}^2(\theta)$ are the mean and variance of the posterior distribution of parameters θ and $p(\theta_i)$ is the probability of the ith parameter set.

GLUE estimate parameters in similar sequence as GENCALC does, first phenology and then growth. At the end of optimization, the set of parameters having maximum likelihood values is selected as final coefficients. GLUE has been applied in the field of hydrology extensively (Beven 2018) and crop sciences (He et al. 2010) for parameter estimation. It has been used to estimate genetic coefficients of major crops including maize (He et al. 2009; Ahmed et al. 2018; Sheng et al. 2019; Jha et al. 2021), rice (Buddhaboon et al. 2018; Prasad and Mailapalli 2018; Tian et al. 2018; Tan and Duan 2019; Gao et al. 2020; Hyun et al. 2021; Jha et al. 2022), wheat (Ji et al. 2014; Ibrahim et al. 2016; Li et al. 2018; Mereu et al. 2019; Yan et al. 2020), soybean (Rodrigues et al. 2012; Salmerón and Purcell 2016; Nath et al. 2017; Memic et al. 2021), and sorghum (Vieira et al. 2019).

10.3.7 Parameter ESTimation (PEST)

Automatic optimization like GLUE takes lot of time to get results due to high number of runs required and of longer duration. To expedite the estimate process, the Parameter ESTimation (PEST) software (Doherty et al. 1994) has been developed and coupled with DSSAT as DSSAT-PEST package (Ma et al. 2020). With an advantage of quick convergence of search space, high efficiency, and transferability of codes in any language, it is easy to use for parameter estimation in crop models. The underlying algorithm of this software is Gauss-Marquardt-Levenberg nonlinear algorithm (Liang et al. 2016) which estimates parameter by reducing the number of objective functions (Eq. 10.9):

$$\phi = (c - Xb)^t Q(c - Xb) \tag{10.9}$$

where X is the model action, b is the desired parameter, c is the observed value of objective function, and Q is the cofactor matrix which weighs parameters based on observation. This PEST software runs with DSSAT input (cultivar, parameter output, and simulation control) and output files (cultivar coefficient and error) with control file of optimization (Ma et al. 2020). Ma et al. (2020) extensively applied PEST for maize, rice, wheat, soybean, and cotton (*Gossypium hirsutum* L.). Song et al. (2015) used PEST for parameter estimation and compare it with GLUE for maize. Maize coefficients are estimated for simulating irrigation strategies using PEST software (Fang et al. 2019).

10.3.8 Evolutionary Algorithm: Multi-objective Evolutionary Algorithm

The optimization involves multiple objective functions during the process, for example, anthesis and maturity date and yield in case of crop modeling. Cultivar's genetic coefficients control the objective function in synchrony rather than in silo. To simplify in terms of mathematical equation (Eq. 10.10),

$$F(x) = (f1(x), \ldots, fm(x))T \tag{10.10}$$

where main function $F(x)$ consists of m number of objective functions in the decision search space.

The single objective in Eq. (10.10) often intersects or complements to generate final result and hence conflicts with other objective functions. Calibrating one objective function may disturb other objective functions. Hence, a single solution cannot be achieved by optimizing all objective functions altogether. To overcome this problem, the best trade-off is designed and called as the Pareto optimality concept of Edgeworth and Pareto (Stadler 1979). It involves the principle of population-based nature and hence is considered as evolutionary algorithm. A powerful yet simple algorithm, a non-dominated sorting genetic algorithm-II (NSGA-II) (Deb et al. 2002), has become popular in the last two decades for multi-objective optimization for crop models. It employs non-dominated ranking rule to set objective functions and diversified population through crowding distance ranking. Sarker and Ray (2009) used this algorithm for crop models to estimate parameters. However, all these methods are used to optimize resource use at the field for best set of management practices. Recently it was used for parameter estimation for crop model (Kropp et al. 2019). Despite that it is not popular in crop modeling community, it has immense potential to explore for optimizing genetic coefficients of the cultivar. It needs a programmer to rearrange codes to design the Pareto fronts for optimizing coefficients.

10.3.9 Noisy Monte Carlo Genetic Algorithm (NMCGA)

Genetic algorithm (GA; Goldberg et al. 1989), a multidimensional, a multimodal, a discontinuous search algorithm having vast search space, outperforms other optimization techniques (Wu et al. 2006). The noisy Monte Carlo genetic algorithm (NMCGA; Ines and Mohanty 2008) earlier used in hydrology was first used in crop modeling to estimate genetic coefficients of maize (Jha et al. 2021). It estimates fitness of set of parameters based on the prior distribution and range from dataset (set of cultivar coefficients of all cultivars for the given crop in the model) using Monte Carlo resampling (Ines and Mohanty 2008). Based on lowest RMSE between simulated and observed values, the resampled parameter sets are evaluated under a noisy space (Wu et al. 2006). For optimal solution, fittest parameters go through crossover and mutation with several generations.

The objective function of the parameter set for the ith ensemble is formulated as Eq. 10.11:

$$
\text{Obj}(K)_i = \text{Min} \left(\frac{1}{T} \sum_{t=1}^{T} \left| \frac{1}{N_{\text{resample}}} \left(\sum_{r=1}^{N_{\text{resample}}} \text{Sim} \left(K^r \right)_{\text{ti}} \right) - \text{Obs}_t \right| \right) \forall_i \quad (10.11)
$$

where K^r is the set of K parameters combinations with r realizations generated from Monte Carlo resampling, N_{resample} is the total number of realizations for simulated (Sim (K^r)) and observed variables (Obs$_t$), and t_i is the running index for time T (Ines and Mohanty 2008). Noisy fitness is calculated using the inverse of the modified-penalty approach of Hilton and Culver (2000) (Eqs. 10.12 and 10.13):

$$
Z(K)_i = \text{Obj}(K)_i \left(1 + \text{Penalty} \left(K \right)_i \right) \forall_i \quad (10.12)
$$

$$\text{fitness}(p^*)_i = \frac{1}{Z(K)_i} \, \forall_i \qquad (10.13)$$

where $p*$ is the chromosome and fitness ($p*$) is the noisy fitness of that chromosome sampled from each ensemble i from the Monte Carlo resampling. A chromosome realization is penalized (Penalty (K)) if its predicted variables violate some preset rules against the goodness-of-fit evaluation (Ines and Mohanty 2008). Sampling fitness is calculated based on Eq. 10.14 to reduce the noise in fitness:

$$\text{Sfitness } (p^*) = \frac{1}{R} \sum_{i=1}^{R} \text{fitness}(p^*)_i \qquad (10.14)$$

where R is the total number of ensemble i. The arrays of parameter set (chromosome) of means and standard deviations undergo through the search process until the best chromosome is generated.

Jha et al. (2021) employed sequential optimization, first for phenology and then for growth coefficients for maize cultivars. Pabico et al. (1999) used GA to determine genetic coefficients of soybean cultivars. Xu et al. (2016) have used genetic algorithm to calibrate parameters of the soil-water-atmosphere-plant (SWAP)–Environmental Policy Integrated Climate (EPIC) coupled model.

10.3.10   Markov Chain Monte Carlo (MCMC)

A formal Bayesian approach, Monte Carlo, is a computational technique for sampling independent random sequence with a defined probability distribution function. However, Markov chain Monte Carlo (MCMC) draws sample from a distribution where the next sample is dependent on the previous sample, hence forming a chain called Markov chain (Shapiro 2003). It is capable of distinguishing the effect of input, output, model structure, and parameter. Comparison of formal Bayesian, MCMC, and pseudo-Bayesian, GLUE, underlies in the difference in estimating model residual error. The latter has no strong assumptions on residual error distributions (Tan et al. 2019). Iizumi et al. (2009) employed MCMC to estimate model parameters for rice. Sexton et al. (2016) used MCMC and GLUE to estimate parameters for sugarcane (*Saccharum officinarum* L.) and found both could be able to simulate biomass accurately. A modified MCMC, Metropolis-Hastings algorithm (López-Cruz et al. 2016), used for greenhouse crop models and differential evolution adaptive Metropolis (DREAM) algorithm have been used to estimate model parameters (Dumont et al. 2014).

10.4 Other New Promising Parameter Estimation Methods

There are several evolving algorithms which are used in global optimization of parameters in the field of crop resource planning and hydrology and can be used for genetic coefficient estimation and optimization after carefully revising same basic codes and testing. Some of them are highlighted here.

10.4.1 Differential Evolution (DE) Algorithm

DE algorithm is a global optimization method which focuses on multi-sampling objective function (target: phenology and yield) for optimizing the population (parameter sets) starts with random selection from the initial population (Storn and Price 1997). Zúñiga et al. (2014) used this algorithm to calibrate SUCROS model (van Ittersum et al. 2003) and later used for husk tomato crop (*Physalis ixocarpa* Brot. ex Horm.). Recently, Martínez-Ruiz et al. (2021) used DE algorithm to calibrate HORTSYST model (Martínez-Ruiz et al. 2012).

10.4.2 Covariance Matrix Adaptation Evolution Strategy (CMA-ES)

A special numerical optimization method for nonlinear problems is based on biological evolution where new individuals are generated by variation and selection in each generation. A maximum likelihood and covariance matrix of each generation is updated, and new evolution path is generated till the final solution is achieved (Hansen and Kern 2004). Zúñiga et al. (2014) used CMA-ES for husk tomato and compared with other methods.

10.4.3 Particle Swarm Optimization (PSO)

Inspired by social psychology, in this method (Kennedy and Eberhart, 1995), particles (here parameter) are placed in search space with defined objective function, and it evaluates the objective function at each location (Kennedy and Eberhart, 1995). Movement of particle is determined by current and best location (solution). Once all particle is optimized individually, then swarm like birds flock move for optimal solution. Jin et al. (2017) used PSO algorithm to feed AquaCrop model (Vanuytrech et al. 2014) for winter wheat yield estimation. Kaleeswaran et al. (2021) used PSO to inform crop selection based on resource availability.

10.4.4 Artificial Bee Colony (ABC)

Based on flying and dancing communication pattern of honeybees, food location represents an optimal solution, and nectar represents fitness of the solution. The total number of bees for food search is equivalent to number of optimal solutions. The artificial bee colony (ABC) algorithm generated a randomly distributed population for all the employed and onlooker bees, and they pass information about food source to other bees. Similarly, optimal solution is fitted based on food source, and nectar amount represents solution and fitness, respectively (Karaboga and Akay 2009). Chen et al. (2016) employed ABC for designing irrigation scheduling for multiple crops. Zúñiga et al. (2014) used ABC compared to other bioinspired algorithm explained in previous sections.

10.4.5 Ensembling Approach

Every method has its own advantages and disadvantages when it comes to measuring uncertainty in simulated values. Parameters estimated by individual method can simulate phenology in a better way than the growth simulation and vice versa. Empirically, it is evident that ensemble averages have better results than even the best single method (Chen et al. 2015; Martre et al. 2015). In the crop modeling community, after successful results from climate ensembling, scientists have started ensembling model results to get ensembled simulations through Agricultural Modeling Intercomparison and Improvement Project (AgMIP, Rosenzweig et al. 2013). However, a very few researchers have started ensembling parameter estimation methods instead of ensembling model itself. The basic questions that arise while doing ensembling are (1) relatedness and target of parameter estimation methods, (2) assigning weights to each method, (3) ensemble based on single vs multiple model input and output, (4) evaluating uncertainty estimates of all methods, and (5) compatibility of methods with models.

Several researchers have tried to compare parameter estimates and highlighted advantages and disadvantages of individual method (Ibrahim et al. 2016; López-Cruz et al. 2016; Buddhaboon et al. 2018; Tan et al. 2019; Gao et al. 2020). Jha et al. (2021) employed ensemble approach in parameter estimation for maize cultivar for the first time rather than ensembling model output. The detailed approach of ensembling by weighted average and simple average is explained in Jha et al. (2021). They compared GENCALC, GLUE, and NMCGA (two variants, with standard deviation and without standard deviation: NMCGA_SD and NMCGA_NO_SD). The results of genetic coefficients of maize cultivar are shown in Table 10.1; and the model performances are shown in Fig. 10.2.

10 Estimation of Crop Genetic Coefficients to Simulate Growth and Yield... 297

Table 10.1 Genetic coefficients estimated by different methods. GENCALC, GLUE, NMCGA_SD, NMCGA_NO_SD, and ensembling approach in 2017 and 2018

Methods	P1	P2	P5	G2	G3
GENCALC	143.8	0.54	780.0	750	8.5
GLUE	133.2 (30.7)	1.7 (0.5)	767.5 (40.1)	762 (176)	12.6 (2.6)
NMCGA_SD	134.4 (8.4)	1.714 (0.2)	758.6 (73.1)	779.7 (20.6)	13.2 (0.2)
NMCGA_NO_SD	134.9	1.7	666.4	806.6	14.8
Arithmetic average	136.6	1.4	743.1	774.6	12.3
Weighted average	137.5	1.4	749.0	777.4	11.4

Source: Jha et al. (2021)
Note: P's are phenology parameters and G's are growth parameters; values in () are standard deviation of parameter estimates. NMCGA_SD (noisy Monte Carlo genetic algorithm with standard deviation); NMCGA_NO_SD (noisy Monte Carlo genetic algorithm without standard deviation). P1 = juvenile phase coefficient (°C-d); P2 = photoperiod sensitivity coefficient (days); P5 = grain-filling duration coefficient (°C-d); G2 = potential kernel number coefficient; G3 = kernel filling rate (mg/day)

10.5 Statistical Evaluation of Performance of Genetic Coefficients

Crop models are based on empirical equations, and a set of hypotheses describing dynamic growth and development can be resulted in biased simulation or error as compared to the observed values. It is advisable to have in season observed value in addition to end season observed data for statistical evaluation (Sinclair and Seligman 2000). Hence, the performance of the model should be evaluated statistically with the observed data (Willmott 1982). R^2 is a measure of the correlation of simulated and observed values and used to evaluate the fitness of the linear model (Correndo et al. 2021). It misrepresents the under- or overestimation of the observed data as it is insensitive to proportional difference between observed and simulated data (Legates and McCabe 1999; Krause et al. 2005). Hence deviation and test statistics are required to evaluate the model performances.

Test statistics includes coefficient of determination (R^2; Eq. 10.15), and deviation statistics include mean bias error (MBE; Eq. 10.16), root mean square error (RMSE; Eq. 10.17), and index of agreement (d-index; Eq. 10.18) (Willmott 1982) to measure the performances of the calibration methods:

$$R^2 = \frac{\left[\sum_{i=0}^{n}\left(O - \overline{O}\right)\left(M - \overline{M}\right)\right]^2}{\sum_{i=0}^{n}\left(O - \overline{O}\right)^2 \sum_{i=0}^{n}\left(M - \overline{M}\right)^2} \tag{10.15}$$

$$\mathrm{MBE} = \frac{1}{n}\sum_{1}^{n}(M - O) \tag{10.16}$$

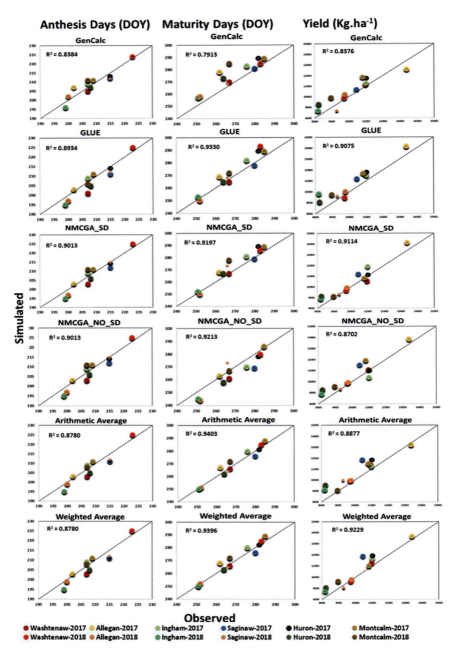

Fig. 10.2 Comparison of simulated and observed phenology and yield of maize for all the methods and ensemble for different validated sites. (Source: Jha et al. 2021)

$$\text{Root Mean Square Error} = \sqrt{\frac{\sum_1^n (M - O)^2}{n}} \qquad (10.17)$$

$$\text{Index of Agreement } (d - \text{index}) = 1 - \left[\frac{\sum_1^n (O - M)^2}{\sum_{i=0}^n \left(|M - \overline{O}| + |O - \overline{O}| \right)^2} \right] \qquad (10.18)$$

where M and O are simulated and observed variables (e.g., ADAP (anthesis date), MDAP (maturity date), or HWAM (yield)), respectively.

These objective functions are determined by crop genetic coefficients and help in simulating crop growth, development, and yield and help in assessing impact of climate change. Jha (2019) and Jha et al. (2021) compared the performance of CERES-Maize (Attia et al. 2021) using different parameters estimated by selected methods (e.g., GENCALC, GLUE, and NMCGA) and compared with ensembling approaches. They found that ensembling of genetic coefficients improved phenology and yield predictions once calibrated over multiple seasons rather than using an individual method. Better MBE, RMSE, and d-index for ensembling method have more effectiveness in simulating phenology and yield as compared to other individual method as shown in Table 10.2 (Jha et al. 2021). Further details on the pros and cons of different metrics for model performance and evaluation can be found at Correndo et al. (2021).

10.6 Conclusions

Increasing food demand of growing population must be met by enhancing food production to synchronize the dimension of food security by the end of the century. Climate vulnerability along with other major global issues impedes the target of food security globally. With limited resources, we need to produce more food with climate-resilient cultivars. Crop models play a vital role in testing cultivars under varying G x E x M scenarios. New cultivars need to be updated with their genetic coefficients to simulate their growth and development and hence prediction of phenology and yield under different environments. Field experiments are scarce with current limited extent of land resources, and hence estimating genetic coefficients is laborious, costly, and therefore a daunting task. Different optimization methods for parameter estimation play a crucial role in meeting these requirements. The selection of methods to estimate genetic coefficients also requires careful cataloguing of input data and protocols. To avoid biasness on accounting uncertainties, we should emphasize on ensemble methods rather than using the individual method of parameter estimation as discussed above in this chapter. The additional benefit of applying ensemble approach is to improve the prediction performance by reducing variance error of different methods. The performance and robustness are two critical components which are desirable for all model users in predicting

Table 10.2 Performance of CERES-Maize using parameters estimated by GENCALC, GLUE, NMCGA, and ensembling approach during calibration in 2017 and 2018

	ADAP (DOY)			MDAP (DOY)			HWAM (kg.ha^{-1})		
	MBE	RMSE	d-index	MBE	RMSE	d-index	MBE	RMSE	d-index
GENCALC	−1	4	0.93	6	12	0.84	604	784	0.96
GLUE	−2	5	0.89	4	12	0.84	1065	1093	0.93
NMCGA_SD	−2	5	0.88	2	10	0.87	81	665	0.97
NMCGA_NO_SD	−2	5	0.88	−8	11	0.84	594	833	0.95
Arithmetic average	−2	4	0.91	−1	9	0.90	861	1107	0.90
Weighted average	−2	4	0.91	−1	9	0.90	801	937	0.94

Source: Jha et al. (2021)

Note: ADAP (anthesis day after planting), DOY (day of year), MDAP (maturity day after planting), HWAM (yield at harvest maturity (kg/ha))

phenology and yield. Fine-tuned and evaluated model can be used to assess crop potential yield analysis, yield gap assessment, projection of climate, and economic and other decision support analysis which helps growers to enhance profitability and strengthen environmental stewardships.

Acknowledgments Authors thank the Feed the Future Sustainable Intensification Innovation Lab and its Digital Tools, Geospatial, and Farming Systems Consortium funded by the United States Agency for International Development (grant number AID-OAA-L-14-00006) and the College of Agriculture at Kansas State University for its support. Contribution number 22-241-B from Kansas Agricultural Experiment Station.

References

Adnan AA, Diels J, Jibrin JM, Kamara AY, Craufurd P, Shaibu AS , ... Tonnang, ZEH (2019) Options for calibrating CERES-maize genotype specific parameters under data-scarce environments. PLoS One 14(2):e0200118

Ahmed I, Rahman MH, Ahmed S, Hussain J, Ullah A, Judge J (2018) Assessing the impact of climate variability on maize using simulation modeling under semi-arid environment of Punjab, Pakistan. Environ Sci Pollut Res 25(28):28413–28430

Alagarswamy G, Ritchie JT (1991) Phasic development in CERES-sorghum model. In: Hodges T (ed) Predicting crop phenology. CRC Press, Boca Raton, pp 143–152

Alsajri FA, Wijewardana C, Irby JT, Bellaloui N, Krutz LJ, Golden B, Gao W, Reddy KR (2020) Developing functional relationships between temperature and soybean yield and seed quality. Agron J 112(1):194–204

Anothai J, Patanothai A, Jogloy S, Pannangpetch K, Boote KJ, Hoogenboom G (2008) A sequential approach for determining the cultivar coefficients of peanut lines using end-of-season data of crop performance trials. Field Crop Res 108(2):169–178

Arjona JM, Villegas D, Ammar K, Dreisigacker S, Alfaro C, Royo C (2020) The effect of photoperiod genes and flowering time on yield and yield stability in durum wheat. Plan Theory 9(12):1723

Aslam MA, Ahmed M, Stöckle CO, Higgins SS, Hayat R (2017) Can growing degree days and photoperiod predict spring wheat phenology? Front Environ Sci 5:57

Attia A, El-Hendawy S, Al-Suhaibani N, Tahir MU, Mubushar M, dos Santos Vianna M, Ullah H, Mansour E, Datta A (2021) Sensitivity of the DSSAT model in simulating maize yield and soil carbon dynamics in arid Mediterranean climate: effect of soil, genotype and crop management. Field Crop Res 260:107981

Baker JT (2004) Yield responses of southern US rice cultivars to CO_2 and temperature. Agric For Meteorol 122(3–4):129–137

Bao Y, Hoogenboom G, McClendon RW, Paz JO (2015) Potential adaptation strategies for rainfed soybean production in the South-Eastern USA under climate change based on the CSM-CROPGRO-soybean model. J Agric Sci 153(5):798–824

Bao Y, Hoogenboom G, McClendon R, Vellidis G (2017) A comparison of the performance of the CSMCERES-maize and EPIC models using maize variety trial data. Agric Syst 150:109–119

Beven, K (2018) Environmental modelling: an uncertain future?. CRC press

Birch CJ, Hammer GL, Rickert KG (1998) Temperature and photoperiod sensitivity of development in five cultivars of maize (*Zea mays* L.) from emergence to tassel initiation. Field Crop Res 55(1–2):93–107

Boote KJ, Prasad PVV, Allen LH Jr, Singh P, Jones JW (2018) Modeling sensitivity of grain yield to elevated temperature in the DSSAT crop models for peanut, soybean, dry bean, chickpea, sorghum, and millet. Eur J Agron 100:99–109

Brooks SP, Morgan BJ (1995) Optimization using simulated annealing. J R Stat Soc Ser D (Statist) 44(2):241–257

Bu T, Lu S, Wang K, Dong L, Li S, Xie Q, Xu X, Cheng Q, Chen L, Fang C, Li H (2021) A critical role of the soybean evening complex in the control of photoperiod sensitivity and adaptation. Proc Natl Acad Sci 118(8):e2010241118

Buddhaboon C, Jintrawet A, Hoogenboom G (2018) Methodology to estimate rice genetic coefficients for the CSM-CERES-Rice model using GENCALC and GLUE genetic coefficient estimators. J Agric Sci 156(4):482–492

Calmon MA, Jones JW, Shinde D, Specht JE (1999) Estimating parameters for soil water balance models using adaptive simulated annealing. Appl Eng Agric 15(6):703

Cammarano D, Rötter RP, Asseng S, Ewert F, Wallach D, Martre P, Hatfield JL, Jones JW, Rosenzweig C, Ruane AC, Boote KJ (2016) Uncertainty of wheat water use: simulated patterns and sensitivity to temperature and CO_2. Field Crop Res 198:80–92

Candela A, Noto LV, Aronica G (2005) Influence of surface roughness in hydrological response of semiarid catchments. J Hydrol 313(3–4):119–131

Chen W, Huang C, Shen H, Li X (2015) Comparison of ensemble-based state and parameter estimation methods for soil moisture data assimilation. Adv Water Resour 86:425–438

Chen S, Shao D, Li X, Lei C (2016) Simulation-optimization modeling of conjunctive operation of reservoirs and ponds for irrigation of multiple crops using an improved artificial bee colony algorithm. Water Resour Manag 30(9):2887–2905

Clerget B, Dingkuhn M, Chantereau J, Hemberger J, Louarn G, Vaksmann M (2004) Does panicle initiation in tropical sorghum depend on day-to-day change in photoperiod? Field Crop Res 88(1):21–37

Clerget B, Sidibe M, Bueno CS, Grenier C, Kawakata T, Domingo AJ, Layaoen HL, Palacios NG, Bernal JH, Trouche G, Chantereau J (2021) Crop-photoperiodism model 2.0 for the flowering time of sorghum and rice that includes daily changes in sunrise and sunset times and temperature acclimation. Ann Bot 128:97–113

Correndo AA, Hefley TJ, Holzworth DP, Ciampitti IA (2021) Revisiting linear regression to test agreement in continuous predicted-observed datasets. Agric Syst 192:103194

Craufurd PQ, Mahalakshmi V, Bidinger FR, Mukuru SZ, Chantereau J, Omanga PA, Qi A, Roberts EH, Ellis RH, Summerfield RJ, Hammer GL (1999) Adaptation of sorghum: characterization of genotypic flowering responses to temperature and photoperiod. Theor Appl Genet 99(5): 900–911

Craufurd PQ, Vadez V, Jagadish SVK, Prasad PVV, Zaman-Allah M (2013) Crop science experiments designed to inform crop modeling. Agric For Meteorol 170:8–18

Cutforth HW, Shaykewich CF (1990) A temperature response function for corn development. Agric For Meteorol 50(3):159–171

Deb K, Pratap A, Agarwal S, Meyarivan TAMT (2002) A fast and elitist multiobjective genetic algorithm: NSGA-II. IEEE Trans Evol Comput 6(2):182–197

Dingkuhn M, Kouressy M, Vaksmann M, Clerget B, Chantereau J (2008) A model of sorghum photoperiodism using the concept of threshold-lowering during prolonged appetence. Eur J Agron 28(2):74–89

Doherty J, Brebber L, Whyte P (1994) PEST: model-independent parameter estimation. Watermark Computing, Corinda, Australia 122:336

Dumont B, Leemans V, Mansouri M, Bodson B, Destain JP, Destain MF (2014) Parameter identification of the STICS crop model, using an accelerated formal MCMC approach. Environ Model Softw 52:121–135

Eeswaran R, Nejadhashemi AP, Kpodo J, Curtis ZK, Adhikari U, Liao H, Li SG, Hernandez-Suarez JS, Alves FC, Raschke A, Jha PK (2021) Quantification of resilience metrics as affected by conservation agriculture at a watershed scale. Agric Ecosyst Environ 320:107612

10 Estimation of Crop Genetic Coefficients to Simulate Growth and Yield. . .

Elias AA, Robbins KR, Doerge RW, Tuinstra MR (2016) Half a century of studying genotype × environment interactions in plant breeding experiments. Crop Sci 56(5):2090–2105

Erskine W, Ellis RH, Summerfield RJ, Roberts EH, Hussain A (1990) Characterization of responses to temperature and photoperiod for time to flowering in a world lentil collection. Theor Appl Genet 80(2):193–199

Evans LT, Fischer RA (1999) Yield potential: its definition, measurement, and significance. Crop Sci 39(6):1544–1551

Fang Q, Ma L, Harmel RD, Yu Q, Sima MW, Bartling PNS, Malone RW, Nolan BT, Doherty J (2019) Uncertainty of CERES-maize calibration under different irrigation strategies using PEST optimization algorithm. Agronomy 9(5):241

Ferreyra RA (2004) A faster algorithm for crop model parameterization by inverse modeling: simulated annealing with data reuse. Trans ASAE 47(5):1793

Folliard A, Traoré PCS, Vaksmann M, Kouressy M (2004) Modeling of sorghum response to photoperiod: a threshold–hyperbolic approach. Field Crop Res 89(1):59–70

Forrester JW (1961) Industrial dynamics. Pegasus Communications. Inc., Waltham

Gallagher JN (1979) Field studies of cereal leaf growth: I. Initiation and expansion in relation to temperature and ontogeny. J Exp Bot 30(4):625–636

Gao Y, Wallach D, Liu B, Dingkuhn M, Boote KJ, Singh U, Asseng S, Kahveci T, He J, Zhang R, Confalonieri R (2020) Comparison of three calibration methods for modeling rice phenology. Agric For Meteorol 280:107785

Gilardelli C, Stella T, Confalonieri R, Ranghetti L, Campos-Taberner M, García-Haro FJ, Boschetti M (2019) Downscaling rice yield simulation at sub-field scale using remotely sensed LAI data. Eur J Agron 103:108–116

Goldberg DE, Korb B, Deb K (1989) Messy genetic algorithms: motivation, analysis, and first results. Complex systems 3(5):493–530

Grimm SS, Jones JW, Boote KJ, Hesketh JD (1993) Parameter estimation for predicting flowering date of soybean cultivars. Crop Sci 33(1):137–144

Guo T, Mu Q, Wang J, Vanous AE, Onogi A, Iwata H, Li X, Yu J (2020) Dynamic effects of interacting genes underlying rice flowering-time phenotypic plasticity and global adaptation. Genome Res 30(5):673–683

Hadley P, Roberts EH, Summerfield RJ, Minchin FR (1984) Effects of temperature and photoperiod on flowering in soya bean [*Glycine max* (L.) Merrill]: a quantitative model. Ann Bot 53(5): 669–681

Hammer GL, Vanderlip RL, Gibson G, Wade LJ, Henzell RG, Younger DR, Warren J, Dale AB (1989) Genotype-by-environment interaction in grain sorghum. II. Effects of temperature and photoperiod on ontogeny. Crop Sci 29(2):376–384

Han F, Chen H, Li XJ, Yang MF, Liu GS, Shen SH (2009) A comparative proteomic analysis of rice seedlings under various high-temperature stresses. Biochim Biophys Acta, Proteins Proteomics 1794(11):1625–1634

Hansen N, Kern S (2004) Evaluating the CMA evolution strategy on multimodal test functions. In: International conference on parallel problem solving from nature. Springer, Berlin/Heidelberg, pp 282–291

Hassanien MK, Medany MA (2007, April) The impact of climate change on production of maize (Zea mays L.). In: Proc. of the international conference on climate change and their impacts on costal zones and River Deltas, Alexandria-Egypt, pp. 23–25

He J, Dukes MD, Jones JW, Graham WD, Judge J (2009) Applying GLUE for estimating CERES-maize genetic and soil parameters for sweet corn production. Trans ASABE 52(6):1907–1921

He J, Jones JW, Graham WD, Dukes MD (2010) Influence of likelihood function choice for estimating crop model parameters using the generalized likelihood uncertainty estimation method. Agric Syst 103(5):256–264

Henderson CR (1985) Best linear unbiased prediction of nonadditive genetic merits in noninbred populations. J Anim Sci 60(1):111–117

Hilton ABC, Culver TB (2000) Constraint handling for genetic algorithms in optimal remediation design. J Water Resour Plan Manag 126(3):128–137

Hodges T, French V (1985) Soyphen: soybean growth stages modeled from temperature, daylength, and water availability. Agron J 77(3):500–505

Hoogenboom G, Porter CH, Shelia V, Boote KJ, Singh U, White JW, Hunt LA, Ogoshi R, Lizaso JI, Koo J, Asseng S, Singels A, Moreno LP, Jones JW (2019) Decision support system for agrotechnology transfer (DSSAT) Version 4.7.5. DSSAT Foundation, Gainesville. https://DSSAT.net

Hunt LA, Pararajasingham S, Jones JW, Hoogenboom G, Imamura DT, Ogoshi RM (1993) GENCALC: software to facilitate the use of crop models for analyzing field experiments. Agron J 85(5):1090–1094

Hyles J, Bloomfield MT, Hunt JR, Trethowan RM, Trevaskis B (2020) Phenology and related traits for wheat adaptation. Heredity 125(6):417–430

Hyun S, Kim TK, Kim KS (2021) Comparison of the weather station networks used for the estimation of the cultivar parameters of the CERES-Rice model in Korea. Korean J Agric For Meteorol 23(2):122–133

Ibrahim OM, Gaafar AA, Wali AM, Tawfik MM, El-Nahas MM (2016) Estimating cultivar coefficients of a spring wheat using GenCalc and GLUE in DSSAT. J Agron 15(3):130–135

Iizumi T, Yokozawa M, Nishimori M (2009) Parameter estimation and uncertainty analysis of a large-scale crop model for paddy rice: application of a Bayesian approach. Agric For Meteorol 149(2):333–348

Ines AV, Mohanty BP (2008) Parameter conditioning with a noisy Monte Carlo genetic algorithm for estimating effective soil hydraulic properties from space. Water Resour Res 44(8):W08441

Jagadish SVK, Craufurd PQ, Wheeler TR (2007) High temperature stress and spikelet fertility in rice (*Oryza sativa* L.). J Exp Bot 58(7):1627–1635

Jha PK (2019) Agronomic management of corn using seasonal climate predictions, remote sensing and crop simulation models. Doctoral Dissertation, Michigan State University

Jha PK, Kumar SN, Ines AV (2018) Responses of soybean to water stress and supplemental irrigation in upper Indo-Gangetic plain: field experiment and modeling approach. Field Crop Res 219:76–86

Jha PK, Ines AV, Singh MP (2021) A multiple and ensembling approach for calibration and evaluation of genetic coefficients of CERES-maize to simulate maize phenology and yield in Michigan. Environ Model Softw 135:104901

Jha PK, Ines AV, Han E, Cruz R, Prasad PV (2022) A comparison of multiple calibration and ensembling methods for estimating genetic coefficients of CERES-Rice to simulate phenology and yields. Field Crop Res 284:108560

Ji J, Cai H, He J, Wang H (2014) Performance evaluation of CERES-wheat model in Guanzhong plain of Northwest China. Agric Water Manag 144:1–10

Jin X, Li Z, Yang G, Yang H, Feng H, Xu X, Wang J, Li X, Luo J (2017) Winter wheat yield estimation based on multi-source medium resolution optical and radar imaging data and the AquaCrop model using the particle swarm optimization algorithm. ISPRS J Photogramm Remote Sens 126:24–37

Jones JW, Boote KJ, Jagtap SS, Mishoe JW (1991) Soybean development. Model Plant Soil Syst 31:71–90

Kaleeswaran V, Dhamodharavadhani S, Rathipriya R (2021) Multi-crop selection model using binary particle swarm optimization. In: Innovative data communication technologies and application. Springer, Singapore, pp 57–68

Karaboga D, Akay B (2009) A comparative study of artificial bee colony algorithm. Appl Math Comput 214(1):108–132

Kennedy J, Eberhart R (1995) Particle swarm optimization. In: Proceedings of ICNN'95-international conference on neural networks, vol 4. IEEE, pp 1942–1948

Kiniry JR (1991) Maize phasic development. Model Plant Soil Syst 31:55–70

10 Estimation of Crop Genetic Coefficients to Simulate Growth and Yield...

Kiniry JR, Ritchie JT, Musser RL (1983) Dynamic nature of the photoperiod response in maize. Agron J 75(4):700–703

Krause P, Boyle DP, Bäse F (2005) Comparison of different efficiency criteria for hydrological model assessment. Adv Geosci 5:89–97

Kropp I, Nejadhashemi AP, Deb K, Abouali M, Roy PC, Adhikari U, Hoogenboom G (2019) A multi-objective approach to water and nutrient efficiency for sustainable agricultural intensification. Agric Syst 173:289–302

Kumar SR, Hammer GL, Broad I, Harland P, McLean G (2009) Modelling environmental effects on phenology and canopy development of diverse sorghum genotypes. Field Crop Res 111(1–2):157–165

Legates DR, McCabe GJ Jr (1999) Evaluating the use of "goodness-of-fit" measures in hydrologic and hydroclimatic model validation. Water Resour Res 35(1):233–241

Li Z, He J, Xu X, Jin X, Huang W, Clark B, Yang G, Li Z (2018) Estimating genetic parameters of DSSAT-CERES model with the GLUE method for winter wheat (*Triticum aestivum* L.) production. Comput Electron Agric 154:213–221

Liang H, Hu K, Li B (2016) Parameter optimization and sensitivity analysis of soil-crop system model using PEST. Trans Chin Soc Agric Eng 32(3):78–85

Liang X, Hoogenboom G, Voulgaraki S, Boote KJ, Vellidis G (2021) Deriving genetic coefficients from variety trials to determine sorghum hybrid performance using the CSM–CERES–Sorghum model. Agron J 113:251–2606

Lin X, Fang C, Liu B, Kong F (2021) Natural variation and artificial selection of photoperiodic flowering genes and their applications in crop adaptation. aBIOTECH 1–1

López-Cruz IL, Ruiz-García A, Fitz-Rodríguez E, Salazar-Moreno R, Rojano-Aguilar A (2016) A comparison of Bayesian and classical methods for parameter estimation in greenhouse crop models. In: V international symposium on models for plant growth, environment control and farming management in protected cultivation, vol 1182, pp 241–248

Lobell DB, Cassman KG, Field CB (2009) Crop yield gaps: their importance, magnitudes, and causes. Annu Rev Environ Resour 34:179–204

Ma H, Malone RW, Jiang T, Yao N, Chen S, Song L, Feng H, Yu Q, He J (2020) Estimating crop genetic parameters for DSSAT with modified PEST software. Eur J Agron 115:126017

Maiorano A, Martre P, Asseng S, Ewert F, Müller C, Rötter RP, Ruane AC, Semenov MA, Wallach D, Wang E, Alderman PD (2017) Crop model improvement reduces the uncertainty of the response to temperature of multi-model ensembles. Field Crop Res 202:5–20

Makowski D, Hillier J, Wallach D, Andrieu B, Jeuffroy MH (2006) Parameter estimation for crop models. In: Working with dynamic crop models. Elsevier, Amsterdam, pp 101–149

Martínez-Ruiz A, López-Cruz IL, Ruiz-García A, Ramírez-Arias A (2012) Calibración y validación de un modelo de transpiración para gestión de riegos de jitomate (*Solanum lycopersicum* L.) en invernadero. Revista Mexicana de Ciencias Agrícolas 3(SPE4):757–766

Martínez-Ruiz A, Ruiz-García A, Prado-Hernández J, López-Cruz IL, Valencia-Islas J, Pineda-Pineda J (2021) Global sensitivity analysis and calibration by differential evolution algorithm of HORTSYST crop model for fertigation management. WaterSA 13(5):610

Martre P, Wallach D, Asseng S, Ewert F, Jones JW, Rötter RP, Boote KJ, Ruane AC, Thorburn PJ, Cammarano D, Hatfield JL (2015) Multimodel ensembles of wheat growth: many models are better than one. Glob Chang Biol 21(2):911–925

Masle J, Doussinault G, Sun B (1989) Response of wheat genotypes to temperature and photoperiod in natural conditions. Crop Sci 29(3):712–721

Matsumoto T, Du H, Lindsey JS (2002) A parallel simplex search method for use with an automated chemistry workstation. Chemom Intell Lab Syst 62(2):129–147

Mavromatis T, Boote KJ, Jones JW, Irmak A, Shinde D, Hoogenboom G (2001) Developing genetic coefficients for crop simulation models with data from crop performance trials. Crop Sci 41(1):40–51

Mavromatis T, Boote KJ, Jones JW, Wilkerson GG, Hoogenboom G (2002) Repeatability of model genetic coefficients derived from soybean performance trials across different states. Crop Sci 42(1):76–89

Mehrabi Z, Ramankutty N (2019) Synchronized failure of global crop production. Nat Ecol Evol 3(5):780–786

Memic E, Graeff S, Boote KJ, Hensel O, Hoogenboom G (2021) Cultivar coefficient estimator for the cropping system model based on time-series data-a case study for soybean. Trans ASABE 64:1391–1402

Mereu V, Gallo A, Spano D (2019) Optimizing genetic parameters of CSM-CERES wheat and CSM-CERES maize for durum wheat, common wheat, and maize in Italy. Agronomy 9(10):665

Mertens J, Madsen H, Feyen L, Jacques D, Feyen J (2004) Including prior information in the estimation of effective soil parameters in unsaturated zone modelling. J Hydrol 294(4):251–269

Miralles DJ, Slafer GA (1999) Wheat development. In: Wheat: ecology and physiology of yield determination. CRC Press, Boca Raton, pp 13–43

Nakagawa H, Yamagishi J, Miyamoto N, Motoyama M, Yano M, Nemoto K (2005) Flowering response of rice to photoperiod and temperature: a QTL analysis using a phenological model. Theor Appl Genet 110(4):778–786

Nath A, Karunakar AP, Kumar A, Yadav A, Chaudhary S, Singh SP (2017) Evaluation of the CROPGRO-soybean model (DSSAT v 4.5) in the Akola region of Vidarbha, India. Ecol Environ Conserv 23:153–159

Nelder JA, Mead R (1965) A simple method for function minimization. Comput J 7(4):308–313

Nico M, Miralles DJ, Kantolic AG (2019) Natural post-flowering photoperiod and photoperiod sensitivity: roles in yield-determining processes in soybean. Field Crop Res 231:141–152

Nuttall JG, Barlow KM, Delahunty AJ, Christy BP, O'Leary GJ (2018) Acute high temperature response in wheat. Agron J 110(4):1296–1308

Ohigashi K, Mizuguti A, Nakatani K, Yoshimura Y, Matsuo K (2019) Modeling the flowering sensitivity of five accessions of wild soybean (*Glycine soja*) to temperature and photoperiod, and its latitudinal cline. Breed Sci 69:15–136P

Pabico JP, Hoogenboom G, McClendon RW (1999) Determination of cultivar coefficients of crop models using a genetic algorithm: a conceptual framework. Trans ASAE 42(1):223

Parenti A, Cappelli G, Zegada-Lizarazu W, Sastre CM, Christou M, Monti A, Ginaldi F (2021) SunnGro: a new crop model for the simulation of sunn hemp (*Crotalaria juncea* L.) grown under alternative management practices. Biomass Bioenergy 146:105975

Piper EL, Smit MA, Boote KJ, Jones JW (1996) The role of daily minimum temperature in modulating the development rate to flowering in soybean. Field Crop Res 47(2–3):211–220

Porter JR, Gawith M (1999) Temperatures and the growth and development of wheat: a review. Eur J Agron 10(1):23–36

Prasad PVV, Djanaguiraman M (2011) High night temperature decreases leaf photosynthesis and pollen function in grain sorghum. Funct Plant Biol 38(12):993–1003

Prasad PVV, Djanaguiraman M (2014) Response of floret fertility and individual grain weight of wheat to high temperature stress: sensitive stages and thresholds for temperature and duration. Funct Plant Biol 41(12):1261–1269

Prasad LRV, Mailapalli DR (2018) Evaluation of nitrogen fertilization patterns using DSSAT for enhancing grain yield and nitrogen use efficiency in rice. Commun Soil Sci Plant Anal 49(12): 1401–1417

Prasad PVV, Boote KJ, Allen LH Jr, Sheehy JE, Thomas JMG (2006) Species, ecotype and cultivar differences in spikelet fertility and harvest index of rice in response to high temperature stress. Field Crop Res 95(2–3):398–411

Prasad PVV, Pisipati SR, Ristic Z, Bukovnik U, Fritz AK (2008) Impact of nighttime temperature on physiology and growth of spring wheat. Crop Sci 48(6):2372–2380

Prasad PVV, Bheemanahalli R, Jagadish SVK (2017) Field crops and the fear of heat stress – opportunities, challenges, and future directions. Field Crop Res 200:114–121

Puteh AB, Rosli R, Mohamad RB (2010) Dormancy and cardinal temperatures during seed germination of five weedy rice (*Oryza spp.*) strains. Pertanika journal of tropical agricultural. Science 33(2):243–250

Ritchie JT, Nesmith DS (1991) Temperature and crop development. Model Plant Soil Syst 31:5–29

Rodrigues RDÁ, Pedrini JE, Fraisse CW, Fernandes JMC, Justino FB, Heinemann AB, Costa LC, Vale FXRD (2012) Utilization of the CROPGRO-soybean model to estimate yield loss caused by Asian rust in cultivars with different cycle. Bragantia 71:308–317

Román-Paoli E, Welch SM, Vanderlip RL (2000) Comparing genetic coefficient estimation methods using the CERES-maize model. Agric Syst 65(1):29–41

Rood SB, Major DJ (1981) Diallel analysis of the photoperiodic response of maize 1. Crop Sci 21(6):875–878

Rosenzweig C, Jones JW, Hatfield JL, Ruane AC, Boote KJ, Thorburn P, Antle JM, Nelson GC, Porter C, Janssen S, Asseng S (2013) The agricultural model intercomparison and improvement project (AgMIP): protocols and pilot studies. Agric For Meteorol 170:166–182

Sacks WJ, Kucharik CJ (2011) Crop management and phenology trends in the US Corn Belt: impacts on yields, evapotranspiration and energy balance. Agric For Meteorol 151(7):882–894

Salmerón M, Purcell LC (2016) Simplifying the prediction of phenology with the DSSAT-CROPGRO-soybean model based on relative maturity group and determinacy. Agric Syst 148:178–187

Sánchez B, Rasmussen A, Porter JR (2014) Temperatures and the growth and development of maize and rice: a review. Glob Chang Biol 20(2):408–417

Saravi B, Nejadhashemi AP, Jha P, Tang B (2021) Reducing deep learning network structure through variable reduction methods in crop modeling. Artif Intell Agric 5:196–207

Sarker R, Ray T (2009) An improved evolutionary algorithm for solving multi-objective crop planning models. Comput Electron Agric 68(2):191–199

Setiyono TD, Weiss A, Specht J, Bastidas AM, Cassman KG, Dobermann A (2007) Understanding and modeling the effect of temperature and daylength on soybean phenology under high-yield conditions. Field Crop Res 100(2–3):257–271

Sexton J, Everingham Y, Inman-Bamber G (2016) A theoretical and real-world evaluation of two Bayesian techniques for the calibration of variety parameters in a sugarcane crop model. Environ Model Softw 83:126–142

Shapiro A (2003) Monte Carlo sampling methods. In: Handbooks in operations research and management science, vol 10, pp 353–425

Sheng M, Liu J, Zhu AX, Rossiter DG, Liu H, Liu Z, Zhu L (2019) Comparison of GLUE and DREAM for the estimation of cultivar parameters in the APSIM-maize model. Agric For Meteorol 278:107659

Sinclair TR, Seligman NA (2000) Criteria for publishing papers on crop modeling. Field Crop Res 68(3):165–172

Sinclair TR, Kitani S, Hinson K, Bruniard J, Horie T (1991) Soybean flowering date: linear and logistic models based on temperature and photoperiod. Crop Sci 31(3):786–790

Slafer GA, Rawson HM (1996) Responses to photoperiod change with phenophase and temperature during wheat development. Field Crop Res 46(1–3):1–13

Song LB, Chen S, Yao N, Feng H, Zhang TB, He JQ (2015) Parameter estimation and verification of CERES-maize model with GLUE and PEST methods. Trans Chin Soc Agric Machine 46(11):95–111

Stadler W (1979) A survey of multicriteria optimization or the vector maximum problem, part I: 1776–1960. J Optim Theory Appl 29(1):1–52

Stewart DW, Dwyer LM, Carrigan LL (1998) Phenological temperature response of maize. Agron J 90(1):73–79

Storn R, Price K (1997) Differential evolution–a simple and efficient heuristic for global optimization over continuous spaces. J Glob Optim 11(4):341–359

Tan J, Duan Q (2019) Parameter estimation and uncertainty analysis of ORYZA_V3 model using the GLUE method. Trans ASABE 62(4):941–949

Tan J, Cao J, Cui Y, Duan Q, Gong W (2019) Comparison of the generalized likelihood uncertainty estimation and Markov chain Monte Carlo methods for uncertainty analysis of the ORYZA_V3 model. Agron J 111(2):555–564

Tao F, Zhang Z (2010) Adaptation of maize production to climate change in North China Plain: quantify the relative contributions of adaptation options. Eur J Agron 33(2):103–116

Therond O, Hengsdijk H, Casellas E, Wallach D, Adam M, Belhouchette H, Oomen R, Russell G, Ewert F, Bergez JE, Janssen S (2011) Using a cropping system model at regional scale: low-data approaches for crop management information and model calibration. Agric Ecosyst Environ 142(1–2):85–94

Tian Z, Niu Y, Fan D, Sun L, Ficsher G, Zhong H, Deng J, Tubiello FN (2018) Maintaining rice production while mitigating methane and nitrous oxide emissions from paddy fields in China: evaluating tradeoffs by using coupled agricultural systems models. Agric Syst 159:175–186

UN (2015) Resolution adopted by the General Assembly on 25 September 2015. Transforming our world: the 2030, United Nations

Van Bussel LGJ, Stehfest E, Siebert S, Müller C, Ewert F (2015) Simulation of the phenological development of wheat and maize at the global scale. Glob Ecol Biogeogr 24(9):1018–1029

van Ittersum MK, Leffelaar PA, van Keulen H, Kropff MJ, Bastiaans L, Goudriaan J (2003) On approaches and applications of the Wageningen crop models. Eur J Agron 18(3–4):201–234

Van Oort PAJ, Zhan T, De Vries ME, Heinemann A, Meinke H (2011) Correlation between temperature and phenology prediction error in rice (*Oryza sativa* L.). Agric For Meteorol 151(12):1545–1555

Vanuytrech E, Raes D, Steduto P, Hsiao C, Fereres E, Heng LK, Vila MG, Moreno PM (2014) AquaCrop: FAO's crop water productivity and yield response model. Environ Model Softw 62: 351–360

Vilayvong S, Banterng P, Patanothai A, Pannangpetch K (2015) CSM-CERES-Rice model to determine management strategies for lowland rice production. Sci Agric 72:229–236

Vieira PVD, de Freitas PSL, Rezende R, Dallacort R, Barbieri JD, Daniel DF (2019) Calibration and simulation of the CERES-Sorghum and CERES-maize models for crops in the central-west region of Paraná State. J Agric Sci (Toronto) 11(18):140–154

Wang JY (1960) A critique of the heat unit approach to plant response studies. Ecology 41(4): 785–790

Wang E, Martre P, Zhao Z, Ewert F, Maiorano A, Rötter RP, Kimball BA, Ottman MJ, Wall GW, White JW, Reynolds MP (2017) The uncertainty of crop yield projections is reduced by improved temperature response functions. Nat Plant 3(8):1–13

Wang N, Wang E, Wang J, Zhang J, Zheng B, Huang Y, Tan M (2018) Modelling maize phenology, biomass growth and yield under contrasting temperature conditions. Agric For Meteorol 250:319–329

Wang X, Zhao C, Müller C, Wang C, Ciais P, Janssens I, Peñuelas J, Asseng S, Li T, Elliott J, Huang Y (2020) Emergent constraint on crop yield response to warmer temperature from field experiments. Nat Sustain 3(11):908–916

Warrington IJ, Kanemasu ET (1983a) Corn growth response to temperature and photoperiod I. seedling emergence, tassel initiation, and anthesis. Agron J 75(5):749–754

Warrington IJ, Kanemasu ET (1983b) Corn growth response to temperature and photoperiod II. Leaf-initiation and leaf-appearance rates. Agron J 75(5):755–761

Wei J, Messina C, Langton S, Qin Z, Perdomo A, Loeffler C (2009) Predictability of CERES-Maize for flowering date. International Annual Meeting of Crop Science Society of America, American Society of Agronomy and Soil Science Society of America, November 1–5, 2009, Pittsburgh, PA, USA. Abstract 702–9

Wilkerson GG, Jones JW, Boote KJ, Ingram KT, Mishoe JW (1983) Modeling soybean growth for crop management. Trans ASAE 26(1):0063–0073

Willmott CJ (1981) On the validation of models. Phys Geogr 2(2):184–194

Willmott CJ (1982) Some comments on the evaluation of model performance. Bull Am Meteorol Soc 63(11):1309–1313

Wolabu TW, Tadege M (2016) Photoperiod response and floral transition in sorghum. Plant Signal Behav 11(12):e1261232

Wu J, Zheng C, Chien CC, Zheng L (2006) A comparative study of Monte Carlo simple genetic algorithm and noisy genetic algorithm for cost-effective sampling network design under uncertainty. Adv Water Resour 29(6):899–911

Xu X, Sun C, Huang G, Mohanty BP (2016) Global sensitivity analysis and calibration of parameters for a physically-based agro-hydrological model. Environ Model Softw 83:88–102

Yan L, Jin J, Wu P (2020) Impact of parameter uncertainty and water stress parameterization on wheat growth simulations using CERES-wheat with GLUE. Agric Syst 181:102823

Yang Z, Wilkerson GG, Buol GS, Bowman DT, Heiniger RW (2009) Estimating genetic coefficients for the CSM-CERES-maize model in North Carolina environments. Agron J 101(5): 1276–1285

Yin X, Kropff MJ, Horie T, Nakagawa H, Centeno HG, Zhu D, Goudriaan J (1997) A model for photothermal responses of flowering in rice I. model description and parameterization. Field Crop Res 51(3):189–200

Zha H, Lu J, Li Y, Miao Y, Kusnierek K, Batchelor WD (2021) In-season calibration of the CERES-Rice model using proximal active canopy sensing data for yield prediction. In: Precision agriculture'21, vol 263. Academic Publishers, Wageningen

Zong W, Ren D, Huang M, Sun K, Feng J, Zhao J, Xiao D, Xie W, Liu S, Zhang H, Qiu R (2021) Strong photoperiod sensitivity is controlled by cooperation and competition among Hd1, Ghd7 and DTH8 in rice heading. New Phytol 229(3):1635–1649

Zúñiga ECT, Cruz ILL, García AR (2014) Parameter estimation for crop growth model using evolutionary and bio-inspired algorithms. Appl Soft Comput 23:474–482

Chapter 11
Climate Change Impacts on Animal Production

Raman Jasrotia, Menakshi Dhar, and Seema Langer

Abstract Change in climate presents a serious peril to the animal species. Long-term deviations in the global or regional climate patterns have evident repercussions on the environment. Variance in the climatic pattern has a direct and indirect impact on animal production, so for this reason, it is requisite to perceive the appropriate way out not only to maintain the economy but also to reduce the hazardous environmental pollutants that will mitigate the negative impacts of climate change. The science of climate change signifies an increase in temperature of the sea surface, plummeting of air quality, and disruption of the natural systems due to elevation in the emission of greenhouse gases. Climatic variations are the utmost stressors of animal production as it exerts great influence on the forage quality, water accessibility, breeding, milk production, and the overall cattle farming sector. Salination of freshwater river systems due to the upsurge in sea level lessens the hygienic status of the production. Any transition in the temperature threatens the fish resources equally. Besides warming, climatic variability generates acidic conditions in the water bodies, which in turn curtail the global fish supply. Rising temperature hastens the growth of parasites that intensifies the potential for morbidity and death. Augmentation in heat stress reduces the yield in the dairy, beef, and poultry industry and thus induces heavy economic loss. The animal industry in the USA witnessed a loss of between 1.69 and 2.36 billion dollars annually due to heat stress. Animal products are the principal agricultural products of food security across the globe. These products provide 17% of worldwide consumption of energy in kilocalories and 33% of protein consumption globally. Climate change has adverse implications on animal production and productivity which accordingly influence food security.

Keywords Animal industry · Climatic pattern · Food security · Heat stress · Morbidity

---

R. Jasrotia (✉) · M. Dhar · S. Langer
Department of Zoology, University of Jammu, Jammu, India

© The Author(s), under exclusive license to Springer Nature Switzerland AG 2022
M. Ahmed (ed.), *Global Agricultural Production: Resilience to Climate Change*,
https://doi.org/10.1007/978-3-031-14973-3_11

11.1 Introduction

11.1.1 Global and Country Scenario of Climate Change

Climate change has a great influence on animal and plant lives, in every continent of the world. Variation in the degree of warming by every small fraction makes a difference, and any climate change is a serious threat to biological diversity in the succeeding years. Global warming is considered the serious cause of the extinction of species. Loss of species due to climatic changes may range from 0% to 54% (Urban 2015). There is a reduction in the viability of species due to climate changes. According to the Intergovernmental Panel on Climate Change, 2013 rise in global temperature due to an increase in the concentration of greenhouse gases will lead to a decrease in the snow and glaciers, and eventually sea level will also rise. There has been a decline in Arctic sea ice extent by 7.4% per decade, and in both the Southern and Northern Hemisphere, snow cover and glaciers have lessened (Yatoo et al. 2012). According to the United Nations Intergovernmental Panel on Climate Change, there will be an increase of 1.8 to 4.0 °C in temperature, and sea level is expected to rise between 18 and 59 cm in the next 90 years. Rising levels of greenhouse gases, i.e., CO_2, CH_4, and N_2O, in the atmosphere because of the activities of humans is the key factor of climate change. The last 6 years, i.e., from 2014 to 2020, are recorded as the 6 warmest years. There is a surge in the sea level, which further increases by the melting of glaciers. With the increasing carbon dioxide concentration in the atmosphere, the concentration of carbon dioxide also increases in the ocean which decreases the pH level of the water body, and the phenomenon is called ocean acidification. All these climatic changes have an impact on the biotic components present on the Earth's surface. According to IPCC, an average rise of 1.5 °C increases the risk of extinction of about 20–30% species. Various plant and animal species will not be able to adapt themselves to climate change. Climate change has pernicious repercussions on animal life, which can prove disastrous in the upcoming times (Fig. 11.1). According to Food and Agriculture Organization (2020), there is a dire need to intumesce the livestock sector globally owing to the escalating demand for animal-origin foods. Change in climatic conditions poses a serious threat to animal production.

11.1.2 Animal Production Under Climate Variability

Livestock production plays a significant role in the maintenance of the food supply. Change in climate conditions vitiates the production and quality of meat, milk, and eggs as it influences the reproductive behavior, metabolism, health conditions, and immunity of an animal. Conversion of forest land into barren lands due to drought and deforestation decreases the food availability for grazing animals. In developing countries, the livestock sector is growing expeditiously because of the elevated

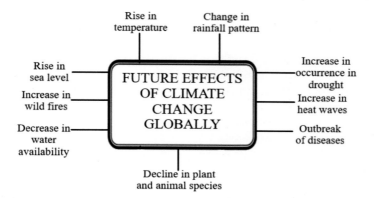

Fig. 11.1 Effect of alterations in climatic conditions

demand for animal products. However, in developed countries, this sector is endeavoring to become more efficient. It is predicted that in the near future, animal production will get adversely affected in view of competition for land, water, food, feed, and other changes looming in the environment. In developing countries, the livestock sector is one of the rapidly thriving agricultural subsectors. Demand for animal products in such countries is soaring at a rate of knots due to an increase in the population growth, movement of people from the rural to urban areas, and increase in per capita income (Delgado 2005). Animal production is the engine of development in various countries across the globe. The majority of the people, especially those dwelling in the developing countries, depend on animal production to boost up the several attributes of their livelihoods (Thornton et al. 2006; Thornton and Gerber 2010). Approximately, 30% of the Earth's ice-free land surface area is occupied by the livestock system (Steinfeld et al. 2006). The livestock sector proffers employment to 1.3 billion people across the globe, and in the developing countries, this sector directly augments the sustenance of 600 million poor farmers (Thornton et al. 2006). Globally, animal products accord 17% to kcal consumption and 33% to the consumption of proteins, although striking differences exist between the poor and rich countries (Rosegrant et al. 2009). Fisheries form the primary source of food for the increasing population across the world. They contribute to 17% of the world's total animal protein. They are important in developing tropical countries that depend on the fish for 70% of their nutrition. Loss of fish as a source of protein will put up an increased pressure on forests and other croplands.

11.1.3 Demand for Animal Products

There is an increased demand for animal productivity due to various reasons as follows.

11.1.3.1 Population Growth

According to the UNDP Annual Report (2008), it has been estimated that in the year 2050, the human population would be in the range of 7.96 to 10.46 billion, and much increase in population will be espied in developing countries. This alacritous surge in the population enunciates an increase in the food supply, which can be accomplished by improving the production of animal products. Animal products will provide nutrition security to the surging population. According to a report generated by Alexandratos and Bruinsma (2002), over the next 40 years, it is expected that the world population will increase by 2.25%, and so the global food production needs to be increased by 70% with doubling the production from developing countries.

11.1.3.2 Growth in per Capita Income

In a country, an increase in per capita income by 1% effectuates growth in the output of animal production by 0.21% (Chand and Raju 2008). Food preferences have been changed owing to the rise in per capita income in developing nations. World GDP revealed an annual increase of 3.85% between 1950 and 2002, which according to Maddison 2003 resulted in an increase in the per capita income growth rate by 2.1%. Across the globe, over the period of 40 years, global real per capita is expected to augment by over 10,000 US dollars per capita.

11.1.3.3 Urbanization

Across the globe, more than four billion people reside in urban areas, and it has been estimated that by the year 2050, approximately seven billion people will live in urban areas. With the rise in income, people begin to migrate from rural to urban areas. According to Yitbarek (2019), migration of people from rural space to urban centers will continue at a rapid pace, and it is expected that 70% of the world's total population will be living in urban areas in the near future. In developing nations it is prophesied that urbanization will continue at a swift rate, which in turn will influence the consumption habits of the people, and evidence support that an increase in the rate of urbanization may lead to an increase in consumption of animal products (Rae 1998; Delgado 2003). According to the studies done by Delgado (2005), urbanization often whets improvements in technologies like cold chains, to allow the trade of perishable animal products more widely and easily. In developing nations, due to rapid urbanization, animal production plays an indispensable role in accomplishing food security (Godber and Wall 2014).

Worldwide, more than 60 billion land animals are utilized for the production of meat, egg, and dairy products. According to Yitbarek (2019), animal production will depict a significant increase by the year 2050, viz., pig meat by 290%, egg meat by 90%, poultry meat by 700%, milk by 180%, sheep and goat meat by 200%, and buffalo and beef meat by 180%. Approximately, one-third of the global human protein consumption is met by the food obtained from animals and other animal products (Popp et al. 2010). The livestock sector acts as the source of livelihood across the world for around one billion of the poorest people (Hurst et al. 2005). According to the International Fund for Agricultural Development (2007) and Kabubo-Mariara (2009), whenever there is a failure in crop production, at that time animal products come to the rescue of the people by acting as an important food source. Yawson et al. (2017) reported that the average per capita consumption of meat is prognosticated to upsurge from about 34 kg in 2015 to 49 kg in 2050. Demand for animal products is predicted to rise considerably in the near future. According to the data provided by the Agricultural and Processed Food Products Export Development Authority (2018), India accounts for approximately 5.65% of egg production and 3% of the meat production over the world. India has the largest population of milk-producing animals in the world. Various animal species are important as they form the important food source having high nutritive value; some species are important for industrial purposes as they supply hides, skin, and fiber. Even some valuable by-products such as dung for fuel and manure and the horns are also obtained for the production of fancy items. Animal production can be a small-scale cottage industry or large-scale manufacturing industry and so helps in providing part-time or full-time employment to the people. The livestock sector is the source of regular income because of the quotidian production of dairy and poultry products. Fluctuations in climatic conditions have a tremendous effect on the fisheries sector. In the next few years, the air temperature and water temperature will continue to rise, due to which the level of the sea will surge up as the glacial mass will begin to melt. This will lead to acidification of water bodies owing to increased absorption of carbon dioxide emissions (Bindoff et al. 2007). Climate change even affects the distribution of fish in water bodies.

11.1.4 Institutes Working on Animal Production Under Changing Climate

The Indian Council of Agricultural Research (ICAR)-National Institute of Animal Nutrition and Physiology (NIANO), set up on November 24, 1995, at Bangalore, plays a pivotal role in conducting elementary analysis with respect to resource management of animal forage using various physiological-nutritional perspectives to ameliorate the animal productivity. Animal Production Research Institute (APRI) was established in the year 1908. Since then it is working to increase per capita animal productivity and profitability of farmers involved in livestock production.

This institute also aims to optimize the utilization of natural resources such as land and water to safeguard and preserve the environment. The National Research Institute of Animal Production was set up in Poland in 1950 and is authorized to carry out development and research work related to genetics and breeding of animals and all the issues related to animal production. Animal Production Research Institute-Giza situated in Egypt facilitates innovative and effective research on agri-food issues to achieve sustainable development outcomes. The Institute of Animal Sciences and Pastures (IZ) at Sau Paulo State, Brazil, works with an aim to research increasing animal productivity by using new technologies. This institute is committed to face any kind of challenges in the near future. Post Graduate Institute of Animal Sciences, Kattupakkam, situated in Chennai city, Tamil Nadu, was founded in the year 1957. The institute aims to improve livestock productivity by using various scientific techniques in the management of livestock. National Dairy Research Institute-National Innovations on Climate Resilient Agriculture (NDRI-NICRA), in Karnal, Haryana, effectuates pioneering research for animal welfare while sustaining the animal productivity in changing climate conditions. The institute is striving hard for increasing livestock production by fighting against both biotic and abiotic stress conditions. International Livestock Research Institute (ILRI), a global research center based in Kenya, was established in the year 1994. This institute is a member of the Consultative Group on International Agricultural Research (CGIAR). The research work focuses on various livestock challenges such as the vaccine for animal diseases, animal genetics, changing climatic conditions adaptation and mitigation, rapidly emerging infectious diseases, and markets for animal products. The Institute of Animal Husbandry was founded in 1948, in Belgrade (Zemun), and it carries out research activities in the areas of animal breeding, feeding, genetics, and physiology to enhance the productivity of animal products. The National Animal Production Research Institute was set up in Zaria (Nigeria) to develop new appropriate technologies for increasing animal production to assure food security to the growing population.

11.1.4.1 Livestock Census

The 20th livestock census was set in motion during October 2018 in both the rural and urban cities. This census was performed in approximately 6.6 lakh villages and 89,000 urban places across India and included more than 27 crore households and non-households:

- Total livestock population = 535.78 million.
- Total bovine population = 302.79 million.
- Total cattle population = 192.49 million.
- Total cow population = 145.12 million.

11.2 Quantification of Climate Change

11.2.1 Overview of Responses to Temperature, Drought, and Carbon Dioxide

11.2.1.1 Temperature

According to the report generated, the US livestock industry suffered a loss of 1.69 to 2.36 US billion dollars due to warm conditions of the environment. Increased temperature reduces the sperm quality and concentration in bulls, poultry, and pigs (Karaca et al. 2002; Kunavongkrita et al. 2005). Temperature increases between 1 and 5 °C can whip up the mortality rate in grazing cattle (Howden et al. 2008). An increase in the temperature of water alters the physiology and male-female ratio of the fish species. Increasing temperature accelerates the rate of transmission of communicable diseases. According to Tubiello et al. (2008), forage supply gets affected by high temperature as it shifts C3 grasses to C4 grasses. Howden et al. (2008) reported that the temperature rise has shifted *Kobresia* communities, the highly productive alpine, to the *Stipa* communities that are less productive. In the swine industry, Mayorga et al. (2019) reported huge loss linked with heat stress as this decreases feed efficiency, carcass quality, and reproductive performance and increases infection and death rate. Above a certain maximum limit of temperature, intake of feed, production of poultry, milk, reproduction, hormonal activity, and the immunity of an animal get suppressed (Das et al. 2016). Temperature changes decrease the production of dairy and beef products that incur a striking loss in the economy (Nardone et al. 2010).

11.2.1.2 Drought

Besides being affected by an increase in temperature due to changing climate, livestock is susceptible to extreme events such as drought (Kanwal et al. 2020). Drought poses a serious risk to the environment that influences the production of livestock negatively. This prolonged period of scanty rainfall is considered a momentous natural menace and is generally acknowledged as one of the dominant causes of damage to the environment, farming, and ecosystem (Vicente-Serrano et al. 2010). Dzavo et al. (2019) recorded water shortage as the most common cause for the loss of cattle in semiarid and subhumid areas. Starvation was found to trigger cattle loss due to lack of food. Fodder supply becomes sparse due to lack of rainfall as a result of which the price of fodder also rises. In India, approximately 68% of the sown area is at the risk due to drought, and every year it affects about 50 million people. The deficiency of nutrition in the diet of livestock is balanced by the fat resources in the body. Drought leads to fluctuations in the populations of livestock by increasing death rate and decreasing birth rate (Ellis and Swift 1988; Oba and Kotile 2001). According to the United Nations Environment Programme (1989),

India is vulnerable to utmost events due to changing climate. The effect of a dry spell is noticeable even in lactating animals (Kanwal et al. 2020). The scarcity of rainfall has a strong influence on the sheep. Research studies have shown that drought leads to depletion in offspring production and lessens milk production, and infertility issues even cause serious diseases and death of an animal in certain cases. Studies conducted by Salmoral et al. (2020) revealed that the drought that occurred in the UK in the year 2018 imposed a remarkable impact on the growth of grass that affects the availability of feed, prices, the income of farmers, and thus animal welfare. Nanson et al. (2002) reported that more than 50% of the world's surface area is drained by the dryland rivers. The abundance of fish in these dryland rivers is affected by the drought conditions as the water flow stops and most of the river channels dry up (Knighton and Nanson, 2000). The drought conditions threaten the resistance of the fish population which eventually leads to mass mortality in fish (Hopper et al. 2020; Vertessy et al. 2019).

A decrease in abundance and biomass of trout in streams was observed in water systems near Western Cascade Mountains during the drought year (Kaylor et al. 2019). Hakala and Hartman (2004) reported that in response to drought-like conditions, the abundance of adult brook trout decreased by 60%. On similar lines, James et al. (2010) observed a decline in population biomass of adult brown trout following drought. Drought also presents an acute risk to the livestock sector as such condition lowers the production of hay and fodder (Schaub and Finger 2020). Smit et al. (2008) and Webber et al. (2018) had observed considerable diminution in the production of grassland and feed crops. Changing climatic conditions have an indirect effect on the production of poultry as it greatly affects the maize yield production. Availability and the price of poultry feed get affected due to climate change as reported by Liverpool-Tasie et al. (2019).

11.2.1.3 Carbon Dioxide

The livestock population is facing a serious challenge due to changing atmospheric conditions. Over the last previous 200 years, levels of carbon dioxide in the atmosphere have been increased by approximately 30%. Semple (1970) reported that natural ecosystems act as the source of the majority of food supply to ruminants and 95% of the livestock food is supplied by the rangelands (Holochek et al. 1989). Plants produce their food by the process of photosynthesis and so act as the primary producers. During this process, carbon dioxide is transformed into sugars such as glucose; thus CO_2 is vital for the growth of plants. But the increased levels of CO_2 drop the level of nitrogen in the leaves, which is considered as a most crucial nutrient for animals that depend on plant-based food (Ehleringer et al. 2005). Under elevated concentrations of carbon dioxide in the atmosphere, it has been reported that the plants elevate the release of secondary metabolites due to which animals feeding on such plants show a decrease in growth rate and increase in death rate (Percy et al.

2002). Roughly, one-third of the CO_2 that is produced due to human activities dissolves in the oceans which causes ocean acidification. Elevated levels of CO_2 lead to difficulty in breathing in marine fishes, and as a result, it inhibits their food-capturing ability and they become prone to predators. The most drastic effects of the elevated CO_2 concentration are prophesied in oxygen minimum zones in the oceans, where oxygen is found at very low concentrations (Brewer and Peltzer, 2009).

The quality of forages has been reduced due to morphological changes linked with elevated CO_2 (Owensby et al. 1996). Due to the increased concentration of carbon dioxide, more waxes get deposited in the plant leaves, which further lessen the forage quality for livestock (Thomas and Harvey, 1983). In the future, the production of livestock will most likely get distressed by increasing temperature and increasing CO_2 levels as they modify the growing conditions of plants that are used by animals for feeding purposes (Loholter et al. 2012). Preliminary analysis has revealed that in 2020, the average concentration of carbon dioxide in the atmosphere all over the globe was 412.5 ppm, which indicates a surge of 2.6 ppm over the levels of CO_2 recorded in the year 2019. Levels of CO_2 have depicted an increase of 12% since the year 2000.

11.2.2 Overview of Responses to Biotic Stress Such as Parasites

Livestock animals such as sheep and goats act as the vital component of the dairy farming section. Various helminths act as parasites in these animals and thus affect the farming systems across the world. These parasites lessen the productivity of these animals as they feed on the body or the blood of the host. Greer (2008) reported that *Haemonchus contortus* absorbs nutrients from the gastrointestinal tract of the host species, and this way the parasite damages the lining of their GI tract. As a result, the host shows various symptoms such as a decrease in weight, hyperoxia, and death in certain cases. Climate affects the copiousness and survival rate of infective stages of parasites, thus increasing the infection rate of animals (O'Connor et al. 2006). Stress triggered by the direct and indirect effects of bacteria, viruses, insects, and nematodes is referred to as biotic stress. This stress leads to loss due to pathogenicity and death in animals (Jaya et al. 2016). Changing climatic conditions have a great influence on the infectious diseases in animals as they alter their spatial distribution, disturb the seasonal and annual cycles, modify the vulnerability of animals to diseases, and also change the prevalence and severity of diseases in them (Patterson and Guerin, 2013; Bagath et al. 2019 and Filipe et al. 2020). Various transmissible disease-causing organisms responsible for causing various diseases in animals are sensitive to climate change especially rainfall, temperature, and moisture. Pathogens transmitted through food, water, and soil are most probably affected by the change in climatic conditions (McIntyre et al. 2017).

11.3 Impact of Climate Change on Livestock Production Systems

Long-term change in the climate of the Earth due to an increase in the average temperature of the atmosphere is called climate change. Animal production is an indispensable resource for the people living in poorly developed communities. Any change in the environment of an animal affects the efficaciousness of the animal production system as these changes markedly influence the growth, development, and reproduction of all animals (Fig. 11.2).

11.3.1 Quality of Feed

Change in the climatic conditions such as fluctuating temperature, intense heat waves, wind, precipitation, etc. in a certain region presents a great threat to the animals. Animal production gets affected because of the decreased quality of the forage available for feeding. Decrease in the production of herbs and increase in lignification of plant tissues vitiate the forage digestibility by animals. Furthermore, the area under the shrub cover is increasing with the change in climate that tends to diminish both the quality and quantity of feed available to the animals (Hidosa and Guyo 2017). The research findings have suggested that with the increase in temperature and carbon dioxide levels, the primary productivity of greensward and grazing lands decreases. Climate change decreases the productivity and grazing capacity of pasture lands. Moreover, it changes the pasture composition and also increases the offset of biomass yield (Attia-Ismail 2020). Plants growing on pasturelands entirely rely upon rainfall, so any change in the pattern of rainfall will affect the plants. Climatic changes such as reduced rainfall and the increase in drought-like conditions will decrease the primary productivity of rangelands/pastures, which will lead to overgrazing which may result in conflict over the scarce food resources. There is a growing probability of an increase in weather events, and that will have a great impact on the grazing systems in arid and semiarid areas especially at altitudes (Hoffman and Vogel 2008). Similar kinds of effects can be expected in the

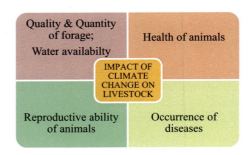

Fig. 11.2 Effect of climate change on animals

non-grazing systems where the animals are confined to climate-controlled buildings. Decreased agricultural production and the increase in the competition for food resources will surge the prices of oilcake and grains, which are considered major feed sources in non-grazing systems. In various regions of the world, wide fluctuations in the pattern of rainfall will have a great impact on forage production (Sejian et al. 2016). Studies done by Giridhar and Samireddypalle (2015) suggested that any climatic change has an adverse impact on productivity, quality of species, production of forage, and also the ecological roles of grasslands.

A dry spell over a long period also poses a great threat to pasture and feed supplies, as this leads to a decrease in the availability of quality forage to the grazing animals. Decreased precipitation and high temperature in the summer season in certain areas cause intense droughts, which may affect crop production and thus pose a significant problem for the animals that rely on grains for their food. So, it is evident that climate change has a negative impact on the animal production system.

11.3.2 Health of Animals

Change in climate may have a direct or indirect influence on animal health. Studies conducted by the National Research Council revealed that at a temperature above 30 °C, feed intake of cattle, sheep, goats, pigs, and chickens lessens by 3–5% with a single-degree rise in temperature. The secretion of stress hormones is also provoked by the temperature change. Reduced intake of feed due to prolonged exposure to high air temperature dwindles the production of catecholamines, growth hormones, and glucocorticoids. Studies done by Itoh et al. (1998a, b), Moore et al. (2005), and Sano et al. (1983, 1985) depicted the change in the metabolism of glucose, lipids, and proteins in animals that were under heat-stressed conditions. A decrease in the intake of feed and availability of forage leads to acute rumen acidosis, which increases the risk of laminitis and milk fat depression in animals. Heat stress impairs the protective value of the colostrum in cows and pigs. Animals require different types of nutrients such as minerals, vitamins, protein, and energy which vary with the region and the type of animal (Thornton et al. 2009). Any disruption in the availability of these nutrients due to heat stress affects both the process of digestion and metabolism in animals (Mader 2003). The deficiency of sodium and potassium in dairy cattle engenders metabolic alkalosis and increases the rate of respiration (Chase 2012). The reproductive capability of hens decreases because of heat stress, which has a significant effect on the production of eggs due to interference in the process of ovulation. Change in climatic conditions in the different regions of the world presents a great threat to the sustainability of animal production systems. Under cold stress conditions, animals overfeed on the protein-rich feed to increase the production of heat; howbeit it causes complications in the gastrointestinal tract. Increased temperature reduces the activity of chymotrypsin, trypsin, and amylase which decreases the nutrient digestibility in poultry (Amundson et al. 2006). An increase in the temperature of water jeopardizes the existence of various fish species.

Le Quesne and Pinnegar (2012) reported that ocean acidification decreases the development of otolith and calcified structures in fishes.

11.3.3 Reproduction in Animals

Unpredictable changes in the rainfall pattern and temperature influence the maturity and gonadal development of fishes during the breeding season. An increase in temperature influences the spawning and maturation of fishes. So the overall productivity of marine and freshwater ecosystems gets decreased due to any change in climatic conditions. The transfer of energy between the animal and its surrounding gets altered due to extreme changes in the climate which has an adverse effect on the reproduction in animals. The time period of the estrous cycle varies due to seasonal fluctuations in the environment of any animal. Heat and cold stress conditions bring down the rate of conception. Moreover, the functioning of the endocrine system also gets disrupted. Singh et al. (2013) reported that heat stress induces an increase in the secretion of adrenocorticotrophin hormone and cortisol that results in obstruction of sexual behavior induced by estradiol. According to Roth et al. (2000), ovarian follicles get damaged and are not able to survive when the temperature of the body surpasses 40 °C. Bilby et al. (2008) reported that high-temperature conditions lead to infertility due to an increase in the production of uterine PGF (2 alpha). In the cold season, the rate of conception was recorded to be 40–60%, whereas it decreases to 10–20% in hotter months (Cavestany et al. 1985). Balic et al. (2012) reported that an increase in temperature alters hormonal balance, sexual behavior, and quality of semen that has a significant impact on the overall reproductive performance of bulls. Seasonal infertility has also been reported in pigs because of the changes in photoperiod and temperature conditions (Auvigne et al. 2010), due to which the swine industry suffers a lot. Change in climate affects the process of reproduction in most of the fishes (Pankhurst and Munday 2011). According to Pankhurst and King (2010), in autumn-spawning fish species, increased temperature impedes the inception of ovulation, thus swaying the process of reproduction.

11.3.4 Diseases in Animals

The risk for the outbreak of diseases increases due to changes in the temperature of water systems; thus this may incur huge economic losses in the aquaculture sector. Prathap et al. (2017) reported that the temperature of the udder in dairy cows increases due to heat stress which is recognized as the fons et origo of mastitis disease. Animal productivity across the globe gets decreased by 25% due to various livestock diseases (Grace et al. 2015). Heat stress can lead to acidic conditions in the rumen of animals that cause lameness in dairy and beef cows (Cook and Nordlund 2009). A biting midge species, *Culicoides imicola*, serves as a vector for

11 Climate Change Impacts on Animal Production

Schmallenberg virus and bluetongue virus in ruminants, and the studies done by Wittmann et al. (2001) revealed that 2 °C rise in air temperature spreads this species tremendously. These animal viruses are proliferating at a faster rate due to change in climatic conditions. According to Caminade et al. (2019), with ascend in humidity to about 85%, reproduction in ticks increases; thus climate change accelerates tick infestation in animals. Clearing away of forests and decreasing the area under vegetation lead to an imbalance in the ecosystem due to an increase in humidity and temperature that augment the spread of vector-borne diseases. Fox et al. (2012) reported that the larvae of *Haemonchus contortus*, a nematode, show an increase in the development with the increase in temperature, thus causing severe anemic conditions in sheep as this worm is responsible for the bloodsucking from the stomach of the sheep. Animal diseases caused by the helminths are known to increase with climate change. According to data generated by WHO (2008), alterations in the climatic condition such as an increase in rainfall, temperature, and humidity can augment the spread of spores of *Bacillus anthracis* that cause anthrax disease in animals. Salinity affects the water that animals use for drinking purpose, thus causing diarrhea in animals. Alam et al. (2017) revealed that changes in the salinity of water bodies cause malfunctioning of the immune system and various diseases related to the skin in animals, thus having a negative impact on the health of animals. White et al. (2003) performed studies on Australian livestock and concluded that outbreak of ticks leads to an 18% decrease in the bodyweight of animals. In sheep, cutaneous myiasis increases with elevation in humid conditions and rainfall during the summer season (Sutherst 1990). Due to a surge in humidity and temperature, the developmental rate of parasites and the disease-causing organisms increases as reported by Mashaly et al. (2004). Thus, it can be concluded that the economy of the nation gets disturbed due to decreases in animal production owing to various diseases with climatic changes. The aquaculture sector gets equally affected by the change in the climate. Altered weather conditions have a negative influence on both the wild and cultured fish population due to an increase in susceptibility to sundry diseases. Elevated water temperature increases the risk of furunculosis and white spot disease in fishes (Lopez et al. 2010). Alteration in climatic conditions has a proclivity for various diseases in animals.

11.4 Impact of Climate Change on Animal Productivity

11.4.1 Milk Production

Heat stress has a great impact on animal productivity. Temperature-humidity index lesser than 68 is apt for the performance of cattle in a temperate climate (Gauly et al. 2013). The temperature-humidity index of approximately 72 is desirable for high milk-producing cows in the subtropical and tropical climate. Panting, sweating, and standing for long periods indicate heat stress in dairy cows (Koirala and Bhandari 2019) due to which the cows eat less forage. Both composition and the quality of milk decrease due to climatic changes. Various constituents of milk such as percentage of fat, amino acids, lactose, and casein content change due to an increase in the temperature of the body that influences the synthesis of fat in the mammary gland. Prathap et al. (2017) reported the production of milk is affected by the increase in temperature as it causes an imbalance of various hormones such as lactotropin, estrogen, birth hormone, growth hormone, and progesterone hormone. There is a decrease in milk production in the animals when the temperature increases above 35 °C (Wheelock et al. 2010). Valtorta et al. (2002) recorded a 10–14% reduction in the production of milk in dairy cows in response to heatwave conditions. Heat stress has a negative effect on the production of milk and meat. According to Bernabucci (2019), the hot environment negatively affects the quality of animal products besides its quantity. Summer et al. (2018) pointed out that both the organic and inorganic constituents of milk get affected by heat stress.

11.4.2 Wool Production

Unevenness in the rainfall pattern and concentration of carbon dioxide in the atmosphere affects the quantity and quality of forage available to the animals. The amount of water resources are declining, and so it is envisaged that the health of animals will be badly affected by increasing temperature. Alterations in the forage quality will lessen the productivity of clean wool. Reduction in the availability of pasturelands will affect the diameter and strength of wool fiber (Howden et al. 2004).

11.4.3 Poultry Production

Climate change has a similar impact on the poultry industry. Tankson et al. (2001) reported that an increase in temperature will decrease the body and carcass weight of poultry which has a significant impact on the energy and the protein content of the birds. Moreover, the rate of reproduction also declines due to climate changes. Obtrusion of ovulation and decrease in the feed intake affect egg production (Nardone et al. 2010). An increase in temperature also reduces the quality of eggs.

11.4.4 Meat Production

The findings of Nardone et al. (2010) have revealed that beef cattle with thick and dark color coats are at more risk of increased temperature. In ruminants, global warming can lessen down the size of the body, the thickness of fat, and the weight of the carcass. Lucas et al. (2000) observed that the survival rate of the young ones of pigs decreases when the temperature rises above 25 °C. Moreover, there will be a reduction in feed intake and carcass weight due to changes in climatic conditions.

11.5 Climate Change and Mortality

When the body temperature of an animal increases by 3 to 4 °C above normal, then it may lead to heatstroke, heat cramps, and organ dysfunction in animals. Extreme weather conditions increase the death rate among animals (Vitali et al. 2015). In the year 2003, during the summer season in Europe, thousands of poultry, pigs, and rabbits died due to severe heat waves. According to Howden et al. (2008), a rise in temperature between 1 °C and 5 °C above-average levels leads to high mortality in grazing animals. An increase in the death rate in Mecheri sheep was observed by Purusothaman et al. (2008) in India during the summer months due to thermal stress or heat stress conditions. Various events are on the record that depicts that extreme weather conditions increase the mortality rate in animals. In Ethiopia, a drought occurred in the years 1973–1974, which leads to mortality of 30% goats, 50% sheep, and 90% cattle due to a decrease in the availability of water and feed (Kidus, 2010). Elevated carbon dioxide concentration in water bodies has a detrimental impact on the growth and viability of early life stages of fishes that inhabit the bottom of water bodies as they do not possess a regulatory system for the maintenance of pH (Frommel et al. 2014).

11.6 Modeling and Simulation

Changing climate leads to precariousness in livestock production. Climate models apprise humans about the rising unevenness in the climate patterns. Climate change adaptation has gained huge attention, and it is managed by making high-tech innovations and new policies (Crane et al. 2011). Based on different climate scenarios, various models such as regional circulation models (RCMs), general circulation models (GCMs), economic models, etc. are used to depict the impact of changing climate in the near future (Hein et al. 2009; Olson et al. 2008). General circulation models figure out the potential causes of climate variability and project climatic variations in the coming decades. GCMs are also called global climate models. Sutherst et al. (1999) and Sutherst (2000) described CLIMEX, a bioclimatic modeling software that validates the evolution of models which outline the abundance and distribution of any species based on climate. Regional climate modeling (RCM) is another alternative for global modeling, which simulates smaller portions instead of the entire globe. According to Maure et al. (2018), CORDEX regional climate models predicted that the western part of South Africa will receive less rainfall and heat waves will increase that have a negative impact on various productivity sectors like utilization of wildlife, apiculture, the fisheries sector, and livestock as the effective temperature for living species may surpass. Harrison et al. (2016) utilized farm systems and economic modeling for predicting the effects of climate change on the production and economy of dairy products. They used historical climate data and regional climate change projections for the years 2040 and 2080 to determine the upcoming climate conditions. Biophysical modeling has been used to predict the impact of climate change on consumption of pasturelands, additional feeding, and milk productivity and also determines the risks to the corporate sectors that are related to varying prices of milk and other input costs (Harrison et al. 2017). Global Livestock Environment Assessment Model (GLEAM) has been developed by the Food and Agriculture Organization (2020) that quantifies the productivity and utilization of natural resources in the animal production sector. This model identifies the impact of environmental changes on the animals, thus contributing toward the evaluation of alteration and reduction scenarios to develop a more sustainable animal sector. This modeling framework can be used both at the regional and global levels.

11.7 Adaptation Options

Changing climate conditions undoubtedly have a negative impact on the health of animals. Under the conditions of heat stress, modifications in the diet composition in such a way that it either increases the feed intake by animals or compensates for the less consumption of feed can help in improving animal productivity. Alteration in the frequency and time of feeding can help in eluding excessive load of heat and thus increases the chances of survival, particularly in poultry (Renaudeau et al. 2012). Efficient cooking systems can be applied to decrease heat stress in animals. A combination of cooling with other treatments can be used to ameliorate the fertility rate in heat-stressed livestock (Bernabucci 2019). Climate change induces heat stress, increases the incidence of disease, and brings a reduction in the availability of the pasturelands, and the livestock tolerates these environmental constraints through morphological, behavioral, hormonal, biochemical, and cellular adaptation (Sejian et al. 2017). Adaptation strategies include modification both in the production and management systems, breeding practices, amendment in policies, advancement in technologies, and modifying the perception of farmers (Rowlinson et al. 2008; USDA 2013). According to IFAD (2010), integrating livestock animals with crop production and forestry and altering the time and site of farm operations acts as an adaptative measure for livestock production. Diverseness of livestock and variety of crops can surge the tolerance for heatwaves and dry spell which intensifies the production of livestock even when the animals are vulnerable to stresses of temperature and rainfall. Besides this, crop and livestock animal diversity are effectual in combating the diseases related to climate change (Batima et al. 2005; Kurukulasuriya and Rosenthal 2003). According to the studies conducted by Renaudeau et al. (2012), Thornton and Herrero (2010), and Havlík et al. (2013), changes in feeding practices such as alteration of diet composition, modification of

11 Climate Change Impacts on Animal Production

feeding time, and inclusion of agro-sylviculture species in the diet of animals can help them to adapt in the changing climate conditions. All these practices lessen the risk of changing climate by reducing feed insecurity during drought conditions, decreasing extreme heat load, and reducing malnutrition and death rate in animals. Transition in breeding practices can surge the tolerance for heat stress and diseases in animals by ameliorating their breeding and growth (Henry et al. 2012). The development of genebanks can enhance the breeding programs which will act as an insurance policy for livestock animals (Thornton et al. 2008).

11.8 Conclusion

Certain steps are required to be taken by the government by focusing on the advancement to lessen the effect of climate change on the livestock and aquaculture sector. Climate change is viewed as a substantial threat to the continuance of life on the earth, and it is one of the serious challenges of this century. The cognizance of change in climate conditions and their impact on animal health is very limited across the world. Climatic events have a serious impact on the biotic components of the ecosystem. It is necessary to understand the alterations in climate, and certain policies should be developed in response to these climatic variations. Varieties of fodder that are resistant to drought-like conditions need to be developed so that good-quality feed remains available to the animals. Shelter for animals should be designed in such a way, keeping in mind the heat stress, comfort, and behavior of animals (Ali et al. 2020). Climate alterations jeopardize the existence of the livestock system. Adaptation to climate changes and framing various policies at the regional, national, and international levels are ultra-critical to defend animal production. One of the most propitious adaptations is to use various crop varieties as feed for the livestock (Downing et al. 2017). Diversification of feed increases the tolerance toward the alterations in climate changes. Advanced technologies can be utilized to link data on climate change with the outbreak of various diseases.

Acknowledgments The authors would like to thank the Government of India (GOI) for providing necessary facilities under FIST, PURSE, and RUSA programs. The valuable suggestions and help provided by the Head, Department of Zoology, University of Jammu, are duly acknowledged.

References

Alam MZ, Carpenter-Boggs L, Mitra S, Haque M, Halsey J, Rokonuzzaman M, Saha B, Moniruzzaman M (2017) Effect of salinity intrusion on food crops, livestock, and fish species at Kalapara Coastal Belt in Bangladesh. J Food Qual:1–23
Alexandratos N, Bruinsma J (2002) World agriculture towards 2030/2050: the 2012 revision. ESA working paper No. 12-03

Ali MZ, Carlile G, Giasuddin M (2020) Impact of global climate change on livestock health: Bangladesh perspective. Open Veterinary J 10(2):178–188

Amundson JL, Mader TL, Rasby RJ, Hu QS (2006) Environmental effects on pregnancy rate in beef cattle. J Anim Sci 84:3415–3420

Attia-Ismail SA (2020) Influence of climate changes on animal feed production, the problems and the suggested solutions. In: EwisOmran ES, Negm A (eds) Climate change impacts on agriculture and food security in Egypt. Springer Water. Springer, Cham

Auvigne V, Leneveu P, Jehannin C, Peltoniemi O, Sallé E (2010) Seasonal infertility in sows: a five year field study to analyze the relative roles of heat stress and photoperiod. Theriogenology 74: 60–66

Bagath M, Krishnan G, Devaraj C, Rashamol VP, Pragna P, Lees AM, Sejian V (2019) The impact of heat stress on the immune system in dairy cattle: a review. Res Vet Sci 126:94–102

Balic IM, Milinkovic-Tur S, Samardzija M, Vince S (2012) Effect of age and environmental factors on semen quality, glutathione peroxidase activity and oxidative parameters in Simmental bulls. Theriogenology 78(2):423–431

Batima P, Bat B, Tserendash L, Bayarbaatar S, Shiirev-Adya S, Tuvaansuren G, Natsagdorj, L, Chuluun T (2005) Adaptation to climate change, vol. 90. ADMON Publishing, Ulaanbaatar

Bernabucci U (2019) Climate change: impact on livestock and how can we adapt. Anim Front 9(1): 3–5. https://doi.org/10.1093/af/vfy039

Bilby TR, Baumgard LH, Collier RJ, Zimbelman RB, Rhoads ML (2008) Heat stress effects on fertility: consequences and possible solutions. The proceedings of the 2008 South Western nutritional conference

Bindoff NL, Willebrand J, Artale V et al (2007) Observation, oceanic climate change and sea level. In: Solomon S, Qin D, Manning M, Chen Z, Marquis M, Averyt KB, Tignor M, Miller HL (eds) Climate change 2007: the physical science basis. Contribution of working group I to the fourth assessment report of the Intergovernmental Panel on Climate Change. Cambridge University Press, Cambridge, pp 385–432

Brewer PG, Peltzer ET (2009) Limits to marine life. Science 324:347–348

Caminade C, McIntyre KM, Jones AE (2019) Impact of recent and future climate change on vector-borne diseases. Ann N Y Acad Sci 137:119–129

Cavestany D, El-Whishy AB, Foot RH (1985) Effect of season and high environmental temperature on fertility of Holstein cattle. J Dairy Sci 68(6):1471–1478

Chand R, Raju SS (2008) Livestock sector composition and factors affecting its growth Ind. Jn of Agri Econ 63(2):1–13

Chase LE (2012) Climate change impacts on dairy cattle. Climate change and agriculture: Promoting practical and profitable responses. http://www.climateandfarming.org/pdfs/FactSheets/III.3 Cattle.pdf. Accessed 12 Feb 2013

Cook NB, Nordlund KV (2009) The influence of the environment on dairy cow behavior, claw health and herd lameness dynamics. Vet J 179:360–369

Crane TA, Roncoli C, Hoogenboom G (2011) Adaptation to climate change and climate variability: the importance of understanding agriculture as performance. NJAS Wageningen J Life Sci 57: 179–185

Das R, Sailo L, Verma N, Bharti P, Saikia J, Imtiwati KR (2016) Impact of heat stress on health and performance of dairy animals: a review. Vet World 9(3):260–268

Delgado C (2003) Rising consumption of meat and milk in developing countries has created a new food revolution. J Nutr 133:3907S–3910S

Delgado C (2005) Rising demand for meat and milk in developing countries: implications for grasslands-based livestock production. In: McGilloway DA (ed) Grassland: a global resource. Wageningen Academic Publisher, The Netherlands, pp 29–39

Downing MMR, Nejadhashemi AP, Harrigan T, Woznicki SA (2017) Climate change and livestock: impacts, adaptation, and mitigation. Clim Risk Manag 16:145–163

11 Climate Change Impacts on Animal Production

Dzavo T, Zindove TJ, Dhliwayo CM (2019) Effects of drought on cattle production in sub-tropical environments. Trop Anim Health Product Health 51:669–675. https://doi.org/10.1007/s11250-018-1741-1

Ehleringer JR, Cerling TE et al (eds) (2005) A history of atmospheric CO_2 and its effects on plants, animals, and ecosystems. Springer, New York

Ellis JE, Swift DM (1988) Stability of African pastoral ecosystems: alternate paradigms and implications for development. Rangeland Ecol Manage/J Range Manage Arch 41(6):450–459

FAO (2020) Global Livestock Environmental Assessment Model (GLEAM). http://www.fao.org/gleam/en/

Filipe JF, Herrera V, Curone G, Vigo D, Riva F (2020) Floods, hurricanes, and other catastrophes: a challenge for the immune system of livestock and other animals. Front Vet Sci 7:1–8

Fox NJ, Marion G, Davidson RS, White PC, Hutchings MR (2012) Livestock helminths in a changing climate: approaches and restrictions to meaningful predictions. Animals 2:93–107

Frommel AY, Maneja R, Lowe D, Pascoe CK, Geffen AJ, Folkvord A, Piatkowski U, Clemmesen C (2014) Organ damage in Atlantic herring larvae as a result of ocean acidification. Ecol Appl 24:1131–1143

Gauly M, Bollwein H, Breves G, Brugemann K, Danicke S, Das G, Demeler J, Hansen H, Isselstein J, Knnig S, Loholter M, Martinsohn M, Meyer U, Potthoff M, Sanker C, Schroder B, Wrage N, Meibaum B (2013) Future consequences and challenges for dairy cow production systems arising from climate change in Central Europe. Animal 7:843–859

Giridhar K, Samireddypalle A (2015) Impact of climate change on forage availability for livestock. In: climate change impact on livestock: adaptation and mitigation

Godber OF, Wall R (2014) Livestock and food security: vulnerability to population growth and climate change. Glob Chang Biol 20(10):3092–3102

Grace D, Bett B, Lindahl J, Robinson T (2015) Climate and livestock disease: assessing the vulnerability of agricultural systems to livestock pests under climate change scenarios. CCAFS Working Paper no. 116. Copenhagen, Denmark: CGIAR Research Program on Climate Change, Agriculture and Food Security (CCAFS)

Greer AW (2008) Trade-offs and benefits: implications of promoting a strong immunity to gastrointestinal parasites in sheep. Parasite Immunol 30:123–132

Hakala JP, Hartman KJ (2004) Drought effect on stream morphology and brook trout (*Salvelinus fontinalis*) populations in forested headwater streams. Hydrobiologia 515:203–213

Harrison MT, Cullen BR, Rawnsley RP (2016) Modelling the sensitivity of agricultural systems to climate change and extreme climatic events. Ag.Sys 148:135–148. https://doi.org/10.1016/j.agsy.2016.07.006

Harrison MT, Cullen BR, Armstrong DP (2017) Management options for Australian dairy farms under climate change: effects of intensification, adaptation and simplification on pastures, milk production and profitability. Ag Sys 155:19–32. https://doi.org/10.1016/j.agsy.2017.04.003

Havlík P, Valin H, Mosnier A, Obersteiner M, Baker JS, Herrero M, Rufino MC, Schmid E (2013) Crop productivity and the global livestock sector: implications for land use change and greenhouse gas emissions. Am J Agric Econ 95:442–448

Hein L, Metzger MJ, Leemans R (2009) The local impacts of climate change in the Ferlo, Western Sahel. Clim Chang 93:465–483

Henry B, Charmley E, Eckard R, Gaughan JB, Hegarty R (2012) Livestock production in a changing climate: adaptation and mitigation research in Australia. Crop Pasture Sci 63:191–202

Hidosa D, Guyo M (2017) Climate change effects on livestock feed resources: a review. J Fisheries Livest Prod 5(4):1–4

Hoffman MT, Vogel C (2008) Climate change impacts on African rangelands. Rangelands 30:12–17

Holochek JL, Peiper RD, Herbel CH (1989) Range management: principles and practices, 501 p. Prentice-Hall, Inc., Englewood Cliffs

Hopper GW, Gido KB, Pennock CA, Hedden SC, Frenette BD, Barts N, et al. (2020). Nowhere to swim: Interspecific responses of prairie stream fishes in Isolated Pools during severe drought. AquatSci 82. https://doi.org/10.1007/s00027-020-0716-2

Howden SM, Harle KJ, Dunlop M, Hunt L (2004) The potential impact of climate change on wool growing in 2029 a research brief conducted by CSIRO sustainable ecosystems for future Woolscapes 1–27

Howden SM, Crimp SJ, Stokes CJ (2008) Climate change and Australian livestock systems: impacts, research and policy issues. Aust J Exp Agric 48:780–788

Hurst P, Termine P, Karl M (2005) Agricultural workers and their contribution to sustainable agriculture and rural development. FAO, Rome

IFAD (International Fund for Agricultural Development) (2010) Livestock and climate change. http://www.ifad.org/lrkm/events/cops/papers/climate.pdf

International Fund for Agricultural Development (2007) Livestock and climate change. In: Rota A (ed) Livestock thematic papers: tools for project design. International Fund for Agricultural Development, Rome, pp 2–4

Itoh F, Obara Y, Rose MT, Fuse H, Hashimoto H (1998a) Insulin and glucagon secretion in lactating dairy cows due to heat exposure. J Anim Sci 76:2182–2189

Itoh F, Obara Y, Rose MT, Fuse H (1998b) Heat influence on plasma insulin and glucagon in response to secretogogues in non-lactating dairy cows. Dom Anim Endocrinol 15:499–510

James DA, Wilhite JW, Chipps SR (2010) Influence of drought conditions on brown trout biomass and size structure in the Black Hills, South Dakota. N Am J Fish Manag 30:791–798

Jaya KS, Sinha B, Sinha SK, Paswan JK (2016) Focusing biotic stress in livestock. Indian Farmer 3(11):812–814

Kabubo-Mariara J (2009) Global warming and livestock husbandry in Kenya: impacts and adaptations. Ecol Econ 68:1915–1924

Kanwal V, Sirohi S, Chan P (2020) Effect of drought on livestock enterprise: evidence from Rajasthan. Ind J Anim Sci 90(1):94–98

Karaca AG, Parker HM, Yeatman JB, McDaniel CD (2002) Role of seminal plasma in heat stress infertility of broiler breeder males. Poult Sci 81:1904–1909

Kaylor MJ, VerWey BJ, Cortes A, Dana R (2019) Warren Drought impacts to trout and salamanders in cool, forested headwater ecosystems in the western Cascade Mountains, OR. Hydrobiologia 833:65–80

Kidus M (2010) The negative impact of climate change on Ethiopia

Knighton AD, Nanson GC (2000) Waterhole form and process in the Anastomosing Channel system of Cooper Creek, Australia. Geomorphology 35:101–117. https://doi.org/10.1016/S0169-555X(00)00026-X

Koirala A, Bhandari P (2019) Impact of climate change on livestock production. Nepalese Vet J 36: 178–183

Kunavongkrita A, Suriyasomboonb A, Lundeheimc N, Learda TW, Einarsson S (2005) Management and sperm production of boars under differing environmental conditions. Theriogenology 63:657–667

Kurukulasuriya P, Rosenthal S (2003) Climate change and agriculture: a review of impacts and adaptations. Climate change series paper no. 91. World Bank, Washington DC

Le Quesne WJF, Pinnegar JK (2012) The potential impacts of ocean acidification: scaling from physiology to fisheries. Fish Fish 13(3):333–344

Liverpool-Tasie LSO, Sanou A, Tambo JA (2019) Climate change adaptation among poultry farmers: evidence from Nigeria. Clim Chang 157:527–544. https://doi.org/10.1007/s10584-019-02574-8

Lohölter M, Meyer U, Döll S, Manderscheid R, Weigel HJ, Erbs M, Höltershinken M, Flachowsky G, Dänicke S (2012) Effects of the thermal environment on metabolism of deoxynivalenol and thermoregulatory response of sheep fed on corn silage grown at enriched atmospheric carbon dioxide and drought. Mycotoxin Res 28(4):219–227. https://doi.org/10.1007/s12550-012-0137-8

Lopez MM, Gale P, Oidtmann B, Peeler E (2010) Assessing the impact of climate change on disease emergence in freshwater fish in the United Kingdom. Transbound Emerg Dis 57(5): 293–304

Lucas EM, Randall JM, Meneses JF (2000) Potential for evaporative cooling during heat stress periods in pig production in Portugal. J Agric Eng Res 76:363–371

Mader TL (2003) Environmental stress in confined beef cattle. J Anim Sci 81:110–119

Mashaly MM, Hendricks GL, Kalama MA (2004) Effect of heat stress on production parameters and immune responses of commercial laying hens. Poult Sci 83:889–894

Maure G, Pinto I, Ndebele-Murisa M, Muthige M, Lennard C, Nikulin G, Dosio A, Meque A (2018) The southern African climate under 1.5°C and 2°C of global warming as simulated by CORDEX regional climate models environ. Res. Lett 13:065002

Mayorga EJ, Renaudeau D, Ramirez BC, Ross JW, Baumgard LH (2019) Heat stress adaptations in pigs. Anim Front 9(1):54–61

McIntyre KM, Setzkorn C, Hepworth PJ, Morand S, Morse AP, Baylis M (2017) Systematic assessment of the climate sensitivity of important human and domestic animals pathogens in Europe. Sci Rep 7:1–10. https://doi.org/10.1038/s41598-017-06948-9

Moore CE, Kay JK, VanBaale MJ, Collier RJ, Baumgard LH (2005) Effect of conjugated linoleic acid on heat stressed Brown Swiss and Holstein cattle. J Dairy Sci 88:1732–1740

Nanson GCGC, Tooth S, Knighton AD (2002) A global perspective on dryland rivers: perceptions, misconceptions and distinctions. In Bull L, Kirby M (eds) Dryland rivers: hydrology and geomorphology of semi-arid channels. Wiley, Chichester, pp. 17–54. Available at: https://books.google.gr/books?id=qjHoYZXQee0C

Nardone A, Ronchi B, Lacetera N, Ranieri MS, Bernabucci U (2010) Effects of climate change on animal production and sustainability of livestock systems. Livest Sci 130:57–69

O'Connor LJ, Walkden-Brown SW, Kahn LP (2006) Ecology of the free-living stages of major trichostrongylid parasites of sheep. Vet Parasitol 142:1–15

Oba G, Kotile DG (2001) Assessments of landscape level degradation in southern Ethiopia: pastoralists versus ecologists. Land Degrad Dev 12(5):461–475

Olson JM, Alagarswamy G, Andresen JA, Campbell DJ, Davis AY, Ge J, Huebner M, Lofgren BM, Lusch DP, Moore NJ (2008) Integrating diverse methods to understand climate-land interactions in East Africa. Geoforum 39:898–911

Owensby CE, Cochran RM, Auen LM (1996) Effects of elevated carbon dioxide on forage quality for ruminants. In: Koerner C, Bazzaz F (eds) Carbon dioxide, populations, and communities. Academic Press, Physiologic Ecology Series, pp 363–371

Pankhurst NW, King HR (2010) Temperature and salmonid reproduction: implications for aquaculture. J Fish Biol 76:69–85

Pankhurst NW, Munday PL (2011) Effects of climate change on fish reproduction and early life history stages. Mar Freshw Res 62:1015–1026

Patterson CD, Guerin MT (2013) The effects of climate change on avian migratory patterns and the dispersal of commercial poultry diseases in Canada-Part I. Worlds Poultry Sci J 69:17–26. https://doi.org/10.1017/S0043933913000020

Percy KE, Awmack CS et al (2002) Altered performance of forest pests under atmospheres enriched by CO_2 and O_3. Nature 420:403–407

Popp A, Lotze-Campen H, Bodirsky B (2010) Food consumption, diet shifts and associated non-CO_2 greenhouse gases from agricultural production. Glob Environ Chang 20:451–462

Prathap P, Archana PR, Joy A, Veerasamy S, Krishnan G, Bagath M, Manimaran V (2017) Heat stress and dairy cow: impact on both milk yield and composition. Int J Dairy Sci 12:1–11

Purusothaman MR, Thiruvenkadan AK, Karunanithi K (2008) Seasonal variation in body weight and mortality rate in Mecheri adult sheep. Livest Res Rural Dev 20(9):1–6

Rae AN (1998) The effects of expenditure growth and urbanisation on food consumption in East Asia: a note on animal products. Agric Econ 18:291–299

Renaudeau D, Collin A, Yahav S, de Basilio V, Gourdine JL, Collier RJ (2012) Adaptation to hot climate and strategies to alleviate heat stress in livestock production. Animal 6(5):707–728. https://doi.org/10.1017/S1751731111002448

Rosegrant MW, Fernandez M, Sinha A, Alder J, Ahammad H, de Fraiture Charlotte, Eickhour, B, Fonseca J, Huang J, Koyama O, Omezzine AM, Pingali P, Ramirez R, Ringler C, Robinson S, Thornton P, van Vuuren D, Yana-Shapiro H (2009) Looking into the future for agriculture and AKST. In: McIntyre BD, Herren HR, Wakhungu J, Watson RT (eds) International assessment of agricultural knowledge, science and Technology for Development (IAASTD): agriculture at a crossroads, global report. Island Press, Washington, DC, pp 307–376

Roth Z, Meidan R, Braw-Tal R, Wolfenson D (2000) Immediate and delayed effects of heat stress on follicular development and its association with plasma FSH and inhibin concentration in cows. J Reprod Fertil 120(1):83–90

Rowlinson P, Steele M, Nefzaoui A (2008) Livestock and global climate change: adaptation I and II. In: Rowlinson P, Steel M, Nefzaoui A (eds) Livestock and global climate change conference proceeding. Cambridge University Press, Tunisia, pp 56–85

Salmoral G, Ababio B, Holman IP (2020) Drought impacts, coping responses and adaptation in the UK outdoor livestock sector: insights to increase drought resilience. Land 9:202. https://doi.org/10.3390/land9060202

Sano H, Takahashi K, Ambo K, Tsuda T (1983) Turnover and oxidation rates of blood glucose and heat production in sheep exposed to heat. J Dairy Sci 66:856–861

Sano H, Ambo K, Tsuda T (1985) Blood glucose kinetics in whole body and mammary gland of lactating goats exposed to heat. J Dairy Sci 68:2557–2564

Schaub S, Finger R (2020) Effects of drought on hay and feed grain prices. Environ. Res. Lett.15: 034014

Sejian V, Hyder I, Maurya VP, Bagath M, Krishnan G, Aleena J, Archana PR, Lees AM, Kumar D, Bhatta R, Naqvi SMK (2017) Adaptive mechanisms of sheep to climate change. In: Sejian V, Bhatta R, Gaughan J, Malik P, Naqvi S, Lal R (eds) Sheep production adapting to climate change. Springer, Singapore, pp 117–147. https://doi.org/10.1007/978-981-10-4714-5_5

Sejian V, Gaughan JB, Bhatta R, Naqvi SMK (2016) Impact of climate change on livestock productivity. Broadening Horizons, Feedipedia

Semple AT (1970).Grassland improvement. CRC Press, Cleveland pp 1–400

Singh M, Chaudhari BK, Singh JK, Singh AK, Maurya PK (2013) Effects of thermal load on buffalo reproductive performance during summer season. J Biol Sci 1(1):1–8

Smit HJ, Metzger MJ, Ewert F (2008) Spatial distribution of grassland productivity and land use in Europe. Agric Syst 98:208–219

Steinfeld H, Gerber P, Wassenaar T, Castel V, Rosales M, de Haan C (2006) Livestock's long shadow: environmental issues and options. FAO, Rome

Summer A, LoraI FP, Gottardo F (2018) Impact of heat stress on milk and meat production. Anim Front 9(1):39–46

Sutherst RW (1990) Impact of climate change on pests and diseases in Australasia. Search 21(7): 230–232

Sutherst RW (2000) Climate change and invasive species—a conceptual framework," in Invasive species in a changing world, H. A. Mooney and R. J. Hobbs, Eds., pp. 211–240, Island Press, Washington, DC

Sutherst RW, Maywald GF, Yonow T, Stevens PM (1999) CLIMEX® predicting the effects of climate on plants and animals. CSIRO Publishing, Collingwood

Tankson JD, Vizzier-Thaxton Y, Thaxton JP, May JD, Cameron JA (2001) Stress and nutritional quality of broilers. Poult Sci 80:1384–1389

Thomas JF, Harvey CN (1983) Leaf anatomy of four species grown under continuous CO_2 enrichment. Bot Gaz 144:303–309

Thornton PK, Gerber P (2010) Climate change and the growth of the livestock sector in developing countries. Mitigation Adapt Strateg Glob Change 15:169–184

Thornton PK, Herrero M (2010) The inter-linkages between rapid growth in livestock production, climate change, and the impacts on water resources, land use, and deforestation. World Bank policy research working paper, WPS 5178. World Bank, Washington, DC

Thornton PK, Jones PG, Owiyo TM, Kruska RL, Herrero M, Kristjanson P, Notenbaert A, Bekele N, Orindi V, Otiende B, Ochieng A, Bhadwal S, Anantram K, Nair S, Kumar V, Kulkar U (2006) Mapping climate vulnerability and poverty in Africa. 200p. Nairobi (Kenya): ILRI

Thornton PK, Herrero M, Freeman A, Mwai O, Rege E, Jones P, McDermott J (2008) Vulnerability, climate change and livestock: research opportunities and challenges for poverty alleviation. International Livestock Research Institute (ILRI), Kenya

Thornton PK, Van de Steeg J, Notenbaert A, Herrrero M (2009) The impacts of climate change on livestock and livestock systems in developing countries: a review of what we know and what we need to know. Agric Syst 101(3):113–127

Tubiello F, Schmidhuber J, Howden M, Neofotis PG, Park S, Fernandes E, Thapa D (2008) Climate change response strategies for agriculture: challenges and opportunities for the 21st century. The World Bank, Washington, DC

UNDP (United Nations Development Programme) (2008) Human development report 2007/2008: fighting climate change: human solidarity in a divided world. New York, USA

Urban MC (2015) Accelerating extinction risk from climate change. Science 348:571–573

USDA (United States Department of Agriculture) (2013) Climate change and agriculture in the United States: effects and adaptation. USDA Technical Bulletin, Washington, DC. http://www.usda.gov/oce/climate_change/effects_2012/CC%20and%20Agriculture%20Report%20%2802-04-2013%29b.pdf

Valtorta SE, Leva PE, Gallardo MR, Scarpati OE (2002) Milk production responses during heat wave event in Argentina. 15th conference on biometereology and aerobiology – 16th international congress on biometeorology, Kansas City, MO. American Meteorological Society, Boston, pp 98–101

Vertessy R, Barma D, Baumgartner L, Mitrovic S, Sheldon F, Bond N (2019) Independent assessment of the 2018–19 fish deaths in the lower darling. Australian Government, Canberra

Vicente-Serrano SM, Beguería S, Lopez J, Moreno I (2010) A multiscalar drought index sensitive to global warming: the standardized precipitation evapotranspiration index. J Clim 23:01696–01718. https://doi.org/10.1175/2009JCLI2909.1

Vitali A, Felici A, Esposito S, Bernabucci U, Bertocchi L, Maresca C, Nardone A, Lacetera N (2015) The impact of heat waves on dairy cow mortality. J Dairy Sci 98:4572–4579

Webber H et al (2018) Diverging importance of drought stress for maize and winter wheat in Europe. Nat Commun 9:4249

Wheelock JB, Rhoads RP, Van Baale MJ, Sanders SR, Baumgard LH (2010) Effect of heat stress on energetic metabolism in lactating Holstein cows. J Dairy Sci 93(2):644–655

White N, Sutherst RW, Hall N, Whish-Wilson P (2003) The vulnerability of the Australian beef industry to impacts of the cattle tick (*Boophilus microplus*) under climate change. Clim Chang 61:157–190

WHO (2008) Anthrax in humans and animals. World Health Organization, Geneva

Wittmann EJ, Mellor PS, Baylis M (2001) Using climate data to map the potential distribution of *Culicoides imicola* (Diptera: Ceratopogonidae) in Europe. Rev Sci Tech 20:731–740

Yatoo MI, Kumar P, Dimri U, Sharma MC (2012) Effects of climate change on animal health and diseases. Intl J Livestock Res 2(3):15–24

Yawson DO, Mulholland BJ, Ball T, Adu MO, Mohan S, White PJ (2017) Effect of climate and agricultural land use changes on UK feed barley production and food security to the 2050s. Land 6(74):1–14

Yitbarek MB (2019) Livestock and livestock product trends by 2050: review. Intl J Anim Res 4:1–30

Chapter 12
Climate Change and Global Insect Dynamics

Raman Jasrotia, Menakshi Dhar, Neha Jamwal, and Seema Langer

Abstract Diversification of insects has occurred through 450 million years of earth's fluctuating climate, yet swiftly deviating patterns of temperature and rainfall present unexpected obstacles along with the anthropogenic stresses. Climate variance and extreme weather events have a considerable impact on insect population dynamics. Insects are very sensitive to the ongoing climate warming. The temperature has a direct impact on the maintenance of essential life functions in insects such as survival, growth, development, metabolism, voltinism, and even availability of the host. A decrease in precipitation leads to drought-like conditions, which affect the abundance and diversity of soil insects. Global warming supports the manifestation of insect-transmitted plant diseases, and the population of the insect vectors gets increased. Research findings suggest that with a rise of temperature by 2 °C, insects experience more than the expected life cycles in a season. Elevation of carbon dioxide levels affects the behavior and production of insects as the host plant grown in such conditions is less nutritious for the insects. Alteration in the pattern of precipitation influences the insect pest predators, parasites, and diseases emanating in complex dynamics. Climate change incites the change in insect dynamics across the globe, and every day about 45–275 species of insects are becoming extinct. Beetle incidence in a protected forest in New Hampshire, USA, has decreased by 83% in a resampling project spanning 45 years, apparently as a function of warmer temperatures and reduced snowpack. In a subarctic forest in Finland, negative associations with a warming climate were detected for subsets of the moth fauna to name a few. Climate change is itself not one phenomenon but includes a shift in limits (both maxima and minima), average condition, and variance. Hence, multidisciplinary actions are required to be taken for solving the menace of climate change that has a direct or indirect effect on insect diversity.

Keywords Climate variance · Extinct · Global warming · Insect dynamics · Metabolism

---

R. Jasrotia (✉) · M. Dhar · N. Jamwal · S. Langer
Department of Zoology, University of Jammu, Jammu, Jammu & Kashmir, India

© The Author(s), under exclusive license to Springer Nature Switzerland AG 2022
M. Ahmed (ed.), *Global Agricultural Production: Resilience to Climate Change*,
https://doi.org/10.1007/978-3-031-14973-3_12

12.1 Introduction

Global climatic alteration has created chaos all over the world, threatening not only plants or animals but also entire life forms on this planet. From declining polar ice caps to dwindling biodiversity, everything on earth has started receding at an unimaginable rate. It has been estimated that the global average temperature will hit 1–4.5 °C hike in the coming 100 years (IPCC 2014) mainly due to increased surface temperature, variable precipitation, increase in carbon dioxide (CO_2) concentration, and their interactions among them (Nayak et al. 2020).

The change in climate due to several natural and anthropogenic factors (Fig. 12.1) has led to various discernible changes like floods and droughts all across the globe, and it has been estimated that the growing rate of climate change will have a very strong impact on agriculture mostly in agro-based countries, for instance, India where almost one-third of the population is reliant on agriculture. According to the Economic Survey of India (2018) report, a reduction in annual agricultural income by 15–18% due to change in agricultural productivity as a result of climate change is foreseen. In these changing climatic circumstances, knowledge about insect dynamics is cardinal to draw up effectual strategies to counter the impact of climate change. Insects belong to that particular group of organisms that most likely do not utilize their metabolism for the maintenance of body temperature but depend upon surrounding temperature conditions for their successful development, reproduction, and survival, i.e., poikilothermic (Bale et al. 2002). Insects are highly responsive to even slight changes in temperature conditions as it dominates certain life events like growth and development, physiology, behavior, and relationship with other species as well. These climatic changes may not always be harmful to insects, but in some

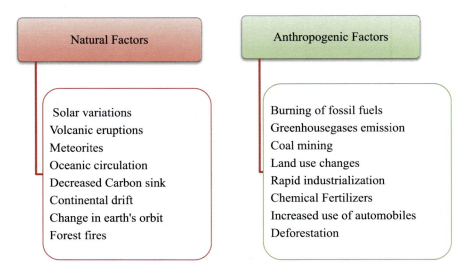

Fig. 12.1 Factors responsible for climate change

12 Climate Change and Global Insect Dynamics

cases, these also prove beneficial for the insect populations depending upon their role in animal, plant, or human health (Sharma 2010; War et al. 2016).

Since insects have a variably shorter life span and high reproductive rate than other animals and plants, they show significant responses toward altering climate including contraction of geographical distribution besides all the developmental and behavioral changes. Climate change bears direct (Samways 2005; Parmesan 2007, Merrill et al. 2008; Nayak et al. 2020) as well as indirect (Harrington et al. 2001; Bale et al. 2002) effects on insect populations, and continuous monitoring of all the sensitive arthropod species gives the scientists an upper hand to understand the constant changes in biodiversity (Gregory et al. 2009). Climate change has been presumed to be the vital element for the wiping out of arthropod species (Butchart et al. 2005). Highly vulnerable are the species inhabiting cold regions (high altitude) because temperature warming has led to their forced shift uphill. Due to inhabitable conditions in high-altitude areas, eventually, many species have become extinct which is not easily detected until several hundred years (Sharma 2014). According to a report by Franco et al. (2006), climate change resulted in the extermination of four species of butterflies from lower reaches in the UK in over 25 years. In this global sixth extinction phase, driven largely due to anthropogenic activities, the current rate of extinction is 100–1000 times much more as compared to previous times. This climate change will soon devour the remaining species as nearly 45–275 species are vanishing each day (Sharma 2014). Habitat loss and the introduction of alien species, apart from extinction, are among the distinct drivers for the loss of species. The expected 80% pollination by insects (Pudasaini et al. 2015) considerably suffers from the hands-on climate change leading to poor yields and, ultimately, a threat to global food security. Global warming and climate alterations will highly dominate some important parameters in insect development and association (Fig. 12.2).

12.2 Insect Production Under Climatic Variability

Raising, breeding, and harvesting of insects as livestock are known as insect farming, microstock, or ministock. Insect farming is done to obtain various insect products. Honeybees belonging to the genus *Apis* are found across the globe even in different climatic conditions. There is an uneven distribution of these species. At present, the natural population of honeybees has shown a steep decline, and it has become a matter of great concern as this has led to a decrease in the production of various products that are obtained by the honeybees such as beeswax, honey, royal jelly, etc. Various factors as listed by Potts et al. (2010) such as the loss of habitat, use of pesticides, insecticides in agriculture, the introduction of invasive species, and climate change are responsible for the decline in the bee population. Changing climate poses a great risk even to the pollination services (Hegland et al. 2009; Schweiger et al. 2010). It is expected that because of the climatic change that occurs due to various anthropogenic activities, there will be an extinction of various insect

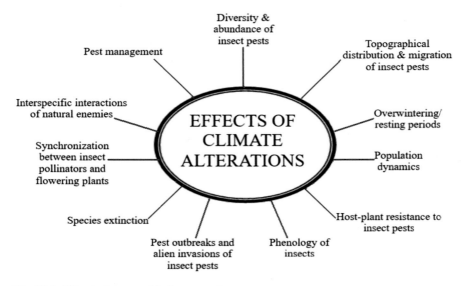

Fig. 12.2 Climate change and its impact on insects

species as both their survival and reproduction get hampered (Reddy et al. 2012). The most apt temperature for the rearing of the silkworm is about 24–28 °C. An increase in temperature and carbon dioxide concentration has a direct impact on the life cycle of the silkworm. To balance the declined levels of nutrition in the leaves of mulberry, silkworm feeds on a large number of such leaves, which may lead to an increase in its life cycle. Silkworm, being poikilotherms, is more sensitive to atmospheric temperature. Due to changes in climate and agricultural activities, insect pest scenario has also depicted huge changes (Neelaboina et al. 2018). Production of raw silk is more vulnerable to changing climate as it affects both the host plants and silkworm rearing technologies. It has been predicted that climate change will have a severe impact on the productivity of the silkworm host, rearing of a silkworm, and post-cocoon technology, which will further have a great influence on the country's economy. An increase of 20 °C or more mean temperature annually will have a severe impact on the sericulture practices in tropical regions. There will be a net revenue loss of 10–20% in sericulture across the temperate regions (Ram et al. 2016). Abiotic factors such as temperature, rainfall, and humidity have a great influence on the production of lac (Bhagat and Mishra 2002). Sharma (2007) and Thomas (2010) concluded that lac production is mainly affected by the change in temperature. In the years 2003–2004, 20,050 tonnes of lac was produced, but this production declined to 16,978 tonnes in 2014–2015 because of high temperature during summers (Pal 2009; Yogi et al. 2017). The occurrence of frequent droughts affects the lac sector equally. Changing climate creates a stressful environment, and it has been predicted to have a negative impact on the abundance and diversity of insect pests that will ultimately affect the extent of damage in crops that are economically important (Fand et al. 2012). Thus, across the world, the rate of biodiversity loss is increasing due to the negative effect of climate change.

12.3 Institutes Working on Insect Production Under Changing Climate

The International Platform of Insects for Food and Feed (IPIFF), which was created in 2012, has the main objective of promoting the broad use of insects as a protein-source alternative for consumption by humans and as animal feed. The organization actively supports the insect sector development. The main aim of IPIFF is to provide information regarding the benefits of eating insects by the general public. The Centre of Environment Sustainability through insect farming aims to achieve the goals of the growth of the insect industry. According to its leaders, insect farming provides an economical and sustainable path for the production of high-value protein. GREEiNSECT, a research project funded by Danida, Ministry of Foreign Affairs, works to investigate the use of selected species in insect farming which can play an important role in sustainable food security. They carry out research on mass rearing of insects and their contribution toward food security and generation of income. ICAR-National Bureau of Agricultural Insect Resources is a leading institution located in Bangalore that is involved in the collection, characterization, authentication, preservation, exchange, exploration, and application of insects that are important for the agricultural sector. The Institute of Entomology, Biology Centre, Czech Academy of Sciences (CAS), aims to work out the taxonomy, genetics, physiology, and ecology using a wide range of insects and model ecosystems. This institute aims to understand the effect of climate change on the composition and structure of arthropod species.

12.4 Quantification of Climate Change

Climate change is expected to bring about remarkable responses from various species of insects. In recent years, such responses have been detected already as reported by Hill et al. (2002), Battisti et al. (2005), and Netherer and Schopf (2010a, b). Any climatic change beyond the species tolerance leads to a shift in the life cycle events, individual density, and morphological forms, and some may even become extinct (Rosenzweig et al. 2007).

12.4.1 High Temperature

The biggest threat pounded by climate change is the rapid change in the relative abundance of insect species since they are unable to oppose harsh and stressful climatic conditions that may lead to their peril (Jump and Penuelas 2005). With the increase in temperature, the high-latitude or mountain resident insects are most likely to be coerced toward further high altitudes from their native places (Parmesan 2006; Menéndez 2007). Even after moving toward high altitude, they will eventually run out of the habitable area and may inescapably become extinct. Climate change has a significant impact in determining the geographical distribution of insect pests, and according to Hill (1987), low temperatures are more dominant than high temperatures in the distribution pattern. Increasing temperatures tend to impart greater ability in extending the geographical range of insect species that are inhibited by low temperatures at high latitudes to overwinter (Elphinstone and Toth 2008). Butterflies of North America and Europe have shown a range shift in their distribution as many species have shifted at high altitudes and toward the north due to climate change and global warming (Konvicka et al. 2003; Wilson et al. 2005). The same kind of northward and high-altitude distribution shift has been witnessed in the case of butterflies, beetles, aquatic bugs, dragonflies, and grasshoppers in the UK (Hickling et al. 2006) and corn earworm, *Helicoverpa zea*, in North America. Range expansion of pink bollworm, *Pectinophora gossypiella*, is sought due to warmer areas which will aid in its reach to colder areas which were otherwise intolerable to the pest (Gutiérrez et al. 2006). An expected movement of pod borers, *Helicoverpa armigera*, and *Maruca vitrata* from present tropical distribution in Asia, Africa, and Latin America to northern Europe and North America in the next 50 years is also predicted (Sharma 2010). Range expansion has more often been recorded than range contractions. Northward migration of *Nizara viridula* (green stinkbug) was studied by Musolin (2007), in Japan.

Insects going through winter diapause will be the ones that are likely to undergo major changes. Higher temperatures will lead to increased metabolism, consuming their reserved nutrient source much early, thereby leading to shortening of the duration of diapause or overwintering period. Delayed onset of diapause would be seen due to warming in winter periods, while early summer may lead to early cessation of diapause, thereby extending the life cycles of the insect pests. Every 2 °C rise in temperature is estimated to add one to five additional life cycles per season (Pandi et al. 2018) which will lead to agricultural damage and yield loss. With each degree of temperature rise, the yield loss would increase to another 10–25% (Shrestha 2019). This will ultimately lead to higher insect populations, thereby threatening food security to a wider extent. A study by Ouyang et al. (2016) deciphered up to 7 days earlier emergence in *Helicoverpa armigera* due to an increase in temperature. The rapid increase in the insect pest population may be attributed to the higher temperatures due to the considerable reduction of reproductive maturity in insects. The phenological changes in insects can be easily monitored since a slight climate change can lead to behavioral changes. For instance, high temperatures will lead to early adult emergence in insects, and the flight period will increase to significant levels (Menéndez 2007). Lepidopterans are known to exhibit the best examples of changes in phenology. A study by Roy and Sparks (2000) revealed that 26 species out of 35 species of butterflies in the UK showed early initial emergence. In Spain, 17 butterfly species proceeded their first appearance by

1–7 weeks in barely 15 years (Stefanescu et al. 2003). Similarly, 16 species of butterflies out of 23 (~70%) in California, USA, had advanced emergence by almost 8 days per 10 years (Forister and Shapiro 2003). Apart from butterflies, aphids were also reported to advance their emergence much prior to their actual period of emergence in the UK (Harrington et al. 2007). The increase in the temperature will aid in the early emergence of insects, leading to a higher number of life cycles per season and perhaps more damage to crops annually. Berg et al. (2006) reported that an increase in temperature has decreased the reproduction time by half in the spruce beetle, which has led to the damage of spruce forests.

12.4.2 Carbon Dioxide

Increased concentration of carbon dioxide has a marked influence on the plant phenotype (Curtis and Wang 1998). Elevated carbon dioxide concentration leads to an increase in photosynthesis rate, growth rate, and biomass (Norby et al. 1999; Owensby et al. 1999). This results in an increased ratio of carbon and nitrogen in the tissues as nitrogen concentration becomes diluted by 15–25% (Hughes and Bazzaz 1997). An increase in the concentration of carbon dioxide also lessens the water content of leaves and augments the rate of senescence in plants (Sicher and Bunce 1997), thus affecting the insects feeding on them. Insects having powerful and sharp mandibles such as crickets, grasshoppers, and larvae of the caterpillar are classified as leaf-chewing insects. It has been observed that such insects eat up more areas of the leaf when they feed on the plants that are cultivated under elevated carbon dioxide concentrations (Lindroth et al. 1995). On similar lines, the insects that feed within the leaf are called leaf miners, and they also damage more area of the leaf which is grown under elevated carbon dioxide concentration due to a decrease in nitrogen concentration (Salt et al. 1995). Thus in response to elevated concentration of carbon dioxide, the consumption level of insects rises. Coviella and Trumble (1999) reported that due to elevated atmospheric carbon dioxide levels, insects feeding on plants will tackle host plants that are less nutritious, and this will lead to an increase in the larval developmental period and may even surge the death rate in some cases. Moreover, it also lessens the efficiency of ingestion of food in insects as reported by Fajer (1989). Performance of herbivore insects as investigated by Zvereva and Kozlov (2010) shows a positive correlation with a nitrogen concentration of the leaf, and under elevated carbon dioxide, nitrogen, and water content, this decreases both in collard and mustard plants. Cabbage white butterfly causes more damage to the leaf structure of the plant grown under increased carbon dioxide concentration (Hamilton et al. 2005). Fewer herbivore insects were found on the plants that were not grown in ambient carbon dioxide concentration. Thus, it can be concluded that the plants grown under elevated carbon dioxide levels provide less nutrition to the insects, which has a direct effect on their performance and behavior. Elevation in CO_2 decreases the nutritional content of plant leaves by decreasing the concentration of proteins and amino acids (Johnson et al. 2020). The performance of

Helicoverpa armigera declines when exposed to elevated CO_2 concentration due to a decrease in the nutritional chemistry of the host plant. Tocco et al. (2021) found that the dung beetle, *Euoniticellus intermedius*, on exposure to elevated atmospheric carbon dioxide shows an increase in the developmental period and death rate of the beetle. The rise in CO_2 levels also reduces the size and mass of an adult beetle which affects its fitness. Elevated levels of carbon dioxide have an indirect effect on the leaf chemistry due to which the palatability of the leaves also decreases (Bezemer and Jones 1998). The meta-analysis of the effect of elevated carbon dioxide concentration on the insects was done by Stiling and Cornelissen (2007), and they found that under elevated carbon dioxide concentration, an abundance of insects declines by approximately 22.0%, the consumption rate of plants by insects increases by almost 17.0%, the development time increases by about 4.0%, the relative growth rate depicted a decline of 9.0%, and pupal weight decreased by 5.0%. Elevated carbon dioxide raise the mean annual temperature from 10.5 to 20.1 °C, and the damage to plant leaves increase the levels of leaf sugars by 31% which led to a significant rise in the density (DeLucia et al. 2008). At elevated carbon dioxide, the levels of leaf sugars increase by 31% that leads to a significant rise in the density of Japanese beetle. Hematophagous insects show a direct response to carbon dioxide (Guerenstein and Hildebrand 2008), whereas herbivore arthropods are affected by the altered leaf chemistry that occurs due to a rise in carbon dioxide levels (Cornelissen 2011). In addition to increasing temperatures and humidity, increased CO_2 levels also greatly influence the host-plant interaction. Gregory et al. (2009) deciphered that a high level of CO_2 will, no doubt, increase plant growth and productivity, but it may tend to increase the level of damage caused by herbivorous insects. However, in the case of enriched CO_2 environments, nitrogen-based defenses will tend to decrease, while carbon-based defense will increase slightly (Sharma 2014). This host-plant interaction is detrimental for insects practicing monophagy (single host plant) since depletion of a single host will lead to questionable sustenance of monophagous insects. For instance, the gypsy moth *Lymantria dispar* feeds on *Quercus rubra* (red oak) and *Quercus velutina* (black oak). If the eggs of gypsy moth hatch before budding in the oak plant, the larvae will end up starving, and if eggs hatch extremely late after budding, it will lead to reduced fecundity as the foliage quality will reduce sharply (Ward and Masters 2007).

12.4.3 Drought

Drought is one of the biggest challenges for the production of cereals under the current scenario of climate change, and this has a huge impact on the outbreaks of insect pests. Climate change not only includes the increases in temperature. The intensity and frequency of drought have raised, and it has been estimated that in the near future, this condition will increase which will have an alarming effect on the mortality of trees (Diffenbaugh et al. 2017; Lehner et al. 2017; Hartmann et al. 2018). Extreme alterations in rainfall patterns will inevitably pose a detrimental

12 Climate Change and Global Insect Dynamics

influence on the abundance and diversity of insects. Sardana and Bhat (2016) elucidated that deviating or fluctuating weather conditions cause an upsurge of various insect pests like heavy rains might lead to the emergence of red hairy caterpillar, while long dry conditions followed by severe rainfall will lead to the eruption of cutworms. Water stress in sorghum leads to great damage by *Chilo partellus* (spotted stem borer) and *Melanaphis sacchari* (sugarcane aphid) than the plants in well-irrigated regions. Hence, an increase or decrease in insect damage may be attributed to a change in the moisture content of the host plant. According to Sharma et al. (1999), humid conditions also meddle with the interactions between host plants and insects. The more humid the conditions, the more easy it would be for insects to detect odors to build a relationship with host plants. Lack of rainfall accompanied by swift growth of vegetation sets off significant changes in the brains of these insects that lead to the secretion of serotonin, which stimulates locusts to breed profusely, and they become densely populated. In recent years, change in environmental parameters such as drought has led to the outbreak of locusts.

Deficit rainfall for a prolonged time affects the growth and survival of trees which leads to a severe outbreak of insects in forest areas (Netherer and Schopf 2010a, b). It has been found by Dai et al. (2004) that drought-like conditions have tend to increase since the mid-1950s in the land areas of the Northern Hemisphere. Under the conditions of drought stress, more infections tend to develop. Drought provokes the outbreak of insects. Herms and Mattson (1992) proposed that drought-like conditions increase the fitness and abundance of herbivore insects due to an increase in the nutritional status of plants. Pests feeding on the plant sap depict a positive response to the drought condition. Drought increases the concentration of sugar and nitrogen in the leaves of plants, and the insects feeding on such leaves show increased fecundity rate, development, and abundance (Herms 2002). McClure (1980) demonstrated that the abundance, survival, and fecundity of *Fiorinia externa* got increased with an increase in the nitrogen content of eastern hemlock trees.

Drought has a deleterious effect on the insects feeding on the tree trunk; however, the leaf-eating, gall-making, and sap-feeding insects are benefited from the drought-like conditions. Under acute drought, outbreaks of the bark beetles occur as observed by Netherer et al. (2019). Recent investigations carried out by Ahmed et al. (2017) and Nguyen et al. (2018) revealed that the rate of parasitism is low in aphids that are fed on the water-stressed plants due to a reduction in the abundance and size of the host. Temperature, along with other variables such as humidity, rainfall, carbon dioxide (CO_2) concentration, and radiations, also aids in influencing pest status (Harrington et al. 2001).

12.4.4 Biotic Stress

Due to the complete sedentary lifestyle of the lac insect, they are more prone to the attack of predators, which results in considerable damage to the lac crop (Singh et al. 2011). Both vertebrate and invertebrate species act like the predators of the lac insect

(Mohanta et al. 2014; Shah et al. 2015). Among vertebrates, rats and squirrels are the most common enemies of the lac insect. Invertebrate enemies destroy 30–40% of the lac cells and thus have an adverse effect on the yield and fecundity of lac insects (Sarvade et al. 2018).

12.5 Modeling and Simulation

According to the production model as given by Valashedi and Pichaghchi (2019), the production of insect products is significantly related to temperature, and even a half-degree increase in temperature due to climate change will decrease the production of honey by approximately 40 tonnes per year. Trait-based models suggest that insect populations inhabiting the low-to-mid-latitude areas are at more risk due to climate change (Kellermann and Heerwaarden 2019). Experimental simulation of climate change due to elevated temperature and carbon dioxide concentration was carried out in laboratory conditions by Schneider et al. (2020). They found that increased temperature favors the survival and development of pests, from eggs to adult stages. The relationship between microclimate, ecophysiology, and vital rates can be determined by using the mechanistic models of the effects of climate change on insects. Such models depict responses specific to the developmental stages and carryover effects between the consecutive stages (Maino et al. 2016). Lobo (2016) suggested the use of species distribution models or SDMs for predicting the presence of insect species under different climatic conditions. This model relies on the information of the presence of species.

To determine the relationship among pests, plants, and their environment, crop and forestry population system models act as useful tools. Tang and Cheke (2008) proposed that optimal strategies to achieve the goals at the societal and individual level can be found using simulation models. With climatic variations determined by NASA-Goddard Institute of Space Studies (GISS) general circulation models, it has been estimated that European corn borer will shift up to 1220 km in a northward direction and the future generations will even continue to occur in that region (Porter et al. 1991). Using various models, it has been estimated that an increase in temperature by 2 °C could increase the life cycles per year. Various correlative models such as MaxEnt, Bioclim, and random forest are used to predict the possibly appropriate regions for a particular species (Kumar et al. 2014). According to Evans et al. (2015) and Gillson et al. (2013), correlative modeling is the most common method used for forecasting the climate change effects on the wide range of insect species, and it has become the basis of climate change policy. Correlative modeling serves as an important tool for assessing the alteration in species distribution and their rate of extinction. Results of these models are given in the form of maps that depict the regions that are adequate for the survival of any species. Another type of model, i.e., the mechanistic model, involves the understanding of environmental variables and the ability of an insect species to tolerate these environmental conditions (Kumar et al. 2014). Both correlative modeling and mechanistic modeling are categorized as ecological niche models (ENMs). Thus, the analysis of climate changes along with the development of various models facilitates the prediction of risks of pests.

12.6 Adaptation Options

Insects express different types of adaptability toward the changing climatic conditions. Insect communities respond to climate changes due to sensitiveness to temperature and the short time between the consecutive generations. In Europe, heritable changes in the dates of egg hatching have been reported by Asch et al. (2012) that occurred due to disturbance in the phenological rhythmicity between the winter moth and the oak tree because of increasing atmospheric temperature. Insects are retorting to the changing climatic conditions by the shift in the process of voltinism or by adaptation to the local environmental conditions. An alteration in the timing of the emergence of adults is another way of responding to the changing climate (Maurer et al. 2018). Buckley et al. (2015) have found that over the last few years, rocky mountain grasshoppers inhabiting the higher altitudes show setbacks in their development and those living in lower altitudes manifest early development. Certain insects respond to climatic changes by proliferating their number of generations in a year (Altermatt 2010). Alteration in the temperature and rainfall pattern decreases the availability of host plant which forces the insects to shift to the new host plant for feeding as reported by Bush (1969) in apple maggot that changed its host plant from hawthorn fruit to apple trees. Lehmann et al. (2020) assessed the 31 insect pests and observed that among them 29 species showed some kind of response to climate change by changing their geographic range, duration of life cycle stages, and food web interactions. According to Diamond (2018), insect pests depict an evolutionary response to global warming. Being cold-blooded, they are more responsive to climate warming and thus show response to climate change in various ways; some may undergo alteration in the periodic events of their life cycle, and some may even alter their distribution pattern. Climate crisis greatly influences the insect pests that use specified host plants in their life cycle and dwell in a narrow range of the habitat. Insects living in tropical regions are more sensitive to increasing temperature, and adaptation, dispersal, and phenotypic and genotypic plasticity can lessen the impact of this elevated temperature on these insect species (Deutsch et al. 2008). Atmospheric warming, particularly in high latitudes, increases the phenomenon of multivoltinism in organisms that rely on external sources for maintaining their body temperature. To cope up with water loss in insects, cockroaches depict aggregation (Dambach and Goehlen 1999). For the reduction of water loss, during summers, clumping behavior is seen in *Chironomus* larvae. In Finland, Pöyry et al. (2011) reported an increase in multi-voltinism in moths due to a temperature rise. Insects living in montane forests buffer against the rapidly changing climatic conditions by shifting to higher altitudes or toward the poleward aspect of the slope. They express different phenotypes in response to the environmental conditions including the alterations in the global climate. This phenotypic plasticity helps the insects in their survival and adaptability (Bonamour et al. 2019; Sgrò et al. 2016).

12.7 Conclusion

The worldwide climate change crisis has triggered crucial changes in the association of insect pest and their host. Climate change has led to change in the geographical reach of various insect species, thereby altering their diversity and abundance. This change in topography has resulted in more crop loss, thereby imposing a burden on agricultural output and food security. The phenomenon of insect evolution has been estimated to be as long as 500 million years ago which is still an ongoing process. Insects have managed to co-evolve along with the host and numerous abiotic factors to ensure sustainability, therefore making them a highly resilient group of animals in the entire animal kingdom. Climate change has vastly influenced extinction, synchronous pollination, pest outbreaks, phenology, host-plant resistance, and a series of uncountable and interrelated associations among insects and plants. Most of the implications of climate change are attributed to human activities so the solution also lies in curbing human activities. Therefore, proper inspection of anthropogenic activities is required to understand and address future and long-term implications of climate change.

Acknowledgments The authors would like to thank the Government of India (GOI) for providing necessary facilities under FIST, PURSE, and RUSA programs. The valuable suggestions and help provided by the Head, Department of Zoology, University of Jammu, are duly acknowledged.

References

Ahmed SS, Liu D, Simon J-C (2017) Impact of water-deficit stress on tritrophic interactions in a wheat-aphid-parasitoid system. PLoS One 12(10):e0186599. https://doi.org/10.1371/journal.pone.0186599

Altermatt F (2010) Climatic warming increases voltinism in European butterflies and moths. Proc Biol Sci 277:1281–1287

Asch MV, Salis L, Holleman LJM, Lith BV, Visser ME (2012) Evolutionary response of the egg hatching date of a herbivorous insect under climate change. Nat Clim Chang 3:244–248

Bale JS, Masters GJ, Hodkinson ID, Awmack C, Bezemer TM, Valerie K, Brown VK, Butterfield J, Buse A, Coulson JC, Farrar J, Good JEG, Harrington R, Hartley S, Jones TH, Lindroth RL, Press MC, Symmioudis I, Watt AD, Whittaker JB (2002) Herbivory in global climate change research: direct effects of rising temperature on insect herbivores. Glob Change Biol 8:1–16

Battisti A, Stastny M, Netherer S et al (2005) Expansion of geographic range in the pine processionary moth caused by increased winter temperatures. Ecol Appl 15:2084–2096

Berg EE, Henry JD, Fastie CL, De Volder AD, Matsuoka SM (2006) Spruce beetle outbreaks on the Kenai Peninsula, Alaska, and Kluane National Park and Reserve, Yukon Territory: relationship to summer temperatures and regional differences in disturbance regimes. For Ecol Manag 227: 219–232

Bezemer TM, Jones TH (1998) Plant-insect herbivore interactions in elevated atmospheric CO_2: quantitative analyses and guild effects. Wiley on behalf of Nordic Society. Oikos 82(2):212–222

Bhagat ML, Mishra YD (2002) Abiotic factors affecting lac productivity. In: Recent advances in lac culture. ILRI, Ranchi

Bonamour S, Chevin LM, Charmantier A, Teplitsky C (2019) Phenotypic plasticity in response to climate change: the importance of cue variation. Philos Trans R Soc B Biol Sci 374:20180178. https://doi.org/10.1098/rstb.2018.0178

Buckley LB, Nufio CR, Kirk EM, Kingsolver JG (2015) Elevational differences in developmental plasticity determine phenological responses of grasshoppers to recent climate warming. Proc Biol Sci 282:20150441–20150446

Bush GL (1969) Sympatric host race formation and speciation in frugivorous flies of the genus Rhagoletis (Diptera, Tephritidae). Evolution 23:237–251

Butchart SH, Stattersfield AJ, Baillie J, Bennun LA, Stuart SN, Akçakaya HR, Hilton-Taylor C, Mace GM (2005) Using Red List Indices to measure progress towards the 2010 target and beyond. Philos Trans R Soc Lond B Biol Sci 360(1454):255–268

Cornelissen T (2011) Climate change and its effects on terrestrial insects and herbivory patterns. Neotrop Entomol 40:155–163

Coviella CE, Trumble JT (1999) Effects of elevated atmospheric carbon dioxide on insect-plant interactions. Conserv Biol 13(4):700–712

Curtis PS, Wang X (1998) A meta-analysis of elevated CO_2 effects on woody plant mass, form and physiology. Oecologia 113:299–313

Dai AG, Trenberth KE, Qian T (2004) A global dataset of Palmer Drought severity index for 1870–2002: relationship with soil moisture and effects of surface warming. J Hydrometeorol 5: 1117–1130

Dambach M, Goehlen B (1999) Aggregation density and longevity correlate with humidity in first-instar nymphs of the cockroach (Blattella germanica L., Dictyoptera). J Insect Physiol 45(5): 423–429. https://doi.org/10.1016/s0022-1910(98)00141-3

DeLucia EH, Casteel CL, Nabity PD, O'Neill BF (2008) Insects take a bigger bite out of plants in a warmer, higher carbon dioxide world. Proc Natl Acad Sci U S A 105(6):1781–1782. https://doi.org/10.1073/pnas.0712056105

Deutsch CA, Tewksbury JJ, Huey RB, Sheldon KS, Ghalambor CK, Haak DC, Martin PR (2008) Impacts of climate warming on terrestrial ectotherms across latitude. Proc Natl Acad Sci 105(18):6668–6672

Diamond SE (2018) Contemporary climate-driven range shifts: putting evolution back on the table. Funct Ecol 32:1652–1665

Diffenbaugh NS, Singh D, Mankin JS, Horton DE, Swain DL, Touma D et al (2017) Quantifying the influence of global warming on unprecedented extreme climate events. Proc Natl Acad Sci U S A 114:4881–4886

Economic survey of India (2018) Chapter 6: Climate, climate change and agriculture, vol I. Ministry of finance, Government of India, pp 88–101

Elphinstone J, Toth IK (2008) Erwinia chrysanthemi (Dikeya spp.)-The facts. Potato Council, Oxford

Evans TG, Diamond SE, Kelly MWX (2015) Mechanistic species distribution modelling as a link between physiology and conservation. Conserv Physiol 03:1–56

Fajer ED (1989) The effects of enriched carbon dioxide atmospheres on plant insect herbivore interactions: growth responses of larvae of the specialist butterfly, Junonia coenia (Lepidoptera: Nymphalidae). Oecologia (Berlin) 81:514–520

Fand BB, Kamble AL, Kumar M (2012) Will climate change pose serious threat to crop pest management: a critical review? Int J Sci Res Publ 2(11):1–14

Forister ML, Shapiro MA (2003) Climatic trends and advancing spring flight of butterflies in lowland California. Glob Chang Biol 9:1130–1135

Franco AM, Hill JK, Kitschke C, Collingham YC, Roy DB, Fox RI, Huntley BR, Thomas CD (2006) Impacts of climate warming and habitat loss on extinctions at species' low-latitude range boundaries. Glob Chang Biol 12(8):1545–1553

Gillson L, Dawson TP, Jack S, McGeoch MA (2013) Accommodating climate change contingencies in conservation strategy. Trends Ecol Evol 28:135–142

Gregory PJ, Johnson SN, Newton AC, Ingram JS (2009) Integrating pests and pathogens into the climate change/food security debate. J Exp Bot 60(10):2827–2838

Guerenstein PG, Hildebrand JG (2008) Roles and effects of environmental carbon dioxide in insect life. Annu Rev Entomol 53:161–178

Gutiérrez AP, D'Oultremont T, Ellis CK, Ponti L (2006) Climatic limits of pink bollworm in Arizona and California: effects of climate warming. Acta Oecol 30:353–364

Hamilton JG, Orla D, Mihai A, Arthur RZ, Alistair R, May RB, Evan HD (2005) Anthropogenic changes in tropospheric composition increase susceptibility of soybean to insect herbivory. Environ Entomol 34(2):479–485

Harrington R, Fleming R, Woiwood I (2001) Climate change impacts on insect management and conservation in temperate regions: can they be predicted? Agric For Entomol 3:233–240

Harrington R, Clark SJ, Weltham SJ, Virrier PJ, Denhol CH, Hulle M, Maurice D, Rounsevell MD, Cocu N (2007) Environmental change and the phenology of European aphids. Glob Chang Biol 13:1556–1565

Hartmann H, Moura CF, Anderegg WR, Ruehr NK, Salmon Y, Allen CD et al (2018) Research frontiers for improving our understanding of drought-induced tree and forest mortality. New Phytol 218:15–28

Hegland SJ, Nielsen A, Lázaro A, Bjerknes AL, Totland Ø (2009) How does climate warming affect plant pollinator interactions? Ecol Lett 12:184–195

Herms DA (2002) Effects of fertilization on insect resistance of Woody ornamental plants: reassessing an entrenched paradigm. Environ Entomol 31(6):923–933

Herms DA, Mattson WJ (1992) The dilemma of plants: to grow or defend. Q Rev Biol 67(3): 283–335

Hickling R, Roy DB, Hill JK, Fox R, Thomas CD (2006) The distributions of a wide range of taxonomic groups are expanding polewards. Glob Chang Biol 12:450–455

Hill DS (1987) Agricultural insect pests of temperate regions and their control. Cambridge University Press, New York

Hill JK, Thomas CD, Fox R et al (2002) Responses of butterflies to twentieth century climate warming: implications for future ranges. Proc R Soc Lond B 269:2163–2171

Hughes L, Bazzaz FA (1997) Effect of elevated CO_2 on interactions between the western flower thrips, *Frankliniella occidentalis* (Thysanoptera: Thripidae) and the common milkweed, *Asclepias syriaca*. Oecologia 109:286–290

IPCC (2014) Impacts, adaptation and vulnerability. In: Field CB, Barros VR, Dokken DJ, Mach KJ, Mastrandrea MD, Bilir TE, Chatterjee M, Ebi KL, Estrada YO, Genova RC, Girma B, Kissel ES, Levy AN, MacCraken S, Mastrandrea PR, White LL (eds) Working group II contribution to the fifth assessment report of intergovernmental panel on climate change. Cambridge University Press, Cambridge, p 1132

Johnson SN, Waterman JM, Hall CR (2020) Increased insect herbivore performance under elevated CO_2 is associated with lower plant defence signalling and minimal declines in nutritional quality. Sci Rep 10:14553. https://doi.org/10.1038/s41598-020-70823-3

Jump AS, Penuelas J (2005) Running to stand still: adaptation and the response of plants to rapid climate change. Ecol Lett 8:1010–1020

Kellermann V, Heerwaarden BV (2019) Terrestrial insects and climate change: adaptive responses in key traits. Physiol Entomol 44(2):99–115

Konvicka M, Maradova M, Venes J, Fric Z, Kepka P (2003) Uphill shifts in distribution of butterflies in the Czech Republic: effects of changing climate detected on a regional scale. Glob Ecol Biogeogr 12:403–410

Kumar S, Neven LG, Yee WL (2014) Evaluating correlative and mechanistic niche models for assessing the risk of pest establishment. Ecosphere 5:1–23

Lehmann P, Ammunét T, Barton M, Battisti A, Eigenbrode SD, Jepsen JU, Kalinkat G, Neuvonen S, Niemelä P, Terblanche JS, Økland B, Björkman C (2020) Complex responses of global insect pests to climate warming. Front Ecol Environ 18:141–150

Lehner F, Coats S, Stocker TF, Pendergrass AG, Sanderson BM, Raible CC, Smerdon JE (2017) Projected drought risk in 1.5 °C and 2 °C warmer climates. Geophys Res Lett 44:7419–7428

Lindroth RL, Arteel GE, Kinney KK (1995) Responses of three saturniid species to paper birch grown under enriched CO_2 atmospheres. Funct Ecol 9:306–311

Lobo JM (2016) The use of occurrence data to predict the effects of climate change on insects. Curr Opin Insect Sci 17:62–68. https://doi.org/10.1016/j.cois.2016.07.003

Maino JL, Kong JD, Hoffmann AA, Barton MG, Kearney MR (2016) Mechanistic models for predicting insect responses to climate change. Curr Opin Insect Sci 17:81–86. https://doi.org/10.1016/j.cois.2016.07.006

Maurer JA, Shepard JH, Crabo LG, Hammond PC, Zack RS, Peterson MA (2018) Phenological responses of 215 moth species to interannual climate variation in the Pacific Northwest from 1895 through 2013. PLoS One 13:e0202850. https://doi.org/10.1371/journal.pone.0202850

McClure MS (1980) Foliar nitrogen: a basis for host suitability for elongate hemlock scale, Fiorinia externa (Homoptera: Diaspididae). Ecology 61(1):72–79

Menéndez R (2007) How are insects responding to global warming? Tijdschrift voor Entomologie 150:355–365

Merrill R, Gutiérrez D, Lewis O, Gutiérrez J, Diez S, Wilson R (2008) Combined effects of climate and biotic interactions on the elevational range of a phytophagous insect. J Anim Ecol 77:145–155

Mohanta J, Dey DG, Mohanty N (2014) Studies on lac insect (Kerria lacca) for conservation of biodiversity in Similipal Biosphere Reserve, Odisha, India. J Entomol Zool Stud 2(1):1–5

Musolin DL (2007) Insect in a warmer world: ecological, physiological and life history responses of true bugs (Heteroptera) to climate change. Glob Chang Biol 13:1565–1585

Nayak SB, Rao KS, Ramalakshmi V (2020) Impact of climate change on insect pests and their natural enemies. Int J Ecol Environ Sci 2(4):579–584

Neelaboina BK, Khan GA, Kumar S, Gani M, Ahmad MN, Ghosh MK (2018) Impact of climate change on agriculture and sericulture. J Entomol Zool Stud 6(5):426–429

Netherer S, Schopf A (2010a) Potential effects of climate change on insect herbivores in European forests – general aspects and the pine processionary moth as specific example. For Ecol Manag 259:831–838

Netherer S, Schopf A (2010b) Potential effects of climate change on insect herbivores – general aspects and a specific example (Pine processionary moth, Thaumetopoea pityocampa). For Ecol Manag 259:831–838

Netherer S, Panassiti B, Pennerstorfer J, Matthews B (2019) Acute drought is an important driver of bark beetle infestation in Austrian Norway spruce stands. Front For Glob Change 2:39. https://doi.org/10.3389/ffgc.2019.00039

Nguyen LTH, Monticelli LS, Desneux N, Metay-Merrien C, Amiens-Desneux E, Lavoir AV (2018) Bottom-up effect of water stress on the aphid parasitoid. Aphidius ervi Entomologia Generalis 38(1):15–27

Norby RJ, Willschleger SD, Gunderson CA, Johnson DW, Ceulemans R (1999) Tree responses to rising CO_2 in experiments: implications for the future forest. Plant Cell Environ 22:683–714

Ouyang F, Hui C, Men X, Zhang Y, Fan L, Shi P, Zhao ZH, Ge F (2016) Early eclosion of overwintering cotton bollworm moths from warming temperatures accentuates yield loss in wheat. Agric Ecosyst Environ 217:89–98

Owensby CE, Ham JM, Knapp AK, Allen LM (1999) Biomass production and species composition change in a tall grass prairie ecosystem after long-term exposure to elevated atmospheric CO_2. Glob Chang Biol 5:497–506

Pal G (2009) Impact of scientific lac cultivation training on lac economy: a study in Jharkhand. Agric Econ Res Rev 22:139–143

Pandi GG, Chander S, Singh MP, Pathak H (2018) Impact of elevated CO_2 and temperature on brown planthopper population in Rice ecosystem. Proc Natl Acad Sci India Sect B Biol Sci 88: 57–64

Parmesan C (2006) Influences of species, latitudes and methodologies on estimates of phenological response to global warming. Glob Chang Biol 13:1860–1872

Parmesan C (2007) Ecological and evolutionary responses to recent climate change. Annu Rev Ecol Evol Syst 37:637–669

Porter JH, Parry ML, Carter TR (1991) The potential effects of climatic change on agricultural insect pests. Agric For Meteorol 57(1–3):221–240

Potts SG, Jacobus CB, Kremen C, Neumann P, Schweiger O, William EK (2010) Global pollinator declines: trends, impacts and drivers. Trends Ecol Evol 25(6):345–353

Pöyry J, Leinonen R, Söderman G, Nieminen M, Risto KH, Carter TR (2011) Climate-induced increase of moth multivoltinism in boreal regions. Glob Ecol Biogeogr 20(2):289–298

Pudasaini R, Chalise M, Poudel PR, Pudasaini K, Aryal P (2015) Effect of climate change on insect pollinator: a review. N Y Sci J 8(3):39–42

Ram RL, Maji C, Bindroo BB (2016) Impact of climate change on sustainable Sericultural development in India. Int J Agric Innov Res 4(6):1110–1118

Reddy PVR, Verghese A, Rajan VV (2012) Potential impact of climate change on honeybees (*Apis spp.*) and their pollination. Pest Management in Horticultural. Ecosystems 18(2):121–127

Rosenzweig C, Casassa G, Karoly DJ et al (2007) Assessment of observed changes and responses in natural and managed systems. In: Parry ML et al (eds) Climate change 2007: impacts, adaptation and vulnerability. Contribution of working group II to the fourth assessment report of the intergovernmental panel on climate change. Cambridge University Press, Cambridge, pp 79–131

Roy DB, Sparks TH (2000) Phenology of British butterflies and climate change. Glob Chang Biol 6: 407–416

Salt DT, Brooks GL, Whittaker JB (1995) Elevated carbon dioxide affects leaf-miner performance and plant growth in docks (*Rumex* spp.). Glob Chang Biol 1:153–156

Samways M (2005) Insect diversity conservation. Cambridge University Press, Cambridge, p 342

Sardana HR, Bhat MN (2016) Pest scenario, plant protection approaches in the current context of changing climate. In: Chattopadhyay C, Prasad D (eds) Dynamics of crop protection and climate change. Studera Press, New Delhi, pp 167–186

Sarvade PRKS, Rajak SK, Upadhyay VB (2018) Impact of biotic and abiotic factors on lac production and peoples livelihood improvement in India-An overview. J Appl Natl Sci 10(3): 894–904

Schneider D, Ramos AG, Córdoba-Aguilar A (2020) Multigenerational experimental simulation of climate change on an economically important insect pest. Ecol Evol 10(23):12893–12909

Schweiger O, Biesmeijer JC, Bommarco R, Hickler T, Hulme P, Klotz S, Kuhn I, Moora M, Nielsen A, Ohlemuller R, Petandou T, Potts SG, Pysek P, Stout JC, Sykes M, Tscheulin T, Vila M, Wather GR, Westphal C (2010) Multiple stressors on biotic interactions: how climate change and alien species interact to affect pollination. Biol Rev 85:777–795

Sgrò CM, Terblanche JS, Hoffmann AA (2016) What can plasticity contribute to insect responses to climate change? Annu Rev Entomol 61:433–451. https://doi.org/10.1146/annurev-ento-010715-023859

Shah TH, Thomas M, Bhandari R (2015) Lac production, constraints and management: a re-view. Int J Curr Res 7(3):13652–13659

Sharma KK (2007) Lac insect-host plant interaction: implications on quantity and quality of lac. In: Model training course on advanced lac production, storage and application technology for employment and income generation. ILRI, Ranchi

Sharma HC (2010) Global warming and climate change: impact on arthropod biodiversity, pest management and food security. In: Thakur R, Gupta PR, Verma AK (eds) Perspectives and challenges of integrated Pest Management for Sustainable Agriculture. Souven Natn Symp Nauni, Solan, pp 1–14

Sharma HC (2014) Climate change effects on insects: implications for crop protection and food security. J Crop Improv 28(2):229–259. https://doi.org/10.1080/15427528.2014.881205

Sharma HC, Mukuru SZ, Manyasa E, Were J (1999) Breakdown of resistance to sorghum midge, *Stenodiplosis sorghicola*. Euphytica 109:131–140

Shrestha S (2019) Effects of climate change in agricultural insect Pest. Acta Sci Agric 3(12):74–80

Sicher RC, Bunce JA (1997) Relationship of photosynthetic acclimation to changes of Rubisco activity in field-grown winter wheat and barley during growth in elevated carbon dioxide. Photosynth Res 52:27–38

Singh JP, Jaiswal AK, Monobrullah MD (2011) Safety evaluation of some newer pesticides against lac insect (*Kerria lacca*) for managing predators. Indian J Agric Sci 81:465–469

Stefanescu C, Penuelas J, Filella I (2003) Effects of climatic change on the phenology of butterflies in the Northwest Mediterranean Basin. Glob Chang Biol 9:1494–1506

Stiling P, Cornelissen T (2007) How does elevated carbon dioxide (CO_2) affect plant-herbivore interactions? A field experiment and a meta-analysis of CO_2-mediated changes on plant chemistry and herbivore performance. Glob Change Biol 13:1823–1842

Tang S, Cheke RA (2008) Models for integrated pest control and their biological implications. Math Biosci 215:115–125

Thomas M (2010) Madhya Pradesh: current status of lac production, issues, remedial measures and support system for development. In: Current issues related to lac production. 35–37 pp

Tocco C, Foster J, Venter N, Cowie B, Marlin D, Marcus Byrne M (2021) Elevated atmospheric CO_2 adversely affects a dung beetle's development: another potential driver of decline in insect numbers? Glob Chang Biol 27(19):4592–4600

Valashedi NR, Pichaghchi BH (2019) Effect of global warming on honey production in Shahindej area. Honeybee Sci J 10(18):36–43. https://doi.org/10.22092/hbsj.2019.120081

War AR, Tagger GK, War MY, Hussain B (2016) Impact of climate change on insect pests, plant chemical ecology, tritrophic interactions and food production. Int J Biol Sci 1:16–29

Ward NL, Masters GJ (2007) Linking climate change and species invasion: an illustration using insect herbivores. Glob Chang Biol 13:1605–1615

Wilson RJ, Gutiérrez D, Gutiérrez J, Martinez D, Aguado R, Montserrat VJ (2005) Changes to the elevational limits and extent of species ranges associated with climate change. Ecol Lett 8:1138–1146

Yogi RK, Alok K, Jaiswal AK (2017) Lac, plant resins and gums statistics 2015: at a glance. ICAR-Indian Institute of Natural Resins and Gums, Ranchi, pp 1–72

Zvereva EL, Kozlov MV (2010) Responses of terrestrial arthropods to air pollution: a meta-analysis. Environ Sci Pollut Res Int 17:297–311

Chapter 13
Sustainable Solutions to Food Insecurity in Nigeria: Perspectives on Irrigation, Crop-Water Productivity, and Antecedents

Abdulazeez Hudu Wudil, Asghar Ali, Hafiz Ali Raza, Muhammad Usman Hameed, Nugun P. Jellason, Chukwuma C. Ogbaga, Kulvir Singh, Fatih Çiğ, Murat Erman, and Ayman El Sabagh

Abstract Improving living standards by enhancing agricultural productivity is mandatory to resolve Nigeria's socioeconomic problems as more than 50% of the country's population is dependent on agriculture for a living. Irrigation might offer huge potential in Nigerian agriculture, owing to the country's vast water resources. This review seeks to provide an overview of Nigeria's poverty and food insecurity situation and also proposes a long-term solution based on irrigated agriculture. This investigation utilized data from the past 20 years from more than 100 studies on food security, irrigation, and crop-water productivity between 2000 and 2020. The results elucidated that 92% of the evaluated studies opined that improvements in irrigation schemes enhanced the living standards of farming communities, reduced poverty, and improved food security status. Maintaining the current rise in the agriculture sector and its substantial contribution to poverty reduction seems to be indispensable in enhancing agricultural productivity. Therefore, agriculture equipped with better irrigation facilities is necessary for achieving the desired agricultural productivity. It is also crucial to increase the quality and efficacy of social services at all agrarian

A. H. Wudil · A. Ali
Institute of Agricultural and Resource Economics, University of Agriculture, Faisalabad, Punjab, Pakistan

H. A. Raza · M. U. Hameed
Institutes of Agricultural Extension, Education and Rural Development, University of Agriculture, Faisalabad, Punjab, Pakistan

N. P. Jellason
Teesside University International Business School, Middlesbrough, UK

C. C. Ogbaga
Department of Biology and Biotechnology, Nile University of Nigeria, Abuja, Nigeria

K. Singh
Department of Agronomy Punjab Agricultural University, Regional Research Station, Faridkot, India

F. Çiğ · M. Erman · A. El Sabagh (✉)
Faculty of Agriculture, Department of Field Crops, Siirt University, Siirt, Turkey

© The Author(s), under exclusive license to Springer Nature Switzerland AG 2022
M. Ahmed (ed.), *Global Agricultural Production: Resilience to Climate Change*,
https://doi.org/10.1007/978-3-031-14973-3_13

353

levels. In summary, enhancing food security, increasing irrigation efficiency, and crop-water productivity by improvement in social participation, facilitation of technical training, research and development promotion, intensification of governance, and public-sector management are of utmost importance for Nigeria. Appropriate access to high-quality marketing opportunities and the adoption of contemporary agricultural technologies would be key to the next level of success.

Keywords Food security · Livelihood · Irrigation · Nigeria · Poverty

13.1 Introduction

Agricultural productivity, especially in low-income nations, is critical to global food security and the battle against hunger and poverty (von Braun et al. 2008). Rapid population growth and lower per capita agricultural output in Sub-Saharan Africa have increased the demand for improvised irrigation facilities in the region (Oldeman 1997; Angelakıs et al. 2020b). Although the amount of freshwater available for agriculture in the world is rapidly diminishing (Cai and Rosegrant 2002), there is potential in Sub-Saharan Africa, particularly Nigeria, owing to the large surface as well as groundwater resources (Xu et al. 2019). Irrigated acreage and efficiency should be improved to meet the food and fiber demand of the ever-increasing African population (Gebrehiwot and Gebrewahid 2016). The global population in the next 30 years might be growing by additional two billion people. Feeding such a huge population and reducing hunger significantly could only be possible by boosting agricultural production. This, in turn, will be dependent on expanding irrigation acreage coupled with efficient water management, even though a rising number of countries are experiencing water scarcity. According to the FAO, the irrigated area in developing nations would increase by nearly 20% by 2030. FAO predicts that using irrigation water more efficiently and planting several crops each year on irrigated land can expand the effective irrigated area by 34% by just consuming 14% higher water (FAO 2018). The most remarkable growth rate of 44% is predicted in Sub-Saharan Africa, where only 4% of the cultivable area is now irrigated (Pavelic et al. 2013).

Nigeria is the most populous country in the African continent and the seventh most populated nation on the globe (Adekola 2016). The country's population in 2019 was 203 million of which the rural population constituted 51.4% of the total and a population density of 212 inhabitants per square kilometer (Oluwatayo et al. 2019). The country's population has grown from 41 million in 1963 to 140 million in 2006 and recently touched 213 million (Anaele 2014a, b; Statista 2022). Most of the policymakers often doubt that with a growth rate of 2.59% from 2019 (Nzediegwu and Chang 2020), the country's resources can maintain pace with the growing population. The agricultural sector which provided employment to 36.55% of nation's economically active people remains the country's largest employer in 2017 (Akoteyon 2018). Low-cost techniques and small landholdings of between 0.5 and 2.5 ha characterize the farming system of Nigeria, leading to lowland and labor productivity (FAO 2018; Jellason et al. 2020; Jellason et al. 2021b). In addition, Nigeria is also afflicted by extreme poverty and food scarcity (Otaha 2013; Adebayo and Ojo 2012).

Food access is one of the most critical aspects of food security. Nigeria's enormous rainfed agricultural industry has been unable to maintain pace with the country's rapid population increase (Byerlee et al. 2014). And the simplest method to gain such access is to raise food production, which can be accomplished by cropping intensification (Byerlee et al. 2014), land area expansion (Gibbs et al. 2010), productivity, or a combination of these factors (Chamberlin et al. 2014). Irrigation is critical for enhancing cropping intensity and production (Carruthers et al. 1997). However, there is less understanding of the relationship between food production, food security, irrigation agriculture, and environmental sustainability in most Sub-Saharan African countries (Qadir et al. 2010). Maximizing the productive potential of irrigation water is critical to achieving growth, sustainable development, poverty reduction, and maintaining food security (Grey and Sadoff 2007). Many low-income countries continue to prioritize water and water management (Grey et al. 2016). Nigeria has 71 million hectares of agricultural land, accounting for 77% of the country's total geographical area. Out of this, 40.5 million hectares are arable land with around one million hectares of internal water bodies. Despite these potentials, high food import bills continue to plague the country (Onuka 2017). Prevalence of malnutrition is a concern in all sections of the country, particularly with rural areas being more vulnerable. Food shortages, hunger, poor food quality, high food costs, and even a complete absence of food are all too common, particularly in north-central and northeast regions (Akinyele 2009; Matemilola and Elegbede 2017). Inequality, food insecurity, and poverty are persistent challenges which bedevil the country despite the strength of the economy (Grant et al. 2012). This study aims to overview the prevalence of poverty and food insecurity in Nigeria and provides long-term remedies based on irrigation agriculture.

13.1.1 Conceptual Framework for Effective Irrigation System

The authors developed a conceptual framework as illustrated in Fig. 13.1 to show the development pathway toward sustainable food security, poverty reduction, and economic growth in Nigeria.

Figure 13.1 shows how the availability of irrigation water, along with adequate water management and better agronomic techniques, can lead to increased productivity, poverty reduction, and long-term food security. Conceptually, increasing productivity translates to higher producer income, better work wages, more affordable food prices for consumers, and economic growth. This could lead to improved natural resource management and environmental protection, achieving the cardinal Millennium Development Goal of reducing poverty and food insecurity while protecting ecological health.

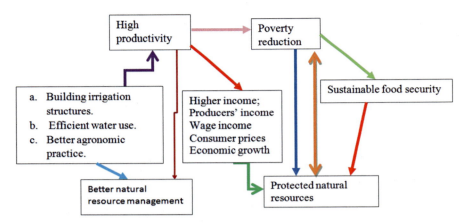

Fig. 13.1 The link between access to irrigation and poverty reduction: a conceptual framework

13.2 Methodology

The research collected secondary data from over 80 studies on food security, irrigation, water efficiency, and crop-water production. We used FAO statistics, Web of Science, and Google Scholar. The information gathered was evaluated in order to reach a reasonable conclusion about Nigeria's food insecurity issue, which has been a source of concern for stakeholders in the food subsector in recent years (Eme et al. 2014). In addition, the same databases were utilized to analyze the literature and empirical findings on irrigation agriculture's contribution to food security and poverty alleviation in developing nations, focusing on Sub-Saharan Africa. The keywords used in the search included irrigation water use efficiency, food security, water productivity, and irrigated agriculture.

13.3 Food Insecurity and Poverty in Nigeria

Food security prevails if people have access to safe, healthy, and ample food at all times to keep them active and healthy (McGuire 2015). Nigeria's food insecurity is worrying, with the situation worsening in the north (Adebayo and Ojo 2012; Babatunde et al. 2008) and nearly 62% of the total population living in extreme poverty (Astou 2015; Benatar 2016). In 2018, Sub-Saharan Africa had the highest percentage of undernourished persons (22.80%) in the world (Boliko 2019). Although global food insecurity declined from 14.8% in 2000 to 10.8% in 2018, hunger in Nigeria has increased since 2007, rising from 6.1% in 2007 to 13.4% in 2015 (Fawole and Adeoye 2015). Food insecurity in the country is alarming and shocking (Fawole and Özkan 2017). From 2009 to 2017, food insecurity continued to climb, with minor fluctuations in all three generally used metrics: the prevalence of undernourishment, food insecurity, and the number of undernourished persons (FAO 2019).

Nigeria was named the country with the most significant poverty rate globally by the World Poverty Clock in June 2018. According to data from the World Bank, 87 million people live in extreme poverty, accounting for 46.55% of the entire population (World Poverty Clock 2018). Nearly, four million Nigerians have fallen into poverty since June 2018, a trend hastened by unemployment, insecurity, low crop yield, and high food costs (World Poverty Clock 2018). Nigeria had the most significant stunting frequency in Africa, at 43.6% in 2018, while the prevalence of undernourishment increased from 9.3% to 11.5% between 2000 and 2018 (Otekunrin et al. 2019a).

Specifically, in Kwara State, Akinde et al. (2016) conducted a study on the food security determinants among rural families. According to the findings, over one-third of the rural farming households surveyed were food insecure. Another study on the determinants of poverty among crop farmers in Nigeria (Olawuyi 2012) found that only 69.2% of farm households were food secure. Similarly, Okunmadewa et al. (2007) investigated the food security condition among Nigerian urban families and discovered a 49% incidence of food insecurity in the study area. Food insecurity among women and children has been a severe and recurring problem (Sasson 2012). Food insecurity in Sub-Saharan Africa is caused by a mismatch between food production and population growth (Khan et al. 2014). The increase in agricultural production is 3.7%, but it is not keeping up pace with the 6.5% increase in food consumption (Ebele Mary et al. 2014). A map of Nigeria with the distribution of food insecurity by states and regions is given (Fig. 13.2).

13.3.1 Irrigation, Poverty, and Food Insecurity Nexus

Irrigated area must be doubled from 12 to 24 million hectares, and water productivity from irrigated and rainfed agriculture must rise by at least 60% to meet future food demand in Africa (Wright and Cafiero 2011; Shrestha 2017). Irrigation water investment is a tool for Africa's long-term development (Mwanza 2003; Adela et al. 2019). Access to irrigation water is critical for farmers to access modern farm inputs though an increase in efficiency and income, improving production and income while reducing poverty (Zewdie et al. 2019). Alternative water sources for home usage include irrigation water and crop yield growth (Usman et al. 2019). Farmers can use irrigation to get out of the "multi-scale poverty trap" (Burney and Naylor 2012; Porter et al. 2014; Lundqvist and Unver 2018). Irrigation enhances equality in the favor of resource-poor farmers (Prasad et al. 2006).

The Malabo Proclamation endorsed by the African Union's state chiefs and government in June 2014 states that "efficient and effective water management systems, particularly through irrigation," is the key to sustainable food production in Sub-Saharan Africa (Bjornlund et al. 2017). According to Wang et al. (2019), in 1900, the irrigated land area was 40 million hectares globally. However, by 1998, the figure had risen to 271 million hectares, with much of the growth occurring after the 1950s (Döll and Siebert 2000). The apparent influence on crop yield has been the

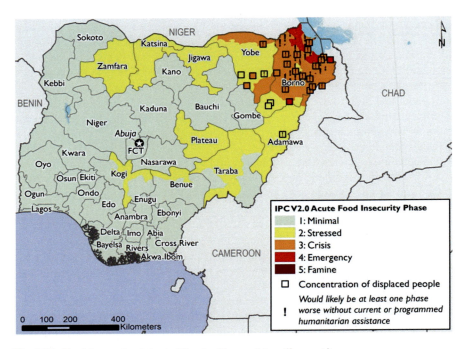

Fig. 13.2 Food insecurity status in Nigeria. (Source: https://fews.net/)

primary driver of this unprecedented intensification in irrigated agriculture (Angelakıs et al. 2020a). Rainfed agriculture covers around 80% of the world's farmed land and accounts for roughly 60% of crop production. In contrast, irrigated agriculture covers approximately 275 million hectares, or about 20% of cultivated land, and produces 40% of the world's food (Bjornlund et al. 2017; Angelakıs et al. 2020a).

Irrigation investments, poverty alleviation, and food security have a strong positive association (Chapagain 2006). In comparison to non-irrigated farmland, irrigated land provides 2–2.5 times the yield and 3 times the crop value per hectare, despite irrigation accounting for only one-sixth of the world's total production area, which includes cropland, rangeland, and pasture (Xie and Zhou 2014). According to Smith (2004), agricultural intensification through irrigation is a catalyst for poverty alleviation and food security, particularly in developing countries. Income, inequality, and poverty reduction are all influenced by irrigation (Bhattarai and Narayanamoorthy 2003). Another study found that non-irrigated households had a higher incidence and degree of poverty than irrigation households (Meliko and Oni 2011).

Furthermore, a study by Adebayo et al. (2018) discovered that irrigation agriculture is positively connected with enhanced crop productivity, income, and household food security, especially when combined with superior agronomic techniques.

13.3.2 Irrigation Development as the Cornerstone of Food Security in Nigeria

If Nigeria alleviates rural poverty and food insecurity while still meeting rising food demand, it would need to invest in irrigation or enhance current production systems. Insurgencies, adverse climatic conditions, and low production are significant causes of Nigeria's food insecurity, poverty, and hunger (Otekunrin et al. 2019a; Jellason et al. 2021a). Irrigation agriculture remains an important alternative to fulfil increasing food demand due to partial and temporal variations in rainfall (Otekunrin et al. 2019b). Nevertheless, any effort to expand agriculture must be complemented by the development of irrigation systems (Kadigi 2012; Akinde et al. 2016; Easter and Welsch 2019). In Sub-Saharan Africa, Nigeria has the most irrigation potential which is estimated to be more than 2.5 million hectares (Xie et al. 2014). Climate change, population increase, and other factors have necessitated making irrigation crucial for Nigeria's food security strategy. Sub-Saharan Africa has the smallest planted irrigation area and the lowest irrigation efficiency, resulting in the highest hunger levels (Smith 2004; Adebayo et al. 2018). Data presented in Fig. 13.3 supports this assertion by demonstrating a negative relationship between irrigation, irrigation efficiency, and malnourishment. Malnourishment is minimal in the region with high agricultural and irrigation efficiency. Irrigation-enhanced agriculture is a catalyst for poverty reduction, particularly in developing nations (Bhattarai and Narayanamoorthy 2003; Smith 2004).

Low staple food production and the continued effect of fuel oil on Nigeria's economy are two reasons contributing to the country's high degree of food insecurity (Osabohien et al. 2018). According to Omorogiuwa et al. (2014), just 40% of the country's agricultural land is farmed, despite being suitable for agriculture. However, there are 84 million hectares of arable land, besides the availability of 267 billion cubic meters of surface water (Davies et al. 2010) and three of Africa's eight major rivers in the country. Irrigated agriculture accounts for merely 2% of total

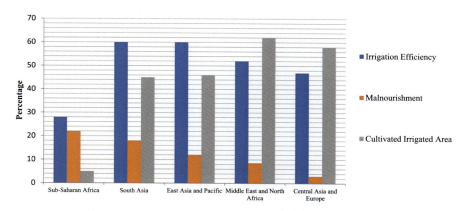

Fig. 13.3 Irrigation and malnourishment data from different regions. (Source: Domenech 2015)

cultivable land (Bahri et al., 2011). Irrigated farms in the country's dry savanna agroecological zones provide higher returns than non-irrigated farms in the exact location (Oni et al. 2009). Irrigated agricultural regions are 2.5 times more productive than rainfed agrarian areas (Stockle 2001). Furthermore, an estimate by FAO (2001) indicated that irrigation can increase the productivity of most crops by 100 to 400% compared to rainfed agriculture.

Several authors (Irz et al. 2001; Christiaensen 2007; Otsuka and Kijima 2010) argue that irrigation is critical for global productivity growth, poverty reduction, and food security. Rainfed rice yields have rarely exceeded 3 tons/ha, even in nations with better production systems such as China, Japan, Indonesia, and Sri Lanka, where irrigated rice yields have averaged 5–10 tons/ha (Seck et al. 2012). This elucidates that irrigation is a critical component in alleviating food scarcity and lowering poverty levels in many Sub-Saharan African countries (Mkavidanda and Kaswamila 2001; REPOA 2004; Sokoni and Shechambo 2005). Nigeria's water resources are abundant enough to support year-round rice production. As evidence, the ten plot states irrigation project produced an additional yearly production of one million metric tonnes in 2012 (Uduma et al. 2016).

In Sub-Saharan Africa (SSA), rapid population increase and shifting food consumption patterns necessitate doubling food output by 2050 (Leimbach et al. 2018). Due to the limited tendency of land expansion, around 85% of the increase in output would have to come from increased crop yields and greater crop intensity, both of which are the result of irrigation (Edgerton 2009). Furthermore, Yang and Zehnder (2001) demonstrate that water scarcity is a severe impediment to expanding agricultural production. Due to rising obstacles to the expansion of the farming output, insufficient or absence of water in some regions of the globe has slowed the poverty reduction strategy (Brown and Halweil 1998, Felloni et al. 1999, Liu et al. 2000, Yang and Zehnder 2001). If a country's internal renewable water resource is less than 1000 cubic meters per inhabitant per year, it is considered water-stressed. Nigeria's average internal renewable water resources per capita were 1158 cubic meters in 2017. Irrigation has many promises, especially if combined with solid agronomic methods that save water and are environmentally benign. Nigeria aims to produce more food sustainably which is a good initiative. However, there is enormous potential for changing production methods, agricultural water management, technologies, and practices. Before beginning new initiatives, it is critical to understand the restrictions, what can be fixed in the future, and what new models might be available to unlock various irrigation potentials of Nigeria. As Africa's most populous country, there is a surge in demand for water and food. Nigeria's predicament exemplifies the water and food situation broadly in Africa.

13.3.3 *Irrigation Potential in Nigeria*

Nigeria's usable surface water resources have been approximately 80% of the total natural flow (Frenken 2005) (Table 13.1). It has a volume of over 267 billion cubic

13 Sustainable Solutions to Food Insecurity in Nigeria: Perspectives...

Table 13.1 Surface water irrigation potential in Nigeria

	Uplands (ha)	River Valleys (ha)	Inland swamp (ha)	Delta swamp (ha)	Total	%
North	343,000	578,000	154,100	–	1,075,600	68
Middle belt	82,000	28,000	28,000	–	138,000	9
South	180,000	11,000	93,400	78,000	362,400	23
Total (ha)	605,000	617,500	275,500	78,000	1,576,000	100
Percentage (%)	**38**	**39**	**18**	**5**	**100**	

Source: Aquastat (2005)

Table 13.2 Groundwater resources in Nigeria by region

Region	Basement type	Average yield per second
Sokoto Basin	Sedimentary rock	1–5 l/s
Chad Basin zone	Sedimentary rock	1.6–2 l/s
Middle Niger Basin	Sandstone aquifers	0.7–5 l/s
Niger Valley	Alluvium	7.5–37 l/s
Benue Basin	Sandstone aquifers	1.00–8 l/s
South west zone	Sedimentary rock	–
South central	Sedimentary rock	3–7 l/s
South-eastern	Cretaceous sediment	–
Basement complex	Cretaceous sediment	1–2 l/s

Source: Umara (2014)

meters (Bm^3). Surface water from Niger, Cameroon, and Benin provides 65.2 km^3 per year of external water resources (Umara 2014). The country's groundwater potential is around 57.9 km^3, with an average production of 3.5–10 l per second (Umara 2014). Irrigation is practiced on less than 7% of farmed land, and merely 12% of the irrigation capacity is only utilized (Bahri et al. 2010). In addition, there are 149 dams around the country. Among them, the states own 81, while 59 are owned by the federal government, and 9 by private companies. There are 107 major dams of which 59 are intended for irrigation and 20 for hydropower generation. Only 15 of the country's 34 small and medium dams are being used for irrigation (Adedeji 2008).

Nigeria's irrigation potential ranges from 1.5 to 3.2 million hectares. According to the most recent estimate, over 2.1 million hectares of land can be irrigated with around 1.6 million hectares via surface water and 0.5 million hectares via groundwater (Bashir and Kyung-Sook 2018).

Though available extractable water resources in Northern Nigeria are enough for at least 0.5 million ha, regions suitable for irrigation with groundwater are yet to be examined and identified. The region-specific basement aquifers and average groundwater removal yield per second are depicted in Table 13.2.

Low-lying land flooded by rainwater during the rainy season is known as "Fadama areas." They are found across the ecological zones of the Sahel, Sudan, and sections of the Guinea savanna. These wetlands are also crucial for agriculture's grazing and irrigation.

13.3.4 Role of Irrigation in Agricultural Production, Poverty Alleviation, Food Security, and Economy

The relationship between agricultural output increase, poverty reduction, and food security has been established (Mellor 1995; Thirtle et al. 2003; Koledoye and Deji 2015). Nigeria's irrigation potential demonstrates a great possibility, particularly in the north, where food insecurity and poverty are more acute. However, since irrigated land accounts for less than 1% of total cropland, its contribution to total crop production is negligible (Bashir and Kyung-Sook 2018). For example, only 2.8% of farm home plots were irrigated in the 2010–2011 cropping season, while the value in the following year was still low (1.6%) (Tashikalma et al. 2014). Irrigation is primarily being used in the northwest, with 6% irrigated plots compared to only 1.3% in the southwest (Thirtle et al. 2001). For each percentage increase in agricultural productivity, the headcount measure of poverty declined by nearly 1% in a sample of 40 nations (Thirtle et al. 2001). Agricultural productivity increase is more likely to favor the poor and consequently expand the economy (Thirtle et al. 2001).

Adugna et al. (2014) conducted a study in Ethiopia and found that based on a sample of 313 rainfed and irrigated farmers, poverty incidence was 37.3% higher on rainfed-only farms. Based on data collected from 200 farmers in Ethiopia's Ada Liben district, a related study examined the influence of small-scale irrigation on household food security (Tesfaye et al. 2008). Rice, maize, tomatoes, and other vegetables are cultivated under Nigeria's public irrigation programs. Rainfed (lowland and upland) rice accounted for 77% of the 3.2 million hectares of crop harvested in 2018/2019. Contrarily, irrigation systems account for only 17% of cultivated land and 27% of domestic production (Adekoyeni et al. 2018). Irrigated land in Nigeria can provide a significantly higher yield of 3.5–4 tons per hectare, as compared to rainfed land, which produces only 1.9 tons per hectare (Adekoyeni et al. 2018). However, there is a difference in yield between lowland cultivars that yield 2.2 tons per hectare and highland rainfed cultivars that produce 1.7 tons per hectare (Uduma et al. 2016) (Fig. 13.4). For instance, the Bakalori irrigation system is one of the country's operational irrigation projects, with yields of up to 4.6–5.2 tons per hectare, comparable to Asian rice yields of 5.5 tons per hectare in well-managed farmland (Breisinger et al. 2015) (Table 13.3).

Table 13.4 shows that the Sudan and Savanna zones have a higher yield potential than the Guinea savanna and forest zones. As a result, we may infer that the Savanna zone, which has the highest level of food insecurity, has more potential for rice production, though it is the cornerstone of poverty reduction and food security.

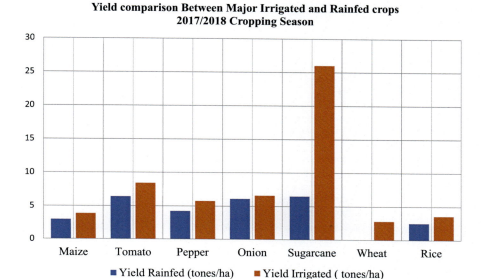

Fig. 13.4 Average yield of irrigated and rainfed agriculture in Nigeria. (Source: Tashikalma et al. 2014)

Table 13.3 Average yield per hectare of irrigated rice in some irrigation scheme in Nigeria

Location	Zone	Average yield (t/ha)	State located
Kadawa	Sudan	3.54	Kano
Watari	Sudan	8.03	Kano
Marte	Sahel	4.68	Borno
Bakalori	Sudan	4.50	Sokoto
Ngala	Sahel	5.00	Borno
Bedeggi	Guinea Savanna	2.78	Niger
Bende	Equatorial Forest	1.75	Abia

Source: Kebbeh et al. (2003)

13.4 Priorities for Sustainable Irrigation

Irrigation practices alone will not be enough to alleviate Nigeria's food insecurity and poverty.

Therefore specific priorities should be considered for it to be sustainable which can successfully improve the farming community's livelihood and also exert a multiplier effect on society as a whole. Several studies have been undertaken and published on the importance of infrastructure development, education, access to input, a sound marketing system, training, and research and development to increase productivity, reduce poverty, improve food security, and grow the economy. There

Table 13.4 Priorities for sustainable irrigation

Priorities	References
1. Road, pipe-borne water, and electricity are essential in improving agricultural productivity, hence accelerating the poverty reduction process and improving the food security of rural poor	Smith (2004), Fanadzo et al. (2010), Nadeem et al. (2011) and Llanto (2012)
2. Investments in agriculture and technology. Policies and institutional and economic reforms need to be redirected toward agricultural transformation	Hussain et al. (2004)
3. The technical skills of farmers should accompany irrigation as prioritized area	Fanadzo (2012), Beyene and Engida (2013) and Adekunle et al. (2015)
4. An increase in productivity of agricultural water use reduces the cost of production and helps conserve natural biomass	Turral et al. (2010)
5. Improving output marketing, postharvesting handling, value additions, and technologies	Namara et al. (2011), Shiferaw et al. (2011), Ali et al. (2015) and Gibbs et al. (2010)
6. For sustainability, application of critical inputs, seeds, fertilizers, herbicides, etc., in the correct quantity assurance of affordable cost and timeliness in their supply is essential for transformation	Namara et al. (2011), Ragasa et al. 2013, Ali et al. (2015), Gibbs et al. (2010) and Aloyce et al. (2019)
7. Encouragement of private-sector involvement	Arigor et al. (2015) and Ogundere (2007)
8. Research and development and favorable policies related to water management and social protection policies to protect shock and risk associated with agriculture	Rockström (2010), Ugalahi et al. (2016), Osabohien et al. (2018) and Tashikalma et al. (2014)

are a few studies which indicate priority areas in addition to irrigated agriculture investment.

13.5 Conclusion

In Nigeria, food insecurity and poverty are widespread, and the situation has worsened which demands urgent action. This poses a severe threat to Nigeria's long-term growth plan besides complexities in achieving food security. However, to reclaim the country's glory as a leading food producer in Sub-Saharan Africa, productivity must be increased, and opportunities must be created for the country's growing youth population. The simplest way to achieve this is to invest heavily in irrigation agriculture and its precursors. Improving irrigation projects will surely enhance the farming community's and customers' living conditions by lowering food prices resulting in high dividends. Irrigated agriculture would help to alleviate poverty and improve food security, national security, and economic progress.

Nigeria has enormous potential, particularly in locations with relatively abundant land and water resources for the expansion of irrigated agriculture. Nevertheless, a higher level of farmer participation in irrigation development programs is urgently required to promote accessible and sustainable irrigation production systems. This could improve the efficiency of water resource management. Farmers must be protected by policies that provide them with possibilities for better and assured produce pricing. Furthermore, farmers' access to subsidized inputs and a viable credit system which allows them to borrow money without putting up their assets at the disposal of funding agencies must be prioritized. The government should prioritize more research on the irrigation sector and also organize farmer training on better agronomic techniques to conserve the natural environment and fulfil the Millennium Development Goals (MDGs) of zero hunger.

Conflict of Interest Authors declare no conflict of interest.

References

Adebayo PF, Ojo EO (2012) Food security in Nigeria: an overview. Eur J Sustain Dev 1(2):199–199
Adebayo O, Bolarin O, Oyewale A, Kehinde O (2018) Impact of irrigation technology use on crop yield, crop income and household food security in Nigeria: a treatment effect approach. AIMS Agric Food 3:154–171. https://doi.org/10.3934/agrfood.2018.2.154
Adedeji AA (2008) Seismic analysis of earth wall gravity dams using decoupled modal approach. Int Egyp J Eng Math Theory Appl 5:19–34
Adekola PO (2016) Unemployment in Nigeria; a challenge of demographic change? Int J Sci Res Multidiscip Stud 1:1–9
Adekoyeni O, Fagbemi S, Ismaila A (2018) Ofada Rice identity, physical qualities and processing technology options for upgrading: a review. Annu Res Rev Biol 23:1–9. https://doi.org/10.9734/arrb/2018/38938
Adekunle C et al (2015) Effect of industrial externalities on technical efficiency among cassava-based farming households in Ewekoro local government area, Ogun State, Nigeria. Niger J Agric Food Environ 11:82–89
Adela FA, Aurbacher J, Abebe GK (2019) Small-scale irrigation scheme governance - poverty nexus: evidence from Ethiopia. Food Secur 11:897–913. https://doi.org/10.1007/s12571-019-00953-8
Adugna E, Ermias A, Mekonnen A, Mihret D (2014) The role of small scale irrigation in poverty reduction. J Dev Agric Econ 6:12–21. https://doi.org/10.5897/jdae2013.0499
Akinde SB, Sunday AA, Adeyemi FM, Fakayode IB, Oluwajide OO, Adebunmi AA, Oloke JK, Adebooye CO (2016) Microbes in irrigation water and fresh vegetables: potential pathogenic bacteria assessment and implications for food safety. Appl Biosaf 21:89–97. https://doi.org/10.1177/1535676016652231
Akinyele IO (2009) Ensuring food and nutrition security in rural Nigeria: an assessment of the challenges, information needs, and analytical capacity. International Food Policy Research Institute, pp 1–90
Akoteyon IS (2018) Transformation towards sustainable and resilient wash services analysis of household access to water and sanitation in rural communities in Southwest, Nigeria, pp 1–5
Ali A, Wei YZ, Mustafa MA (2015) Exploiting Propolis as an antimicrobial edible coating to control post-harvest anthracnose of bell pepper. Packag Technol Sci 282:173–179

Aloyce A, Ndakidemi PA, Mbega ER (2019) Survey and conventional management methods of bacterial wilt disease in open fields and greenhouses in Tanzania. J Plant Pathol 101:1107–1114. https://doi.org/10.1007/s42161-019-00346-y

Anaele C (2014a) Governance and under-development of sub-Sahara Africa. Hist Res Lett 11:41–46

Anaele C (2014b) Slave-trade, Christianity and European imperialism in Nigeria: a study of the ante and post abolition periods. Can Soc Sci 10:78–82. https://doi.org/10.3968/4261

Angelakıs AN, Zaccaria D, Krasilnikoff J, Salgot M, Bazza M, Roccaro P et al (2020a) Irrigation of world agricultural lands: evolution through the millennia. Water 12(5):1285

Angelakıs AN, Antoniou G, Voudouris K, Kazakis N, Dalezios N, Dercas N (2020b) History of floods in Greece: causes and measures for protection. Nat Hazards 101:833–852. https://doi.org/10.1007/s11069-020-03898-w

AQUASTAT F (2005) AQUASTAT database

Arigor AJ, Nyambi NI, Obuo PO (2015) Analysis of effect of governments trade policy on rice supply in three local government areas of Cross River State, Nigeria. Afr J Agric Res 10:829–834. https://doi.org/10.5897/ajar2014.8642

Astou D (2015) Food imports as a Hindrance to food security and sustainable development: the cases of Nigeria and Senegal 61. City University of New York

Babatunde RO, Omotesho OA, Olorunsanya EO, Owotokit GM (2008) Determinants of vulnerability to food insecurity: a gender-based analysis of farming households in Nigeria. Indian J Agric Econ 63:116–125. https://doi.org/10.22004/ag.econ.204567

Bahri A, Sally H, Namara RE, McCartney M, Awulachew SB, van Koppen B, Van Rooijen D (2010) Water for food in a changing world, Contributions to the Rosenberg international forum on water policy. Routledge, London

Bahri A, Sally H, McCartney M, Namara R, Awulachew SB, van Koppen B, van Rooijen D (2011) Integrated watershed management. In: Water for food in a changing world, vol 2. Routledge, London, p 50

Bashir A, Kyung-Sook C (2018) A review of the evaluation of irrigation practice in Nigeria: past, present and future prospects. Afr J Agri Res 13(40):2087–2097

Benatar SR (2016) The poverty of the concept of 'poverty eradication'. S Afr Med J 106:16–17. https://doi.org/10.7196/SAMJ.2016.v106i1.10417

Beyene LM, Engida E (2013) Public Investment in Irrigation and Training for an agriculture-led development: a CGE approach for Ethiopia. SSRN Electron J. https://doi.org/10.2139/ssrn.2352907

Bhattarai M, Narayanamoorthy A (2003) Impact of irrigation on rural poverty in India: an aggregate panel-data analysis. Water Policy 5:443–458

Bjornlund H, van Rooyen A, Stirzaker R (2017) Profitability and productivity barriers and opportunities in small-scale irrigation schemes. Int J Water Resour Dev 33:690–704. https://doi.org/10.1080/07900627.2016.1263552

Boliko MC (2019) FAO and the situation of food security and nutrition in the world. J Nutr Sci Vitaminol 65:S4–S8. https://doi.org/10.3177/jnsv.65.S4

Breisinger C, Ecker O, Trinh Tan J-F (2015) Conflict and food insecurity: how do we break the Links? Conflict and food security. International Food Policy Research Institute (IFPRI), pp 50–59

Brown LR, Halweil B (1998) China's water shortage could shake world food security. World Watch 11:10–21

Burney JA, Naylor RL (2012) Smallholder irrigation as a poverty alleviation tool in sub-Saharan Africa. World Dev 40:110–123. https://doi.org/10.1016/j.worlddev.2011.05.007

Byerlee D, Stevenson J, Villoria N (2014) Does intensification slow crop land expansion or encourage deforestation? Glob Food Sec 3(2):92–98

Cai X, Rosegrant MW (2002) Global water demand and supply projections: part 1. A modeling approach. Water Int 27:159–169. https://doi.org/10.1080/02508060208686989

13 Sustainable Solutions to Food Insecurity in Nigeria: Perspectives... 367

Carruthers I, Rosegrant MW, Seckler D (1997) Irrigation and food security in the 21st century. Irrig Drain Syst 11:83–101. https://doi.org/10.1023/A:1005751232728

Chamberlin J, Jayne TS, Headey D (2014) Scarcity amidst abundance? Reassessing the potential for cropland expansion in Africa. Food Policy 48:51–65

Chapagain AK (2006) Globalisation of water: opportunities and threats of virtual water trade; Dissertation, UNESCO-IHE Institute for Water Education, Delft and Delft University of Technology

Christiaensen LJ (2007) Down to earth: agriculture and poverty reduction in Africa. World Bank Publications

Davies KW, Petersen SL, Johnson DD, Davis DB, Madsen MD, Zvirzdin DL, Bates JD (2010) Estimating juniper cover from National Agriculture Imagery Program (NAIP) imagery and evaluating relationships between potential cover and environmental variables. Rangel Ecol Manag 63:630–637

Döll P, Siebert S (2000) A digital global map of irrigated areas. ICID J 49:55–66

Domenech L (2015) Is reliable water access the solution to undernutrition? A review of the potential of irrigation to solve nutrition and gender gaps in Africa South of the Sahara. International Food Policy Research Institute (IFPRI), Washington, DC

Easter KW, Welsch DE (2019) Implementing irrigation projects: operational and institutional problems. In: Irrigation investment, technology, and management strategies for development. Routledge, pp 33–56

Ebele Mary O, Kelechi Enyinna U, Agwu Ukpai K (2014) The effect of policy measures on entrepreneurship development analysis of Nigeria's experience. Eur J Bus Manag (Online) 6: 2222–2839

Edgerton MD (2009) Increasing crop productivity to meet global needs for feed, food, and fuel. Plant Physiol 149:7–13. https://doi.org/10.1104/pp.108.130195

Eme OI, Onyishi AO, Uche OA, Uche IB (2014) Food insecurity in Nigeria: a thematic exposition. Oman Chapter Arab J Bus Manag Rev 34(2361):1–14

Fanadzo M (2012) Revitalisation of smallholder irrigation schemes for poverty alleviation and household food security in South Africa: a review. Afr J Agric Res 7:1956–1969. https://doi.org/10.5897/ajarx11.051

Fanadzo M, Chiduza C, Mnkeni PNS, van der Stoep I, Stevens J (2010) Crop production management practices as a cause for low water productivity at Zanyokwe irrigation scheme. Water SA 36:27–36. https://doi.org/10.4314/wsa.v36i1.50904

FAO. 2001. The state of food and agriculture 2001. Food & Agriculture Org

FAO (2018) Small family farms country factsheet – Nigeria. Food and Agriculture Organisation of the United Nations. http://www.fao.org/3/I9930EN/i9930en.pdf

FAO (2019) The state of food security and nutrition in the world: safeguarding against economic slowdowns and downturns. FAO, Rome

Fawole OI, Adeoye IA (2015) Women's status within the household as a determinant of maternal health care use in Nigeria. Afr Health Sci 15:217–225. https://doi.org/10.4314/ahs.v15i1.28

Fawole WO, Özkan B (2017) Identifying the drivers of food security based on perception among households in South Western Nigeria. Eur J Interdiscip Stud 9:49. https://doi.org/10.26417/ejis.v9i1.p49-55

Felloni F, Wahl T, Wandschneider P (1999) Evidence of the effect of infrastructure on agricultural production and productivity: implications for China. Chinese Agriculture and the WTO, Proceedings of WCC, 101

Frenken K (2005) Irrigation in Africa in figures: AQUASTAT survey, vol 29. Food & Agriculture Org

Gebrehiwot KA, Gebrewahid MG (2016) The need for agricultural water management in Sub-Saharan Africa. J Water Resour Protect 08:835–843. https://doi.org/10.4236/jwarp.2016.89068

Gibbs HK, Ruesch AS, Achard F, Clayton MK, Holmgren P, Ramankutty N, Foley JA (2010) Tropical forests were the primary sources of new agricultural land in the 1980s and 1990s. Proc Natl Acad Sci 107(38):16732–16737

Grant SB, Saphores JD, Feldman DL, Hamilton AJ, Fletcher TD, Cook PL, Marusic I (2012) Taking the "waste" out of "wastewater" for human water security and ecosystem sustainability. Science 337:681–686

Grey D, Sadoff CW (2007) Sink or swim? Water security for growth and development. Water Policy 9:545–571

Grey D, Sadoff C, Connors G (2016) Effective cooperation on transboundary waters: a practical perspective. World Bank, Washington, DC, pp 15–20. https://doi.org/10.1596/24047

https://www.statista.com/statistics/1122838/population-of-nigeria/

Hussain I, Mudasser M, Hanjra MA, Amrasinghe U, Molden D (2004) Improving wheat productivity in Pakistan: econometric analysis using panel data from Chaj in the upper Indus basin. Water Int 29:189–200. https://doi.org/10.1080/02508060408691768

Irz X, Lin L, Thirtle C, Wiggins S (2001) Agricultural productivity growth and poverty alleviation. Dev Policy Rev 19:449–466. https://doi.org/10.1111/1467-7679.00144

Jellason NP, Conway JS, Baines RN (2020) Exploring smallholders' cultural beliefs and their implication for adaptation to climate change in North-Western Nigeria. Soc Sci J:1–16. https://doi.org/10.1080/03623319.2020.1774720

Jellason NP, Conway JS, Baines RN, Ogbaga CC (2021a) A review of farming challenges and resilience management in the Sudano-Sahelian drylands of Nigeria in an era of climate change. J Arid Environ 186:104398

Jellason NP, Robinson EJ, Ogbaga CC (2021b) Agriculture 4.0: is sub-Saharan Africa ready? Appl Sci 11(12):5750

Kadigi RMJ (2012) Supporting policy research to inform agricultural policy in Sub-Saharan Africa and South Asia irrigation and water use efficiency in Sub-Saharan Africa, pp 1–36

Kebbeh M, Haefele S, Fagade S, Abidjan CDI (2003) Challenges and opportunities for improving irrigated rice productivity in Nigeria. West Africa Rice Development Association (WARDA), Bouake

Khan ZR, Midega CA, Pittchar JO, Murage AW, Birkett MA, Bruce TJ, Pickett JA (2014) Achieving food security for one million sub-Saharan African poor through push–pull innovation by 2020. Philos Trans R Soc B Biol Sci 369(1639):20120284

Koledoye GF, Deji OF (2015) Gender analysis of technology utilisation among small scale oil palm fruits processors in Ondo state, Nigeria. Acta Agronomica 64:36–47. https://doi.org/10.15446/acag.v64n1.42908

Leimbach M, Roming N, Schultes A, Schwerhoff G (2018) Long-term development perspectives of sub-Saharan Africa under climate policies. Ecol Econ 144:148–159. https://doi.org/10.1016/j.ecolecon.2017.07.033

Liu J, Qiu C, Xiao B, Cheng Z (2000) The role of plants in channel-dyke and field irrigation systems for domestic wastewater treatment in an integrated eco-engineering system. Ecol Eng 16:235–241. https://doi.org/10.1016/S0925-8574(00)00061-6

Llanto GM (2012) The impact of infrastructure on agricultural productivity 2012–12. PIDS discussion paper series

Lundqvist J, Unver O (2018) Alternative pathways to food security and nutrition – water predicaments and human behavior. Water Policy 20:871–884. https://doi.org/10.2166/wp.2018.171

Matemilola S, Elegbede I (2017) The challenges of food security in Nigeria. Open Access Lib J 04:1–22. https://doi.org/10.4236/oalib.1104185

McGuire S (2015) FAO, IFAD, and WFP. The state of food insecurity in the world 2015: meeting the 2015 international hunger targets: taking stock of uneven Progress. Rome: FAO, 2015. Adv Nutr 6:623–624. https://doi.org/10.3945/an.115.009936

Meliko MO, Oni SA (2011) Effect of irrigation on poverty among small-scale farmers in Limpopo Province of South Africa. J Agric Sci 3:190–195. https://doi.org/10.5539/jas.v3n3p190

Mellor, 1995.pdf, n.d.

Mkavidanda TAJ, Kaswamila AL (2001) The role of traditional irrigation systems (Vinyungu) in alleviating poverty in Iringa rural district, Tanzania. Mkuki na Nyota Publishers, Dar es Salaam

Mwanza DD (2003) Water for sustainable development in Africa. Environ Dev Sustain 5:95–115. https://doi.org/10.1023/A:1025380217316

Nadeem N, Mushtaq K, Javed MI (2011) Impact of social and physical infrastructure on agricultural productivity in Punjab, Pakistan-A production function approach. Pak J Life Soc Sci 9:153–158

Namara RE, Horowitz L, Nyamadi B, Barry B (2011) Irrigation development in Ghana: past experiences, emerging opportunities, and future directions. Ghana Strategy Support Program (GSSP) GSSP Working Paper No. 0027 41

Nzediegwu C, Chang SX (2020) Since January 2020 Elsevier has created a COVID-19 resource centre with free information in English and Mandarin on the novel coronavirus COVID-19. The COVID-19 resource centre is hosted on Elsevier Connect, the company's public news and information, pp 19–21

Ogundere F (2007) Trade liberalization and import demand for rice in Nigeria: a dynamic modelling. J Econ Rural Dev 16:34–45

Okunmadewa FY, Yusuf SA, Omonona BT (2007) Effect of social capital on rural poverty in Nigeria. Pak J Soc Sci 4:331–339

Olawuyi S (2012) Determinants of poverty among crop farmers: a case of Ogo-Oluwa local government, Oyo State. Br J Econ Manag Trade 2:340–352. https://doi.org/10.9734/bjemt/2012/2121

Oldeman LR (1997) Soil degradation: a threat to food security? Paper presented at the international conference on time ecology: time for soil culture – temporal perspectives on sustainable use of soil

Oluwatayo IB, Timothy O, Ojo AO (2019) Land acquisition and use in Nigeria: implications for sustainable food and livelihood security. In: Land use-assessing the past, envisioning the future. IntechOpen

Omorogiuwa O, Zivkovic J, Ademoh F (2014) The role of agriculture in the economic Development of Nigeria. Eur Sci J 10:133–147

Oni O, Nkonya E, Pender J (2009) Trends and drivers of agricultural productivity in Nigeria The Nigeria Strategy Support Program (NSSP) about nssp/apsf

Onuka OI (2017) Reversing Nigeria's food import dependency – agricultural transformation. Agric Dev 2:1–12. https://doi.org/10.20448/journal.523.2017.21.1.12

Osabohien R, Osabuohien E, Urhie E (2018) Food security, institutional framework and technology: examining the nexus in Nigeria using ARDL approach. Curr Nutr Food Sci 14:154–163. https://doi.org/10.2174/1573401313666170525133853

Otaha I (2013) Food insecurity in Nigeria: way forward. Afr Res Rev 7:26. https://doi.org/10.4314/afrrev.v7i4.2

Otekunrin OA, Otekunrin OA, Momoh S, Ayinde IA (2019a) Assessing the zero hunger target readiness in Africa: global hunger index (GHI) patterns and its indicators. In: Proceedings of the 33rd annual National Conference of the farm management association of Nigeria (FAMAN), 7th–10th October, 2019, pp 456–464. https://doi.org/10.13140/RG.2.2.16210.09926

Otekunrin OA, Otekunrin OA, Momoh S, Ayinde IA (2019b) How far has Africa gone in achieving the zero hunger target? Evidence from Nigeria. Global Food Secur 22:1–12

Otsuka K, Kijima Y (2010) Technology policies for a green revolution and agricultural transformation in Africa. J Afr Econ 19:ii60–ii76

Pavelic P, Villholth KG, Shu Y, Rebelo LM, Smakhtin V (2013) Smallholder groundwater irrigation in sub-Saharan Africa: country-level estimates of development potential. Water Int 38:392–407. https://doi.org/10.1080/02508060.2013.819601

Porter JR, Xie L, Challinor AJ et al (2014) Chapter 7: Food security and food production Systems. In: Climate Change 2014: impacts, adaptation, and vulnerability. Part A: Global and sectoral aspects. Contribution of Working Group II to the Fifth Assessment Report of the Intergovernmental Panel on Climate Chan. Cambridge University Press, p 485–533

Prasad AS, Umamahesh NV, Viswanath GK (2006) Optimal irrigation planning under water scarcity. J Irrig Drain Eng 132:228–237

Qadir M, Wichelns D, Raschid-Sally L, McCornick PG, Drechsel P, Bahri A, Minhas PS (2010) The challenges of wastewater irrigation in developing countries. Agric Water Manag 97:561–568. https://doi.org/10.1016/j.agwat.2008.11.004

Ragasa C, Dankyi A, Acheampong P, Wiredu AN, Chapoto A, Asamoah M, Tripp R (2013) Patterns of adoption of improved rice technologies in Ghana. IFPRI Working paper N 35

REPOA (2004) The use of sustainable irrigation for poverty Alleviation in Tanzania: the case of Smallholder Shadrack Mwakalila the use of sustainable irrigation for poverty, 69

Rockström J, Karlberg L, Wani SP, Barron J, Hatibu N, Oweis T, Bruggeman A, Farahani J, Qiang Z (2010) Managing water in rainfed agriculture-the need for a paradigm shift. Agric Water Manag 97:543–550. https://doi.org/10.1016/j.agwat.2009.09.009

Sasson A (2012) Food security for Africa: an urgent global challenge. Agric Food Secur 1:1–16. https://doi.org/10.1186/2048-7010-1-2

Seck PA, Diagne A, Mohanty S, Wopereis MCS (2012) Crops that feed the world 7: Rice. Food Secur 4:7–24. https://doi.org/10.1007/s12571-012-0168-1

Shiferaw B, Prasanna BM, Hellin J, Bänziger M (2011) Crops that feed the world 6. Past successes and future challenges to the role played by maize in global food security. Food Secur 3:307–327. https://doi.org/10.1007/s12571-011-0140-5

Shrestha PK (2017) Economic liberalization in Nepal: evaluating the changes in economic structure, employment and productivity. J Dev Innov 1(1):60–83

Sokoni C, Shechambo T (2005) Changes in the upland irrigation system and implications for rural poverty alleviation: a case of the Ndiwa irrigations system, west Usambara mountains. Tanzania 5(44)

Smith LED (2004) Assessment of the contribution of irrigation to poverty reduction and sustainable livelihoods. Int J Water Resour Dev 20:243–257. https://doi.org/10.1080/0790062042000206084

Statista (2022) Population of Nigeria in selected years between 1950 and 2021

Stockle CO (2001) Environmental impact of irrigation: a review. In: IV international congress of agricultural engineering

Tashikalma A, Sani R, Giroh D (2014) Comparative profitability analysis of selected rainfed and irrigated food crops in Adamawa state, Nigeria. Global J Pure Appl Sci 20:77. https://doi.org/10.4314/gjpas.v20i2.1

Tesfaye A, Bogale A, Namara RE, Bacha D (2008) The impact of small-scale irrigation on household food security: the case of Filtino and Godino irrigation schemes in Ethiopia. Irrig Drain Syst 22:145–158. https://doi.org/10.1007/s10795-008-9047-5

Thirtle C, Irz X, Lin L, Mckenzie-Hill V, Wiggins S (2001) Relationship between changes in agricultural productivity and the incidence of poverty in developing countries. Department for International Development, London, pp 1–33

Thirtle C, Lin L, Piesse J (2003) The impact of research-led agricultural productivity growth on poverty reduction in Africa, Asia and Latin America. World Dev 31:1959–1975. https://doi.org/10.1016/j.worlddev.2003.07.001

Turral H, Svendsen M, Faures JM (2010) Investing in irrigation: reviewing the past and looking to the future. Agric Water Manag 97:551–560. https://doi.org/10.1016/j.agwat.2009.07.012

Uduma BU, Samson OA, Mure UA (2016) Irrigation potentials and rice self-sufficiency in Nigeria: a review. Afr J Agri Res 11(5):298–309

Umara B (2014) The state of irrigation development in Nigeria. Irrigation in West Africa: current status and a view to the future, 243

Usman MA, Gerber N, von Braun J (2019) The impact of drinking water quality and sanitation on child health: evidence from rural Ethiopia. J Dev Stud 55:2193–2211. https://doi.org/10.1080/00220388.2018.1493193

Von Braun J, Fan S, Meinzen-Dick RS, Rosegrant MW, Nin Pratt A (2008) International agricultural research for food security, poverty reduction, and the environment: what to expect from scaling up CGIAR investments and "Best Bet" programs (No. 594-2016-39951). International Food Policy Research Institute (IFPRI), Washington, DC

Wang W, Zhuo L, Li M, Liu Y, Wu P (2019) The effect of development in water-saving irrigation techniques on spatial-temporal variations in crop water footprint and benchmarking. J Hydrol 577:123916. https://doi.org/10.1016/j.jhydrol.2019.123916

World Poverty Clock (2018) World Poverty Clock

Wright B, Cafiero C (2011) Grain reserves and food security in the Middle East and North Africa. Food Secur 3:61–76. https://doi.org/10.1007/s12571-010-0094-z

Xie Y, Zhou X (2014) Income inequality in today's China. Proc Natl Acad Sci 111(19):6928–6933

Xie H, You L, Wielgosz B, Ringler C (2014) Estimating the potential for expanding smallholder irrigation in sub-Saharan Africa. Agric Water Manag 131:183–193. https://doi.org/10.1016/j.agwat.2013.08.011

Xu Y, Seward P, Gaye C, Lin L, Olago DO (2019) Preface: groundwater in Sub-Saharan AfricaPréface: les eaux souterraines en Afrique Sub-SahariennePrefacio: Agua subterránea en el África Subsahariana前言: 撒哈拉以南非洲地区的地下水Prefácio: Águas subterrâneas na África Subsaariana. Hydrogeol J 27:815–822

Yang H, Zehnder A (2001) China's regional water scarcity and implications for grain supply and trade. Environ Plan 33:79–95

Zewdie MC, van Passel S, Cools J, Tenessa DB, Ayele ZA, Tsegaye EA, Minale AS, Nyssen J (2019) Direct and indirect effect of irrigation water availability on crop revenue in Northwest Ethiopia: a structural equation model. Agric Water Manag 220:27–35. https://doi.org/10.1016/j.agwat.2019.04.013

Chapter 14
Functions of Soil Microbes Under Stress Environment

Sana Zahra, Rifat Hayat, and Mukhtar Ahmed

Abstract All the functions carried out in an ecosystem are due to the action of several microbial species present in the earth. So, any kind of stress can alter their proper functioning and force them into stress conditions. However, microbes have the ability to reduce the intensity of stress by several acclimation mechanisms. In this review, the type of stressors like drought, temperature (freezing, high), soil type, heavy metals, nutrient status, etc., which affect the functions of microbes and the acclimation mechanisms to respond such stress conditions, was discussed. In addition, some techniques which were used by researchers to identify the population of microbes and their action toward stress were also discussed. Also, this review highlights how microbes play a role in reducing stress conditions from plants. This is because in a soil ecosystem, plants and microbes rely on each other, and any sort of stress that affects microbes will also influence physiology of plants as well. Among all the type of microbes, bacteria and fungi are discussed briefly because of their abundance in soil ecosystem and their beneficial role in enhancing plant growth under stress environments.

Keywords Soil microbes · Drought · Temperature · Moisture · Heavy metals

14.1 Introduction

Microbes are unicellular or multicellular, either prokaryotic or eukaryotic tiny organisms that can only be seen under microscope. However, they are present in a huge amount in the different ecosystems. In a soil ecosystem, they are almost present everywhere; specially their amount is considerable in the area of rhizosphere due to

---

S. Zahra · R. Hayat (✉)
Institute of Soil & Environmental Sciences, Pir Mehr Ali Shah Arid Agriculture University, Rawalpindi, Pakistan
e-mail: hayat@uaar.edu.pk

M. Ahmed
Department of Agronomy, PMAS Arid Agriculture University, Rawalpindi, Pakistan

© The Author(s), under exclusive license to Springer Nature Switzerland AG 2022
M. Ahmed (ed.), *Global Agricultural Production: Resilience to Climate Change*,
https://doi.org/10.1007/978-3-031-14973-3_14

the presence of root exudates, as it will serve as food for them. Out of so many types discovered until now, five main types of microbes include bacteria, fungi, protozoa, algae, and viruses. Bacteria are unicellular organisms categorized into different types based on their shapes which are *cocci, bacilli, spirilla*, etc. Fungi are basically plants like unicellular or multicellular small organisms that do not contain chlorophyll; common types include *Agaricus, Rhizopus, Penicillium*, etc. Protozoa are unicellular organisms; common types include *Paramecium, Amoeba*, etc. Algae are plantlike organisms mainly green in color mostly found at wet ecosystems; its types include *Fucus, Laminaria*, and *Spirogyra*. Electron microscope is used for viruses because of its small size among all other types of microbes. *Bacteriophage* is a common type of virus. Microbes are widely studied because of their abundance and importance in soil ecosystem functioning. All the processes in a soil environment are due to the different functions of microbes (Kennedy and Gewin 1997).

Soil microbes take part in cycling of nutrients and waste and thus prevent the ecosystem. They fix atmospheric nitrogen for plants, thus improving soil nutrient status; they recycle the synthetic chemicals applied to soil. In this review functions of two types of microbes, i.e., bacteria and fungi, are discussed mainly because of their abundance in soil as compared to the other ones and due to the beneficial roles they play in stress environment (Aislabie et al. 2013).

14.1.1 Effect of Different Stress Environments on Microbes and Functions of Microbes in Mitigating That Stress

Stress is defined as something which can alter the functioning of organisms. It can be biotic and abiotic, both of which causes retardation in the functioning of microbes, which not only leads to the reduced agricultural productivity but also causes disturbance in the plant and microbial functioning. Importantly, a stress environment can be detrimental for microbes present in soil. Accordingly, in this review paper, I have discussed several stress environments and their effects on microbial functioning and the mechanisms adopted by microbes to cope with such conditions. The type of stress ranges from environmental to anthropogenic and from stress caused by chemical to physical modifications. Each type of the stress will affect them in several ways. A type of stress that is tolerable for one species will be detrimental for other, for example, a high temperature which is bearable or favorable for thermophilic bacteria can be detrimental for other species of bacteria or cause dormancy of some species. Consequently, there will be varying acclimation mechanisms based on varying stressors faced by different microbial species. Death of any of microbial species will add nutrients into the soil which is either used by plants or by microbes to perform their functions for survival under stress environments (Farrar and Reboli 2006; Schimel and Bennett 2004).

The adaptability to the stress conditions by microbes is a long-term achievement that can be achieved by genetic alterations after several years or even decades.

14 Functions of Soil Microbes Under Stress Environment

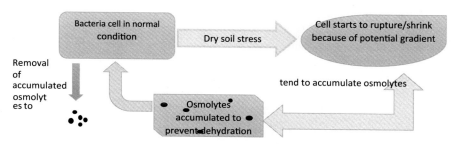

Fig. 14.1 Conceptual diagram of bacterial cell in drought and rewetting stress

Several direct and indirect mechanisms help microbes to overcome stress condition that come one after another like drought stress and rewetting of soil because in drought condition soil becomes drier and there is a chance of dehydration, while rewetting after it can cause cell rupture (Kieft 1987). In drought condition where the soil is dryer, solute concentration in surrounding environment rises and hence creates a potential gradient which causes cell rupture. So, bacteria tend to accumulate osmolytes like amino compounds to maintain an equilibrium with the surrounding to avoid dehydration. After getting rid of drought stress, it will face another stress in the form of rewetting of soil which again can cause cell rupture, so bacterial species tend to remove those accumulated osmolytes for their survival (Fig. 14.1) (Koujima et al. 1978).

Everything in excess and less both have beneficial and harmful effects; likewise increased temperature and a too cold or freezing temperature will be a stressor to microbes because in such condition, the microbial cell membrane will get rupture due to the formation of ice crystals in it. Acclimation mechanisms adopted by microorganisms under such conditions are modifying their membrane to avoid making crystals, stability in membrane fluidity, and adopting such proteins which resist freezing (Walker et al. 2006).

Heavy metals that are dumped or deposited in the soil either naturally or through anthropogenic activities create worst conditions by causing stress to the microbes. Several researches have been held to figure out the main sources of emission/discharge of heavy metals and to know their impact on microbial community within soil because in a soil ecosystem, the microbes drastically get affected by heavy metals and it causes a shift of microbial community from a particular ecosystem (Singh et al. 2014). Furthermore, different soil type and soil structure causes both a favorable and stress condition for microbes. The research studies based on experimentations revealed that the stable soil microaggregates provide a favorable environment for microbes and serve as best habitat for microbes. Clayey soil having smaller particles contains considerable amount of different species of microbes than the sandy soils having comparatively large soil particles. However, it may also cause a stress environment. For example, clayey soils have more pore volume than sandy soils, but the pores are smaller because of the smaller particle size of clay; it will retain more water for longer time which causes oxygen-deficient situation and causes stress environment for aerobic microbes. The nutrient are either provided through fertilizers or occurs naturally will define the population of microbes and microbial population in a soil is randomly distributed based on the type and amount of nutrient. However, microbes are present in a considerably huge amount at the place, where roots are present in soil (Burdman et al. 2000).

14.1.2 Functions of Microbes in Mitigating Stress for Plants

Soil-plant-microbe ecosystems are interlinked to one another, so any sort of stresses that influence the functions of microbes will also cause a negative impact on plants and physiological and metabolic mechanisms. Therefore, in this review, I have discussed the stresses faced by plants in an ecosystem along with microbes and the microbial functions in mitigating that stress. As mentioned above, stress may be biotic and abiotic. Biotic stress includes pathogens, weeds, and pest infestation, while abiotic stress includes salinity, drought, metal toxicity, temperature, etc. In salinity stress, an uprising concentration of ethylene is reported; however, reduced root activity and reduced chlorophyll content are witnessed under drought stress (Zapata et al. 2003).

14.1.3 Functions of Microbes Under Nutrient Deficiency Stress

A stress condition marked with oxygen deficiency and arid climate poses a great challenge to the macronutrient (P, S, and others) and micronutrient (Fe and others) cycling which can cause a stressful condition because of the crucial role of these nutrients in plant functioning and development, such as protein synthesis, root and shoot growth, and cell wall and organelle formation. So, fungi and bacteria are considered the main microbial communities that coexist in the soils with nutrients and expedite the process of nutrient fixing through redox reactions, for example, the *Thiobacillium* and *Metallogenium* species of bacteria are known for the dissolution of Fe through weathering processes, such as sorption, solubilization, chelation, accumulation, transformation, and precipitation. *Pseudomonas* species of bacteria was found to have performed well under aerobic conditions, whereas other microbes, such as *Desulfotomaculum*, under anaerobic conditions in degraded soils helped in the mobility of Fe nutrients. The fungi improve the availability and translocation of Fe by releasing siderophores (chelators). It helps in the mineralization and decomposition of Fe and enhancing soil fertility. Sulfur up to 95% is usually bound in organic form. Under stress environments, microbes can help to convert this crude form of sulfur to more utilizable inorganic form through microbial desulfurization. An experimental study identified several species of bacteria, such as *Pseudomonas*

14 Functions of Soil Microbes Under Stress Environment

brassicacearum, Stenotrophomonas rhizophila, and *others from Arthrobacter* genus. All such varieties of microbes were proved to be able to coexist with organic sulfur for its transformation under such conditions.

Furthermore, in anaerobic conditions, acidophilic microbes (e.g., *Acidithiobacillus ferrooxidans*) enhanced Fe and S nutrient mineralization through being capable of performing aerobic respiration. Phosphorus in soil is present in organic and an inorganic form (Hayat et al. 2010). Many microorganisms undertake the responsibility of converting organic phosphate or P esters to inorganic P. The inorganic P is solubilized by microorganisms called PSM that released different acids in soil and lower soil pH. The solubility of P can be increased by the respiration of microbes as this will release CO_2 which reacts with the water available in soil pores thus forming carbonic acid, which in turn will solubilize P in the soil (Berg 2009).

Although microbial population also get affected by stress environment, they have adopted certain strategies as discussed above, to overcome these stress environments. However, they also take part in mitigating that stress from plants. Microbes like plant growth-promoting bacteria and mycorrhizal fungi seem beneficial in several research studies.

14.1.3.1 Bacteria

Bacteria are the unicellular prokaryotic organisms that are too small which are only seen under microscope. They are present almost everywhere. In the rhizosphere the bacterial species are in huge amount as compared to the other microbes present in soil (Kaymak 2010). A spoon of soil contains millions of bacteria. They may be beneficial or harmful. Some types of bacteria have been found to be effective for plants in stress environment. The activity of PGPR can result in better performance or survival of plants under stress environment, as they took part in several mechanisms to cope up with stress conditions. For example, plant growth-promoting bacteria are present in the root nodules which benefit the plants in their growth even under stress conditions by fixing the atmospheric nitrogen for them (Kloepper and Schroth 1978). In the saline condition when there is risk of reduced crop productivity, due to decrease in nitrogen fixation, the plant growth-promoting bacteria fix the atmospheric nitrogen and provide it to the plants by converting it into plants available form, thus reducing the risk under such environment. Many bacteria in the soil secrete enzymes which solubilize the phosphorus and make it available to plants also by various enzymatic secretions; they make a barrier to the stressor (Berg 2009; Hayat et al. 2010).

High Concentration of Na^+ and Functioning of PGPR in Minimizing Its Negative Impact

Na toxicity is thought to be an important factor which has drastic effect in plants because it causes retardation in nutrient uptake by plants, so microbes like PGPR seem effective in this regard. They have potential to cope with such stress environments by producing exopolysaccharides which not only reduce Na^+ uptake but also bind it, so that their concentration will be reduced thoroughly; this will create a maximum K^+/Na^+ condition which is effective in salinity stress conditions (Geddie and Sutherland 1993; Hamdia et al. 2004).

Water-Deficit Stress Condition and Functioning of PGPR in Minimizing Its Negative Impact

As discussed above, in a soil environment, there is close interaction between plant, soil, and microbes so a stress condition in soil affects both microbes and plants. We know that the plant body constitutes of more than 90% of water, so water serves as a building block for plants. From seedling to germination stages, all the processes like process of photosynthesis, etc. involve water molecule; hence, a low water content/supply to plants can cause reduced plant growth and plant yield, decreased photosynthetic process, membrane damage, etc. Similarly, a water-deficit condition can cause reduction in leaf area in plants and cause severe stress condition for plants. Such kind of stress may cause reduced physiological and biochemical characteristics. So, plant growth-promoting bacteria have the potential to cope with such conditions and minimize that stress condition from plants. In a water-deficit situation, the PGPR produces exopolysaccharides which gives protection to them from dehydration and making them survive under such condition (Sandhya et al. 2009).

Functions of PGPR in Minimizing Stress Caused by Pathogens

Plant pathogens are the organisms which cause several diseases in plants and cause alterations in their physiology because not all plants are vulnerable to pathogenic attacks. The effects caused by pathogens (like destruction of entire plant species) are not only related to plants, but it has severe impacts on the economy of country. In such situation, the plant growth-promoting bacteria seem beneficial in minimizing the stress from plants, by several mechanisms such as:

(a) Induced systematic resistance in plants: It is a mechanism which is triggered in plants when a pathogen is attacking; it is basically a physical or chemical barrier of the host plant.
(b) Reducing pathogens in plants by producing iron-chelating compounds: To minimize the pathogen population, they produce certain iron-chelating compounds to create iron-deficit condition for pathogens (Arora et al. 2001; Bhattacharyya and Jha 2012).

14 Functions of Soil Microbes Under Stress Environment

14.1.3.2 Arbuscular Mycorrhizal Fungi

A symbiotic association in which both partners get benefitted is accomplished by plant roots and fungi which are known as mycorrhizae. All types of the soils around the world have fungi; in fact, it is most abundantly present in soils after bacteria. From all the types of fungi discovered until now, the *arbuscular mycorrhizae* and *ectomycorrhizae* are abundantly found in symbiotic associations in a soil ecosystem.

It plays function such as in making plants able to absorb more water by increasing its root surface area, so that water can easily be accessible to plants in a deficient condition. In a symbiotic association, the mycorrhizae not only benefit the plant with supplying sufficient amount of nutrients and water by increasing its root surface area but also shield them from various other stresses (Evelin et al. 2009).

It involves several steps:

1. Penetration of fungi into the roots
2. The multiplication of fungal hyphae into soil
3. Absorption of nutrient and water

Functions of Arbuscular Mycorrhizal Fungi in Different Stress Environments

The functions of arbuscular mycorrhizal fungi are useful in minimizing stress environments faced by plants during their growth stages and also play a significant role in stress environment caused by water-deficit condition. Due to increase in root surface area and small projections, it is effective in absorbing more water in a scarce condition (Khalvati et al. 2005). It helps to overcome pathogenic attacks. It is not only involved in making water and nutrients available to the plants but also regulates the defense mechanism in plants against pathogenic attacks (Azcón-Aguilar and Barea 1997). The arbuscular mycorrhizal fungi provide tolerance to the plants in a drought stress condition; also it is found useful in making plants survive under salinity stress.

The maintenance of K^+/Na^+ ratio is accomplished by the mycorrhizal fungi as it seems effective in saline conditions because an increase K^+/Na^+ tells us about the tolerance level in most plants (Zhang et al. 2011). Arbuscular mycorrhizal fungi have potential to increase nodulation under salinity stress. VAM plays a major role in nitrogen fixation in a salinity stress condition.

14.2 Techniques to Study Microbial Functions

Because of the very small size of microbes, it is unable to witness their functions by naked eye, so there are several techniques invented to study their function in soil environment. To well understand the microbial population in a soil ecosystem and to know their functions, both in normal and under stress conditions flow cytometry or single cell analysis technique seems effective. In this technique different chemicals are used which indicates about the microbial activity. Methods based on rRNA and rDNA analyses seems effective in knowing the microbial population and the functions performed by microbes under stress and normal conditions (Torsvik and Øvreås 2002). Genomic methods such as metagenomics and microarrays are used to study the population and types of microbes. Bacterial artificial chromosomes seem beneficial in getting information regarding functions of several types of bacteria in a soil ecosystem. However, the changes that occurred in the microbial communities as a result of different stressors can also be detected. A changing environment can cause shifting of microbial community. However, functional analyses of environmental DNA tell about the processes that occur in soil and within different microbial communities (Xu 2006).

14.3 Conclusion

Different stress environments have a different range of negative effects on functions of microbes as well as on the plants in a soil-plant-microbe ecosystem. However, it can be mitigated by microorganisms for their survival using different strategies based on type and intensity of stress. Under drought and rewetting stress, the microbes survive first by accumulating osmolytes in drought stress while removing them in rewetting stress. After which they help in mitigating the stress environment faced by plants; mainly it can be mitigated by the action of PGPR and mycorrhizal fungi. So, their functions under stress environments were identified by using several techniques, which are highlighted in this review.

References

Aislabie J, Deslippe JR, Dymond J (2013) Soil microbes and their contribution to soil services. In: Ecosystem services in New Zealand–conditions and trends, vol 1, no 12. Manaaki Whenua Press, Lincoln, pp 143–161

Arora NK, Kang SC, Maheshwari DK (2001) Isolation of siderophore-producing strains of Rhizobium meliloti and their biocontrol potential against Macrophomina phaseolina that causes charcoal rot of groundnut. Curr Sci:673–677

Azcón-Aguilar C, Barea JM (1997) Arbuscular mycorrhizas and biological control of soil-borne plant pathogens–an overview of the mechanisms involved. Mycorrhiza 6(6):457–464

Berg G (2009) Plant–microbe interactions promoting plant growth and health: perspectives for controlled use of microorganisms in agriculture. Appl Microbiol Biotechnol 84(1):11–18

Bhattacharyya PN, Jha DK (2012) Plant growth-promoting rhizobacteria (PGPR): emergence in agriculture. World J Microbiol Biotechnol 28(4):1327–1350

Burdman S, Jurkevitch E, Okon Y (2000) Recent advances in the use of plant growth promoting rhizobacteria (PGPR) in agriculture. Microb Interact Agric Forestry II:229–250

Evelin H, Kapoor R, Giri B (2009) Arbuscular mycorrhizal fungi in alleviation of salt stress: a review. Ann Bot 104(7):1263–1280

14 Functions of Soil Microbes Under Stress Environment

Farrar WE, Reboli AC (2006) The genus Bacillus–medical. Prokaryotes 4:609–630

Geddie JL, Sutherland IW (1993) Uptake of metals by bacterial polysaccharides. J Appl Bacteriol 74(4):467–472

Hamdia MAE-S, Shaddad MAK, Doaa MM (2004) Mechanisms of salt tolerance and interactive effects of Azospirillum brasilense inoculation on maize cultivars grown under salt stress conditions. Plant Growth Regul 44(2):165–174

Hayat R, Ali S, Amara U, Khalid R, Ahmed I (2010) Soil beneficial bacteria and their role in plant growth promotion: a review. Ann Microbiol 60(4):579–598

Kaymak HC (2010) Potential of PGPR in agricultural innovations. In: Plant growth and health promoting bacteria, pp 45–79

Kennedy AC, Gewin VL (1997) Soil microbial diversity: present and future considerations. Soil Sci 162(9):607–617

Khalvati MA, Hu Y, Mozafar A, Schmidhalter U (2005) Quantification of water uptake by arbuscular mycorrhizal hyphae and its significance for leaf growth, water relations, and gas exchange of barley subjected to drought stress. Plant Biol 7(6):706–712

Kieft TL (1987) Microbial biomass response to a rapid increase in water potential when dry soil is wetted. Soil Biol Biochem 19(2):119–126

Kloepper JW, Schroth M (1978) Plant growth-promoting rhizobacteria on radishes. In: Proceedings of the 4th International Conference on Plant Pathogenic Bacter, Station de Pathologie Vegetale et Phytobacteriologie, INRA, Angers, France, vol 2, pp 879–882

Koujima I, Hayashi H, Tomochika K, Okabe A, Kanemasa Y (1978) Adaptational change in proline and water content of Staphylococcus aureus after alteration of environmental salt concentration. Appl Environ Microbiol 35(3):467–470

Sandhya V, Grover M, Reddy G, Venkateswarlu B (2009) Alleviation of drought stress effects in sunflower seedlings by the exopolysaccharides producing Pseudomonas putida strain GAP-P45. Biol Fertil Soils 46(1):17–26

Schimel JP, Bennett J (2004) Nitrogen mineralization: challenges of a changing paradigm. Ecology 85(3):591–602

Singh BK, Quince C, Macdonald CA, Khachane A, Thomas N, Al-Soud WA et al (2014) Loss of microbial diversity in soils is coincident with reductions in some specialized functions. Environ Microbiol 16(8):2408–2420

Torsvik V, Øvreås L (2002) Microbial diversity and function in soil: from genes to ecosystems. Curr Opin Microbiol 5(3):240–245

Walker VK, Palmer GR, Voordouw G (2006) Freeze-thaw tolerance and clues to the winter survival of a soil community. Appl Environ Microbiol 72(3):1784–1792

Xu J (2006) Invited review: microbial ecology in the age of genomics and metagenomics: concepts, tools, and recent advances. Mol Ecol 15(7):1713–1731

Zapata PJ, Serrano M, Pretel MT, Amorós A, Botella MÁ (2003) Changes in ethylene evolution and polyamine profiles of seedlings of nine cultivars of Lactuca sativa L. in response to salt stress during germination. Plant Sci 164(4):557–563

Zhang YF, Wang P, Yang YF, Bi Q, Tian SY, Shi XW (2011) Arbuscular mycorrhizal fungi improve reestablishment of Leymus chinensis in bare saline-alkaline soil: implication on vegetation restoration of extremely degraded land. J Arid Environ 75(9):773–778

Chapter 15
Modeling Impacts of Climate Change and Adaptation Strategies for Cereal Crops in Ethiopia

A. Araya, P. V. V. Prasad, P. K. Jha, H. Singh, I. A. Ciampitti, and D. Min

Abstract Teff, maize, wheat, sorghum, and barley are the five major food crops in Ethiopia. This chapter provides a summary of the work investigating the effect of climate change and potential adaptation strategies to mitigate their effects for the abovementioned major field crops in Ethiopia. Climate change studies were carried out using an in silico approach via the utilization of crop growth [AquaCrop, Decision Support System for Agrotechnology Transfer (DSSAT), Agricultural Production Systems sIMulator (APSIM)] and global climate models. Maize varieties, Melkasa-1, BH-660, and BH-540, resulted in a significant change in yield during the midcentury by -13 to -8%, $+3$ to $+13\%$, and -10 to $+4\%$, respectively. For maize, the use of optimal planting date, nitrogen (N) fertilization, and irrigation contributed to improve yield under future climates. For wheat, cross-location average yield could slightly increase during the midcentury when simulated under RCP8.5 (elevated CO_2 scenario) when accompanied with optimal N fertilization management. In contrast, barley yield during the midcentury is projected to decline by 6 to 11% relative to baseline yield. Optimal planting date, tied ridging, rotation with legumes, and N fertilization along with elevated CO_2 could minimize the negative impacts of climate change on the productivity of barley. For sorghum, simulation studies showed that the crop is highly responsive to time of planting, with yields negatively impacted during the midcentury by up to 9.1% for March and 12.2% for April planting. Planting time could be considered as an effective adaptation strategy for

---

A. Araya · P. K. Jha
Sustainable Intensification Innovation Lab, Kansas State University, Manhattan, KS, USA

P. V. V. Prasad (✉)
Sustainable Intensification Innovation Lab, Kansas State University, Manhattan, KS, USA

Department of Agronomy, Kansas State University, Manhattan, KS, USA
e-mail: vara@ksu.edu

H. Singh
Department of Agronomy, Kansas State University, Manhattan, KS, USA

West Florida Research and Education Center, University of Florida, FL, USA

I. A. Ciampitti · D. Min
Department of Agronomy, Kansas State University, Manhattan, KS, USA

© The Author(s), under exclusive license to Springer Nature Switzerland AG 2022
M. Ahmed (ed.), *Global Agricultural Production: Resilience to Climate Change*,
https://doi.org/10.1007/978-3-031-14973-3_15

sorghum in Ethiopia. For teff, yield during the midcentury could decline by up to 12% when sown after the top 10 cm soil is wet and no extended dry spells of more than 7 days occur afterward for over 25 days. This indicates the importance of precipitation quantity and seasonal distribution for sowing teff. In addition, optimal N fertilization (64 kg/ha) could increase productivity of teff while reducing the negative impacts of climate change. Higher N above this level (64 kg/ha) causes issues related to lodging. Thus, for teff crop, yield losses could be reduced due to the effect of climate change by planting early and providing optimal N fertilization.

Keywords Maize · Wheat · Teff · Sorghum · Ethiopia · DSSAT · AquaCrop · APSIM

15.1 Introduction

Teff (*Eragrostis tef*), wheat (*Triticum aestivum*), maize (*Zea mays*), sorghum (*Sorghum bicolor*), and barley (*Hordeum vulgare*) are the major cereal crops in Ethiopia (Taffesse et al. 2011). Enhancing cereal productivity under the increasing population growth is critically needed in order to reduce hunger and malnutrition. Elevated temperatures, rainfall variabilities, and occurrence of other extreme events (i.e., flood and drought stress) could pose critical threat to crop production (IPCC 2013, 2021). Many cereals are sensitive to temperature increase and water stress, especially if the stress occurs during the flowering period (Prasad et al. 2008a, 2015, 2017; Lizaso et al. 2018). Climate-related stress in Ethiopia is projected to reduce the yield of the cereal crops under future scenarios (Kassie et al. 2014a, b; Araya et al. 2015b, 2020b, 2021a; Gebrekiros et al. 2016; Abera et al. 2018). Climate change is a threat to food security, although the overall impacts are yet to be understood, and adaptation management strategies need to be identified in order to reduce the risk. In addition, as available resources are limited, the adaptation management strategies need to be quantified in order to address the threat timely and cost-effectively. Crop growth simulation models have been used to quantify the impacts of climate change and evaluate optimal adaptation management strategies at various spatial scales to support decisions (Araya et al. 2020a, b, 2021c; Silungwe et al. 2018). Individual quantitative information on components of climate change factors is available at various scales in scientific studies and reports. However, the quantitative information on the impact of climate change and adaptation strategies for the above major cereal crops in Ethiopia have not been adequately summarized. This synthesis can provide useful insights on future research investments and for guiding new policies at the regional and country scales. This study mainly focuses on midcentury period (2040–2069) to understand and quantify the yield deviation due to climate change and discusses the management strategies that can be used to reduce the risk. Therefore, the objective of this chapter is to present a summary of individual studies relevant to the impact of climate change and adaptation strategies for major cereal crops (teff, wheat, maize, sorghum, and barley) in Ethiopia.

15.2 Methods

15.2.1 Study Sites, Data Sources, and Scenarios

The analysis was carried out based on the information obtained from previous studies (Akinseye et al. 2020; Araya et al. 2015a, b, 2020a, b, 2021a, b, c; Gebrekiros et al. 2016; Thomas et al. 2019; Zewdu et al. 2020) that were focused on future climate change and adaptation for major cereal crops in Ethiopia (Table 15.1). However, some other studies that were focused on crop management data based on present or past climate were also included. These investigations were conducted at different scales and locations (from site specific to country scale), and many of the management scenarios evaluated differ among all the different field crops. Climate change studies were conducted using different crop growth models such as Decision Support System for Agrotechnology Transfer (DSSAT), Agricultural Production Systems sIMulator (APSIM), and AquaCrop along with global climate models (GCM). Most of the simulation studies on the selected five major crops were conducted for the midcentury (2040–2069) relative to the baseline (1980–2005/2009) period. Table 15.1 shows the locations, crops, and various scenarios and treatments used for assessing the impacts of climate change and adaptation strategies. Since the climate change studies differ in time and spatial scale as well as in terms of management treatment for each crop, the data is summarized and presented by crop type.

15.2.2 Maize

Climate change and adaptation management strategies presented and discussed by Araya et al. (2021a) are summarized. The climate data (daily maximum and minimum temperature and radiation data) based on the Coordinated Regional Downscaling Experiment (CORDEX) for midcentury (2040–2069) period (Endris et al. 2013; Mascaro et al. 2015) under high Representative Concentration Pathways (RCP8.5) was extracted for 21 Ethiopian locations and entered in DSSAT model. Maize was exposed to three worst case scenarios: (i) the climate extracted under high-emission scenario, (ii) maize grown in soils with low water-holding capacity (sandy loam soils), and (iii) under unchanged rainfall [[although future rainfall based on GCMs was expected to increase (Vizy and Cook 2012; Thomas et al. 2019)]. The baseline (1981–2010) rainfall was extracted from the Climate Hazards Group Infrared Precipitation with Station data (CHIRPS) (Funk et al. 2014, 2015; Dinku et al. 2018). Three maize varieties (Melkasa-1, BH-660, and BH-540), three irrigation treatments (0, 60, and 150 mm), four N fertilizer treatments (64, 96, 128, and 160 kg N/ha), and three planting dates (April 25, May 25, and June 25) were evaluated for identifying adaptation options for the midcentury period (Araya et al. 2021a).

Table 15.1 The locations, crops, and various scenarios and treatments used for assessing the impacts of climate change and adaptation strategies

Country	No of locations	Crop model / No. of varieties	Baseline period	Baseline rainfall	GCM	Period	RCP	CO$_2$ con. / ppm	Soil type	Irrigation / mm	Nitrogen / kg/ha	Planting date/ density	References (source)
Ethiopia	22 locations	Maize (3 varieties) DSSAT	1980–2005	CHRIPS	CORDEX	2040–2069	8.5	571	Sandy loam	0, 60, and 150 mm	64, 96, 128, 160	April 25; May 25; June 25	Araya et al. (2021a)
Ethiopia	Bako	Maize	1980–2009	MS	20GCM (CMIP5)	2010–2039	4.5 and 8.5	380, 432, 571	Clay	–	Vary by farmers/ survey	May 25	Araya et al. (2015a)
						2040–2069							
		DSSAT and APSIM				2070–2099		801					
Ethiopia	21 locations	Wheat DSSAT	1980–2005	CHRIPS	CORDEX	2040–2069	8.5	571, 380	Clay and sandy clay loam	0, 60, and 150 mm	64, 96, 128, 160	–	Araya et al. (2020a)
Ethiopia	Kulumsa	3 wheat varieties APSIM	1980–2009	MS	3GCM (CMIP5)	2040–2069	8.5	571	Clay	Rainfed	32, 64, 96, 128	July 10; Density: 100, 200, and 300 p/m^2	Araya et al. (2020b)
Ethiopia	Kulumsa	3 wheat varieties APSIM	1980–2009	+20% and −20% rain	1, 2, 4, 6 °C	–	–	360, 432, 571 801	Clay	Rainfed	32, 64, 96, 128	June 25– July 10; July 10–30; Aug 1–15	Araya et al. (2020b)
Ethiopia	Adigudom	Barley DSSAT	1980–2009	MS	3GCM (CMIP5)	2040–2069	8.5	571	Clay, loam, and sandy clay loam	Rainfed	32, 64, 96, 128	June 20– Aug 20	Araya et al. (2021b)

Country	Location	Crop / Model	Period	Climate data	Scenario/GCMs	Future period	RCP	CO_2	Soil	Water	Fertilizer	Planting date	Reference
Ethiopia	Adigudom	Barley DSSAT	1980–2009	MS	1, 2, 4, 6 °C	–	–	360, 432, 571 801	Clay, loam, and sandy clay loam	Rainfed	32, 64, 96, 128	June 20–Aug 20	Araya et al. (2021b)
Ethiopia	Adigudom and Kulumsa	Barley DSSAT	1980–2019	MS	–	–	–	–	Clay, loam, and sandy clay loam	Rainfed and tied ridging	64 kg N/ha and rotation with chickpea	July 20, plt. density: 250 plants/ m^2	Araya et al. (2021c)
Ethiopia	Srinka and Kobo	2 sorg. var. DSSAT	1980–2009	MS	20 CIMP5 GCMs	2040–2069 and 2070–2099	4.5 and 8.5	–	Silt loam and clay	Rainfed	–	–	Zewdu et al. (2020)
Ethiopia	Alamata	1 sorg. var. APSIM	1980–2009	MS	1 GCM HadGEM2-ES	2010–2039 2040–2069 and 2070–2099	4.5 and 8.5	–	–	Rainfed	64 kg N/ha	Mar, Apr, May, June	Gebrekiros et al. (2016)
Ethiopia	6 agro-ecologies	1 sorg. DSSAT	1960–1990		HadGEM2_ES	2035, 2055 and 2085	RCP8.5		Grid scale	Rainfed			Thomas et al. (2019)
W. Africa (Nigeria and Mali)	Bamako and Kano	2 sorg. var. APSIM	1980–2009	MERRA	5 CMIP5 GCMs	2010–2039 2040–2069	4.5 and 8.5	360 and 571	–	Rainfed	NPK 60: 30:30	June 14, July 9, and August 5	Akinseye et al. (2020)
Ethiopia	Debrezeit	1 teff var. AquaCrop	1980–2009	MS	5 CMIP5 GCMs	2010–2039 2040–2069	4.5 and 8.5	–		Rainfed	64 kg N/ha	July 18, July 28, Aug 19	Araya et al. (2015b)

CMIP5 coupled model intercomparison project phase 5, *CORDEX* coordinated regional downscaling experiment, *CHIRPS* climate hazards group infrared precipitation with station data, *GCM* global climate model, *MERRA* modern-era retrospective analysis for research and applications, *MS* measured, *Sorg.* sorghum, *var.* variety

15.2.3 Wheat

The impacts of climate change and adaptation strategies for wheat were conducted from site specific to national scale on various soils (clay and sandy clay loam soils) based on climate change scenarios described above for maize (Araya et al. 2020a, b). While only one wheat variety was used when conducting national-scale studies, three wheat varieties (early-, medium-, and late-maturing varieties) were evaluated at two selected locations (Araya et al. 2017, 2020b). Separate studies were conducted using either DSSAT or APSIM model. The future climate data for 21 locations was extracted based on methods described for maize. Climate change adaptation strategies that include three irrigation rates (0, 60, and 150 mm) and four N fertilizer rates (64, 96, 128, and 160 kg N/ha) under elevated and baseline carbon dioxide (CO_2) scenarios were evaluated as presented for maize (Table 15.1). Furthermore, responses of three wheat varieties to various combinations of elevated temperatures (1, 2, 3, 4, 5, and 6 °C), changed rainfall (-20% and $+20\%$), N rates (32, 64, 96, and 128 kg N/ha), plant densities (100, 200, and 300 plants m^{-2}), and CO_2 levels (360, 432, 571, and 801 μmol mol^{-1}) were evaluated (Table 15.1). The results of the combination of these factors were extracted, discussed, and summarized.

15.2.4 Barley

Climate change impact assessment and adaptation strategies for barley were conducted in Northern Ethiopia for two selected locations (Araya et al. 2021b). The main study was conducted using DSSAT model. Climate data from three GCMs ensembles were extracted for the midcentury period (under elevated CO_2 (RCP8.5; 571 μmol mol^{-1})) and entered into the crop model (Table 15.1). In addition, sensitivity analysis was carried out to understand the response of barley to the combination of climatic factors such as elevated temperatures (baseline temperature +1, 2, 4, and 6 °C), CO_2 (360, 432, 571, and 801 μmol mol^{-1}), different N rates (32, 64, 96, and 128 kg N/ha), and soil types (clay, loam, and sandy clay loam). In a separate study, the impact of tied ridging and different crop rotations with wheat and chickpea (*Cicer arietinum*) (wheat-barley, wheat-chickpea-barley, chickpea-barley) in improving barley yield was evaluated as a climate change adaptation strategy in Northern Ethiopia (Araya et al. 2021c). Furthermore, information on optimal planting date for barley was also reviewed from Araya et al. (2012), Gessesse and Araya (2015), and Araya et al. (2021c). The results of the impacts of climate change and agronomic management practices for reducing the negative impacts of climate change on barley yield were reanalyzed, extracted, discussed, and summarized.

15.2.5 Sorghum

Climate change impact assessment reports were reviewed for Ethiopian sorghum from Gebrekiros et al. (2016), Thomas et al. (2019), and Zewdu et al. (2020). These authors used different GCMs and crop models such as APSIM and DSSAT to conduct the simulation studies at different temporal and spatial scales. Zewdu et al. (2020) used 20 GCMs under RCP4.5 and RCP8.5 for the periods 2040–2069 and 2070–2099. The climate data was entered in DSSAT, and climate change impact results were generated for two sorghum cultivars at two locations in Northern Ethiopia (Table 15.1). Gebrekiros et al. (2016) used APSIM model, and descriptions of treatments and scenarios are presented in Table 15.1. Similarly, information on the contribution of N fertilization, planting date, and irrigation in reducing climatic risk on sorghum yield was reviewed and summarized based on information presented in Hegano et al. (2016), Shamme et al. (2016), Mebrahtu and Tamiru (2019), Wale et al. (2019), Abera et al. (2020), Kotharia et al. (2020), Mehari et al. (2020), and Getachew et al. (2021).

15.2.6 Teff

The impact of climate change on teff productivity was assessed for major teff-growing area in Central Ethiopia (Debrezeit). The study was conducted using AquaCrop model based on five Coupled Model Intercomparison Project Phase 5 (CMIP5) GCMs under RCP4.5 and RCP8.5 scenarios (Araya et al. 2015b) (Table 15.1). Araya et al. (2015b) evaluated suitable sowing times to reduce drought risks under climate change for the near-term (2010–2039), midterm (2040–2069), and end-term (2070–2099) periods. In addition, information on the impact of management practices such as N fertilizer and irrigation on teff yield was discussed and summarized based on the information presented in Araya et al. (2011, 2019), Haileselassie et al. (2016), and Tsegay et al. (2015).

15.3 Results and Discussion

15.3.1 Maize

Short-maturing maize variety, Melkasa-1, yield decreased by 8.7 to 15% during the midcentury period (Table 15.2 and Fig. 15.1a, b and c). Under rainfed condition, Melkasa-1 yield increased by 168–207 kg/ha^{-1} for every additional 32 kg N above the 64 kg N/ha up to 160 kg N/ha (Fig. 15.1a). Similarly, under irrigated conditions (150 mm), Melkasa-1 produced additional yield gain over the 64 kg N/ha by 248, 213, and 301 kg/ha due to the application of 96, 128, and 160 kg N/ha,

Table 15.2 Comparison of baseline against the future (midcentury) yield for three maize varieties under different N and water management strategies for Ethiopia

Crop variety	Irrigation treatment	Nitrogen (kg/ha)			
		64 Dev. (%)	96 Dev. (%)	128 Dev. (%)	160 Dev. (%)
Melkasa-1	Rainfed	−8.7	−8.9	−8.0	−11.2
	60 mm	−7.6	−9.9	−12.3	−11.0
	150 mm	−7.4	−7.5	−12.3	−14.9
BH−660	Rainfed	20.0	16.0	13.1	10.9
	60 mm	10.9	10.0	5.0	7.6
	150 mm	6.2	7.7	4.0	2.4
BH−540	Rainfed	8.0	1.3	−5.8	−5.8
	60 mm	−0.4	−3.9	−7.0	−9.7
	150 mm	0.0	−4.6	−7.4	−13.9

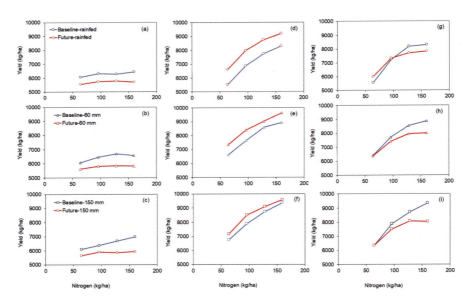

Fig. 15.1 The relationship between maize yield and N fertilizer and irrigation under baseline (1980–2005) and future (2040–2069) climate for (**a–c**) Melkasa-1, (**d–f**) BH-660, and (**g–i**) BH-540 for as averaged for 21 locations in Ethiopia

respectively (Fig. 15.1c). This shows that the increase beyond 64 kg N/ha did not improve maize yield substantially, which implies that Melkasa-1 yield could be optimized with the application of 64 kg N/ha. Araya et al. (2021a) reported the right amount of N rate for Melkasa-1 was 64 kg N/ha. Climate characteristics (Kassie et al. 2014a, b), yielding potential and N use efficiency (Tolessa et al. 2007; Abera et al. 2018), seeding rate (Zeleke et al. 2018), and soil characteristics (USDA, 2014a, b) could affect the N application rate (Araya et al. 2021a). For example, the recommended N fertilizer for dryland rift valley of Ethiopia was less than 64 kg N/ha (Kassie et al. 2014a).

Midcentury maize (variety BH-660) yield increased significantly with the increase in N fertilizer from 64 to 160 kg N/ha (Table 15.1). However, the rate of yield increase was decreasing up to 160 kg N/ha. The increase in maize yield during the midcentury due to the application of 96, 128, and 160 kg N/ha when compared to maize grown (under the rainfed) with 64 kg N/ha generated yield advantages of 1360, 2148, and 2588 kg/ha, respectively. This shows that there was an increase in maize yield by 1360, 788, and 440 kg/ha for each additional application of 32 kg N beyond 64 kg/ha up to 160 kg N/ha (Fig. 15.1d). Similarly, the yield gains with irrigated condition during the midcentury climate could range from 14 to 18.5% (1042–1329 kg/ha) at 92 kg N/ha, 22.8 to 26.8% (1682–1923 kg/ha) at 128 kg N/ha, and 30.8 to 33.4% (2269–2400 kg/ha) at 160 kg N/ha, respectively, relative to their corresponding 64 kg N/ha. The lowest and highest increase corresponded to 60 and 150 mm irrigation water application, respectively (Fig. 15.1e, f). Experimental studies in Ethiopia showed higher yield of maize BH-660 at the rate of 92–115 kg N/ha (Mandefro et al. 2001; Abebe and Feyisa 2017). Similarly, Araya et al. (2021a) reported the application of 128–160 kg N/ha could enhance midcentury maize yield. Considering all these management practices, BH-660 under midcentury climate change increased by up to 20%, compared to the corresponding baseline yield. This shows optimal application of N could be considered as a potential agronomic climate change adaptation strategy for maize in Ethiopia. Thomas et al. (2019) reported that climate change during the midcentury might not significantly decrease the yield of maize in Ethiopia due to the expected increased future rainfall along with improved agronomic practices (e.g., application of N at optimal level).

The yield of the maize variety BH-540 under climate change varied compared to the corresponding baseline. Under midcentury climate scenario, there was an additional increase in maize yield under rainfed condition by 1346, 373, and 117 kg/ha with the increase in N rate from 64 to 96, 96 to 128, and 128 to 160 kg N/ha, respectively (Fig. 15.1g). Similarly, the yield increases for irrigated midcentury maize due to each 32 kg increment in N rate from 64 to 96, 96 to 128, and 128 to 160 kg N/ha were 1168, 561, and −32 kg/ha, respectively. These results portrayed that increasing N beyond 128 kg N/ha has no positive contribution to yield enhancement. Araya et al. (2021a) reported the optimal N application for the variety BH-540 was 128 kg/ha.

Choice of planting time is one of the most important and less costly adaptation strategies for maize crop under climate change. Araya et al. (2021a) showed that the optimal planting date for Melkasa-1 for most part of Ethiopian locations was around May 25 with some exception in the eastern and southern parts such as Jijiga, Harar, A. Minch, and Dilla (Fig. 15.2a), whereas the optimal planting date for BH-660 and BH-540 was around April 25 to May 25 but still with some exception like Dilla, Asela, Jijiga, and A. Minch (Fig. 15.2b). As maize is sensitive to water stress, other reports from Ethiopia showed that planting time could significantly affect maize yield (Balem et al. 2020). This study showed that the choice of planting date could impact maize yield between −13% and 21% for Melkasa-1 and −32% and 21% for

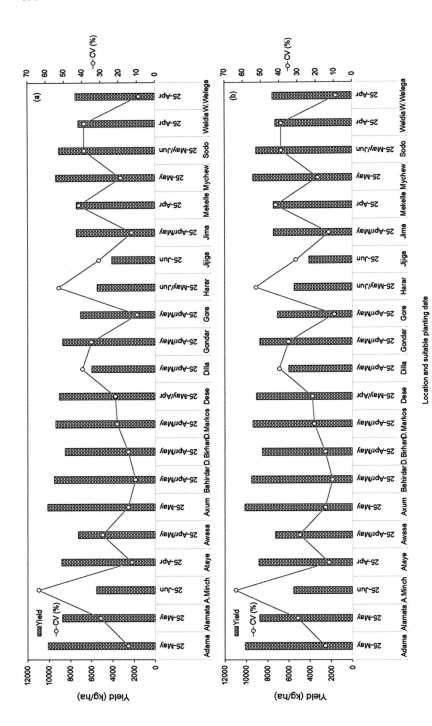

Fig. 15.2 Optimal planting dates selected based on inter-seasonal yield variabilities (CV %) and yield for Melkasa-1 (**a**) and BH-660 (**b**) maize varieties for different Ethiopian locations

BH-660. Dolapo et al. (2019) and Balem et al. (2020) reported the optimal interaction of planting date and fertilizer application could significantly contribute to maize yield improvement and economic benefit.

Irrigation slightly improved cross-location maize yield under both the baseline and climate change scenario. Melkasa-1 maize yield increased by 9 and 4% during the baseline and midcentury period when supplied with 150 mm, respectively. Yield of BH-660 increased by 8–23% and 4–8%, under the baseline and midcentury climate scenario, respectively, when 150 mm irrigation was applied, compared to the corresponding rainfed (Araya et al. 2021a) (Table 15.3). However, the baseline maize performs better under higher irrigation due to relatively longer growing period. Similarly, Araya et al. (2015a) projected a decrease by 9–13% in days to maturity for midcentury maize in southwestern Ethiopia. Days to maturity shortened due to increased temperature would mean grain filling could be shortened, which could have a substantial negative impact on yield especially for those short-maturing varieties like Melkasa-1. In the case of BH-660, yield did not seem to reduce under climate change among other factors because of its relative longer maturity period and increased rainfall. Other similar studies on maize indicated that median maize yield could slightly increase by 1.4–5.5% for the period 2035–2085 relative to 2013 (Thomas et al. 2019). For BH-540, yield increased by 6.6–14.5% due to the application of 150 mm irrigation water during the baseline when compared to the corresponding baseline management (rainfed and 64 kg N/ha), whereas the yield increase for the midcentury maize was between 2.8 and 6% with 150 mm irrigation water (Table 15.3 and Fig. 15.1i). Overall, BH-660 performed best under climate change scenario followed by BH-540 and least was for Melkasa-1. With the use of improved variety, N management, and irrigation practices, there is great potential for enhancing maize yield in Ethiopia during the midcentury period. Although future

Table 15.3 Comparison of rainfed against their corresponding irrigated scenario for the baseline and midcentury maize yield under different N management strategies

		Baseline (1980–2005)				Midcentury (2040–2069)			
		N kg/ha							
		64	96	128	160	64	96	128	160
Crop variety	Irrig. Trt.	Dev. (%)	Dev. (%)	Dev. (%)	Dev. (%)	Dev. (%)	Dev. (%)	Dev. (%)	Dev. (%)
	Rainfed								
Melkasa-1	60 mm	0.0	2.0	7.0	2.0	1.0	1.0	2.0	2.0
	150 mm	1.0	1.0	7.0	9.0	2.0	3.0	2.0	4.0
	Rainfed								
BH-660	60 mm	20.0	11.0	11.0	8.0	11.0	5.0	3.0	5.0
	150 mm	23.0	15.0	13.0	13.0	8.0	7.0	4.0	4.0
	Rainfed								
BH-540	60 mm	15.0	6.0	4.0	7.0	6.0	1.0	3.0	2.0
	150 mm	14.5	8.8	6.6	12.4	6.0	2.4	4.8	2.8

Dev. percent of deviation

rainfall distributions are uncertain, it is anticipated that rainfall in Ethiopia is expected to increase, which might maintain maize yield levels (Thomas et al. 2019).

15.3.2 Wheat

Wheat is sensitive to elevated temperature although most wheat-growing Ethiopian locations are within the optimal range (<21 °C) (Araya et al. 2020a). Some studies showed temperatures beyond 30 °C could reduce yield due to floret sterility (Farooq et al. 2011). Other reports indicated that the reproductive and grain-filling periods of crops are sensitive to high temperatures (Prasad et al. 2008a, 2017 Prasad and Djanaguiraman 2014). Araya et al. (2020b) conducted sensitivity analysis for wheat grown within optimal ranges of temperature and reported an increase in wheat yield by 37% at 432 μmol/mol CO_2 and by 49% at 571 μmol/mol CO_2, compared to baseline CO_2 scenario (360 μmol/mol). On the other hand, assuming baseline CO_2 (360/380 μmol/mol) and increased temperature by 2 °C, wheat yield decreased by 1.7 to 10%, while under elevated CO_2 scenario (571 μmol/mol), wheat yield increased between 3.8 and 7.0% (Araya et al. 2020b). Similarly, some studies showed that median wheat yield in Ethiopia could slightly decrease by 0.3 to 2.7% for the period 2035–2085 relative to 2013 (Thomas et al. 2019). Furthermore, considering an increase in temperature by 4 °C under baseline CO_2 scenario (unchanged CO_2), wheat yield was simulated to decrease by 10 to 28.5%, whereas wheat yield slightly improved (-6.9 to $+4.5\%$) under elevated CO_2 (571 μmol/mol) when compared to baseline yield. The same authors reported an increase in wheat yield in Central Ethiopia during the midcentury by 0.3 to 9.1% under elevated CO_2 with N supply of 64 to 128 kg/ha. Elevated CO_2 might have positive impacts on yield because simulated temperatures are within the optimal range (the optimal temperature for grain-filling period is within the range of 15 to 25 °C; Nuttall et al. 2017), whereas, for locations that are beyond the optimal temperature limit, less beneficial effect of CO_2 was simulated (Araya et al. 2020a). Thus, climate change may not substantially decrease wheat yield during the midcentury period as long as temperatures are not beyond the requirement limit along with optimal management practices and elevated CO_2 scenarios. However, there could be some level of variation among wheat varieties in response to climate change (Sommer et al. 2013). Araya et al. (2020b) studied the response of three wheat varieties (early, medium, and late maturing) to climate change under elevated CO_2 scenario with improved N management (64 to 128 kg N/ha). They reported that the yield of all three varieties slightly varied. However, yield of the varieties remained unchanged or improved (-0.4 to $+9\%$) under near-future, midcentury, and end-century period although the response of the varieties to CO_2 and N slightly differs. For example, under improved management, the yield of an early-, medium-, and late-maturing cultivar slightly increased by 3.4 to 4.3, 0.3 to 9.1, and 1.1 to 3.5% during the midcentury period, respectively (Araya et al. 2020b).

In Ethiopia, wheat-planting date could vary depending on the locations due to difference in climatic (onset of rain) and topographic factors. For example, 75% onset of rain for Adet (northwestern Ethiopia) occurs around mid-June (Abera et al. 2019). Similarly, Gari et al. (2019) reported that farmers in the central highland of Ethiopia plant wheat in early to late June. In contrast, in Northern Ethiopia, planting of wheat is conducted around early to end of July. Therefore, use of location-specific optimal planting date could increase resilience to climatic risks, reduce the impacts of climate change, and improve rainwater use efficiency and yield (Araya et al. 2010, 2011; Araya and Stroosnijder 2011). Adjusting planting date (by matching the water stress-sensitive growth stages with the main rainy season) could help to reduce drought stress, improve water use efficiency, and increase yield (Araya and Stroosnijder 2011).

The response of wheat to N fertilizer could differ by location, water availability, and CO_2 concentration or combinations of the three factors (Fig. 15.3). Araya et al. (2020a) reported most of the locations in Ethiopia showed an increase in yield with increase in N, while some dry locations did not respond well to the increase in N fertilizer. For example, Fig. 15.3 shows a strong linear relationship between yield and N rate. The same authors reported a yield increase of 4.7 kg/ha for every unit increase in N rate (kg/ha) considering rainfed yield at zero N of 2581 kg/ha during the midcentury period under elevated CO_2 scenario (Fig. 15.3). In contrast, for every unit of increase in N rate, there was a wheat yield increase by 5.5% under 60 mm and 6.1% under 150 mm irrigation level (Araya et al. 2020a). The simulated yield levels for zero N under 60 and 150 mm irrigation during the midcentury were 2481 and 2328 kg/ha, respectively (Araya et al. 2020a). Araya et al. (2020b) reported an increase in wheat yield by at least 36% due to increase in N from 64 to 128 kg/ha during the baseline period. Cross-location average yield increased by 16 to 21% due to increased N (160 kg/ha) when compared to 64 kg N/ha (Araya et al. 2020a). Thus, increase in N fertilizer could be considered as an effective and suitable climate change adaptation practice under climate change.

Irrigation did not substantially contribute to cross-location yield increment because of:

(i) Diversity of climate locations, which might have masked the contribution of irrigation. Wheat was responsive to irrigation only in drier locations.
(ii) Improved water use efficiency, photosynthesis, and yield under elevated CO_2 (Hsiao and Jackson 1999).

Figure 15.3 indicated the yield increase due to irrigation is negligible when averaging cross-location yield values although not all locations produced similar level of yield. Araya et al. (2020a) reported irrigation improves wheat yield for drier areas (locations), but the impacts of irrigation were limited when averaged across the locations because most of them receive adequate rainfall for growing wheat. Simulation studies in Central Ethiopia showed that a decrease in rainfall by 20% under elevated temperature (2 °C) and CO_2 (571 µmol/mol) did not reduce yield (Araya et al. 2020b). This could be due to the positive effect of CO_2 on enhancing water use efficiency during drought years (Leakey et al. 2006; Kimball 2016).

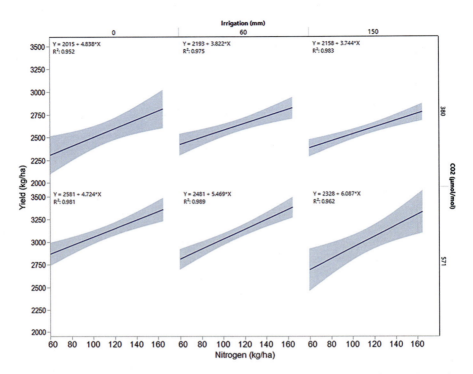

Fig. 15.3 Wheat yield as affected by N fertilizer, CO_2, and irrigation under future climate for elevated and baseline CO_2 in Ethiopia

15.3.3 Barley

Barley is sensitive to temperature changes. An increase in temperature by 2 and 4 °C with baseline CO_2 (360 μmol/mol) could decrease barley yield by 14 to 20% and 29 to 33%, respectively (Araya et al. 2021b). Projections for midcentury based on three global climate model (GCM) ensembles under RCP8.5 showed that barley yield could decrease by 6 to 11% during the midcentury (Araya et al. 2021b) (Table 15.4). Many studies showed that elevated CO_2 under future climate scenarios could benefit C3 crops (like wheat and barley) when temperatures are not beyond the optimal limit (Prasad et al. 2002, 2003, 2005, 2006, 2017; Ainsworth and Long 2021). In conditions where reproductive and grain-filling periods are not limited by high temperatures (heat), elevated CO_2 could increase wheat yield by enhancing N and water use efficiency and stimulating carbon assimilation (Leakey et al. 2006). Kimball (2016) reported that exposure of C3 crops to an elevated CO_2 of 550 μmol/mol could decrease evapotranspiration (10%) and increase yield (19%), compared to a baseline CO_2 scenario of 353 μmol/mol. Ainsworth and Long (2021) reported increased CO_2 by 200 μmol/mol under optimal condition (no stress) could increase yield of C3 crops by 18%, while the yield gain could be limited to 10% under N-deficient conditions or further increase in temperature.

15 Modeling Impacts of Climate Change and Adaptation Strategies for...

Table 15.4 Summary of impacts of midcentury climate change and management practices on major cereals grown in Ethiopia

Crops	Changes from the baseline (Percent)	Variety characteristics			Planting date			Irrigation (mm)			N fertilizer (kg/ha)				References
		Early	Medium	Late	Early	Normal	Late	0	60	150	64	96	128	160	
Maize	(−13 to −8%)	×				×	×	×	×	×	×				Araya et al. (2021a)
	(2.4 to 20%)			×	×				×	×				×	
	(−14 to +8%)		×			×		×	×	×			×		
Wheat	(4.3 to 6.2%)	×			×	×		×			×		×		Araya et al. (2020b)
	(0.3 to 5.2%)		×		×	×		×			×		×	×	
	(1.1 to 5.9%)			×	×	×		×			×		×		
Barley	(−11 to −6%)	×			×	×	×		×	×	×				Araya et al. (2021b)
Sorghum	(−9.1 to −3.4)		×		×			×	×		×				Gebrekiros et al. (2016)
	(−22 to −10%)		×			×		×	×		×				
	(−6 to 1.4%)	×	×	×		×									Thomas et al. (2019)
Sorghum	(−4 to 5%)	×			×			×			×				Zewdu et al. (2020)
	(−6 to 2%)	×			×			×			×				
Teff	(2 to 5%)		×		×			×			×				Araya et al. (2015b)
	(−8 to −6%)		×			×		×			×				

The dry planting (sowing in dry soil before the start of rain) practice of barley in Northern Ethiopia is one of the traditional practices used for coping with drought (Araya et al. 2012). However, dry planting (that occurs around June 20–25) technique increases the prevalence of weeds as weed seeds emerge faster than barley. Araya et al. (2012) reported early planting after the emergence of weeds would be the best strategy for farmers in the Northern Ethiopia in order to kill weeds, reduce risk of sowing failure (false start), and increase barley rainwater use efficiency and yield. Araya et al. (2021b) showed that the start of barley planting in northern semi-arid Ethiopia could slightly vary by soil type with earlier (July 1) and later (July 20) planting for coarse- and fine-textured soils, respectively. Similarly, Araya et al. (2010) reported planting of barley around July 4–12 in Northern Ethiopia improves water use efficiency and yield. Barley yield improved with early planting, although there are possibilities of sowing failure (false start) occurs by up to 20% (Araya et al. 2012). Similarly, Araya et al. (2021b) projected a decline in barley yield during the midcentury by 20 to 25% assuming unchanged (baseline) CO_2 scenario. Kebebe et al. (2019) studied the impact of midcentury climate change on barley yield (in Lemu Bilbilo district of Oromia region in Ethiopia) and reported a yield decline by at least by 13.8 and 5.8% under RCP4.5 and RCP8.5, respectively. Silungwe et al. (2018) highlighted that sowing date strategies and fertilizer application (micro-dose fertilization) are suitable practices for enhancing food security under rainfed condition.

The optimal N fertilizer for barley can vary with soil types. Araya et al. (2021b) reported that the optimal N fertilizer in Northern Ethiopia was 64 kg N/ha for coarse- and 32 kg N/ha for fine- and medium-textured soils. Nitrogen fertilizer management along with the inclusion of legumes in rotations could be considered as an adaptation crop management strategy for adding N to the system via N fixation in legumes and enhancing barley yield under climate change. For example, barley rotations after chickpea were reported to enhance barley yield due to N addition (Araya et al. 2021c).

Irrigation needs of crops depend on climate condition, crop type, growth stage, and soil factors (Doorenbos and Pruitt 1977; Doorenbos and Kassam 1979; Allen et al. 1998; Araya et al. 2011). Barley in Northern Ethiopia is moderately affected by irrigation. Araya et al. (2010) reported that full irrigation did not significantly change the barley yield when compared to the control. However, the irrigation needs depend on the distribution of the rainfall at the location during the season. Ararssa et al. (2019) reported a decrease in yield with increase in irrigation. They reported that some level of water stress of about 20% less than full irrigation might be beneficial for enhancing barley yield. In Northern Ethiopia, more irrigations are needed with delayed planting because of the short rainy season (Araya and Stroosnijder 2011). Similarly, other reports also showed that delayed planting could lead to increased relying of the crop on irrigation (Carter and Stoke 1985).

Tied ridging conserves the rainwater and improves soil water storage throughout the growing season (Wiyo et al. 2000; Araya and Stroosnijder 2010; Biazin and Stroosnijder 2012; Silungwe et al. 2018). Tied ridging improved soil water by more than 13 and 44%, respectively, when compared to the control (Araya and

Stroosnijder 2010). Tied ridge prolongs the retention of soil moisture, enhances nutrient uptake by crops, and provides suitable environment to crops especially in areas where there are agrometeorological challenges such as temporal and spatial rainfall variability (Silungwe et al. 2018). Okeyoa et al. (2014) evaluate the impact of mulching, tied ridging and minimum tillage on maize yield in Central Highlands of Kenya proved the importance of mulching and tied ridging for increasing yield and reducing runoff and improving soil water. The same authors reported that during short rains in 2011, tied ridging and mulching increased maize grain yields by 94 and 75%, respectively, compared with control. However, tied ridging might have negative impact in places where there is good supply of water and where soils are dominated by clay with shallow characteristics due to sensitivity of barley to water logging (aeration stress) (Araya et al. 2021c).

15.3.4 Sorghum

Sorghum as one of the major crops in Ethiopia is projected to be impacted by climate change. Zewdu et al. (2020) conducted simulation study on the impact of climate change on sorghum yield using CERES-sorghum for two sorghum varieties at two locations (Kobo and Srinka) in Northern Ethiopia. They reported a decrease by 4 to 6% for Kobo area whereas an increase by 2 to 5% for Srinka area during the midcentury under RCP8.5 (Zewdu et al. 2020). Under midcentury RCP4.5, sorghum yield decreases by 5 and 2% for Kobo and Srinka locations, respectively. The two varieties slightly varied in terms of yield performance under climate change (Zewdu et al. 2020) (Table 15.4). Similarly, Misganaw and Mohammed (2021) reported an increase in yield for early- and late-maturing sorghum varieties during the midcentury climate scenario. Summary of impacts of midcentury climate change and management practices on major cereals grown in Ethiopia is presented in Table 15.4. Akinseye et al. (2020) reported that sorghum yield declines by 4.8 and 6.2% at Bamako and Kano for early-maturing sorghum variety, respectively, and an increase by 12.3% at Bamako and 2% at Kano for medium-maturing varieties during the midcentury period. As described in sections above, increased temperatures might have contributed to the decrease in yield. Upper threshold temperature limit for crops might vary depending on crop type and crop growth stage. The optimal temperature for the time of flowering period is in the range of 25 to 28 °C (Prasad et al. 2006, 2008b, 2015, 2017). However, short time exposure to high temperature above 31 °C could significantly decrease pollen and floret fertility (Prasad et al. 2006, 2008b, 2015; Prasad and Djanaguiraman 2011). Negative effects of elevated temperatures could include decreased floret fertility, increased pollen sterility, decreased seed set, and reduced grain number (Prasad et al. 2008b, 2015; Djanaguiraman et al. 2014, 2018; Prasad and Djanaguiraman 2011). In addition, yield reduction could also be attributed to shortening growing period (Hasanuzzaman et al. 2013; Hatfield and Prueger 2015).

In Northern Ethiopia, use of optimal planting time and varietal choice are keys to successful sorghum production. Gebrekiros et al. (2016) studied the impact of climate change on sorghum yield at one of the locations (Alamata) in Northern Ethiopia. They reported that sorghum yield during the midcentury climate could decline more when planted late relative to the baseline scenario. Gebrekiros et al. (2016) concluded that April and March planting could be used to reduce the negative impact of climate change on sorghum yield during the midcentury period. Eggen et al. (2019) reported change in the onset of rain under future climate could decrease Ethiopian sorghum yield. Early planting and irrigation were found to increase sorghum yield under future climate in semi-arid regions of Ethiopia (Kobo and Meisso; Getachew et al. 2021). However, there might be some difference in planting date depending on cultivar/variety characteristics. For example, Akinseye et al. (2020) reported that use of optimal planting date could reduce yield loss although may vary by variety and location.

A study in Northern Ethiopia showed that sorghum gives the highest yield when 69 kg N/ha was applied in three split applications each receiving 1/3 at sowing, 1/3 at mid-vegetative, and 1/3 at booting (Abera et al. 2020). Shamme et al. (2016) conducted field experiments in Western Ethiopia and reported that N rate of 92 kg/ha was optimal for sorghum production. Simulation studies showed that sorghum responds well to N application of 69 kg N/ha in Senegal although the response differs by climate condition (Araya et al. under review). Other studies also showed that N rate of 46 kg/ha could result in high yield (Hegano et al. 2016).

In Northern Ethiopia, flood irrigation is used to reduce drought risk during vegetative and mid-growth stages in sorghum (Mebrahtu and Tamiru 2019; Wale et al. 2019; Mehari et al. 2020). These studies showed that irrigated sorghum produces higher yield compared to those in non-irrigated fields. Climate change adaptation strategies for sorghum might vary by agro-ecology and cultivar characteristics (Akinseye et al. 2020). In dryland Raya and Wag Hemra areas of Northern Ethiopia, supplementary irrigation has been used as an effective way for enhancing yield of sorghum (Mebrahtu and Tamiru 2019; Wale et al. 2019; Mehari et al. 2020). Kotharia et al. (2020) reported that irrigation requirement for sorghum decreases under climate change due to the shortening of the growing period. This decrease in growing period could contribute to reduce the assimilate gains due to the shortening of the grain-filling period. In semi-arid Cameron, sorghum yield could reduce by rainfall variability and drought (Abou et al. (2021). In addition, drought tolerance and heat tolerance and yield-enhancing traits were identified as the most important traits for climate change adaptation in sorghum (Singh et al. 2014; Kotharia et al. 2020). Low income, small farm size, poor access to yield-enhancing factors (e.g., irrigation and improved varieties), and other socioeconomic factors contributed to their vulnerability. Climate change adaptation strategies for sorghum should include the improvement of socioeconomic conditions (Abou et al. 2021).

15.3.5 Teff

Climate change could reduce teff yield during the midcentury if suitable adaptation measures are not implemented (Araya et al. 2015b). Suitability studies under climate change for teff were presented by Yumbya et al. (2014) and Zewudie et al. (2021). Studies showed that teff distribution under future climate is expected to increase in some areas while could decrease in other areas of Ethiopia (Zewudie et al. 2021). By the midcentury, teff area in Ethiopia is projected to decrease by 24% mainly due to climate change (Yumbya, et al. 2014). Many of the warmer areas in Ethiopia are projected to be lost as unsuitable for teff (Zewudie et al. 2021). Zewudie et al. (2021) reported that temperature, precipitation, and slope are land suitability determining factors for teff under future climate. For example, in Northern Ethiopia, teff production has been limited by climate variability (Araya and Stroosnijder 2011). Studies on other grain crops showed that increased temperatures and water stress are expected to affect crop development and yield under current and future climates (Prasad et al. 2008a, 2017; Prasad and Djanaguiraman 2014; Hatfield and Prueger 2015).

Studies showed that teff is sensitive to sowing date strategies under the present and climate change scenarios (Araya et al. 2015b). Teff responded well to early sowing mainly due to the matching of the critical stages of teff with the length of rainy period (Araya et al. 2015b) (Table 15.4). According to Araya et al. (2015b), teff yield during the midcentury could decline by up to 9% when normal sowing time is used, while no yield decline was simulated for teff sown early in the season (Table 15.4). Similarly, Haileselassie et al. (2016) reported early sowing was found to reduce irrigation application, enhance water use efficiency, and improve yield. Early sowing of teff without irrigation could yield as high as late sown teff that received four irrigations (from flowering to maturity period). If normal planting has to be used, one irrigation at the time of flowering could yield as high as that which received four irrigations for late sown teff (Haileselassie et al. 2016). Overall, this indicates that use of optimal sowing time in teff could be considered as an adaptation management strategy under future climate.

Similarly, use of optimal plant density is key for enhancing yield. Mengie et al. (2021) reported optimal plant density could contribute to yield enhancement. The same authors reported seed rate of 5 kg/ha in row and broadcasting sowing method yielded 2300 and 2160 kg/ha, respectively, which is higher than the other seeding rates tested in their experiment (Mengie et al. 2021). This shows use of optimal seeding rate could be considered as a yield-enhancing strategy for teff under climate change.

Araya et al. (2011) presented teff crop coefficient and irrigation water requirement. Teff studies in semi-arid Ethiopia suggested that (i) teff's early seedling establishment requires moist/wet topsoil, (ii) teff is likely to give significantly higher grain yield when a nearly optimal water supply is provided, and (iii) teff can tolerate moderate water stress, but yield and biomass could reduce under severe water stress (Araya et al. 2011). Tsegay et al. (2015) reported optimal sowing of teff with one irrigation at flowering along with optimal N fertilizer could help to achieve stable yield in Northern Ethiopia. Applied irrigation should match with N fertilizer supply. For example, applying irrigation without adequate supply of N or vice versa may not enhance yield (Araya et al. 2019).

Nitrogen fertilizer application of up to 64 and 32 kg N/ha improved teff yield by up to 91 and 42%, respectively, compared to teff without N fertilizer (Haileselassie et al. 2016). Teff yield could improve by up to 119% with optimal N fertilizer application rate and irrigation management compared to that without irrigation and N fertilizer (Haileselassie et al. 2016). Araya et al. (2019) reported N fertilizer application rate of 64 kg/ha could be optimal under adequate water supply; however, increasing N fertilizer beyond this level may cause lodging. In addition, increasing N fertilizer application rate without adequate water supply has little yield benefit (Araya et al. 2019).

15.4 Conclusions

Under climate change, maize yield could reduce due to the shortening of the grain-filling period. Although temperature has increased during the midcentury relative to the baseline, it is not beyond the optimal limit of the required for the growth and development of maize for most highlands of Ethiopia. Use of optimal planting date, application of N fertilizer, and irrigation contributed to yield increment under future climate. Different varieties of maize in Ethiopia responded differently to climate change. Melkasa-1, BH-660, and BH-540 yield changed by -13 to -8%, +3 to +13%, and -10 to +4%, respectively, compared to their corresponding baseline yield with the same management.

Wheat yield in highlands of Ethiopia is expected to slightly increase by up to 6% during the midcentury. Optimal N management is an effective climate adaptation practice. However, drier locations were less responsive to N but were more responsive to irrigation. There was an increase in wheat yield by 4.7 kg/ha for every unit increase in N rate (kg/ha) considering rainfed yield at zero N of 2581 kg/ha during the midcentury period (under elevated CO_2 scenario). The rate of increase did not change substantially when irrigation of 150 mm was applied. This indicates that N substantially improved wheat yield when average cross-location was considered, while irrigation did not substantially improve wheat yield. Only drier locations were responsive to irrigation.

Some of the major sources of barley yield losses in Northern Ethiopia during the baseline scenario were associated with use of inappropriate planting date and N rates. Barley yield during the midcentury could decline by 6 to 11% when compared to the corresponding baseline yield. Use of optimal planting date, N, crop rotation, and tied ridging along with elevated CO_2 scenario were beneficial for growing barley under the midcentury climate. Tied ridging could minimize drought risks under the present and future climate change through improving soil water availability in the root zone, enhanced barley yields, and increased rainwater use efficiency. In addition, the inclusion of legumes like chickpea could enhance the biological fixation of N, which could be beneficial for resource-poor farmers in Ethiopia under future climate.

The use of optimal planting date and N fertilizer management are among the best management strategies for reducing the impact of climate change on sorghum yield. Many studies showed N rate of 46 to 92 kg/ha was suitable for enhancing sorghum yield depending on water availability. Studies showed sorghum yield in Northern Ethiopia could reduce due to midcentury climate change by up to 9.1% for March, up to 12.2% for April, or up to 22.2% for May planting. Thus, use of optimal planting time and N fertilizer could be considered as an adaptation strategy for sorghum in Ethiopia.

Teff yield could decline due to climate change during the midcentury period by up to 12%. Rainfall distribution and amount play substantial role on yield performance of teff during the midcentury period. Studies showed that teff yield losses could be minimized by using early planting strategies. Elevated CO_2 also improved teff yield probably due to improved water use efficiency, resulting from reduced transpiration (limited stomatal conductance under elevated CO_2).

Acknowledgments We thank the Feed the Future Sustainable Intensification Innovation Lab funded by the United States Agency for International Development (grant number AID-OAA-L-14-00006) and Department of Agronomy at Kansas State University for supporting their research. Contribution number 22-239-B from the Kansas Agricultural Experiment Station.

References

Abebe Z, Feyisa H (2017) Effects of nitrogen rates and time of application on yield of maize: rainfall variability influenced time of N application. Hindawi Int J Agron:1545280. https://doi.org/10.1155/2017/1545280

Abera K, Crespo O, Seid J, Mequanent F (2018) Simulating the impact of climate change on maize production in Ethiopia, East Africa. Environ Syst Res 7:4–12. https://doi.org/10.1186/s40068-018-0107-z

Abera EA, Getnet M, Nigatu L (2019) Impacts of climate change on bread wheat (*Triticum aestivum* L) yield in adet, Northwestern Ethiopia. J Pet Environ Biotechnol 10:396. https://doi.org/10.35248/2157-7463.19.10.396

Abera K, Tana T, Takele A (2020) Effect of rates and time of nitrogen fertilizer application on yield and yield components of sorghum [*Sorghum bicolor* (L.) Moench] at Raya Valley, Northern Ethiopia. Int J Plant Breed Crop Sci 7(1):598–612

Abou S, Ali M, Wakponou A, Sambo A (2021) Sorghum farmers' climate change adaptation strategies in the semiarid region of Cameroon. In: Leal FW, Oguge N, Ayal D, Adeleke L, da Silva I (eds) African handbook of climate change adaptation. Springer, Cham. https://doi.org/10.1007/978-3-030-45106-6_41

Ainsworth EA, Long SP (2021) 30 years of free-air carbon dioxide enrichment (FACE): what have we learned about future crop productivity and its potential for adaptation? Glob Chang Biol 27:27–49. https://doi.org/10.1111/gcb.15375

Akinseye FM, Ajeigbe HA, Traore PCS, Agelee SO, Zemadim B, Whitbread A (2020) Improving sorghum productivity under changing climatic conditions: a modelling approach. Field Crop Res 246:107685. https://doi.org/10.1016/j.fcr.2019.107685

Allen RG, Periera LS, Raes D, Smith M (1998) Crop evapotranspiration. Guidelines for computing crop water requirement, FAO irrigation and drainage paper no. 56. FAO, Rome

Ararssa A, Gebremariam A, Mulat W, Mekonnen M (2019) Effects of irrigation management on yield and water productivity of barley *Hordeum vulgare* in the Upper Blue Nile basin: case study in northern Gondar. Water Conserv Sci Eng 4. https://doi.org/10.1007/s41101-019-00071-8

Araya A, Stroosnijder L (2010) Effects of tied ridges and mulch on barley (*Hordeum vulgare*) rainwater use efficiency and production in Northern Ethiopia. Agric Water Manag 97:841–847. https://doi.org/10.1016/j.agwat.2010.01.012

Araya A, Stroosnijder L (2011) Assessing drought risk and irrigation need in northern Ethiopia. Agric For Meteorol 151:425–436. https://doi.org/10.1016/j.agrformet.2010.11.014

Araya A, Habtu S, Hadgu KM, Kebede A, Dejene T (2010) Test of AquaCrop model in simulating biomass and yield of water deficient and irrigated barley (*Hordeum vulgare*). Agric Water Manag 97:1838–1846. https://doi.org/10.1016/j.agwat.2010.06.021

Araya A, Stroosnijder L, Girmay G, Keesstra SD (2011) Crop coefficient, yield response to water stress and water productivity of teff (*Eragrostis tef* (Zucc.)). Agric Water Manag 98:775–783. https://doi.org/10.1016/j.agrformet.2011.11.001

Araya A, Stroosnijder L, Habtu S, Deesstra SD, Berhe M, Hadgu KM (2012) Risk assessment by sowing dates for barley (Hordeum vulgare) in Ethiopia. Agric For Meteorol 154–155:30–37. https://doi.org/10.1016/j.agrformet.2011.11.001

Araya A, Hoogenboom G, Luedeling E, Hadgu KM, Kisekka I, Martorano LG (2015a) Assessment of maize growth and yield using crop models under present and future climate in southwestern Ethiopia. Agric For Meteorol 214–215:252–265. https://doi.org/10.1016/j.agrformet.2015.08.259

Araya A, Girma A, Demelash T, Martorano LG, Haileselassie H, Abraha AZ (2015b) Assessing impacts of climate change on teff (*Eragrostis teff*) productivity in Debrezeit area, Ethiopia. Int J Agric Sci Res 4(3):039–048

Araya A, Kisekka I, Girma A, Hadgu KM, Beltrao NES, Ferreira H, Afewerk A, Birhane A, Tsehaye Y, Martorano LG (2017) The challenges and opportunities for wheat production under future climate in Northern Ethiopia. Camb Agric Sci 155:379–393. https://doi.org/10.1017/S0021859616000460

Araya A, Habtu SM, Aklilu M, Kiros MH, Foster AJ, Lucieta GM (2019) Climate smart water and nitrogen management for local teff (*Eragrostis teff*) in northern Ethiopia. In: Climate-smart agriculture: enhancing resilient agricultural systems, landscapes and livelihoods in Ethiopia and beyond. World Agroforestry (ICRAF), Nairobi. ISBN:978-9966-108-24-1

Araya A, Prasad PVV, Zambreski Z, Gowda PH, Ciampitti IA, Assefa Y, Girma A (2020a) Spatial analysis of the impact of climate change factors and adaptation strategies on productivity of wheat in Ethiopia. Sci Total Environ 731:139094. https://doi.org/10.1016/j.scitotenv.2020.139094

Araya A, Prasad PVV, Gowda PH, Djanaguiraman M, Kassa AH (2020b) Potential impacts of climate change factors and agronomic adaptation strategies on wheat yields in central highlands of Ethiopia. Clim Chang 159:461–479. https://doi.org/10.1007/s10584-019-02627-y

Araya A, Prasad PVV, Gowda PH, Zambreski Z, Ciampitti IA (2021a) Management options for mid-century maize (*Zea mays* L.) in Ethiopia. Sci Tot Environ 758:143635. https://doi.org/10.1016/j.scitotenv.2020.143635

Araya A, Prasad PVV, Gowda PH, Djanaguiraman M, Gebretsadkan Y (2021b) Modeling the effects of crop management on food barley production under midcentury changing climate in northern Ethiopia. Clim Risk Manag 32:100308. https://doi.org/10.1016/j.crm.2021.100308

Araya A, Prasad PVV, Ciampitti IA, Jha PK (2021c) Using crop simulation model to evaluate influence of water management practices and multiple cropping systems on crop yields: a case study for Ethiopian highlands. Field Crop Res 260:108004. https://doi.org/10.1016/j.fcr.2020.108004

Balem T, Kebede M, Golla B, Tufa T, Chala G, Abera T (2020) Phenological and grain yield response of hybrid maize varieties, released for differing agro-ecologies, to growing temperatures and planting dates in Ethiopia. Afr J Agric Res 16:1730–1739. https://doi.org/10.5897/AJAR2020.15103

Biazin B, Stroosnijder L (2012) To tie or not to tie ridges for water conservation in Rift Valley drylands of Ethiopia. Soil Tillage Res 124:83–94. https://doi.org/10.1016/j.still.2012.05.006

Carter KE, Stoke R (1985) Effects of irrigation and sowing date on yield and quality of barley and wheat. N Z J Exp Agric 13:77–83

Dinku T, Funk C, Peterson P, Maidment R, Tadesse T, Gadain H, Ceccato P (2018) Validation of the CHIRPS satellite rainfall estimates over eastern Africa. Q J R Meteorol Soc 144(Suppl. 1): 292–312. https://doi.org/10.1002/qj.3244

Djanaguiraman M, Prasad PVV, Murugan M, Perumal R, Reddy UK (2014) Physiological differences among sorghum (*Sorghum bicolor* L. Moench) genotypes under high temperature stress. Environ Exp Bot 100:43–54. https://doi.org/10.1016/j.envexpbot.2013.11.013

Djanaguiraman M, Perumal R, Jagadish SVK, Ciampitti IA, Welti R, Prasad PVV (2018) Sensitivity of sorghum pollen and pistil to high temperature stress. Plant Cell Environ 41:1065–1082. https://doi.org/10.1111/pce.13089

Dolapo B, Akinnuoye-Adelabu MT, Modi AT (2019) Interactive effect of planting date and fertiliser application on maize growth and yield under dryland conditions. S Afr J Plant Soil 36:189–198. https://doi.org/10.1080/02571862.2018.1525772

Doorenbos J, Kassam AH (1979) Yield response to water, FAO irrigation and drainage paper no. 33. FAO, Rome

Doorenbos J, Pruitt WO (1977) Crop water requirements, Irrigation and drainage paper no. 24. Food and Agricultural Organization, Rome

Eggen M, Ozdogan M, Zaitchik B, Ademe D, Foltz J, Simane B (2019) Vulnerability of sorghum production to extreme, sub-seasonal weather under climate change. Environ Res Lett 14:045005

Endris HS, Omondi P, Jain S et al (2013) Assessment of the performance of CORDEX regional climate models in simulating east African rainfall. J Clim 26:8453–8475. https://doi.org/10.1175/JCLI-D-12-00708.1

Farooq M, Bramley H, Palta JA, Siddique KHM (2011) Heat stress in wheat during reproductive and grain-filling phases. Crit Rev Plant Sci 30(6):491–507. https://doi.org/10.1080/07352689.2011.615687

Funk C, Peterson P, Landsfeld M, Pedreros D, Verdin J, Rowland J, Romero B, Husak G, Michaelsen J, Verdin A (2014) A quasi-global precipitation time series for drought monitoring. US Geol Surv Data Ser 832(4). https://doi.org/10.3133/ds832

Funk C, Peterson P, Landsfeld M, Pedreros D, Verdin J, Shukla S, Husak G, Rowland J, Harrison L, Hoell A, Michaelsen J (2015) The climate hazards group infrared precipitation with stations – a new environmental record for monitoring extremes. Sci Data 2:150066. https://doi.org/10.1038/sdata.2015.66

Gari AT, Getnet M, Nigatu L (2019) Modeling climate change impacts on bread wheat (*Triticum aestivum* L.) production in Central Highlands of Ethiopia. J Agric Sci Food Res 10(56). https://doi.org/10.35248/2593-9173.19.10.256

Gebrekiros G, Araya A, Yemane T (2016) Modeling impact of climate change and variability on sorghum production in Southern Zone of Tigray, Ethiopia. J Earth Sci Clim Chang 7:322. https://doi.org/10.4172/2157-7617.1000322

Gessesse AT, Araya A (2015) Effect of in-situ rainwater conservations and sowing date on barley yield and weed infestation: a case study at Maychew and Mekelle, Northern Ethiopia. Malay J Med Biol Res 2:41–48. https://doi.org/10.18034/mjmbr.v2i1.387

Getachew F, Bayabil HK, Hoogenboom G, Teshome FT, Zewdu E (2021) Irrigation and shifting planting date as climate change adaptation strategies for sorghum. Agric Water Manag 255: 106988. https://doi.org/10.1016/j.agwat.2021.106988

Hasanuzzaman M, Nahar K, Alam MM, Roychowdhury R, Fujita M (2013) Physiological, biochemical, and molecular mechanisms of heat stress tolerance in plants. Int J Mol Sci 14(5): 9643–9684. https://doi.org/10.3390/ijms14059643

Hatfield JL, Prueger JH (2015) Temperature extremes: effect on plant growth and development. Weather Clim Extremes 10(A):4–10. https://doi.org/10.1016/j.wace.2015.08.001

Hegano A, Adicha A, Tessema S (2016) Economic analysis of the effect of nitrogen and phosphorous fertilizer application for sorghum production at Alduba, South Omo, Southwestern Ethiopia. Int J Agric Econ 1(2):26–30. https://doi.org/10.11648/j.ijae.20160102.11

Hsiao TC, Jackson RB (1999) Interactive effects of water stress and elevated CO_2 on growth, photosynthesis, and water use efficiency. In: Luo Y, Mooney HA (eds) Carbon dioxide and environmental stress. Academic, San Diego, pp 3–31

IPCC (2013) Summary for policymakers. In: Stocker TF, Qin D, Plattner GK et al (eds) Climate change 2013: the physical science basis. Contribution of Working Group I to the Fifth Assessment Report of the Intergovernmental Panel on Climate Change. Cambridge University Press, Cambridge/New York

IPCC (2021) Summary for policymakers. In: Climate change 2021: the physical science basis. Contribution of Working Group I to the Sixth Assessment Report of the Intergovernmental Panel on Climate Change. Cambridge University Press, Cambridge/New York

Kassie BT, Van Ittersum MK, Hengsdijk H, Asseng S, Wolf J, Rotter RO (2014a) Climate induced yield variability and yield gap of maize (Zea mays L.,) in the central rift valley of Ethiopia. Field Crop Res 160:41–53. https://doi.org/10.1016/j.fcr.2014.02.010

Kassie BT, Rotter RP, Hengsdijk H, Asseng S, Van Ittersum MK, Kahiluoto H, Van Keulen H (2014b) Climate variability and change in the central Rift Valley of Ethiopia: challenges for rainfed crop production. Agric Sci 152:58–74. https://doi.org/10.1017/S002185961200098

Kebebe B, Korecha D, Mamo G, Dandesa D, Yibrah M (2019) Modeling climate change and its impacts on food barley (Hordeum vulgare L.) production using different climate change scenarios in Lemu-Bilbilo district, Oromia regional state, Ethiopia. Int J Res Environ Sci 5(3): 33–40. https://doi.org/10.20431/2454-9444.0503005

Kimball BA (2016) Crop responses to elevated CO_2 and interactions with H_2O, N, and temperature. Curr Opin Plant Biol 31:36–43. https://doi.org/10.1016/j.pbi.2016.03.006

Kotharia K, Alea S, Bordovskya JP, Portera DO, Munstera CL, Hoogenboom G (2020) Potential benefits of genotype-based adaptation strategies for grain sorghum production in the Texas High Plains under climate change. Eur J Agron 117:126037. https://doi.org/10.1016/j.eja.2020. 126037

Leakey ADB, Uribelarrea M, Ainsworth EA, Naidus AL, Rogers A, Ort DR, Long SP (2006) Photosynthesis, productivity, and yield of maize are not affected by open-air elevation of CO_2 concentration in the absence of drought. Plant Physiol 140:779–790

Lizaso JI, Ruiz-Ramos M, Rodríguez L, Gabaldon-Leal C, Oliveira JA, Lorite IJ, Sánchez D, García E, Rodríguez A (2018) Impact of high temperatures in maize: phenology and yield components. Field Crop Res 126:129–140. https://doi.org/10.1016/j.fcr.2017.11.013

Mandefro N, Tanner D, Twumasi-Afriyie S (2001) Enhancing the contribution of maize to food security in Ethiopia: proceedings of the second national maize workshop of Ethiopia. Ethiopian Agricultural Research Organization (EARO) and International Maize and Wheat Improvement Center (CIMMYT), Addis Ababa

Mascaro G, White DD, Westerhoff P, Bliss N (2015) Performance of the CORDEX-Africa regional climate simulations in representing the hydrological cycle of the Niger River basin. J Geophys Res-Atmos 120(12):425–444. https://doi.org/10.1002/2015JD023905

Mebrahtu Y, Tamiru H (2019) Response of sorghum to supplementary irrigation in Raya Valley, Northern Ethiopia. Int J Agric Biosci 8(1):1–5

Mehari H, Bedadi B, Abegaz F (2020) Maximizing water productivity of maize using alternate furrow irrigation at clay-loam soil, Raya Valley, Ethiopia. Int J Plant Breed Crop Sci 7(2): 771–778

Mengie Y, Assefa A, Jenber AJ (2021) Sowing methods and seeding rates effects on yield and yield components of Teff (*Eragrostis teff* [Zucc.] Trotter) at Adet, Northwest Ethiopia. Heliyon 7(3): e06519. https://doi.org/10.1016/j.heliyon.2021.e06519

Misganaw A, Mohammed A (2021) Simulation study on climate change impact and management options for sorghum [*Sorghum bicolor* (L.) Moench] production in the Semi-Arid Northeastern Ethiopia. Agrotechnology 10(204)

Nuttall JG, O'Leary GJ, Panozzo JF et al (2017) Models of grain quality in wheat – a review. Field Crop Res 202:136–145. https://doi.org/10.1016/j.fcr.2015.12.011

Okeyoa AI, Mucheru-Munaa M, Mugwea J, Ngeticha KF, Mugendi DN, Diels J, Shisanya CA (2014) Effects of selected soil and water conservation technologies on nutrient losses and maize yields in the central highlands of Kenya. Agric Water Manag 137:52–58

Prasad PVV, Djanaguiraman M (2011) High night temperature decreases leaf photosynthesis and pollen function in grain sorghum. Funct Plant Biol 38:993–1003. https://doi.org/10.1071/FP11035

Prasad PVV, Djanaguiraman M (2014) Response of floret fertility and individual grain weight of wheat to high temperature stress: sensitive stages and thresholds for temperature and duration. Funct Plant Biol 41:1261–1269. https://doi.org/10.1071/FP14061

Prasad PVV, Boote KJ, Allen LH Jr, Thomas JMG (2002) Effects of elevated temperature and carbon dioxide on seed-set and yield of kidney bean (*Phaseolus vulgaris* L.). Glob Chang Biol 8:710–721. https://doi.org/10.1046/j.1365-2486.2002.00508.x

Prasad PVV, Boote KJ, Allen LH Jr, Thomas JMG (2003) Super-optimal temperatures are detrimental to peanut (*Arachis hypogaea* L.) reproductive processes and yield at both ambient and elevated carbon dioxide. Glob Chang Biol 9:1775–1787. https://doi.org/10.1046/j.1365-2486.2003.00708.x

Prasad PVV, Allen LH Jr, Boote KJ (2005) Crop responses to elevated carbon dioxide and interaction with temperature: grain legumes. J Crop Improv 13:113–155. https://doi.org/10.1300/J411v13n01_07

Prasad PVV, Boote KJ, Allen LH Jr, Thomas JMG (2006) Adverse high temperature effects on pollen viability, seed-set, seed yield and harvest index of grain sorghum (*Sorghum bicolor* L.) are more severe at elevated carbon dioxide due to higher tissue temperatures. Agric For Meteorol 139:237–251. https://doi.org/10.1016/j.agrformet.2006.07.003

Prasad PVV, Pisipati SR, Mutava RN, Tuinstra MR (2008a) Sensitivity of grain sorghum to high temperature stress during reproductive development. Crop Sci 48:1911–1917. https://doi.org/10.2135/cropsci2008.01.0036

Prasad PVV, Staggenborg SA, Ristic Z (2008b) Impacts of drought and/or heat stress on physiological, development, growth and yield process of crop plants. Adv Agric Syst Model 1:301–355. https://doi.org/10.2134/advagricsystmodel1.c11

Prasad PVV, Djanaguiraman M, Perumal R, Ciampitti IA (2015) Impact of high temperature stress on floret fertility and individual grain weight of grain sorghum: sensitive stages and thresholds for temperature and duration. Front Plant Sci 6:820. https://doi.org/10.3389/fpls.2015.00820

Prasad PVV, Bhemanahalli R, Jagadish SVK (2017) Field crops and the fear of heat stress: opportunities, challenges and future directions. Field Crop Res 200:114–121. https://doi.org/10.1016/j.fcr.2016.09.024

Shamme SK, Raghavaiah CV, Balemi T, Hamza I (2016) Sorghum (*Sorghum bicolor* L.) growth, productivity, nitrogen removal, N-use efficiencies and economics in relation to genotypes and nitrogen nutrition in Kellem Wollega Zone of Ethiopia, East Africa. Adv Crop Sci Technol 4(218). https://doi.org/10.4172/2329-8863.1000218

Silungwe FR, Graef F, Bellingrath-Kimura SD, Tumbo SD, Kahimba FC, Lana MA (2018) Crop upgrading strategies and modelling for rainfed cereals in a semi-arid climate – a review. Water 10:356. https://doi.org/10.3390/w10040356

Singh P, Nedumaran S, Traore SP, Boote KJ, Rattunde HFW, Prasad PVV, Singh NP, Srinivas K, Bantilan C (2014) Quantifying potential benefits of drought and heat tolerance in rainy season sorghum for adapting to climate change. Agric For Meteorol 185:37–48. https://doi.org/10.1016/j.agrformet.2013.10.012

Sommer R, Glazirina M, Yuldashev T, Otarov A, Ibraeva M, Martynova L, Bekenov M et al (2013) Impact of climate change on wheat productivity in Central Asia. Agric Ecosyst Environ 178:78–99. https://doi.org/10.1016/j.agee.2013.06.011

Taffesse AS, Dorosh P, Asrat S (2011) Crop production in Ethiopia: Regional Patterns and Trends Development Strategy and Governance Division, International Food Policy Research Institute, Ethiopia Strategy Support Program II, Ethiopia ESSP II working paper no. 016

Thomas T, Dorosh P, Robertson R (2019) Climate change impacts on crop yields in Ethiopia. IFPRI and EDRI. Strategy support program, working paper 130, Washington, DC

Tolessa D, Du Preez CC, Ceronio GM (2007) Comparison of maize genotypes for grain yield, nitrogen uptake and use efficiency in Western Ethiopia. S Afr J Plant Soil 24:70–76. https://doi.org/10.1080/02571862.2007.10634784

Tsegay A, Vanuytrecht E, Abrha B, Deckers J, Gebrehiwot K, Raes D (2015) Sowing and irrigation strategies for improving rainfed teff (*Eragrostis teff* (Zucc.) Trotter) production in the water scarce Tigray region, Ethiopia. Agric Water Manag 150:81–91

USDA (2014a) Soil quality indicators. https://www.nrcs.usda.gov/wps/portal/nrcs/detail/soils/health/assessment/?cid=stelprdb1237387. Accessed Apr 2020

USDA (2014b) Soil health – nitrogen. Guide for educators. https://www.nrcs.usda.gov/Internet/FSE_DOCUMENTS/nrcs142p2_051575.pdf

Vizy EK, Cook KH (2012) Mid-twenty-first-century changes in extreme events over northern and tropical Africa. J Clim 25:5748–5767. https://doi.org/10.1175/JCLI-D-11-00693.1

Wale A, Sebnie W, Girmay G, Beza G (2019) Evaluation of the potentials of supplementary irrigation for improvement of sorghum yield in Wag-Himra, Northeastern, Amhara, Ethiopia. Cogent Food Agric 5:1664203. https://doi.org/10.1080/23311932.2019.1664203

Wiyo KA, Kasomekera ZM, Feyen J (2000) Effect of tied-ridging on soil water status of a maize crop under Malawi conditions. Agric Water Manag 45:101–125. https://doi.org/10.1016/S0378-3774(99)00103-1

Yumbya J, de Vaate MDB, Kiambi D, Kebebew F, Rao KPC (2014) Assessing the effect of climate change on teff in Ethiopia: implication for food security. African Biodiversity Conservation and Innovations Centre (ABCIC). ISBN:978-9966-072-34-4

Zeleke A, Alemayehu G, Yihenew GS (2018) Effects of planting density and nitrogen fertilizer rate on yield and yield related traits of maize (*Zea mays* L.) in northwestern, Ethiopia. Adv Crop Sci Technol 6(352). https://doi.org/10.4172/2329-8863.1000352

Zewdu E, Hadgu G, Nigatu N (2020) Impacts of climate change on sorghum production in Northeastern Ethiopia. Afr J Environ Sci Technol 14(2):49–63. https://doi.org/10.5897/AJEST2019.2803

Zewudie D, Ding W, Rong Z, Zhao C, Chang Y (2021) Spatiotemporal dynamics of habitat suitability for the Ethiopian staple crop, *Eragrostis teff* (teff), under changing climate. Peer J 9:e10965. https://doi.org/10.7717/peerj.10965

Chapter 16
Strategies for Mitigating Greenhouse Gas Emissions from Agricultural Ecosystems

H. Singh, P. V. V. Prasad, B. K. Northup, I. A. Ciampitti, and C. W. Rice

Abstract Climate change, driven by rising greenhouse gas (GHG) concentrations in the atmosphere, poses serious and wide-ranging threats to human societies and natural ecosystems all over the world. Agriculture and forestry account for roughly one-third of global emissions, including 9 to 14% of GHGs from crop and livestock activities. Due to increasing demand based on human population and income growth and dietary change, GHG emissions are likely to increase by about 76% by 2050 relative to the levels in 1995. Nitrous oxide (N_2O) and methane (CH_4) are the major GHGs contributed from the agricultural sector, contributing 50 and 70%, respectively, to the total levels. However, carbon dioxide (CO_2) emissions are mainly contributed by a change in land use patterns and decomposition of organic materials. Global emission pathways that would limit warming to 1.5 °C or less, in line with the Paris Agreement's temperature goal, depend on significant reductions in agricultural GHGs (N_2O and CH_4) as well as net zero CO_2 emissions from fossil fuels. As the agricultural sector mainly contributes to N_2O and CH_4, 4.8 Gt CO_2-eq reduction in direct global agricultural non-CO_2 emissions below baseline by 2050 is needed. These ambitious targets of mitigation pathways present an enormous challenge, and accomplishment of these goals is only possible by the implementation of effective GHG mitigation strategies to the agricultural sector. Mitigation measures in the agricultural sector include increasing C sequestration as well as reduction in the GHGs from livestock and agricultural processes. In this chapter, we discussed mitigation strategies for GHG emissions from the agricultural sector at the global scale.

Keywords Agricultural systems · Carbon sequestration · Climate change · Ecosystems · Greenhouse gas · Livestock

---

H. Singh · P. V. V. Prasad (✉) · I. A. Ciampitti · C. W. Rice
Department of Agronomy, Kansas State University, Manhattan, KS, USA
e-mail: vara@ksu.edu

B. K. Northup
Agronomy Department, West Florida Research and Education Center, Institute of Food and Agricultural Sciences, University of Florida, Jay, FL, USA

© The Author(s), under exclusive license to Springer Nature Switzerland AG 2022
M. Ahmed (ed.), *Global Agricultural Production: Resilience to Climate Change*,
https://doi.org/10.1007/978-3-031-14973-3_16

16.1 Introduction

Over the last several decades, an increase in agricultural GHG emissions has been reported, along with the growing global agricultural production. Agriculture and forestry, which together account for roughly one-third of global emissions, have received much attention in recent years. According to the Intergovernmental Panel on Climate Change (IPCC 2014), the agricultural sector is the second highest GHG contributor after electricity and heat production sector, with this last sector contributing about 24% of the global GHG emissions. However, crop and livestock production are expected to increase by 48% and 80% by 2050, respectively, as the human population grows and shifts toward a more animal-based diet (Bennetzen et al. 2016). Thereby, this scenario for increasing crop and livestock production poses the risk to increase by 76% in agricultural GHG emissions by 2050 relative to 1995 (Popp et al. 2010). The global trends in total GHG emissions from agriculture, forestry, and other land use activities between 1970 and 2010 are presented in Fig. 16.1 (Smith et al. 2014). According to GlobAgri-WRR model, it is projected that GHG from the agricultural sector alone would fill about 70% of the allowable "emissions budget" in 2050 (15 of 21 Gt), leaving almost no space for emissions from other economic sectors and making the achievement of even the 2 °C target

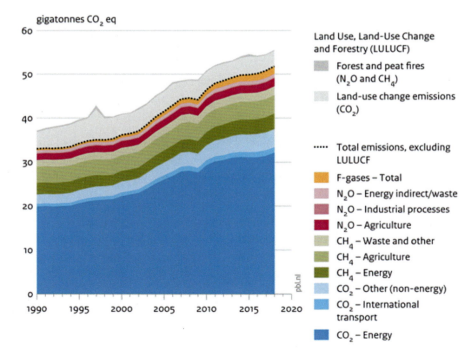

Fig. 16.1 Global trends in total GHG emissions from agriculture, forestry, and other land use activities between 1990 and 2018. (Adapted from Olivier and Peters 2020)

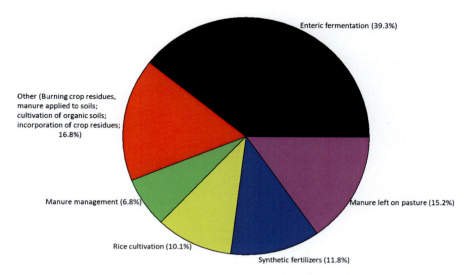

Fig. 16.2 Different sources responsible for these agricultural GHG emissions and their percent contribution. (Source: Data adapted from FAO)

impossible (Searchinger et al. 2018). Agricultural lands have a significant impact on the earth's C and nitrogen (N) cycles due to their large size and intensive management, and agricultural activities result in releases of all three GHGs. The land use changes mainly result in the emission of CO_2, while agricultural management practices are the major contributor to N_2O (50%) and CH_4 (70%) emissions of the total anthropogenic emissions of these gases. Both are potent GHGs: N_2O has a global warming potential 296 times that of CO_2, and CH_4 has a global warming potential 23 times that of CO_2. The different sources responsible for these agricultural GHG emissions and their percent contribution are listed in Fig. 16.2 (FAO 2010).

These agricultural GHG emissions can be divided into two categories based on their production: (i) crops and (ii) livestock. The sectors are interlinked as some crops are grown for animal feed, while at the same time, the animal manure can be used as fertilizer for crops. Thereby, the allocation of the emissions to these categories is complicated and depends on accounting methodologies. Agricultural activities are the main source of the global N_2O emissions, with the share of almost 65%. For the livestock category, animal dung and urine on pastures, rangeland, and paddocks are the largest global source of N_2O emissions, accounting for 23% of the total N_2O and 4% of the total N_2O from manure management. For the crop category, synthetic N fertilizer use is the largest source, accounting for 13% of the total N_2O emissions, followed by the 11% share from decomposition of crop residues. Additionally, manure management accounts for 9% of the total N_2O emissions. Therefore, all these sources account for 74% of global N_2O emissions, with 32% share from livestock, 24% share from the crop, and 18% share from fossil fuel combustion (Fig. 16.3). Additionally, indirect N_2O emissions from agricultural activities account for another 9% of the total N_2O emissions (Fig. 16.3) (Olivier and

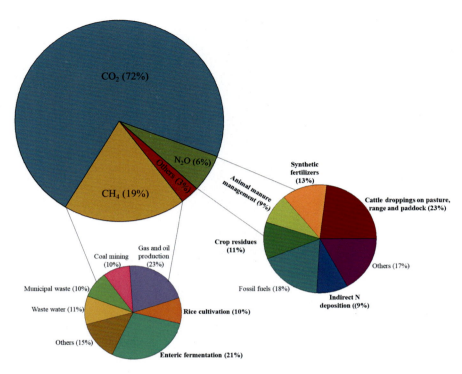

Fig. 16.3 Key drivers of nitrous oxide (N_2O) and methane (CH_4) emissions from the agricultural sector. Sections with bold letters represent agricultural sources. (Data adapted from Olivier and Peters 2020)

Peters 2020). Similarly, enteric fermentation from ruminants and rice production in flooded conditions contributes to CH_4 emissions for the livestock and crop, respectively. Cattle alone are responsible for 21% of current global CH_4 emissions, accounting for 75% of all ruminant-related CH_4 emissions (31%), followed by buffalo, sheep, and goats that have contributions of about 10%, 7%, and 5%, respectively. Rice cultivation on flooded rice fields accounts for 10% of CH_4 emissions due to the anaerobic decomposition of organic material resulting in the production of CH_4 (Fig. 16.3) (Olivier and Peters 2020). However, the CO_2 emissions are mainly derived from land use changes such as clearing of forests for agricultural development. The conversion of soil carbon (C) to CO_2 by soil microbes is accelerated in response to cultivation and growing annual crops (Verge et al. 2007). However, after few decades of soil cultivation, the soil C content is stabilized at low levels and loss as CO_2 decrease (Hutchinson et al. 2007). In addition, the use of fossil fuels for farming operations is also a source of CO_2 emissions in agriculture (Dyer and Desjardins 2003). Other sources of CO_2 emissions from agricultural lands include (a) transformations between croplands and pasture; (b) peat drainage and burning; (c) wood harvesting; (d) regrowth of forest and other natural

16 Strategies for Mitigating Greenhouse Gas Emissions from... 413

vegetation after agricultural abandonment and harvest; and (e) soil CO_2 flux due to grassland and cropland management (Hansis et al. 2015; Houghton and Nassikas 2017; Gasser et al. 2020).

Global N_2O emissions were reported to increase to 1.1% in 2019 to a total of 2.8 $GtCO_2$-eq, similar to the annual average reported since 2014, when growth rates ranged between 0.8 and 1.3%. The different sources that were the main role players for the increase in N_2O emissions in 2019 were application of synthetic N fertilizers (+2.7%); manure deposited in pastures, rangeland, and paddocks (+1.3%); indirect N_2O from agriculture (+2.1%); and other agricultural sources (+1.1%), accounting for more than 75% of the total net increase in N_2O emissions. The countries with the largest increase in N_2O emissions in 2019 were Brazil (+2.9%), Australia (+5.9%), China (+0.9%), India (+1.6%), and the Russian Federation (+2.1%), whereas the countries with decreased N_2O emissions in 2019 were Sudan, Zaire, the Central African Republic, and the United States. Similarly, global CH_4 emissions were reported to increase at 1.3% to a total of 9.8 $GtCO_2$-eq, which was lower than the 1.8% increase in 2018. This was significantly greater than years 2015 and 2016, with an overall increase of 0.3% and 0.1%, respectively, but similar to the increase reported in years 2012, 2014, and 2017 of around 1.4%, which is also the average annual increase since 2010. Among the different sources of CH_4 emissions, livestock farming (particularly non-dairy cattle) was the second largest contributor after coal production. Among different countries that contributed most to the 1.3% growth were notably China (+2.2%) and the United States (+2.5%), with increases also seen in (in decreasing order of absolute changes) Indonesia, Brazil, the Russian Federation, Pakistan, and India. Notably, decreases were seen in Turkey, Sudan, Canada, Venezuela, Germany, and Zaire.

Global emission pathways that would limit warming to 1.5 °C or less, in line with the Paris Agreement's temperature goal, depend on significant reductions in agricultural GHGs (N_2O and CH_4) as well as net zero CO_2 emissions from fossil fuels (Leahy et al. 2020). Similarly, Wollenberg et al. (2016) also suggested a global target of reducing non-CO_2 emissions from agriculture by 1 Gt CO_2-eq below baseline by 2030 to restrict warming to about 2 °C above pre-industrial levels in 2100. The most magnificent scenarios evaluated by the IPCC (2018), which limit warming to 1.5 °C with limited or no overshoot, reduce global agricultural emissions by 16–41% (interquartile range) in 2050 compared to 2010, whereas baseline emissions increase by 24–54% over the same period. This % reduction equates to 4.8 Gt CO_2-eq in direct global agricultural non-CO_2 emissions below baseline by 2050 (Huppmann et al. 2018; Frank et al. 2019). These ambitious targets of mitigation pathways represent a large challenge, and accomplishing these targets is only possible by the implementation of effective GHG mitigation strategies from the agricultural sector.

As a major source of global emissions, the agricultural sector may also provide relatively low-cost opportunities for GHG mitigation. Agricultural GHG fluxes are complex due to interaction with other factors and variation in fluxes on spatial (varied fluxes at different places on piece of land) and temporal (variation based on time of the day) basis. However, the active management of agricultural systems offers possibilities for GHG mitigation (Smith et al. 2008). Mitigation measures in the agricultural sector include increasing C sequestration and reducing the emissions from both livestock and agricultural processes. There are two ways to achieve mitigation in the agricultural sector, i.e., through supply-side measures and demand-side measures. Supply-side measures include reducing emissions via livestock management, land management, and land use change and increasing C sequestration from afforestation. Demand-side measures include changes in eating habits and reducing food wastes; however, quantitative measures for demand-side measures are more uncertain (Smith et al. 2014). In this chapter, we will discuss mitigation strategies for GHG emissions from the agricultural sector at a global scale.

16.2 Mitigation Opportunities: Increased Sinks and Reduced Emissions

16.2.1 Increasing Carbon Sequestration

According to the recent IPCC reports, even if we can substantially reduce anthropogenic C emissions in the near future, it is necessary to make efforts to sequestering previously emitted C to ensure atmospheric C to safe levels and mitigate climate change (Smith et al. 2014). Carbon sequestration can be defined as a sustained increase in C storage (in soil or plant material or in the sea). Among these sources of C sequestration, the soil's usefulness as a C sink and drawdown solution are essential, based on global estimates of historic C stocks and projections of rising emissions (Lal 2004, 2008). Since more than one-third of the world's arable land is under agriculture (World Bank 2015) and soil C pool (2500 Gt) being 3.3 times the size of the atmospheric pool (760 Gt) and 4.5 times the size of the biotic pool (560 Gt) (Lal 2004), increasing soil C in agricultural systems will be a key component of using soils as a C sink. The C sequestration potential of global soil is estimated between 0.4 and 1.2 Gt C year^{-1} or 5–15% (1 Pg $= 1 \times 10^5$ g) (Lal 2004). Various crop management techniques have been suggested for increasing C sequestration in soils (Janzen et al. 1998). However, large uncertainties have been reported with quantifying the impact of different crop management techniques on C sequestration and GHG mitigation. Increasing soil C sequestration could potentially remove between 0.79 and 1.54 Gt C year^{-1} from the atmosphere in a feasible manner, recognizing the large potential of soils mitigating CO_2 emissions (Laborde et al. 2021).

Due to the historical expansion of agriculture and pastoralism (Sanderman et al. 2017) and subsequent land use conversion from native ecosystems (e.g., peatlands, forests, grasslands) to arable land, 33% of the soils around the globe have been degraded and have lost much of their soil C (FAO 2019). The average amount of soil organic carbon (SOC) in the top 30 cm of native soil worldwide is about 15 Mg ha^{-1}

(Hutchinson et al. 2007). However, within the first 20 years of cultivation, about 20–30% and 50–75% of this C are lost to the atmosphere as CO_2 in temperate and tropical regions, respectively (Dumanski 2004). However, Lal (2013) reported that prolonged intensive cultivation decreases the soil C stock at the rate of 0.1–1.0% $year^{-1}$. The extent of C loss ranges from 10 to 30 Mg C ha^{-1}, depending on the soil type and historic land use, which is higher in soils prone to erosion, salinization, and nutrient mining than the C loss from least or undegraded soils (Lal 2013). The historical C losses from global soils are estimated to be 78 ± 12 Pg (Lal 2004; Buragohain et al. 2017). Globally, the soils of Africa are relatively low in soil organic C content with about 58% of soils containing less than 0.5% organic C and only 4% containing more than 2% organic C (Du Preez et al. 2011).

Different management practices reported to increase C sequestration include (i) reduced and zero tillage, (ii) perennial and deep-rooting crops, (iii) more efficient use of organic amendments (animal manure, sewage sludge, cereal straw, compost), (iv) improved rotations, (v) irrigation, (vi) bioenergy crops, (vii) intensification, (viii) including cover crops, and (ix) conversion of arable land to grassland or woodland (Smith 2004). The potential of these management practices for sequestering C is presented in Table 16.1. It has been estimated that implementation of appropriate management practices could help to sequester approximately 0.4–0.8 Pg C $year^{-1}$ (Watson et al. 1996). Similarly, Lal (2010) reported that adopting suitable management practices for C sequestration at agricultural soils and restoring of degraded soils can help in sequestering about 0.6–1.2 Pg C $year^{-1}$ for about 50 years with a cumulative sink capacity of 30–60 Pg. The potential of different management practices in sequestering C and mitigating CO_2 emissions is described below; however, prudent combination of these management practices would result in enhanced C sequestration.

Table 16.1 Carbon sequestration potential by different management practices

Management practice	Soil carbon sequestration potential (t C ha^{-1} $year^{-1}$)
No tillage	0.38
Reduced tillage	<0.38
Set-aside	<0.38
Permanent crops	0.62
Deep-rooting crops	0.62
Animal manure application	0.38
Cereal straw application	0.69
Sewage sludge	0.26
Composting	0.38
Bioenergy crops	0.62
Organic farming	0–0.54
Extensification	0.54

All estimates are adapted from the figures in Smith et al. (2000)

16.2.1.1 Tillage Methods and Residue Management

Conventional tillage can be defined as a plow-based method which includes successive operations of plowing or turning over of soil, whereas conservation tillage is a generic term indicating at tillage methods that reduce runoff and loss of soil by erosion as compared to conventional tillage practices. Conservation tillage practices reported to increase C sequestration by reducing tillage-induced breakdown of soil aggregates resulting in the slowdown of organic matter decomposition relative to the conventional tillage and adding organic matter as residues to the surface soil (Hati et al. 2020). Different tillage practices impact both soil-aggrading and soil-degrading processes, thereby affecting soil C storage (Lal and Kimble 1997) (Fig. 16.4). Soil-aggrading processes have a positive impact on SOC and include the humification of crop residue, increase in resistant or non-labile fraction of SOC, sequestration of SOC in the formation of organo-mineral complexes, and increase in stable aggregation and deep placement of SOC in sub-soil horizons, while soil-degrading processes have a negative impact on SOC and include erosion, leaching, and mineralization. The effect of tillage on soil processes that affect C dynamic and reserves in soils can be observed in Fig. 16.4.

Several studies have reported that conservation tillage practices help in sequestering soil C in both temperate and tropical regions. Conservation tillage increased SOC by about 8% as compared to conventional tillage on an Ultisol in eastern Nigeria (Ohiri and Ezumah 1990). Several studies emphasize that conservation tillage practices have already increased soil C contents relative to levels that would have existed under conventional farming (e.g., moldboard plowing); they have estimated C sequestration rates of 0.31–0.82 Mg C ha^{-1} year^{-1} in the United States and across the world (West and Post 2002; Spargo et al. 2008; Franzluebbers 2010). However, the capability of no tillage for increasing C sequestration is still debatable. Several authors in recent years found that no-till was capable only of increasing the

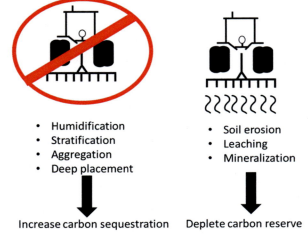

Fig. 16.4 Tillage effects on soil processes that affect C dynamics and reserves in soil

soil C in the top layer of soil, while it was compensated with the greater decrease observed in deeper layers, thereby resulting in no difference among different tillage treatments for the total C in the soil profile. However, long-term experiment results show that switching from plow-till to no-till farming is the most effective factor in crop management for SOC sequestration (Table 16.2). In a recent meta-analysis, Nicoloso and Rice (2021) found that soil C can be increased to a depth of 1 m by the intensification of no-tillage cropping systems which included double cropping, leguminous cover crops.

Crop residue management impacts the SOC dynamics as crop residues are a direct source to SOC pool. Crop residues contain approximately 45% C by dry weight (Lal 1997). Assuming that crop residues contain an average of 45% C and that approximately 15% of residue-derived C is stored as passive C in the soil, aboveground crop residues have a large potential to store SOC in the passive form on a global scale (Lal 1997). The total amount of SOC storage is determined by the quantity and quality of crop residue, plant roots, and other organic material returned to the soil, as well as the rate of their decomposition. Residue retention in combination with reduced-tillage and no-tillage practices is a viable option for increasing SOC storage in soil. In surface soil layers, under no-tillage practices, some of the residue-derived SOC gets converted into passive pool and forms organo-mineral complexes, which takes between 100 and thousands of years for decomposition. SOC accumulates when residue C inputs exceed residue C outputs and soil disturbance is kept to a minimum, while under intensive or conventional tillage practices, the decomposition of crop residues is accelerated due to good aeration, thereby resulting in reduced residue-derived C sequestration. Therefore, no-tillage practices in combination with residue retention help in the formation of the passive SOC pool and are important for long-term C sequestration.

16.2.1.2 Crop Selection and Rotation

Crop rotation refers to a planned sequence of crops grown in a regularly recurring succession on the same area, in contrast to continuous monoculture or growing a variable sequence of crops. Carbon sequestration on agricultural lands can be affected by crop rotations, climates, soils, and management practices. The use of balanced fertilization, application of organic amendments, and similarly application of crop residues in addition to intensive crop rotations can increase C sequestration levels to 5–10 Mg ha^{-1} year^{-1} since those amendments contain 10.7–18% C, which can also be helpful in the sequestration of C (Mandal et al. 2007). Different legume crops, such as peas (*Pisum sativum*), lentils (*Lens culinaris*), alfalfa (*Medicago sativa*), chickpea (*Cicer arietinum*), and sesbania (*Sesbania grandiflora*), can serve as substitute sources for N. Soil structure improvement and increased SOC content in sub-soil horizons are possible by growing deep-rooted plants. Similarly, improvement in SOC content of the sub-soil could improve in response to growing improved pastures in acid savanna soils in South America (Fisher et al. 1994). In West Africa, Lal et al. (1978, 1979) also observed significant positive effects of growing cover

Table 16.2 Impact of adopting no-tillage practices on soil carbon sequestration in different parts of the world

Location	Rotations/soils	Increase in SOC sequestration (kg ha^{-1} year^{-1})	Depth (cm)	Duration (years)	Reference
Brazil (South)	Various rotations	611	30	9	Bayer et al. (2000)
Canada	Average for groups: Gleysolic, brown, dark brown, and black (Century Model prediction)	200	–	10	Desjardins et al. (2005)
Europe	Assessment based on long-term experiments: Europe	387	25	–	Smith et al. (2000)
	United Kingdom	613	25	–	
Spain	Various rotations on Calcic Luvisol	100	30	11	López-Fando and Pardo (2001)
United States:	Various crop rotations on:				
(1) Kansas	Grundy silty clay loam	20	30	15	Havlin et al. (1990)
	Muir silt loam	62	30	15	
(2) Nebraska	Spring wheat-fallow spring	−225	30.4	12	Halvorson et al. (2002)
	Wheat-winter wheat-sunflower	542	30.4	12	
(3) Ohio	Various rotations on clay loam	566	30	30	Dick et al. (1998)
(4) Oregon	Various crops on coarse-silty mixed mesic	94	22.5	44	Rasmussen and Rhode (1988)
	Winter wheat-lentil (*Lens culinaris* Medik.)	587	20	3	Bezdicek et al. (2002)
	Winter wheat-barley with no-till management	166	20	25	
(6) Texas	Continuous corn (4y) followed by continuous cotton (4y) on sandy clay loam	15-20	20	26	Salinas-Garcia et al. (1997)
(7) Miscellaneous regions	39 paired tillage experiments	220	Various depths	5–20	Paustian et al. (1997)
World	Till to no-till 276 paired treatments excluding wheat-fallow treatments	570 ± 140	Various depths	Various time	West and Post (2002)

crops on increase in SOC content. Cover crops help in increasing soil C content only in surface layers; utilizing agroforestry (AF) systems could help in depositing C to deeper layers of soil (Meena et al. 2020; Sarto et al. 2020). The AF consists of mixture of trees, agricultural crops, and livestock to exploit the economic and ecological benefits of agroecosystem. It is a crucial leader of terrestrial C sequestration containing about 12% of the global terrestrial C (Dixon 1995). The roots of forest tress and perennial crops penetrate deeper subsurface horizons, thus placing SOC at deeper horizons far away from the range of tillage implements (Lorenz and Lal 2014). Estimating the C sequestration potential of agroforestry systems under varied ecological and management environments ranged from 0.29 to 15.21 Mg ha^{-1} $year^{-1}$ in aboveground plant biomass and 30 to 300 Mg ha^{-1} $year^{-1}$ in belowground plant parts up to a depth of 1.0 m (Nair et al. 2010). Thereby, the implementation of appropriate crop rotation and utilizing AF can help in sequestering soil C at a rate of 0.15–0.17 Mg C ha^{-1} $year^{-1}$ (Meena et al. 2020).

Bare soil is prone to erosion and nutrient leaching and contains less C than the same field under vegetation. One of the solutions for increasing C sequestration is to plant cover and catch crops that cover the soil between the main crop or in fallow periods. It is estimated that eliminating summer fallow and replacing it with some cover crop would help in sequestering soil C at a rate of approximately 0.05–0.20 Mg C ha^{-1} $year^{-1}$ (Meena et al. 2020). The basic concept of increasing C sequestration on eliminating summer fallow is that it increases soil biomass addition, resulting in increased C deposition. Also, if the soil is left bare (fallow), it is more prone to erosion by wind or water, and as most of the C is deposited in surface layers in croplands, it is more prone to wind and water erosion and decomposition. Soil erosion alone is responsible for the loss of 1.1 Pg C $year^{-1}$ (Meena et al. 2020). Legumes enhance biological diversity, increase N input (via N fixation), and improve crop residue quality and overall soil C flux (Lal 2004). The greater the biodiversity of an ecosystem, the more will be the sequestration capacity. The unique advantage of cover crops over the other management options is that they not only enhance the SOC stock but also reduce the C loss, unlike organic manures. Hence, replacing the fallow period with cover cropping improves the soil quality by enriching SOC through their biomass and promoting soil aggregation and protecting the surface soil from runoff and erosion.

16.2.2 Reducing Nitrous Oxide Emissions

In recent years, there has been a growing interest in the possibility of mitigating climate change by reducing emissions of non-CO_2 GHGs. Agriculture is the largest anthropogenic source of N_2O, one of the most important non-CO_2 GHGs because it is a long-lived GHG (about 114 years) and a major source of NO in the stratosphere (Reay et al. 2012). For the past few decades, the amount of N_2O in the atmosphere has increased almost linearly at approximately 0.7 ppb or 0.26% $year^{-1}$ (Smith 2010). The IPCC (2001) reported that the increased microbial production of N_2O in expanding and fertilized agricultural lands is the main driver of this increase. With a growing human population and the resulting need for more food production, agricultural land area and N_2O emissions are expected to increase in the coming decades. We assume that changes in N cycling in soil systems have influenced increases in atmospheric N_2O over the past century and will help dictate future changes since roughly 70% of the N_2O emitted is derived from soils (Bouwman 1990; Braker and Conrad 2011). Among different continents, Asia is the continent with the largest N_2O emissions, reflecting its large population and agricultural area (Oenema et al. 2014). On a per capita basis, Asia has the lowest estimated N_2O emissions, followed by Africa and Europe. Expressed per surface area of agricultural land, emissions are highest in Asia and Europe and least in Oceania and Africa. The largest source of N_2O emissions in Asia, Europe, and North America is fertilizer N, while manure N from grazing animals is the largest source in Africa, Latin America, and Oceania. Therefore, the main source for N_2O emissions from the agricultural land includes lower efficiency of synthetic N fertilizers applied to croplands and urine and dung excreted by the animals, either in pastures or in confinements (stables, barns, sheds, corrals). In general, management practices that optimize the natural ability of the crop to compete with processes where plant available N is lost from the soil-plant system (i.e., NH_3 volatilization, denitrification, and leaching) and directly lowering the rate and duration of the loss processes can reduce N_2O emissions from synthetic N fertilizers and organic N sources such as crop residue and animal excreta (Doerge et al. 1991). In this section, we have described different management strategies which have the potential for mitigating N_2O emissions from croplands and grazing lands around the world.

16.2.2.1 4R of Fertilizer Management

The major source of N_2O emissions from croplands is the application of N fertilizers. In addition, increasing demands for food around the world would not allow reductions in the usage of N fertilizers to decrease N_2O emissions. Moreover, crop improvement in major crops such as corn (*Zea mays* L.) increases the dependency on N fertilization as yields increase over time (Ciampitti and Vyn 2012). Therefore, the only solution to reduce N_2O emissions from croplands without jeopardizing global food production is to enhance nitrogen use efficiency (NUE) (Ciampitti and Vyn 2014; Singh et al. 2019). The uptake of N fertilizer by crops varies widely across the world, and global cereal NUE is reported to be only 33% (Raun and Johnson 1999). Additionally, the insignificant trend of increase in global cereal NUE from 2002 to 2015 reported by Omara et al. (2019) is a cause of concern. It is estimated that each year, approximately 1.5 Tg of N is lost as N_2O to the atmosphere because of the application of synthetic N fertilizers to agricultural ecosystems (Mosier et al. 1996). This accounted for about 44% of the anthropogenic input and 13% of the total annual N_2O input into the atmosphere. However, the contribution of synthetic N fertilizers to N_2O emissions is still thought to be underestimated. Additionally, N_2O production from other major N sources such as animal manures

16 Strategies for Mitigating Greenhouse Gas Emissions from... 421

and biological N fixation has not been included in the abovementioned estimates. To meet the needs of rapidly expanding population, the use of N fertilizers is also projected to increase in the coming years for increasing global food production. Thereby, it is very important to reduce the loss of N fertilizers as N_2O emissions and increase the N use efficiency. This will result in mitigating GHG emissions from different N fertilizers and will be economically beneficial for the producers. The "4R" approach of using the right source, right rate, right timing, and right placement is an accepted framework for reducing loss of N fertilizers as N_2O and increasing crop N use efficiency. Modifying just one of the 4R components may not be enough to reduce N_2O emissions (Decock 2014). Different studies demonstrated that the use of right time alone (delayed and/or split application) (Phillips et al. 2009; Zebarth et al. 2012) or right source (e.g., urea-containing microbial inhibitors) (Parkin and Hatfield 2013; Sistani et al. 2011) has been not very successful in mitigating N_2O emissions. The 4R technique is effective when you have site-, soil-, and crop-specific knowledge and information, accompanied with appropriate technologies and best management practices. It has been reported that implementation of 4R strategy could help in achieving N uptake more than 70% for many cereals (Snyder and Fixen 2012).

While choosing the best fertilizer source may appear to be a simple task, there are several factors that ultimately influence this decision. Selecting an appropriate fertilizer source starts with an assessment of which nutrients are necessary, and this information comes from some form of site diagnostics such as soil testing. The responses of different N fertilizers (nitrate-, ammonium-, or urea-based) to N_2O emissions are very dynamic depending on soil conditions (well-drained or moist conditions), air temperatures, and other climatic conditions. Therefore, there is possibility of decreasing N_2O emissions from N fertilizers and increasing N use efficiency by choosing specific fertilizers for a particular location. Another option for choosing the right source of N fertilizer is the use of "enhanced efficiency fertilizers" instead of conventional fertilizers. Enhanced efficiency fertilizers have been reported to improve N fertilizer use efficiency by increasing the availability of N to crops while reducing N loss to the environment (Snyder 2017; Zhang et al. 2015) including N_2O emissions (Akiyama et al. 2010; Ju et al. 2011). Experiments have shown that these types of fertilizer can decrease N_2O emissions by 35–38% relative to conventional N fertilizer (Akiyama et al. 2010). Bastos et al. (2021) and Arango and Rice (2021) found a 66% reduction in N_2O emissions with a combination of placement and a nitrification inhibitor.

Nitrous oxide emission from N fertilizer application can be reduced by synchronizing with plant N demand. The N uptake during the beginning of the growing season of the crop is lower, increases exponentially during vegetative growth, and drops sharply at crop maturity. Therefore, applying N fertilizer a few weeks after planting rather than at or before planting increases the likelihood that the N will end up in the crop rather than be lost to the atmosphere as N_2O emissions. Soil moisture is the major driver of the N_2O emissions from soil as it regulates the availability of oxygen to microbes. Impacted by different soil types, the maximum N_2O emissions are emitted when soil water-filled pore space ranges from 60 to 90% (Wang et al.

2021; Bastos et al. 2021). Therefore, application of N fertilizer during high soil moisture levels may also help in reducing N_2O emissions. Split N applications to crops result in reduced concentrations of soil mineral N in the early growth stage of crops. Application of the second portion of N during the active growth phase, when N uptake is at maximum, also reduces the potential for N_2O emissions to occur (Van Groenigen et al. 2010). Split application of N was reported as an effective strategy to reduce N_2O emissions from potato cultivation (Burton et al. 2008). In corn production, a single application of N was reported to emit 35% more N_2O compared to split applications (Fernández et al. 2016).

In addition to the right timing, applying N more than the crop requirement increases soil ammonium and nitrate concentrations in soils (Andraski et al. 2000). As a consequence, relatively higher N_2O emissions can occur when compared with applications at the required rate (McSwiney and Robertson 2005; Ma et al. 2010). To know the amount of N fertilizer application, the proper information about the site soil and crop need is required. Stehfest and Bouwman (2006) also reported the rate of N fertilizer application to be the strongest predictor of N_2O emissions in their extensive review of published articles all over the world. Although the reported mean N_2O emission factor is 1.2%, which means for every 100 kg of N input, 1.2 kg of N is lost as N_2O emissions (Albanito et al. 2017), results from a growing number of field experiments indicate that the fraction of applied N emitted as direct N_2O increases with increasing rate of N application (McSwiney and Robertson 2005; Ma et al. 2010; Hoben et al. 2011; Shcherbak et al. 2014; Millar et al. 2018). Therefore, using the single emission factor across the fertilizer rates may result in an underestimation of fertilizer-induced N_2O emissions when fertilizer addition exceeds crop demand.

Right placement of N fertilizer in the soil also helps to reduce N_2O emissions. For example, the application of urea in a narrow band close to plant roots instead of its application by broadcast helps to reduce N_2O emissions. Also, different crops have exhibited different root growing habits and require specific N fertilizer placement method for the enhancement of N use efficiency. For corn, shallow instead of deep placement of N fertilizers is reported to decrease N_2O emissions and increase N use efficiency (Breitenbeck and Bremner 1986). The precision fertilizer application tools are also reported to help reduce N_2O emissions and increase N use efficiency. This is because precision fertilizer application helps to access the spatial variability in the field, recommending less N fertilizer application in areas of the field with low yield potential, thereby helping to avoid N fertilizer wastage on locations in the field that are not likely to respond to N fertilizer application. Precision fertilizer application reduced the average N fertilizer rate by 25 kg N ha^{-1} in one study, resulting in significant reductions in N_2O emissions (Sehy et al. 2003).

16.2.2.2 Grazing and Manure Management

The relative importance of microbial processes that lead to N_2O emissions from animal manures will be determined by the manure environment, which is influenced by local management practices and climate, both of which vary between regions. A large portion of N_2O emissions resulting from manure are produced in manure-amended soils by microbial nitrification under aerobic conditions and partial denitrification under anaerobic conditions, with denitrification producing more N_2O (Hockstad and Hanel 2018). This manure can be deposited by the grazing animals in grassland-based systems or applied manually after collection and storage from confined-animal feeding systems. Under continuous stocking, specific hotspots of mineral N, or higher overall amounts of mineral N, are expected to appear in soils within grazed paddocks or portions of grazed paddocks. This premise is based on the fact that cattle have more opportunity (more time) to congregate in local areas (e.g., water sources, near to borders, shady areas) of paddocks, resulting in less-even N distributions (Singh et al. 2019). It is reported that animals spend 27% of their time and deposit around 49% of all N in consumed biomass to these areas (Augustine et al. 2013). Additionally, N_2O emissions from the pen surfaces of open-lot dairy or beef feedlot facilities can also be significant due to improper handling and storage of the manure (Montes et al. 2013).

For grassland-based systems, changing the form of grazing management and intensity of grazing pressure are among the strategies available to reduce N_2O emissions. Due to the effects on soil compaction and other physical, chemical, and biological properties of soils, higher stocking rates applied to pastures result in higher N_2O emissions from grazing lands. Also, stocking at high rates may result in the consumption of more low-quality forage by animals, which has an impact on both animal performance and greater N_2O emissions (Wang et al. 2015). Thus, the management of stocking density (animal numbers ha^{-1} $year^{-1}$) applied to graze paddocks is an essential practice for mitigating N_2O emissions. Increased N_2O emissions due to increased deposition of manure and urine could be caused by intensive forms of stocking. Further, the anaerobic conditions caused by increased soil compaction in grazing paddocks help to support N_2O emissions from these deposits. Reduced dietary N and increased mineral content of biomass available for grazing are two other ways to reduce N_2O emissions from grazing lands. N excretion in urine is reduced when dietary N is reduced. Additionally, inhibiting nitrification from N hotspots in grazing lands could be a useful strategy for reducing N_2O emissions. Approximately 55% of the total daily N_2O emissions from grazing paddocks is contributed by N hotspots which include urine patches, dung pats, shaded areas, and areas near water troughs (Cowan et al. 2015). The primary source of significant emissions from these hotspots is cow urine and dung, which enriches the soil with nutrients, particularly N, and moisture, creating ideal conditions for N_2O emissions. Different mitigation strategies for reducing N_2O emissions from these areas have been recommended, including restricted grazing during wet periods that favor denitrification, feeding cattle low-N diets, using stand-off pads, application of soil amendments (i.e., lime) to increase soil pH to shift the balance between N_2O and non-greenhouse N_2, or use of zeolite to capture soil NH_4. The blanket application of nitrification inhibitors like dicyandiamide in combination with urease inhibitors like nBTPT has been recommended as the best approach to reduce N losses from grazing lands among all the abovementioned strategies (Zaman and Nguyen 2012). However, there is a need of research for investigating timing, type, rate, and cost associated with nitrification inhibitor application in different regions for mitigating N_2O emissions from grazing lands.

In confined-animal feeding systems, manure is typically collected and must be managed from the point of excretion through storage, treatment, and finally applying to land. To reduce the N_2O emissions from animal manures during its storage, it is suggested that solid manures need to be kept covered. However, there are some studies with contradicting results reporting increased N_2O emissions of manure covering (Table 16.3) (Petersen et al. 2013). Additionally, the application of nitrification inhibitors to the manures while storage has the potential to reduce N_2O emissions (Petersen 2018). According to one meta-analysis, the reduction in N_2O emissions due to nitrification inhibitor application to stored manures can range from 40 to 50% (Qiao et al. 2015). Likewise for N fertilizer application, different factors such as method, rate, placement, and timing of application according to crop nutrient requirements are crucial for mitigating N_2O emissions from manures.

16.2.3 *Reducing Methane Emissions*

Methane is a GHG currently contributing to about 15 % of global anthropogenic GHGs emitted every year when assuming a greenhouse warming potential of 25 times CO_2 over 100 year and 50.6% of anthropogenic CH_4 emissions are released as a result of agricultural activities. China followed by India, Brazil, the United States, Indonesia, Australia, Russia, Argentina, Thailand, and Nigeria are ten major contributors of the CH_4 emissions from the agricultural sector, constituting about 54.6% of the global emissions. Among different agricultural activities, 59.8% of CH_4 emissions are contributed by the enteric fermentation followed by emissions from rice cultivation, other agricultural activities, and manure management (Karakurt et al. 2012). Enteric fermentation refers to the process of foods being fermented by microbes in an animal's digestive system. As a byproduct of this process, CH_4 is released by animals exhaling (Karakurt et al. 2012). The majority of CH_4 emissions in this sector is contributed by domesticated ruminants like cattle, buffalo, sheep, goats, and camels. However, other domesticated non-ruminants such as swine and horses also contribute to CH_4 emissions through enteric fermentation, but emissions per animal species vary significantly. Another major contributor to CH_4 emissions from the agricultural sector includes rice cultivation which contributes approximately 11% of global anthropogenic CH_4 emissions (IPCC 2013). In a flooded rice field, the decomposition of organic materials in an environment without oxygen results in the release of CH_4. The breakdown of organic components under flooded rice conditions consumes available oxygen in soil and water rapidly, and methanogenic bacteria produce CH_4 when the oxygen in the environment is depleted. Additionally, manure storage from confined-animal feeding systems in liquid form can contribute to CH_4 emissions. Storing manures in liquid systems such as lagoons, ponds, or pits results in anaerobic conditions, resulting in CH_4 emissions (Steed and Hashimoto 1994). However, the amount of CH_4 from manure varies with

16 Strategies for Mitigating Greenhouse Gas Emissions from... 425

Table 16.3 Effects of different management options on CH_4, N_2O, and combined $CH_4 + N_2O$ emissions from manure storage

Type of storage	Management option	Nitrous oxide	Methane	$N_2O + CH_4$	References
Solid manure	Forced v. passive composting	−35	−90	−78	Amon et al. (2001)
		−41	+32	−7	Amon et al. (2001)
		+44	−81	−34	Pattey et al. (2005)
			−28		Hao et al. (2001)
	Straw cover	−42	−45	−42	Yamulki (2006)
		−11	−50	−14	Yamulki (2006)
	Plastic cover	−70	−6	−36	Chadwick (2005)
		+2000	−81	−17	Chadwick (2005)
		−54	+120	+111	Chadwick (2005)
		−99	−87	−98	Hansen et al. (2006)
		−32			Thorman et al. (2006)
		+304			Thorman et al. (2006)
Liquid manure	Straw cover	+57	−25		VanderZaag et al. (2009)
		+100	−27	−23	VanderZaag et al. (2009)
			+37	−24	Guarino et al. (2006)
			+3		Guarino et al. (2006)
			+7		Guarino et al. (2006)
			−28		Guarino et al. (2006)
	Solid cover	+432	+22	+238	Berg et al. (2006)
		+30	−32	+1	Amon et al. (2007)
		−4	−70	−52	Amon et al. (2007)
		−50	−37	−48	Amon et al. (2007)
		−13	−14	−13	Clemens et al. (2006)
		+20	−16	−11	Clemens et al. (2006)
		+2	−29	−4	Clemens et al. (2006)
		−19	−14	−16	Clemens et al. (2006)

"+" represents higher emissions (%) and "−" lower emissions (%) compared with the reference (untreated) manure. The comparison of systems is based on CO_2 equivalents. Data is adapted from Peterson et al. (2013)

respect to the storage type, ambient temperature for storage, and manure composition. Open biomass burning, savanna burning, agricultural residue burning, and open forest clearing burning are other agricultural sources of CH_4 emissions. In this section, we will be discussing strategies to mitigate CH_4 emissions from different agricultural sources.

16.2.3.1 Improving Rumen Fermentation Efficiency and Productivity of Animals

Due to their unique digestive system, which includes a rumen, ruminant animals such as cattle, buffalo, sheep, and goats produce a lot of CH_4. The methanogenic archaebacterium responsible for CH_4 production is located mainly in the rumen, and its growth is affected by diet and other nutritionally related characteristics such as level of intake, feeding strategies, quality of fodder, and fodder concentrate ratios (Karakurt et al. 2012). Therefore, numerous nutritional technologies have been evaluated to increase rumen fermentation efficiency and reduce CH_4 production, such as direct inhibitors, feed additives, propionate enhancers, CH_4 oxidizers, probiotics, defaunation, diet manipulation, and hormones. Up to 40% reduction in CH_4 emissions is reported as a result of dietary manipulation depending on the degree of change and nature of the intervention (Benchaar et al. 2001). Dietary manipulation includes improving forage quality or changing the proportion of diet and dietary supplementation of feed additives that directly either inhibit methanogens or alter the metabolic pathways leading to a reduction of the substrate for methanogenesis. Forage quality can be improved by providing high-quality forage as it contains higher amounts of easily fermentable carbohydrates and less neutral detergent fiber, leading to a higher digestibility and passage rate, thereby resulting in lower CH_4 production, while more mature forage has a higher C:N ratio, which results in decreased digestibility and higher CH_4 production (Beever et al. 1986). Feeding legume forage results in lower CH_4 emissions as it contains condensed tannins, a low fiber content, high dry matter intake, and fast passage rate (Beauchemin et al. 2008). In general, feeding C_3 plant yields less CH_4 emissions than that from C_4 plants (Archimède et al. 2011). Similarly, replacing grass silage with maize silage helps in reducing CH_4 emissions from enteric fermentation. The reason is the same that grass silage is usually harvested at a later stage of maturity and contains lower content of digestible organic matter, lower sugar, and N contents, whereas maize silage provides higher contents of dry matter with readily digestible carbohydrates, e.g., starch, increasing the dry matter intake and animal performance (Beauchemin et al. 2008). Additionally, concentrates, fat supplementation, organic acids, essential oils, ionophores, and probiotics as feed additives reduce CH_4 emissions from enteric fermentation. Another method suggested for increasing rumen fermentation is the possibility of breeding animals with low CH_4 emissions. However, Eckard et al. (2010) suggested that breeding for reduced CH_4 production is unlikely compatible with other breeding objectives. Another way to reduce enteric CH_4 emissions is to increase the milk yield of dairy animals. However, increasing

16 Strategies for Mitigating Greenhouse Gas Emissions from. . .

productivity will only reduce the total enteric CH_4 emissions if the amount of milk produced is kept constant by reducing the number of animals (Sirohi et al. 2007). Diet not only has a direct impact on CH_4 emissions from intestinal fermentation, but it also has an indirect impact on CH_4 emissions during storage by influencing manure composition (Hindrichsen et al. 2005).

16.2.3.2 Manure Management

Methane production is significantly decreased under dry and aerobic conditions; thereby, switching from liquid to dry manure management systems would help minimize CH_4 emissions from manure storage and handling. Methanogenesis is dependent on temperature, being lower under cooler temperatures. Therefore, storing slurry at cooler temperatures (10 °C) could result in 30% to 46% reduction in CH_4 emissions (Table 16.4). In cold and temperate climates, the temperature difference between animal housing and outside manure storage is significant. Therefore, by frequent removal of manure from housing to outside storage could help mitigate CH_4 from manure (Table 16.5). While storage, aeration of the solid manure left for composting also helps reduce CH_4 emissions from manure as it helps maintain aerobic conditions. Similar to N_2O emissions, covering both liquid and solid manures using straw or plastic sheets is also a mitigation strategy for CH_4 emissions from manure. However, some studies also reported contradicting results showing increased CH_4 emissions on manure covering (Chadwick 2005; Berg et al. 2006). Another method reported to mitigate CH_4 emissions from manure is its separation, herein defined as a process whereby a fraction of slurry particles is isolated by one of the several mechanical separation processes. Separate storage of the liquid and solid fractions after manure separation has, in most cases, but not always, resulted in lower CH_4 emissions (Table 16.4). Anaerobic digestion of manure is another strategy for mitigating CH_4 emissions where methanogenesis is optimized for breaking down degradable organic matter in manure and transforming it into biogas. As CH_4 is collected and used as fossil fuel, it reduces CH_4 emissions during storage. The potential of anaerobic digestion for reducing CH_4 emissions from manure reported under different studies can be found in Table 16.4. Additionally, treatment of slurry/manure using sulfuric acid is reported to reduce CH_4 emissions by 67% to 99% during 3-month storage period (Table 16.4). Manure aeration is an efficient way for mitigating CH_4 emissions because aerobic conditions are maintained. Amon et al. (2006) reported a reduction in CH_4 emissions (by 57%), with aeration of cattle slurry, while Martinez et al. (2003) reported reductions in CH_4 emissions of 70% to 99% after aeration of pig slurry. Therefore, using these mitigation strategies alone or in combination with others could help reduce CH_4 emissions during manure storage and handling.

Table 16.4 Effects of different management options on CH_4, N_2O, and combined $CH_4 + N_2O$ emissions from manure treatment

Management option	Type of manure	Nitrous oxide	Methane	$CH_4 + N_2O$	References
Manure separation	Pig slurry (5 °C)	0	−8	−8	Dinuccio et al. (2008)
	Pig slurry (25 °C)		+3	+41	Dinuccio et al. (2008)
	Cattle slurry (5 °C)	0	+4	+4	Dinuccio et al. (2008)
	Cattle slurry (25 °C)	0	−9	−9	Dinuccio et al. (2008)
	Cattle slurry	+1133	−34	−23	Fangueiro et al. (2008)
	Cattle slurry + wooden lid	+10	−42	−39	Amon et al. (2006)
	Pig slurry		−93	−29	López-Mosquera et al. (2011)
	Cattle slurry		−42	+25	López-Mosquera et al. (2011)
	Pig slurry		−18		Martinez et al. (2003)
	Cattle slurry		−40		Martinez et al. (2003)
Anaerobic digestion	Cattle slurry	−9	−32	−14	Clemens et al. (2006)
	Cattle slurry	+49	−68	−48	Clemens et al. (2006)
	Cattle slurry + wooden lid	+41	−67	−59	Amon et al. (2006)
Aeration	Cattle slurry	+144	−57	−43	Amon et al. (2006)
	Pig slurry		−99		Martinez et al. (2003)
	Pig slurry		−70		Martinez et al. (2003)
Dilution	Pig slurry		−35		Martinez et al. (2003)
	Cattle slurry		−57		Martinez et al. (2003)
Additives					
NX_{23}	Pig slurry		−47		Martinez et al. (2003)
Stalosan	Pig slurry		−54		Martinez et al. (2003)
Biosuper	Pig slurry		−64		Martinez et al. (2003)
Sulfuric acid (pH 6)	Cattle slurry		−87		Petersen et al. (2012)
	Pig slurry		−99		Petersen et al. (2012)
	Pig slurry		−94		Petersen et al. (2012)

"+" represents higher emissions (%) and "−" lower emissions (%) compared with the reference (untreated) manure. The comparison of systems is based on CO_2 equivalents

16.2.3.3 Reducing CH_4 Emissions from Flooded Rice Cultivation

Rice is grown on over 140 million hectares around the world and is the world's most widely consumed staple food. About 90% of the world's rice is produced and consumed in Asia, and 90% of rice land is flooded, at least temporarily (Wassmann et al. 2009). During the growing season, the soil redox potential decreases significantly due to flooded and anaerobic conditions, creating an environment conducive to methanogenesis, thereby resulting in CH_4 emissions. Estimates of global CH_4 emissions from paddy soils range from 31 to 112 Tg year^{-1}, accounting for up to 19% of the total emissions, while 11% of global agricultural N_2O emissions come from rice fields (US-EPA 2006; IPCC 2007). Rice production may need to increase to keep pace with the growing demand; efficient and sustainable management is needed to mitigate CH_4 emissions from rice paddy fields while maintaining high rice yields. Water regime and organic inputs determine most CH_4 emissions from rice fields, but soil type, weather, tillage management, residues, fertilizers, and rice cultivar also play a role. Therefore, changing the water management with soil submergence to a limited period seems to be the most promising option for mitigating CH_4 emissions from flooded rice fields. Midseason drainage (a common irrigation practice adopted in major rice-growing regions of China and Japan) and intermittent irrigation (common in northwest India) reduce CH_4 emissions by over 40%. Under midseason drainage, the time under anaerobic conditions is reduced, and most of the CH_4 in the soil is oxidized when exposed to air, which raises the soil redox potential to levels that prevent methanogenesis (Souza et al. 2021). However, the field needs to be reflooded before the soil moisture level falls a critical plant water stress level and prevents yield loss. Also, practicing early-season drainage in combination with midseason drainage is reported to be more effective than only midseason drainage as it helps reduce about 80–90% of CH_4 emissions. As the main solution for reducing CH_4 emissions for flooded rice is to limit soil submergence to a limited period, switching flooded rice cultivation to upland rice cultivation also reduces CH_4 emissions. However, the adoption of upland rice cultivation is not preferred because its production potential is much lower (Neue 1993). Another option for minimizing CH_4 emissions from flooded rice is by the adoption of direct seeding instead of transplanting. However, there are debates about the profitability of direct seeds rice due to the weed problem.

In addition to water management, fertilization management is relevant for mitigating CH_4 emissions from rice cultivation. Soil fertilization using fresh organic matter amendments, such as rice straw and green manures, significantly increases CH_4 production and emissions. Therefore, organic amendments may need to be minimized to reduce CH_4 emissions from wetland rice fields. However, sometimes, use of green manures and crop residues is the only source of soil nutrition for resource-limited farmers. In general, due to the availability of chemical fertilizers and responsive rice cultivars, organic amendments have declined in recent years. Among different chemical fertilizers, sulfate-containing fertilizers mitigate CH_4 emissions (Ro et al. 2011). This is because sulfate-reducing bacteria compete with methanogens for limited hydrogen. Use of urea-encapsulated calcium carbide as an N fertilizer if flooded rice is reported to mitigate CH_4 emissions due to slow release of acetylene (Bronson and Mosier 1991).

16.2.4 Quantifying and Modeling GHG Fluxes

The improvement in accuracy and robustness of the estimates of the GHG implications of the abovementioned practices is necessary as the agricultural sector plays an important role in addressing climate change. Particularly, the capacity to estimate

430   H. Singh et al.

Table 16.5 Effects of different management options on CH_4, N_2O, and combined $CH_4 + N_2O$ emissions from animal housing

Management option	Animal category	Nitrous oxide	Methane	$N_2O + CH_4$	References
Straw bedding	Fatteners	+106	−2	+29	Philippe et al. (2007)
	Gestating sows	+383	−9	+131	Philippe et al. (2007)
	Weaned pigs		−18	+22	Cabaraux et al. (2009)
	Dairy cattle	+85	+33	+48	Edouard et al. (2012)
Sawdust v. straw	Weaned pigs	+286	−51	+195	Nicks et al. (2003)
	Fatteners	+6867	−33	+286	Nicks et al. (2004)
	Fatteners	+7600	+100	+667	Kaiser (1999)
Wood shavings v. straw	Laying hens	+259	+319	+275	Mennicken (1998)
Cooling	Pigs		−31		Sommer et al. (2004)
	Fatteners		−43		Groenestein et al. (2012)
	Nursing sows		−46		Groenestein et al. (2012)
	Gestating sows		−33		Groenestein et al. (2012)
	Weaned pigs		−30		Groenestein et al. (2012)
Frequent manure removal	Pigs	−39	−56	−51	Amon et al. (2007)
	Pigs		−40		Haeussermann et al. (2006)
	Weaned pigs	0	−50	−50	Groenestein et al. (2012)
	Fatteners	0	−86	−86	Groenestein et al. (2012)

"+" represents higher emissions (%) and "−" lower emissions (%) compared with the reference (untreated) manure. The comparison of systems is based on CO_2 equivalents

CH_4 and N_2O emissions and changes in emissions needs to be strengthened, and a global monitoring system to provide measurements of soil C stocks over time should be established. Making informed decisions about the most appropriate mitigation strategies requires a thorough understanding of how much C can be sequestered or how various practices can reduce much GHG emissions. However, significant gaps remain, particularly in developing countries, where there are still many questions about the sources of agricultural emissions, as well as a lack of methods and methodologies for monitoring emissions through supply chains and evaluating the GHG impacts of investments. Additionally, the mathematical models can articulate

16 Strategies for Mitigating Greenhouse Gas Emissions from... 431

the factors that control GHG fluxes and soil C stock changes. Therefore, a combination of field measurements and models considering farming systems is the most effective method for estimating global-scale agricultural emissions and sinks, as well as forecasting changes in emissions due to changes in management practices, environmental and economic conditions, or government policies (Table 16.5).

The rate of GHG emissions from soils and/or uptake can be measured directly using the chamber method and micrometeorological techniques. However, because emission rates are highly variable in both space and time, measuring flows of these gases over areas and time periods of interest poses significant challenges. For example, following a rainstorm or fertilization, N_2O emission rates can change 100-fold or more (Smith et al. 2000), and similar changes in CO_2 emission rates occur after tillage (Reicosky et al. 1997). Therefore, calculating annual flux rates demands frequent sampling to adequately represent large, short-term fluxes and avoid under- or over-estimation of fluxes. Due to the high spatial variability of flux rates, either several small areas within a field must be sampled and averaged, or the measurement technique must integrate fluxes over a relatively large area. In addition, automated chamber systems can be utilized for overcoming the error due to temporal variability.

Mathematical models can be used for articulating the factors that control GHG fluxes and soil C stock changes. There are two basic types of models: (i) empirical and (ii) "process-oriented" models. Empirical models use field measurements to determine statistical relationships between soil C stocks and environmental and management factors (e.g., IPCC 1997; Ogle et al. 2003), whereas more dynamic, "process-oriented" models attempt to simulate the biological, chemical, and physical processes that control GHG dynamics. Process-oriented models are useful to portray the effect of combinations of management practices as well as soil and climate conditions. Several dynamic, process-based models have been developed to simulate soil C stock changes and N_2O and CH_4 fluxes from soil.

16.3 Conclusions

Global agriculture has significant potential to reduce GHG emissions and sequester C in soils using currently available technology. However, because there are so many variables that influence emission and sequestration processes, some practices that reduce one gas emissions may increase emissions of another. Promoting practices that maintain or increase C stocks while also increasing the efficiency of agricultural inputs (e.g., fertilizer, irrigation, pesticides, animal feed, and animal waste) is the key to reducing net GHG emissions from agriculture. To achieve the best overall mitigation results, GHG mitigation practices should address both C stocks and N_2O and CH_4 emissions. The largest potentials for soil C sequestration are associated with adoption of no-till practices, reduced fallow, use of cover crops, and conservation set-asides with perennial grasses and trees on highly erodible cropland. Nitrous oxide emissions from soils constitute the single largest agricultural GHG source. More efficient use of N fertilizer and manure, increasing the overall efficiency of N use for crop improvement, as well as additives that inhibit the formation of N_2O in soils could help in the reduction of N_2O emissions. Methane emissions are mainly contributed through enteric fermentation and emissions from stored manure from livestock production or from flooded rice cultivation. Manure management systems that capture and combust CH_4 can provide a renewable energy source that both is helpful in reducing CH_4 emissions and can displace fossil fuels. Improved production technologies (e.g., improved feed quality, CH_4-suppressing feed additives, and animal breeding) can reduce enteric CH_4 emissions, increase livestock production, and perhaps improve profitability. For rice cultivation, avoiding the use of organic inputs, fertilizer management, using nitrification inhibitors and irrigation management techniques such as midseason drainage or intermittent drainage can help in mitigating CH_4 emissions.

With respect to quantification, this report finds that direct field measurement is viable, although at times expensive, for assessing C sequestration; field measurement of CH_4 and N_2O is not yet ready for wide implementation. Direct measurement appears best suited for programs focused on innovative new practices for which research is lacking. In contrast, modeling will likely be most efficient for scaling up known management practices well supported by research and modeling capacity. Important data gaps remain for program or project implementation particularly management data for establishing baseline conditions. Additional work is needed to assess potential reversal rates for the subset of management practices for which this could be a problem.

Acknowledgments We thank the following entities for supporting research related to mitigating GHG emissions from the agricultural sector: the Department of Agronomy, Kansas State University; Feed the Future Sustainable Intensification Innovation Lab funded by the United States Agency for International Development (grant number AID-OAA-L-14-00006); and funds allocated to the USDA-ARS project 3070-21610-003-00D by the National Institute of Food and Agriculture, United States Department of Agriculture (award number 2019-68012-29888). Contribution number 22-240-B from Kansas Agricultural Experiment Station.

References

Akiyama H, Yan X, Yagi K (2010) Evaluation of effectiveness of enhanced-efficiency fertilizers as mitigation options for N2O and NO emissions from agricultural soils: meta-analysis. Glob Chang Biol 16(6):1837–1846

Albanito F, Lebender U, Cornulier T, Sapkota TB, Brentrup F, Stirling C, Hillier J (2017) Direct nitrous oxide emissions from tropical and sub-tropical agricultural systems – a review and modelling of emission factors. Sci Rep 7(1):1–12

Amon B, Amon T, Boxberger J, Alt C (2001) Emissions of NH3, N2O and CH4 from dairy cows housed in a farmyard manure tying stall (housing, manure storage, manure spreading). Nutr Cycl Agroecosyst 60(1):103–113

Amon T, Amon B, Kryvoruchko V, Zollitsch W, Mayer K, Gruber L (2007) Biogas production from maize and dairy cattle manure—influence of biomass composition on the methane yield. Agric Ecosyst Environ 118(1–4):173–182

Amon B, Kryvoruchko V, Amon T, Zechmeister-Boltenstern S (2006) Methane, nitrous oxide and ammonia emissions during storage and after application of dairy cattle slurry and influence of slurry treatment. Agric Ecosyst Environ 112(2-3):153–162

Andraski TW, Bundy LG, Brye KR (2000) Crop management and corn nitrogen rate effects on nitrate leaching. J Environ Qual 29(4):N1095–N1103

Arango MA, Rice CW (2021) Impact of nitrogen management and tillage practices on nitrous oxide emissions from rainfed corn. Soil Sci Soc Am J 85(5):1425–1436

Archimède H, Eugène M, Magdeleine CM, Boval M, Martin C, Morgavi DP, Lecomte P, Doreau M (2011) Comparison of methane production between C3 and C4 grasses and legumes. Anim Feed Sci Technol 166:59–64

Augustine DJ, Milchunas DG, Derner JD (2013) Spatial redistribution of nitrogen by cattle in semiarid rangeland. Rangel Ecol Manag 66(1):56–62

Bastos LM, Rice CW, Tomlinson PJ, Mengel D (2021) Untangling soil-weather drivers of daily N2O emissions and fertilizer management mitigation strategies in no-till corn. Soil Sci Soc Am J 85(5):1437–1447

Bayer C, Mielniczuk J, Amado TJ, Martin-Neto L, Fernandes SV (2000) Organic matter storage in a sandy clay loam Acrisol affected by tillage and cropping systems in southern Brazil. Soil Tillage Res 54(1–2):101–109

Beauchemin KA, Kreuzer M, O'mara F, McAllister TA (2008) Nutritional management for enteric methane abatement: a review. Aust J Exp Agric 48(2):21–27

Beever DE, Dhanoa MS, Losada HR, Evans RT, Cammell SB, France J (1986) The effect of forage species and stage of harvest on the processes of digestion occurring in the rumen of cattle. Br J Nutr 56(2):439–454

Benchaar C, Pomar C, Chiquette J (2001) Evaluation of dietary strategies to reduce methane production in ruminants: a modelling approach. Can J Anim Sci 81(4):563–574

Bennetzen EH, Smith P, Porter JR (2016) Decoupling of greenhouse gas emissions from global agricultural production: 1970–2050. Glob Chang Biol 22(2):763–781

Berg W, Brunsch R, Pazsiczki I (2006) Greenhouse gas emissions from covered slurry compared with uncovered during storage. Agric Ecosyst Environ 112(2-3):129–134

Bezdicek D, Fauci M, Albrecht S, Skirvin K (2002, January 16–18) Soil carbon and C sequestration under different cropping and tillage practices in the Pacific northwest. Proceedings of the Pacific Northwest Direct Seed Cropping Systems Conference, Spokane, WA

Bouwman AF (1990) Soils and the greenhouse effect

Braker G, Conrad R (2011) Diversity, structure, and size of N2O-producing microbial communities in soils – what matters for their functioning? Adv Appl Microbiol 75:33–70

Breitenbeck GA, Bremner JM (1986) Effects of rate and depth of fertilizer application on emission of nitrous oxide from soil fertilized with anhydrous ammonia. Biol Fertil Soils 2(4):201–204

Bronson KF, Mosier AR (1991) Effect of encapsulated calcium carbide on dinitrogen, nitrous oxide, methane, and carbon dioxide emissions from flooded rice. Biol Fertil Soils 11(2): 116–120

Buragohain S, Sarma B, Nath DJ, Gogoi N, Meena RS, Lal R (2017) Effect of 10 years of biofertiliser use on soil quality and rice yield on an Inceptisol in Assam, India. Soil Res 56(1):49–58

Burton DL, Zebarth BJ, Gillam KM, MacLeod JA (2008) Effect of split application of fertilizer nitrogen on N2O emissions from potatoes. Can J Soil Sci 88(2):229–239

Cabaraux JF, Philippe FX, Laitat M, Canart B, Vandenheede M, Nicks B (2009) Gaseous emissions from weaned pigs raised on different floor systems. Agric Ecosyst Environ 130(3–4):86–92

Clemens J, Trimborn M, Weiland P, Amon B (2006) Mitigation of greenhouse gas emissions by anaerobic digestion of cattle slurry. Agric Ecosyst Environ 112(2–3):171–177

Chadwick DR (2005) Emissions of ammonia, nitrous oxide and methane from cattle manure heaps: effect of compaction and covering. Atmos Environ 39(4):787–799

Ciampitti IA, Vyn TJ (2012) Physiological perspectives of changes over time in maize yield dependency on nitrogen uptake and associated nitrogen efficiencies: a review. Field Crop Res 133:48–67

Ciampitti IA, Vyn TJ (2014) Understanding global and historical nutrient use efficiencies for closing maize yield gaps. Agron J 106(6):2107–2117

Cowan NJ, Norman P, Famulari D, Levy PE, Reay DS, Skiba UM (2015) Spatial variability and hotspots of soil N_2O fluxes from intensively grazed grassland. Biogeosciences 12(5):1585–1596

Decock C (2014) Mitigating nitrous oxide emissions from corn cropping systems in the Midwestern US: potential and data gaps. Environ Sci Technol 48(8):4247–4256

Desjardins RL, Smith W, Grant B, Campbell C, Riznek R (2005) Management strategies to sequester carbon in agricultural soils and to mitigate greenhouse gas emissions. In: Increasing climate variability and change. Springer, Dordrecht, pp 283–297

Dick WA, Blevins RL, Frye WW, Peters SE, Christenson DR, Pierce FJ, Vitosh ML (1998) Impacts of agricultural management practices on C sequestration in forest-derived soils of the eastern Corn Belt. Soil Tillage Res 47(3–4):235–244

Dinuccio E, Berg W, Balsari P (2008) Gaseous emissions from the storage of untreated slurries and the fractions obtained after mechanical separation. Atmos Environ 42(10):2448–2459

Dixon RK (1995) Agroforestry systems: sources of sinks of greenhouse gases? Agrofor Syst 31(2): 99–116

Doerge TA, Roth RL, Gardner BR (1991) Nitrogen fertilizer management in Arizona. College of Agriculture, University of Arizona, Tucson

Du Preez CC, Van Huyssteen CW, Mnkeni PN (2011) Land use and soil organic matter in South Africa 2: a review on the influence of arable crop production. S Afr J Sci 107(5):1–8

Dumanski J (2004) Carbon sequestration, soil conservation, and the Kyoto protocol: summary of implications. Clim Chang 65(3):255–261

Dyer JA, Desjardins RL (2003) The impact of farm machinery management on the greenhouse gas emissions from Canadian agriculture. J Sustain Agric 22(3):59–74

Eckard RJ, Grainger C, De Klein CAM (2010) Options for the abatement of methane and nitrous oxide from ruminant production: a review. Livest Sci 130(1-3):47–56

Edouard N, Charpiot A, Hassouna M, Faverdin P, Robin P, Dollé JB (2012, June) Ammonia and greenhouse gases emissions from dairy cattle buildings. In: International symposium on emission of gas and dust from livestock. (p. np)

Fangueiro D, Senbayran M, Trindade H, Chadwick D (2008) Cattle slurry treatment by screw press separation and chemically enhanced settling: effect on greenhouse gas emissions after land spreading and grass yield. Bioresour Technol 99(15):7132–7142

FAO (2010) Food and agriculture organization of the United Nations statistical databases. See http://faostat.fao.org/

Fernández FG, Venterea RT, Fabrizzi KP (2016) Corn nitrogen management influences nitrous oxide emissions in drained and undrained soils. J Environ Qual 45(6):1847–1855

Fisher MJ, Rao IM, Ayarza MA, Lascano CE, Sanz JI, Thomas RJ, Vera RR (1994) Carbon storage by introduced deep-rooted grasses in the South American savannas. Nature 371(6494):236–238

Food and Agriculture Organization of the United Nations (FAO) (2019) Recarbonization of global soils – a dynamic response to offset global emissions. FAO, Rome. http://www.fao.org/3/i723 5en/I7235EN.pdf

Frank S, Havlík P, Stehfest E, van Meijl H, Witzke P, Pérez-Domínguez I, van Dijk M, Doelman JC, Fellmann T, Koopman JF, Tabeau A (2019) Agricultural non-CO_2 emission reduction potential in the context of the 1.5 C target. Nat Clim Chang 9(1):66–72

Franzluebbers AJ (2010) Achieving soil organic carbon sequestration with conservation agricultural systems in the southeastern United States. Soil Sci Soc Am J 74(2):347–357

Gasser T, Crepin L, Quilcaille Y, Houghton RA, Ciais P, Obersteiner M (2020) Historical CO_2 emissions from land use and land cover change and their uncertainty. Biogeosciences 17(15): 4075–4101

Groenestein K, Mosquera J, Van der Sluis S (2012) Emission factors for methane and nitrous oxide from manure management and mitigation options. J Integr Environ Sci 9(Supp 1):139–146

Guarino M, Fabbri C, Brambilla M, Valli L, Navarotto P (2006) Evaluation of simplified covering systems to reduce gaseous emissions from livestock manure storage. Trans ASABE 49(3):737–747

Haeussermann A, Hartung E, Gallmann E, Jungbluth T (2006) Influence of season, ventilation strategy, and slurry removal on methane emissions from pig houses. Agric Ecosyst Environ 112 (2–3):115–121

Halvorson AD, Wienhold BJ, Black AL (2002) Tillage, nitrogen, and cropping system effects on soil carbon sequestration. Soil Sci Soc Am J 66(3):906–912

Hansen J, Sato M, Ruedy R, Lo K, Lea DW, Medina-Elizade M (2006) Global temperature change. Proc Natl Acad Sci 103(39):14288–14293

Hansis E, Davis SJ, Pongratz J (2015) Relevance of methodological choices for accounting of land use change carbon fluxes. Glob Biogeochem Cycles 29(8):1230–1246

Hao X, Chang C, Larney FJ, Travis GR (2001) Greenhouse gas emissions during cattle feedlot manure composting. J Environ Qual 30(2):376–386

Hati KM, Biswas AK, Somasundaram J, Mohanty M, Singh RK, Sinha NK, Chaudhary RS (2020) Soil organic carbon dynamics and carbon sequestration under conservation tillage in tropical vertisols. In: Ghosh P, Mahanta S, Mandal D, Mandal B, Ramakrishnan S (eds) Carbon management in tropical and sub-tropical terrestrial systems. Springer, Singapore. https://doi.org/10.1007/978-981-13-9628-1_12

Havlin JL, Kissel DE, Maddux LD, Claassen MM, Long JH (1990) Crop rotation and tillage effects on soil organic carbon and nitrogen. Soil Sci Soc Am J 54(2):448–452

Hindrichsen IK, Wettstein HR, Machmüller A, Jörg B, Kreuzer M (2005) Effect of the carbohydrate composition of feed concentrates on methane emission from dairy cows and their slurry. Environ Monit Assess 107(1):329–350

Hoben JP, Gehl RJ, Millar N, Grace PR, Robertson GP (2011) Nonlinear nitrous oxide (N_2O) response to nitrogen fertilizer in on-farm corn crops of the US Midwest. Glob Chang Biol 17(2): 1140–1152

Hockstad L, Hanel L (2018) Inventory of US greenhouse gas emissions and sinks, No. cdiac: EPA-EMISSIONS. Environmental System Science Data Infrastructure for a Virtual Ecosystem

Houghton RA, Nassikas AA (2017) Global and regional fluxes of carbon from land use and land cover change 1850–2015. Glob Biogeochem Cycles 31(3):456–472

Huppmann D, Rogelj J, Kriegler E, Krey V, Riahi K (2018) A new scenario resource for integrated 1.5 C research. Nat Clim Chang 8(12):1027–1030

Hutchinson JJ, Campbell CA, Desjardins RL (2007) Some perspectives on carbon sequestration in agriculture. Agric For Meteorol 142(2-4):288–302

IPCC (1997) In: Watson RT, Zinyowera MC, Moss RH (eds) The regional impacts of climate change: an assessment of vulnerability

IPCC (2013) In: Stocker TF, Qin D, Plattner G-K, Tignor M, Allen SK, Boschung J, Nauels A, Xia Y, Bex V, Midgley PM (eds) Climate change 2013: the physical science basis. Contribution of working group I to the fifth assessment report of the intergovernmental panel on climate change, Cambridge, United Kingdom and New York

IPCC (2014) Contribution of Working Group I to the fifth assessment report of the Intergovern-mental Panel on Climate Change. Cambridge University Press

IPCC (2018) Global warming of 1.5 C. In: Masson-Delmotte V, Zhai P, Pörtner HO, Roberts D, Skea J, Shukla PR, Pirani A, Moufouma-Okia W, Péan C, Pidcock R, Connors S (eds) An IPCC special report on the impacts of global warming, vol 1. Intergovernmental Panel on Climate Change, Cambridge University Press, pp 1–9

IPCC Climate Change (2007) Synthesis Report. In: Pachauri RK, Reisinger A (eds) Contribution of Working Groups I, II and III to the fourth assessment report of the Intergovernmental Panel on Climate Change Core Writing Team. Intergovernmental Panel on Climate Change, Geneva

Janzen HH, Desjardins RL, Asselin JMR, Grace B (1998) The health of our air: toward sustainable agriculture in Canada. Ministry of Public Works and Government Services

Ju X, Lu X, Gao Z, Chen X, Su F, Kogge M, Römheld V, Christie P, Zhang F (2011) Processes and factors controlling N_2O production in an intensively managed low carbon calcareous soil under sub-humid monsoon conditions. Environ Pollut 159(4):1007–1016

Kaiser, S., 1999. Analyse und Bewertung eines Zweiraumkompoststalls für Mastschweine unter besonderer Berücksichtigung der gasförmigen Stoffströme. Arbeitskreis Forschung und Lehre der Max-Eyth-Gesellschaft Agrartechnik im VDI

Karakurt I, Aydin G, Aydiner K (2012) Sources and mitigation of methane emissions by sectors: a critical review. Renew Energy 39(1):40–48

Laborde D, Mamun A, Martin W, Piñeiro V, Vos R (2021) Agricultural subsidies and global greenhouse gas emissions. Nat Commun 12(1):1–9

Lal R (1978) Influence of within-and between-row mulching on soil temperature, soil moisture, root development and yield of maize (*Zea mays* L.) in a tropical soil. Field Crop Res 1:127–139

Lal R (1979) Influence of Six Years of no-tillage and conventional plowing on fertilizer response of maize (*Zea mays* L.) on an Alfisol in the Tropics. Soil Sci Soc Am J 43(2):399–403

Lal R (1997) Residue management, conservation tillage and soil restoration for mitigating greenhouse effect by CO_2-enrichment. Soil Tillage Res 43(1–2):81–107

Lal R (2004) Soil carbon sequestration impacts on global climate change and food security. Science 304(5677):1623–1627

Lal R (2008) Carbon sequestration. Philos Trans R Soc B 363:815–830

Lal R (2010) Managing soils and ecosystems for mitigating anthropogenic carbon emissions and advancing global food security. Bioscience 60(9):708–721

Lal R (2013) Food security in a changing climate. Ecohydrol Hydrobiol 13(1):8–21

Lal R, Kimble JM (1997) Conservation tillage for carbon sequestration. Nutr Cycl Agroecosyst 49(1):243–253

Leahy S, Clark H, Reisinger A (2020) Challenges and prospects for agricultural greenhouse gas mitigation pathways consistent with the Paris agreement. Front Sustain Food Syst 4:69

López-Fando C, Pardo MT (2001) The impact of tillage systems and crop rotations on carbon sequestration in a calcic Luvisol of Central Spain. In: Conservation agriculture, a worldwide challenge. First World Congress on conservation agriculture, Madrid, Spain, 1-5 October, 2001. Volume 2: offered contributions. XUL, pp 135–139

López-Mosquera ME, Fernández-Lema E, Villares R, Corral R, Alonso B, Blanco C (2011) Composting fish waste and seaweed to produce a fertilizer for use in organic agriculture. Procedia Environ Sci 9:113–117

Lorenz K, Lal R (2014) Soil organic carbon sequestration in agroforestry systems. A review. Agron Sustain Dev 34(2):443–454

Ma BL, Wu TY, Tremblay N, Deen W, Morrison MJ, McLaughlin NB, Gregorich EG, Stewart G (2010) Nitrous oxide fluxes from corn fields: on-farm assessment of the amount and timing of nitrogen fertilizer. Glob Chang Biol 16(1):156–170

Mandal B, Majumder B, Bandyopadhyay PK, Hazra GC, Gangopadhyay A, Samantaray RN, Mishra AK, Chaudhury J, Saha MN, Kundu S (2007) The potential of cropping systems and soil amendments for carbon sequestration in soils under long-term experiments in subtropical India. Glob Chang Biol 13(2):357–369

Martinez J, Guiziou F, Peu P, Gueutier V (2003) Influence of treatment techniques for pig slurry on methane emissions during subsequent storage. Biosyst Eng 85(3):347–354

McSwiney CP, Robertson GP (2005) Nonlinear response of N_2O flux to incremental fertilizer addition in a continuous maize (*Zea mays* L.) cropping system. Glob Chang Biol 11(10): 1712–1719

Meena RS, Kumar S, Yadav GS (2020) Soil carbon sequestration in crop production. In: Meena R (ed) Nutrient dynamics for sustainable crop production. Springer, Singapore. https://doi.org/10. 1007/978-981-13-8660-2_1

Mennicken L (1998) Biobett für Legehennen – ein Beitrag zum Umweltschutz? [biobeds for laying hens – a contribution to environmental protection?]. DGS 13:12–20

Millar N, Urrea A, Kahmark K, Shcherbak I, Robertson GP, Ortiz-Monasterio I (2018) Nitrous oxide (N_2O) flux responds exponentially to nitrogen fertilizer in irrigated wheat in the Yaqui Valley, Mexico. Agric Ecosyst Environ 261:125–132

Montes F, Meinen R, Dell C, Rotz A, Hristov AN, Oh J, Waghorn G, Gerber PJ, Henderson B, Makkar HPS, Dijkstra J (2013) SPECIAL TOPICS – mitigation of methane and nitrous oxide emissions from animal operations: II. A review of manure management mitigation options. J Anim Sci 91(11):5070–5094

Mosier AR, Duxbury JM, Freney JR, Heinemeyer O, Minami K (1996) Nitrous oxide emissions from agricultural fields: Assessment, measurement and mitigation. In: Progress in nitrogen cycling studies. Springer, Dordrecht, pp 589–602

Nair PR, Nair VD, Kumar BM, Showalter JM (2010) Carbon sequestration in agroforestry systems. Adv Agron 108:237–307

Neue HU (1993) Methane emission from rice fields. Bioscience 43(7):466–474

Nicks B, Laitat M, Vandenheede M, Désiron A, Verhaeghe C, Canart B (2003) Emissions of ammonia, nitrous oxide, methane, carbon dioxide and water vapor in the raising of weaned pigs on straw-based and sawdustbased deep litters. Anim Res 52(3):299–308

Nicks B, Laitat M, Farnir F, Vandenheede M, Desiron A, Verhaeghe C, Canart B (2004) Gaseous emissions from deep-litter pens with straw or sawdust for fattening pigs. Anim Sci 78(1):99–107

Nicoloso RS, Rice CW (2021) Intensification of no-till agricultural systems: An opportunity for carbon sequestration. Soil Sci Soc Am J 85(5):1395–1409

Oenema O, Ju X, de Klein C, Alfaro M, del Prado A, Lesschen JP, Zheng X, Velthof G, Ma L, Gao B, Kroeze C (2014) Reducing nitrous oxide emissions from the global food system. Curr Opin Environ Sustain 9:55–64

Ogle SM, Jay Breidt F, Eve MD, Paustian K (2003) Uncertainty in estimating land use and management impacts on soil organic carbon storage for US agricultural lands between 1982 and 1997. Glob Chang Biol 9(11):1521–1542

Ohiri AC, Ezumah HC (1990) Tillage effects on cassava (*Manihot esculenta*) production and some soil properties. Soil Tillage Res 17(3-4):221–229

Olivier JG, Peters JA (2020) Trends in global CO_2 and total greenhouse gas emissions: 2020 report. PBL Netherlands Environmental Assessment Agency, The Hague

Omara P, Aula L, Oyebiyi F, Raun WR (2019) World cereal nitrogen use efficiency trends: review and current knowledge. Agrosyst Geosci Environ 2(1):1–8

Parkin TB, Hatfield JL (2013) Enhanced efficiency fertilizers: effect on nitrous oxide emissions in Iowa. United States Department of Agriculture – Agricultural Research Service and University of Nebraska, Lincoln

Pattey E, Trzcinski MK, Desjardins RL (2005) Quantifying the reduction of greenhouse gas emissions as a resultof composting dairy and beef cattle manure. Nutr Cycl Agroecosyst 72(2):173–187

Paustian KAOJH, Andren O, Janzen HH, Lal R, Smith P, Tian G, Tiessen H, Van Noordwijk M, Woomer PL (1997) Agricultural soils as a sink to mitigate CO_2 emissions. Soil Use Manag 13:230–244

Petersen SO, Hoffmann CC, Schäfer CM, Blicher-Mathiesen G, Elsgaard L, Kristensen K, Larsen SE, Torp SB, Greve MH (2012) Annual emissions of CH_4 and N_2O, and ecosystem respiration, from eight organic soils in Western Denmark managed by agriculture. Biogeosciences 9(1):403–422

Petersen SO (2018) Greenhouse gas emissions from liquid dairy manure: prediction and mitigation. J Dairy Sci 101(7):6642–6654

Petersen SO, Dorno N, Lindholst S, Feilberg A, Eriksen J (2013) Emissions of CH_4, N_2O, NH_3 and odorants from pig slurry during winter and summer storage. Nutr Cycl Agroecosyst 95(1):103–113

Philippe FX, Laitat M, Canart B, Vandenheede M, Nicks B (2007) Comparison of ammonia and greenhouse gas emissions during the fattening of pigs, kept either on fully slatted floor or on deep litter. Livest Sci 111(1–2):144–152

Phillips RL, Tanaka DL, Archer DW, Hanson JD (2009) Fertilizer application timing influences greenhouse gas fluxes over a growing season. J Environ Qual 38(4):1569–1579

Popp A, Lotze-Campen H, Bodirsky B (2010) Food consumption, diet shifts and associated non-CO_2 greenhouse gases from agricultural production. Glob Environ Chang 20(3):451–462

Qiao C, Liu L, Hu S, Compton JE, Greaver TL, Li Q (2015) How inhibiting nitrification affects nitrogen cycle and reduces environmental impacts of anthropogenic nitrogen input. Glob Chang Biol 21(3):1249–1257

Rasmussen PE, Rohde CR (1988) Long-term tillage and nitrogen fertilization effects on organic nitrogen and carbon in a semiarid soil. Soil Sci Soc Am J 52(4):1114–1117

Raun WR, Johnson GV (1999) Improving nitrogen use efficiency for cereal production. Agron J 91(3):357–363

Reay DS, Davidson EA, Smith KA, Smith P, Melillo JM, Dentener F, Crutzen PJ (2012) Global agriculture and nitrous oxide emissions. Nat Clim Chang 2(6):410–416

Reicosky DC, Dugas WA, Torbert HA (1997) Tillage-induced soil carbon dioxide loss from different cropping systems. Soil Tillage Res 41(1–2):105–118

Ro S, Seanjan P, Tulaphitak T, Inubushi K (2011) Sulfate content influencing methane production and emission from incubated soil and rice-planted soil in Northeast Thailand. Soil Sci Plant Nutr 57(6):833–842

Salinas-Garcia JR, Hons FM, Matocha JE, Zuberer DA (1997) Soil carbon and nitrogen dynamics as affected by long-term tillage and nitrogen fertilization. Biol Fertil Soils 25(2):182–188

Sanderman J, Hengl T, Fiske GJ (2017) Soil carbon debt of 12,000 years of human land use. Proc Natl Acad Sci 114(36):9575–9580

Sarto MV, Borges WL, Sarto JR, Rice CW, Rosolem CA (2020) Deep soil carbon stock, origin, and root interaction in a tropical integrated crop–livestock system. Agrofor Syst 94:1865–1877

Searchinger T, Waite R, Hanson C, Ranganathan J, Dumas P, Matthews E (2018) World resources report: creating a sustainable food future. World Resources Institute, p 96

Sehy U, Ruser R, Munch JC (2003) Nitrous oxide fluxes from maize fields: relationship to yield, site-specific fertilization, and soil conditions. Agric Ecosyst Environ 99(1-3):97–111

Shcherbak I, Millar N, Robertson GP (2014) Global meta-analysis of the nonlinear response of soil nitrous oxide (N_2O) emissions to fertilizer nitrogen. Proc Natl Acad Sci 111(25):9199–9204

Singh H, Northup BK, Baath GS, Gowda PH, Kakani VG (2019) Greenhouse mitigation strategies for agronomic and grazing lands of the US Southern Great Plains. Mitig Adapt Strateg Glob Chang:1–35

Sirohi S, Michaelowa A, Sirohi SK (2007) Mitigation options for enteric methane emissions from dairy animals: an evaluation for potential CDM projects in India. Mitig Adapt Strateg Glob Chang 12(2):259–274

Sistani KR, Jn-Baptiste M, Lovanh N, Cook KL (2011) Atmospheric emissions of nitrous oxide, methane, and carbon dioxide from different nitrogen fertilizers. J Environ Qual 40(6): 1795–1805

Smith P (2004) Carbon sequestration in croplands: the potential in Europe and the global context. Eur J Agron 20(3):229–236

Smith KA (ed) (2010) Nitrous oxide and climate change. Earthscan

Smith P, Milne R, Powlson DS, Smith JU, Falloon P, Coleman K (2000) Revised estimates of the carbon mitigation potential of UK agricultural land. Soil Use Manag 16(4):293–295

Smith P, Martino D, Cai Z, Gwary D, Janzen H, Kumar P, McCarl B, Ogle S, O'Mara F, Rice C, Scholes B (2008) Greenhouse gas mitigation in agriculture. Philos Trans R Soc B Biol Sci 363(1492):789–813

Smith P, Clark H, Dong H, Elsiddig EA, Haberl H, Harper R, House J, Jafari M, Masera O, Mbow C, Ravindranath NH (2014) Agriculture, forestry and other land use (AFOLU). In: IPCC Working Group III Contribution to AR5 (ed) Climate change 2014: mitigation of climate change. Intergovernmental Panel on Climate Change, Cambridge University Press

Snyder CS (2017) Enhanced nitrogen fertiliser technologies support the '4R'concept to optimise crop production and minimise environmental losses. Soil Res 55(6):463–472

Snyder CS, Fixen PE (2012) Plant nutrient management and risks of nitrous oxide emission. J Soil Water Conserv 67(5):137A–144A

Sommer SG, Petersen SO, Møller HB (2004) Algorithms for calculating methane and nitrous oxide emissions from manure management. Nutr Cycl Agroecosyst 69(2):143–154

Souza R, Yin J, Calabrese S (2021) Optimal drainage timing for mitigating methane emissions from rice paddy fields. Geoderma 394:114986

Spargo JT, Alley MM, Follett RF, Wallace JV (2008) Soil carbon sequestration with continuous no-till management of grain cropping systems in the Virginia coastal plain. Soil Tillage Res 100(1–2):133–140

Steed J Jr, Hashimoto AG (1994) Methane emissions from typical manure management systems. Bioresour Technol 50(2):123–130

Stehfest E, Bouwman L (2006) N_2O and NO emission from agricultural fields and soils under natural vegetation: summarizing available measurement data and modeling of global annual emissions. Nutr Cycl Agroecosyst 74(3):207–228

Thorman RE, Chadwick DR, Boyles LO, Matthews R, Sagoo E, Harrison R (2006, July) Nitrous oxide emissions during storage of broiler litter and following application to arable land. In: International congress series, vol 1293. Elsevier, pp 355–358

US-EPA (2006) Global anthropogenic non-CO_2 greenhouse gas emissions: 1990–2020. United States Environmental Protection Agency, Washington, DC. Online Available at: http://www. epa.gov/nonco2/econ-inv/downloads/GlobalAnthroEmissionsReport.pdf (EPA 430-R-06-003, June 2006)

VanderZaag AC, Gordon RJ, Jamieson RC, Burton DL, Stratton GW (2009) Gas emissions from straw covered liquid dairy manure during summer storage and autumn agitation. Trans ASABE 52(2):599–608

Van Groenigen JW, Velthof GL, Oenema O, Van Groenigen KJ, Van Kessel C (2010) Towards an agronomic assessment of N_2O emissions: a case study for arable crops. Eur J Soil Sci 61(6): 903–913

Verge XPC, De Kimpe C, Desjardins RL (2007) Agricultural production, greenhouse gas emissions and mitigation potential. Agric For Meteorol 142(2–4):255–269

Wang T, Teague WR, Park SC, Bevers S (2015) GHG mitigation potential of different grazing strategies in the United States Southern Great Plains. Sustainability 7(10):13500–13521

Wang C, Amon B, Schulz K, Mehdi B (2021) Factors that influence nitrous oxide emissions from agricultural soils as well as their representation in simulation models: a review. Agronomy 11(4):770

Wassmann R, Hosen Y, Sumfleth K (2009) Reducing methane emissions from irrigated rice (no. 16 (3)). International Food Policy Research Institute (IFPRI), Washington, DC

Watson RT, Zinyowera MC, Moss RH (1996) Climate change 1995. Impacts, adaptations and mitigation of climate change: scientific-technical analyses. IPCC Cambridge University Press

Wollenberg E, Richards M, Smith P, Havlík P, Obersteiner M, Tubiello FN, Herold M, Gerber P, Carter S, Reisinger A, Van Vuuren DP (2016) Reducing emissions from agriculture to meet the 2 C target. Glob Chang Biol 22(12):3859–3864

West TO, Post WM (2002) Soil organic carbon sequestration rates by tillage and crop rotation: a global data analysis. Soil Sci Soc Am J 66:1930–1946

World Bank (2015) Agricultural land (% of land area). Available at: http://data.worldbank.org/ indicator/AG.LND.AGRI.ZS/countries?display=graph. Verified 16 Sept 2015

Yamulki S (2006) Effect of straw addition on nitrous oxide and methane emissions from stored farmyard manures. Agric Ecosyst Environ 112(2–3):140–145

Zaman M, Nguyen ML (2012) How application timings of urease and nitrification inhibitors affect N losses from urine patches in pastoral system. Agric Ecosyst Environ 156:37–48

Zebarth BJ, Snowdon E, Burton DL, Goyer C, Dowbenko R (2012) Controlled release fertilizer product effects on potato crop response and nitrous oxide emissions under rain-fed production on a medium-textured soil. Can J Soil Sci 92(5):759–769

Zhang X, Davidson EA, Mauzerall DL, Searchinger TD, Dumas P, Shen Y (2015) Managing nitrogen for sustainable development. Nature 528(7580):51–59

Chapter 17
Environmental and Economic Benefits of Sustainable Sugarcane Initiative and Production Constraints in Pakistan: A Review

Hafiz Ali Raza, Muhammad Usman Hameed, Mohammad Sohidul Islam, Naveed Ahmad Lone, Muhammad Ammar Raza, and Ayman E. L. Sabagh

Abstract Sugarcane crop has a vital role to play in the economy of developing countries. The crop requires a high amount of water during its development. Therefore, it becomes necessary to adopt innovative, ecofriendly, and water-efficient methods for its cultivation. In this chapter, sugarcane production constraints have been discussed to promote sustainable sugarcane production with special reference to Sustainable Sugarcane Initiative (SSI) techniques. The constraints include high input costs, poor production practices, water scarcity, lack of implementation of modern technologies, less incentives, climate change, and delay in payment to the farmers. Sugarcane production can significantly be increased by using SSI with less input costs, efficient water utilization, reduction of weed losses, and controlling the infestation of pests and diseases. There is a need to take proper steps for increasing the production and profitability of sugarcane by timely irrigation, cost-effective inputs, better-quality seeds, and preventive measures against post-harvest losses. The capacity building of sugarcane farmers is also recommended.

Keywords Sugarcane production · Traditional methods · Input cost · Sustainable Sugarcane Initiative · Economic stability

---

H. A. Raza · M. U. Hameed
Institute of Agricultural Extension, Education and Rural Development, University of Agriculture, Faisalabad, Pakistan

M. S. Islam
Department of Agronomy, Hajee Mohammad Danesh Science and Technology University, Dinajpur, Bangladesh

N. A. Lone · M. A. Raza · A. E. L. Sabagh (✉)
Department of Field Crops, Faculty of Agriculture, Kezer Campus, SIIRT University, Siirt, Turkey

© The Author(s), under exclusive license to Springer Nature Switzerland AG 2022
M. Ahmed (ed.), *Global Agricultural Production: Resilience to Climate Change*,
https://doi.org/10.1007/978-3-031-14973-3_17

17.1 Introduction

Sugarcane is an important economic and commercial crop in the world (Grivet and Arruda 2002). It has a significant role in socioeconomic developments as it improves the income of the growers and creates employment opportunities for masses; It create employment opportunities to more than half a million people globally (Raza et al. 2019a, b). Due to its economic and medicinal value, it is cultivated worldwide and gives high-yielding products. Sugarcane belongs to the family Poaceae; the crop has fibrous, stout, and jointed stalks; it is about 3 m height and rich in sugar (Maloa 2001). The decreasing trend of sugarcane production has been observed from the last couple of years globally. Unfavorable climatic conditions, agricultural transformation, and low returns from the market, as well as decline in planting area, have been expected to lead to the lower production of sugarcane in the upcoming years. The most noticeable decline in production has been recorded in Brazil the leading country in sugarcane production and contributing more than one third of the overall sugarcane production in the world (James 2008). Sugarcane is considered one of the important cash crops, grown all over the world. Among the sugarcane producers, Brazil is the leading sugarcane-producing country with an annual production of 739,300 thousand metric tons (TMTs) and contributes about 39% of the world's total sugarcane production (Walton 2020). India ranks the second-largest producer and contributes almost 19% of the overall sugarcane production in the world with an annual production of 341,200 TMTs (Masuku 2011). China is the third- and Thailand is the fourth-largest sugarcane producers in the world with an annual production of 125,500 and 100,100 TMTs, respectively. Pakistan stands at the fifth position among other sugarcane-producing countries with an annual production of 63,800 TMTs (Aman and Khan 2021). Sugarcane is considered an essential raw material for sugar production in Pakistan, and it is expected to produce 5.9 million metric tons in 2021–2022. Non-availability of minimum support prices, delays in payment dues and water scarcity are prompting some farmers to switch to other crops such as cotton and corn instead of sugarcane.

Sugarcane contributes approximately 60% of foreign exchange earnings and almost 18.9% of the national gross domestic product (GDP) in Pakistan (Chandio et al. 2016). Agriculture provides the basic necessities of life to almost 68% of the total population living in rural areas, and unfortunately, 62% of which is living below the poverty line (Aslam 2016). The total area cultivated in Pakistan is approximately 22 million hectares (Mha) and includes rice 13.14% (2.89 Mha), wheat 41.73% (9.18 Mha), maize 5.14% (1.13 Mha), sugarcane 5.18% (1.14 Mha), and cotton 13.45% (2.96 Mha). These major five crop covers almost 78.64% (17.30 Mha) of the overall cropped area and reflect that these five crops represent a large area of cultivated land (Mari et al. 2011). In Pakistan, among the five major crops, sugarcane occupies the second-largest among the cash crops. It has industrial importance in the sugar industry and other byproducts that are produced from sugarcane.

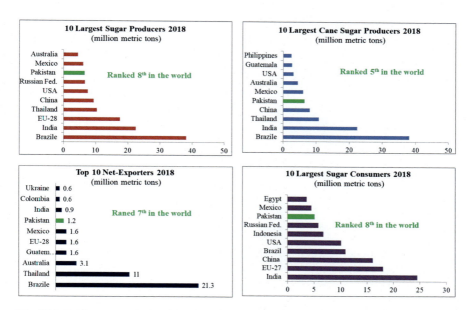

Fig. 17.1 Pakistan sugar in the global perspective. (Adapted from PSMA annual report, 2018)

The total cultivated land area of sugarcane around the world is 27 Mha with a total production of 1333 million tons (Natrajin 2005). In the world ranking, Pakistan is the eighth-largest consumer of white sugar, seventh-largest net sugar exporter, seventh-largest cane sugar producer, and fifth in sugarcane production with an annual production of 83.3 million tons. Figure 17.1 shows the status of the Pakistan sugar industry with reference to the global sugar industry. The total area, production, and yield for sugarcane crops in Pakistan have been shown in Figs. 17.2, 17.3 and 17.4. During 2016–2017, its total cultivated area was 1.217 million hectares with a production of about 73.6 million tons, and its role in GDP and the value addition of agriculture are 0.7% and 3.6%, respectively (Azam and Shafique 2017). In Pakistan, sugarcane is grown in three climatic zones, tropical Sindh, subtropical Punjab, and temperate Peshawar valley. Punjab is the major contributor with almost 62% share in sugarcane production, while Sindh and the North-West Frontier Province (NWFP) also contribute about 26% and 16%, respectively. Sugarcane is the second major provider of sweetness after honey in Pakistan (Qureshi and Afghan 2005), and it provides the raw material for the second agro-based industry after textiles. However, in recent times, sugarcane is recognized for its role in sustainable energy production (Gheewala et al. 2011). Moreover, unprocessed sugarcane is consumed as food and feed for animals in leading producing countries such as Brazil, India, and Cuba (Girei and Giroh 2012). Furthermore, sugarcane juice is used as a raw material and also used for wax (Lamberton and Redcliffe 1960). Wax is a vital part of the cosmetic and pharmaceutical industries, and it is considered as a better substitute for expensive carnauba wax (Singh et al. 2015). However, some

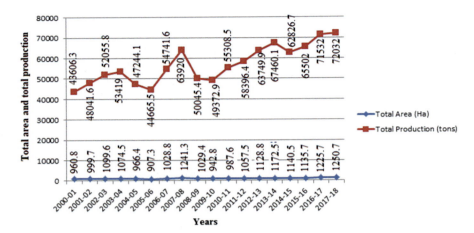

Fig. 17.2 Total area (Ha) and total production (tons) of sugarcane crop in Pakistan

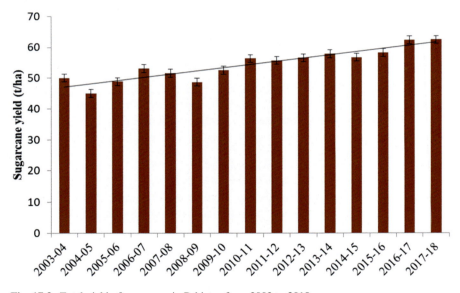

Fig. 17.3 Total yield of sugarcane in Pakistan from 2003 to 2018

important byproducts of sugarcane are refined sugar, molasses, brown sugar, jaggery, biogas production, pulp, biofertilizer, ethanol (Xu et al. 2005), and paper making (Prasara-A and Gheewala 2016). In India, sugarcane is commonly used in the treatment of anuria, hemorrhage, jaundice, dysuria, and other urinary diseases, respectively.

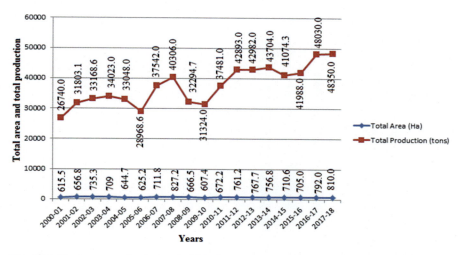

Fig. 17.4 Total area, production, and yield of sugarcane crop in the Punjab province of Pakistan

17.2 Sugarcane as an Energy Source

Pakistan is facing a challenge to energy crises in recent times (Knox et al. 2010). Sugarcane can be used as a reasonable source to overcome the energy crisis in Pakistan (Solangi et al. 2019). Bioenergy has gained better attention as a substitute for fossil fuels. Bioethanol obtained from sugarcane can offer advantages to the environment, human health, and economy of Pakistan (Pereira and Ortega 2010). In the residential region of São Paulo, ethanol replaced gasoline in Brazil resulting in major improvements in air quality. On the basis of lifecycle, it decreases the emissions of greenhouse gases if proper agricultural practices and suitable feedstock are used (Macedo et al. 2008). Ethanol is produced mostly in Brazil from sugarcane and in the USA from corn. In 2008, Brazil produced 22.5 billion liters of ethanol, the European Union 2.7 billion liters, and the USA 34 billion liters mainly from sugar 106 beet (Low and Isserman 2009). For the production of ethanol in 2008, Brazil used 3.4 million hectares of land, while the USA used 8.13 million hectares (Goldemberg and Guardabassi 2010).

17.3 Overview of Sugarcane Production in Pakistan

In Pakistan, ethanol is produced at a very small scale in sugar industries, and it is being used for its own sustainability. Figures 17.5 and 17.6 show the total yield and average recovery of sugarcane in the Punjab province of Pakistan. The average per hectare production of sugarcane is ranging from 620 to 700 maund per acre which is very low in Pakistan as compared to other sugarcane-producing countries (Rai and

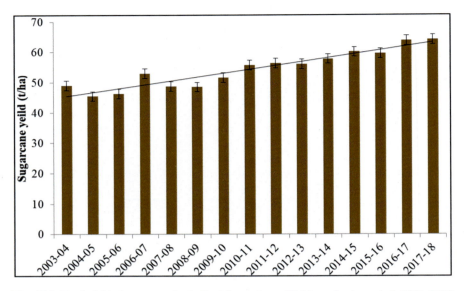

Fig. 17.5 Total yield of sugarcane in the Punjab province of Pakistan for the periods 2003–2018

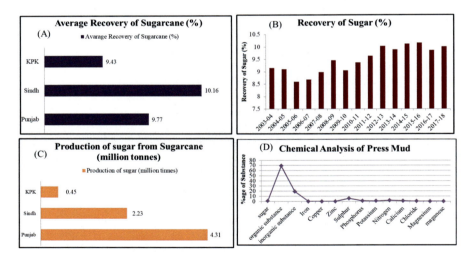

Fig. 17.6 (**a**) Average recovery of sugarcane, (**b**) recovery of sugar, (**c**) production of sugar from sugarcane, and (**d**) chemical analysis of press mud in Pakistan. (Adapted from PSMA annual report, 2018)

Shekhawat 2014). Similarly, its per acre yield is very low in Punjab as compared to other country provinces due to various factors. Among these factors, soil type, soil erosion (Iqbal and Ahmad 2005), cultural practices, plant material, climatic conditions, fertilizer, labor component, pest and disease management, lack of technology, and irrigation water have a considerable impact on sugarcane production (Lahoti

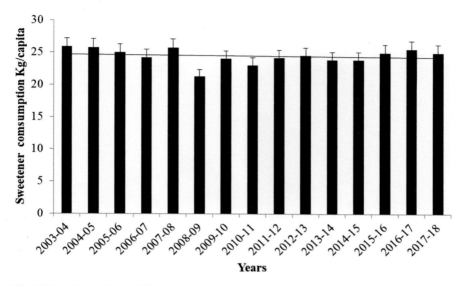

Fig. 17.7 Pakistan Sugar Mills Association (PSMA) sweetener consumption kg/capita. (Adapted from PSMA annual report, 2018)

et al. 2010). Similarly, high input costs like urea, DAP, FYM, irrigation, seed, pesticides, water shortage, and weedicides were also considered important factors in this regard (Sawaengsak and Gheewala 2017). Therefore, high input price directly affects the production of sugarcane. Similarly, distance to sugar mills, the operation of poor management, and post-harvest losses are the gap between potential and actual yield ultimately hampering sugarcane production (Fischer 2015). Sugarcane varieties are also the major factor of low production because these varieties perform effectively in the first year but not performing subsequently ultimately records low yield (Perera et al. 2003). Weeds compete with the crop for the available nutrients, sunlight, and water, which reduces the yield drastically and results in low-quality sugarcane (Girei and Giroh 2012). Hence, farmers are unable to get high sugarcane production due to many causes such as late planting, lack of financial resources, primitive or post-harvest measures, and environmental resistance (Rabelo et al. 2011). Pakistan Sugar Mills Association (PSMA) mentioned that the sweet consumption kg/capita, provincial shares in Pakistan, and area under cultivation are shown in Figs. 17.7, 17.8 and 17.9.

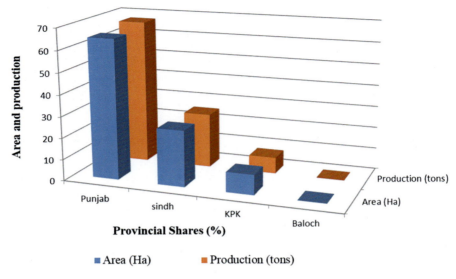

Fig. 17.8 Provincial shares for sugarcane crops in Pakistan

Fig. 17.9 Total area under cultivation for sugarcane in different provinces of Pakistan. (Adapted from Pakistan Sugar Mills Association (PSMA) annual report, 2018)

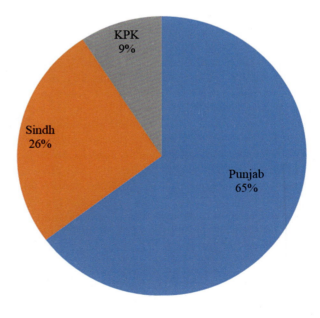

17.4 The Current System of Sugarcane Production in Pakistan

17.4.1 Climate

Sugarcane is grown in tropical or subtropical climates with a minimum of 600 mm rainfall annually. Sugarcane in Pakistan is harvested in the southern, central, and northwestern zones. The range of minimum temperature during December to January is about 4 °C, and the maximum temperature is 38 °C from June to July. During the winter seasons, the minimum temperature hinders or stops the growth of sugarcane. The climate throughout the year normally favors crop productivity. But extreme conditions of weather especially a limited amount of rainfall are a serious concern to produce sugarcane crop interference in Pakistan.

17.4.2 Climate Change and Sugarcane Response

Among many other factors, climate change is one of the emerging issues in the world. It is anticipated that it has a negative impact on sugarcane production, particularly in developing countries due to lack of awareness, ineffectual forecasting, unsuitable vindication strategies on the effects of climate change, and more exposure to natural hazards. It poses a significant threat to farmers due to the lack of proper infrastructure, inappropriate strategies, and the adoption of traditional agronomic practices (Käyhkö 2019). In Pakistan, farmers' livelihoods and agricultural productivity are affected due to the climate change. Therefore, a precise understanding of climate change and adoption of appropriate mitigation strategies can reduce the economic losses of sugarcane. Thus, environmental awareness is an important step as it is responsible for the reduction in cane yield (Abid et al. 2019).

Cane production may have been negatively affected and will continue to be significantly affected by the increased frequency and intensity of extreme environmental conditions due to climate change. Similarly, changes in the environment lead to global warming having increased greenhouse gas emissions. Global warming is believed to be caused by increasing concentrations of CO_2 and other greenhouse gases (GHGs) in the atmosphere (Zhao and Li 2015). Cane is sensitive to rainfall, temperature, sunlight, and soil (Trenberth 2012). Global temperatures are thought to increase by 3–5 °C by the end of the twenty-first century (Chohan 2019). Different climatic conditions can lead to changes in the sea level, precipitation, floods, droughts, abiotic pressures, and above all a rise in temperature. Rising temperatures could be favorable for some crops such as C_3 plants and sugarcane in some parts of the present world.

Cane production in Pakistan is negatively affected by abiotic and biotic factors diseases and pests are important biotic factors. There are many reasons for rising temperatures in the ecosystem, and change in human activities and deforestation, burning of fossil fuels, and industrialization of the ecosystem are the main causes (Chohan 2019). These are the reasons for low or high rainfall, high temperatures, high pest pressure, more favorable environment for pest growth, disease infestation, higher water requirements, reduced soil fertility, and pollination services. According to the previous studies (Nazir et al. 2013; Hussain et al. 2018; Raza et al. 2019a, b; Moitinho et al. 2021; Triques et al. 2021; Singh et al. 2018; Marin et al. 2019; Farooq and Gheewala 2020), several factors are responsible for the lower production of cane, viz., harvesting cost, transportation, high prices of inputs, a number of harvests, burring of the sugarcane residues, increased greenhouse gases, carbon monoxide, global, abnormal rainfall, and drought stresses, and excess use of pesticides and fertilizers which affects the soil organisms, environment, and soil fertility. However, lack of awareness and adoption rate of the latest technologies were identified as the major reasons of these constraints during farm surveys.

Extreme weather conditions, floods, salinity, drought, and frost have been shown to be the major causes for the deterioration of cane production in Pakistan (Chohan 2019). Punjab, especially in southern Punjab has the highest sugarcane production mainly due to suitable ecology in the area for its production. Rahim Yar Khan is the largest sugarcane-growing area in South Punjab. Over the past decade, due to the failure of other crops such as cotton, farmers have been growing sugarcane as they have more availability in sugar mills, sugarcane logistic support, and more profitable products. But in recent years, the trend of growing the cane community has changed due to the effect of climate change, and they have switched to other crops. However, this situation is very worrying and alarming, and Pakistan has no other alternative for sugar production other than the cultivation of cane.

It is, therefore, very important to inform farmers about the negative effects of climate change and the necessity to adopt appropriate mitigation strategies against it. Hence, the level of awareness and adoption of agronomic measures, including resistant varieties; sowing time and planting methods; soil and land preparation; weed, pest, and disease management; water; and nutrient management, appear to be promising measures to increase sugarcane production and boost farmers' income levels and living standards. It has been hypothesized that climate change is causing a decline in the production of sugarcane.

17.4.3 *Preparation of Land*

Sugarcane rigger, cultivator, chisel, and subsoiler are used to get proper germination and better crop growth. The simple plow is significant for the good preparation of seedbed in the sugarcane field. For achieving optimal crop growth, the land is prepared in such a way because the crop of sugarcane is deep-rooted, and proper land preparation plays a vital role in the growth of the root system of cane. Sugarcane rigger, cultivator, chisel, and subsoiler are used to prepare the land which enhances proper germination and better crop growth. Deep plowing with subsoiler should be used to prepare the soil properly one time after every 5 years in order to pulverize and increase the rate of water infiltration in the soil (Memon et al. 2010).

17.4.4 Time of Planting and Seed Rates

Two planting seasons are usually practiced in Pakistan: spring sowing in February to March and September to November sowing for rabi or fall. From the first week of September, planting starts in the fall and continues to mid-October in Sindh and Punjab. In other provinces like Khyber Pakhtunkhwa, planting is done in October and November. Planted crop in September commonly produces 25–35% higher yield. In Pakistan, the planting time of sugarcane is generally carried out in the autumn and spring seasons. Planting of high yield and high sugar recovery is done in autumn compared to planting in spring (Nazir et al. 2013). Sets should be selected merely from the young, cultivated crop as a completed matured crop will have a large of dry scale buds. In the dry scale buds' case, it should be treated with a lime solution. By two to three buds, all the sets should be equal in size and should be cut with a sharp tool.

17.4.5 Methods of Planting

The most commonly planting method of sugarcane are the double-set, end-to-end, and overlapping methods (Nazir et al. 2013). In conventional methods, 3 budded sets of 16,000 or 48,000 buds are directly implanted in the soil to attain 44,000 canes per acre for the normal population, but unluckily, merely 15,000 mill-able canes are attained at the end, and the row space is maintained at 1.5–2.5 ft which is 45–74 cm. For the better improvement of sugarcane yield, healthy seeds are used which increases the cane yield by 20–25%. These varieties contain high sugar content and are mostly planted in Punjab (Table 17.1).

17.4.6 Fertilizers

Fertilizers are the vital component for getting the optimum yield of sugarcane. In Pakistan, most of the farmers are using fertilizers in inadequate, imbalanced, and improper ways in a sugarcane field. In developed countries, only nitrogenous fertilizers are used for sugarcane production, but developing countries, like Pakistan, are utilizing a combination of different fertilizers such as potassium, nitrogen, and phosphate. The appropriate doses of balanced fertilizers are important to achieve the maximum yield of the sugarcane crops. Moreover, the use of

Table 17.1 Recommended varieties of sugarcane for the Punjab province

Varieties	Sugar (%)	Production capacity (maund)	Immunity
CPF-247	12.5	1400	Very good
SPF-245	11	1300	Medium
HSF-242	12.5	1500	Medium
CPF 243	12.55	1300	Medium
CP-77 400	11.90	1300	More
CPF 237	12.50	1400	Less
SPF-213	10.50	1300	Less
CP-72 2086	12.36	1065	More
HSF-240	11.70	1355	Less
SPF-234	11.60	1450	Less

Table 17.2 Duration of irrigation for sugarcane crops

Month	Number of irrigations	Duration of irrigation (days)
March, April	2–3	18–20
May, June	5	10–15
July, August	3–4	13–15
September, October	3	15–22
November–February	2	40–50

potassium is almost neglected in crops of cane. Table 17.1 exhibits fertilizer recommendations with respect to sugarcane crops for the Punjab zone (Nazir et al. 2013).

17.4.7 Irrigation

One of the aspects which are mostly neglected in this region is the application of irrigation methods. Lysimeter studies have exposed that the crop of sugarcane needs 88 to 118 kg water per kg cane and 884 to 1157 kg water per kg sugar produced, respectively (Shrivastava et al. 2011). It is difficult for some farmers to manage the enormous amount of water in fields due to financial weakness. Sugarcane crop gets into flooded conditions, and zones of the root remain merged in water (Giordano et al. 2019). It not only decreases the yield of sugarcane by decreasing sugarcane production but also causes waterlogging (Malik and Gurmani 1999). Furthermore, some areas are water-wracked, which leads to salinity (Watto and Mugera 2015). The mentioned number of irrigation and duration of irrigation for sugarcane crops is shown in Table 17.2.

17.4.8 Harvesting and Transportation

Most of the farmers cultivate sugarcane crops without soil analysis and seed treatment, which results in low yield and high production costs due to the absence of technology and modernization. Sugarcane is harvested when the crop attains the age of 12–14 months. The harvesting of sugarcane is done manually, hand-harvesting of sugarcane requires labor intensively, and one person can harvest on average 10,000 kg of sugarcane per day. When the crop of cane is 12–14 months old, it's the right time for harvesting.

Using a special type of tool, sugarcane is cut at ground level in the form of sticks. When sugarcane is harvested, it has a sugar content of almost 10%. The roots are left in the ground as they will ultimately grow and sprout to form the next crop. For loading, sugarcane is bound, topped, and stripped in bundles of 10 to 15 kg after cutting. Within 24–48 h of cutting, the harvested cane should be sent to the mill because late transportation will result in loss of sugar (Nazir et al. 2013). Figure 17.10 shows the flow sheet diagram of the conventional sugarcane cultivation method.

17.5 Sugarcane Crop: The Highest Consumer of Water

Pakistan has become a water-scarce country due to different reasons which ultimately has affected sugarcane production due to its high water demand. To complete one growth cycle, sugarcane requires 1500 to 2500 mm of rainfall/water. So, the crop needs 1500 to 3000 L of water to make a kilogram of sugarcane. Therefore, there is a need to conserve water for future usage for humans as well as for crop plants through the introduction of the Sustainable Sugarcane Initiative (SSI) for enhancing the production of sugarcane with minimum water requirement (Liu et al. 2018). The idea stands on the base of "more with less."

17.6 Sustainable Sugarcane Initiative (SSI)

The SSI is a method of sugarcane production with less water, fewer seeds, and optimum fertilization. The SSI technology has a definite economic advantage over the conventional method of cultivation. Through this method, the average yield of 118.14 tons per hectare can be obtained, whereas the yield from the conventional method was 64.74 tons per hectare. Farmers can achieve about 20% more productivity while reducing 30% of water and 25% chemical inputs using SSI technology (Gujja et al. 2009). The conventional method of sugarcane cultivation is one of the major issues in Pakistan because it requires more seed rate, less intercropping, high weeds infestation, a smaller number of tillers, and more water requirement throughout the cropping season. So, it is time to change the conventional method of

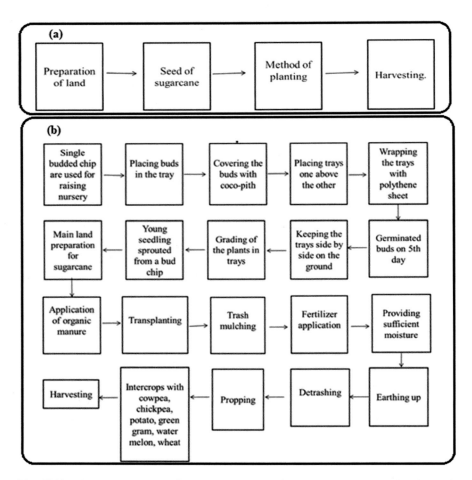

Fig. 17.10 Flow sheet diagram of (**a**) conventional sugarcane cultivation method and (**b**) SSI method for sugarcane cultivation

cultivation to a Sustainable Sugarcane Initiative method because SSI uses less seed, less water, more production, number of tillers, more accessibility to the air and light and optimal land use for higher yields. The major principles of the SSI method are single-budded chips raising nursery; young seedling transplanting (25–35 days old); 5×2 ft wide space-maintaining in the field; avoiding the accumulation of water and providing sufficient moisture; promoting plants protection method and organic measure; effective utilization of land by intercropping practice.

17.6.1 Nursery Planting

In this technique, single-budded chips (5000 buds/acre) are used for raising the nursery. Certain buds are placed in a tray filled with coco pith, and then placed with one another and wrapped with polythene sheets to keep air, water, and sunlight from entering the trays. Chlorpyrifos 50 EC is used as a measure by drenching the soil around the trays to avoid termites of sugarcane. Single-budded seed gives surely a 70% germination percentage when treated with chemicals (Jain et al. 2009).

17.6.2 Transplanting

Then the seedlings are transplanted into the already prepared field after 25–35 days at larger spaces of about 5 ft between rows. It is important to note that in the SSI method, the shot growth rate is much faster than the conventional method.

17.6.3 Wider Spacing

A wider spacing of 5 × 2 ft as recommended in the SSI system allows better yield as more sunlight is penetrating in the crop canopy and intercultural operations become easier. The use of intercultural operations to get rid of weeds is recommended as it reduces the damage caused by weeds by up to 60% (Babu 2015). It was observed that this wider space also enhances the weight and height of individual cane. Conventional methods have the efficiency to produce 10–15 tillers, whereas by using SSI, more than 20–25 tillers/plant can be obtained. The cultural practices made it easier and effectively control weeds without using agrochemicals. This technique allows the movement of farm machinery for multiple operations (Shanthy and Ramanjaneyulu 2016). Therefore, the SSI technique is the best strategy to save water and provide soil moisture by using irrigation-efficient techniques such as drip irrigation (Arthi et al. 2016).

17.6.4 Water-Efficient Utilization

Low production of sugarcane is the major challenge among sugarcane farmers in Pakistan. The low average yield of sugarcane is due to a shortage of water during its production period. However, this problem can be overwhelmed through the adoption of SSI. In Pakistan, the water table is depleting continuously. Therefore, it cannot sustain the traditional methods of sugarcane production, as they need more water (Panghal 2010).

17.6.5 An Organic Method of Cultivation

In the SSI method, farmers should add more biofertilizers and organic manures and follow measures of biocontrol, and this method discourages high uses of weedicides, pesticides, and chemical fertilizers. Sudden shifting to organic farming is not suitable; instead, a steady decrease of the inorganic method and implementation of the organic method can be tried by farmers for long-period profits.

17.6.6 Intercropping with Other Crops

In SSI method intercropping of cane with watermelon, French bean, wheat, chickpea, brinjal, potato and cowpea and in adding to effective use of land, this practice will decrease the growth of the weed up to 60% and give extra income to farmers (Loganandhan et al. 2013).

17.6.7 Overall Benefits of the SSI Method

In SSI method, the seed cost can be decreased up to 75% drastically, the rate of plant mortality decrease, weight, and length of individual sugarcane increase, easily transport the seedling to longer distance due to wider space intercultural with other crops. Table 17.3 displays a comparison between SSI and conventional method of sugarcane cultivation (Arthi et al. 2016).

17.7 Model Application of Sugarcane Crop

Accurate crop simulation models are valuable tools for a wide range of applications, including the evaluation of various crop management strategies and the understanding of potential climate change impacts (Thorburn et al. 2014). Crop models are useful tools for increasing sugarcane productivity since they help with knowledge synthesis and application, as well as yield forecasting (Andrade et al. 2016). Field-scale models, such as ALMANAC (Kiniry et al. 1992), EPIC (Williams et al. 1983), Canegro (Marin et al. 2019; Inman-Bamber 1991), and APSIM (Marin et al. 2019; Keating, et al. 1999), as well as regional-scale ones, such as Agro-IBIS (Kucharik 2003) and LPJmL (Bondea et al. 2007), have been applied to energy crops under a wide range of environments. These models differ in the degree of parameterization needed and in their ability to simulate different cultivars and different stress conditions (Marin and Jones 2014; O'Leary 2000). These complexities can be a barrier to the application of sugarcane crop models, possibly because of the lack of

Table 17.3 Comparison between Sustainable Sugarcane Initiative and conventional method of sugarcane cultivation

Comparison	Sustainable Sugarcane Initiative method	Conventional sugarcane cultivation method
Number of sets for sugarcane cultivation	5000	20,000–30,000
Spacing between two rows	5 ft	2–3.5 ft
Planting	After 20–25 days, transplanting nursery is grown in the main sugarcane field	No need of transplanting
Water requirement	Less water required	More water required
Mortality rate of cane plant	Low rate	High rate
No. of tillers per plant	25–30	10–15
Ease for intercropping	More	Less
Accessibility of light and air	More	Less
No. of plants per clump	9–10	4–5
No. of weeds	Less	More
Uniformity	Grading can be done through nursery	No grading

understanding of their capabilities and limitations and because of the difficulties in using them. Another problem seems to be the general lack of model credibility (Marin and Jones 2014). For crop simulations to be reliable, high-quality field data is required for model development, and more effort is needed in the parameterization and validation of models (Surendran et al. 2012; Andrade et al. 2016). Some of the physiological development and growth parameters that appear in model functions vary among sugarcane cultivars and therefore need to be estimated from data in order to predict growth and yield (Marin and Jones 2014). Region-specific calibrations of models are also essential (Andrade et al. 2016). Model calibration is a fundamental step in achieving high accuracy in crop development and yield estimation. Among the several models available in the literature, the Canegro model (Singels et al. 2008), included in the software DSSAT (Hoogenboom et al. 2018), can be applied to help in the interpretation of experimental results and in long-term simulations, to estimate the internal variability of yield, and thus to recommend management practices for sugarcane (Nassif et al. 2012; Hoffman et al. 2018). Since there are differences in growth among sugarcane cultivars, the accuracy of the model depends on its adequate parameterization, being performed according to each genotype.

17.8 SSI Method of Cultivation

17.8.1 Selection of Bud

For raising a healthy nursery, young mother canes are used in the SSI method, which have a good length of 7–8 in and are 7–9 months old. Canes with spots, fungus, and growth disease can be noticed and spotted. The required quantity of canes is cut, and buds are removed from the certain selected cane by a tool called a bud chipper. Bud chipper contains a fixed blade on the wood plank for cutting and a handle. Adjust a cane on a plank in such a way that cutting blade is over the cane and once the handle is pressed, a single bud chip comes off the canes. In this way, about 150/h can be easily cut off. The chipped buds will be treated through a chemical or organic solution. Per acre, 450–500 canes are required (Jain et al. 2009).

17.8.2 Treatment of Buds

Before planting, it is vital to treat the chipped buds with different chemical and organic solutions to avoid infestation. The buds are taken in a tube made of plastic or aluminum. Pour 10 L of water into the tube, and add 20 mL malathion or 5 g carbendazim and 500 g *Pseudomonas* or *Trichoderma*, 1 to 2 L cow urine, and 100 g lime. Put the bud chip in gunny or plastic bag, and dip the bag for 10 to 15 min in the prepared solution. For 2 to 3 h, the bud chip has to be dried in a shady place and then used for the plantation of the nursery (Jain et al. 2010).

17.8.3 Nursery

Young saplings are raised up in the nursery under the shady net. It is an entirely covered structure meant to make favorable conditions like wind-free, warm environment and provide shades. Well-decomposed coco pith is taken for raising nursery, and in the tray, partly fill each cone with coco pith. In the cone of the tray, put the buds in a slightly oblique or flat site, and don't push/press it too hard. Confirm that the faces of bud side up. In trays, the bud chip is entirely covered with coco pith. After filling all the trays, place them all over each other, and have a vacant tray down and top. Roughly, 100 trays are to be positioned together and covered. To create humidity and high temperature, keep the bundles for 5–8 days in the same position, and put a small weight on them. By soaking the soil with chlorpyrifos 50 EC (5 mL/L), take actions to control the termites near the trays. The nursery area must be free from weeds. Bundles can be kept preferably inside a room or in a shade net and tightly covered. If the climate is too cold, then the electric bulb creates artificial warmth. For nursery management, this is the most critical phase. Within

17 Environmental and Economic Benefits of Sustainable Sugarcane... 459

3 to 5 days, under proper conditions (especially warm temperature), primordia (white roots) will come out, and in the next 2–3 days, shoots appear. Either on the fifth or eighth day, based on the climatic condition, the trays must be removed from the polythene sheet and placed on the ground to facilitate watering. The irrigating trays must be started in the evening on the basis of the moisture content of the coco pith for the next 15 days. Leaves will start sprouting, and shoots will start growing strong. After the appearance of two leaves, the use of water should be gradually increased depending on the moisture level in trays. The grading of plants must be done at about 20-day-old seedlings (during the six-leaf stage). For a day, water should not be given to lose the coco pith that allows the easy lift-up of young seedlings. Plants that have a similar height/age can be lifted and placed in one tray. According to their height, grading of plants is attained, and the dead or damaged plant can be detached (Jain 2011).

17.8.4 Preparation of the Main Field

The preparation of the main field is the same as the conventional method. The following step should be followed for better mainland preparation (Gujja et al. 2009).

17.8.5 Removal of Residues

It is very important to prepare the land for sugarcane crop and it needs to be addressed from the planting of the entire crop up to the harvesting. Stalks are to be docile and detached from the arena, and all the remains can be fused into the soil through a rotavator (Nagendran 2009).

17.8.6 Tillage

Tillage operations by a tractor are quick and effective, and it is advisable that one plow for good and already aerated soil conditions and two plows for rough and hard soil are being applied. After plowing, the soil must be kept for an interval of time under good climate for a week or two before going for more tillage operations (Panghal 2010). By using a rotavator or harrows, tillage operation can be carried out. The operations are to be repeated to make the soil bed free from crop residues, weeds, and clods. By using a tractor, the land should be deeply cultivated after tillage operation. If the land is rough, flattening must be done using a leveler. After leveling, to facilitate the easy movement of irrigation water, a gentle slope can be maintained.

17.8.7 Application of Organic Fertilizers

The SSI method boosts the use of organic fertilizer. It increases the content of macro- and micro-nutrients in the soil in an ecofriendly way. It supports the ideal use of some chemical manure that can protect the soil from hazardous effects and degradation. Organic fertilizer like well-rotten press mud/compost/FYM should be utilized (almost 8–10 tons/acre). The amount of organic fertilizer should be adjusted to supply 112 kg of nitrogen/acre with one or more sources. For every 1 kg/acre of *Pseudomonas* and *Trichoderma*, decaying cultures can be combined with the organic fertilizers. Organic matter provides energy and a food source for biological activity. Many nutrients are held in organic matter until soil microorganisms decompose the materials and release them for plant use. This will increase the fertility of soil to realize higher yields.

17.8.8 Construction of Furrows, Ridges, and Transplanting

The distance between rows must be 5 ft to make the furrows. The soil should be aerated by running a subsoiler installed on the plow. This will sustain in deep plantation, a good combination of the fertilizer and prevention of lodging (Galal 2016). From nursery to the mainland, the ideal age of the young seedlings for transplanting is 25–35 days. It is recommended to stop giving water at least 1 day before transplanting. This will loosen the coco pith in cones and aid in the easy lifting of seedlings for transplantation. The planting method is zigzag which can be followed to attain maximum tillers and use more spaces. For easy penetration of sunlight and profuse tilling, the plant-to-plant distance of 2 ft must be maintained. One or 2 days before transplanting, moisten the soil by irrigating the field. Similarly, after planting, instantly apply appropriate irrigation as required according to the type of soil. If the soil is not properly compacted, water will run and air spaces will fill up adjacent to the plant. If the compaction of soil is not good. It is significant to water the field with a small quantity of water instead of swamping (Gujja et al. 2009). The expected outcomes of the Sustainable Sugarcane Initiative are given in Table 17.4.

17.8.9 Reduction in Weed Loss and Mulching

Generally, weed infestation is high during the initial growth stages when the crop is not well established. Weeds suppress the main crop leading to the loss in the production of sugarcane. In SSI, a nursery of sugarcane is grown which reduces competition at initial stages with weeds, and the incident of weeds is reduced by up to 60%. Seedlings are grown in a controlled environment and provided with optimum nutrients until fully established. SSI supports wider spacing which allows the mechanical destruction of weeds in an organic way. In sugarcane cultivation, trash

17 Environmental and Economic Benefits of Sustainable Sugarcane... 461

Table 17.4 Different points of view for the expected outcomes of the Sustainable Sugarcane Initiative

Farmers	Factory	Government
Saving in seed (sets)	Higher cane recovery	Employment generation in rural area
Higher cane yield with net return	Increase in crushing day	Electricity saved can be used for some other purposes
Bringing additional area under cane	Reduction in production cost	Groundwater exploitation can be reduced
More crops in unit area and time	Potential for cogeneration	Higher returns to the government through tax collection from sugarcane industries
Saving on water, labor, and electricity	Additional ethanol production	
Raising cane crop with poor-quality water		
Cultivation cane in marginal and problem soils		
Timely and need-based fertilizer application		

mulching is vital as it aids in developing a competition-free environment in the absence of weeds. Mulching will grow earthworms which in turn will increase the water infiltration and aeration of the soil. Within 3 days of planting, cane trash can be applied at 1.5 tons/acre (Galal 2016).

17.8.10 Fertilizer Application Doses

In cane cultivation, nutrient management is very necessary for the growth of good crop. It is always better to know the quantity of the needed nutrients by testing soil and improving the soil accordingly. If it is not convenient, then phosphorus, potassium, and nitrogen can be applied at the rate of 25 kg, 48 kg, and 112 kg, respectively, by the organic or inorganic method. Muriate of potash, superphosphate, urea, and ammonium sulfate is applied to attain the requirement of nutrients. Under the presence of mulching, a plant can get efficient NPK amount from the soil and due to having a healthy environment during early sprouting, sugarcane becomes resistant against an attack of certain fungus. The mentioned quantity of manures can be applied in two to three split doses for efficient use. At the time of preparation of land, apply organic fertilizers and incorporate green fertilizers into the soil. Moreover, biofertilizers such as rhizobacteria and *Azospirillum* are used, 2 kg each on the 30th and 60th days after planting by mixing it with FYM (200 kg/acre).

17.8.11 Water Management

Flooding in the field is not preferred compared to providing enough water on the required time. In the conventional methods, flooding is done, which supplies more water than the biological demand of the crop resulting in water excessibility, which may affect the growth of the crop. After transplantation, the irrigation frequency may differ depending on crop age, availability of moisture, rainfall, and type of soil. The frequency will be less for clay, and for sandy soil, it will be more. Irrigation is recommended, during the grand growth period (101–270 days) once in 7 days, during the tilling stage (36–100 days) once in 10 days, and during the maturity period (from 271 days till harvest) once in 15 days. Furrow irrigations help in water conservation hence increase water use efficiency. Alternate furrow irrigation means after 7–15 days as per the age of the crop and the moisture content, irrigating the odd numbers of furrows of initially followed through irrigating the even numbers of furrows. This will ensure up to 50% saving of water. Due to the raising of single seedlings and wider spacing in the SSI method, drip irrigation can be practiced efficiently (Gujja et al. 2009).

17.8.12 Earthing Up, De-trashing, and Propping

Earthing up means strengthening the crop stand using soil at the root zone. Generally during a crop period, full and partial two earthing up followed. Fractional earthing up is prepared after the application of the first fertilization, top dressing basically to cover the manure and to provide waterfront to the newly established roots. In this case, a small amount of soil from each furrow side is taken and placed over the manure band. This can also be prepared by the application of a country plow or bullock-drawn tool. Full earthing up is planned after coinciding with peak tilling the second top dressing. For irrigation, the freshly made furrows will be later used (Shanthy and Ramanjaneyulu 2016).

De-trashing means the elimination of additional and unfruitful leaves from the plants. Many leaves are produced by cane, and on average, a normal stalk bears 30–35 leaves in good condition. But only eight to ten leaves are sufficient for effective photosynthesis and the basal leaves do not participate in the method and finally they get dry. However, they would contest for the nutrients or could be utilized for the growth of stalk. The removal of dry leaves is important in the fifth and seventh months and mulch should be applied in interspaces for proper growth.

Propping means supporting the cane to avoid falling. It is generally done by attaching the cane to the leaves. At SSI, on one side of the field, it is suggested to provide a border such as a wooden structure to support housing products. In this way, it is possible to prevent the attachment of the middle leaves around, and thus the creation of its leaves will help in the growth of the crop and save work.

17.8.13 Protection of Plant

Light earthing up, with better water management besides trash mulching, is done on the 35th day. When the age of the crop is 45–60 days, 50 fertilized *Sturmiopsis* parasites/acre are released. When the age of crop is 4–11 months old, at 20 m' distance, the cards pasted with eggs of *Trichogramma chilonis* at 10 cards/acre should be distributed. Sugarcane can be prevented from moths through a variety of ways such as moth destruction by parasite *Isotima jevensis* Rohn, destruction and picking with hand, and selection of bud chips with resistant and disease-free varieties. Male moths can be trapped and destroyed against the third or fourth broods of the pest, release of parasite *Isotima javensis* Rohn, destruction and picking with hand, and selection of bud chips with resistant varieties and disease-free. Similarly, higher yield can be realized by the destruction of affected clumps, optimization of soil moisture, healthy buds, and crop rotation.

17.8.14 Intercropping and Harvesting

In the SSI method of sugarcane with wide spaces between the rows, intercropping in sugarcane with watermelon, cowpea, wheat, brinjal, chickpea, French bean, green gram, potato, and various other crops can be tried. Intercropping may be tried depending on location-specific factors. In the initial stage, intercropping controls up to 60% of weeds and increases the income of the farmer. They act as active mulch and preserve moisture and decrease the attack of the pest by being substitute hosts in several cases. The addition of green manures results in incresed the soil fertility when intercropping is incorporated. In most cases, the harvesting of sugarcane is done with collaboration in the industry. The desired level of sucrose content in the plants will be reached on the tenth month of 1-year crop duration, and they will be prepared for cutting within the next 2 months (Gujja et al. 2009).

17.9 Benefits of the SSI Method

In the tropics and subtropical part of India, this method of cultivation gives higher yield of almost 20–25%. As compared with the traditional method, maturity will be earlier, and crop growth will be healthy. Between the rows and clumps, equal and sufficient spacing allows air circulation and sufficient light improving the growth of the crop. This method permits a farmer to pay individual attention to the crop's pits or crops. It has been found useful under saline water and saline soil irrigated conditions, and it gives better ratoon crops. Age of all shoots will be the same; therefore, there are uniform accumulation of sugar in cane and growth of cane. An important factor is that the seedlings are placed at depth, which will be always moist;

therefore, the yields will not get affected in drought cases or cases of water non-availability (Loganandhan et al. 2013).

In this method, the cost of seed is reduced up to 75%, by using of optimum inputs, controlling weeds up to 60%, reduces delta of water and increasing revenue by efficient use of land. Sugarcane growers are facing the challenges of the high cost of production due to the conventional methods. There is a dire need to replace the conventional method of production with SSI to ensure high productivity by the sustainable use of resources. It leads to the substantial increase in sugarcane productivity, reduces the cost of production, and increases the farmer's income with cumulative effects of sustainable development (Rao 2014). Thus, the focus should be on increasing the production and proper utilization of agriculture practices for the wellbeing of farmers (Loganandhan et al. 2013). This is applicable by the adoption of new innovative methods such as SSI and the involvement of newly developed biotechnological tools (cultivars, gene enhancement) in sugarcane cultivation. The conceptual framework for sugarcane production is to enhance the income level of sugarcane farmers by utilizing available land resources in a more profitable manner. Alongside the need to improve yield and productivity of sugarcane along with disease resistance, the current scenario demands the resistant varieties to mitigate climate change which induced direct effects on the growth and development of sugarcane (Sundara 2011).

17.10 Conclusions

The focus on sustainable development is increasing worldwide. Certified schemes for SSI have become very popular in developed countries. Different countries are using different methods for sugarcane cultivation like the Roundtable on Sustainable Biomaterials (RSB), Better Sugarcane Initiative (BSI), Renewable Energy Directive (RED), Global Bioenergy Partnership (GBEP), and Sustainability Assessment of Food and Agriculture systems (SAFA). In Pakistan, there is no strategy for the cultivation of sugarcanes. There are different factors which are responsible for the low average production of sugarcane. Presently, Pakistan ranks as the third-largest groundwater consumer, accounting for almost 9% of the global groundwater withdrawals. For competitive water users and policymakers, water scarcity has become an increasingly social and economic concern. Almost 50–70% of water is lost due to surface evaporation, transpiration by weeds, and run-off leaching beyond the root zone. At any time, water becomes a limiting factor; when growth is decreased, it ultimately results in decrease in yield. Climate change and excessive use of pesticides are the main reasons for higher input costs, destroying natural biodiversity and causing threat to human health in developing countries. Sugarcane farmers are facing a myriad of challenges that directly or indirectly impact sugarcane production. So, there is a need to introduce sustainable agricultural techniques using the government to enhance the productivity of sugarcane. For this purpose, SSI should be initiated in Pakistan with the special regard to minimize the input costs by reducing the usage of chemical pesticides on sugarcane crops to make them environmental friendly. Therefore, the possible ways to increase sugarcane production to meet the demand of the increasing population are enhancing the capacity building of farmers regarding the proper utilization of resources, proper awareness regarding production practices, and motivating them to adopt new resistant varieties which are more resistant against sugarcane pests and diseases and to adopt innovative technologies such as SSI.

References

Abid M, Scheffran J, Schneider UA, Elahi E (2019) Farmer perceptions of climate change, observed trends and adaptation of agriculture in Pakistan. Environ Manag 63(1):110–123

Aman R, Khan AR (2021) Strategic alliance within the sugar industry of Pakistan: a resource dependence perspective. Asian J Bus Environ 11(4):31–38

Andrade AS, Santos PM, Pezzopane JRM, de Araujo LC, Pedreira BC, Pedreira CGS et al (2016) Simulating tropical forage growth and biomass accumulation: an overview of model development and application. Grass Forage Sci 71(1):54–65

Arthi K, Saravanakumar V, Balasubramanian R (2016) Is Sustainable Sugarcane Initiative (SSI) technology more profitable than conventional method for sugarcane production? – An economic analysis §. Agric Econ Res Rev 29(1):117–126

Aslam M (2016) Agricultural productivity current scenario, constraints and future prospects in Pakistan. Sarhad J Agric 32(4):289–303

Azam A, Shafique M (2017) Agriculture in Pakistan and its impact on economy. A review. Int J Adv Sci Technol 103:47–60

Babu SC (2015) Private sector extension with input supply and output aggregation: case of sugarcane production system with EID Parry in India. Knowledge Driven Development Elsevier, pp 73–90

Bondea UA, Smith PC, Zaehle S, Schaphof S, Lucht W, Cramer W, Gerten D, Lotze-Campen H, Muller C, Reichstein M et al (2007) Modelling the role of agriculture for the 20th century global terrestrial carbon balance. Glob Chang Biol 13:679–706

Chandio AA, Yuansheng J, Magsi H (2016) Agricultural sub-sectors performance: an analysis of sector-wise share in agriculture GDP of Pakistan. Int J Econ Financ 8(2):156

Chohan M (2012) Impact of climate change on sugarcane crop and remedial measures – a review. Pak Sugar J 34(1):15–22

Farooq N, Gheewala SH (2020) Assessing the impact of climate change on sugarcane and adaptation actions in Pakistan. Acta Geophysica 68:1489–1503

Fischer R (2015) Definitions and determination of crop yield, yield gaps, and of rates of change. Field Crop Res 182:9–18

Galal MOA (2016) A new technique for planting sugarcane in Egypt. IIOAB J 7(4):15–21

Gheewala SH, Bonnet S, Prueksakorn K, Nilsalab P (2011) Sustainability assessment of a biorefinery complex in Thailand. Sustainability 3(3):518–530

Giordano M, Scheierling SM, Tréguer DO, Turral H, McCornick PG (2019) Moving beyond 'more crop per drop': insights from two decades of research on agricultural water productivity. Int J Water Resour Dev:1–25

Girei A, Giroh D (2012) Analysis of the factors affecting sugarcane (Saccharum officinarum) production under the out growers scheme in Numan Local Government Area Adamawa State, Nigeria. J Educ Pract 3(8):195–200

Goldemberg J, Guardabassi P (2010) The potential for first-generation ethanol production from sugarcane. Biofuels Bioprod Biorefin Innov Sustain Econ 4(1):17–24

Grivet L, Arruda P (2002) Sugarcane genomics: depicting the complex genome of an important tropical crop. Curr Opin Plant Biol 5(2):122–127

Gujja B, Loganandhan N, Goud V, Agarwal M, Dalai S (2009) Sustainable sugarcane initiative: improving sugarcane cultivation in India

Hoffman N, Singels A, Patton A, Ramburan S (2018) Predicting genotypic differences in irrigated sugarcane yield using the Canegro model and independent trait parameter estimates. Eur J Agron 96:13–21. https://doi.org/10.1016/j.eja.2018.01.005

Hoogenboom GJW, Jones PW, Wilkens CH, Porter KJ, Boote LA, Hunt U, Singh JI, Lizaso JW, White O, Uryasev R, Ogoshi J, Koo V, Shelia, Tsuji GY (2018) Decision support system for agrotechnology transfer (DSSAT). Version 4.6. DSSAT Foundation, Washington, DC. Accessed Mar 2018

Hussain S, Khaliq A, Mehmood U, Qadir T, Saqib M, Iqbal MA, Hussain S (2018) Sugarcane production under changing climate: effects of environmental vulnerabilities on sugarcane diseases, insects and weeds. Climate Change and Agriculture

Inman-Bamber NG (1991) A growth model for sugar-cane based on a simple carbon balance and the CERES-Maize water balance. S Afr J Plant Soil 8(2):93–99

Iqbal M, Ahmad M (2005) Science & technology based agriculture vision of Pakistan and prospects of growth. In: Proceedings of the 20th annual general meeting Pakistan Society of Development Economics. Pakistan Institute of Development Economic (PIDE), Islamabad, pp 1–27

Jain R (2011) Bud chip nurseries–history, methods of raising, results of germination studies, First National Seminar on sustainable sugarcane initiative. SSI A Methodology to Improve Cane Productivity, pp 13–16

Jain R, Solomon S, Shrivastava A, Lal P (2009) Nutrient application improves stubble bud sprouting under low temperature conditions in sugarcane. Sugar Tech 11(1):83–85

Jain R, Solomon S, Shrivastava A, Chandra A (2010) Sugarcane bud chips: a promising seed material. Sugar Tech 12(1):67–69

James G (2008) Sugarcane. Wiley

Käyhkö J (2019) Climate risk perceptions and adaptation decision-making at Nordic farm scale – a typology of risk responses. Int J Agric Sustain 17:431–444

Keating BA, Robertson MJ, Muchow RC, Huth NI (1999) Modelling sugarcane production systems I. Development and performance of the sugarcane module. Field Crops Res 61:253–271

Kiniry JR, Williams JR, Gassman PW, Debaeke P (1992) A general, process-oriented model for two competing plant species. Trans ASAE 1992(3):801–810

Knox JW, Díaz JR, Nixon D, Mkhwanazi M (2010) A preliminary assessment of climate change impacts on sugarcane in Swaziland. Agric Syst 103(2):63–72

Kucharik CJ (2003) Evaluation of a process-based agro-ecosystem model (Agro-IBIS) across the US corn belt: Simulations of the interannual variability in maize yield. Earth Interact 7:1–33

Lahoti S, Chole R, Rathi N (2010) Constraints in adoption of sugarcane production technology. Agric Sci Dig 30(4):270–272

Lamberton J, Redcliffe A (1960) The chemistry of sugar-cane wax. I. The nature of sugar-cane wax. Aust J Chem 13(2):261–268

Liu T, Bruins RJ, Heberling MT (2018) Factors influencing farmers' adoption of best management practices: a review and synthesis. Sustainability 10(2):432

Loganandhan N, Gujja B, Goud VV, Natarajan U (2013) Sustainable sugarcane initiative (SSI): a methodology of 'more with less'. Sugar Tech 15(1):98–102

Low SA, Isserman AM (2009) Ethanol and the local economy: industry trends, location factors, economic impacts, and risks. Econ Dev Q 23(1):71–88

Macedo IC, Seabra JE, Silva JE (2008) Greenhouse gases emissions in the production and use of ethanol from sugarcane in Brazil: The 2005/2006 averages and a prediction for 2020. Biomass Bioenergy 32(7):582–595

Malik K, Gurmani M (1999) Sugarcane production problems of lower Sindh and measure to combat the problems. Dewan Sugar Mills Limited, Budho Talpur

Maloa MB (2001) Sugarcane: a case as development crop in South Africa, pp 4–5

Mari A, Panhwar R, Kaloi G, Unar G, Junejo S, Chohan M, Jagirani A (2011) Evaluation of some new sugarcane varieties for cane yield and quality in different agro- ecological zones of Sindh. Pak J Sci 63(1)

Marin FR, Jones JW (2014) Process-based simple model for simulating sugarcane growth and production. Sci Agric 7:11–16

Marin FR, Edreira JIR, Andrade J, Grassini P (2019) On-farm sugarcane yield and yield components as influenced by number of harvests. Field Crop Res 240:134–142

Masuku M (2011) Determinants of sugarcane profitability: the case of smallholder cane growers in Swaziland. Asian J Agric Sci 3(3):210–214

Memon A, Khushk A, Farooq U (2010) Adoption of sugarcane varieties in the sugarcane growing areas of Pakistan. Pak J Agric Res 23

Moitinho MR, Ferraudo AS, Panosso AR, Da Silva Bicalho E, Teixeira DDB, De Andrade Barbosa M, Tsai SM, Borges BMF, De Souza Cannavan F, De Souza JAM (2021) Effects of burned and unburned sugarcane harvesting systems on soil CO2 emission and soil physical, chemical, and microbiological attributes. Catena 196:104903

Nagendran K (2009) Farm machinery and implements in sugarcane cultivation. In: Rajula Shanthy T, Nair NV (eds) Sugarcane production technology. NFCSF & SBI, Kalaikathir Printers, Coimbatore, pp 34–45

Nassif DSP, Marin FR, Pallone Filho WJ, Resende RS, Pellegrino GQ (2012) Parametrização e avaliação do modelo DSSAT/Canegro para variedades brasileiras de cana-de-açúcar. Pesquisa Agropecuária Brasileira 47:311–318. https://doi.org/10.1590/S0100-204X2012000300001

Natrajin B (2005) Sugar and sugarcane international and national scenario and the role of sugarcane breeding institute in varietal improvement in India. Int Trg

Nazir A, Jariko GA, Junejo MA (2013) Factors affecting sugarcane production in Pakistan

O'Leary GJ (2000) A review of three sugarcane simulation models with respect to their prediction of sucrose yield. Field Crops Res 68:97–111

Panghal S (2010) Cane production mechanization – a solution for labour problems. Indian Sugar 45:27–32

Pereira CL, Ortega E (2010) Sustainability assessment of large-scale ethanol production from sugarcane. J Clean Prod 18(1):77–82

Perera M, Sivayoganathan C, Wijeratne M (2003) Technical knowledge and adoption of farming practices to farmer level extension communication of outgrower farmers of Sri Lankan sugar industry. Sugar Tech 5(3):121–129

Prasara-A J, Gheewala SH (2016) Sustainability of sugarcane cultivation: case study of selected sites in north-eastern Thailand. J Clean Prod 134:613–622

Qureshi MA, Afghan S (2005) Sugarcane cultivation in Pakistan. Sugar Book Pub. Pakistan Society of Sugar Technologist

Rabelo S, Carrere H, Maciel Filho R, Costa A (2011) Production of bioethanol, methane and heat from sugarcane bagasse in a biorefinery concept. Bioresour Technol 102(17):7887–7895

Rai MK, Shekhawat N (2014) Recent advances in genetic engineering for improvement of fruit crops. Plant Cell Tissue Organ Culture (PCTOC) 116(1):1–15

Rao JN (2014) Small-area estimation. Wiley StatsRef: Statistics Reference Online, pp 1–8

Raza HA, Amir R, Ullah MK, Ali A, Saeed M, Shahbaz SU, Wudil A, Farooq N, Ahmad W, Shoaib M (2019a) Coping strategies adopted by the sugarcane farmers regarding integrated pest management in Punjab. J Glob Innov Agric Soc Sci 7(1):33–37

Raza HA, Amir R, Idrees MA, Yasin M, Yar G, Farah N, Younus M (2019b) Residual impact of pesticides on environment and health of sugarcane farmers in Punjab with special reference to integrated pest management. J Glob Innov Agric Soc Sci 7:79–84

Sawaengsak W, Gheewala SH (2017) Analysis of social and socio-economic impacts of sugarcane production: a case study in Nakhon Ratchasima province of Thailand. J Clean Prod 142:1169–1175

Shanthy TR, Ramanjaneyulu S (2016) Socio-economic performance analysis of sugarcane cultivation under sustainable sugarcane initiative method. Indian Res J Ext Educ 14(3):93–98

Shrivastava AK, Srivastava AK, Solomon S (2011) Sustaining sugarcane productivity under depleting water resources. Curr Sci:748–754

Singels A, Jones M, van der Berg M (2008) DSSAT v.4.5 DSSAT/Canegro: sugarcane plant module: scientific documentation. International Consortium for Sugarcane Modeling: South African Sugarcane Research Institute, Mount Edgecombe, 34p

Singh A, Lal UR, Mukhtar HM, Singh PS, Shah G, Dhawan RK (2015) Phytochemical profile of sugarcane and its potential health aspects. Pharmacogn Rev 9(17):45

Singh, S., H. Singh, M. Kumari and L. Meena. 2018. Assessment of variations in yield gap and constraints analysis in the sugarcane production in Bihar.

Solangi YA, Tan Q, Mirjat NH, Valasai GD, Khan MWA, Ikram M (2019) An integrated Delphi-AHP and fuzzy TOPSIS approach toward ranking and selection of renewable energy resources in Pakistan. Processes 7(2):118

Sundara B (2011) Agrotechnologies to enhance sugarcane productivity in India. Sugar Tech 13(4): 281–298

Surendran NS, Kang S, Zhang X, Miguez FE, Izaurralde RC, Post WM, Dietze MC, Lynd LR, Wullschleger SD (2012) Bioenergy crop models: descriptions, data requirements, and future challenges. GCB Bioenergy 4:620–633

Thorburn P, Biggs J, Jones MR, Singels A, Marin F, Martine JF et al (2014) Evaluation of the APSIM-Sugar model for simulation sugarcane yield at sites in seven countries: initial results. *Proc S Afr Sugar Technol Assoc 87*:318–322

Trenberth KE (2012) Framing the way to relate climate extremes to climate change. Clim Chang 115:283–290

Triques MC, Oliveira D, Goulart BV, Montagner CC, Espíndola ELG, De Menezes-Oliveira VB (2021) Assessing single effects of sugarcane pesticides fipronil and 2, 4-D on plants and soil organisms. Ecotoxicol Environ Saf 208:111622

Walton J (2020) The 5 countries that produce the most sugar. investopedia com, February

Watto MA, Mugera AW (2015) Efficiency of irrigation water application in sugarcane cultivation in Pakistan. J Sci Food Agric 95(9):1860–1867

Williams JR, Jones CA, Dyke PT (1983) The EPIC Model and its application. In: Proceedings of the international symposium on minimum data sets for agrotechnology transfer, Andhra Pradesh, India, 21–26 March 1983

Xu F, Sun R-C, Sun J-X, Liu C-F, He B-H, Fan J-S (2005) Determination of cell wall ferulic and p-coumaric acids in sugarcane bagasse. Anal Chim Acta 552(1-2):207–217

Zhao D, Li Y-R (2015) Climate change and sugarcane production: potential impact and mitigation strategies. Int J Agron 2015:01–10

Chapter 18
Modeling Photoperiod Response of Canola Under Changing Climate Conditions

Ameer Hamza, Fayyaz-ul-Hassan, Mukhtar Ahmed, Emaan Yaqub, Muhammad Iftikhar Hussain, and Ghulam Shabbir

Abstract Disturbance in the photoperiod urged cultivars to show variant behavior regarding their phenology. There is evidence of variability in the sensitivity of cultivars to photoperiod causing pre-anthesis phases to respond to the photoperiod differently among them. A field experiment was conducted with eight canola cultivars (i.e., NARC Sarsoon, Punjab Canola, Faisal Canola, ROHI Sarsoon, Super Canola, Cyclone, Crusher and LG-3295) at two variable sites of rain-fed Pothwar. The study sites included the National Agricultural Research Center (NARC) in Islamabad (latitude 38.78 °N, 73.57 °E and 1632 ft. elevation) and URF-Koont in Chakwal (latitude 32.93 °N, 72.86 °E and 1634 ft. elevation). NARC Sarsoon showed significant results during both years of 2019–2020 and 2020–2021 with a mean photoperiod of 9.95 h^{-1} at NARC-Islamabad. Likewise, ROHI Sarsoon responded significantly during both years of 2019–2020 and 2020–2021 with a mean photoperiod of 10.44 and 10.07 h^{-1} at URF-Koont. Because of genetic characteristics (e.g., better yield potentials, early maturity and optimum usage of environmental conditions), these two varieties show excellence over other varieties. The DSSAT CSM-CROPGRO-Canola model confirmed the field results and accurately reproduced the photoperiodic response of canola cultivars. Based on this work it can be recommended that ideotype designing could be an option to mitigate the impact of climate variability, crop simulation modelling and

---

A. Hamza · Fayyaz-ul-Hassan · M. Ahmed (✉) · E. Yaqub
Department of Agronomy, PMAS Arid Agriculture University, Rawalpindi, Pakistan
e-mail: ahmadmukhtar@uaar.edu.pk

M. I. Hussain
Department of Plant Biology and Soil Science, Universidade de Vigo, Vigo (Pontevedra), Spain

CITACA, Agri-Food Research and Transfer Cluster, Campus da Auga, Universidade de Vigo, Ourense, Spain

Research Institute of Science & Engineering (RISE), University of Sharjah, Sharjah, UAE

G. Shabbir
Department of Plant Breeding and Genetics, Pir Mehr Ali Shah Arid Agriculture University, Rawalpindi, Pakistan

© The Author(s), under exclusive license to Springer Nature Switzerland AG 2022
M. Ahmed (ed.), *Global Agricultural Production: Resilience to Climate Change*,
https://doi.org/10.1007/978-3-031-14973-3_18

effective and sustained implementation of a road map to understand the agricultural environment and climate change. To reduce oilseed imports, governments should offer incentives to farmers for enhancing the production of canola.

Keywords Photoperiod · Climate change · DSSAT CSM-CROPGRO-Canola · Ideotype

18.1 Introduction

The Global Climate Index 2021 survey states that, in a condition of a high susceptibility to climate change, Pakistan is a very low greenhouse gas (GHG) emitting country; however, the vulnerability is because of geographic and diverse climatic conditions, the threat of climatic changes related to water security and food owing to the intrinsic arid climate's association with the high dependency on water from melting glaciers. Climate variability is accepted as a worldwide phenomenon with long-term effects such as growth and change (Ahmed et al. 2022). Therefore, Pakistan is vulnerable to the effects of climate change because of its rapid industrialization.

According to German Watch, Pakistan has been ranked in the top 10 of the countries most affected by climate change during the past 20 years (Economic Survey of Pakistan 2020–2021). The rate of receiving energy from the Sun and its loss into the atmosphere regulates the balance of the world's temperature and climate. This energy is dispersed around the world by the wind and other means that affect the climate of various regions. Variation and increasing temperature throughout the twenty-first century will not be the same, which will cause draught in some countries and floods in other regions that will bring disasters (IPCC 2014). Change in climate is assumed to be troubling for agricultural communities that try to establish a quality yield (Erbs et al. 2015).

Climate change has a damaging effect on canola phenology, resulting in a low seed yield (average 950 kg ha^{-1}) in Punjab, Pakistan. Temperature change has been revealed to be a serious threat to agricultural production systems in developing countries as global studies have shown (Mal et al., 2018). Climate variability results in frequent changes in temperature events. Short-term change in temperature is solid evidence of variations in the flowering of plants, which has been observed by Moss et al. (2022).

Photoperiod refers to the length of the day, which varies with latitude and seasons. It is controlled by the rotation of the earth around the Sun and its tilt. With continuous rotation, the hemisphere is exposed to various amounts of sunlight, thus forming distinct seasons characterized by numerous lengths of day and temperatures. There is no significant difference in day length between years. Therefore, it is a reliable clue for plants to drive their nutritional, metabolic and reproductive behaviors, ultimately leading to regular seasonal rhythms. It is known that climate change has no direct impact on the photoperiod; however, photoperiod can predict environmental factors that directly affect plants' phenology. During evolution, the accuracy of physiological and behavioral photoperiod regulation related to environmental conditions has been selected (Walker et al. 2019).

Environmental conditions that change day and night are essential for the growth and development of plants. The seasonal changes in photoperiod and temperature are segments of the regular rotation of plant growth and reproduction (Shalom et al. 2015). The main factors that influence the flowering of plants are photoperiod and temperature. Long-day plants flower more rapidly as the photoperiod increases. The approach to describing the photoperiod's response of crop species helps breeders accelerate the development of genotypes with the desired responses.

In *Brassica* species, phenological development is altered by photoperiod, temperature and vernalization (Robertson et al. 2002). Photoperiod and temperature are the main abiotic environmental factors that determine the growth and development of crops (Chaturvedi et al. 2018). In view of the observed environmental change trends, it is important to conduct an analysis aimed at describing and selecting plant species that not only have the best performance characteristics but also have the best adaptability to environmental changes (Tchorzewska et al. 2017). In long-day plants, flowering occurs more rapidly because of increases in photoperiod—that is, there is a direct relationship between time to flowering and photoperiod (Torabi et al. 2020).

There is evidence of variability in the sensitivity of cultivars to photoperiod, causing pre-anthesis phases to respond to photoperiod in a different way among them (Pérez et al. 2020). For selecting a suitable environment for a genotype or specie in which it can grow successfully, it is important to determine the photoperiodic parameters of the flowering stage and also for crop growth and yield predictive models' development (Torabi et al. 2020). It is also crucial to estimate the uncertainty, which is related to the results; only considering the crop model results is not enough (Wallach and Thorburns 2017).

Crop simulators have been developed to evaluate the procedures of agronomic management strategies and to help analysts to understand the bridge between ecosystem, production variation, and crop management. To recognize the crop responses, a crop phenological model is a useful tool for accessing plant growth processes that can take years to calculate in the field (Fourcaud et al. 2008). Crop models have been used by many research sponsorships and groups for decision making in the agricultural system (Bannayan and Hoogenboom 2009; Hoogenboom 2000).

To assess the explanation of problems observed in the handling of crops, especially in developing countries where changing climatic conditions prevail, a crop model—that is, a Decision Support System for Agricultural Technology (DSSAT) model—is the best tool to apply in such a situation (Hoogenboom 2000). The crop simulation modeling approach can help quantify the yield of field crops under various climate scenarios. The adoption of the DSSAT model for canola is important to verify crop opportunities in varied climatic conditions. Satisfactory simulated results were observed for the growth parameters of the culture compared to the observed values. Furthermore, it was concluded that the CROPGRO model is an efficient tool for predicting and simulating phenology, growth and crop yield under semi-arid conditions (Boote et al. 1998).

In Pakistan, there are very few studies for assessing the impact of climate change and the adaptability of canola cultivation, which is one of the most important topics in the world. As time goes by, it poses a great threat to food security, so it is necessary to focus on this subject and carry out necessary research work according to the country's climatic conditions. This research was being carried out to simulate the potential impact of climate change on rapeseed in diverse environments, taking into account the importance of it in Pakistan and the topics with the following goals: (1) evaluate of photoperiodic response of canola cultivars, (2) assess the potential impact of climate variability on the growth and yield of canola, (3) apply the DSSAT model in canola evaluation and (4) validate and recommend adaptation strategies using the crop DSSAT model.

18.2 Role of Models in Canola Production

Dreccer et al. (2018) recorded the effects of temperature and water stress on the yield of wheat, barley, canola, chickpea and peas where they were analyzed in four major Australian production areas. In general, canola is the most sensitive to water stress. High temperature in the non-stress range reduces yield because of the specific effects on crops. Jing et al. (2016) reported that the CSM-CROPGRO-Canola model was calculated determining plant and soil data collected from field trials. The model can forecast the attended crop growth and simulate the light-absorption and utilization characteristics of rapeseed.

George and Kaffka (2017) recorded on a *rom,* a multi-environmental Canola variety, experiment to test the ability of the Agricultural Production System Simulator model (APSIM) to simulate canola production in California; it can accurately simulate canola production in various regions. With proper management and variety selection, canola ought to have a higher average yield throughout California. Without other improvements in variety adaptability or management changes, these simulations indicate that California canola production will decline moderately, but that it is still economically viable.

Hoisaini et al. (2012) evaluated that the Lebig–Sprengel (LS) and Mitscherlich–Baule (MB) models were suggested only to clarify the reaction of plants to nutrients and to evaluate the comprehensive response of canola to B and salinity pressure. Water salinity treatment consists of non-saline water—3, 6, 9 and 12 dS m^{-1}. Treatment B is used to add 0, 10, 20 and 30 mg kg^{-1} as H_3BO_3 to the soil. The results show that the improved LS model can satisfactorily predict the dry matter yield of canola. The improved LS model estimates the relative dry matter of the soil B concentration and salinity level; it is near to the consistent relative yield.

Therefore, use of the improved LS model is recommended to estimate the relative yield of canola under salinity and B stress. The threshold of salinity rises with the hike of B consolidation, and the maximum dry-matter yield decreases with the increase of B merging. It was found that excessive B reduced the dry-matter yield of canola. When plants are under both B and salt stress, this effect is inhibited. Irrigation water salinity and B consolidation both impact plant water use efficiency (WUE), but only B concentration affects rapeseed production in the same way.

Qian et al. (2018) recorded that the CSM-CROPGRO-Canola model was used to accept the response of canola to the predicted climate variation of Brandon on the prairies and Sinipishin and Normandine in eastern Canada. Based on the climate variation simulation of the regional climate model, CanRCM4, two representative concentration paths (i.e., RCP4.5 and RCP8.5) were developed for the near (2041–2070) and distant (2071–2100) future climate scenarios. Estimates of the planting dates based on air temperature, precipitation and soil moisture considers the potential of early planting as an adaptation measure.

Compared with the baseline climate, under RCP4.5 the simulated seed production decreases of Brandon, Sinipishin and Normandine are 42%, 21% and 24%, respectively, and in the distant future, respectively, 37%, 27% and 23%. A greater reduction was simulated under RCP8.5, especially with Brandon and Sini Pissin in the distant future. Under the current nitrogen fertilizer application rate, the simulated seed yield reduction is related to the increase of heat and water stress under rain-fed conditions. Barthet et al. (2020) recorded that the Canadian canola samples were harvested in 2016 and 2017 to develop a near infrared (NIR) model of canola quality.

All calibration models were tested for the first time on an external verification sample set in 2017. The handheld NIR spectrometer used in this study had a limited wavelength range of 908.1–1676.2 nm. Yet, the verification results showed that it can be used to predict several important parameters that define the quality of canola. The final test was performed using the calibration model with the fewest number of factors on the second external canola validation sample set (i.e., harvested in 2018). The prediction model of total glucosinolates is not very good, but it still can be used to classify tests into low- or high-glucosinolate samples.

Yordanova et al. (2018) evaluated that the effective analysis carried out by applying accurate models was based on plant growth and yield processes—for example, the feasibility model of canola as a biofuel such as the simulation model of the "Almanac for Agricultural Land Management with Numerical Evaluation Standards." Farre et al. (2007) stated that (1) the canola production history was introduced in the context of long-term climate records; (2) the impact of planting location, rainfall, soil type and soil moisture on yield and oil content was assessed; and (3) a critical sowing date for canola production was determined. He et al. (2015) evaluated that a modeling method was used to assess the canola crop's yield potential and yield gap, that how they are affected by inter-annual climate change and that water requirements using the APSIM-Canola model can narrow the yield gap. Improving water conditions can increase yield and water efficiency.

18.3 Materials and Methods

18.3.1 Study Locations

A field experiment was conducted with eight Canola cultivars (i.e., NARC Sarsoon, Punjab Canola, Faisal Canola, ROHI Sarsoon, Super Canola, Cyclone, Crusher and LG-3295) at two sites of rain-fed Pothwar. The study sites were the National Agricultural Research Center (NARC), Islamabad (latitude 38.78 °N, 73.57 °E and 1632 ft. elevation) and URF-Koont, Chakwal (latitude 32.93 °N, 72.86 °E and 1634 ft. elevation) (Fig. 18.1).

18.3.2 Climatic Conditions During the Canola Growing Seasons

Means of metrological parameters were calculated at NARC-Islamabad during both years, 2019–2020 and 2020–2021. The seasonal rainfall was 555.16 mm during 2019–2020 and 244.86 mm during 2020–2021. Respectively, sunshine hours during 2019–2020 and 2020–2021 were 6.37 h and 6.98 h. Mean maximum temperature was 21.76 °C, whereas mean minimum temperature was 9.31 °C during season 2019–2020. Similarly, during season 2020–2021 mean maximum temperature was 24.28 °C, whereas mean minimum temperature was 8.97 °C. Metrological parameter means were calculated at URF-Koont during both seasons, 2019–2020 and 2020–2021. The seasonal rainfall was 386.4 mm during 2019–2020, whereas seasonal rainfall was 161.4 mm during 2020–2021. Mean hours of sunshine during the growing seasons of 2019–2020 and 2020–2021 was 5.59 h and 5.34 h. Mean maximum temperature was 22.48 °C, whereas mean minimum temperature was 7.7 °C during season 2019–2020. Similarly, during season 2020–2021, mean maximum temperature was 23.85 °C, whereas mean minimum temperature was 7.6 °C.

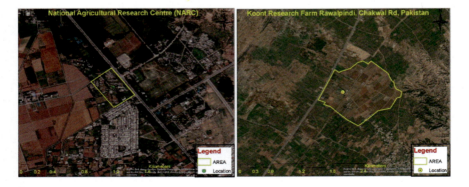

Fig. 18.1 Study sites

18.3.3 Experimental Design and Management Practices

Land preparation was done a week before sowing with some necessary tillage (i.e., 1–2 ploughings). The recommended dose of N-P-K was applied as 90–60–50 kg/hac. The Randomized Complete Block Design (RCBD) with three replications was selected for the experiment. Each plot was consistent on an area of 6 m². Seeds were sown with a hand drill at the depth of 1.5 inch with plant-to-plant distance of 10 cm and row-to-row distance of 30 cm. In total, each experimental plot had six lines. The crop was sown in between 16–20 October in years 2019–2020 and 2020–2021 at NARC-Islamabad after preparing the land well with necessary tillage practices. Whereas at URF-Koont, Chakwal, crop was sown in October during both years, 2019–2020 and 2020–2021.

18.3.4 Crop Measurements

During crop data collection, all the phonological stages including days to emergence, DFF, days of flowering, days to maturity, and the harvest index (H.I) were recorded.

18.3.5 Soil Measurements

The soil analysis at a depth of 0–30 cm showed a silt loam texture with organic carbon of 0.80% and PH of 7.60 in NARC-Islamabad. Whereas for URF-Koont, Chakwal, the soil analysis at the depth of 0–30 cm showed a sandy clay loam texture with organic carbon of 0.65% and PH of 8.1 (Tables 18.1 and 18.2).

Table 18.1 Soil physiochemical variables at NARC-Islamabad

Depth (cm)	Sand %	Silt %	Clay %	O.C	B.D	PH	SLL	SDUL	SSAT	Texture
0–30	34	33	33	0.80	1.30	7.60	0.195	0.360	0.450	Silt loam
30–60	32	33	35	0.60	1.35	8.20	0.195	0.350	0.440	Silt loam
60–90	32	33	35	0.41	1.35	8.40	0.200	0.340	0.430	Silt loam

Table 18.2 Soil physiochemical variables at URF-Koont

Depth (cm)	Sand %	Silt %	Clay %	O.C	B.D	PH	SLL	SDUL	SSAT	Texture
0–30	56	22	22	0.65	1.45	8.1	0.151	0.245	0.417	Sandy clay loam
30–60	56	20	24	0.45	1.45	8.8	0.151	0.245	0.417	Sandy clay loam
60–90	54	20	26	0.31	1.50	8.5	0.145	0.245	0.417	Sandy clay loam

Where *O.C* organic carbon, *B.D* bulk density, *SLL* soil lower limit, *SDUL* soil density upper limit, *SSAT* soil saturation

18.3.6 Modeling Flowering Phase

During the modeling phase, various modifier functions were used to predict flowering. Some of the temperature and photoperiod tasks were used to access the temperature and photoperiod effects on flowering as developed by Torabi et al. (2020). Diverse functions of temperature and photoperiod are described in the following sections.

18.3.6.1 Temperature Function

Segmented Function (S)

$$f(T) = \frac{(T - T_b)}{(T_o - T_b)} \ (\text{if } T_b < T < = T_o)$$

$$f(T) = \frac{(T_c - T)}{(T_c - T_o)} \ (\text{if } T_o < T < = T_c)$$

$$f(T) = 0 \ (\text{if } T < = T_b \text{ or } T = > T_c)$$

where T is the average temperature from emergence to flowering; T_b is the base temperature, which was 5 °C; T_o denotes the optimum temperature, 26 °C; and T_c stands for ceiling temperature, which was 40 °C.

18.3.6.2 Photoperiod Function

$$f(\text{PP}) = 1 - (P_c - \text{PP}) \times P_S$$

Negative Exponential Function

$$f(\text{PP}) = \exp\left[-P_S \times (P_c - \text{PP})\right]$$

In the negative exponential (NE) function, PP denotes photoperiod (hd^{-1}); critical photoperiod is denoted by P_c below which the rate of development decreases because of the short photoperiod. P_S stands for photoperiod sensitivity.

18.3.7 Model Description

The CSM-CROPGRO-Canola model can predict growth and other crop parameters. It also provides templates for species, ecotypes, and cultivar traits. This model has a generic approach that facilitates simulations for the crop and its phonological responses. The model needs input files (e.g., soil, weather, coefficients, eco, and cultivar) to simulate results accurately. The simulated values were compared with observed values. A CSM-CROPGRO-Canola model can predict the phenology and other aspects of a crop (e.g., growth and yield).

18.3.8 Model Calibration

I. *Manual genetic parameter estimations*. Genetic parameters were generated manually based on observed data for each location (i.e., NARC-Islamabad and URF-Koont) during both growing seasons of 2019–2020 and 2020–2021. First, coefficients were generated by GEN for each cultivar then they were manually adjusted for each cultivar according to their respective responses.

II. *Genetic parameter estimations with the DSSAT-GLUE package*. To minimize the error between observed and simulated, data calibration is required. Two tools of the DSSAT model—Generalized Likelihood Uncertainty Estimation (GLUE) and Genetic Coefficient Calculator (GENCALC)—were used for calibration. In the CROPGRO-Canola model, by running these tools, genetic parameters were calibrated and then repeated adjustments were made manually until simulated parameters close to the observed data were reached. Accuracy of the model then was checked with statistical measurers—that is, root mean square error (RMSE), R^2 and d-index.

18.3.8.1 Upscaling Strategies for Cultivar Parameters in Regional Simulation of Canola Growth

On the basis of the two experimental sites, two upscaling strategies for the estimations of cultivar genetic parameters of canola were established and evaluated. To understand these, strategies could be split into two distinct solutions. Based on two different locations' 2 years of crop data (i.e., days to anthesis, days of flowering, days to maturity, leaf area index, biological yield, grain yield, and harvest index) genetic parameters were established directly for the first kind of solution. The second solution mainly focused on the distribution of genetic parameters across the experimental sites—NARC-Islamabad and URF-Koont—in both growing seasons of 2019–2020 and 2020–2021. In simulation of days to anthesis, days of flowering, days to maturity, leaf area index, biological yield, grain yield, and harvest index, these strategies were compared.

18.3.8.2 Strategy 1: Single-Site Parameter

For the single-site parameter (SSP) strategy, the authors used all eight cultivars that were sown at the two different locations of NARC-Islamabad and URF-Koont during two growing seasons, 2019–2020 and 2020–2021. Each cultivar was parameterized to determine simulation uncertainty caused by the eight cultivars. For each site based on 2 years, 2019–2020 and 2020–2021, of observed days to anthesis, days of flowering, days to maturity, leaf area index, biological yield, grain yield, and harvest index, cultivar genetic parameters were estimated with DSSAT-GLUE.

18.3.8.3 Strategy 2: Virtual Cultivar Parameters Generated from Posterior Parameter Distributions

From posterior parameter distributions, virtual cultivar parameters (VCPs) were generated for various scenarios under several climatic condition and for two locations for both growing seasons.

18.3.9 Model Performance Evaluation

In the current study, the DSSAT's CSM-CROPGRO module was tested for canola phenology, days to first flower (DFF), days to anthesis (DTA), days to end of flowering (EOF), days to maturity (DTM), biological yield, grain yield, and harvest index (H.I), which were the main components for optimum crop productivity. These stages were thoroughly scattered around the 1:1 line. The comparison of model performance was measured by using validation skill scores (i.e., R^2, RMSE, d-index).

18.3.10 Statistical Analysis

An analysis of variance (ANOVA) was performed to check the significant differences between means of various parameters for eight cultivar treatments, and two locations for the year 2020–2021 canola growing season. The ANOVA also was performed to find the significance of the effects of Y, L, Cv and all possible interactions on yield and other parameters. Multiple regression analysis and correlation analysis were performed to show the relationship of various parameters with yield and the direct and indirect effects of these parameters on yield.

18.4 Results and Discussion

18.4.1 Climatic Parameters

18.4.1.1 Metrological Characteristics of NARC-Islamabad

Weather conditions prevailing during study seasons were shown earlier in Figs. 18.1 and 18.2. Means of metrological parameters were calculated at NARC-Islamabad during both years 2019–2020 and 2020–2021. The seasonal rainfall was 555.16 mm during 2019–2020, whereas seasonal rainfall was 244.86 mm during 2020–2021. Mean maximum temperature was 21.76 °C, whereas mean minimum temperature was 9.31 °C during season 2019–2020. Similarly, during season 2020–2021 mean maximum temperature was 24.28 °C, whereas mean minimum temperature was 8.97 °C.

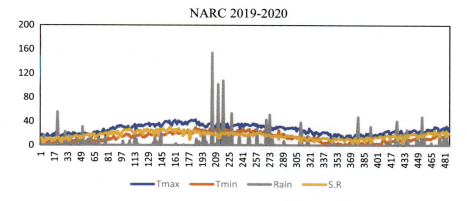

Fig. 18.2 Metrological characteristics of NARC-Islamabad during growing season 2019–2020

18.4.1.2 Metrological Characteristics of URF-Koont

Weather conditions prevailing during the study seasons are shown in Figs. 18.3 and 18.4. Means of metrological parameters were calculated at URF-Koont during both seasons, 2019–2020 and 2020–2021. The seasonal rainfall was 386.4 mm during 2019–2020, whereas seasonal rainfall was 161.4 mm during 2020–2021. Mean

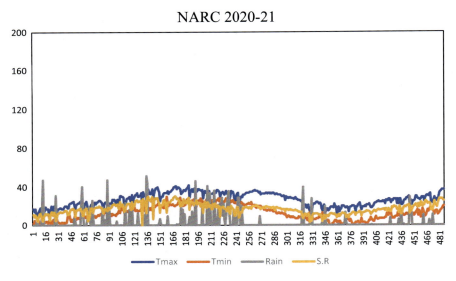

Fig. 18.3 Metrological characteristics of NARC-Islamabad during growing season 2020–2021

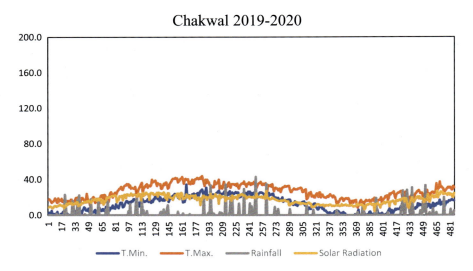

Fig. 18.4 Metrological characteristics of URF-Koont during growing season 2020–2021

maximum temperature was 22.48 °C, whereas mean minimum temperature was 7.7 °C during season 2019–2020. Similarly, during season 2020–2021 mean maximum temperature was 23.85 °C, whereas mean minimum temperature was 7.6 °C.

18.4.2 Agronomic Parameters

18.4.2.1 Days to Emergence

During the 2019–2020 growing season at NARC-Islamabad, seedlings emerged after 4–5 days from sowing; whereas during season 2020–2021 at NARC-Islamabad, seedlings emerged after 5 days from sowing. Similarly, during growing season 2019–2020 at URF-Koont, seedlings emerged above ground level after 7 days from sowing; whereas during growing season 2020–2021 at URF-Koont, seedlings emerged after 6–7 days from sowing.

18.4.2.2 Days to Anthesis

A significant difference was observed in DTAof all cultivars over the locations shown in Table 18.3. Days to anthesis of all eight cultivars had significant differences around the two locations of NARC-Islamabad and URF-Koont. Statistical analysis showed a highly significant difference among L, Y, Cv, L × Cv, whereas all the other interactive effects—namely, L × Y, Y × Cv, L × Y × Cv—were not significant at $p \leq 0.05$. During 2019–2020 and 2020–2021 at NARC-Islamabad, maximum number of DTAwere observed for Cyclone (103 days) and Cyclone (102 days), whereas minimum number of DTAduring both seasons were observed for the cultivars Faisal Canola (78 days) and Faisal Canola (75 days), respectively.

Similarly, during 2019–2020 and 2020–2021 at URF-Koont, minimum number of DFF were recorded for ROHI Sarsoon (57 days) and ROHI Sarsoon (54 days), whereas maximum number of days for the first season were recorded for Faisal Canola (77 days) and Super Canola (77 days); and for the second season, maximum DTAwas for Super Canola (75 days). The photoperiodic response plays an important role in controlling circadian cycles, increasing the expression of *CONSTANS* (*CO*) proteins under long days. In light of these results, there is evidence of variability in the sensitivity of cultivars to photoperiod (Slafer and Rawson 1994; Miralles and Richards 2000; González et al. 2003; Whitechurch et al. 2007), causing pre-anthesis phases to respond to current photoperiod in a different way among them. For visual comparison between cultivars at two different locations over two growing seasons, see Figs. 18.5, 18.6, 18.7 and 18.8.

Table 18.3 Three dependent variables, ANOVA table with DOF, F values and significant levels of fixed effects

| Source | DF | F values and significant levels of fixed effects | | | | | | |
		DFF	DOF	DTM	LAI	B.Y	G.Y	H.I
R	2							
L	1	6989.03***	3216.7***	2192.3***	3313.22***	361.1***	5054.5***	199.9***
Y	1	153.1***	975.9***	189.6***	17823.4***	3509.0***	34196.8***	792.5***
Cv	7	449.8***	530.9***	246.0***	2111.03***	299.4***	4350.6***	184.4***
L × Y	1	2.28NS	20.7***	27.0***	735.64***	74.3***	462.5***	6.6**
L × Cv	7	273.1***	267.0***	224.01***	544.96***	86.7***	1011.5***	56.5***
Y × Cv	7	1.76NS	37.1***	10.90***	131.96***	28.3***	97.5***	17.0***
L × Y × Cv	7	1.65NS	32.2***	13.58***	194.72***	26.92***	92.3***	5.0**
Error	62							

**Significant level at 0.05 level, ***Significant level at 0.01 level, *R* replication, *L* locations, *Y* years, *Cv* cultivars, *L* × *Y* interaction of locations and years, *L* × *Cv* interaction of locations and cultivars, *Y* × *Cv* interaction of years and cultivars, *L* × *Y* × *Cv* interaction of locations, years and cultivars

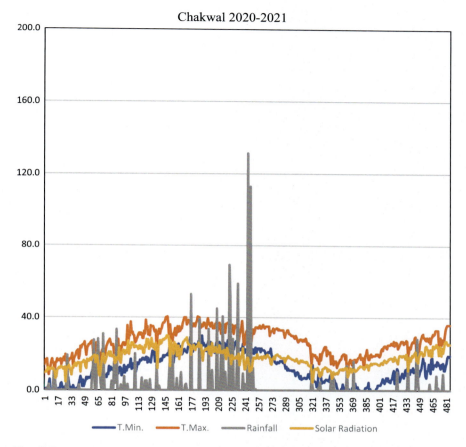

Fig. 18.5 Metrological characteristics of URF-Koont during growing season 2020–2021

18.4.2.3 Days to End of Flowering

Days to EOF varied significantly at two different climatic locations, NARC-Islambad and URF-Koont, over the 2 years shown in Table 18.3. The ANOVA table shows that Y, L, Cv and all the interactions—L × Y, L × Cv, Y × Cv, L × Y × Cv—were significantly different at $P \leq 0.05$, maximum number of days. During the growing seasons 2019–2020 and 2020–2021 at NARC-Islamabad, maximum number of days were observed for LG-32 (126 days) and Cyclone (123 days), whereas minimum number of days was recorded for Faisal Canola (115 days) and ROHI Sarsoon (100 days).

Likewise, during the growing seasons 2019–2020 and 2020–2021 at URF-Koont, maximum number of days to EOF were recorded for Faisal Canola (118 days) and Super Canola (114 days), whereas minimum number of days was

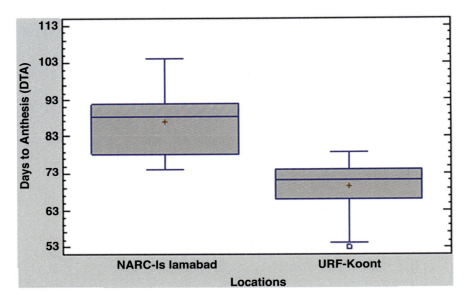

Fig. 18.6 DTA at different locations of NARC-Islamabad and URF-Koont

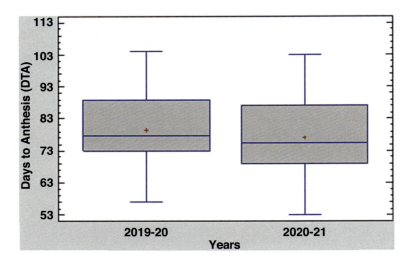

Fig. 18.7 DTA during both growing seasons of 2019–2020 and 2020–2021

observed for ROHI Sarsoon (88 days) and Sarsoon (81 days). Length of the flowering stage and growth period are key grain yield determinants for canola (Diepenbrock 2000). Comparison of two growing seasons at two separate locations are shown in Figs. 18.9, 18.10 and 18.11.

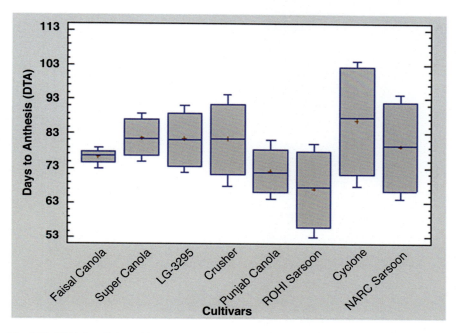

Fig. 18.8 DTA for all the cultivars

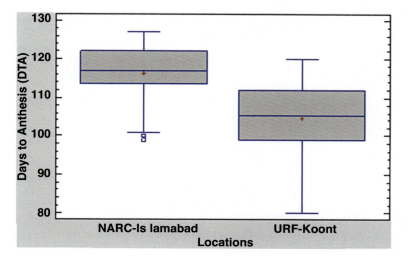

Fig. 18.9 DOF at the two locations of NARC-Islamabad and URF-Koont

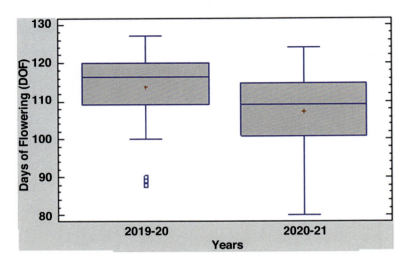

Fig. 18.10 DOF during both growing seasons of 2019–2020 and 2020–2021

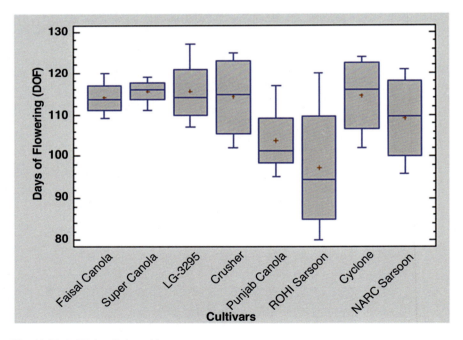

Fig. 18.11 DOF for all the cultivars

18.4.2.4 Days to Maturity

Days to maturity (DTM) was significantly influenced by the treatments. Statistical analysis showed that all treatments, L, Y, Cv and their interactions—L × Y, L × Cv, Y × Cv, L × Y × Cv—were highly significant at $P < 0.05$, as shown in Table 18.3. During 2019–2020 and 2020–2021 at NARC-Islamabad, maximum DTM were observed for cultivars Crusher (186 days) and Cyclone (186 days), whereas minimum DTM were observed for Faisal Canola (172 days) and ROHI Sarsoon (170 days). Similarly, during 2019–2020 and 2020–2021 at URF-Koont, maximum number of DTM were observed for Super Canola (180 days) and two cultivars for the second season, Super Canola (172 days) and Faisal Canola (173 days); whereas minimum number of DTM were observed for cultivars ROHI Sarsoon (156 days) and ROHI Sarsoon (152 days), respectively (see Figs. 18.12, 18.13 and 18.14).

18.4.2.5 Leaf Area Index

An ANOVA table shows that all the treatments, L, Y, Cv and their interactions—L × Y, L × Cv, Y × Cv, L × Y × Cv—were highly significant at $P < 0.05$, as shown in Table 18.3. During both growing seasons 2019–2020 and 2020–2021, maximum leaf area index (LAI) was observed for cultivars NARC-Sarsoon (4.89) and NARC-Sarsoon (4.65), whereas minimum LAI was observed for Faisal Canola (4.04) and Faisal Canola (3.28) for both seasons. In addition, during 2019–2020 and 2020–2021 at URF-Koont, maximum LAI was witnessed for cultivars ROHI Sarsoon (4.75) and ROHI Sarsoon (4.17), whereas minimum LAI for both seasons was observed for Faisal Canola (3.64) and Faisal Canola (3.21) (see Figs. 18.15, 18.16 and 18.17).

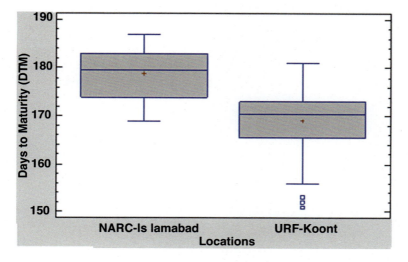

Fig. 18.12 DTM at the two locations of NARC-Islamabad and URF-Koont

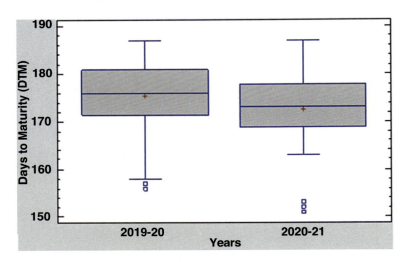

Fig. 18.13 DTM during both growing seasons of 2019–2020 and 2020–2021

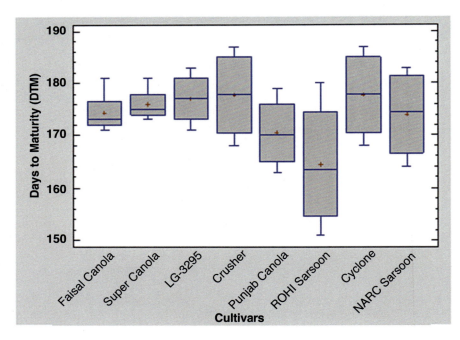

Fig. 18.14 DTM for all cultivars

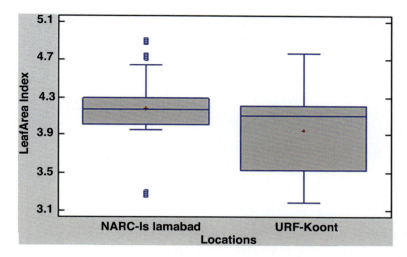

Fig. 18.15 LAI at the two locations of NARC-Islamabad and URF-Koont

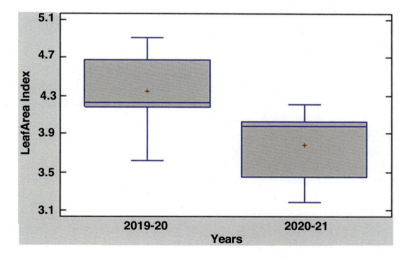

Fig. 18.16 LAI during both growing seasons of 2019–2020 and 2020–2021

18.4.2.6 Biological Yield

Results from data analysis show that all the treatments, L, Y, Cv and their interactions—L × Y, L × Cv, Y × Cv, L × Y × Cv—were highly significant at $P < 0.05$, as shown in Table 18.3. During both growing seasons 2019–2020 and 2020–2021 at NARC-Islamabad, highest biological yield was observed for Super Canola (13,854 kg/hac) and NARC Sarsoon (13,094 kg/hac), whereas lowest

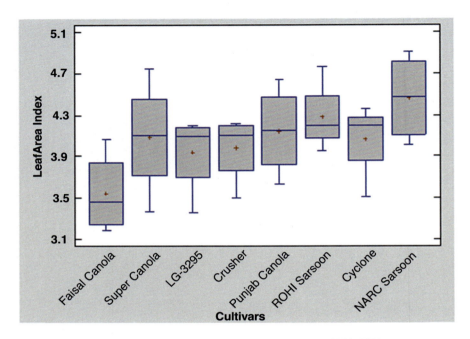

Fig. 18.17 LAI for all cultivars during both seasons 2019–2020 and 2020–2021

biological yield was observed for LG-3295 (12,770 kg/hac) and Faisal Canola (11,034 kg/hac). In the same way, during seasons 2019–2020 and 2020–2021 at URF-Koont, highest biological yield was observed for ROHI Sarsoon (13,768 kg/hac) and NARC-Sarsoon (12,165 kg/hac); whereas lowest biological yield was tracked for Faisal Canola (11,545 kg/hac) and LG-3295 (10,911 kg/hac). Increasing temperature adversely affected crop biomass. Among locations at NARC-Islamabad, there were relatively lower temperatures than in URF-Koont, which accelerated the life cycle. So, biomass production was not good at URF-Koont as compared to NARC-Islamabad (see Figs. 18.18, 18.19 and 18.20).

18.4.2.7 Grain Yield

Grain yield varied considerably among the eight cultivars at varying locations (i.e., NARC-Islamabad and URF-Koont) during both the 2019–2020 and 2020–2021 seasons. An ANOVA table shows that the treatments, L, Y, Cv and their interactions—L × Y, L × Cv, Y × Cv, L × Y × Cv—were significantly different at $p \leq 0.05$ (see Table 18.3). Throughout 2019–2020 and 2020–2021 at NARC-Islamabad, high-yielding cultivars were NARC Sarsoon (2930 kg/hac) and NARC Sarsoon (2670 kg/hac), whereas low-yielding cultivars were Faisal Canola (2230 kg/hac) and Faisal Canola (1860 kg/hac). Correspondingly, during 2019–2020 and

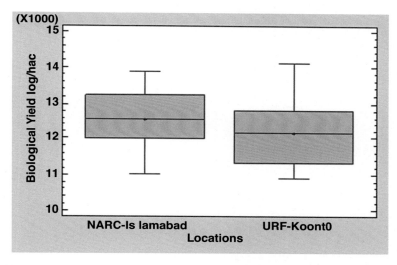

Fig. 18.18 Biological yield at the two locations of NARC-Islamabad and URF-Koont

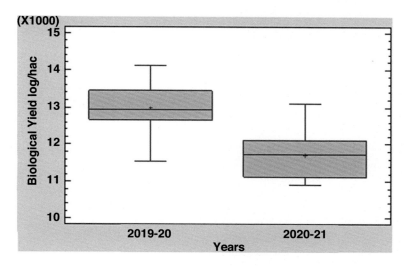

Fig. 18.19 Biological yield during both growing seasons of 2019–2020 and 2020–2021

2020–2021 at URF-Koont, high-yielding cultivars were NARC Sarsoon (2737 kg/hac) and ROHI Sarsoon (2331 kg/hac), whereas low-yielding cultivars were Faisal Canola (2115 kg/hac) and Faisal Canola (1762 kg/hac) (see Figs. 18.21, 18.22 and 18.23). High temperatures significantly reduced the grain yield of canola because of the shortening of the reproductive growth stage (Chaudhary et al. 2020). The length of the flowering stage and growth period are key grain yield determinants for canola (Diepenbrock 2000).

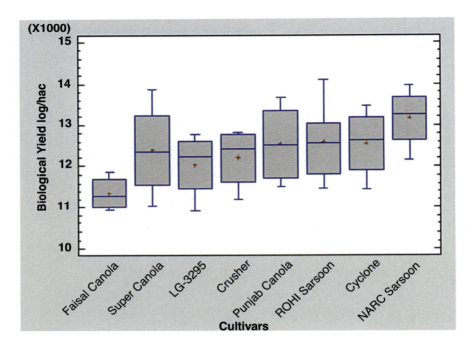

Fig. 18.20 Biological yield for all the cultivars

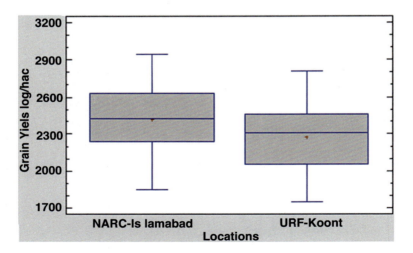

Fig. 18.21 Grain yield at the two locations of NARC-Islamabad and URF-Koont

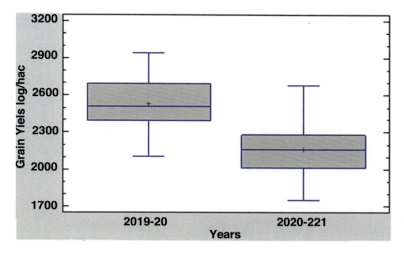

Fig. 18.22 Grain yield during both growing seasons of 2019–2020 and 2020–2021

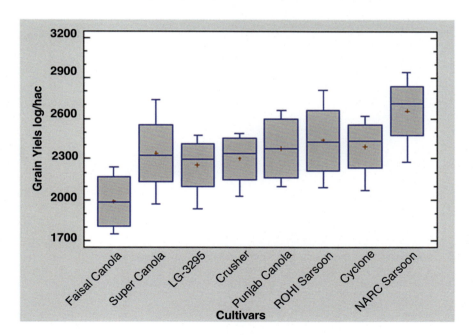

Fig. 18.23 Grain yield of all cultivars

18.4.2.8 Harvest Index

Harvest index (H.I) significantly differs for all the eight cultivars at varying locations (i.e., NARC-Islamabad and URF-Koont) during both seasons (2019–2020 and 2020–2021). An ANOVA table explains that all the treatments, L, Y, Cv and their

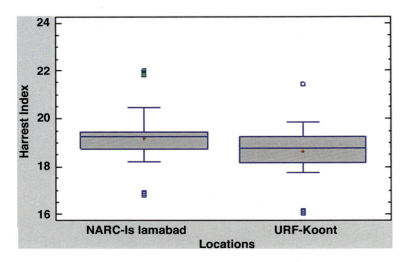

Fig. 18.24 H.I at the two locations of NARC-Islamabad and URF-Koont

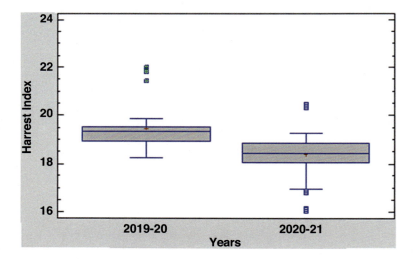

Fig. 18.25 H.I during both growing seasons of 2019–2020 and 2020–2021

interactions—L × Y, L × Cv, Y × Cv, L × Y × Cv—were significantly different at $p < 0.05$ (see Table 18.3). During 2019–2020 and 2020–2021 at NARC-Islamabad, cultivars with maximum H.I were NARC Sarsoon (21.9) and NARC Sarsoon (20.39), whereas cultivars with minimum H.I were Faisal Canola (18.80) and Faisal Canola (16.11).

On the contrary, during 2019–2020 and 2020–2021 at URF-Koont, maximum H.I was observed for ROHI Sarsoon (20.84) and ROHI Sarsoon (19.17), whereas cultivars with minimum H.I were Faisal Canola (18.31) and Faisal Canola (16.11) (see Figs. 18.24, 18.25 and 18.26). Grain size is reduced by increases in temperature.

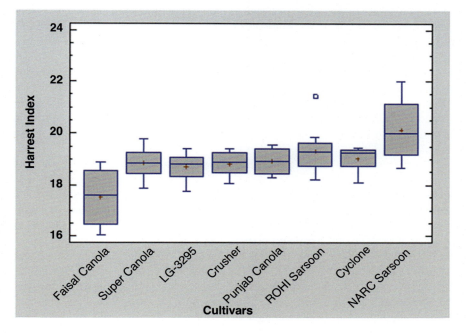

Fig. 18.26 H.I index of all cultivars

By reduction in grain size and weight, H.I decreases. Among the locations, URF-Koont had a higher temperature than NARC-Islamabad. Increases in temperature were observed over the years, resulting in reduction of grain size and weight (i.e., harvest index).

18.4.3 Simulation Outcomes

18.4.3.1 Phenology

Results showed that predicted days to anthesis at Islamabad during the growing season of 2019–2020 were a comparatively close correlation to observed days. At NARC-Islamabad, maximum DTAwere observed for Cyclone (103) and minimum number of DTAwere for ROHI Sarsoon (79). Meanwhile, maximum and minimum simulated days were recorded for Cyclone (103 days) and Faisal Canola (77 days), whereas the average number of stimulated days was 87.8 and observed days was 88. The comparison of model performance was measured by using validation skill scores (R^2, RMSE, d-index). The values for R^2, RMSE and d-index were 0.99, 0.61 and 0.99.

During 2019–2020 at URF-Koont, maximum simulated days for anthesis were counted for two cultivars, Faisal Canola (77 days) and Super Canola (77 days), and maximum observed days were the same as model simulated Faisal Canola (77 days) and Super Canola (77 days). Minimum simulated number of DTAwere for ROHI Sarsoon (57), which is exactly as observed for ROHI Sarsoon (57). The comparison of model performance was measured by using validation skill scores (R^2, RMSE, d-index). The values for R^2, RMSE and d-index were 0.98, 0.57 and 0.99, whereas the average simulated and observed number of days were 70.625 and 70.625. For the growing season 2020–2021 at NARC-Islamabad, maximum and minimum simulated DTAwere for Cyclone (100 days) and Faisal Canola (77 days), whereas maximum and minimum observed DTAwere for Cyclone (102 days) and Faisal Canola (75 days).

The comparison of model performance was measured by using validation skill scores (R^2, RMSE, d-index). The values for R^2, RMSE and d-index were 0.99, 1.19 and 0.99. The average simulated and observed days were 87.25 and 85.625, whereas during the 2020–2021 growing season at URF-Koont, maximum and minimum simulated DTAwere for Super Canola (75 days) and ROHI Sarsoon (56 days); whereas maximum and minimum observed days were for Super Canola (75 days) and ROHI Sarsoon (54 days). The comparison of model performance was measured by using validation skill scores (R^2, RMSE, d-index). The values for R^2, RMSE and d-index were 0.98, 0.93 and 0.99. The average simulated and observed days were 68.5 and 65.75.

Simulated days to EOFwere close to observed days. During 2019–2020 at NARC-Islamabad, maximum and minimum simulated days were for LG-3295 (125 days) and Faisal Canola (114 days), whereas maximum and minimum observed days were for LG-3295 (126 days) and Faisal Canola (115 days). The comparison of model performance was measured by using validation skill scores (R^2, RMSE, d-index). The values for R^2, RMSE and d-index were 0.99, 0.59 and 0.99. Similarly, during 2019–2020 at URF-Koont, maximum and minimum simulated days to EOFwere for Faisal Canola (77 days), Super Canola (77 days) and ROHI Sarsoon (57 days); whereas maximum and minimum observed days to EOFwere the same as the model predicted—Faisal Canola (77 days), Super Canola (77 days) and ROHI Sarsoon (57 days).

The comparison of model performance was measured by using validation skill scores (R^2, RMSE, d-index). The values for R^2, RMSE and d-index were 0.98, 0.57 and 0.99. For the second season, 2020–2021 at NARC-Islamabad, maximum and minimum simulated DOF were for LG-3295 (125 days) and Faisal Canola (114 days); whereas maximum and minimum observed days to EOF were for LG-3295 (126 days) and Faisal Canola (115 days). The comparison of model performance was measured by using validation skill scores (R^2, RMSE, d-index). The values for R^2, RMSE and d-index were 0.99, 0.59 and 0.99. Similarly, during 2020–2021 at URF-Koont, maximum and minimum simulated days to EOFwere for Super Canola (129 days) and ROHI Sarsoon (88 days); whereas maximum and minimum observed days were for Super Canola (130 days) and ROHI Sarsoon (88 days). The comparison of model performance was measured by using validation skill scores (R^2, RMSE, d-index). The values for R^2, RMSE and d-index were 0.99, 0.62 and 0.99. Average simulated and observed values were very close to each other: 108.25 days and 108.62 days.

18 Modeling Photoperiod Response of Canola Under Changing Climate Conditions 497

Comparison between simulated and observed data for DTM showed that there was a close link between the simulated and observed values. During the 2019–2020 growing season at NARC-Islamabad, maximum and minimum simulated days were for Crusher (186 days) and Faisal Canola (169 days), whereas maximum and minimum observed DTM were for Crusher (186 days) and Faisal Canola (172 days). The comparison of model performance was measured by using validation skill scores (R^2, RMSE, d-index). The values for R^2, RMSE and d-index were 0.97, 0.70 and 0.99. Average simulated and observed days were 177.25 and 172.62.

Similarly, during the 2019–2020 growing season at URF-Koont, maximum and minimum simulated number of DTM were for Faisal Canola (174 days), Super Canola (174 days) and ROHI Sarsoon (154 days); whereas maximum and minimum observed DTM were for Super Canola (180 days) and ROHI Sarsoon (154 days). The comparison of model performance was measured by using validation skill scores (R^2, RMSE, d-index). The values for R^2, RMSE and d-index were 0.92, 1.91 and 0.97. Average simulated and observed DTM were 168 and 170.75. During growing season 2020–2021 at NARC-Islamabad, maximum and minimum simulated number of DTM were for Crusher (186 Days) and Faisal Canola (169 days), whereas maximum and minimum observed number of DTM were for Crusher (186 days) and Faisal Canola (172 days). The comparison of model performance was measured by using validation skill scores (R^2, RMSE, d-index). The values for R^2, RMSE and d-index were 0.97, 1.70 and 0.99. Average simulated and observed days were 177.2 and 179.6.

Likewise, at URF-Koont for growing season 2020–2021, maximum and minimum simulated DTM were for Faisal Canola and Super Canola (177 days) and ROHI Sarsoon (156 days); whereas maximum and minimum observed DTM were for Super Canola (180 days) and ROHI Sarsoon (156 days). The comparison of model performance was measured by using validation skill scores (R^2, RMSE, d-index). The values for R^2, RMSE and d-index were 0.92, 1.91 and 0.97. Average simulated and observed DTM were 168 and 170.75 (see Figs. 18.27, 18.28, 18.29, 18.30, 18.31, 18.32, 18.33, 18.34, 18.35, 18.36, 18.37 and 18.38).

18.4.3.2 Leaf Area Index, Biomass and Grain Yield

Simulated leaf area index (LAI) values were exactly as observed for all cultivars during both years; this showed high model accuracy. During 2019–2020 at NARC-Islamabad, maximum and minimum simulated biological yield were for Super Canola (13,828 kg/hac) and Faisal Canola (11,852 kg/hac); whereas observed maximum and minimum biological yield were for Super Canola (13,854 kg/hac) and Faisal Canola (11,861 kg/hac). Average simulated and observed was 13020.1 kg/hac and 13094.7 kg/hac. The comparison of model performance was measured by using validation skill scores (R^2, RMSE, d-index). The values for R^2, RMSE and d-index were 0.99, 74.43 and 0.99.

Similarly, during 2019–2021 at URF-Koont, maximum and minimum simulated biological yield were for NARC Sarsoon (13,971 kg/hac) and Faisal Canola

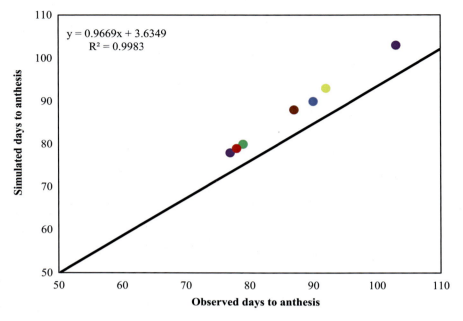

Fig. 18.27 Simulated and observed DTA for NARC-Islamabad during 2019–2020 growing season

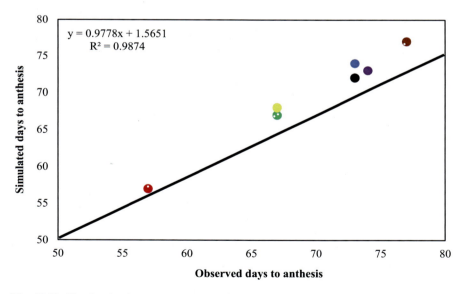

Fig. 18.28 Simulated and observed DTA for URF-Koont during 2019–2020 growing season

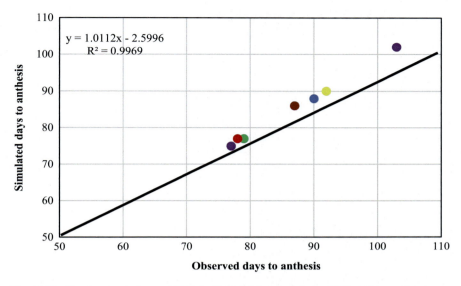

Fig. 18.29 Simulated and observed DTA for NARC-Islamabad during 2020–2021 growing season

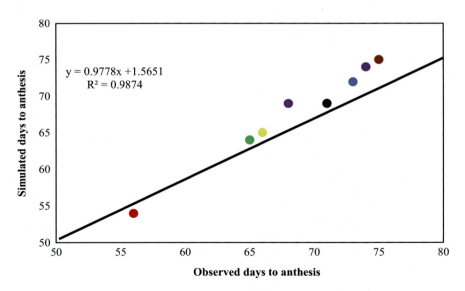

Fig. 18.30 Simulated and observed DTA for URF-Koont during 2020–2021 growing season

(11,500 kg/hac); whereas maximum and minimum observed biological yield were for NARC Sarsoon (13,982 kg/hac) and Faisal Canola (11,545 kg/hac). Average simulated and observed biological yield were 12811.3 kg/hac and 12872.1 kg/hac. The comparison of model performance was measured by using validation skill

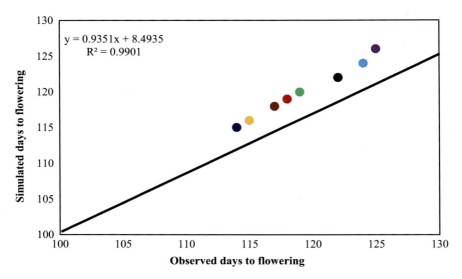

Fig. 18.31 Simulated and observed DOF for NARC-Islamabad during 2019–2020 growing season

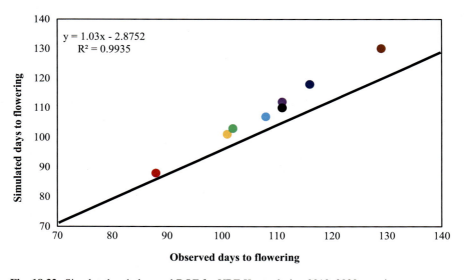

Fig. 18.32 Simulated and observed DOF for URF-Koont during 2019–2020 growing season

scores (R^2, RMSE, d-index). The values for R^2, RMSE and d-index were 0.97, 107.1 and 0.99.

During growing season 2020–2021 at NARC-Islamabad, maximum and minimum simulated biological yield were for NARC Sarsoon (13,095 kg/hac) and Faisal Canola (11,040 kg/hac); whereas maximum and minimum observed biological yield were for NARC Sarsoon (13,094 kg/hac) and Faisal Canola (11,034 kg/hac).

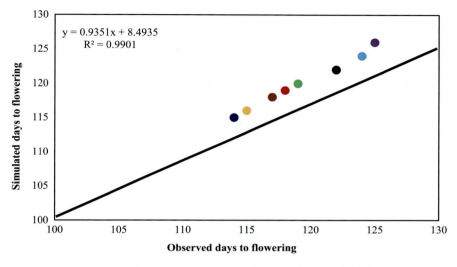

Fig. 18.33 Simulated and observed DOF for NARC-Islamabad during 2020–2021 growing season

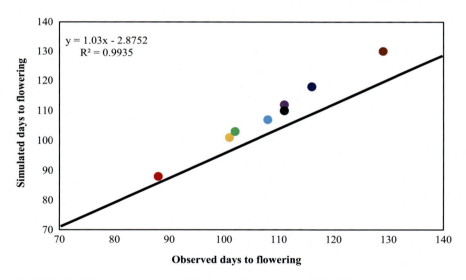

Fig. 18.34 Simulated and observed DOF for URF-Koont during 2020–2021 growing season

Average simulated and observed biological yield were 12019.1 kg/hac and 12,013 kg/hac. The comparison of model performance was measured by using validation skill scores (R^2, RMSE, d-index). The values for R^2, RMSE and d-index were 0.99, 6.73 and 0.99.

Similarly, during 2020–2021 at URF-Koont, maximum and minimum simulated biological yield were for ROHI Sarsoon (12,145 kg/hac) and Faisal Canola

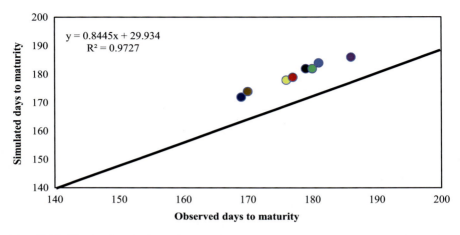

Fig. 18.35 Simulated and observed DTM for NARC-Islamabad during 2019–2020 growing season

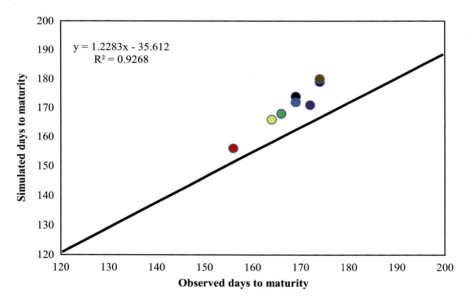

Fig. 18.36 Simulated and observed DOF for URF-Koont during 2019–2020 growing season

(10,932 kg/hac); whereas maximum and minimum observed biological yield were for NARC Sarsoon (12,165 kg/hac) and Faisal Canola (10,936 kg/hac). Average simulated and observed days were 11420.8 kg/hac and 11,423 kg/hac. The comparison of model performance was measured by using validation skill scores (R^2, RMSE, d-index). The values for R^2, RMSE and d-index were 0.99, 20.8 and 0.99.

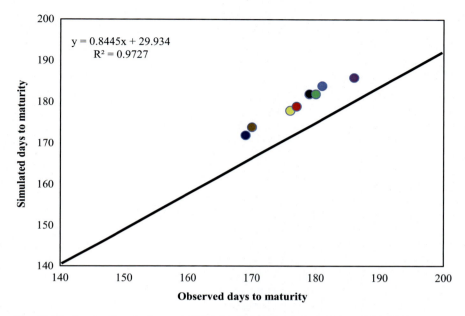

Fig. 18.37 Simulated and observed DTM for NARC-Islamabad during 2020–2021 growing season

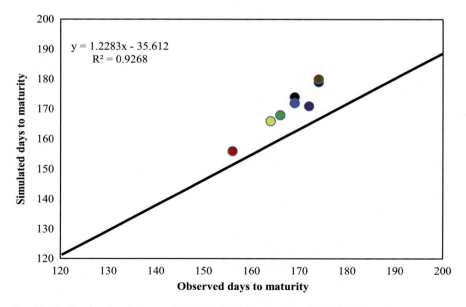

Fig. 18.38 Simulated and observed DOF for URF-Koont during 2020–2021 growing season

Grain yield predicted by the model was close to observed yield. During growing season 2019–2020 at NARC-Islamabad, maximum and minimum grain yield were for NARC Sarsoon (2889 kg/hac) and Faisal Canola (2234 kg/hac); whereas maximum and minimum observed grain yield were for NARC Sarsoon (2930 kg/hac) and Faisal Canola (2230 kg/hac). Average maximum and minimum grain yield were 2564.1 kg/hac and 2577.5 kg/hac. The comparison of model performance was measured by using validation skill scores (R^2, RMSE, d-index). The values for R^2, RMSE and d-index were 0.99, 20.07 and 0.99.

Similarly, at URF-Koont during 2019–2020, maximum and minimum grain yield were for ROHI Sarsoon (2753 kg/hac) and Faisal Canola (2115 kg/hac); whereas maximum and minimum observed grain yield were for ROHI Sarsoon (2798 kg/hac) and Faisal Canola (2115 kg/hac). Average maximum and minimum grain yield were 2458.7 kg/hac and 2478.8 kg/hac. The comparison of model performance was measured by using validation skill scores (R^2, RMSE, d-index). The values for R^2, RMSE and d-index were 0.99, 23.88 and 0.99. During growing season 2020–2021 at NARC-Islamabad, maximum and minimum grain yield were for NARC Sarsoon (2689 kg/hac) and Faisal Canola (1847 kg/hac); whereas maximum and minimum observed days were for NARC Sarsoon (2670 kg/hac) and Faisal Canola (1860 kg/hac). Average maximum and minimum grain yield were 2252 kg/hac and 2251.2 kg/hac. The comparison of model performance was measured by using validation skill scores (R^2, RMSE, d-index). The values for R^2, RMSE and d-index were 0.99, 8.19 and 0.99.

Likewise, at URF-Koont during 2020–2021, maximum and minimum simulated grain yield were for ROHI Sarsoon (2332 kg/hac) and Faisal Canola (1765 kg/hac); whereas maximum and minimum observed grain yield were for ROHI Sarsoon (2331 kg/hac) and Faisal Canola (1762 kg/hac) Average maximum and minimum grain yield were 2067.6 kg/hac and 2066.3 kg/hac. The comparison of model performance was measured by using validation skill scores (R^2, RMSE, d-index). The values for R^2, RMSE and d-index were 0.99, 2.49 and 0.99.

Simulated harvest index was very close to the observed one. During 2019–2020 at NARC-Islamabad, maximum and minimum H.I were for NARC Sarsoon (21.71) and Faisal Canola (18.84); whereas observed maximum and minimum H.I recorded were for NARC Sarsoon (21.9) and Faisal Canola (18.8). Average simulated and observed harvest index were 19.57 and 19.66. The comparison of model performance was measured by using validation skill scores (R^2, RMSE, d-index). The values for R^2, RMSE and d-index were 0.97, 0.13 and 0.99.

Similarly, during 2019–2020 at URF-Koont, maximum and minimum simulated H.I were for ROHI Sarsoon (19.77) and Faisal Canola (18.39); whereas maximum and minimum observed days were recorded for ROHI Sarsoon (20.84) and Faisal Canola (18.31). Average simulated and observed harvest index were 19.15 and 19.28. The comparison of model performance was measured by using validation skill scores (R^2, RMSE, d-index). The values for R^2, RMSE and d-index were 0.84,

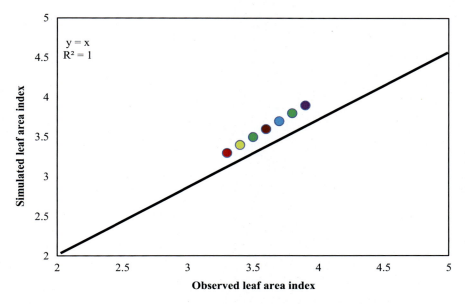

Fig. 18.39 Simulated and observed LAI for NARC-Islamabad during 2019–2020 growing season

0.28 and 0.99. During 2020–2021 at NARC-Islamabad, maximum and minimum H.I were for NARC Sarsoon (20.53) and Faisal Canola (16.73); whereas observed maximum and minimum harvest index recorded were for NARC Sarsoon (20.39) and Faisal Canola (16.85). Average simulated and observed H.I were 18.68 and 18.69. The comparison of model performance was measured by using validation skill scores (R^2, RMSE, d-index). The values for R^2, RMSE and d-index were 0.99, 0.63 and 0.99.

Likewise, during 2020–2021 at URF-Koont, maximum and minimum simulated H.I were for ROHI Sarsoon (19.21) and Faisal Canola (16.14); whereas maximum and minimum observed days were recorded for ROHI Sarsoon (19.17) and Faisal Canola (16.11). Average simulated and observed H.I were 18.07 and 18.05. The comparison of model performance was measured by using validation skill scores (R^2, RMSE, d-index). The values for R^2, RMSE and d-index were 0.99, 0.05 and 0.99 (see Figs. 18.39, 18.40, 18.41, 18.42, 18.43, 18.44, 18.45, 18.46, 18.47, 18.48, 18.49, 18.50, 18.51, 18.52, 18.53 and 18.54).

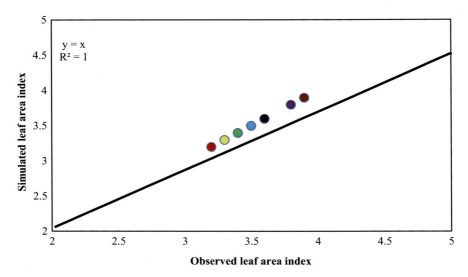

Fig. 18.40 Simulated and observed LAI for URF-Koont during 2019–2020 growing season

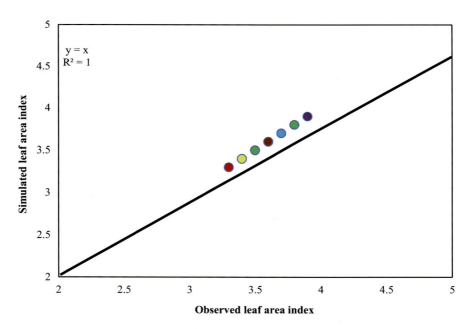

Fig. 18.41 Simulated and observed LAI for NARC-Islamabad during 2020–2021 growing season

18 Modeling Photoperiod Response of Canola Under Changing Climate Conditions

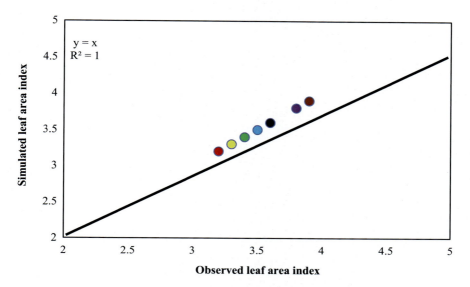

Fig. 18.42 Simulated and observed LAI for URF-Koont during 2020–2021 growing season

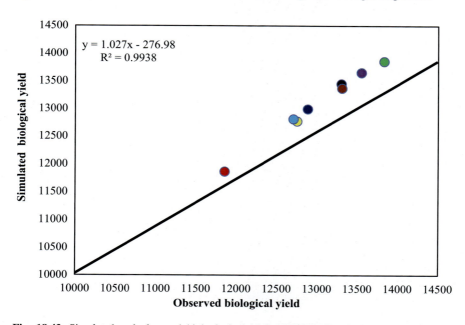

Fig. 18.43 Simulated and observed biological yield for NARC-Islamabad during 2019–2020 growing season

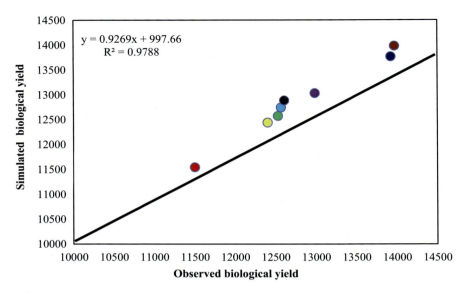

Fig. 18.44 Simulated and observed biological yield for URF-Koont during 2019–2020 growing season

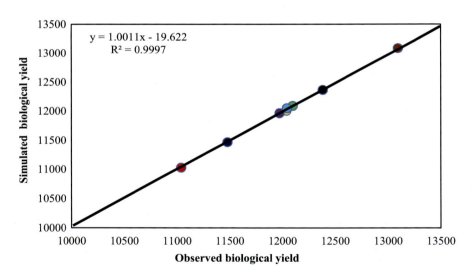

Fig. 18.45 Simulated and observed biological yield for NARC-Islamabad during 2020–2021 growing season

18 Modeling Photoperiod Response of Canola Under Changing Climate Conditions

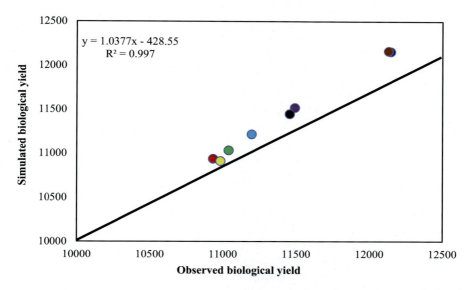

Fig. 18.46 Simulated and observed biological yield for URF-Koont during 2020–2021 growing season

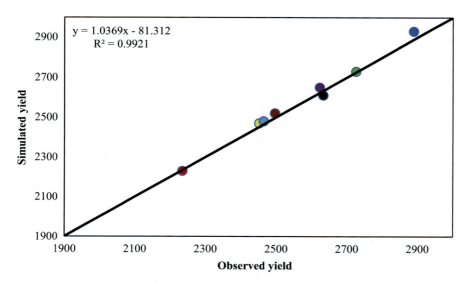

Fig. 18.47 Simulated and observed grain yield for NARC-Islamabad during 2019–2020 growing season

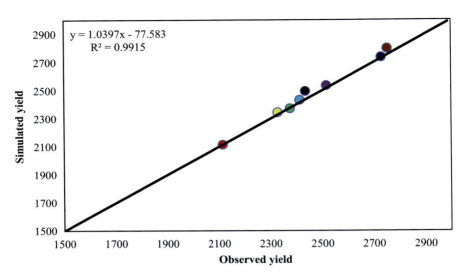

Fig. 18.48 Simulated and observed grain yield for URF-Koont during 2019–2020 growing season

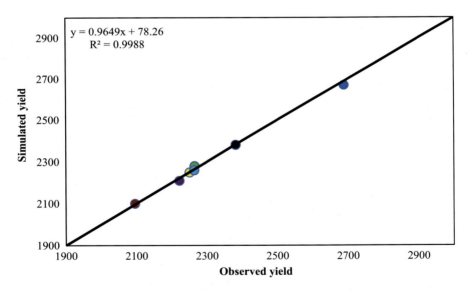

Fig. 18.49 Simulated and observed grain yield for NARC-Islamabad during 2020–2021 growing season

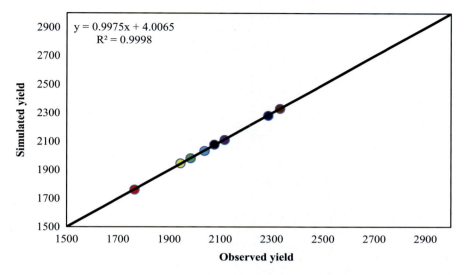

Fig. 18.50 Simulated and observed grain yield for URF-Koont during 2020–2021 growing season

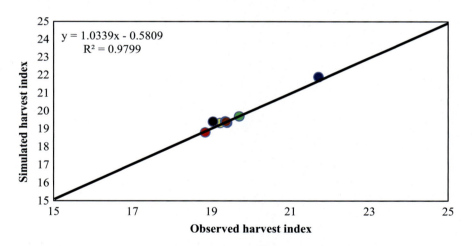

Fig. 18.51 Simulated and observed H.I for NARC-Islamabad during 2019–2020 growing season

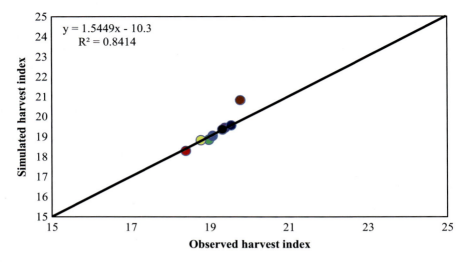

Fig. 18.52 Simulated and observed H.I for URF-Koont during 2019–2020 growing season

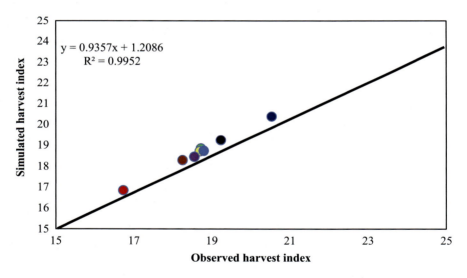

Fig. 18.53 Simulated and observed H.I for NARC-Islamabad during 2020–2021 growing season

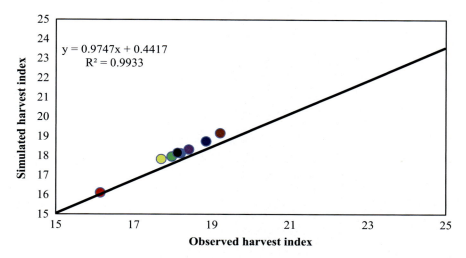

Fig. 18.54 Simulated and observed H.I for URF-Koont during 2020–2021 growing season

18.5 Conclusions

Photoperiod refers to the length of the day, which varies with latitude and seasons. It is controlled by the rotation of the earth around the Sun and its tilt. With the continuous rotation, the hemisphere is exposed to various amounts of sunlight, thus forming distinct seasons characterized by various day lengths and temperatures. There is no significant difference in day length between years. Therefore, it is a reliable clue for plants to drive their nutritional, metabolic and reproductive behaviors, ultimately leading to regular seasonal rhythms; although climate change has no direct impact on photoperiod. Nevertheless, photoperiod can predict environmental factors that directly affect the phenology of plants.

The main factors that influence flowering of plants are photoperiod and temperature. Long day plants flower more rapidly as the photoperiod increases. The approach to describing the photoperiod response of crop species will help breeders accelerate the development of genotypes with the desired photoperiod responses. For selecting a suitable environment for a genotype or specie where it can grow successfully, it is important to determine photoperiodic parameters of the flowering stage and for crop growth and yield predictive model development. The DSSAT CSM-CROPGRO-Canola model has confirmed field results and accurately reproduced the photoperiodic response of canola cultivars.

References

Ahmed M, Hayat R, Ahmad M, ul-Hassan M, AMS K, ul-Hassan F, ur-Rehman MH, Shaheen FA, Raza MA, Ahmad S (2022) Impact of climate change on dryland agricultural systems: a review of current status, potentials, and further work need. Int J Plant Product. https://doi.org/10.1007/s42106-022-00197-1

Bannayan M, Hoogenboom G (2009) Using pattern recognition for estimating cultivar coefficients of a crop simulation model. Field Crop Res 111(3):290–302. https://doi.org/10.1016/j.fcr.2009.01.007

Barthet VJ, Petryk MW, Siemens B (2020) Rapid nondestructive analysis of intact canola seeds using a handheld near-infrared spectrometer. J Am Oil Chem Soc 97:577

Boote KJ, Jones JW, Hoogenboom G, Pickering NB (1998) The CROPGRO model for grain legumes. In: Tsuji G, Hoogenboom G, Thornton P (eds) Understanding options for agricultural production, vol 7. Systems approaches for sustainable agricultural development. Springer, Netherlands, pp 99–128. https://doi.org/10.1007/978-94-017-3624-4_6

Chaturvedi AK, Graubard BI, Broutian T, Pickard RK, Tong ZY, Xiao W, Gillison ML (2018) Effect of prophylactic human papillomavirus (HPV) vaccination on oral HPV infections among young adults in the United States. J Clin Oncol 36(3):262

Chaudhary S, Devi P, Bhardwaj A, Jha UC, Sharma KD, Prasad PV, Siddique KH, Bindumadhava H, Kumar S, Nayyar H (2020) Identification and characterization of contrasting genotypes/cultivars for developing heat tolerance in agricultural crops: current status and prospects. Front Plant Sci 11:587264

Diepenbrock W (2000) Yield analysis of winter oilseed rape (Brassica napus L.): a review. Field Crop Res 67(1):35–49

Dreccer MF, Fainges J, Whish J, Ogbonnaya FC, Sadras VO (2018) Comparison of sensitive stages of wheat, barley, canola, chickpea and field pea to temperature and water stress across Australia. Agric For Meteorol 248:275–294

Erbs M, Manderscheid R, Jansen G, Seddig S, Wroblewitz S, Hüther L, Schenderlein A, Wieser H, Dänicke S, Weigel H-J (2015) Elevated CO2 (FACE) affects food and feed quality of cereals (wheat, barley, maize): interactions with N and water supply. Procedia Environ Sci 29:57–58. https://doi.org/10.1016/j.proenv.2015.07.155

Farré I, Robertson M, Asseng S (2007) Reliability of canola production in different rainfall zones of Western Australia. Aust J Agric Res 58(4):326–334

Fourcaud T, Zhang X, Stokes A, Lambers H, Körner C (2008) Plant growth modelling and applications: the increasing importance of plant architecture in growth models. Ann Bot 101(8):1053–1063. https://doi.org/10.1093/aob/mcn050

George N, kaffka S (2017) Canola as a new crop of California: a stimulation study. Agron J 109(2):496–509

González FG, Slafer GA, Miralles DJ (2003) Floret development and spike growth as affected by photoperiod during stem elongation in wheat. Field Crop Res 81(1):29–38. https://doi.org/10.1016/S0378-4290(02)00196-X

He D, Wang J, Wang E (2015) Modelling the impact of climate variability and irrigation on winter canola yield and yield gap in Southwest China. MODSIM 2015. In: 21st international congress on modelling and simulation. Modelling and simulation society of Australia and New Zealand, pp 389–395

Hoogenboom G (2000) Contribution of agrometeorology to the simulation of crop production and its applications. Agric For Meteorol 103(1–2):137–157

Hosaini Y, Homaee M, Karimian NA, Saadat S (2012) Modeling vegetative stage response of canola (*Brassica napus* L.) to combined salinity and boron tresses. Int J Plant Prod 3(1):91–104

IPCC (2014) Summary for policymakers. In: Field CB, Barros VR, Dokken DJ et al (eds) Climate change 2014: impacts, adaptation, and vulnerability. Part a: global and sectoral aspects. Contribution of working group II to the fifth assessment report of the intergovernmental panel on climate change. Cambridge University Press, Cambridge, United Kingdom and New York, NY, USA, pp 1–32

Jing Q, Shang J, Qian B, Hoogenboom G, Huffman T, Liu J, Walters D (2016) Evaluation of the CSM-CROPGRO-canola model for simulating canola growth and yield at West Nipissing in eastern Canada. Agron J 108(2):575–584

Mal S, Singh RB, Huggel C, Grover A (2018) Introducing linkages between climate change, extreme events, and disaster risk reduction. In: Mal S, Singh RB, Huggel C (eds) Climate change, extreme events and disaster risk reduction: towards sustainable development goals. Springer International Publishing, Cham, pp 1–14. https://doi.org/10.1007/978-3-319-56469-2_1

Miralles DJ, Richards RA (2000) Responses of leaf and tiller emergence and primordium initiation in wheat and barley to interchanged photoperiod. Ann Bot 85(5):655–663. https://doi.org/10.1006/anbo.2000.1121

Moss ED, Evans DM (2022) Experimental climate warming reduces floral resources and alters insect visitation and wildflower seed set in a cereal agro-ecosystem. Front Plant Sci 13. https://doi.org/10.3389/fpls.2022.826205

Pérez-Gianmarco TI, Severini AD, González FG (2020) Photoperiod-sensitivity genes (Ppd-1): quantifying their effect on the photoperiod response model in wheat. J Exp Bot 71(3): 1185–1198

Qian B, Jing Q, Bélanger G, Shang J, Huffman T, Liu J, Hoogenboom G (2018) Simulated canola yield responses to climate change and adaptation in Canada. Agron J 110(1):133–146

Robertson MJ, Asseng S, Kirkegaard JA, Wratten N, Holland JF, Watkinson AR, Farre I (2002) Environmental and genotypic control of time to flowering in canola and Indian mustard. Aust J Agric Res 53(7):793–809

Shalom SR, Gillett D, Zemach H, Kimhi S, Forer I, Zutahy Y, Eshel D (2015) Storage temperature controls the timing of garlic bulb formation via shoot apical meristem termination. Planta 242(4):951–962

Slafer GA, Rawson HM (1994) Does temperature affect final numbers of primordia in wheat? Field Crop Res 39(2–3):111–117. https://doi.org/10.1016/0378-4290(94)90013-2

Tchorzewska D, Bocianowski J, Najda A, Dąbrowska A, Winiarczyk K (2017) Effect of environment fluctuations on biomass and allicin level in Allium sativum (cv. Harnas, Arkus) and Allium ampeloprasum var. ampeloprasum (GHG-L). J Appl Bot Food Qual 90

Torabi B, Adibnya M, Rahimi A, Azari A (2020) Modeling flowering response to temperature and photoperiod in safflower. Ind Crop Prod 151:112474. https://doi.org/10.1016/j.indcrop.2020.112474

Wallach D, Thorburn PJ (2017) Estimating uncertainty in crop model predictions: current situation and future prospects. Eur J Agron 88:201708

Walker WH 2nd, Meléndez-Fernández OH, Nelson RJ, Reiter RJ (2019) Global climate change and invariable photoperiods: a mismatch that jeopardizes animal fitness. Ecol Evol 9(17):10044–10054. https://doi.org/10.1002/ece3.5537

Whitechurch EM, Slafer GA, Miralles DJ (2007) Variability in the duration of stem elongation in wheat genotypes and sensitivity to photoperiod and vernalization. J Agron Crop Sci 193(2): 131–137

Yordanova MM, Loughran G, Zhdanov AV, Mariotti M, Kiniry SJ, O'Connor P, Gladyhev V (2018) M 1 mR employ ribosome stalling as a mechanism for molecular memory formation. Nature 553(7688):356–360

Chapter 19
Modelling and Field-Based Evaluation of Vernalisation Requirement of Canola for Higher Yield Potential

Emaan Yaqub, Mukhtar Ahmed, Ameer Hamza, Ghulam Shabbir, Muhammad Iftikhar Hussain, and Fayyaz-ul-Hassan

Abstract The climate is getting changed around the world, and it is influencing the agricultural production and agronomic practices. The agriculture sector is highly vulnerable to the phenomena of climate change. In Pakistan, the phenomena of climate change have been witnessed from decades and affecting the agriculture production and management practices, but no serious steps have been taken to minimise the problems of climate change and to reduce the effects of climate change on agriculture production and agronomic practices. Hence, the current study was carried out during canola growing seasons of 2019–2020 and 2020–2021 at both sites under rainfed conditions of Pothwar by keeping in view the circumstances of climate change aided with simulation modelling. The experiment was conducted with eight cultivars of canola arranging with the randomised complete block design with three replications at both sites with different sowing dates to form variable conditions of climate change during different phenological stages of crop specifically at flowering stage and grain filling stage. The Decision Support System for Agrotechnology Transfer (DSSAT) was used to simulate crop phenology, leaf area index (LAI), biomass, and yield. Days to the end of flowering was predicted by DSSAT with close association with observed days. The model predicted the days to

---

E. Yaqub · M. Ahmed (✉) · A. Hamza · Fayyaz-ul-Hassan
Department of Agronomy, PMAS Arid Agriculture University, Rawalpindi, Pakistan
e-mail: ahmadmukhtar@uaar.edu.pk

G. Shabbir
Department of Plant Breeding and Genetics, Pir Mehr Ali Shah Arid Agriculture University, Rawalpindi, Pakistan

M. I. Hussain
Department of Plant Biology and Soil Science, Universidade de Vigo, Vigo, Pontevedra, Spain

CITACA, Agri-Food Research and Transfer Cluster, Campus da Auga, Universidade de Vigo, Ourense, Spain

Research Institute of Science & Engineering (RISE), University of Sharjah, Sharjah, UAE

© The Author(s), under exclusive license to Springer Nature Switzerland AG 2022
M. Ahmed (ed.), *Global Agricultural Production: Resilience to Climate Change*,
https://doi.org/10.1007/978-3-031-14973-3_19

maturity with close association with our observed days to maturity with R^2, RMSE and d-index of 0.99, 0.55 and 0.99, respectively. The model simulated LAI with good accuracy with R^2, RMSE and d-index value of 1, 0 and 1, respectively. The simulation outcomes for the biological yield depicted good performance of model with R^2, RMSE and d-index values of 0.99, 67.46 kg ha^{-1} and 0.99, respectively. Furthermore, grain yield simulation was close to observed data with R^2, RMSE and d-index of 0.98, 29.39 kg ha^{-1} and 0.99, respectively. The findings of our studies confirm that DSSAT is a good research tool that can be used to evaluate different managements and cultivars under multiple environments and furthermore can be used to design crop ideotypes as per changing requirements of the climate.

Keywords Climate changeDSSAT · Crop phenology · Leaf area index · Biomass · Yield · Ideotypes

19.1 Introduction

Climate change has harmed agricultural production and ecological systems in both developed and developing countries (Ahmed 2020; IPCC 2018), as the mean temperature is expected to increase by 0.3–4.8 °C at the end of the twenty-first century across the globe (IPCC 2013). It is expected that the crop growth, phenology and particularly yield are altered due to the increase in temperature and uncertainty in extreme events such as dry days, wet days, floods and droughts (Fatima et al. 2020; Babel et al. 2019; Kheir et al. 2022; Rahman et al. 2018). Since the Industrial Revolution, the global mean temperature has risen by 0.85 °C, and Pakistan ranked in the top ten countries globally which is effected due to climate change in the last 20 years, according to Germanwatch. Pakistan witnessed 152 extreme weather events and lost 0.53% per unit GDP (Global Climate Risk Index 2020). Extreme event in the form of flood (e.g. 2022 flood) resulted to almost $10 billion damage to the economy of Pakistan. The agriculture industry of Pakistan is considered to be vulnerable to climate change (Tariq et al. 2018; Ahmed et al. 2019). The impact of climate change on the agricultural production in Pakistan will vary across agricultural regions, based on direct/abiotic (climate warming) and indirect/biotic (augmented by pest and pathogen pressure) effects on crop production. Climate change in Pakistan is resulting in the shortage of food, and it is directly impacting the crop production (Abbas et al. 2017; Rasul and Sharma 2016). In Punjab, Pakistan, climate change has had a negative impact on canola phenology, leading to a little seed output (Zahoor et al. 2022). Many recent global climate change studies have found that climate change poses a severe danger to agricultural production systems in poor countries (IPCC 2019). This temperature trend has been documented in Punjab, Pakistan, for three decades, the start of the 1980s and primarily in the 2000s (Wang et al. 2011). The average temperature in Punjab, Pakistan, has risen by 0.78–1.5 °C over the last three decades and is anticipated to rise from 2 to 4 °C by the termination of the era, potentially affecting agricultural production (Naz et al. 2022; Ahmad et al. 2015). The average annual increase in surface temperature has had an impact on Pakistan's socio-economic sector (Akram and Hamid 2015).

Climate and agronomic managing strategies, such as sowing dates and cultivar selection, influence the phenology of all crops (Afzal et al. 2021; Ahmad et al. 2016). The long-term response of crop phenology to heating drifts has been difficult to quantify due to constant changes in sowing dates and the introduction of new cultivars (Ahmad et al. 2017). Crop improvement rates are boosted in most environments as temperatures rise (Ahmad et al. 2016), and increase in temperature has a direct impact on the length of phenological phases and, as a result, on seed output (Sommer et al. 2013). To develop improved adaptation techniques, like enhanced agronomic practices and better cultivars, which can lessen the potential harmful influence of climate change, it is essential to understand the phenological reactions of a crop as a result of variations in local temperature (Ahmad et al. 2016; Ahmed et al. 2022; Ali et al. 2022). An increase in temperature may be causing the duration of the phenological phases to shorten and the phenological phases of crop cycles to advancement. Later sowing dates and the introduction of new cultivars with a longer thermal time need could lessen these effects (Li et al. 2016). Vernalisation is the process in which flowering of a fully hydrated seed or a growing plant is developing by the cold treatment. The vegetative period of the plant is short, leading to an early flowering because of vernalisation. Plants requiring vernalisation show a delayed flowering or a vegetative flora without cold treatment. Often, these plants become rosettes with no elongation of the stem. Vernalisation involves the production of a hormone called vernalin; Melcher (1939) discovered it. Vernalisation is a process of aerobics which requires metabolic energy. Since all genotypes of canola appear to be commonly vernalised, it has been considered in many phenological models to affect phenological development (Wang et al. 2012). Vernalisation of germinated seeds or seedlings, just above freezing, is affected by the phenological development of canola. Seedlings exposed to these conditions are more responsive to the temperature and photoperiod effects than to those not vernalised seedlings. Vernalisation is process by which plants use a prolonged cold period (winter) to promote flowering. Many plants are vernalised and actively repress flora until after a prolonged cold exposure. This synchronises seed production with the favourable spring environment. It is equally important to have certain photoperiods and ambient temperatures following vernalisation. The growing degree days (GDD) approach was the first approach of assessing the influence of temperature on phenological development. A base temperature is assumed in this system, and the rate of development is a linear function of temperature above this temperature. GDDs are computed by taking the average of the day's maximum and minimum temperatures and deducting the base temperature. Growing degree days are accumulated during the growing season, usually starting from planting date, and a GDD need for each stage of development is determined using field observations (Aslam et al. 2017).

Crop simulation models were developed to evaluate agronomic management options and to help analysts understand the relationship between ecosystem, production variance and management. Crop phenological modelling is effective for simulating plant growth processes that could take years in the field to quantify (Fourcaud et al. 2008). These models have been utilised by several research organisations to make judgments in the agricultural system (Hoogenboom et al. 2019;

Bannayan et al. 2003). Crop models use high and low temperature, average rainfall and solar radiation per day as inputs to estimate daily growth and development. Crop models, such as the Decision Support System for Agrotechnology Transfer (DSSAT), are a useful tool for assessing and determining the causes of crop management issues, mostly in developing nations where climatic circumstances are changing (Hoogenboom et al. 2015). The objectives of this study were to evaluate the vernalisation requirement of canola cultivars under the specific regions of the University Research Farm Koont (URF-Koont) and National Agricultural Research Centre Islamabad (NARC-Islamabad) and to identify the ideotypes to inform breeders which varieties have less vernalisation requirement for the selected regions. We used the DSSAT-CROPGRO simulation model as a tool to predict the likely performance of selected canola cultivars under the range of selected locations and its environments. We hypothesised that the vernalisation requirement of canola cultivars will be less, and we will find out the short-duration varieties with high yield potential. However, in Pakistan, the evaluation of vernalisation requirement of canola has not been reported yet. Therefore, in Pakistan, it was needed to conduct an experiment on the evaluation of vernalisation requirement of canola to increase its yield potential.

19.2 Crop Modelling and Canola Production Under Changing Climate

Cristy et al. (2019) concluded that field experimentation and crop simulation studies were used over the potential cropping zone of Southern Australia to determine the yield potential of winter-spring canola crosses compared to currently available spring-type and winter-type cultivars. According to analyses, the four evaluated winter-spring crosses had a variety of vernalisation requirements, ranging from minor spring-type requirements to high winter-type requirements. The Catchment Analysis Tool (CAT) spatial modelling framework was used in this study to evaluate the expected canola yields of four cultivars across the entire cropping region of Southern Australia. Whish et al. (2020) performed a thorough phenological study of Australian canola cultivars at three locations with different vernal temperatures and photoperiods combined with a synthetic light system to extend the light system to 16 h. Only a few commercial Australian cultivars demonstrated substantial photoperiod responses, but the majority showed large vernal responses. Furthermore, the method for calculating vernal time (using the average daily temperature determined from the maximum and minimum temperatures or the sub-daily temperature estimate) altered the conclusions of how vernal exposure shortened flowering time. Waalen et al. (2014) performed an experiment to examine if there was a relation between the maintenance of cultivar-specific freezing tolerance levels and vernalisation saturation in winter rapeseed (*Brassica napus* L.) under field circumstances. Two cultivars, 'Banjo' and 'Californium', with varying vernalisation requirements, were chosen after a controlled screening of 18 cultivars. The vernalisation response and freezing tolerance of the two cultivars under field conditions were evaluated on five different dates throughout the winter of 2010/2011. Californium reached vernalisation saturation on October 11, but 'Banjo' took 13 days longer. The maximum freezing tolerance of the two cultivars was reached in early December, and it was sustained for 31 days in 'Californium' and 67 days in 'Banjo'. The results of the experiment suggested that freezing tolerance and vernalisation saturation do not have a straightforward relationship. Matar et al. (2021) investigated the effect of photoperiod and developmental age on flowering time and vernalisation responsiveness in winter rapeseed, as well as the timing of vernalisation-driven floral transition. Floral transition is initiated within a few weeks of vernalisation, according to microscopy and whole transcriptome investigations of shoot apical meristems of plants maintained under controlled conditions. The presence of some Bna.SOC1 and Bna.SPL5 homoeologs among the induced genes suggests that they are involved in the timing of cold-induced floral transition. Furthermore, the blooming response of plants with a shorter pre-vernalisation time was linked to Bna.SOC1 and Bna.SPL5 gene expression delays. Nikoubin et al. (2009) conducted an experiment to see how vernalisation affects the phenology and development rates of canola types in a split plot; the experiment was set up as a randomised complete block design with four replications. The results revealed that increasing the vernalisation time from 0 to 50 days resulted in a reduction in the number of days spent at each stage of development (the commencement of green and yellow buds, as well as the beginning and end of flowering) and an increase in growth rate. The response of all cultivars to vernalisation was quantitative, showing that no-vernalisation treatment did not prevent flowering. The cultivars could flower if they developed at 85–94% of their maximum development rate. In Hyola308, the demand for vernalisation was 30 days, whereas in other varieties, it was 50 days. A basic vernalisation model was developed as a result of this research, which might be utilised in canola phenological development simulation models.

Schiessl et al. (2015) concluded that climate and day length adaptation influence flowering period, plant height and seed yield in crop plants. To evaluate these features under widely different field circumstances in the essential oilseed crop *Brassica napus*, they undertook a genome-wide association research using data from multiple agro-ecological environments spanning three continents. The Brass genome project genotyped 158 European winter-type *B. napus* inbred lines with 21,623 distinct single-locus single-nucleotide polymorphism (SNP) markers. Over the years 2010–2012, the panel calculated phenotypic relationships for blooming time, plant height and seed yield in 5 highly diverse locales in Germany, China and Chile, a total of 11 distinct environments. Rapacz and Markowski (1999) reported that there was a strong link between winter hardiness and frost resistance in both rape groups. In oilseed rapes grown in the late 1970s, cultivars with low erucic acid, particularly double zero, were less winter hardy than cultivars with high erucic acid. Double-zero cultivars have lesser frost resistance and reduced vernalisation requirements. There's also a relationship between the need for vernalisation and frost tolerance and field survival. Frost resistance of double-zero cultivars in the 1990s was higher than double-low cultivars in the late 1970s. The decline in glucosinolate concentration in the 1970s was found to be associated with a decrease in the requirement for winter hardiness and vernalisation of cultivars. Over the next 20 years, the winter hardiness of double-low cultivars improved, but the vernalisation requirements remained the same. As a result, there was no link found between winter hardiness and the need for vernalisation in modern canola cultivars. Wang et al. (2012) reported that the APSIM-Canola model was calibrated and tested from the data of three field trial locations. In these tests, several cultivars and planting dates were used, and the main phenological phases, biomass and grain production were recorded. The model was able to simulate the commencement of phenological phases with varied sowing dates after the calibration of phenological parameters and explain the difference in biomass and yield induced by late sowing. The model, on the other hand, overestimated canola production under late sowing dates. Canola production dropped linearly with later sowing time, owing to reduced vegetative growth stages, and fluctuated greatly due to inter-annual climate variability, according to the data. On average, the yield potential in the studied region is 3 tonnes/ha. He et al. (2015) concluded that by using the APSIM-Canola model, we can estimate canola crop yield potential and yield gap. Similarly, APSIM can help to quantify the impact of inter-annual climate variability and irrigation water requirement to close the yield gap. The future canola production was totally irrigated, according to the results of a single hybrid cultivar simulation (3452 kg ha^{-1}). Irrigation boosts production and water productivity, especially in dry seasons. Raman et al. (2019) conducted an experiment to improve the resilience of canola to climate change; an integrated approach for breeding climate-smart varieties is required. Although the majority of the current breeding targets for canola improvement programs remain largely unchanged, emerging climate uncertainties reinforced the development of high-yielding resilient varieties for tolerance to excessive drought, frost, heat and waterlogging. Ecological and evolutionary adaptation and selective breeding processes have provided a range of natural variation in 'climate-smart traits' in canola and its closely related species.

19.3 Materials and Methods

Field experiment was conducted at two variable study sites, i.e. NARC-Islamabad (33.6701° N and 73.1261° E) and URF-Koont (32.9328° N and longitude 72.8630° E) (Figs. 19.1 and 19.2). Eight cultivars of canola were used as a plant material. This includes Punjab Canola, Faisal Canola, Super Canola, NARC Sarsoon, LG-3295, Rohi Sarsoon, Cyclone and Crusher during 2019–2020 and 2020–2021. The total area of the field selected was 325 m^2 for each site, and the size of each plot was 2×3 m. Daily weather data of study sites were collected from the Pakistan Meteorological Department (PMD) for the years 2019–2020 and 2020–2021. At both sites (NARC-Islamabad and URF-Koont) during years 2019–2020 and 2020–2021, the seasonal mean maximum temperature was 21.17 °C and 23 °C and 22.3 °C and 23.7 °C, respectively, and the seasonal minimum temperature was 8.7 °C and 8 °C

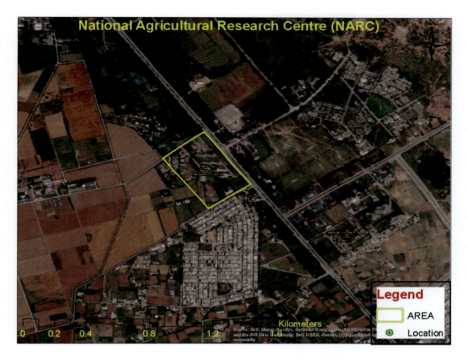

Fig. 19.1 Study site 1, i.e. the National Agricultural Research Centre (NARC) Islamabad

and 7.43 °C and 7.4 °C, respectively. The seasonal rainfall was 555.16 mm and 244.86 mm and 386.4 mm and 161.4 mm, respectively. The seasonal solar radiation was 13.55 and 14.98 and 14.54 and 15.74 MJ/m^2/d, respectively. On the basis of the collected weather data, we observed that the seasonal mean maximum temperature was high at URF-Koont than NARC-Islamabad and the temperature increase ranged between 0.7 and 1.83 °C during both growing seasons at both sites.

Growing degree days (GDD) were calculated as given by McMaster and Wilhelm (1997) using daily Tmin and Tmax and a base temperature of 5 °C as:

$$\text{Accumulative GDD} = \Sigma\,[(T\max + T\min)/2 - Tb]$$

where Tmax was the maximum daily temperature; Tmin, the minimum daily temperature; and Tb, the base temperature, which was taken as 5 °C.

The land was prepared with disc plough, and tillage practices at both sites were done to make the selected area well prepared. Crop was sown with the hand drill at a depth of 1.5 inch with plant-to-plant and row-to-row distance of 10 cm and 30 cm, respectively. The total area of the field selected was 325 m^2 for each site, and the size of each plot was 2×3 m. The recommended doses of fertilisers N-P-K were added at the time of sowing 90-60-50 kg h^{-1}, respectively. The experiment was designed with the randomised complete block design (RCBD) with three replications. Six

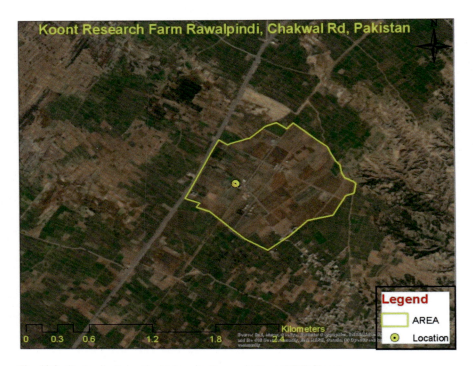

Fig. 19.2 Study site 2, i.e. the University Research Farm (URF) Koont

lines for each cultivar were maintained within each experimental plot at both locations during both growing seasons. The sowing of canola crop was done in between October 16 and 20 at NARC-Islamabad for years 2019–2020 and 2020–2021, while at URF-Koont, the sowing was done in between October 10 and 20 for both years. Different crop parameters were measured at different crop growth stages; crop measurement parameters were days to emergence, days to anthesis, days to end of flowering, leaf area index (LAI), days to maturity, biological yield and grain yield. We measured and observed all the crop parameters for both sites during both growing seasons. To check the soil physio-chemical properties, soil samples were collected from different layers of the experimental fields from 0 to 90 cm at every 30 cm depth intervals at both sites. The soil physio-chemical properties such as texture, sand%, silt%, clay%, organic carbon (OC), bulk density (BD), pH, SNH_4 mg kg^{-1}, SNO_3 mg kg^{-1}, soil lower limit (SLL), soil density upper limit (SDUL) and soil saturation (SSAT) were determined at each depth. The soil samples' analysis results showed that the soil texture was silt loam at NARC-Islamabad and sandy clay loam at URF-Koont. The soil profile at 30 cm depth contained 34% sand, 33% silt, 33% clay, 0.8% OC, 1.3% BD, 7.6 pH, 0.6 SNH4 mg kg^{-1}, 5.2 SNO_3 mg kg^{-1}, 0.195 SLL cm cm^{-1}, 0.36 SDUL cm cm^{-1} and 0.45 SSAT cm cm^{-1} at NARC and 56% sand, 22% silt, 22% clay, 0.65% OC, 1.45% BD, 8.1 pH, 0.5 SNH_4 mg kg^{-1}, 4.2 SNO_3 mg kg^{-1}, 0.1512 SLL cm cm^{-1}, 0.245 SDUL

19 Modelling and Field-Based Evaluation of Vernalisation Requirement... 525

Table 19.1 Soil physio-chemical variables at NARC-Islamabad

Depth	Sand %	Silt %	Clay %	O.C	B.D	PH	SLL	SDUL	SSAT	Texture
0–30 cm	34	33	33	0.80	1.30	7.60	0.195	0.360	0.450	Silt loam
30–60 cm	32	33	35	0.60	1.35	8.20	0.195	0.350	0.440	Silt loam
60–90 cm	32	33	35	0.41	1.35	8.40	0.200	0.340	0.430	Silt loam

Table 19.2 Soil physio-chemical variables at URF-Koont

Depth	Sand %	Silt %	Clay %	O.C	B.D	PH	SLL	SDUL	SSAT	Texture
0–30 cm	56	22	22	0.65	1.45	8.1	0.151	0.245	0.417	Sandy clay loam
30–60 cm	56	20	24	0.45	1.45	8.8	0.151	0.245	0.417	Sandy clay loam
60–90 cm	54	20	26	0.31	1.50	8.5	0.145	0.245	0.417	Sandy clay loam

cm cm^{-1} and 0.417 SSAT cm cm^{-1} at URF-Koont. All physio-chemical properties of soil for both locations have been shown in Tables 19.1 and 19.2.

19.3.1 Phenological Modelling

The phenological growth of canola cultivars from emergence to maturity was measured at two different sites in response to different sowing dates for research studies. A phenological model with distinct sensitivities to vernalisation was applied to the measured phenological data for canola cultivars in these crop experiments at two different locations. The phenological model was updated using optimisation to minimise the least square difference between the measured and predicted dates for canola phenological stages (generalised reduced gradient nonlinear method). Day length, temperature and vernalisation are used to determine the time it takes for two developmental stages in the phenological model, being emergence-start of flowering (SOF) and from start of flowering-end of flowering (EOF). To calculate the daily phenological growth rate (TT_{PP}), the accumulated photo-thermal sum including base temperature (PTT_B), photoperiod (F_{PP}) and vernalisation (F_{vern}) criteria is used, as follows:

$$TT_{PP} = \sum (PTT_B \times F_{PP} \times F_{vern})$$

Temperature growth rate is dependent on the daily average temperature (TT) ranging from 5 °C to an ideal temperature of 26 °C, where development occurs at a rapid rate. The effect of photoperiod (PP_{hr}) on the duration of thermal time was considered through a calculation of day length using the site-specific latitudes for each day.

$$PTT_B = \sum \left(TT_{BO} \times PP_{hr} \times 24^{-1}\right)$$

The effect of photoperiod among cultivars was calculated by using day length and photoperiod sensitivity (PP_{sen}). A daily photoperiod factor was calculated as:

$$F_{PP} = 1 - (0.01 \times PP_{sen}) \times (20 - PP_h)^2$$

The effect of vernalisation was integrated into the model by using a daily vernalisation factor (F_{vern}). Using the technique described by White et al. (2008), the total number of vernalisation days ($Vern_{sen}$, d) needed to achieve full vernalisation was estimated to be between -4 and 18 °C, where average daily temperatures between 2 and 12 °C allocated a vernalisation unit (VD) of 1. VD decreases linearly from 9 to 18 °C for temperatures greater than 12 °C, where it reaches zero. VD decreases linearly from 2 to -4 °C, where its value is zero, for temperatures less than 2 °C.

$$V\nabla = \sum VD - Devern$$

According to the work of Ritchie and Nesmith (1991), if the daily maximum temperature exceeds 25 °C, devernalisation (Devern) was assumed to occur. Using this $V\Delta$ (d) and $Vern_{sen}$ (d), a daily vernalisation factor (F_{vern}, dd^{-1}) is calculated.

$$F_{vern} = \frac{V\nabla}{Vernsen}$$

The phenological phases of emergence-SOF and SOF-EOF were achieved by using the specific parameters of $Vern_{sen}$ when the cultivar-specific TT_{PP} was reached for that phase.

19.3.2 Model Description

For DSSAT model simulation, the inputs required were comprehensive physical and hydraulic properties of soil. The model was not set with autovalidation and calibration. To validate the model for conditions of any locality, changes are made in its parameters. Different new files are created for different management zones to precise agriculture using DSSAT. Assessment of simulations with observed results evaluates the model's value and suitability for accurate prediction and area (Porter et al. 2010). The inputs required under different situations for the application of model are soil properties, genotype information, weather data and experimental condition. These application software aid to prepare these databases and to compare simulated results with observed values and to improve the model's efficiency and accuracy. Proper crop management for risk valuation can be simulated with DSSAT model.

19.3.3 Model Calibration

19.3.3.1 Genetic Parameter Estimations with the DSSAT-GLUE Package

The generalised likelihood uncertainty estimation (GLUE) is a latest method which is used for sensitivity and uncertainty analysis (Yan et al. 2020). On the basis of experimental data, for estimating cultivar parameters, the GLUE method has been integrated into DSSAT (Hoogenboom et al. 2020). In DSSAT, the GLUE method doesn't determine parameters like dry biomass or leaf area, but it can determine parameters related to growth stages and grain characteristics (Li et al. 2018). Experimental data file (T-file) was added to DSSAT and GLUE tool was used to get the best fit. This procedure was repeated for both sites during both growing seasons.

19.3.3.2 Upscaling Strategies for Cultivar Parameters in Regional Simulation of Canola Growth

For cultivar genetic parameter estimations of canola, two upscaling strategies were established and evaluated for two experimental datasets. Split of these upscaling strategies into two types of solutions could be done. On the basis of recorded data for days to anthesis, days to end of flowering, days to maturity, leaf area index, biological yield, grain yield and harvest index, the first type of solution estimated genetic parameters of canola cultivars. The second type attempted to quantify the distribution of genetic parameters for canola cultivars. On the basis of observations for the conducted experiments at both sites NARC-Islamabad and URF-Koont for years 2019–2020 and 2020–2021, this type of solution was established for canola cultivars. In simulations of days to anthesis, days to end of flowering, days to maturity, leaf area index, biological yield, grain yield and harvest index, the upscaling strategies were compared.

19.3.3.3 Strategy 1: Single-Site Parameters (SSPs)

In this strategy, the different canola cultivars were assumed to be sown at both sites NARC-Islamabad and URF-Koont during years 2019–2020 and 2020–2021. Each cultivar was parameterised and validated to explore the uncertainties caused by cultivars during simulation. With the DSSAT-GLUE package, the cultivar genetic parameters were estimated for each site by using observed days to anthesis, days to end of flowering, days to maturity, leaf area index, biological yield, grain yield and harvest index of both years 2019–2020 and 2020–2021. During the study, we focused on uncertainties of SSPs in simulations of phenology.

19.3.3.4 Strategy 2: Virtual Cultivar Parameters (VCPs) Generated from the Posterior Parameter Distributions

Based on observations of eight canola cultivars sown at both sites, the genetic parameters were estimated for each cultivar during both growing seasons 2019–2020 and 2020–2021. The validation of estimated genetic parameters was done for both sites during both growing seasons. In model calibration, we input the required files in the model for its calibration, and the model does not provide automated procedure for its calibration. To validate the model, changes in the input parameters must be done. In DSSAT application, several types of files are generated to get simulated results which includes file X, file A, file T, soil file, climate file and genetic coefficients file. In the optimisation process for each cultivar, the two parameters that were changed $Vern_{sen}$ and TT_{PP}. Vernalisation sensitivity is the $Vern_{sen}$ needed for vernalisation saturation, a sum near 0 being insensitive and a sum near 50 d being very sensitive. These parameters were calculated for both emergence-start of flowering (SOF) and start of flowering-end of flowering (SOF-EOF). The goodness of fit of the model can be judged by the model's ability to predict the saturation from emergence-SOF and SOF-EOF at each site. A root mean square error (RMSE) of 5 days between the measured and predicted flowering dates on a national basis is similar to other canola models (Habekotté 1997; Deligios et al. 2013).

19.3.4 Model Performance Evaluation

During the canola growing season of 2019–2020 and 2020–2021 field experiments, the model was evaluated on the basis of collected data. Genotypic coefficient was changed until the simulation results were different at 10% of observed data for major development stages of canola. Comparison between observed and simulated values was developed for parameters regarding the growth and development of canola to improve cultivar coefficient and for sensitivity analysis of the model.

19.3.5 Statistical Analysis

Analysis of variance (ANOVA) was performed to test the significant difference between means of various parameters for eight varieties at two locations (Islamabad and Chakwal) for the year 2019–2020 and 2020–2021 growing seasons using Statistics 8.1. To find all possible interactions of varieties and locations, the ANOVA was performed. The collected data was statistically analysed and used to parameterise the DSSAT model to run simulating long-term daily climatic data (1988–2021) for selected sites.

19.4 Results and Discussion

19.4.1 Climatic Specifications

The weather conditions that prevailed during both growing seasons at URF-Koont have been shown in Figs. 19.3 and 19.4. The mean values of different climatic parameters were calculated at URF-Koont during the study years of 2019–2020 and 2020–2021. The seasonal mean maximum temperature was 22.3 °C and 23.7 °C, and the seasonal mean minimum temperature was 7.43 °C and 7.4 °C during years 2019–2020 and 2020–2021, respectively. The seasonal rainfall was 386.4 mm and 161.4 mm during growing seasons 2019–2020 and 2020–2021. The seasonal solar radiation was 14.54 and 15.74 MJ/m^2/d during growing seasons 2019–2020 and 2020–2021, respectively. The daily weather data was collected from the Pakistan

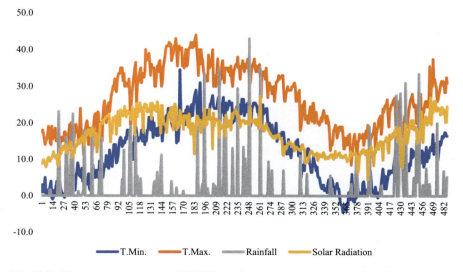

Fig. 19.3 Climatic characteristics of URF-Koont during growing season 2019–2020

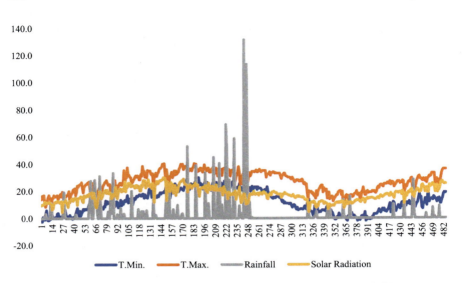

Fig. 19.4 Climatic characteristics of URF-Koont during growing season 2020–2021

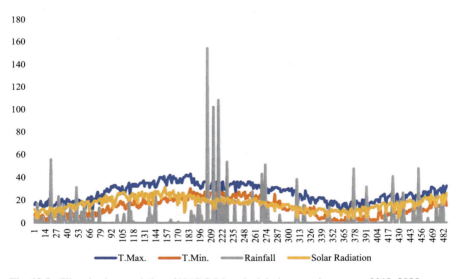

Fig. 19.5 Climatic characteristics of NARC-Islamabad during growing season 2019–2020

Meteorological Department (PMD). The weather conditions that prevailed during both growing seasons at NARC-Islamabad have been presented in Figs. 19.5 and 19.6. The mean values of different climatic parameters were calculated at NARC-Islamabad during study years of 2019–2020 and 2020–2021. The seasonal mean maximum temperature was 21.17 °C and 23 °C, and the seasonal mean minimum temperature was 8.7 °C and 8 °C during years 2019–2020 and 2020–2021,

19 Modelling and Field-Based Evaluation of Vernalisation Requirement... 531

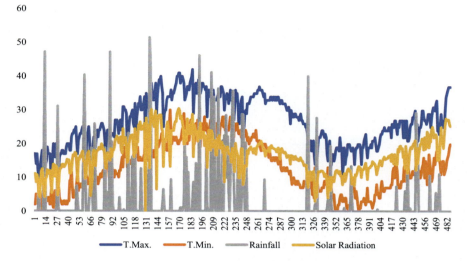

Fig. 19.6 Climatic characteristics of NARC-Islamabad during growing season 2020–2021

respectively. The seasonal rainfall was 555.16 mm and 244.86 mm during growing seasons 2019–2020 and 2020–2021, respectively. The solar radiation was 13.55 and 14.98 MJ/m^2/d during growing seasons 2019–2020 and 2020–2021, respectively. The daily weather data was collected from the Pakistan Meteorological Department (PMD).

19.4.2 Agronomic Parameters

19.4.2.1 Phenology

In the growing season of years 2019–2020 and 2020–2021 at NARC-Islamabad, days to emergence were 5 days after sowing (DAS) during both years, respectively, while at URF-Koont, days to emergence were 6–7 DAS during both years, respectively. According to our observed data, canola cultivars showed variation in days to anthesis at both locations during both growing seasons. At NARC-Islamabad during years 2019–2020, Cyclone took a maximum of 103 days and Faisal Canola took a minimum of 78 days to give the first flower after sowing. At URF-Koont, we observed that Faisal Canola took a maximum of 77 days and ROHI Sarsoon took a minimum of 57 days to give the first flower after sowing, respectively. During years 2020–2021 at NARC-Islamabad, we observed that Cyclone took a maximum of 102 and Faisal Canola took a minimum of 75 days to give the first flower after sowing. At URF-Koont, we observed that Super Canola took a maximum of 75 days and ROHI Sarsoon took a minimum of 54 days to give the first flower after sowing, respectively (Figs. 19.7, 19.8 and 19.9). Statistical analysis showed highly

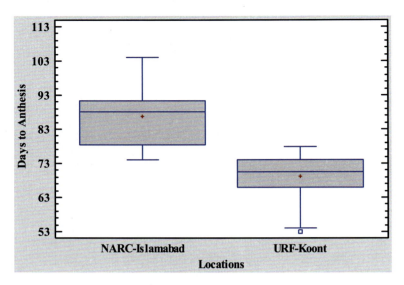

Fig. 19.7 Days to anthesis for both sites

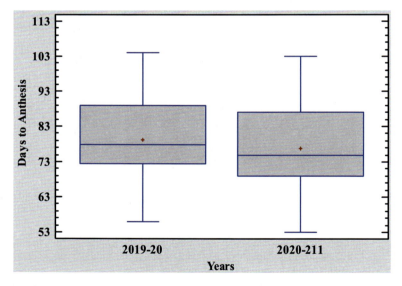

Fig. 19.8 Days to anthesis for growing seasons 2019–2020 and 2020–2021

significant results for locations (L), years (Y), cultivars (CUL) and L × CUL, while all other interactive effects, viz. L × Y, Y × CUL and L × Y × CUL, were non-significant at $p \leq 0.05$ (Table 19.3). The days to anthesis was less at URF-Koont during both years than NARC-Islamabad because the temperature was high at URF-Koont than at NARC-Islamabad during emergence to anthesis due to

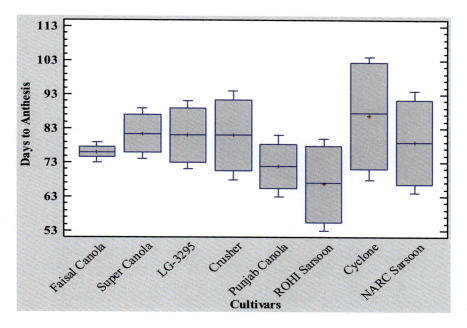

Fig. 19.9 Days to anthesis for cultivars

which the cultivars induce flowering in less days at URF-Koont. Crop growth and development rates are accelerated with an increase in temperature for most environments (Ahmad et al. 2016; Faraji et al. 2009). This increase in temperature has a direct effect on the duration of the phenological phases and ultimately impacts seed yield (Sommer et al. 2013; Tao et al. 2014; Xiao et al. 2016). Advancement of the phenological stages and a decrease in the duration of the phenological phases of crop cycles may occur due to an increase in temperature. Observed data showed variation in days to end of flowering for all cultivars at both sites during both growing seasons. We observed that during years 2019–2020 at NARC-Islamabad, the maximum and minimum days to end of flowering were taken by LG-3295 126 days and 79 days by ROHI Sarsoon. At URF-Koont, we observed that the maximum and minimum days to end of flowering were taken by Faisal Canola 118 days and 88 days by ROHI Sarsoon, respectively. During years 2020–2021, we observed that at NARC-Islamabad, the maximum and minimum days to end of flowering were taken by Crusher 122 days and 100 days by ROHI Sarsoon. At URF-Koont, we observed that the maximum and minimum days to end of flowering were taken by Super Canola 114 days and 81 days by ROHI Sarsoon, respectively (Figs. 19.10, 19.11 and 19.12). Statistical analysis showed highly significant results for L, Y, CUL, treatments and their interactions L × Y, L × CUL, Y × CUL and L × Y × CUL are highly significant. Increasing temperature resulted in variations in the duration of different phenological phases (Table 19.3). Therefore, an early shift in phenology will result in curtailed growth season under contemporary hop of increasing temperature. This

Table 19.3 For the three dependent variables, ANOVA table with degree of freedom with F values and significant levels are shown below

Source	DF	F values and significant level of fixed effects						
		DFF	DOF	DTM	LAI	B.Y	G.Y	H.I
R	2							
L	1	10672.1***	4947.12***	3350.15***	3313.22***	212.32***	4023.86***	48.90***
Y	1	236.73***	1451.50***	283.97***	17823.4***	2587.49***	36429.0***	234.47***
CUL	7	673.30***	779.74***	357.35***	2111.03***	203.42***	5440.39***	124.38***
LxY	1	2.15NS	34.35***	34.35***	735.64***	50.52***	470.17***	0.90**
LxCUL	7	384.27***	379.75***	311.88***	544.96***	74.38***	1432.30***	54.32***
YxCUL	7	0.84NS	52.76***	12.50***	131.96***	22.55***	295.15***	24.81***
LxYxCUL	7	1.23NS	42.94***	21.17***	194.72***	13.87***	139.59***	13.07***
Error	62							

R replication, *L* locations, *Y* years, *CUL* cultivars, *LxY* interaction of locations and years, *LxCUL* interaction of locations and cultivars, *YxCUL* interaction of years and cultivars, *LxYxCUL* interaction of locations, years and cultivars

**Significant level at 0.05 level

***Significant level at 0.01 level

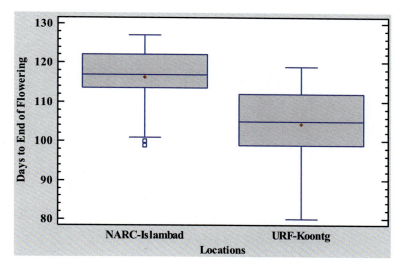

Fig. 19.10 Days to end of flowering for both sites

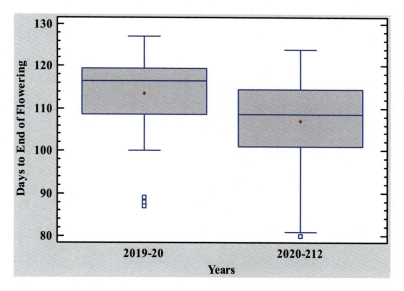

Fig. 19.11 Days to end of flowering for growing seasons 2019–2020 and 2020–2021

variability in phenological development under varying temperature regimes is confirmed by earlier findings (Roetzer et al. 2000; Hatfield et al. 2011; He et al. 2015). On the basis of our observed data, we conclude that during years 2019–2020 at NARC-Islamabad, the maximum and minimum days to maturity were taken by Crusher 186 days and by Faisal Canola 172 days. At URF-Koont, the maximum and minimum days to maturity were taken by Faisal Canola 180 days and by ROHI

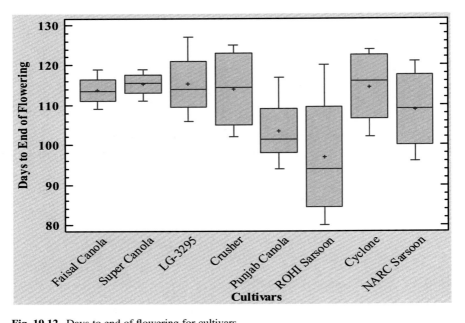

Fig. 19.12 Days to end of flowering for cultivars

Sarsoon 156 days, respectively. During years 2020–2021, we observed that at NARC-Islamabad, the maximum and minimum days to maturity were taken by Cyclone 186 days and by ROHI Sarsoon 170 days. At URF-Koont, we observed that the maximum and minimum days to maturity were taken by Faisal Canola 173 days and by ROHI Sarsoon 152 days, respectively (Figs. 19.13, 19.14 and 19.15). Analysis of variance showed highly significant results for L, Y, CUL, treatments and their interactions L × Y, L × CUL, Y × CUL and L × Y × CUL are highly significant (Table 19.3). The phenology of canola was highly influenced by varying climatic conditions of two selected study sites. The changes in canola phenology was caused by due to increase in temperature during growing seasons and at URF-Koont temperature was high during both growing seasons which results in shortening of phenological phases. Among different growth stages, start of flowering, anthesis and maturity are particularly found sensitive, and their durations were reduced under warming climate (Tao et al. 2013; Ahmad et al. 2015). Increasing temperature caused advancement in anthesis and maturity dates of crop and consequently shortened these phenological phases. This is in line with previous reports about different crops (Tao et al. 2012).

19.4.2.2 Biological and Grain Yield

During years 2019–2020 at NARC-Islamabad, the highest and lowest biological yield was observed in Super Canola 13842 kg h^{-1} and Faisal Canola 11860 kg ha^{-1}.

19 Modelling and Field-Based Evaluation of Vernalisation Requirement...

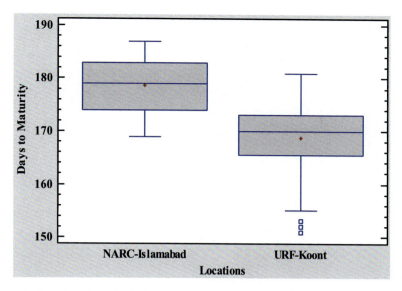

Fig. 19.13 Days to maturity for both sites

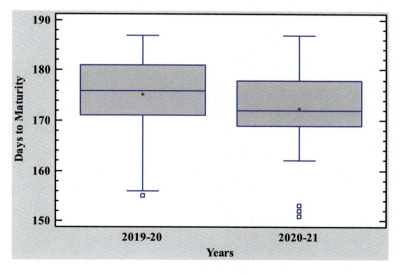

Fig. 19.14 Days to maturity for growing seasons 2019–2020 and 2020–2021

At URF-Koont, we observed the highest and lowest biological yield in ROHI Sarsoon 14100 kg ha^{-1} and Faisal Canola 11540 kg h^{-1}, respectively. During years 2020–2021 at NARC-Islamabad, the highest and lowest biological yield was observed in NARC Sarsoon 13092 kg ha^{-1} and Faisal Canola 11037 kg ha^{-1}. At URF-Koont, the highest and lowest biological yield was observed in NARC Sarsoon

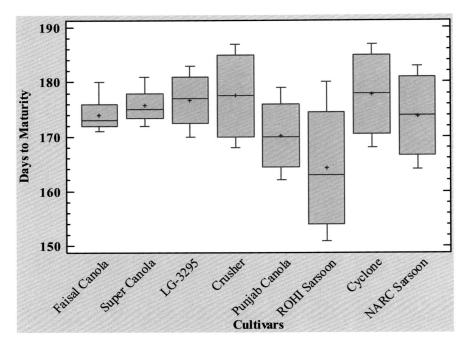

Fig. 19.15 Days to maturity for all cultivars

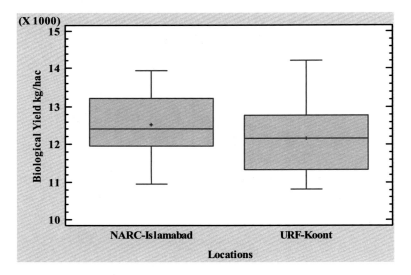

Fig. 19.16 Biological yield at both sites

19 Modelling and Field-Based Evaluation of Vernalisation Requirement... 539

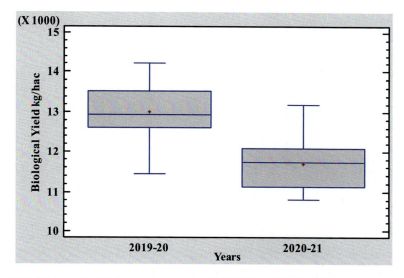

Fig. 19.17 Biological yield for growing seasons 2019–2020 and 2020–2021

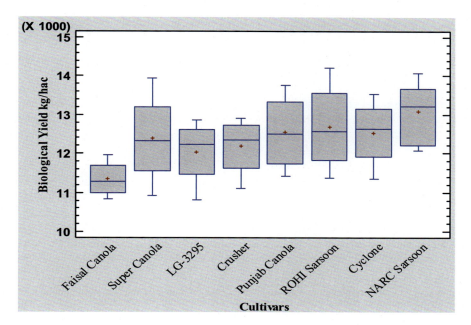

Fig. 19.18 Biological yield for cultivars

12166 kg ha^{-1} and LG-3295 10912 kg ha^{-1}, respectively (Figs. 19.16, 19.17 and 19.18). Biological yield showed variation among study sites. Analysis of variance table described those effects of L, Y, CUL, L × Y, L × CUL, Y × CUL and

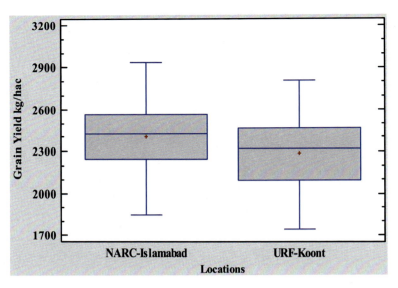

Fig. 19.19 Grain yield of both sites

L × Y × CUL were highly significant (Table 19.3). The growth and development of crop effected by temperature, which directly influences crop age and thus affects the biological and grain yield. Varying climatic parameters have their critical impact on yield. Challinor et al. (2009) also pointed that crop biomass was expressively affected due to change in environments. If the total period of growth and development of crop cultivars is short, then, consequently, there is a reduction of crop production because of the shorter time for total dry matter accumulation during the vegetative phase, particularly for high-input crops (Rezaei et al. 2015; Zhang et al. 2013). At NARC-Islamabad during years 2019–2020, the highest and lowest grain yield was observed for NARC Sarsoon 2926 kg h^{-1} and Faisal Canola 2231 kg h^{-1}. At URF-Koont, the highest and lowest grain yield was observed for ROHI Sarsoon 2796 kg h^{-1} and Faisal Canola 2112 kg h^{-1}, respectively. During years 2020–2021 at NARC-Islamabad, we noted the highest and lowest grain yield was observed for NARC Sarsoon 2667 kg h^{-1} and Faisal Canola 1862 kg h^{-1}. At URF-Koont, we noted the highest and lowest grain yield was observed for ROHI Sarsoon 2330 kg h^{-1} and Faisal Canola 1760 kg h^{-1}, respectively (Figs. 19.19, 19.20 and 19.21). Analysis of variance table showed that the effects of L, Y, CUL, L × Y, L × CUL, Y × CUL and L × Y × CUL were highly significant (Table 19.3). Climatic parameters had great influence on the production of canola crop. The temperature increased during years 2020–2021 at both sites which adversely affected the crop phenology and resulted in the shortening of crop duration, which further affected the grain yield negatively. Change in seasonal temperature impacted the crop production, and reduction in yield during 2020–2021 might be due to higher temperature. Due to warming trends, the biological and grain yield is reduced with early anthesis and maturity (Xiao and Tao 2014). By early anthesis and delayed

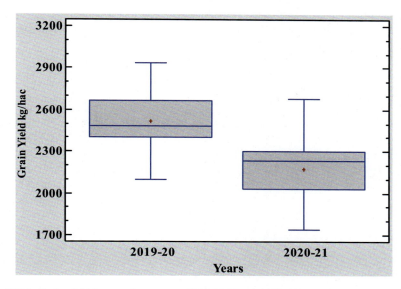

Fig. 19.20 Grain yield for growing seasons 2019–2020 and 2020–2021

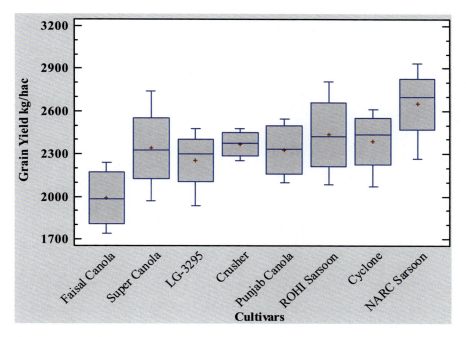

Fig. 19.21 Grain yield for cultivars

maturity, the production of several crops increased due to extended grain filling stage (He et al. 2015). The crop production is less if the duration of crop growth and development is short (Rezaei et al. 2015).

19.4.2.3 Harvest Index

At NARC-Islamabad during years 2019–2020, the highest and lowest harvest index was observed for NARC Sarsoon 21.91 and Faisal Canola 18.81. At URF-Koont, the highest and lowest harvest index was observed for ROHI Sarsoon 19.82 and Faisal Canola 18.30, respectively. During 2020–2021 at NARC-Islamabad, the highest and lowest harvest index was observed for NARC Sarsoon 20.37 and Faisal Canola 16.87. At URF-Koont, the highest and lowest harvest index was observed for ROHI Sarsoon 19.16 and Faisal Canola 16.1, respectively (Figs. 19.22, 19.23 and 19.24). Analysis of variance table explained that the main effects of L, Y, CUL, L × Y, L × CUL, Y × CUL and L × Y × CUL were highly significant (Table 19.3). Harvest index is the ratio between grain yield and biological yield. Variations in harvest index at both sites during growing seasons were observed due to climate change. At NARC-Islamabad, the temperature was lower than URF-Koont, and climatic conditions were favourable for better crop stand which resulted in the proper translocation of photosynthate into grains. Andarzian et al. (2015) also reported that under favourable climate, crop translocates its photosynthate into grains.

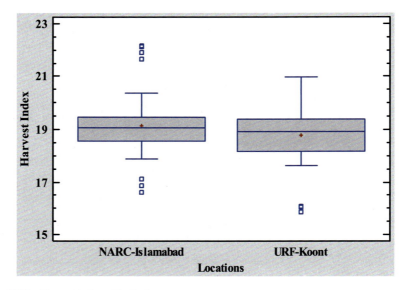

Fig. 19.22 Harvest index of both sites

19 Modelling and Field-Based Evaluation of Vernalisation Requirement...

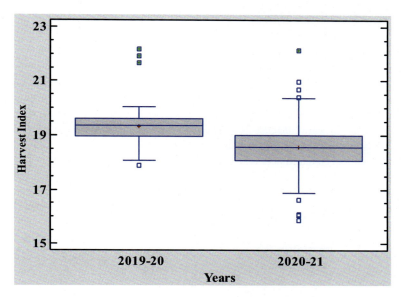

Fig. 19.23 Harvest index for growing seasons 2019–2020 and 2020–2021

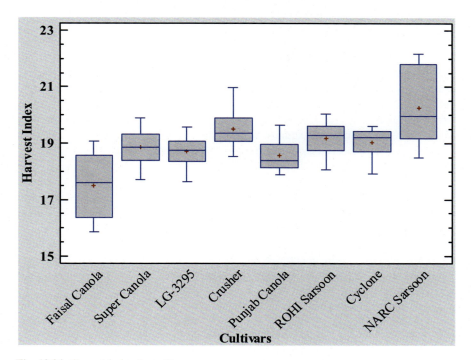

Fig. 19.24 Harvest index for cultivars

19.4.3 Phenology Modelling

For the eight cultivars of canola, a phenological model was established with varying sensitivities to vernalisation for both sites and growing seasons. All the cultivars show different vernalisation requirements under varying climatic conditions of both study sites during both growing seasons. At NARC-Islamabad during years 2019–2020 and 2020–2021, the vernalisation days required to achieve vernalisation for Faisal Canola were 29d and 26d, Super Canola 39d and 35d, LG-3295 41d and 37d, Crusher 44d and 39d, Punjab Canola 31d and 28d, ROHI Sarsoon 30d and 28d, Cyclone 54d and 51d and NARC Sarsoon 44d and 39d, respectively (days = d). At URF-Koont during years 2019–2020 and 2020–2021, the vernalisation days required to achieve vernalisation for Faisal Canola were 26d and 25d, Super Canola 26d and 26d, LG-3295 23d and 23d, Crusher 21d and 20d, Punjab Canola 16d and 15d, ROHI Sarsoon 10d and 9d, Cyclone 22d and 20d and NARC Sarsoon 17d and 16d, respectively (days = d). All the cultivars show weak sensitivities to vernalisation at URF-Chakwal and strong sensitivities to vernalisation at NARC-Islamabad during both growing seasons.

19.4.4 Simulation Outcomes

19.4.4.1 Phenology

We validated the DSSAT model for our experimental data; the model was used to extend our understandings for various crop parameters. Thus, the eight canola cultivars were simulated in our two different experimental locations with different sowing dates during years 2019–2020 and 2020–2021 using historical climate data. Model predicted that days to anthesis at both sites during growing seasons very close association with observed days to anthesis. The performance of DSSAT was compared by using validation skill scores (R^2, RMSE and d-index). During years 2019–2020 at NARC-Islamabad, the model predicted the maximum days to anthesis for Cyclone 103 and minimum days for Faisal Canola 77, and our observed data showed the maximum days for Cyclone 103 and minimum days for Faisal Canola 78. The values for R^2, RMSE and d-index were 0.99, 0.61 and 0.99, respectively, while at URF-Koont, the model predicted the maximum days to anthesis for Faisal Canola 77 and minimum days for ROHI Sarsoon 57, and our observed data showed the maximum days for Faisal Canola 77 and minimum days for ROHI Sarsoon 57. The values for R^2, RMSE and d-index were 0.99, 0.57 and 0.98, respectively, for years 2019–2020. During years 2020–2021 at NARC-Islamabad, the model predicted the maximum days to anthesis for Cyclone 101 and minimum days for Faisal Canola 74, and our observed data showed the maximum days for Cyclone 102 and minimum for Faisal Canola 75. The values for R^2, RMSE and d-index were 0.99, 0.63 and 0.99, respectively, while at URF-Koont, the model predicted the

19 Modelling and Field-Based Evaluation of Vernalisation Requirement...

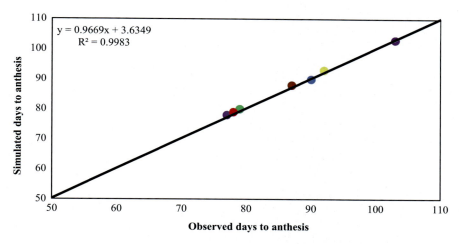

Fig. 19.25 Observed and simulated days to anthesis for NARC-Islamabad during years 2019–2020

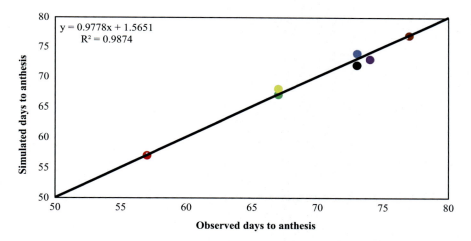

Fig. 19.26 Observed and simulated days to anthesis for URF-Koont during years 2019–2020

maximum days to anthesis for Super Canola 75 and minimum days for ROHI Sarsoon 54, and our observed days to anthesis was maximum for Super Canola 75 and minimum for ROHI Sarsoon 54. The values for R^2, RMSE and d-index were 0.99, 0.81 and 0.97, respectively. DSSAT shows performance with great accuracy and prediction of days to anthesis was close to observed days to anthesis. The model could predict better crop phenology under climate change and study sites by exhibiting the validation skill scores, viz. R^2, RMSE and d-index (Figs. 19.25, 19.26, 19.27 and 19.28).

Days to end of flowering was predicted by DSSAT with close association with observed days to end of flowering. During years 2019–2020 at NARC-Islamabad,

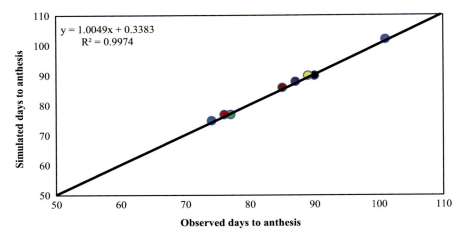

Fig. 19.27 Observed and simulated days to anthesis for NARC-Islamabad during years 2020–2021

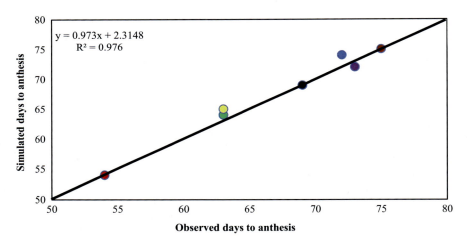

Fig. 19.28 Observed and simulated days to anthesis for URF-Koont during years 2020–2021

the model predicted the maximum days to end of flowering for LG-3295 125 and minimum days for Faisal Canola 114, and our observed maximum days to end of flowering was for LG-3295 126 and minimum days for Faisal Canola 115. The values for R^2, RMSE and d-index were 0.99, 0.59 and 0.99, respectively, while at URF-Koont, the model predicted the maximum days to end of flowering for Super Canola 129 and minimum days for ROHI Sarsoon 88, and our observed maximum days was for Super Canola 130 and minimum days for ROHI Sarsoon 88. The values for R^2, RMSE and d-index were 0.99, 0.62 and 0.99, respectively. During years 2020–2021 at NARC-Islamabad, the model predicted the maximum days to end of flowering for Cyclone 122 and minimum days for ROHI Sarsoon 99, and our

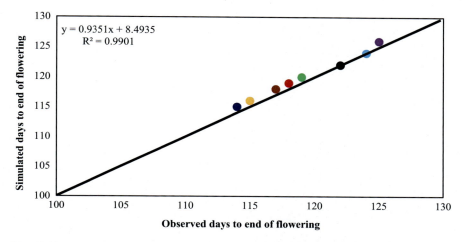

Fig. 19.29 Observed and simulated days to end of flowering for NARC-Islamabad during years 2019–2020

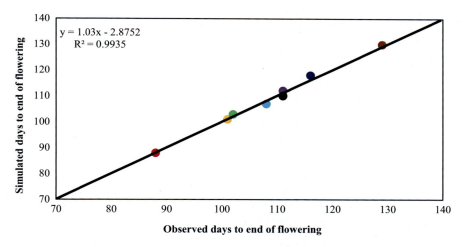

Fig. 19.30 Observed and simulated days to end of flowering for URF-Koont during years 2019–2020

observed maximum days was for Cyclone 123 and minimum days for ROHI Sarsoon 100. The values for R^2, RMSE and d-index were 0.99, 0.64 and 0.99, respectively, while at URF-Koont, the model predicted the maximum days to end of flowering for Super Canola 114 and minimum days for ROHI Sarsoon 81, and our observed maximum days was for Super Canola 114 and minimum days for ROHI Sarsoon 81. The values for R^2, RMSE and d-index were 0.99, 0.52 and 0.99, respectively. DSSAT shows performance with great accuracy and prediction of days to end of flowering was close to observed days to end of flowering. The performance of

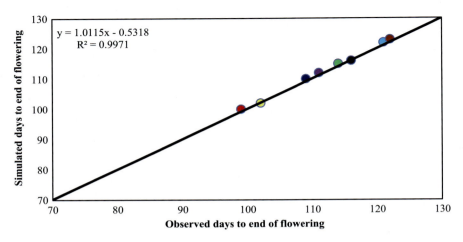

Fig. 19.31 Observed and simulated days to end of flowering for NARC-Islamabad during years 2020–2021

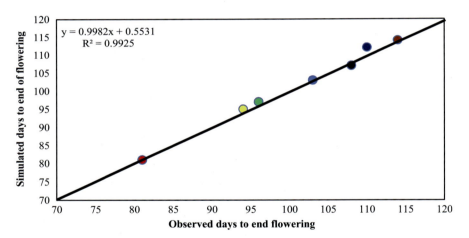

Fig. 19.32 Observed and simulated days to end of flowering for URF-Koont during years 2020–2021

DSSAT was compared by using validation skill scores (R^2, RMSE and d-index) (Figs. 19.29, 19.30, 19.31 and 19.32).

The model predicted the days to maturity with close association with our observed days to maturity. During years 2019–2020 at NARC-Islamabad, the model predicted the maximum days to maturity for Crusher 186 and minimum days for Faisal Canola 169, and our observed data showed the maximum days to maturity for Crusher 186 and minimum days for Faisal Canola 172. The values for R^2, RMSE and d-index were 0.97, 1.70 and 0.99, respectively, while at URF-Koont, the model predicted the maximum days to maturity for Faisal Canola 174 and

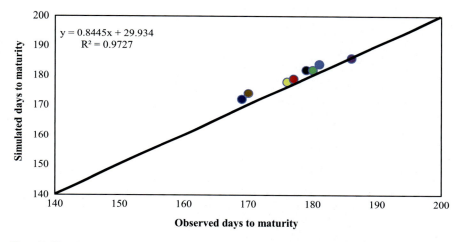

Fig. 19.33 Observed and simulated days to maturity for NARC-Islamabad during years 2019–2020

minimum days for ROHI Sarsoon 156, and our observed data showed the maximum days to maturity for Super Canola 180 and minimum days for ROHI Sarsoon 156. The values for R^2, RMSE and d-index were 0.92, 1.91 and 0.97, respectively. During years 2020–2021 at NARC-Islamabad, the model predicted the maximum days to maturity for Cyclone 184 and minimum days for ROHI Sarsoon 167, and our observed data showed the maximum days to maturity for Cyclone 186 and minimum days for ROHI Sarsoon 170. The values for R^2, RMSE and d-index were 0.97, 1.69 and 0.99, respectively, while at URF-Koont, the model predicted the maximum days to maturity for Super Canola 175 and minimum days for ROHI Sarsoon 151, and our observed data showed the maximum days to maturity for Super Canola 173 and minimum days for ROHI Sarsoon 152. The values for R^2, RMSE and d-index were 0.99, 0.55 and 0.99, respectively. DSSAT shows performance with great accuracy and prediction of days to maturity was close to observed days to maturity. The performance of DSSAT was compared by using validation skill scores (R^2, RMSE and d-index) (Figs. 19.33, 19.34, 19.35 and 19.36).

19.4.4.2 Leaf Area Index

The model predicted the leaf area index (LAI) with very close association with our observed leaf area index. During years 2019–2020 at NARC-Islamabad, the model predicted the maximum LAI for NARC Sarsoon 3.9 and minimum LAI for Faisal Canola 3.3, and observed data for the maximum and minimum LAI was the same for the same cultivars as the model predicted. The values for R^2, RMSE and d-index were 1, 0 and 1, respectively, while at URF-Koont, the model predicted the maximum LAI for ROHI Sarsoon 3.9 and minimum LAI for Faisal Canola 3.2, and our

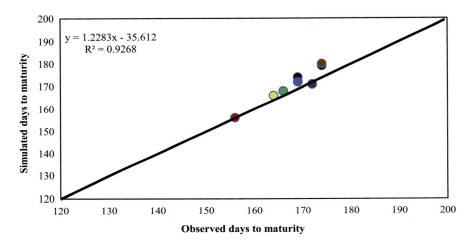

Fig. 19.34 Observed and simulated days to maturity for URF-Koont during years 2019–2020

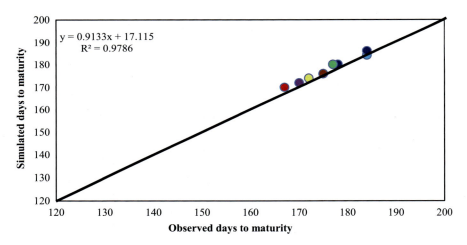

Fig. 19.35 Observed and simulated days to maturity for NARC-Islamabad during years 2020–2021

observed data showed the maximum and minimum LAI was the same for the same cultivar as the model predicted. The values for R^2, RMSE and d-index were 1, 0 and 1, respectively. During years 2020–2021 at NARC-Islamabad, the model predicted the maximum LAI for NARC Sarsoon 3.9 and minimum LAI for Faisal Canola 3.2, and our observed maximum and minimum LAI was the same for the same cultivars as the model predicted. The values for R^2, RMSE and d-index were 1, 0 and 1, respectively, while at URF-Koont, the model predicted the maximum LAI for ROHI Sarsoon 3.7 and minimum LAI for Faisal Canola 3.1, and our observed maximum and minimum LAI was the same for the same cultivars as the model

19 Modelling and Field-Based Evaluation of Vernalisation Requirement...

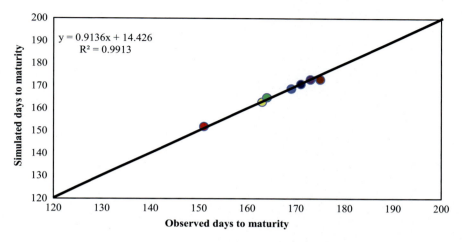

Fig. 19.36 Observed and simulated days to maturity for URF-Koont during years 2020–2021

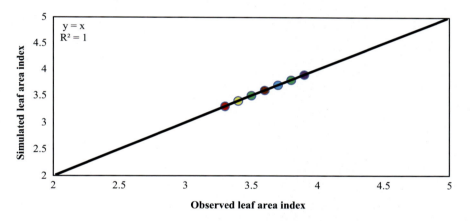

Fig. 19.37 Observed and simulated leaf area index for NARC-Islamabad during years 2019–2020

predicted. The values for R^2, RMSE and d-index were 1, 0 and 1, respectively. DSSAT shows performance with great accuracy and prediction of LAI was the same as the observed LAI for all cultivars during both years. The performance of DSSAT was compared by using validation skill scores (R^2, RMSE and d-index) (Figs. 19.37, 19.38, 19.39 and 19.40).

19.4.4.3 Biological Yield

The model predicted the biological yield with close association with our observed biological yield. At NARC-Islamabad during years 2019–2020, the model predicted

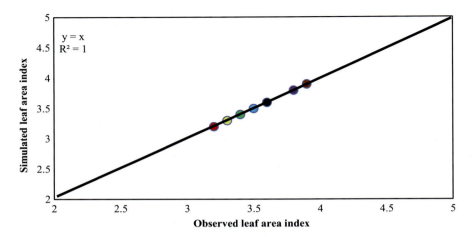

Fig. 19.38 Observed and simulated leaf area index for URF-Koont during years 2019–2020

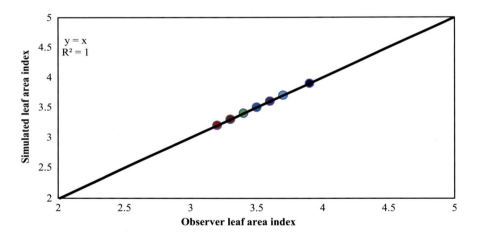

Fig. 19.39 Observed and simulated leaf area index for NARC-Islamabad during years 2020–2021

the maximum biological yield for Super Canola 13828 kg h^{-1} and minimum biological yield for Faisal Canola 11852 kg h^{-1}, and our observed data showed the maximum biological yield for Super Canola 13842 kg h^{-1} and minimum biological yield for Faisal Canola 11860 kg h^{-1}. The values for R^2, RMSE and d-index were 0.99, 67.46 and 0.99, respectively, while at URF-Koont, the model predicted the maximum biological yield for NARC Sarsoon 13971 kg h^{-1} and minimum biological yield for Faisal Canola 11500 kg h^{-1}, and our observed data showed the maximum biological yield for ROHI Sarsoon 14100 kg h^{-1} and minimum biological yield for Faisal Canola 11540 kg h^{-1}. The values for R^2, RMSE and d-index were 0.98, 108.37 and 0.99, respectively. During years 2020–2021 at

19 Modelling and Field-Based Evaluation of Vernalisation Requirement... 553

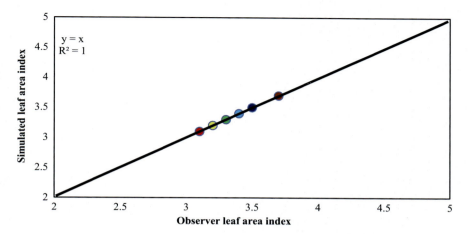

Fig. 19.40 Observed and simulated leaf area index for URF-Koont during years 2020–2021

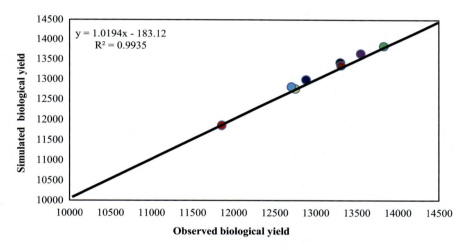

Fig. 19.41 Observed and simulated biological yield for NARC-Islamabad during years 2019–2020

NARC-Islamabad, the maximum biological yield was predicted for NARC Sarsoon 13079 kg h^{-1} and minimum biological yield for Faisal Canola 11014 kg h^{-1}, and our observed data showed the maximum biological yield for NARC Sarsoon 13092 kg h^{-1} and minimum biological yield for Faisal Canola 11037 kg h^{-1}. The values for R^2, RMSE and d-index were 0.99, 11.55 and 0.99, respectively, while at URF-Koont, the model predicted the maximum biological yield for ROHI Sarsoon 12382 kg h^{-1} and minimum biological yield for LG-3295 10886 kg h^{-1}, and our observed data showed the maximum biological yield for NARC Sarsoon 12166 kg h^{-1} and minimum biological yield for LG-3295 10912 kg h^{-1}. The values for R^2, RMSE and d-index were 0.92, 127.46 and 0.99, respectively. DSSAT shows

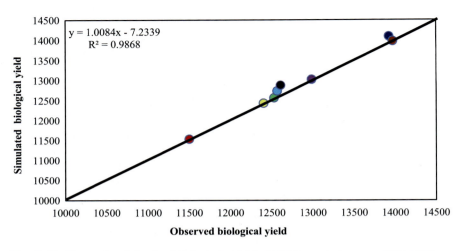

Fig. 19.42 Observed and simulated biological yield for URF-Koont during years 2019–2020

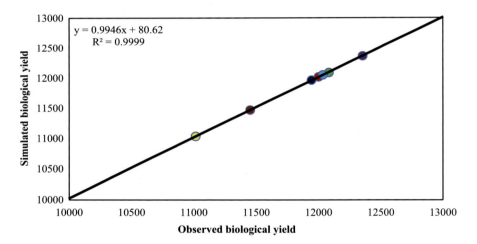

Fig. 19.43 Observed and simulated biological yield for NARC-Islamabad during years 2020–2021

performance with great accuracy and prediction of the biological yield was close to observed biological yield. The performance of DSSAT was compared by using validation skill scores (R^2, RMSE and d-index) (Figs. 19.41, 19.42, 19.43 and 19.44).

19.4.4.4 Grain Yield

Grain yield was predicted by DSSAT with close association with observed grain yield. Predicted grain yield was different for all cultivars, and the model predicted

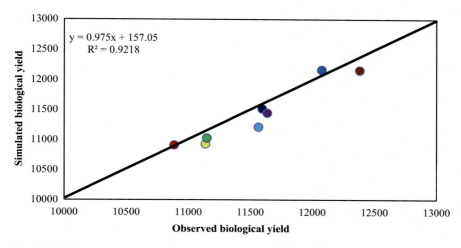

Fig. 19.44 Observed and simulated biological yield for URF-Koont during years 2020–2021

high grain yield for some cultivars and low grain yield for some cultivars than our observed grain yield for both sites during both years, respectively. During years 2019–2020 at NARC-Islamabad, the model predicted the maximum grain yield for NARC Sarsoon 2889 kg h^{-1} and minimum grain yield for Faisal Canola 2234 kg h^{-1}, and our observed data showed the maximum grain yield for NARC 2926 kg h^{-1} and minimum grain yield for Faisal Canola 2231 kg h^{-1}. The values for R^2, RMSE and d-index were 0.98, 29.39 and 0.99, respectively, while at URF-Koont, the model predicted the maximum grain yield for ROHI Sarsoon 2753 kg h^{-1} and minimum grain yield for Faisal Canola 2115 kg h^{-1}, and our observed data showed the maximum grain yield for ROHI Sarsoon 2796 kg h^{-1} and minimum grain yield for Faisal Canola 2112 kg h^{-1}. The values for R^2, RMSE and d-index were 0.99, 23.57 and 0.99, respectively. During years 2020–2021 at NARC-Islamabad, the model predicted the maximum grain yield for NARC Sarsoon 2652 kg h^{-1} and minimum grain yield for Faisal Canola 1853 kg h^{-1}, and our observed data showed the maximum grain yield for NARC Sarsoon 2667 kg h^{-1} and minimum grain yield for Faisal Canola 1862 kg h^{-1}. The values for R^2, RMSE and d-index were 0.99, 11.22 and 0.99, respectively, while at URF-Koont, the model predicted the maximum grain yield for ROHI Sarsoon 2380 kg h^{-1} and minimum grain yield for Faisal Canola 1800 kg h^{-1}, and our observed data showed the maximum grain yield for ROHI Sarsoon 2330 kg h^{-1} and minimum grain yield for Faisal Canola 1760 kg h^{-1}. The values for R^2, RMSE and d-index were 0.97, 27.11 and 0.99, respectively. DSSAT shows performance with great accuracy and prediction of the biological yield was close to observed biological yield. The performance of DSSAT was compared by using validation skill scores (R^2, RMSE and d-index) (Figs. 19.45, 19.46, 19.47 and 19.48).

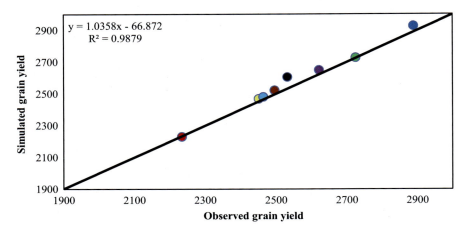

Fig. 19.45 Observed and simulated grain yield for NARC-Islamabad during years 2019–2020

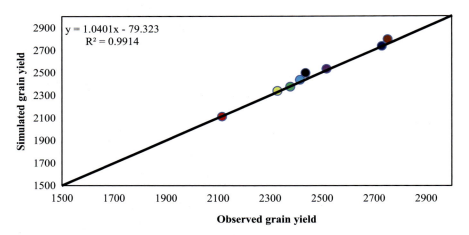

Fig. 19.46 Observed and simulated grain yield for URF-Koont during years 2019–2020

19.4.4.5 Harvest Index

Harvest index (HI) was predicted by DSSAT with close association with observed harvest index. During years 2019–2020 at NARC-Islamabad, the model predicted the maximum HI for NARC Sarsoon 21.71 and minimum HI for Faisal Canola 18.84, and our observed data showed the maximum HI for NARC Sarsoon 21.91 and minimum HI for Faisal Canola 18.81. The values for R^2, RMSE and d-index were 0.98, 0.139 and 0.99, respectively, while at URF-Koont, the model predicted the maximum HI for ROHI Sarsoon 19.77 and minimum HI for Faisal Canola 18.39, and our observed data showed the maximum HI for ROHI Sarsoon 19.56 and minimum HI for Faisal Canola 18.30. The values for R^2, RMSE and d-index were

19 Modelling and Field-Based Evaluation of Vernalisation Requirement...

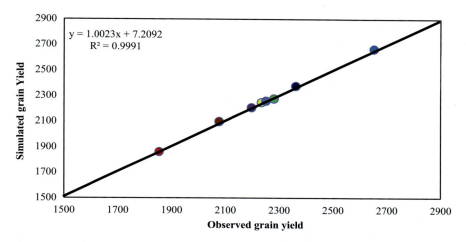

Fig. 19.47 Observed and simulated grain yield for NARC-Islamabad during years 2020–2021

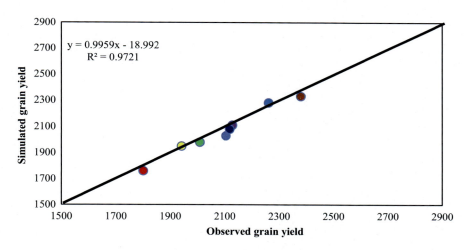

Fig. 19.48 Observed and simulated grain yield for URF-Koont during years 2020–2021

0.99, 0.03 and 0.99, respectively. During years 2020–2021 at NARC-Islamabad, the model predicted the maximum HI for NARC Sarsoon 20.27 and minimum HI for Faisal Canola 16.82, and our observed data showed the maximum HI was for NARC Sarsoon 20.37 and minimum HI was for Faisal Canola 16.87. The values for R^2, RMSE and d-index were 0.99, 0.07 and 0.99, respectively, while at URF-Koont, the model predicted the maximum HI for ROHI Sarsoon 19.22 and minimum HI for Faisal Canola 16.16, and our observed data showed the maximum HI was for ROHI Sarsoon 19.16 and minimum HI was for Faisal Canola 16.10. The values for R^2, RMSE and d-index were 0.99, 0.03 and 0.99, respectively. DSSAT shows performance with great accuracy and prediction of HI was the same as the observed HI for

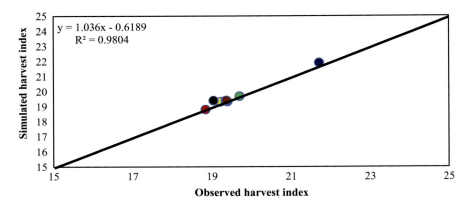

Fig. 19.49 Observed and simulated harvest index for NARC-Islamabad during years 2019–2020

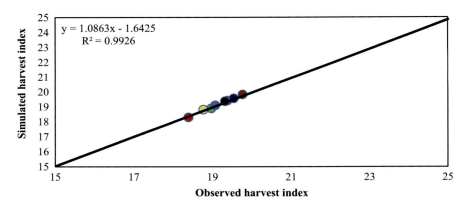

Fig. 19.50 Observed and simulated harvest index for URF-Koont during years 2019–2020

all cultivars during both years. The performance of DSSAT was compared by using validation skill scores (R^2, RMSE and d-index) (Figs. 19.49, 19.50, 19.51 and 19.52).

19.5 Conclusion

The phenology of canola was influenced by temperature at both sites during both growing seasons. The temperature was high at URF-Koont than at NARC-Islamabad during both growing seasons which directly influences the phenological phases of crop. Advancement of the phenological stages and a decrease in the duration of the phenological phases of crop cycles may occur due to an increase in temperature. Therefore, an early shift in phenology will result in curtailed growth season under

19 Modelling and Field-Based Evaluation of Vernalisation Requirement... 559

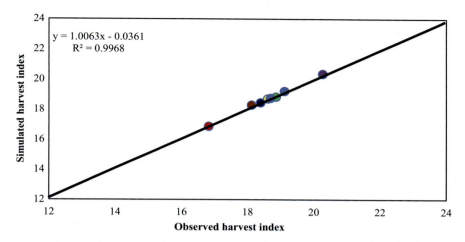

Fig. 19.51 Observed and simulated harvest index for NARC-Islamabad during years 2020–2021

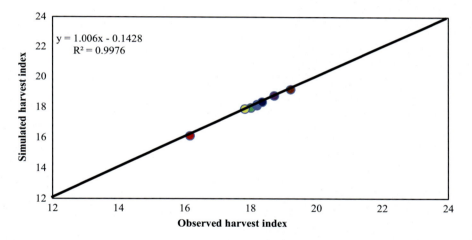

Fig. 19.52 Observed and simulated harvest index for URF-Koont during years 2020–2021

contemporary hop of increasing temperature. A phenological model was established with varying sensitivities to vernalisation for both sites and growing seasons. All the cultivars showed different vernalisation requirements under varying climatic conditions of both study sites during both growing seasons. All the cultivars showed weak sensitivities to vernalisation at URK-Chakwal and strong sensitivities to vernalisation at NARC-Islamabad during both growing seasons. The cultivars required more days to achieve their vernalisation requirement was strong sensitive to vernalisation and the cultivars required less days to achieve their vernalisation requirement was weak sensitive to vernalisation. During years 2019–2020 and 2020–2021 at URF-Koont, we observed that ROHI Sarsoon showed flowering in less days than other cultivars and gave the maximum yield among all the cultivars. So we can conclude that ROHI Sarsoon is an ideal variety for the study site URF-Chakwal and under its climatic conditions. However, NARC Sarsoon is an ideal variety for the study site NARC-Islamabad and under its climatic conditions.

References

Abbas G, Ahmad S, Ahmad A, Nasim W, Fatima Z, Hussain S, Hoogenboom G (2017) Quantification the impacts of climate change and crop management on phenology of maize-based cropping system in Punjab, Pakistan. Agric For Meteorol 247:42–55

Afzal O, Hassan F-U, Ahmed M, Shabbir G, Ahmed S (2021) Determination of stable safflower genotypes in variable environments by parametric and non-parametric methods. Journal of Agriculture and Food Research 6:100233. https://doi.org/10.1016/j.jafr.2021.100233

Ahmad A, Ashfaq M, Rasul G, Wajid SA, Khaliq T, Rasul F, Valdivia RO (2015) Impact of climate change on the rice–wheat cropping system of Pakistan. In: Handbook of climate change and agroecosystems: the agricultural model intercomparison and improvement project integrated crop and economic assessments, part 2, pp 219–258

Ahmad S, Nadeem M, Abbas G, Fatima Z, Khan RJZ, Ahmed M, Khan MA (2016) Quantification of the effects of climate warming and crop management on sugarcane phenology. Clim Res 71(1):47–61

Ahmad S, Abbas Q, Abbas G, Fatima Z, Naz S, Younis H, Rasul G (2017) Quantification of climate warming and crop management impacts on cotton phenology. Plan Theory 6(1):7

Ahmed I, Ullah A, Rahman MH, Ahmad B, Wajid SA, Ahmad A, Ahmed S (2019) Climate change impacts and adaptation strategies for agronomic crops. In: Climate change and agriculture. IntechOpen, pp 1–14

Ahmed M (2020) Introduction to modern climate change. Andrew E. Dessler: Cambridge University Press, 2011, 252 pp, ISBN-10: 0521173159. Sci Total Environ 734, 139397. https://doi.org/10.1016/j.scitotenv.2020.139397

Ahmed M, Hayat R, Ahmad M, ul-Hassan M, Kheir AMS, ul-Hassan F, ur-Rehman MH, Shaheen FA, Raza MA, Ahmad S (2022) Impact of climate change on dryland agricultural systems: a review of current status, potentials, and further work need. Int J Plant Product. https://doi.org/10.1007/s42106-022-00197-1

Akram N, Hamid A (2015) Climate change: a threat to the economic growth of Pakistan. Prog Dev Stud 15(1):73–86

Ali MGM, Ahmed M, Ibrahim MM, El Baroudy AA, Ali EF, Shokr MS, Aldosari AA, Majrashi A, Kheir AMS (2022) Optimizing sowing window, cultivar choice, and plant density to boost maize yield under RCP8.5 climate scenario of CMIP5. Int J Biometeorol. https://doi.org/10.1007/s00484-022-02253-x

Andarzian B, Hoogenboom G, Bannayan M, Shirali M, Andarzian B (2015) Determining optimum sowing date of wheat using CSM-CERES-wheat model. J Saudi Soc Agric Sci 14(2):189–199

Aslam MA, Ahmed M, Stöckle CO, Higgins SS, Hassan Fu, Hayat R (2017) Can growing degree days and photoperiod predict spring wheat phenology? Front Environ Sci 5. https://doi.org/10.3389/fenvs.2017.00057. ISSN: 2296-665X

Babel MS, Deb P, Soni P (2019) Performance evaluation of AquaCrop and DSSAT-CERES for maize under different irrigation and manure application rates in the Himalayan region of India. Agric Res 8(2):207–217

Bannayan M, Crout NMJ, Hoogenboom G (2003) Application of the CERES-wheat model for within-season prediction of winter wheat yield in the United Kingdom. Agron J 95(1):114–125

Challinor AJ, Ewert F, Arnold S, Simelton E, Fraser E (2009) Crops and climate change: progress, trends, and challenges in simulating impacts and informing adaptation. J Exp Bot 60:2775–2789

Christy B, Berger J, Zhang H, Riffkin P, Merry A, Weeks A, O'Leary GJ (2019) Potential yield benefits from increased vernalisation requirement of canola in Southern Australia. Field Crop Res 239:82–91

Deligios PA, Farci R, Sulas L, Hoogenboom G, Ledda L (2013) Predicting growth and yield of winter rapeseed in a Mediterranean environment: model adaptation at a field scale. Field Crop Res 144:100–112

Faraji A, Latifi N, Soltani A, Rad AHS (2009) Seed yield and water use efficiency of canola (*Brassica napus* L.) as affected by high temperature stress and supplemental irrigation. Agric Water Manag 96(1):132–140

Fatima Z, Ahmed M, Hussain M, Abbas G, Ul-Allah S, Ahmad S, Ahmed N, Ali MA, Sarwar G, Haque EU, Iqbal P, Hussain S (2020) The fingerprints of climate warming on cereal crops phenology and adaptation options. Sci Rep 10:18013. https://doi.org/10.1038/s41598-020-74740-3

Fourcaud T, Zhang X, Stokes A, Lambers H, Körner C (2008) Plant growth modelling and applications: the increasing importance of plant architecture in growth models. Ann Bot 101(8):1053–1063

Habekotté B (1997) A model of the phenological development of winter oilseed rape (*Brassica napus* L.). Field Crop Res 54(2–3):127–136

Hatfield JL, Boote KJ, Kimball BA, Ziska LH, Izaurralde RC, Ort DR, Wolfe D (2011) Climate impacts on agriculture: implications for crop production. Environ Res Lett 17:053001

He L, Asseng S, Zhao G, Wu D, Yang X, Zhuang W, Yu Q (2015) Impacts of recent climate warming, cultivar changes, and crop management on winter wheat phenology across the Loess Plateau of China. Agric For Meteorol 200:135–143

Hoogenboom G, Jones JW, Wilkens PW, Porter CH, Boote KJ, Hunt US, Lizaso JI, White JW, Uryasev O, Ogoshi R, Koo J, Shelia V, Tsuji GY (2015) Decision support system for agrotechnology transfer (DSSAT). DSSAT Foundation

Hoogenboom G, Porter CH, Shelia V, Boote KJ, Singh U, White JW, Hunt LA, Ogoshi R, Lizaso JI, Koo J, Asseng S, Singels A, Moreno LP, Jones JW (2019) Decision support system for agrotechnology transfer (DSSAT) version 4.7.5. DSSAT Foundation, Gainesville. https://DSSAT.net

Hoogenboom G, Jones JW, Wilkens PV, Porter CH, Boote KJ, Hunt LA, Singh U, Lizaso JL, White JW, Uryasev O et al (2020) Decision support system for agrotechnology transfer (DSSAT) version 4.5. University of Hawaii, Honolulu

IPCC (2013) Climate change 2013: the physical science basis. Contribution of Working Group I to the Fifth Assessment Report of the Intergovernmental Panel on Climate Change (Stocker TF, Qin D, Plattner GK, Tignor M, Allen SK, Boschung J, Nauels A, Xia Y, Bex V, Midgley PM (eds))

IPCC (2018) Global warming of 1.5°C. An IPCC Special Report on the impacts of global warming of 1.5°C above pre-industrial levels and related global greenhouse gas emission pathways, in the context of strengthening the global response to the threat of climate change, sustainable development, and efforts to eradicate poverty (Masson-Delmotte V, Zhai P, Pörtner HO, Roberts D, Skea J, Shukla PR, Pirani A, Moufouma-Okia W, Péan C, Pidcock R, Connors S, Matthews JBR, Chen Y, Zhou X, Gomis MI, Lonnoy E, Maycock T, Tignor M, Waterfield T (eds))

IPCC (2019) Climate Change and Land: an IPCC special report on climate change, desertification, land degradation, sustainable land management, food security, and greenhouse gas fluxes in terrestrial ecosystems (Shukla PR, Skea J, Calvo Buendia E, Masson-Delmotte V, Pörtner HO, Roberts DC, Zhai P, Slade R, Connors S, van Diemen R, Ferrat M, Haughey E, Luz S, Neogi S, Pathak M, Petzold J, Portugal Pereira J, Vyas P, Huntley E, Kissick K, Belkacemi M, Malley J (eds))

Kheir AMS, Hoogenboom G, Ammar KA, Ahmed M, Feike T, Elnashar A, Liu B, Ding Z, Asseng S (2022) Minimizing trade-offs between wheat yield and resource-use efficiency in the Nile Delta – a multi-model analysis. Field Crop Res 287:108638. https://doi.org/10.1016/j.fcr.2022.108638

Li K, Yang X, Tian H, Pan S, Liu Z, Lu S (2016) Effects of changing climate and cultivar on the phenology and yield of winter wheat in the North China Plain. Int J Biometeorol 60(1):21–32

Li Z, He J, Xu X, Jin X, Huang W, Clark B, Li Z (2018) Estimating genetic parameters of DSSAT-CERES model with the GLUE method for winter wheat (*Triticum aestivum* L.) production. Comput Electron Agric 154:213–221

Matar S, Kumar A, Holtgräwe D, Weisshaar B, Melzer S (2021) The transition to flowering in winter rapeseed during vernalization. Plant Cell Environ 44(2):506–518

McMaster GS, Wilhelm WW (1997) Growing degree-days: one equation, two interpretations. Agric For Meteorol 87(4):291–300

Melchers G (1939) Die bluhhormone. Ber Dtsch Bot Ges 57:29–48

Naz S, Ahmad S, Abbas G, Fatima Z, Hussain S, Ahmed M, Khan MA, Khan A, Fahad S, Nasim W, Ercisli S,Wilkerson CJ, Hoogenboom G (2022) Modeling the impact of climate warming on potato phenology. Eur J Agron 132:126404. https://doi.org/10.1016/j.eja.2021.126404

Nikoubin M, Latifi N, Soltani A, Faraji AA, Mirdavar DF (2009) The effect of vernalization on phenology and development rate in canola. Electron J Crop Prod 2(1):123–135

Porter R, Liu F, Pourkashanian M, Williams A, Smith D (2010) Evaluation of solution methods for radiative heat transfer in gaseous oxy-fuel combustion environments. J Quant Spectrosc Radiat Transf 111(14):2084–2094

Rahman MH, Ahmad A, Wang X, Wajid A, Nasim W, Hussain M, Hoogenboom G (2018) Multi-model projections of future climate and climate change impacts uncertainty assessment for cotton production in Pakistan. Agric For Meteorol 253:94–113

Raman H, Uppal RK, Raman R (2019) Genetic solutions to improve resilience of canola to climate change. In: Genomic designing of climate-smart oilseed crops, pp 75–131

Rapacz M, Markowski A (1999) Winter hardiness, frost resistance and vernalisation requirement of European winter oilseed rape (*Brassica napus* var. oleifera) cultivars within the last 20 years. J Agron Crop Sci 183(4):243–253

Rasul G, Sharma B (2016) The nexus approach to water–energy–food security: an option for adaptation to climate change. Clim Pol 16(6):682–702

Rezaei EE, Webber H, Gaiser T, Naab J, Ewert F (2015) Heat stress in cereals: mechanisms and modelling. Eur J Agron 64:98–113

Ritchie JT, Nesmith DS (1991) Temperature and crop development. In: Modeling plant and soil systems, vol 31. American Society of Agronomy, Inc, pp 5–29

Roetzer T, Wittenzeller M, Haeckel H, Nekovar J (2000) Phenology in Central Europe–differences and trends of spring phenophases in urban and rural areas. Int J Biometeorol 44(2):60–66

Schiessl S, Iniguez-Luy F, Qian W, Snowdon RJ (2015) Diverse regulatory factors associate with flowering time and yield responses in winter-type Brassica napus. BMC Genomics 16(1):737

Sommer R, Glazirina M, Yuldashev T, Otarov A, Ibraeva M, Martynova L, De Pauw E (2013) Impact of climate change on wheat productivity in Central Asia. Agric Ecosyst Environ 178:78–99

Tao F, Zhang Z, Zhang S, Zhu Z, Shi W (2012) Response of crop yields to climate trends since 1980 in China. Clim Res 54(3):233–247

Tao F, Zhang Z, Shi W, Liu Y, Xiao D, Zhang S, Liu F (2013) Single rice growth period was prolonged by cultivars shifts, but yield was damaged by climate change during 1981–2009 in China, and late rice was just opposite. Glob Chang Biol 19(10):3200–3209

Tao F, Zhang Z, Xiao D, Zhang S, Rötter RP, Shi W, Zhang H (2014) Responses of wheat growth and yield to climate change in different climate zones of China, 1981–2009. Agric For Meteorol 189:91–104

Tariq M, Ahmad S, Fahad S, Abbas G, Hussain S, Fatima Z, Hoogenboom G (2018) The impact of climate warming and crop management on phenology of sunflower-based cropping systems in Punjab, Pakistan. Agric For Meteorol 256:270–282

Waalen WM, Stavang JA, Olsen JE, Rognli OA (2014) The relationship between vernalisation saturation and the maintenance of freezing tolerance in winter rapeseed. Environ Exp Bot 106: 164–173

Wang SY, Davies RE, Huang WR, Gillies RR (2011) Pakistan's two-stage monsoon and links with the recent climate change. J Geophys Res Atmos 116:D16

Wang S, Wang E, Wang F, Tang L (2012) Phenological development and grain yield of canola as affected by sowing date and climate variation in the Yangtze River Basin of China. Crop Pasture Sci 63(5):478–488

Whish JPM, Lilley JM, Morrison MJ, Cocks B, Bullock M (2020) Vernalisation in Australian spring canola explains variable flowering responses. Field Crop Res 258:107968

White JW, Herndl M, Hunt LA, Payne TS, Hoogenboom G (2008) Simulation-based analysis of effects of Vrn and Ppd loci on flowering in wheat. Crop Sci 48:678–687

Xiao D, Tao F (2014) Contributions of cultivars, management and climate change to winter wheat yield in the North China Plain in the past three decades. Eur J Agron 52:112–122

Xiao D, Tao F, Shen Y, Qi Y (2016) Combined impact of climate change, cultivar shift, and sowing date on spring wheat phenology in Northern China. J Meteorol Res 30(5):820–831

Yan L, Jin J, Wu P (2020) Impact of parameter uncertainty and water stress parameterization on wheat growth simulations using CERES-wheat with GLUE. Agric Syst 181:102823

Zahoor A, Ahmed M, ul Hassan F, Shabbir G, Ahmad S (2022) Ontogeny growth and radiation use efficiency of canola (Brassica napus L.) under various nitrogen management strategies and contrasting environments. Int J Plant Product. https://doi.org/10.1007/s42106-022-00183-7

Zhang X, Cai J, Wollenweber B, Liu F, Dai T, Cao W, Jiang D (2013) Multiple heat and drought events affect grain yield and accumulations of high molecular weight glutenin subunits and glutenin macropolymers in wheat. J Cereal Sci 57(1):134–140

Chapter 20
Integrated Crop–Livestock System Case Study: Prospectus for Jordan's Climate Change Adaptation

Muhammad Iftikhar Hussain, Abdullah J. Al-Dakheel, and Mukhtar Ahmed

Abstract The integrated crop–livestock system (ICLS) is a multifaceted farming system in which various agricultural practices are combined for sustainable management of available natural resources (i.e., plant, soil, water), reducing the impact of climate change to improve soil properties, crop productivity, animal sector development and farmers' profit in an integrated way. Climate change poses considerable challenges for development, food security and poverty alleviation, particularly in Jordan. The chapter reviews the agricultural practices package adopted by farmers to enhance soil fertility, water use efficiency, resiliency to climate changes and putting more marginal lands and water resources into use in Jordan. These milestones were achieved through provision of distinct integrated plant production packages and distributing them to more marginalized farmers with poor economic conditions. In the livestock sector of Jordan, sustainable production and development of the forage sector is crucial for upscaling of quests with good nutritive value. Several factors were responsible for poor livestock productivity and include low-yield forage genotypes with low quality under marginal environments. To save the freshwater resources, reuse of nonconventional water (NCW), such as treated wastewater (TWW), low-quality saline water and rain harvesting, were vital alternate resources for the agriculture and forestry sectors in Jordan. The

---

M. I. Hussain (✉)
Department of Plant Biology and Soil Science, Universidade de Vigo, Vigo (Pontevedra), Spain

CITACA, Agri-Food Research and Transfer Cluster, Campus da Auga, Universidade de Vigo, Ourense, Spain

Research Institute of Science & Engineering (RISE), University of Sharjah, Sharjah, UAE

A. J. Al-Dakheel
United Arab Emirates University, Al Ain, Abu Dhabi, United Arab Emirates

M. Ahmed
Department of Agricultural Research for Northern Sweden, Swedish University of Agricultural Sciences, Umeå, Sweden

Department of Agronomy, PMAS Arid Agriculture University, Rawalpindi, Pakistan

© The Author(s), under exclusive license to Springer Nature Switzerland AG 2022
M. Ahmed (ed.), *Global Agricultural Production: Resilience to Climate Change*,
https://doi.org/10.1007/978-3-031-14973-3_20

565

ICLS has been adopted in several countries but this concept still has not been adopted in the North African marginal environment. The farmers there are particularly vulnerable to climate change perturbations that include salinity and drought. This challenge requires adaptation of drought- and salt-tolerant genotypes of various forage crops with a high nutritive value. Among them, several forage crops (e.g., sorghum, Pearl millet and triticale) have been adopted by local farming communities in saline and marginal environments of Jordan where livelihood depends on agriculture. It has been concluded that farmers should adopt salt-tolerant forage crops and use NCW and marginal lands to elevate the agricultural and livestock sectors in the region, which will significantly support the local economy, food security and profit of the farmers.

Keywords Crop–livestock integration · Forage crops · Sorghum · Pearl millet · Triticale · Safflower · Dual-purpose crops · Wastewater · Nonconventional water resources · Marginal lands

20.1 Introduction

Jordan has a Mediterranean-style climate with drought episodes and very scarce water availability. The existing renewable freshwater resources have dropped drastically to a per capita share of 144 m^3 per year in 2007 compared to 3400 m^3 per year in 1946. The country is highly affected because of various drought episodes that ruined agriculture, forestry and landscaping activities. Those conditions reflected negatively on the farming community's stability, income and food security. On the other hand, the remaining 80% of the area that received less than 200 mm of annual rainfall per year either had abundant agricultural activities or were under stress from irrational grazing systems—that is, where in April many places converted naked to natural vegetation and warnings became obvious from numerous biodiversity studies.

The available crop options under the prevailing environment are limited, and knowledge about alternative profitable modified crops to alternative water resources for many farmers is lacking. Under the present situation of water shortage, government officials, policymakers and planners are considering nonconventional water resources (e.g., saline and TWW) to bridge the gap between water supply and demand. In Jordan, there is a real need to effectively use all the available nontraditional water resources—that is, TWW, saline and semi-saline water.

A shift toward nontraditional water resources to alleviate the shrinking of the agricultural production system in Jordan has beenobserved. Both treated wastewater and saline water are emphasized. Reclaimed wastewater and saline water are available in many areas, but they only are partially used. There are 22 wastewater treatment plants in Jordan that produce about 90 MCM of treated wastewater yearly from which 93% is used for restricted and unrestricted agriculture, after mixing with freshwater, and for industrial purposes. Introducing salt- and drought-tolerant crops to currently uncultivated areas will provide local residents with an economic base

20 Integrated Crop–Livestock System Case Study: Prospectus for Jordan's. . .

and reduce land degradation. In several parts of Jordan, saving freshwater resources and using alternate water (e.g., TWW, rainwater and desalinated water) are getting attention.

In Jordan, fertile and marginal land resources have not been fully studied. In recent research, it has been reported that there are about 67 natural saline water springs; of which 23 are at the Jordan River basin, 23 are in the Dead Sea basin, 8 are in the Wadi Arabah basin, 2 are in the Al-Jafer basin and 1 is in the Al-Azraq basin. Each year such natural saline springs discharge roughly 46 MCM. Additionally, because of excessive pumping, several subsurface wells changed from producing freshwater to saltwater.

Previous research findings in Jordan have shown plant adaptations to the nontraditional water resources. In this phase, efforts are focused on spreading the knowledge attained from previous phases on crop–forages adapted to saline and reclaimed wastewater in Jordan's agricultural system. The main objective of the work includes research and the extension of services; both produced knowledge transfer to the farmers at marginal environments including the women. Those farmers are using the nontraditional water sources; however, many left their jobs owing to unprofitable production when using the conventional crop genotypes and improper production packages. Improvements are tangible and better crops have been widely adapted to limits defined key farmers who took responsibility for production and dissemination of the adapted genotypes.

An average of five tons of adapted crop grains are produced annually; these include winter crops (e,g., barley, triticale and oats) and summer crops (e.g., Pearl millet and sorghum). Grain multiplication was concentrated at the Al-Khaledyiah Saline Research Station. Framers using nonconventional water sources were receiving the improved grains and cooperated with extension services in data availability for inputs and incomes. The project in Jordan built a new irrigation system of 12 hectares (ha) for the winter crops and developed a 2000 m^{-2} of covered land to produce the summer crops and to protect them from birds, as well as to establish a properly equipped seed store.

The target land area (140 ha) was employed in the project, which helped to achieve a final production of 12,500 kg of grain over a three-year period. This quantity was dispersed to > 250 regional farmers of the target area. Winter crop yields varied from 3.5–5.0 tons per ha and from 8.0–11.0 tons per ha for grain and straw, respectively. "Farmers' field schools" events were planned and used through extension services' efforts to disseminate the production packages either at the farmers' fields or inside the research stations. Flyers, posters and pamphlets were created to aid in explaining the new crops that have been adapted and the alternate water sources.

Conventional and nonconventional are the two types of water resources. Conventional resources include water available from snowmelt and rainfall; this water may be used at the site or taken from streams, lakes, aquifers and rivers. Moreover, this resource can be recycled through a natural hydrological phase. Water resources other than natural, which are obtained from various sources by human intelligence (e.g., desalinated seawater, TWW, and rainfall water captured by water harvesting) are termed nonconventional resources.

Nonconventional water resources, in addition to conventional sources, provide efficient complementary supplies to alleviate water shortages in areas with depleted natural water resources. These sources of water can be used for agriculture and many other purposes through advanced techniques (e.g., harvest of rainwater; desalination of brackish and seawater; capture and reuse of agricultural drainage water; treatment, collection, and use of wastewater; and pumping of groundwater having multiple types of salt). In the present study, diverse means were followed to reach the farmers through field days, seminars and planned visits; and training courses as well as participating in social events. Besides, key farmers were involved in large events on advanced levels, as well as participated in external training courses.

20.2 Description and Characterization of Study Site

Jordan is located at the crossroads of climatic and botanic regions at the junction of three continents (e.g., Europe, Asia and Africa). The country has a Mediterranean climate and four major phyto-geographical regions—the subtropical valley, the highland mountains, the Badia and the Aqaba gulf regions. It harbors several rainfed areas—arid ($<$200 mm), marginal (200–300 mm), semi-arid (300–500 mm) and semi-humid ($\geq$500). Similarly, Jordan has four vegetation regions—Mediterranean, Irano-Turanian, Shahro-Arabian and Sudanian-tropical (Al-Eisawi 1996). This gives Jordan its vast range of diversity in weather, topography and geology which in turn reveal parallel diversity in plant habitats, starting from the Mediterranean to the Shahro-Arabian.

20.2.1 Animal Products

Adaptation of the ICLS should be integrated, which will enhance forage productivity that is a key for ruminant production (Carvalho et al. 2010). Tradition in Jordan's culture is built on growing sheep and goats for their meat, milk and dairy products (e.g., "Jameed," which used in the preparation of the famous local food the "Manssaf"). In addition, dairy cows play a vital role in the animal production sector for milk products (e.g., yogurt, cheese, skim milk). Other secondary products from animals include leather, wool, hair and organic manure. Despite extensive migration from rural areas to cities, demand and consumption habits for animal products increased with the population's increase.

Available statistics for the number of animal species in Jordan totals 67,590 cows, 752,250 goats and 2,262,630 sheep (Abu-Ashour et al. 2010; Tarawneh et al. 2022). Self-sufficiency in fresh cow's milk is 100%, whereas for cow's meat sufficiency it is only 13.8%. The adequacy in other milk products are 99.9%, 100%, 35.5%, 100% and 49.5% for yoghurt, yogurt, cheese, skim milk and Jameed, respectively (Abu-Ashour et al. 2010). Contribution of animal farming to the total agriculture is 55%, with a total income of 376 JOD in 2012. This vital sector requires a sustainable forage supply to meet the population's needs.

20.2.2 Types of Animal Farms

Animal farms in Jordan could be classified as organized (i.e., registered) and nonorganized (i.e., sporadic in rural areas) farms. The amount of sheep and goat farming is not as easy to study as the case of cow farms because cows are stable on farms, whereas sheep and goats, in most cases, are subjected to moves from one place to another—that is, looking for natural grazing lands. The total number of organized cow farms are 1293; 63% of these are classified as small-scale ones (5–50 head/farm), whereas the remaining have > 50 head/farm. These farms are concentrated in four main cities—Zarka (26,810 heads), Mafraq (18,230 heads), Irbid (11,200 heads) and Amman (7690 heads) (Abu-Ashour et al. 2010; Tarawneh et al. 2022).

The nonorganized farms are important components in the animal farms' production; this type of farm is not reflected clearly by statistics. Still, it occupies a large size in total production. In the rural and at city margins, it is traditional to find small herds of sheep or goats in the family yard; similarly, for the crazing cow, families could have only one or two cows. Owners of these farms find their consumers either at their specific locality or abroad; in many cases, they develop a "family" brand name for their high-quality products that find its consumers beyond their locale (i.e., in the big cities). Also, there are small-scale farms with a holding of 5–50 head. In most cases, the women are responsible for growing, feeding, milking and selling the products with the help of family members while the man is working at urban job— that is, all individuals cooperate with each other to manage the family's life.

The number of people in the animal production sector is estimated to be about 50,000 workers (Tarawneh et al. 2022). This number is obtained from a survey of organized farms; however, the actual figure seems larger than this when the nonorganized farms' workers are added. The nonorganized farms are encouraged and supported by the government in the rural areas, where the owners are poor and vulnerable to any market instability—among which the shortage in forage supply, which equals between 60–70% of total animal production costs—adds to the entire effect of climate change. These are the most critical events that lead to terminating many projects.

20.2.3 Forage Production: Demand and Supply

To keep pace with the ICLS integration, it is imperative to have a sustainable forage supply. It also is important to maintain a supply of required quantity and quality of forages in the market. Because of insufficient fertile agricultural land in Jordan, only 8% has been devoted to forage production. There is a large lack in forage supply in the market and its price fluctuates. Available forages for animals in the local market are fresh green plants, dried green plants, dry straw and fermented plants (i.e., silage). Forage prices in tons, average 50, 120, 250 and 400 in Jordan Dinar (JOD) for green plants, silage, straw and dried green plants (alfalfa), respectively (personal communication).

Green plants are grown locally and include corn, alfalfa, sorghum, pearl millet and ray grass. Dry plants (i.e., straw and dried-green alfalfa) are grown locally as well as imported; they include wheat, barley, lentil, chickpea and alfalfa. Other forage sources are the low-quality natural weeds collected in spring from the roadside and from empty land inside the vegetables and fruit's tree farms; those forages prices in average 30 JOD/ton. In addition, the native range lands are limited in area as well as in time available (i.e., early spring only). The market of forage depends on the local production and on imports (Abu-Ashour et al. 2010; Tarawneh et al. 2022). The bill that allows importing has increased importation significantly during the last few years.

20.2.4 Plans Undertaken at a National Level

To rehabilitate the marginal and degraded lands is very much essential to fulfilling the ever-increasing demand of food, feed and fiber of the increasing population. This rehabilitation can be achieved with good management practices by using the nonconventional water resources, forage crops (i.e., resistance to salinity and drought stress) and marginal lands. The degraded lands are used for food, forest, pasture and bioenergy production. Many countries are using the degraded lands for production of biomass and bioenergy. To convert the degraded lands into a productive one with the nonconventional water resources are a good option on the eve of declining freshwater resources. There are opportunities to use this nonconventional water resource for degraded lands by means of physical water movement from the source point to the point of need after treating.

In Jordan, there is a real need to effectively use all the available nontraditional water resources (e.g., wastewater, saline and semi-saline water). Shifting toward nontraditional water resources to alleviate the shrinking of the agricultural production system in Jordan has been noticed. The Jordanian Ministry of Agriculture has adopted several plans to increase forage production and processing. In this regard, it has various packages and training schedules for increasing the capacity-building of farmers and selecting suitable forage species. The Ministry also is putting efforts into expanding the planted area under forage cultivation and to bringing more marginal areas under forage production through employing nonconventional water resources.

The government has encouraged investment in silage production by local companies. One of these investments is the Rum Agricultural Company at Dessah (South 100 km to Aqaba). Rum is investing in a governmental grains and forages project and is producing 20-thousand tons of silage (40% of local need) yearly (Sada et al. 2015; De Pauw et al. 2015). Still, activities of Rum will be stopped because their contract with the government to use the land and water at their project was terminated; this will increase the effect of silage shortage in the market.

Another investment has been initiated by the government at AL-Muhamadyah (South 20 km to Ma'an) and is now under development with a focus on barley and green forage production as well as silage production (personal communications). In 2011, an investment was started at Al-Safee Valley (South 50 km to Karak) by a local farmers' association in partnership with a privet agricultural company. Large areas of land were cultivated to produce silage from green forages but, unfortunately, after one season the farmers stopped the project because they were not able to produce quality silage as they lacked the proper production information. Other minor projects have been started at various locations, such as Al-Azraq (East 80 km to Zarka) and Dulyel (Center 20 km to Zarka).

20.2.5 Climatic Change Impact

Changes in the climate are considered to affect crop and livestock productivity as well as impacting negatively on water supply and soil conditions. The impact of climate change in Jordan is obvious because of frequent dry years, sporadic rain, greater winter and summer temperatures, dams' reserves, wells' salinity and range lands' degradation, particularly in the marginal dry areas. Development of alternative agricultural systems is one of the key adaptation measures to minimize climate change's impact in Jordan. Considerable efforts have been undertaken by the National Center for Agricultural Research and Extension in collaboration with international research centers.

The goal is to develop alternative plant production systems in marginal areas of Jordan that can cope with the impact of climate changes and provide sustainable systems to support the livelihood of poor farmers in the region. Forage–livestock-based systems are one of the most resilient ones in the dry environments and are key to supporting the livelihood of the farmers and Bedouins in the region. To develop resilient forage systems for the marginal areas, where saline and brackish water resources are the main source for supplementary irrigation, extensive number of forage species, varieties and genotypes were evaluated at various locations throughout the dry areas of Jordan under irrigation with saline water up to 8 dS/m.

The ICLS has several vital features (e.g., economic and environmental) that might differ from one region to another. Depending on the regional climatic situation, agricultural systems are organized in such a way as to get maximum benefit from

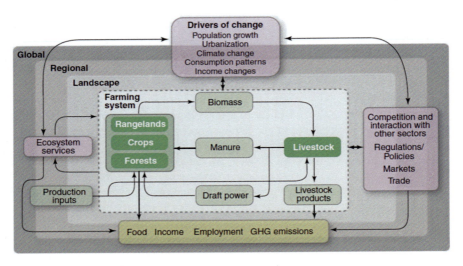

Fig. 20.1 Illustration to demonstrate the various components of the interaction of crop–livestock integration

crop genotypes, cropping systems and crop rotations, as well as integration of suitable livestock into the farming system (Carvalho et al. 2010; Salton et al. 2014). A general interaction of crop–livestock integration is illustrated in Fig. 20.1 to demonstrate all the players and stakeholders on one platform. The ICLS has several benefits over the traditional farming systems and includes enhancing forage and pasture crops' cultivation, increasing soil fertility, organic matter accumulation, increasing nutrient cycling and soil physical and biological properties (Carvalho et al. 2010; Salton et al. 2014).

This chapter contains an overview of the constraints and opportunities of integrated crop–livestock diversification for climate change adaptation in Jordan. It highlights the background, implementation and achievements of the Jordan project, "Adaptation to Climate Change in WANA Marginal Environments through Sustainable Crop and Livestock Diversification." This is important because marginal environment communities (rainfall < 200 mm), extensively subjected to the climate changes to improve their livelihood using nontraditional waters and forage crops.

20.2.6 Site Description

At the Al-Khalediyah Saline Agronomy Research Station in Central-Eastern Jordan, forage species were assessed. The area has a Mediterranean climate with warm winters and summers marked by dry, hot weather.

20.2.7 Species Adaptation and Production Potential

The selected forage crops attainment (about 25) was evaluated to study their adaptation potential under the prevailing environment. Based on this extensive work, promising genotypes were identified from most of the species evaluated that are environmentally and economically feasible under marginal and saline conditions in Jordan. The selected genotypes were tested with the forage–livestock production systems by several farmers. The components of the integrated forage production systems included summer and winter annual and perennial forages.

20.2.8 Farmers' Preference

The productivity of marginal environment and its contribution to the economy, food security and poverty reduction depends on the services provided by functioning of degraded marginal ecosystems, including maintaining soil fertility, freshwater delivery, pollination and pest control. Farmers using nontraditional water sources, primarily saline and TWW, were involved in the selection of appropriate forages. Farmers were invited to the research station because the best genotypes are grown on the farmers' fields; collaborative field days were held and extension service providers followed up. Barley, triticale, sorghum, Pearl millet and sesbania were among the forages that could be easily introduced to the framers' fields with a range of weights.

Saline-tolerant barley was the forage that farmers were most willing to use. Their understanding of the fodder, its growth characteristics and the assurance of a market for the grains and straw were credited with this. Triticale, on the other hand, was initially unwelcome because farmers were uncertain about its market appeal and the challenges of growing on treated soil. It is known locally as "forage wheat," and wheat growing was restricted and prohibited with the treated wastewater.

Farmers were confused about the market acceptance and the complications of growing conditions using TWW. When triticale eventually makes it to the market as animal feeds, farmers welcome it similar to how they would barley (i.e., grains and straw). Sorghum and pearl millet both performed well and were well-liked by farmers, in particular because several cuts could be used to ensure a high yield while also lowering the expense of the irrigation system. Farmers, however, were unable to produce their own seeds and constantly must rely on others. The research findings extracted from the previous phases and projects funded by the in-kind sponsors, with help from the extension servicers, were brought to the farmers' fields gradually. Many genotypes with high-yield potential (i.e., grain or forage), under saline conditions and treated wastewater irrigation, are the target materials to reach the farmers' fields using nontraditional water resources.

20.2.9 Adaptation Strategies

Increasing the quantities of promising grains distributed through each farmer affected the efficiency of the genotypes adopted and released by the project. This increase was from about 20 kg per farmer to reach 150 kg and, in certain cases, to 250 kg at a forerunner farmer. This action was started in the 2013–2014 season and reached acceptance at farmers' levels and thereafter proceeded with this action and distributed bigger quantities for the upcoming seasons.

1. The amount of production was concentrated at the saline research station (i.e., Al-Khlaediyah) by following the optimal production package as sowing date, seeding rate, seed drilling, optimal irrigation, harvesting date and proper threshing that have two major merits:

    (a) The total production increased by up to 5 tons per year, with yield ranging from 450–520 kg per dounoum from triticale and barley genotypes.
    (b) This helped farmers to compare the researcher's field outputs with their farms. This action was an acceptable "farmer's school" learning method with occasional and arranged visits; however, the researchers and extension servicers were always welcomed farmers regardless of their numbers.

    The visit of progressive farmers, researchers, agricultural experts and extension services (Figs. 20.2 and 20.3) were the major means for being in touch with the farmers frequently to answer their questions and to teach them the proper production techniques. Also, the researchers with extension services used to visit the farmers, which included the conduct of field days, general lectures, showing plant samples and conversations with certain pioneer key farmers at their farms.

2. The working team tends to expand their activities to new farmers and to new areas using the nonconventional water sources. The new areas included Shoubak, Karak and Wadi Arabah in the southern parts of Jordan and Al-Halabat in the middle of the country. Farmers agreed to grow the released genotypes in small areas and other farmers were encouraged to grow the crops gradually.

3. Triticale is now a well-known crop among the farmers in the northeast and middle of Jordan. At the beginning, they refused the crop as usual—they did not know it; they did not know whether it is marketable. Now the focus of farmers is on triticale because they found a good market for the grains at a price of 350 JOD per ton with a high-yield straw too.

4. A permanent field was established to multiply the promising grains of sorghum and millet using bird nets. The look of the project encouraged many farmers to test the potential of the adopted crops at rain-fed cultivation sites where the number of farmers received the grain during the winter season to test its potential under rainfall cultivation.

5. The number of farmer's benefits from this project increased gradually from only 15 in the first year to 882,014.

6. A poster was issued on successful farms' stories; they were used as models for other farmers and for new areas.

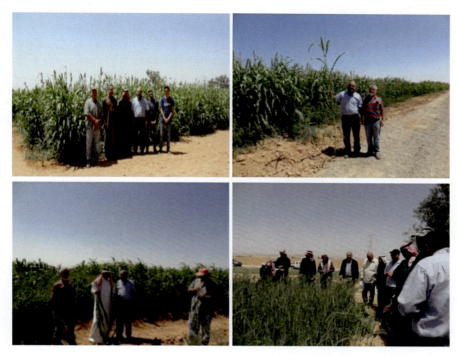

Fig. 20.2 Farmers, researchers and extension service officials visiting research station fields and farmers' fields

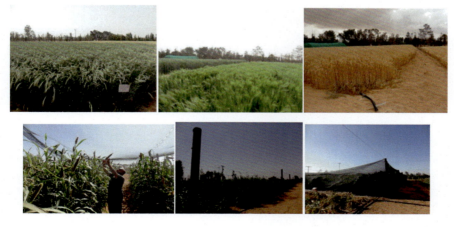

Fig. 20.3 Seed multiplication for winter grains and summer crops at the Khalediyah saline research station

7. To highlight the potential of the promising genotypes from their perspectives, the three pillars (i.e., researchers, extension service providers and farmers) were questioned and recorded in a movie clip during the growing season. These clips were reproduced and showed in the farms' fields or during farmers' visits to the research stations to increase the awareness and to get their viewpoints.

20.3 Integration of the Farming Community in Seed-Production Technologies

20.3.1 Growth, Advancement and Dissemination of Seed-Production Facilities and Genotype Adoption

Al-Khalediyah Saline Agriculture Research Station is one of the most important agricultural stations that belongs to the National Center for Agricultural Research and Extension (NCARE). It is situated in the target areas—Marfaq (TWW), Zarka stream (TWW), Al-Khalediyah (saline) and Azraq (saline). The latter areas are the places where the cooperated farmers grow their crops using the nontraditional water resources (e.g., mainly treated wastewater and saline water).

20.3.2 Seed Store

The research station had seed stored, but it lacked walls, doors, seed shelves, cracked ground and sufficient isolation. A digital scale (150 kg), shelves for small grains, painting, addition of electrical fans for aeration, wall and ground isolation and door modifications are all part of this seed store project's upgrade. Through this project, a seed coating unit, deep freeze, refrigerator and temperature and humidity controller also were added.

20.3.3 Machines

Various types of agricultural machines were available to serve the yield trials and seed production inside the station and for upcoming farmers' services. The potential in the near future was to authorize the machines' movement to cooperative farmers either at low or no cost; therefore to encourage the wide adoption of new and promising genotypes to be released through this project and by the future research findings. The collection of machines included harvesters, various sizes of cultivators, disc plows, tractors, mowers, threshers and sprayers. A forage shopper and a drill machine for seed drilling were donated to the station by the Al-Mafraq Agriculture Department. The cooperative's farmers can benefit from seed drilling during the sowing season.

20.4 Landscape Scale Analysis of Crop Diversification and Effects on the Climate Change Scenario in the Crop–Livestock Farming Context

Most of the West Asia–North Africa (WANA) area contains arid and semi-arid tropical regions with limited water resources. The situation is becoming worse for agricultural production because of the climate change scenario. According to reports of the Intergovernmental Panel on Climate Change (IPCC), greenhouse gasses CO_2, ozone ($[O_3]$), methane, nitrous-oxide and temperature are predicted to increase in the atmosphere (Collins et al. 2013). Nevertheless, drought episodes could occur in the region (Nyasimi et al. 2014). Therefore, screening, selection and development of salt- and drought-tolerant varieties and genotypes have been major adaptation strategies for better use of available arable land and water resources for agricultural growth (Hussain et al. 2018, 2019, 2020; Hussain and Qureshi 2020; Hussain and Al-Dakheel 2018).

In this context, climate resilient crops that can better adapt to marginalized lands in the WANA, especially cultivars and varieties with good yield potential, should be developed, upscaled and disseminated among the regional farming communities for better adaptation and to cope with climate change's impact. The productivity of the traditional farming system should be enhanced through integrated crop-livestock diversification using high-yield crop cultivars and employing nonconventional water resources (e.g., low-quality saline water and TWW). These production packages can enhance the agricultural crops' yield in Al-Zarka and Al-Mafraq (Northeast). Development, advancement and dissemination of seed production packages and identifying genotypes (i.e., 20) with better production potential, which can tolerate salinity and drought stress, under marginal lands of WANA is progressing (Hussain et al. 2018, 2019, 2020; Hussain and Qureshi 2020; Hussain and Al-Dakheel 2018).

Suitable genotypes were obtained from ICBA and screened, evaluated and selected through specific breeding programs at research stations (Table 20.1). Research and a field-based studies were conducted to evaluate the most appropriate crop cultivars and to identify a list of annual and summer salt-tolerant forage crops as integrated feed that can provide food resources throughout the growing season for multiplication and distribution to farmers (Hussain et al. 2018, 2019, 2020; Hussain and Qureshi 2020; Hussain and Al-Dakheel 2018). The higher yield potential varieties were multiplied at local research stations and farmers' fields for enhancing distribution among small and large farms (Hussain et al. 2018, 2019, 2020; Hussain and Qureshi 2020; Hussain and Al-Dakheel 2018).

Various regional and international crop science and breeding research centers and study groups have achieved significant success in the improvement of salt- and drought-tolerant genotypes of food crops, forages and cash crops such as sorghum, maize, Pearl millet, cowpea, buffelgrass, groundnut and sorghum (Hussain and Al-Dakheel 2018; Al-Rifaee 2015; Al-Dakheel et al. 2012; Massimi et al. 2015, 2016). Barley, safflower, quinoa, Pearl millet and sorghum are important forage and grain crops with the capacity to tolerate drought and water insufficiency (Nelson

Table 20.1 Mean Yield for Forage Species Under Saline Conditions in Jordan

	Forage crop	Accession name	Grain yield (t ha^{-1})	Herbage yield (t ha^{-1})
Winter forages	Triticale	Syria-1	4.5	8.0 (dry)
	Barley	Rum	3.3	11.1 (dry)
	Barley	Martin	2.9	17.0 (dry)
	Barley	Saida	3.2	12.3 (dry)
	Barley	Giza-125	2.8	7.2 (dry)
	Barley	Manel	2.9	12.3 (dry)
	Oat	F199084D4	1.5	7.5 (dry)
	Quinoa	NSL-106398	–	15 (dry)
	Egyptian clover	*	–	45 (green cuts)
	Fodder brassica	Hyola 61	1.4	63.4 (green cuts)
	Fodder beet	TINTIN	37.8 (tubers)	112.3 (green)
Summer forages	Sorghum	ICSR 93034	2.5	54 (green)
	Pearl millet	HHVBC tall	2.5	50 (green)
	Corn	White	1.9	72.5 (green)
	Sun flower	Carslien	2.6	18.1 (dry)
	Sudan grass	Sioux	1.9	44 (green)
	Broom corn	Reef1	1.1	52.1 (green)
	Safflower	–	3.5	25 (green)
Perennial forages	Cenchrus	–	–	95 (green)
	Atriplex halimus	–	–	125 (green)
	Cactus	–	–	350 (green)
	Sesbania	–	–	10.9 (green)
	Alfalfa	–	–	18 (green)
	Medicago arboria	–	–	5.2 (green)

et al. 2009) and are well suited to marginal environments of North Africa, especially Jordan. The farmers in North Africa are particularly vulnerable to climate change perturbations that include salinity and drought (Jarvis et al. 2011). Owing to yield losses in diverse field crops and forages, it was a challenge that needed to be addressed for developing, screening, selection and upscaling of drought- and salt-tolerant genotypes of sorghum and Pearl millet, as well as delivering them to the WANA region's farmers whose livelihood depends on agriculture.

Throughout this project thousands of tons of seeds of salt- and drought-tolerant genotypes of sorghum and Pearl millet have been provided to partners in WANA regions since 2011. Currently, several North African seed companies are engaged in research and breeding programs that are producing and marketing seed of the selected genotypes for further distribution to local farmers on demand. According to one estimation, about a million ha of land is planted with these varieties; consequently, they benefit millions of farmers in the target areas of Jordan. The drought- and salt-tolerant crops can be a good source of quality forage for livestock. Because of elevated water-use efficiency, sorghum can be grown under limited amounts of water from germination, early growth stages and up to maturity.

20 Integrated Crop–Livestock System Case Study: Prospectus for Jordan's. . .

From long-term, field-based screening, selection and evaluation of various genotypes and cultivars of barley, Pearl millet, sorghum, triticale, fodder beet, sunflower and thistle have been selected and distributed among small-scale farmers and farmers' associations in Jordan for seed multiplication and further distribution to more marginalized farms. Several genotypes of rapeseed, quinoa and Pearl millet have been extensively tested and produced in the farmers' fields to produce excellent seed production. In the towns of Al-Zarka (Middle) and Al-Mafraq (Northeast), two nurseries have been set up to train and distribute fodder shrubs' seedlings to farmers.

The fodder shrubs were Sesbania, *Medicago arborium*, Kochia and *Acacia saligna*. They were produced and distributed to the participating farmers. According to research and development trials conducted by several colleagues (Hussain et al. 2018, 2019, 2020; Hussain and Qureshi 2020; Hussain and Al-Dakheel 2018; Al-Rifaee 2015; Al-Dakheel et al. 2012; Massimi et al. 2015, 2016; Nelson et al. 2009), the studies showed that sorghum, safflower, buffelgrass, Pearl millet and barley were preferred by farmers as forages. In this context, alfalfa also was liked by several small-scale farmers as a suitable perennial forage nutritive crop. Yet, some large-scale farmers and farmers' associations also promoted several other crops as forages, including barley, fodder beet, triticale and berseem.

20.4.1   Farmers' Field School

Progressive farmers were found and given training in seed production at chosen benchmark sites. Farmers accessing and using the nontraditional water resources (i.e., TWW and saline water) were contacted by the extension services in Al-Mafraq, Al-Kalediays, Al-Azraq and Al-Hashimiyah (along the Zarqa stream). To guide the local farmers in adopting and disseminating the best genotypes suited to their regions, forerunner key farmers were identified. Triticale dry grains could give 4–5 t/ha, which is a desirable yield for farmers. The average yields harvested from the promising barley grown were in the range of 3–4.5 t ha^{-1} of dry grains. The activities were arranged through extension services' programs, where several events were conducted.

The information was disseminated through publication of leaflets that described the major crops' growing packages as barley and triticale, which were tolerant for saline conditions and suitable for TWW irrigation. Farmers' training programs included special sessions related to triticale production technology, soil and water management strategies, forage crops, fertilizer recommendations, sunflower as an oil seed-crop cultivation technology and sugar beet production know-how (in English and Arabic). Information also included feeding schedules for Awasi lams with alfalfa produced under treated wastewater (Arabic).

20.5 Developing Seed Production Technology Packages: Guidelines and Application at the NARS and Farmers' Level (Cultural Practices, Purity Maintenance and Post-Harvest Handling)

20.5.1 Grain Purity Maintenance

To ensure the physical and genetic purity of the accepted genotypes, several hundred spikes of the winter crops (i.e., triticale and barley) that represent the mother crop were individually chosen from seed multiplication fields to retain the purity of the grains. In the following growing season, those individual spikes were cultivated in single rows to eliminate the impurities. The cultivated rows underwent new selection, whereas the others were bulked up and increased as foundational resources for the upcoming seasons. According to the following tables and figure, the project produced and distributed 12,424 kg of adapted forage grains in total between the years 2012 and 2014 (Tables 20.2, 20.3, 20.4 and 20.5).

Table 20.2 Detailed Grain Production during the Period from 2012 to 2014

	2011	2012	2013	2014	Total
Barley	Stock	2423	1875	2765	7063
Triticale	*	1800	890	1920	4610
Oat	*	216	170	270	656
Sorghum	*	*	30	40	70
Pearl millet	*	*	10	15	25

Table 20.3 Cultivated Areas (ha) for Varied Forage Crops

	2011	2012	2013	2014	2015	Total
Barley	3	20.5	31.4	14.3	18.9	88.1
Triticale	*	1.3	16.4	11.9	17	46.6
Oat	*	*	1	0.4	2.1	3.5
Pearl millet	*	*	*	0.8	0.5	1.3
Sorghum	*	*	*	*	0.8	0.8

Table 20.4 Cultivated Areas (ha) by Adapted Forage Crops at Various Sites

	2011	2012	2013	2014	2015	Total
Mafraq (NE)	3	20.5	34.5	12.5	20.1	90.6
Zarka (C)	*	1.3	14.4	12.7	16.1	44.5
Karak (SW)	*	*	*	1.3	0.7	2.0
Ma'an (SE)	*	*	*	0.2	1.8	2.0
Wadi Arabah (SW)	*	*	*	*	0.9	0.9

20 Integrated Crop–Livestock System Case Study: Prospectus for Jordan's... 581

Table 20.5 Average Farm Size (ha) Cultivated by Adapted Forage Crops

	2011	2012	2013	2014	2015	Total
Barley	0.2	1.7	1.1	0.51	0.5	4.01
Triticale	*	0.2	0.5	0.66	0.5	1.86
Oat	*	*	0.02	0.4	0.21	0.63

20.5.2 Role of NARS's Formal Seed System, and Extension, and Dissemination of Conventional and Nonconventional Crops: Continuation of Screening and Evaluation

From the very beginning, farmers preferred barley as a fodder. Triticale initially was rejected, but thanks to the work of the extension specialists, farmers are increasingly beginning to accept this crop. Only educated farmers agree to grow oats because conventional farmers believe the enhanced variety will act like the wild types and invade their fields as weeds. To introduce the oat to local cultivation, more time is required. Over time, the size of the farms for each adapted forage changed. According to Tables 20.3, 20.4 and 20.5, triticale is grown in the second-largest areas after barley.

20.5.3 Integrated Crop Management Packages to Improve Livestock Production

The ICLS plays a vital role in agricultural development of both large- and small-scale farmers and thus also enhancement of the livestock sector (Salton et al. 2014). The availability of suitable forages (e.g., barley, sorghum and Pearl millet) can secure 60–75% of feed for livestock that will ultimately help in the ICLS. This also enhanced the importance and benefits of the production system and farmers' wealth. The project also achieved its goals through providing technical services to farmers to increase their capacity to convert forage crops into high-quality feed. Various forages were screened and chosen to include in diverse nutritive ration programs for livestock. The ICBA has provided them with salt- and drought-tolerant genotypes of sorghum, Pearl millet, barley and other forages (e.g., lucerne, saltbush, sesbania and kochia) that have demonstrated good yield potential at various farmers' fields.

Several morphological, physiological and quality-based experiments were conducted at the designated experimental research station and suitable varieties were identified that have excellent potential for inclusion in ruminant feeds (Massimi et al. 2015, 2016; Abu et al. 2017). Several authors and project partners observed that for a high-quality nutrient and balanced rations, various crops (e.g., alfalfa and berseem including fodder beets) should be thoroughly mixed with other forages (i.e., sorghum, barley) and forage grasses.

Other crops (e.g., Pearl millet and *Panicum turgidum*) should to be tested on an alternative basis that will provide energy, nutrition and crude protein substances (Massimi et al. 2015, 2016). The project demonstrated on-farm techniques for feed processing and usages to improve storage capacity and feed values. The main methods used were silage treatment, treatment of food blocks, production of food in covered piles and biological treatments; these technologies have been demonstrated for a total of more than 1500 farmers (Massimi et al. 2015, 2016; Abu et al. 2017).

20.5.4 Socioeconomic Impact of Improved Production Systems on Farmers' Livelihoods in Marginal Environments

The project showed significant impact on livelihood and socioeconomic characteristics of the farmers of the target WANA marginal lands. The economic viability of integrated crop management packages (ICMPs) introduced into the marginal environment has been assessed, while production and information on soils and water also was documented. The costs and benefits of feed production packages are based on the use of various types of noncoventional water (Hussain et al. 2019, 2020; Hussain and Al-Dakheel 2018; Massimi et al. 2015, 2016; Nelson et al. 2009; Jarvis et al. 2011; Abu et al. 2017).

Demonstration areas for efficient production systems have been built with the full participation of farmers, as well as gender-based participation (i.e., women farmers). A 25–35% increase was observed in farmers' income following adoption of improved production packages, highly nutritive genotypes, higher yield potential varieties and farm management practices. Socioeconomic indicators, production and information on soils and water were collected after reconstitution and adoption by farmers to test whether the candidate technologies were viable, sustainable and value-added.

The results of the assessment of the economic value of crop systems operating on salt-tolerant yields increased agricultural incomes by 70% compared to traditional practices (Massimi et al. 2015, 2016). Farmers who have been involved in genotype testing with experiments at their farms have demonstrated the superiority of the selected millet and sorghum types, which have a feed yield at least 30% higher than their conventional crops. A survey of several farms showed that the introduction of salt-tolerant staples into farmers' "farming systems improves farmers" incomes by 50% compared to traditional practices (Massimi et al. 2015, 2016; Nelson et al. 2009; Jarvis et al. 2011; Abu et al. 2017). One of the major achievements of the project was the rapid growth in the number of participants who delivered and deployed new technologies.

20.5.5 Improving Knowledge and Skills of Farmers and Agricultural Extension Staff in Marginal Environments

Separate training activities and capacity-building programs were started by the project team to enhance the technical skills of farmers and extension staff in farm production (e.g., variety selection, conservation practices for water, seed multiplication) and management actions. Such capacity-building activities were carried out through farmers' field schools and training workshops.

20.6 Summary

The ICLS climate change is greatly influencing ecosystem services, agriculture and water resources. Therefore, various crop production packages, integrated with suitable forage species and livestock, should be given opportunities to prevail to combat the awful consequences of climate change. Several salt- and drought-tolerant forage crops (e.g., barley, sorghum, Pearl millet, fodder beets, lucerne, kochia, saltbush and sesbania) were selected and distributed among the farming communities for seed multiplication and further provision to other small and large farms for better adaptation in the marginal lands of Jordan.

It is necessary to save freshwater resources and use alternate water sources (e.g., TWW and low-quality saline water) to avoid further land degradation and to protect fragile land resources that are resilient to climate change. Sustainable livestock production should be adapted through breeding of salt- and drought-tolerant crops and producing climate-resilient animals. This will also provide an opportunity to increase income, livelihood and socioeconomic situations for owners of small farms. The present model of the ICLS can be further improved and adapted in other degraded marginal environments with similar problems and that are under threat of climate change to get maximum benefits from the crop–livestock integration.

Funding and Acknowledgements This work was implemented as part of the project, "Adaptation to Climate Change in WANA Marginal Environments Through Sustainable Crop and Livestock Diversification," that was a five-year project (2011–2016) jointly supported by the International Fund for Agriculture Development (IFAD), the Arab Fund for Economic and Social Development (AFESD), the OPEC Fund and the Islamic Development Bank (IDB). From North Africa, project partners include: the Desert Research Center (DRC), Cairo, Egypt; the National Center for Agricultural Research and Extension (NCARE), Amman, Jordan; the Ministry of Agriculture & Fisheries, Oman, Jordan; the Ministry of Agriculture, Palestine; the General Commission for Scientific Agricultural Research (GCSAR), Syria; the Arab Center for the Study of Arid Zones and Dry Lands (ACSAD), Tunisia; the Agricultural Research and Extension Authority, Yemen. Senior Scientist, Dr. Abdullah J. Al-Dakheel, from The International Center for Biosaline Agricultural, Dubai, UAE, served as primary investigator.

References

Abu OA, Ismael FM, Al-Abdullah MJ, Jamjum K, Al-Rifaee MK, Tawaha AM, Al-Dakheel AJ (2017) Impact of different levels of salinity on performance of triticale that is grown in Al-Khalidiyah (Mafraq), Jordan. Am Eurasian J Sustain Agri 11:1–6

Abu-Ashour J, Qdais HA, Al-Widyan M (2010) Estimation of animal and olive solid wastes in Jordan and their potential as a supplementary energy source: an overview. Renew Sust Energ Rev 14:2227–2231

Al-Dakheel AJ, Fraj MB, Shabbir GM, Al Gailani AQM (2012) Evaluation of Batini barley landraces from Oman and breeding lines under various irrigation salinity levels. Agri Sci Res J 2:42–50

Al-Eisawi D (1996) Vegetation of Jordan

Al-Rifaee MK (2015) Adaptation of winter crops for summer cultivation and salinity stresses in Mediterranean region: selection for double-cropping and crop rotation. Adv Environ Biol 9: 163–166

Carvalho KCC, Mulinari DR, Voorwald HJC, Cioffi MOH (2010) Chemical modification effect on the mechanical properties of hips/coconut fiber composites. Bioresources 5:1143–1155

Collins M, Knutti R, Arblaster J, Dufresne JL, Fichefet T, Friedlingstein P, Gao X, Gutowski WJ, Johns T, Krinner G, Shongwe M (2013) Long-term climate change: projections, commitments and irreversibility. In: Climate change 2013-the physical science basis: contribution of working group I to the fifth assessment report of the intergovernmental panel on climate change. Cambridge University Press, Cambridge, pp 1029–1136

De Pauw E, Saba M, Ali SH (2015) Mapping climate change in Iraq and Jordan. International Center for Agricultural Research in the dry areas, 27

Hussain MI, Al-Dakheel AJ (2018) Effect of salinity stress on phenotypic plasticity, yield stability and signature of stable isotopes of carbon and nitrogen in safflower. Environ Sci Pollut Res 25: 23685–23694

Hussain MI, Qureshi AS (2020) Health risks of heavy metal exposure and microbial contamination through consumption of vegetables irrigated with treated wastewater at Dubai. UAE Environ Sci Pollut Res 27:11213–11226

Hussain MI, Al-Dakheel AJ, Reigosa MJ (2018) Genotypic differences in agro-physiological, biochemical and isotopic responses to salinity stress in quinoa (*Chenopodium quinoa* Willd.) plants: prospects for salinity tolerance and yield stability. Plant Physiol Biochem 129:411–420

Hussain MI, Muscolo A, Farooq M, Ahmad W (2019) Sustainable use and management of non-conventional water resources for rehabilitation of marginal lands in arid and semiarid environments. Agric Water Manag 221:462–476

Hussain MI, Farooq M, Muscolo A, Rehman A (2020) Crop diversification and saline water irrigation as potential strategies to save freshwater resources and reclamation of marginal soils—a review. Environ Sci Pollut Res 27:28695–28729

Jarvis A, Lau C, Cook S, Wollenberg E, Hansen J, Bonilla O, Challinor A (2011) An integrated adaptation and mitigation framework for developing agricultural research: synergies and trade-offs. Exp Agric 47:185–203

Massimi M, Al-Rifaee MK, Alrusheidat J, Al-Dakheel A, Al-Qawaleet K, Al-Adamat A (2015) Yield response of fodder sorghum (*Sorghum bicolor* L.) to seed rate under non-conventional water conditions. Conference proceedings: Regional symposium on the scientific outcomes of the project: Adaptation to climate change in WANA marginal environments through sustainable crop and livestock diversification, Amman, Jordan

Massimi M, Al-Rifaee M, Alrusheidat J, Al-Dakheel A, Ismail F, Al-Ashgar Y (2016) Salt-tolerant triticale (X Triticosecale Witt) cultivation in Jordan as a new forage crop. Am J Exp Agri 12:1–7

Nelson GC, Rosegrant MW, Koo J, Robertson R, Sulser T, Zhu T, Ringler C, Msangi S, Palazzo A, Batka M, Magalhaes M (2009) Climate change: impact on agriculture and costs of adaptation (Vol. 21). Intl Food Policy Res Inst. Climate Change Impact on Agriculture and Costs of Adaptation. International Food Policy Research Institute, Food Policy Report no. XX, ISBN: 978–0–89629-535-4. Washington, DC, USA, 30 p

Nyasimi M, Amwata D, Hove L, Kinyangi J, Wamukoya G (2014) Evidence of impact: climate-smart agriculture in Africa. CCAFS Working Paper

Sada AA, Abu-Allaban M, Al-Malabeh A (2015) Temporal and spatial analysis of climate change at Northern Jordanian Badia. Jordan J Earth Environ Sci 7:87–93

Salton JC, Mercante FM, Tomazi M, Zanatta JA, Concenco G, Silva WM, Retore M (2014) Integrated crop-livestock system in tropical Brazil: toward a sustainable production system. Agric Ecosyst Environ 190:70–79

Tarawneh RA, Tarawneh MS, Al-Najjar KA (2022) Agricultural policies among advisory and cooperative indicators in Jordan. Int J Res 10:10

Chapter 21
Effect of Salinity Intrusion on Sediments in Paddy Fields and Farmers' Adaptation Initiative: A Case Study

Prabal Barua, Anisa Mitra, and Mazharul Islam

Abstract Bangladesh, with a population of 150 million, is the most overcrowded nation on the Earth. The agricultural sector is facing the effect of congestion at various levels and ways because of climate change-induced disaster. The study for this chapter was conducted to analyze the impact of saline water intrusion on the production and soil conditions in paddy fields of the Southeastern coast of Bangladesh. It reveals that surface water salinity was high everywhere and soil quality was alarming. Communities in the study area stated that the salinity problem in the crop fields led to low production and economic loss for the farmers of Banshkhali upazila of the Chittagong district. The authors found that the salinization process guided not only changing of crop rotation but also discouraged farmers from cultivating food crops in the area. Repairing levees, producing a native high-yield variety, using organic fertilizer and executing Integrated Coastal Zone Management (ICZM) could raise the production of crops and the fertility of sediments there. The study helped to establish that farmers' adaptation practices for reducing the salinity level of agricultural fields could be useful for controlling climate change in the vulnerable areas and worldwide, while addressing the salinization problem.

Keywords Climate change · Agricultural land · Salinization · Adaptation practices

---

P. Barua (✉)
Department of Knowledge Management for Development, Young Power in Social Action, Chittagong, Bangladesh

A. Mitra
Department of Zoology, Sundarban Hazi Desarat College, Pathankhali, West Bengal, India

M. Islam
Coastal and Ocean Management Institute, Xiamen University, Fujian, China

© The Author(s), under exclusive license to Springer Nature Switzerland AG 2022
M. Ahmed (ed.), *Global Agricultural Production: Resilience to Climate Change*,
https://doi.org/10.1007/978-3-031-14973-3_21

587

21.1 Introduction

Changing climate is among the most dreaded troubles during the new millennium. The effects of it are visible everywhere internationally. One of the extremely severe outcomes of weather change is that human beings are being forced to leave their homes, lands and livelihood because the of consequences of climate change which has destroyed some areas. Such factors stand to displace many thousands and thousands of people in the coming years. The coast of Bangladesh is at risk of intense herbal failures, which include cyclones, typhoon surges and floods in aggregate with other natural and humanmade threats, including erosion, excessive arsenic content in groundwater, saline water intrusion, water logging and water and soil salinity; these breakdowns have made coastal dwellers especially susceptible and threatens the entire coast and marine environment (Islam 2004). Regions of the coast constitute approximately 2.5 million hectares (ha), which amounts to about 25% of the total cropland of Bangladesh. Nearly 0.84 million ha have been affected by various intensities of salinity, ensuring exceptionally negative land utilization (Barua and Rahman 2017; Barua et al. 2017).

Among the 181 vulnerable nations that experience a changing climate, Bangladesh is positioned at 165, as well as being the 30th susceptible nation to climate change (IDMC 2021). The geographical and landscape position of Bangladesh makes it particularly susceptible to tremendous weather changes (e.g., cyclone, flood, coastal erosion and storm surges). Its susceptibility is generated not only through its biophysical location but also by its poor socioeconomic conditions (Barua et al. 2017; Barua and Rahman 2020).

Bangladesh is an agricultural sector-dependent nation. Agriculture, however, is surprisingly predisposed to weather changes. It is expected that a changing climate will have a worse effect on agriculture and manufacturing in the new millennium, besides the hassle of excessive temperatures, abnormal rainfall and severe weather patterns brought about by activities such as floods, cyclones, droughts and increasing sea levels (Shameem and Momtaz 2015; Hazbavi et al. 2018).

Soil salinity is a significant land degradation problem in Bangladesh's agriculture sector, which adversely affects the productivity of the land. The Chittagong district, located in the Southeastern coastal area, is susceptible to cyclones, storms and tidal surges, tidal floods, water logging and other natural disasters. There have been 30 devastating cyclones and storm surges in Chittagong and the Cox's Bazar coastal area between 1960 and 2016. The most damaging and powerful cyclone of the last century hit Chittagong on 1991; after that another one ravaged the area in July 2016 when *Ruano* hit the coast of Banshkhali—the Anwara upazila Subdistrict of Chittagong. Saline water (i.e., salinization) is the main associated calamity; its source and process are from various natural disasters, which cause tidal fluctuations because a huge amount of saline water comes ashore inundating coastal areas (Barua et al. 2016; Barua and Rahma 2018, 2019).

Rice is the most significant and demanded agricultural crop product required for feeding and survival of global communities (Shimono et al. 2010). Almost 60% of the world's population completely depends on production in rice paddies (Maclean et al. 2002). In Bangladesh, a paddy is the fastest yielding among all other products in developing countries. Nearly 80% of all fertile land is now used for rice production. Therefore, several declines in paddy production because of a changing climate becomes grave, spoiling food security of the nation (Islam et al. 2020). Therefore, measuring the influence of changing climate on paddy cultivation, and appraising the agricultural cultivators' coping capability, has become a theme of imperative research.

21.2 Effect of Changing Climate on Crop Production

The most susceptible sectors to climate change are recognized to be agricultural activities because of their enormous size and consideration of the weather-related variabilities, causing gigantic economic effects (Mendelsohn 2009). The changes in climate behavior (e.g., rainfall and temperature) drastically impact crop yield. The influence of increasing temperatures, variation in precipitation and fertilization of CO_2 diverges according to the characteristics of the crop, place, zone and degree of the change in the factors. The increasing pattern of temperature rise has verified a decline in crop production, even as the rise in precipitation is expected to counterbalance or decrease the effect of increasing temperature (Adams 1998).

As predicted by the climatic variables observed in Iran, productivity of the crops varied based on adaptation capacities and types of crop, climate condition and CO_2 fertilization's impact (Karimi et al. 2018). Farmers' net profits were found to decline considerably with a reduced level in rainfall or temperature rise in the African nation of Cameroon which faced an absence of a standard approach to responsive policymaking; this was followed by a small necessity for export of agricultural products of the country, thereby resulting in fluctuations in national revenue (Molua 2017). High temperatures affect coffee production in Mexico, and it has been found that yields might not remain cost-effective. Continued coffee-growing may not be feasible for producers in coming years because there is an indication of a 34% decline in production (Gay et al. 2016).

Although climate change affects various economic segments, the damage is significant for rain-fed agriculture (Ochieng et al. 2016, 2017) that predicts a decline on the African continent in major crop yields of 9–25% by 2050 (Schlenker and Lobell 2010). Since the 1964 to 2014 period, 12 droughts and 20 major floods have occurred in Kenya, which affected five million people because of low crop production and food insecurity (Parry et al. 2012). In addition, three million people of Malawi have been impacted by floods in 2015–2016 because of fluctuation in climate factors as a consequence of droughts, floods and other disasters, as well as increased climate variability. Since 2015–2018, six million people have been affected owing to significant drought and resulting food production decline (Katengeza et al. 2019).

As a result of raised monsoon unpredictability and melting of Himalayan glaciers, even an unassuming moderate 1.5–2 °C temperature rise could insensitively affect the accessibility and steadiness of the water assets in South Asia (Vinke et al. 2017); it is predicted that large areas of the countries in South Asia will become used to a reduction in crop productivity (IPCC 2014; Vinke et al. 2017). Aryal et al. (2020) stated that temperature increase has pessimistically influenced India's crop production—5–30% for wheat production, 6–8% for rice production and 10–30% for maize yield.

Consequently, without taking any measures for sustainable climate adaptation, South Asia is expected to drop nearly 2% of its yearly GDP by 2050 and approximately 9% during the twenty-first century (Ahmed and Suphachalasai 2014). In South Asian countries, 70% of the people completely depend on agricultural activities, which ensures 22% of the gross domestic product (GDP), and any reduced rate of GDP will damage the livelihood and economic situation of the substantial number of agricultural farmers (Wang et al. 2019; Aryal et al. 2020).

The influence of climate change recorded on agricultural crop production depends on the location and application of the irrigation activities in the fields. Production could be raised by increasing irrigated places, which could have a damaging effect on the surrounding environment (Kang et al. 2019). The increasing pattern of temperature rise is expected to decrease the production of various crops through abandoning their traditional cycle (Mahato 2014). The collective production of maize, rice and wheat are anticipated to decrease if both the tropical and temperate regions experience warming of 20 °C; generally, climate change has substantial effects on temperate zones because the tropical agriculture products mature earlier than their ideal growth period. Temperature is a problem, thus knowledge of high-temperature stress is important at higher limits of heat (Challinor et al. 2014).

Furthermore, diseases and various species of insect pests are more widespread in warmer and humid regions of the Earth (Rosenzweig 2018). Other variables (e.g., wind speed and humidity, besides rainfall and temperature) also affect crops' production, and when these climatic variables are nonexistent, there is a probability of overforecasting the value of climate change. In addition, it has been recorded that changing climate is expected to decrease China's wheat, corn and rice production from 19%, 13% and 45% to 12%, 36% and 11% by 2100 (Zhang et al. 2017).

Severe weather-related natural hazards have turned out to be more recurrent since the early 1900s in the Netherlands and have drastically impacted the production of wheat in the country. Li et al. (2019) stated that there will be occurrences of long-duration droughts in the upcoming years becasuse of climate change in almost all regions of the Earth, and a raise in the drought-impact placement area from 15.5–45.0% is projected by 2100. Among the most affected continent, Africa will be a more vulnerable region for drought conditions soon. The production of commercially important crops in drought regions is expected to decrease by a rate of 50% by 2050 and nearly 90% by 2100 (Stevanovic et al. 2016).

Loss of production of agricultural crops could increase the price of foods and could have a ridiculous impact on agriculture's benefit around the world, with annual losses of 0.3% of future GDP by 2100 (Barua and Rahman 2020). Yet, Kumar and

Gautam (2014) mentioned that climate change has an inadequate influence on the global food supply, although developing nations could tolerate harsh negative effects. Temperature is forecast to increase by 2.33 °C and 4.78 °C in India along with a replication in CO_2 level and permanence of the heat waves, which could have a harmful impact on agricultural activities.

In Pakistan, farmers could loose US$300 per acre annually by 2100 with an increase of 1 °C in temperature, whereas the average income could be raised by US$120 and US$250 with an increase in rainfall of 9% and 15%, respectively (Shakoor et al. 2019). The loss of production for three different cereal grains (e.g., rice, wheat and maize) are predicted to deteriorate by 10–25% with a 1 °C raise in the global average of surface temperature (Deutsch et al. 2018). Average crop production is anticipated to drop by 6–25% because of climate change in Southern Africa (Waha et al. 2019).

Malhi et al. (2021) stated that climate change is a universal risk to the nutritional and food security of the planet; this is because of the increasing rate of global temperature leading to a raised crop respiration rate and evapotranspiration, elevated pest invasion, changing trends in weed flora and decreased length of crop growth. Climate change is responsible for impacts on the increasing of microbial population and their enzymatic actions in sediments. Population growth has created a massive pressure on agriculture to ensure the safekeeping of food, livelihood and nutrition for the global population—that is, prevent further deterioration because of climate change. With the rate of increasing climate change factors, the study explored the reduction of agricultural production in Bangladesh during the coming years.

21.3 Climate Change and Agriculture Sectors

Changing climate and its consequences for the impact on rice production is not the newest incident in the situation. Mean values of the temperature rise with steady dry spells at the moment before and during the rainy season, superior seasonal rainfall factors and serious consecutive downpours during the last moment of a monsoon are regularly recorded (Kabir et al. 2017). Temperatures have increased over the last three centuries, particularly at the period of the monsoon season, and they have increased by 0.7 °C per decade all over Bangladesh (Ahsan and Islam 2011). It is predicted that by 2030, the mean temperature will increase by 1 °C and by 1.4 °C by 2050 (FAO 2016). Rainfall is awfully erratic and the allocation has been increasing at a jagged rate (Ahsan and Islam 2011). The number of days without rain has raisen, even though the total yearly rainfall remains approximately the same. Rainfall creates intense events (e.g., floods and droughts) that have perceptibly unfavorable effects on rice, and Aman rice production was reduced by 20–30% in the North-western areas of the country in 2006 during the time of drought. The possibility for tropical cyclones, erosion and tidal floods continues to rise in the coastal salinity-prone areas of Bangladesh, where 10% of the zone is 1 m above mean sea level and has more exposure to the tidal inundation problem (Alam et al. 2020).

The intrusion of salinity presents substantial danger to sparkling groundwater bodies as well as sparkling herbal water aquatic wetlands (Talukder et al. 2015). The World Bank said that a converting climate was grounds for sizeable submergence inside the low mendacity areas and enhanced the increased cost of salinity intrusion. Climate change has brought about worldwide warming, which is the main reason for the rise in seawater temperature (IPCC 2013). Except, clean water glide from the upstream vicinity has steadily declined, in particular during the summer and winter seasons. Such incidents are responsible for the additional occurrences of excessive salinity interference in the coastal regions of Bangladesh.

The forecast is that the area of freshwater locations could decrease from 46% to 35%, and that the moderate region of a saline area could decline from 51% to 46% because of the oceans' temperature rise. Additionally, it is a noteworthy statistic that the area of salt water in surrounding areas will rise from 6% to 18% by 2030 (Barua and Rahman 2021). As a result of growing salinity, 21% of the greater land area in comparison to 1990 could be gravely impacted, and the intensity of salinity could be amplified by 15% (Barua et al. 2020, 2021). Alam et al. (2020) showed that the increasing cost of the salinity stage in the sediment should be set at 0.95%, in line with the year. There are exclusive sources of salinity intrusion around the coastal areas, which are a part of the Southeastern coastal sector of Bangladesh.

Paddy land becomes salty as it comes into contact with seawater and continues to be flooded during high tides and intrusion of water from the Sangu River and its streams; as a result salinization processes reduce soil fertility, alter original or old agricultural practices and discourage farmers from cultivating. The primary objectives of the study were to determine soil and water salinity and the current soil fertility status of the rice land and to begin some measures to reduce the salinization processes and improve the study area's fertility status.

21.4   Case Study

Chittagong is a coastal district situated in Southerneastern shore of Bangladesh and is a natural combination of hills and sea. The study was done in the Anwara upazila (Subdistrict), which is under the Division of Chittagong. Among the 11 unions of the Anwara subdistricts, the study concentrated mainly on two areas (i.e., Gohira and Bottali) affected by climate change.

The authors took the sediment samples from the 11 study areas from November 2019 to August 2020 to estimate the fertility circumstances and surface water salinity level. They also used the Global Positioning System (GPS) to document the absolute locations of the samples (Table 21.1).

The major livelihood of the people depends on agriculture, fishing, small-scale business or shopkeeping. Most of the rice fields are suitable for three crops.

Table 21.2 summarizes the selected parameters of surface water salinity, soil quality and fertility status in paddy fields.

21 Effect of Salinity Intrusion on Sediments in Paddy Fields and Farmers'... 593

Table 21.1 Sampling location of the study area

S. No	Sampling station	GPS value
Site 1	Gohira Hill (valley area)	21°255′50.9″–91°59′13.2″
Site 2	Jakulia Hill (valley area)	21°25′22.2″–91°59′30.7″
Site 3	EPZED area (valley area)	21°25′50.8″–91°59′18.5″
Site 4	KAFCO area (valley area)	21°24′09.3″–91°59′31.3″
Site 5	College area (Plain land)	21°24′23.4″–92°01′2.5″
Site 6	Parkee Ghona (P. area)	21°24′40.4″–92°01′71″
Site7	Chandro pahar (P. area)	21°24′42.5″–92°01′9.9″
Site 8	South Rubber Dam (P. area)	21°25′2.6″–92°01′10.7″
Site 9	North Rubber Dam (P. area)	21°25′7.7″–92°01′12.8″
Site 10	Khurulia (P. area)	21°24′52.3″–92°01′44.6″
Site 11	Link road (P. area)	21°24′6.6″–92°01′38.8″

Table 21.2 Summary of surface water salinity, soil quality and fertility status

Water qualityfactors	No. of sample	Minimum	Maximum	Mean	Std. deviation
Salinity (%$_0$)	11	0.42	45.10	24.8291	14.65116
Soil quality					
Ph	11	1.80	3.60	2.8955	0.54150
Color	11	Reddish	Blackish		
Temperature (°C)	11	26.00	35.00	31.8182	2.60070
Salinity (%$_0$)	11	1.00	30.50	19.1727	12.01491
Fertility status					
Structure and textural class	11	Sandy	Sandy loam		
Bulk density (g/cm^3)	11	1.51	1.66	1.5809	0.04949
OC (%)	11	0.13	0.77	0.4473	0.18347
OM (%)	11	0.22	1.32	0.7718	0.31654

The authors found a maximum salinity level of 45.10 ds/m at study area 5 and an average salinity of 24.83 ds/m and a minimum salinity of 0.42 ds/m at site 4, with a standard deviation of 14.65 ds/m (see Table 21.1). Temperature affects soil biota activity directly by determining the level of physiological activity (e.g., enzyme activity) and indirectly by affecting physicochemical properties (e.g., nutrient diffusion and solubility, mineral weathering, evaporation rate and so on). The authors found that the maximum temperature is 26 °C at study area 2, the minimum temperature is 35 °C at study area 6 and the mean temperature is 31.8 °C, with a standard deviation of 2.6 °C (see Table 21.2).

The authors explored the soil color condition in the study areas and found the black or blackish, brown and red or reddish color of sediments in the crop fields. About 54.54% of the samples were black or blackish, 36.36% were brown and 9.09% were red or reddish in the study area (Table 21.3).

Table 21.3 Soil color in the paddy fields of the study areas

Range of limit	Number of samples	Percentage (%)
Black or blackish	6	54.54
Brown	4	36.36
Red or reddish	1	9.09
Total	11	100.0

Table 21.4 Findings of soil structure and texture in the study areas

Site no.	Soil structure or separation				Soil texture	
	% sand	% silt	% clay	Fertility status	Textural class	Fertility status
Site 1	92.9	2.5	4.6	Poor	Sandy	Poor
Site 2	62.9	30	7.1	Poor	Sandy loam	Medium good
Site 3	37.9	52.5	9.6	Good	Silt loam	Good
Site 4	57.9	35	7.1	Medium good	Sandy loam	Medium good
Site 5	60.4	35	4.6	Poor	Sandy loam	Medium good
Site 6	75.4	17.5	7.1	Poor	Sandy loam	Medium good
Site 7	75.4	17.5	7.1	Poor	Sandy loam	Medium good
Site 8	50.4	40	9.6	Good	Loam	Very good
Site 9	32.9	60	7.1	Very good	Silt loam	Very good
Site 10	35.4	57.5	7.1	Very good	Silt loam	Very good
Site 11	45.4	45	9.6	Very good	Loam	Very good

Table 21.4 indicates that the soil textures in the study areas and that flat surface (i.e., plane) land soil was more fertile than hill soil because the portion of silt loam particles was high in the plane soil; on the other hand, the portion of sandy loam and sand particles was high in the hill soil. It is important that in some flat surface land, soil status was sandy loam and the fertility status was medium good.

From these findings, the authors observed that the bulk density of sediment shifts in the total pore space present in the soil; it provides a good estimate of soil porosity. Table 21.5 shows that the authors found the mean soil density in bulk to be 1.5 gm/cc, which indicated that the present level of density was moderate for paddy cultivation in the study areas. The table shows that soil bulk density was poor in valley area soil and soil bulk density was good in flat surface land soils. This highlighted that study sites 5 and 6 both were plane areas but their bulk density was poor.

It was discovered that salinity created a degraded environment and imbalance of the hydrological situation that hampered the regular agricultural crops' production throughout the study areas—that is , the range of salinity level. Maximum salinity content was calculated at 30.5 ds/m in study site 5 and minimum content was found to be 1.0 ds/m at sites 2, 3 and 4. For the other sites, soil salinity was very good because these areas were active with tidal fluctuations and inundation of paddy land by saline water; at site 5, along with tidal creeks, was directly active with the Bay of Bangle and the Sangu River (Table 21.6).

Soil electircal conductivity (EC) was found to be low with respect to the referring level (2.0–4.0 ds/m) (see Table 21.6). According to the findings, it was discovered

21 Effect of Salinity Intrusion on Sediments in Paddy Fields and Farmers'... 595

Table 21.5 Findings of soil bulk density in the study areas

Sample location	Bulk density (g/cm^3)	Fertility status
Site 1	1.66	Poor
Site 2	1.60	Poor
Site 3	1.51	Good
Site 4	1.59	Poor
Site 5	1.61	Poor
Site 6	1.63	Poor
Site7	1.63	Poor
Site 8	1.53	Good
Site 9	1.55	Good
Site 10	1.55	Good
Site 11	1.53	Good

Table 21.6 Findings of soil factors in the study areas' sample sites

Sample No	pH	Salinity	EC mS/cm	% O.C	% O.M	Total % N	Total % P	Total % K	Total % Ca	Total %Mg
1	3.0	22.3	0.08	0.13	00.22	0.06	0.3075	0.20	0.0037	0.110
2	3.5	1	0.05	0.31	00.53	1.00	0.28	0.54	0.0009	0.434
3	1.8	1	0.01	0.62	10.07	1.02	1.135	1.04	0.0000	0.532
4	2.3	1	0.05	0.49	00.85	0.98	0.69	0.56	0.0002	0.160
5	2.8	30.5	0.10	0.53	00.91	1.04	1.0225	0.51	0.0003	0.115
6	3.0	25.5	0.09	0.27	00.47	0.73	1.03	0.33	0.0001	0.061
7	3.0	23.2	0.08	0.47	00.82	0.78	0.7875	0.26	0.0006	0.078
8	2.8	29.4	0.15	0.58	00.01	1.00	1.51	0.64	0.0001	0.313
9	2.6	22	0.12	0.77	00.32	1.23	0.3425	1.05	0.0003	0.584
10	3.5	29.4	0.05	0.46	00.79	0.88	0.7975	0.78	0.0003	0.614
11	3.6	25.6	0.01	0.29	00.50	0.31	0.8325	0.70	0.0001	0.029

that the percentage of the total nitrogen status was good and very good in the study areas but only site 1 was in the hill area. From the findings, it is revealed that nitrogen levels in the agricultural crop fields indicate that they are fertile, and farmers used various types of organic and inorganic fertilizers, especially urea on paddy land.

Potassium (K) is another important nutrient; it is not only important for the increase of fertility status but also it directly involves plants' growth. Optimum limit of the percentage of total K is for four categories—that is, low (< 0.15), medium (0.150–0.30), high (0.30–0.375) and very high (> 0.375) (SRDI 2010; Chowdhury et al. 2011). Minimum percentage of total K was found to be 0.20, maximum was 1.05 and mean was 0.6009; this shows that the percentage of total K was good and very good for crop cultivation.

Islam (2004) reported that many coastal areas, including Chittagong, are facing increased salinity levels in agricultural fields. Nearly 1.5 million ha of arable land in Bangladesh are affected by salinity intrusion caused by slow-onset and fast-onset events (SRDI 2010). It also points out that 71% of the cultivated areas in Banshkhali upazila are affected by high levels of salinity ($>$ 12 dS/m). According to BBS, the net cultivated area in Chittagong decreased by about 7% from 1996 to 2015 (BBS 2016). It has been found that in the immediate aftermath of cyclone *Mahasen*, which hit the Southeastern coast on June 13, 2013, total rice production in Chittagong decreased from 0.70 million tons in 2013 to 0.40 million tons in 2015 (BBS 2013, 2015). The report also stated that the production of the main rice crop (i.e., Aman) in Chittagong declined substantially, from about 0.8 million tons in 2013 to 0.4 million tons in 2015.

Salinity infiltration allegedly increased significantly during the previous 10 years, particularly over the last 5 years, according to focus group participants and survey responders. Cyclone *Mahasen*, which struck the region in 2013, is mostly to blame for the current high salinity in rice fields. When the fieldwork was conducted in 2016, high salinity in rice fields was a problem for roughly 65% of agricultural households. All saline-free and low-salinity farmland has been discovered to have changed into medium- or high-salinity farmland, which has a detrimental impact on crop output.

The majority of the rice grown by farmers in the research areas is an Aman variety, which blooms from April to August. Khankhanabad Union's Aman production pattern has been highly erratic over the last 20 years. The results indicate that between 2000 and 2005, the overall production of Aman was more than 10,000 tons, whereas between 2006 and 2011, it was less than 7500 tons. Aman production was roughly 6800 tons in 2012. Since then, it has significantly fallen by 25% and 15%, respectively, in the study union in 2013 and 2014 (UAO 2015). A similar tendency has been seen in the other studied unions, according to UAO statistics. Farmers reported that in 2013, "zero production" of rice occurred in all four study villages in both of the previously mentioned unions.

Farmers said that in 2013, shortly following the impact of *Mahasen*, all four study villages in both of the unions had "zero production" of rice. More precisely, according to local farmers, the high salinity in the rice fields caused the yield of the Aman crop to change from an average of 3.5 tons per ha in 2012 to 0 tons per ha in 2013 in all the research villages. Despite high saline levels in the years following *Mahasen*, several farmers in the study villages tried Aman farming once more, even though their yields were less than 1 ton per ha. Farmers were able to raise Aman yields marginally in 2015 to an average of 1.5 tons per ha in all four villages; however, the yield was lower before cyclone *Mahasen*.

Regarding the modifications in rice production throughout the previous 20 years, there were many reactions. In the study communities, roughly 76% of farmers thought that rice production had declined over time. In the research areas, rice output has "decreased a lot" over the previous 20 years, according to 51% of respondents. According to the findings of the survey, 98% of households cited saline intrusion as the primary factor contributing to reduced rice output, followed by a lack of rainfall (65%). Other issues mentioned included pest infestation, too much or too little fertilizer, water logging, expensive cultivation costs and a lack of irrigation water. Excessive rainfall over short periods of time, also known locally as "sky floods," was also listed. Other factors cited included pest attack, not having fertilizer at the right time and high cost of cultivation.

All the farmers firmly believed that salinity intrusion into soil and water is the main challenge to rice farming in the study areas. The study also revealed that loss and damage associated with salinity intrusion in rice production affects income groups (e.g., extremely poor, poor and non-poor) in different ways. The income of extremely poor households from rice cultivation was affected the most. In 2013, the loss incurred by the extremely poor was about 70% of their past annual household income, whereas other households lost 40–45% of their previous annual income. In addition, from 2013 to 2016, all the sampled households were gradually adapting in some way to reduce the shortfall in rice production. But the poor and extremely poor households were recovering their situation at a slower rate than non-poor families. The results of correlations among soil salinity levels and studied physicochemical properties of agriculture and field soils of the study areas are shown in Table 21.7.

21.5 Farmers' Adaptation Practices for Reducing the Salinization Problem

Farmers in the study areas noted that climate change and variability directly affected the agricultural sector, especially crops, fisheries and livestock production. That situation led the people to adaptation strategies to mitigate the risk. Based on their experiences, knowledge and resources, they looked for strategies to cope with the changing climatic conditions. The changes in rainfall pattern and temperature rise resulted in changes to crops' emergence, germination and insect pests.

In the research areas, farmers claimed that they were unfamiliar with the idea of preemptive adaptation. They usually waited until a problem occurred before making any preparations; only then did they make adjustments. Then they considered how they were farming and looked at areas farther South. As a potential adaptation strategy, new tree plantations (i.e., quick-growing timber) were of interest to participants in the Southern section. They started paying attention because they believed the trees could change the microclimate and bring more rain. In addition, it would be possible to cultivate watermelon and pumpkin (on a limited scale) if they could prevent the salinity increase. New sesame cultivars that can withstand unexpected stagnant water are needed. The medium highland produces the best yield from sesame, whereas the medium lowland produces the worst yield.

Women have become better educated, and they pass their knowledge on to offspring (future generations) so that they can change with the times. Concerns about local control over tidal water drainage are shared by both genders. Larger farms block canals for their fish farming operations (i.e., reduction of drainage pathways). Coasal embankments could give way at any moment. Farmers in Banshkhali, including the Southeastern coast of Bangladesh, suggested some

Table 21.7 Relationships among the soil salinity and soil physiochemical properties

Physicochemical properties	1	2	3	4	5	6	7	8	9	10
1. Soil pH	–									
2. Soil temperature (°C)	.783[**]	–								
3. EC (dS/m)	**.917**[**]	**.808**[**]	–							
4. Bulk density (g/cm^3)	−.427	−.158	**−.326**	–						
5. OM (%)	−.775[**]	−.896[*]	**−.712**[*]	.251	–					
6. Total N (%)	−.875[**]	−.809[**]	**−.830**[**]	.500	.853[**]	–				
7. Total P (%)	.848[**]	.624[*]	**.762**[**]	−.298	−.480	−.601	–			
8. Exchangeable K (%)	.808[**]	.828[**]	**.653**[*]	−.291	−.738[**]	−.738[**]	.833[**]	–		
9. Exchangeable ca (%)	.115	.289	**−.101**	.041	−.579	−.244	−.159	.250	–	
10. Exchangeable mg (%)	.884[**]	.800[**]	**.785**[**]	−.510	−.879[**]	−.870[**]	.597	.714[*]	.435	–

Note. *p = .05, **p = .01.

21 Effect of Salinity Intrusion on Sediments in Paddy Fields and Farmers'...

adaptation options for reducing the salinization in their agricultural fields, as can be found in Table 21.8.

Table 21.8 Adaptation practices in the study areas: responses of men and women

Proposed adaptation option	Responses of women	Responses of men
Substituting a short-duration variable (125–130 day) for the long-duration *T. Aman* rice variety (BR-23, 150 day) to increase intensity or lower risk.	(i) Superior for early harvest, which may lower the risk of damage to sesame from water logging with rainwater and may enable the risk of heavy rainfall for stormy weather throughout BR23 maturity. (ii) By August 20, short-term Aman rice transplants must receive the ideal amount of rainfall.	In the study areas, men gave the same responses as women, but they placed more emphasis on easy harvesting, proper drainage of rain or tidal water, and a community approach to rodent damage.
The authors found that cowpea and grass pea replanting with *T. Aman* rice in a single *T. Aman* cropping area.	It is possible in the medium highlands.	The concept is good for the medium highlands, but it must be a community-based operation to protect open grazing.
Direct dry seeded/dibbled or transplanted rice cultivation in the rice Aus season.	There was no response.	(i) Farms could be tried in the medium highland areas after sesame or mungbean production, but requires cultivars with short duration. (ii) Rice Aus is dependent on early Kharif-1 bathe.
Deepening existing inner side canal of the rice–fish culture under gher to store more surface water for irrigation.	Absence of rejoinder.	(i) It is possible to go 30–60 cm deeper in an existing canal that is 120–150 cm wide and 60 cm deep. (ii) If there are more, the canal's width must be increased, but they are concerned about taking up too much land.
Ponds designed specifically for irrigating the dry season crop.	Absence of reply.	(i) Ponds with an area of 80–100 m^2 and a depth of 180–210 cm could be used to store fresh surface water for irrigating rabi crops. (ii) They are concerned about cost and area expansion.
The authors recommended special fertilizer application to combat salinization in the crop field.	Lacking of reply.	In the coastal areas, few crop farmers use a solution of gypsum and sugar to decrease salt level in the paddy seedbed.
Paddy field preparation.	Women support men for paddy field preparation.	Tillage of rice fields on a frequent basis to decrease the salt level during cultivation.

21.6 Climate-Smart Agriculture in Bangladesh

Because crop land has shifted to urban, peri-urban and industrial purposes, the country is behind by around 85,000 ha of cultivable land every year. The annual loss of crop land during 1976–2020 was 50,240 ha and accessibility of crop land was in a decreasing pattern, with much larger rates since 2000–2020 (Rahman et al. 2020). Nearly 22% of the country's GDP comes from agricultural sectors, which turns out to be the source for 65% of the nation's labor force. It was estimated that more than 50% of the cultivable land of Bangladesh has been impacted by salinity interference, water logging and drought-related natural events. The nation requires immediate assistance in adopting the climate-smart crop production if its communities are to stay alive and flourish for longer periods.

Changing climate is influencing socioeconomic development of Bangladesh in many ways. For example, increasing sea level is the significant reason for crop lands in coastal zones to become salty and infertile for the long term. The effect of climate change for the agricultural sector becomes indisputable and would definitely depreciate with climate-tolerant cultivation options, not the traditional and resilient ones. In the Southeastern coastal areas of Bangladesh, anywhere the soil is the merely elevated compared to the Eastern water, huge swathes of the crop land are getting parched. Production of the crops is retreating because of increased salinity and as a result of the rising level of the water in the Bay of Bengal. The authors observed that in the coastal zones, the common commercially important plants (i.e., betel nut and coconut trees) were not harvested 60% of the time over two decades, whereas the fruit of banana trees will be disappearing completely within 100 years.

Farmers in the study areas produced various vegetables that are available in the local trade centers of Chaittagong, Dhaka, Rajshahi and Khuln; they are absolutely flavorless and bring in little value compared to the production in zero-salinity areas of the other parts of the country. Nearly 90% of families in communities live in rural areas; it is for this reason that Bangladesh always has required assistance in promoting climate-resilient agriculture as the best options of climate change adaptation (Barua et al. 2021). This will help to prime activation to facilitate crop farmers to raise food security by adaption. To solve the climate change-induced problem, agricultural farmers absolutely need to increase their vegetable beds, keep up the soil's moist condition by encasing the nursery—using leaves and straw to put off excessive loss of water and the threat of coastal erosion. In addition, they need to increase the quantity of the sediments' bioorganic composting ingredients and diversify the patterns of crop rot in their fields.

Developed in 2013, the National Agriculture Policy also considered it necessary to include part of each of the following: Environment Policy of 1992, Fisheries Policy of 1998, Agricultural Land Use Policy of 2001, Policy of 1994, National Jute Policy of 2002, National Livestock Development Policy of 2007, National Food Policy of 2008, Livestock Resources Policy and Action Plan 2005 and National Poultry Development Policy 2008. The major goals and objectives of these policies were to develop sustainable and climate-resilient agricultural activities for

Bangladesh; they were in response to the vulnerability to climate change through increasing crop production. This has continued to place importance on surveys, research, extension facilities, modern technology transfer and updated information-sharing to make this happen. Although this is limited, there are no definite action plans, according to the country's agro-ecological zones (Fig. 21.1).

The authors found that 31.3% of the crop farmers of the Southeastern coast of Bangladeh have typical or adapted substitute land-use options (e.g., coastal farming)

Photographs of Some Climate Smart Agriculture Practice in Bangladesh

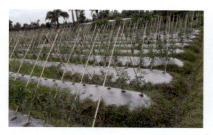

Picture: Heat Tolerant Tomatoo and Brinjal production using marching paper

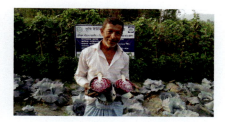

Picture: Climate Resilient High Yielding Red Cabbage Production

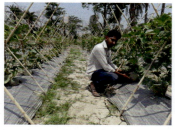

Picture: Production of High nutrient short duration crop Rock Melon

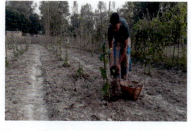

Picture : Using Trico-Compost for high yielding crop production

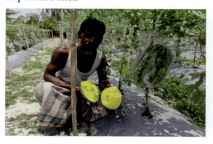

Picture : Climate resilience all year round watermelon production through using marching paper and rotation cropping

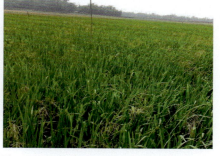

Picture : Disaster resilient high yielding disease free rice production (BRRI-87)

Fig. 21.1 Some of the farmers' adaptation practices in the study areas

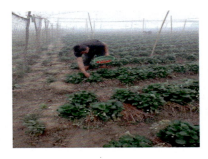
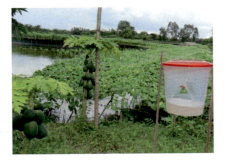

Picture : Production of high yielding rich nutrient Dragon Fruits

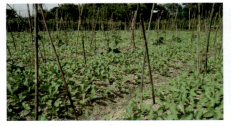
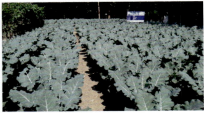

Picture: Disaster Resilient Rich Nutrient Vegetables production

Picture: Short duration, high nutrient Brocoli production

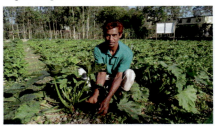
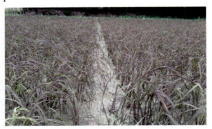

Picture: Climate Resilient high nutrient Scouas production

Picture: Flood Resilient high nutrient black rice production

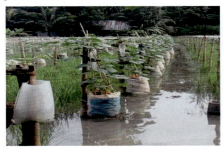
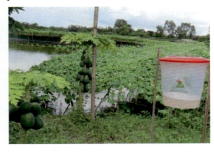

Picture: Climate Resilient Vegetable production with plastic shed

Picture: Climate Resilient Integratted Pesticide free pond dyke farming

Fig. 21.1 (continued)

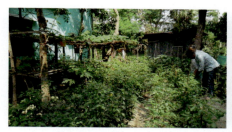
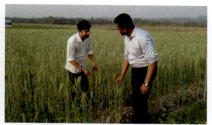

Picture: Climate Resilient all year round multilayerd Vegetable production around the homestead

Picture: Salinity Resilient Wheat Production

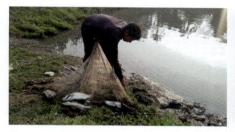
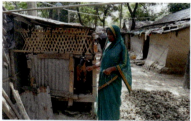

Picture: Salinity Tolerant Fish Farming in sweet pond

Picture: Platform shed goat rearing as climate resilient livestock technology

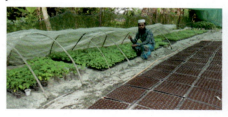
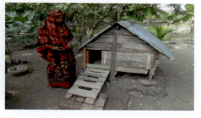

Picture: Vegetables and fruits plant production without soil through using COCODUST

Picture: Platform shed duck rearing as climate resilient livestock technology

Fig. 21.1 (continued)

as an alternative to agricultural crop production. Although the crops' farming land is declining steadily, there are various alternative opportunities for the agriculture (e.g., coastal embankment cropping practices, coastal affoestation, relay crop patterns, farming of salinity-resilient grass, mulching, application of pheromone traps, farming of saline- and flood-resilient rice and so on). Table 21.9 lists of some significant climate-resilient agricultural practicesfor the coastal areas of Bangladesh.

Farmers of the coastal areas of Bangladesh are practicing the following production strategies: salinity-resilient rice, cage fishing, mele (reed), farming through floating dhap, changing the time of planting, high-yield and short-duration rice, methos of Sorjan, raising plums and sunflowers, floating bed vegetables, organic fertilizers, urea deep placement, integrated cultivation, feeding crabs and small

604   P. Barua et al.

Table 21.9 Agro-based resilient practices in the study areas

Resilient sector	Options
Salinity resilient *T. Aman*	Farmers culitvating Bina shail, BR-22 (Kiran) and BR-23 (Dishari).
Salinity resilient BRRI paddy crop	Farmers familiar to cultivating BRRI-33, 34, 35, 56, 57 and 62
Salinity resilient BINA rice	Farmers producing BINA-7, 8, 10 and 16
Salinity resilient Aus rice	Farmers cultivating BRRI-65
Salinity resilient alternate cultivating	Farmers' experiences of producing salinity-resilient grass production, multistage farming
Cultivation of vegetables	Farmers cultivating vegetables through floating stages, farming in homestead areas and farming in pond and road dykes
Climate-resilient livestock farming	Farmers are practicing goat, duck, hen and sheep semi-scavenger housing
Aquaculture	Fish farmers using cage culture, net culture approach for fish farming
Wheat tolerant to salt	BAU-1059, BARI wheat-25, Bijoy
Potato tolerant to salt	Farmers cultivating BARI Alo-22, CIP clone-86, 88 and 163 for production
Salinity resilient sweet potato	Farmers using BARI Mishti Alo-7, 8 and 9 for high yield
Pulses tolerant to salt	Farmers cultivating BARI-2, 3, 4, 5, 6, BM-01, BM-08 BARI Falon-1, BARI Sola-9 for high yield
Quick-acting oilseeds	Farmers cultivating various species of oil seeds like BARI Sharisha-14, 15; BARI Chinabadam-9, BINA China badam-1, BINA China badam-2, BARI Soybean-6 BARI Til-2, 3, 4
Salt-resilient jute production	Farmers now cultivating HC-2, HC 95, CVL 1 species for jute production
Salt-resilient sugarcane production	ISWARDI-40 is cultivated by sugarcane farmers
Climate-resilient other crops	Farmers trying for land use changing practice, integrated farming, crab patenting, shifting plantation timing

indigenous fish, use of nearby dykes, net fishing, salt-resilient wheat (e.g., Bijoy, BAU-1059 line, BARI Gom-25), tomatoes, potatoes and sweet potatoes, heat- and salt-resilient pulsations, salt-resilient and short-time tolerant oilseeds, salt- and heat-salt-resilient jute cultivation, high-yield and salt-resilient sugarcane, platform shed or semi-scavenger rearing processes for livestock (e.g., goats, sheep, ducks and chickens), salinity-resilient fish culture, short-duration fish and vegetable integrated farming, crab farming and so forth. These are all ways to practice climate change adaptation in the coastal communities.

It is also significant that coastal area farmers are cultivating vegetables in crop fields year-round to cope with salinity, brief duration and small cultivation spaces. Some have the support of government and non-governmental organizations that deal with crop production—for example, homestead cultivation; roadside, embankment and dyke farming; dhap/gher and pesticide-free cultivation; storage capacity increase of paddy seeds; guti uria application in rice fields; and organic biocomposting or integrated farming. This also assesses vegetable and crop production that do not have large-scale potential in Bangladesh's coastal areas—that is, farmers who practice crop production only for household consumption and small-scale usage.

21.7 Conclusions and Recommendations

From the findings in the study areas, it has been observed that the relationship between every climate-smart agriculture practice, with per capita food expenditures, the most significant options for coastal farmers' household food security are: flood- and salinity-resilient crop species, production near roads, pond-side vegetable husbandry and various water-harvesting techniques. The results covered in this book's chapter appears steady, allowing for the geographical location on the Southeastern coast of Bangladesh, where salinity intrusion has become the major catastrophe for the coastal communities. Agricultural fields stay waterlogged for long periods of time and pond areas have increased the ease of production of diverse short-duration and high-yield vegetables, especially during the rainy season. Throughout the dry season (November–February), crop farmers can supply water to their crops and vegetable-producing lands by using water they preserved in ponds or canals during the rainy season (July–September). So, it has been found that various salinity- and flood-resilient crops, as well as road, pond and dyke vegetable production options for distinct types of water-harvesting processes were positively correlated with per capita food security in coastal Bangladesh (Fig. 21.2).

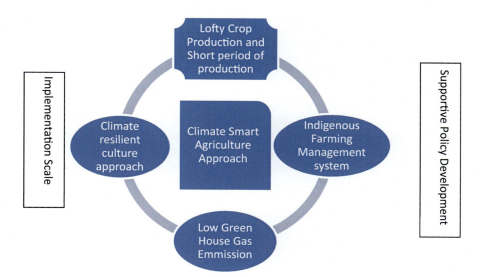

Fig. 21.2 Climate-smart agricultural practices in response to climate change

In this book's chapter, the authors pointed out a poor connection between the climate-smart agriculture coping approach and food security of agricultural households in coastal Bangladesh according to the per capita yearly food costs. Farmers' existing adaptation strategies are insufficient to deal with the rising salinity levels, especially those brought on by extreme events. Along with these climate-related dangers, the level of poverty, low resilience and lack of alternative livelihoods result in significant losses for not just the study communities but also residents of the entire coast.

People are leaving the shore in greater numbers, mostly because of decreased prospects for employment. As sea levels rise and extreme weather events become more common, and if adaption choices are insufficient, this internal movement (i.e., rural–urban, coastal–central) will escalate. Underprivileged families' final destination is an urban slum. Such migration brought on by numerous climatic variables (e.g., saline intrusion) would make it more difficult for the Capital and neighboring cities and towns to provide both former and new city residents with adequate utilities and other services.

Constant research studies, field observations, monitoring, crop and weather information management and technology-related innovative ideas and applications are urgently required for adaptation to climate change and its effects. An exhaustive training program for climate-displaced populations is necessary to increase the ability to cope with new circumstances. The climate change issue is understood to have special significance because of the accumulation of global-warming evidence; currently, this turns out to be a great challenge for the world. Almost all countries have been impacted, and it has become a large threat for global development and food security. Because of low agricultural production and land becoming infertile owing to salinity intrusion a country like Bangladesh is one of the most hands-on of the developing nations.

A universal scenario is needed to tackle the challenges induced by climate change. Climatic changes and their significant effects have been deemed hampered through some oppositions created, together with attempts to reduce the impacts of the national poverty condition and to achieve sustainable development goals (MDG). Besides, a cooperative land execution management process should be formed wherever coastal aquacultural production is to be carried out. Under the approach of community-based management methods, it will permit minor landholders to navigate through the deteriorating political nexus of the bulky and the influential. The salinity-resilient rice varieties or other vegetables, crops, floating gardening and integrated cultivating systems (i.e., shrimp/prawn plus rice) could be applied in a more widespread process to decrease the climate change impact and earnings weaknesses in the coastal areas of Bangladesh. Furthermore, the government should take on programs to set up and reinforce shore embankments so that marginalized communities can return to their own cultural technologies that could reduce susceptibility to climate change and food deficiency in coastal areas.

References

Adams RMB (1998) The effects of global warming on agriculture: an interpretative review. J Climate Res 11(1):19–30

Ahmed M, Suphachalasai S (2014) Assessing the costs of climate change and adaptation in South Asia. Climate Change 40(3):50–65

Ahsan DA, Islam S (2011) Farmers' motivations, risk perceptions and risk management strategies in a developing economy: Bangladesh experience. J Risk Res 14(3):325–349

Alam GMM, Alam K, Shahbaz M, Sarker MNI (2020) Hazards, food insecurity and human displacement in rural riverine Bangladesh: implications for policy. Int J Disaster Risk Reduc 43:34–45

Aryal JP, Rahut DB, Sapkota TB, Khurana R, Khatri-Chhetri A (2020) Climate change mitigation options among farmers in South Asia. Environ Dev Sustain 20(4):120–135

Barua P, Rahman SR (2017) Indigenous knowelge practices for adaptation of climate change in the southern coast of Bangladesh. IUP J Knowl Manage 15(1):88–105

Barua P, Rahman SH (2018) Community-based rehabilitation attempt for sustainable solution of climate displacement crisis in coastal Bangladesh. Int J Migrat Resident Mobility 4:45–60

Barua P, Rahman SH (2019) Indigenous knowledge for sustainabale value chain as climate change adaptation for vegetables product for the coastal communitues. IUP J Supply Chain Manage 19:20–45

Barua P, Rahman SH (2020) Relationship between climate change adaptation and vulnerability aspects for the coastal Bangladesh. Asian Profile 48:47–57

Barua P, Rahman SH (2021) Livelihood Vulnerability and changing pattern of livelihood of climate displaced people in the coastal area of Bangladesh. Rethinking Govern 1:65–91

Barua P, Shahjahan M, Simperingham E (2016) Climate displacement in Bangladesh: legal and policy responses for rights-based solution. Social Change 6:85–100

Barua P, Rahman SH, Molla MH (2017) Sustainable adaptation for resolving climate displacement issues of south eastern islands in Bangladesh. Int J Clim Change Strat Manage 15:60–80

Barua P, Rahman SH, Barua S, Ismail MMR (2020) Climate change vulnerability and responses of Fisherfolk communities in the south-eastern coast of Bangladesh. Water Conserv Manage 4:20–31

Barua P, Rahman SH, Eslamian S (2021) global climate change and inequalities, reduced inequalities. Encyclopedia of the UN Sustainable Development Goals. Springer

BBS (2013) Yearbook of Agricultural Statistics of Bangladesh 2013–2014, Statistics Division, Bangladesh Bureau of Statistics, Ministry of Planning, Government of Bangladesh

BBS (2015) Yearbook of Agricultural Statistics of Chittagong, Statistics Division, Bangladesh Bureau of Statistics , Ministry of Planning, Dhaka, Bangladesh

BBS (2016) Yearbook of Agricultural Statistics of Bangladesh, Statistics Division, Bangladesh Bureau of Statistics, Ministry of Planning, Government of Bangladesh

Challinor AJ, Watson J, Lobell DB, Howden SM, Smith DR, Chhetri N (2014) A meta-analysis of crop yield under climate change and adaptation. Nat Clim Chang 4(4):287–291

Chowdhury MAZ, Banik S, Uddin B, Moniruzzaman M, Karim N, Gan SH (2011) Organophosphorus and carbamate pesticide residues detected in water samples collected from paddy and vegetable fields of the Savar and Dhamrai Upazilas in Bangladesh. Int J Environ Res Public Health 9(9):3318–3329

Deutsch CA, Tewksbury JJ, Tigchelaar M, Battisti DS, Merrill SC, Huey RB, Naylor RL (2018) Increase in crop losses to insect pests in a warming climate. Science 361(5):916–919

FAO (2016) Migration, agriculture and rural development: addressing the root causes of migration and harnessing its potential for development, Rome, Italy

Gay O, Cerdan V, Mardhel M (2016) Application of an index of sediment connectivity in a lowland area. J Soils Sediments 16(1):280–293

Hazbavi Z, Keesstra SD, Nunes JP, Baartman JE, Gholamalifard M, Sadeghi S (2018) Health comparative comprehensive assessment of watersheds with different climates. Ecol Indic 93: 781–790

IDMC (2021) Global report on internal displacement index 2020. Internal Displacement Monitoring Center, Geneva

IPCC (2013) Climate change 2013: the physical science basis. In: Stocker TF, Qin D, Plattner G-K, Tignor M, Allen SK, Boschung J, Nauels A, Xia Y, Bex V, Midgley PM (eds) Contribution of working group I to the fifth assessment report of the intergovernmental panel on climate change. Cambridge University Press, Cambridge, United Kingdom and New York, NY, USA, 1535 pp

IPCC (2014) Climate change 2014: impacts, adaptation, and vulnerability. Part a: global and sectoral aspects. In: Field CB, Barros VR, Dokken DJ, Mach KJ, Mastrandrea MD, Bilir TE, Chatterjee M, Ebi KL, Estrada YO, Genova RC, Girma B, Kissel ES, Levy AN, MacCracken S, Mastrandrea PR, White LL (eds) Contribution of working group II to the fifth assessment report of the intergovernmental panel on climate change. Cambridge University Press, Cambridge, United Kingdom and New York, NY, USA, 1132 pp

Islam AKMS (2020) Mechanized cultivation increases labour efficiency. Bangladesh Rice J 24 (2):49–66

Islam MR (2004) Where land meets the sea: a profile of the coastal zone of Bangladesh. The University Press Limited, Dhaka

Kabir MJ, Alauddin M, Steven S (2017) Farm-level adaptation to climate change in Western Bangladesh: an analysis of adaptation dynamics, profitability and risks. Land Use Policy 64 (2):212–224

Kang S-M, Khan AL, Waqas M, Asaf S, Lee K-E, Park Y-G (2019) Integrated phytohormone production by the plant growth-promoting rhizobacterium *bacillus tequilensis* SSB07 induced thermotolerance in soybean. J Plant Interact 14(1):416–423

Karimi V, Karami E, Keshavarz M (2018) Climate change and agriculture: impacts and adaptive responses in Iran. J Integr Agric 17(2):1–15

Katengeza SP, Holden ST, Lunduka RW (2019) Adoption of drought tolerant maize varieties under rainfall stress in Malawi. J Agric Econ 70(1):198–214

Kumar R, Gautam HR (2014) Climate change and its impact on agricultural productivity in India. J Climatol Weather Forecast 2(1):109–112

Li XF, Huang D, Wu LP (2019) Study on grain harvest losses of different scales of farms – empirical analysis based on 3251 farmers in China. China J Agric Sci 8(1):184–192

Maclean JL, Dawe DC, Hardy B, Hettel GP (2002) Rice almanac. Los Baños (Philippines): international Rice research institute; Bouaké (Côte d'Ivoire): West Africa Rice development association: Cali (Colombia): International Center for Tropical Agricolture: Rome (Italy): food and agriculture organization, pp 11–29

Mahato A (2014) Climate change and its impact on agriculture. Int J Sci Res Publ 4(4):1–6

Malhi GS, Kaur M, Kaushik P (2021) Impact of climate change on agriculture and its mitigation strategies: a review. Sustainability 13(2):1318–1325

Mendelsohn R (2009) The impact of climate change on agriculture in developing countries. J Nat Resour Policy Res 1(1):5–19

Molua EL (2017) Technical efficiency of smallholder tomato production in semi-urban farms in Cameroon: a stochastic frontier production approach. J Manag Sustain 7(4):27–35

Ochieng J, Kirimi L, Makau J (2017) Adapting to climate variability and change in rural Kenya: farmer perceptions, strategies and climate trends. Nat Res Forum 41(9(2)):195–208

Ochieng J, Kirimi L, Mathenge M (2016) Effects of climate variability and change on agricultural production: the case of small scale farmers in Kenya. NJAS Wagening J Life Sci 77(1):71–78

Parry GD, Cooper CL, Moore JM, Yadegarfar G, Campbell MJ, Esmonde L, Morice AH, Hutchcroft BJ (2012) Cognitive behavioural intervention for adults with anxiety complications of asthma: prospective randomised trial. Respir Med 20(4):30–50

Rahman MC, Pede V, Balie J, Pabuayon IM, Yorobe JM, Mohanty S (2020) Assessing the market power of millers and wholesalers in the Bangladesh rice sector. J Agric Dev 30(3):80–95

Rosenzweig MS (2018) Assessing the politics of neo-Assyrian agriculture. Archeological Pap Am Anthropol Assoc 29(1):30–50

Schlenker W, Lobell DB (2010) Robust negative impacts of climate change on African agriculture. Environ Res Lett 5(1):140–150

Shakoor U, Rashid M, Iftikh-Ul-Husnain M, Arif T (2019) Vulnerability of sugarcane crop production to climate change in Pakistan: an empirical investigation. Clim Dev 5(1):60–80

Shameem MIM, Momtaz S (2015) Local perceptions of and adaptation to climate variability and change: the case of shrimp farming communities in the coastal region of Bangladesh. Clim Chang 133:253–266

Shimono H, Suzuki K, Aoki K, Hasegawa T, Okada M (2010) Effect of panicle removal on photosynthetic acclimation under elevated CO_2 in rice. Photosynthetica 48(4):530–536

SRDI (2010) Saline soils of Bangladesh. SRDI, Soil Resource Development Institute, Ministry of Agriculture, Dhaka

Stevanović M, Popp A, Lotze-Campen H, Dietrich JP, Müller C, Bonsch M, Schmitz C, Bodirsky BL, Humpenöder F, Weindl I (2016) The impact of high-end climate change on agricultural welfare. Sci Adv 2(8):50–70

Talukder RK, Alam F, Islam M, Anik AR (2015) Background paper on food security and nutrition prepared for seventh five year plan preparation, Bangladesh. Food Sec 10(2):34–45

UAO (2015) Rice production data for 1990–2015. Upazilla Agriculture Office, Chittagong

Vinke K, Martin MA, Adams S, Baarsch F, Bondeau A, Coumou D (2017) Climatic risks and impacts in South Asia: extremes of water scarcity and excess. Reg Environ Chang 17(2):1569–1583

Waha K, van Wijk MT, Fritz S, See L, Thornton PK, Wichern J, Herrero M (2019) Agricultural diversification as an important strategy for achieving food security in Africa. Glob Chang Biol 24(2):390–400

Wang P, Han Y, Zhang Y (2019) Characteristics of change and influencing factors of the technical efficiency of chemical fertilizer use for agricultural production in China. Resour Sci 42(9):1764–1776

Zhang Y, Min Q, Zhang C, He L, Zhang S, Yang L, Xiong Y (2017) Traditional culture as an important power for maintaining agricultural landscapes in cultural heritage sites: a case study of the Hani terraces. J Cult Herit 25(2):170–179

Chapter 22
Climatic Challenge for Global Viticulture and Adaptation Strategies

Rizwan Rafique, Touqeer Ahmad, Tahira Kalsoom, Muhammad Azam Khan, and Mukhtar Ahmed

Abstract Climate change has posed mammoth challenges for the global viticulture, and almost all the growing regions are facing the mounting pressure exerted owing to this unchecked climatic challenge. Pedo-climatic and topographic features largely affect the production and quality of table and wine. Climatic variability in the form of rising CO_2 and elevated global temperature with increased intensity of water scarcity during the growing season has contributed to the unsustainability of global viticulture. Early phenological development, shortening of phenophases, poor berry development, early maturity with lower yield and inferior quality are the consequences of these challenges. Moreover, the physiological activities of vines, e.g. photosynthetic activity, transpiration and stomatal conductance, are negatively affected along lower water use efficiency (WUE), hence higher irrigation demands.

Keywords Viticulture · Climate change · Temperature · CO_2 · Water deficit · Phenology · Physiology · Berry quality

22.1 Introduction

Grapevines of *Vitis vinifera* are a distinct crop belonging to family Vitaceae. They are a non-climacteric fruit species, commonly used as table grapes and dried raisins and in vinification (wine production) and distillation to produce liquors (Kuhn et al. 2013; Ruel and Walker 2006). Grapes contribute about 16 percent of global fruit production (Bhat et al. 2017). Grapevines are cultivated on an area of 7.4 million hectares with an annual production of 77.8 million tons globally in 2018 with five countries, Spain (13%), China (12%), France (11%), Italy (9%) and Turkey (6%),

---

R. Rafique (✉) · T. Ahmad · T. Kalsoom · M. A. Khan
Department of Horticulture, Pir Mehr Ali Shah Arid Agriculture University, Rawalpindi, Pakistan

M. Ahmed
Department of Agronomy, PMAS Arid Agriculture University, Rawalpindi, Pakistan

© The Author(s), under exclusive license to Springer Nature Switzerland AG 2022
M. Ahmed (ed.), *Global Agricultural Production: Resilience to Climate Change*,
https://doi.org/10.1007/978-3-031-14973-3_22

contributing about 51% of the viticulture industry. The major share of viticulture industry is occupied by the wine industry (246 mhl consumption) with 57% production of wine grapes (OIV 2019). Bordeaux, Burgundy, California, Champagne, La Mancha, Cape/South Africa, Porto/Douro, La Rioja, Mendoza, South Australia, Mosel and Tuscany are home to major wineries globally (Fraga et al. 2012). Table and dried grapes contribute 36% and 7% (Fig. 22.1), respectively, in the total grape production, and now there is a rising popularity of table grapes with fresh grape's juice and dried grapes or raisins with 1.3 million tons production (OIV 2019).

Grape cultivation originated in Armenia near the Caspian Sea region, and gradually, it spread westwards to Europe and eastwards particularly in Iran and Afghanistan (Creasy and Creasy 2018). Viticulture regions are widespread, but usually concentrated in temperate climatic zones. Europe consists of the largest viticulture zones in the world (about 40%), although many areas in Asia, such as India, China, Turkey, Afghanistan, Iran and Pakistan, are emerging as the new high-quality table grape-producing regions. China, in Asia, has recorded major increase in grape production over the last few years. Similarly, viticulture has made inroads in US regions, e.g. California, Georgia, Washington and Florida, with good fruit quality for wine and fresh consumption. In the southern hemisphere, Argentina, Australia, New Zealand, Chile, Brazil and South Africa are among the rapidly flourishing viticulture regions. The major grape producers and global viticulture distribution in different regions are given in Figs. 22.2 and 22.3.

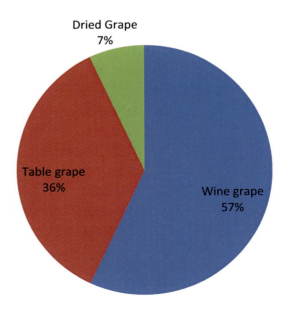

Fig. 22.1 Global viticulture with respect to usage as wine, table and dried grapes

22 Climatic Challenge for Global Viticulture and Adaptation Strategies

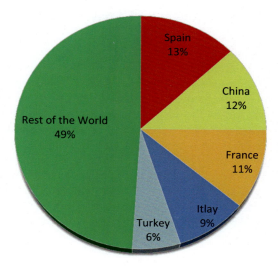

Fig. 22.2 Global grapevine production trends and share of five leading producers

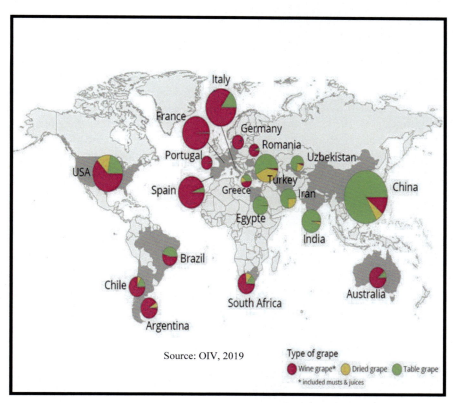

Fig. 22.3 Global distribution of grapevine in different climatic zones of the world

22.2 Botanical and Anatomical Characteristics

Like all other members of Dicotyledoneae, grapevines start their life cycle with two cotyledons. Family Vitaceae's members are termed grapevines, and it contains about 1000 species with 17 genera. Although most members of this family belong to in the tropics or subtropics, even then a species (*Vitis vinifera*) from the temperate zones has become the world's chief fruit producer in about 90 countries. Cultivated grapes belong to either genus *Vitis* (2n 38 chromosomes) or genus *Muscadinia* (2n 40 chromosomes) and have distinct floral morphology (Fig. 22.4). Roots of this family are generally fibrous and well branched and can grow to several metres in length. Vines climb through tendrils which act to provide support, and leaves grow alternatively on branches (Creasy and Creasy 2018; Mullins et al. 1992). There are about 24,000 named cultivars, but there is often more than 1 name for the same cultivar; the number of different and distinguishable cultivars is about 4000 (OIV 2013).

22.3 Factors Influencing Viticulture

Grapevine development is affected by a highly intricate system, consisting of soil characteristics, climate features and vineyard management (Magalhaes 2015). The concept of terroir emerged in this system of interacting factors such as physical, biological and environmental components along with viti-vinicultural techniques which give distinctive characteristics to the products (OIV 2010; Van Leeuwen et al. 2004; Fraga et al. 2013). All the elements in the terroir strongly affect the growth and development of grapevine cultivars. Moreover, these factors also influence the wine type, fruit yield and berry quality. A brief description of these factors is given in Sects. 22.3.1 and 22.3.2.

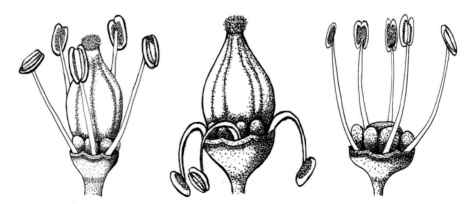

Fig. 22.4 Flower types in the genus *Vitis*: perfect (left), female (centre) and male flower (right). (Keller 2010)

22 Climatic Challenge for Global Viticulture and Adaptation Strategies

22.3.1 Climate

Grapes are cultivated between 50°N and S, where suitable areas lie in small limits. Vines need cool winter and warm to hot and dry summer for good quality of fruit. Subtropics with winter rains are the most suitable areas for viticulture. Rains and cloudy weather at flowering adversely affect the fruit set, while excessive rains during berry ripening lead to berry and bunch rot. Raisins are produced by sun-drying between the vine rows in areas with at least 1 warm, sunny month without rain after harvest is essential (FAOSTAT 2016). Regional climate is the key element of terroir affecting grape production (OIV 2010; Jones and Davis 2000). Base temperature of 10 °C is one of the most important climatic thresholds for budburst in grapevines (Winkler 1974).

Climate is a key factor driving phenology, vine growth and physiological development, thereby affecting the production and quality of grapevine (OIV 2010; Keller 2010; Costa et al. 2019). Furthermore, vineyard's geographical distribution is affected by climatic variables (Fraga et al. 2019). Weather parameters such as temperatures, solar radiation, rainfall pattern and inter-annual seasonal variability affect vine productivity as discussed by Fraga and Santos (2017). Extreme weather events, e.g. heat waves, hailstorms, excessive rainfall and late spring frost, have detrimental impacts on grapevine productivity (Greer and Weedon 2013; Mosedale et al. 2015).

22.3.2 Topographic Features

Topographic features such as land elevation and slope are of significant importance for viticulture (Jones et al. 2004; Yau et al. 2013). Surface elevation affects the temperature in vineyards at farm scale as vertical temperature gradient, and it exerts a strong influence on the site suitability and varietal selection (Magalhaes 2008). Solar exposure to vines is affected by the degree of slope; thus, it has a main impact on canopy microclimate, viticultural management, water drainage and soil erosion in vineyards (Zsofi et al. 2011).

22.3.3 Soil Requirements

Soil consists of organic and inorganic matter, and it is a source for providing water and nutrients which are critical for grapevine growth, physiology and yield responses. It is a key part of terroir and an important factor for viticulture (Magalhaes 2008). In fact, the composition of berries is influenced by the soil's physical and chemical properties and hence affects wine quality (Mackenzie and Christy 2005). Grapevines are well adapted to a wide range of soils; however, poorly drained soils and areas with exceptionally high salinity levels are considered as unsuitable. Light soils with high water-holding capacity are preferred for grape cultivation. Similarly, the water-holding capacity of soils is also essential and has a direct effect on vine performance (Yau et al. 2013; Field et al. 2009). Grapevines are moderately sensitive to salinity, and yield is affected by it. Nevertheless, vine yield is not affected up to 1.5 mmhos/cm, while 10% reduction at 2.5, 25% at 4.1, 50% at 6.7 and 100% at 12 mmhos/cm have been observed. Deep fertile soils result in high yields, but in less fertile soil or soil with limited depth, yield is usually poor. Nutrient requirements of grapevine are 100–160 kg/ha N, 160–230 kg/ha K and 40–60 kg/ha P. More nitrogen is required during early spring when the vines are undergoing rapid vegetative and inflorescence development. Nevertheless, nitrogen level must be low during ripening to prevent excessive vegetative growth (FAOSTAT 2016).

22.4 Climate Change and Viticulture

Climate change is no doubt the major challenge that the viticulture industry has to deal with in the coming decades. Significant changes in temperature have been observed during the past century which include, surface temperature increase of 1.06 °C over a period of more than 100 years, however major increased, i.e. 0.85 °C occurred over the past two decades (IPCC 2014a). Air temperature variations were prominent, i.e. 2–5 °C increase in traditional viticulture zones in different parts of Europe (Christensen et al. 2007). Climatic projections for the twenty-first century indicate temperature increase in different ranges, i.e. stabilization at 1.5 °C higher than the current reference period to more than 4 °C increase in the mean global temperature (IPCC 2014b). The key driver of the temperature increase has been the emission of greenhouse gases; among these, CO_2 is more pertinent in terms of volume and effect (IPCC 2014b). Atmospheric CO_2 levels have increased from 280 μL L^{-1} (preindustrial) to more than 400 μL L^{-1} in 2016, with predicted a rapid increase for the end of century, i.e. 421–936 μL L^{-1} (Meinshausen et al. 2011). Furthermore, a decrease in rainfall has been observed in major viticulture regions, particularly, Southern Europe (IPCC 2014a; Christensen et al. 2007), and it is expected to decrease further in the future.

22.4.1 Elevated CO_2 and Impacts on Viticulture

The global concentration of CO_2 has increased from 280 to 400 ppm; this increase was more rapid after 1950 as indicated in Fig. 22.5. The rise in CO_2 levels may change the global viticulture outlook. As an outcome of elevated CO_2 levels in the future, grapevine physiological activity and growth may be affected.

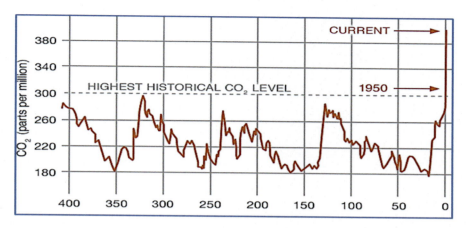

Fig. 22.5 Historical and current atmospheric CO2 level. (Courtesy of NASA)

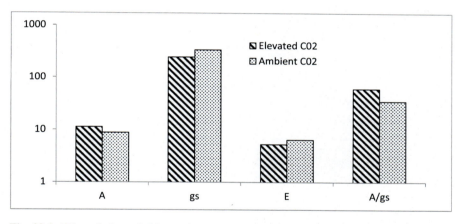

Fig. 22.6 Effect of elevated CO_2 on the rate of photosynthesis (A), stomatal conductance (gs), transpiration rate (E) and photosynthesis/stomatal conductance (A/gs) in vine leaves. (Moutinho-Pereira et al. 2009)

22.4.1.1 Effect of Elevated CO_2 on Vine Physiology

The effect of elevated CO_2 on physiological responses of table grape cultivars is shown in Fig. 22.6. Leaf physiological and anatomical characteristics and vine productivity were accessed for grapevine (*V. vinifera* L.) cultivar Touriga Franca under high CO_2 level of 500 ppm compared to ambient CO_2 level, i.e. 365 ppm. Photosynthetic rate, water use efficiency (WUE), leaf thickness and Mg concentration with C/N, K/N and Mg/N ratios were increased under elevated CO_2; however, stomatal density and N concentration were decreased. On the other hand, transpiration rate (E), stomatal conductance (gs), leaf water potential, photochemical efficiency (Fv/Fm), SPAD value and transmitted red/far-red light were not significantly

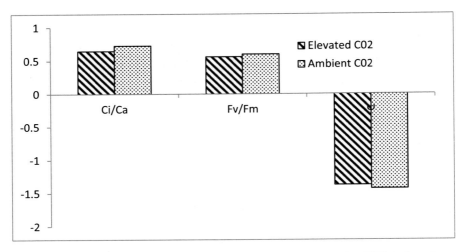

Fig. 22.7 Effect of elevated CO_2 on internal CO_2/ambient CO_2 concentration (Ci/Ca), photochemical efficiency (Fv/Fm) and water potential. (Moutinho-Pereira et al. 2009)

affected by higher CO_2 levels (Moutinho-Pereira et al. 2006, 2009). It is obvious that the photosynthetic activity (A) in grapevine will increase in the future in response to rising CO_2 levels, while stomatal conductance (gs) and transpiration would decrease; however, the ratio of photosynthetic activity to stomatal conductance will increase (Fig. 22.6). Rising CO_2 will also affect Ci/Ca ratio and Fv/Fm ratio negatively, while water potential levels will slightly increase as shown in Fig. 22.7. These trends depict that the climate challenge would have a profound impact on the physiological responses of grapevine.

22.4.1.2 Vine Growth, Yield and Anatomical Characteristics

Elevated atmospheric CO_2 levels affect the growth and anatomical characteristics of grapevine. Data presented in Fig. 22.8 show that elevated atmospheric CO_2 levels resulted in the decreased thickness of total parenchyma, palisade parenchyma, spongy parenchyma and palisade/spongy parenchyma ratio. Despite significant changes in anatomical characteristics along with leaf mass per unit area, may be due to higher light red/far-red light ratio, the stomatal conductance and SPAD values were not much affected as indicated in Table 22.1. Enriched CO_2 also increased vine yield, number of clusters, cluster weight, number of shoots per vine, pruning weight, shoot weight and Ravaz index (Table 22.2) as indicated by Moutinho-Pereira et al. (2009) and Wohlfahrt et al. (2019). The yield gain due to elevated CO_2 was demonstrated under free air carbon dioxide enrichment (FACE) experiments. Recently, increased vine growth and vigour owing to higher rates of photosynthesis under elevated CO_2 have also been noticed (Wohlfahrt et al. 2018). Available records from literature also indicate that higher photosynthetic activity owing to

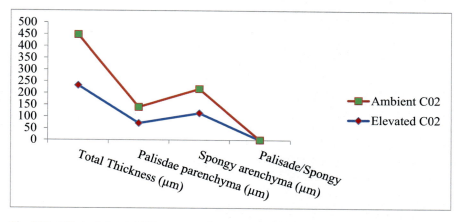

Fig. 22.8 Effect of elevated CO_2 on grapevine anatomical features

Table 22.1 Effect of elevated CO_2 on grapevine stomatal density, SPAD value, infrared light and leaf mass per unit area

CO_2 scenario	Stomatal density	SPAD	Red/far-red	LMA (g·m^{-2})
Elevated CO_2	147.85	45.25	0.202	83.6
Ambient CO_2	147.85	44.45	0.187	72.6

Table 22.2 Effect of elevated CO_2 on grapevine yield, vegetative growth, light interception, leaf mass and Ravaz index

CO_2 scenario	Vine yield (kg)	Clusters per vine	Cluster weight (g)	Shoots per vine	Pruning weight (Kg)	Shoot weight (g)	Ravaz index
Elevated CO_2	5.22	15.57	336.23	14.83	0.75	52.13	8.13
Ambient CO_2	7.28	17.97	403.33	17.90	1.04	64.73	7.13

Table 22.3 Effect of elevated CO_2 on main elements (g kg^{-1}) in grapevine leaves

CO_2 scenario	C	N	P	K	Ca	Mg	Fe
Elevated CO_2	507	21.5	1.56	6.80	17.0	3.94	158
Ambient CO_2	497	23.7	1.63	5.78	19.2	2.01	152

elevated CO_2 would favour yield with higher biomass accumulation (Goncalves et al. 2009; Kizildeniz et al. 2015; Edwards et al. 2016, 2017). The main leaf elements, i.e. N, P, K, Ca, Mg and Fe, were also affected as indicated in Table 22.3. Hence, the effect of CO_2 enrichment on vine phenology will be positive if not complicated by other factors (Moutinho-Pereira et al. 2006, 2009). But, it may not be so in the future due to rising temperature, berry ripening in hot summer and drought effects coupled with rising CO_2. It is obvious here that grapevine leaf anatomical and growth characteristics are affected by rising CO_2. Among quality traits, sugars, acids and berry size were more affected, while juice, wine quality, anthocyanins and proanthocyanidins were not affected by eCO_2 (Martinez-Luscher et al. 2015; Bindi et al. 2001; Salazar-Parra et al. 2012; Wohlfahrt et al. 2021). Recently, it is indicated that elevated CO_2, i.e. 700 ppm, in combination with elevated temperature, i.e. +4 °C, decreased anthocyanin and sugar decoupling due high temperature for cv. Tempranillo (Arrizabalaga-Arriazu et al. 2020).

22.4.2 Effect of Water Stress on Viticulture

Precipitation is an important climatic factor, which affects water availability and use by grapevine (Ferreira et al. 2015). Moderate water stress has some positive effects, e.g. wines of high quality are associated with slight water stress during berry ripening. Dry weather conditions during ripening are favourable for high-quality wine production (Greenspan 2005; Munitz et al. 2017). Severe water stress during early developmental stages may considerably delay the growth and development of grapevine. On the other hand, excessive soil water during the growing season results in vigourous vines, more disease incidence and connected problems which negatively affect wine quality (Magalhaes 2008; Vanden and Centinari 2021). Contrarily, excessive rainfall near maturity is unfavourable, as it causes sugar dilution and diseases (Keller 2010; Munitz et al. 2018; Pellegrino et al. 2005). The impact of water stress depends on vine development stage, e.g. optimal soil moisture levels during budburst, shoot growth stages and inflorescence development are crucial for better vine growth (Poni et al. 1994). Water stress at these stages negatively affects shoot growth, floral cluster development and berry set as discussed in the next sections.

22.4.2.1 Phenology, Growth and Yield Under Water Stress

Water deficit in the beginning of active growth period after dormancy break negatively affects budburst as the rate of mobilization is affected. Rapid shoot growth occurs after budbreak mainly at the expense of stored food reserves in vine during the preceding vegetative cycle (Keller 2005). However, water deficit at active growth phase reduces vine growth, e.g. reduction in shoot growth 20 days after budbreak was noticed for cvs. Cabernet Sauvignon, Pinot Gris and Merlot when midday leaf water potential reached 1.0 MPa (Greenspan 2005; Shellie 2006). Similar reduction in leaf area of cv. Merlot due to water stress was observed by Munitz et al. (2017). Relatively prolonged exposure to moderate water deficit increases root-to-shoot ratio (Chaves et al. 2010). The most active period for vine growth is between budbreak and veraison, and a maximum growth is reached during the early growth cycle usually 60 days after budbreak (Junquera et al. 2006;

Ben-Asher et al. 2006; Munitz et al. 2016; Intrigliolo and Castel 2010). Vine growth then progressively decreases until a vegetative standstill is reached near veraison.

Similarly, reproductive growth correlates with water availability at different developmental stages of the vine. The relationship between yield and water availability from budbreak to harvest was observed in cv. Cabernet Sauvignon (Junquera et al. 2006). Reduced vine yield may be associated with intense and persistent water deficit as it reduces bud fertility along with poor inflorescence development. Vine fertility is reduced by both limited and excessive water availability. Water deficits near flowering limit ovary growth, leading to smaller berries, but the effects on pollen formation and germination and pollen tube growth are even more severe. For instance, sugar uptake and starch accumulation in developing pollen grains are limited under water deficit conditions, causing sterility and poor inflorescence development and fruit set (Keller 2010, 2005; McCarthy 2005).

22.4.2.2 Effects on Vine Physiological Processes

Water stress causes physiological changes, such as reduced leaf photosynthetic activity in response to stomatal closure. Leaf stomatal closure acts as the first line of defence for vines from withering due to heat and drought stress. However, transpiration is a unique component of the radiation energy which is converted into latent heat through the regulation of stomatal closure (Lovisolo et al. 2010). Under high vapour pressure deficit (VPD) levels, stomatal conductance declines up to a threshold. For instance, stomatal conductance of cv. Chardonnay significantly declined at temperatures above 30 °C and high VPD (Poni et al. 1994; O'Neill 1983). Transpiration is the main component of energy balance and provides a cooling mechanism through leaves in plants (Naor et al. 1993) and helps keep leaf temperatures in permissible limits. Even a relatively lower leaf transpiration may lower the leaf temperature by a few degrees and help maintain growth and avoid wilting to a limited extent.

22.4.2.3 Effects on Grape Berry Quality and Composition

Berry total soluble solids (TSS) give an estimation of berry ripening. Rapid TSS as Brix accumulation takes place under water deficit conditions. For example, higher TSS levels per berry weight have been recorded for rainfed vines compared to irrigated vines as indicated by Intrigliolo and Castel (2010) and Esteban et al. (2002). During berry ripening, acid contents of the berry decrease with an increase in pH. A positive relationship between water availability and total acidity was indicated by Intrigliolo and Castel (2010) and Junquera et al. (2012). Increases in titratable acidity due to water stress regardless of the developmental stage were indicated by Girona et al. (2009) for cv. Tempranillo. Higher tartaric acid and lower malic contents were recorded in water deficit vines of cv. Doña Blanca under warm conditions (Uriarte et al. 2017). Similarly, for cv. Tempranillo/110R, (Santesteban et al. 2011) obtained higher titratable acidity values in the higher irrigation treatments. Contrarily, insignificant effects of irrigation treatments on acidity, pH, malic acid and tartaric acid were noticed in cvs. Monastrell/1103 Pa, Cabernet Sauvignon and Merlot as indicated by Munitz et al. (2016). Romeroz et al. (2013) and Acevedo-Opazo et al. (2010).

Water stress early in the season negatively affects vigour, berry size and photosynthetic rate which ultimately lowers acidity and phenolic contents (Esteban et al. 2002; Salon et al. 2005). Controlled deficit irrigation is used to improve berry ripening and wine quality (Uriarte et al. 2015), e.g. elevating the levels of terpenes by modulating structural and regulatory genes (Cramer et al. 2013). Water deficit stimulated the biosynthesis of anthocyanins and phenolic contents (Rogiers et al. 2011). Moreover, the timing and intensity of water deficit affect the metabolism, colour, aroma and flavour compounds of berries. Certainly, water deficit increases the skin-to-pulp ratio in berries compared to well-watered grapevines (Zufferey et al. 2012) while enhancing skin tannin and anthocyanin contents. Increased biosynthesis of anthocyanins in response to water deficit causes differences in colour development (Rossouw et al. 2017).

22.5 Effect of Elevated Temperature on Viticulture

Higher temperature during the active growing season strongly affects grapevines because it is a major driver of developmental stages of grapevine (Parker et al. 2013) and global warming is expected to accelerate phenological events. The phenological shifts at key developmental stages have a strong influence on vineyard management. Moreover, heat events during maturation period will affect wine quality and typicity. Extreme heat stress during the ripening period abruptly reduces grapevine metabolism. It may result in higher sugar levels and lower acidity with potential increase in chances of wine spoilage, hence affecting grapevine production and quality attributes (De Orduna 2010; Fraga et al. 2018) as discussed in Sects. 3.3.1, 3.3.2, and 3.3.3.

22.5.1 Phenology, Growth and Yield Under High Temperature

Grapevine phenology is a good indicator of heat stress and may be used to evaluate the effects of climate change on vine developmental stages like flowering, veraison and grape ripening (Greer and Weston 2010; Bernardo et al. 2018). Air temperature is the key factor driving the timing of phenological stages (Fig. 22.9) along with the duration of phenophases in grapevine (Kose 2014); hence, it affects the inter-annual variability in vine yield and berry quality (De Orduna 2010; Fraga et al. 2014).

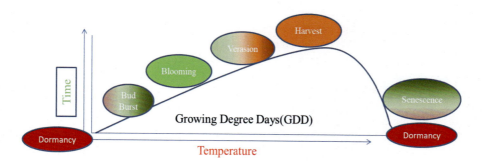

Fig. 22.9 Thermal time model for studying the growth stages of temperate perennial crops

Rising temperature trend is expected to advance grapevine phenology and derive berry ripening during the warmest period of the year (Webb et al. 2007; Duchene et al. 2010) interferes with the quality traits (Van Leeuwen and Seguin 2006). Phenological shifts of 10–24 days from 1975 until 2015 have been noticed in south-west Germany give an alarming situation for global viticulture (Koch and Oehl 2018). Shortening trends for the periods budburst to flowering, flowering to veraison and veraison to maturity have been recorded due to elevated temperatures, e.g. flowering to veraison interval shortened about 1 day for every 5 years (Jones and Davis 2000; Tomasi et al. 2011; Duchene and Schneider 2005). A similar trend with strong correlations between maturity timing and the maximum springtime temperatures under Australian conditions was noticed (Jarvis et al. 2017). The most obvious phenological shifts recorded are for blooming and veraison (Caffarra and Eccel 2011). Similarly, grapevine harvest dates are associated with maximum air temperatures (Koufos et al. 2020). However, significant trends were not observed for the shortening of the veraison to maturity period (Cameron et al. 2021). Previously, it was indicated that among a range of temperature variables, maximum temperature for March–April influenced flowering and veraison timings (Malheiro et al. 2013).

A significant advance is expected in the onset timings of grapevine phenological stages; however, the phenophase duration depends on soil type and grape variety (Fraga et al. 2013; Bernardo et al. 2018). Phenological advancement for 2–3 weeks is expected until 2050, and this advancement is more apparent for the northern hemisphere vineyards (Neethling et al. 2017; Van Leeuwen et al. 2019). In a related study, it was depicted that in the future, many areas presently considered suitable for grapevine production would be eliminated with 81% reduction in acreage for premium quality grape at temperature above 35 °C (White et al. 2006).

Moreover, elevated temperatures are considered detrimental for the reproductive performance and consequently yield of grapevine (Keller et al. 2010), and for temperature at 40 °C, reduction in flowers per inflorescence under warmer conditions was by one-third. Previously, it has been established that day temperature of 35–40 °C near flowering is highly detrimental for good fruit set with lower ovule fertility, hence fewer berries per cluster (Ebadi et al. 1995; Ewart and Kliewer 1977;

Kliewer 1977). Furthermore, pollen germination is also highly temperature sensitive, e.g. in grapevines (Staudt 1982), less pollen germination was noticed at 15 °C, while temperature at 28 °C is considered optimum for better pollen germination and pollen tube growth (Rajasekaran and Mullins 1985). High temperature near flowering negatively affects the carbohydrate contents of pistil and pollen tube growth with lower fruit set (Snider et al. 2011; Pagay and Collins 2017). Furthermore, short periods of extreme temperatures are considered highly detrimental particularly for key developmental stages, e.g. flowering and fruit set, which may negatively affect vine yield and berry quality (Ferris et al. 1998; Hedhly et al. 2005; Prasad et al. 1999).

22.5.2 Fruit Quality and Composition

Rising temperature owing to global warming is expected to change the composition of grape berries. The rate metabolism of grape berries depends on air temperature, whereas elevated temperatures beyond ambient level perturb metabolic pathways and cause changes in the biosynthesis of several important metabolic compounds crucial for maintaining quality (Blancquaert et al. 2018). Elevated air temperatures promote berry sugars coupled with the degradation of berry organic acids. In a rising temperature scenario, juice and wine acidity would be more drastically affected compared to sugar contents as indicated in Fig. 22.10. Such weather conditions would result in unbalanced wines having higher alcohol contents due to high sugars and lower acidity and deprived of essential aromatic compounds (Kose 2014; Van Leeuwen and Destrac-Irvine 2016). Relatively lower titratable acidity has been observed at 30 °C compared to 20 °C (Poudel et al. 2009). Under heat stress

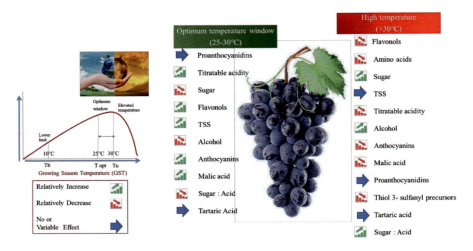

Fig. 22.10 Key quality traits of grape berries under ambient and elevated temperatures

22 Climatic Challenge for Global Viticulture and Adaptation Strategies

conditions, potassium concentration of berries increases near maturity along with high pH value and lower total acidity (Bernardo et al. 2018). Moreover, malic acid is metabolized relatively faster than tartaric acid at elevated temperature, and the optimum temperature for malate biosynthesis is 20–25 °C; however, a major decrease in its biosynthesis has been noticed at 40 °C (Keller 2010).

For most of the grapevine varieties, optimum temperature at maturation stage for the biosynthesis of aroma compounds is 20–22 °C (Van Leeuwen and Destrac-Irvine 2016). Berry colour development is reduced when air temperature exceeds 30 °C, and higher temperatures (above 37 °C) cause major decline in berry colour along with higher volatilization of aroma compounds (Bernardo et al. 2018; Neethling et al. 2017). Total sugars of grapes and ethanol contents of wines have also increased, e.g. wines with ethanol levels have increased by 3% during the last few weeks (Neethling et al. 2012). Anthocyanins are the main pigment-imparting compounds in berries largely found in the skins of coloured varieties, e.g. red grapes. Elevated temperatures lower anthocyanin contents and flavour compounds of berries grown in temperate areas (Poudel et al. 2009; Yamane et al. 2006). Moreover, reduction in delphinidins, anthocyanins, peonidin and petunidins based anthocyanins contents of grape berries was noticed, however biosynthesis of malvidin derivatives was less affected under high temperature conditions (Bernardo et al. 2018).

22.5.3 *Elevated Temperature and Grapevine Physiology*

Among physiological functions, photosynthesis is directly affected by temperature variations as highlighted by Sharma et al. (2019) and Luo et al. (2011), and it is reduced earlier before the onset of other symptoms of high temperature beyond optimum limits. The optimum temperature window differs among species (Xiao et al. 2017; Kun et al. 2018), and for grapevine, it lies between 25 and 35 °C (Ferrandino and Lovisolo 2014). When temperature goes below 10 °C, most of the physiological processes are weakened. On the other hand, heat acclimation mechanisms are activated when the temperature reaches 35 °C, (Bernardo et al. 2018; Greer and Weedon 2012). Similarly, extremely high temperatures, e.g. 40 °C or above, may cause the disruption of the photosynthetic apparatus of plants. Reduction in photosynthetic activity at 45 °C compared to 25 °C has been quantified up to 60% by Lamaoui et al. (2018). Similarly, it was observed (Xiao et al. 2017) that photosynthetic activity does not decrease up to 35 °C; however, it is limited above 40 °C, and this reduction in photosynthesis may be attributed to 15–30% lower stomatal conductance (Lamaoui et al. 2018). The discussion also bears forth that heat and drought stresses are related to each other and reduced stomatal conductance may increase the effects of heat stress due to rise in leaf temperature (Costa et al. 2012). The effects of heat stress on vine stomatal conductance vary among cultivars, and it was noticed that for a common wine cultivar Touriga Nacional, under mild heat stress conditions, leaf stomata remained open which might be beneficial for lowering the leaf temperature to retain normal photosynthesis (Wang et al. 2010).

The lower leaf photosynthetic activity under high temperature might be attributed to disturbed vine biochemical processes, e.g. reduction in ribulose-1,5-bisphosphate (RuBP) regeneration along with the activation of ribulose bisphosphate carboxylase oxygenase (Rubisco) activity (Wen et al. 2005). Under heat stress, photosystem II (PSII) is suspended earlier, and other cellular functions are disrupted as it is highly temperature sensitive (Ferrandino and Lovisolo 2014; Bensalem-Fnayou et al. 2011). Thermal stress even for short periods, e.g. 15 min at 40 °C, may cause irreparable damage to thylakoid membrane permeability and functioning of PSII in grapevines (Ferrandino and Lovisolo 2014; Liu and Fang 2011). Recently, it was revealed that for heat treatments at 35 °C and 40 °C, photosynthetic activity was reduced significantly; however, total chlorophyll contents, chlorophyll fluorescence and thylakoid membrane leakage were not much affected for cvs. Cabernet Sauvignon and Junzi vines (Nievola et al. 2017). For more elevated temperature at 45 °C, lower total chlorophyll contents and increased fluidity of thylakoid membrane were observed along with other obvious stress symptoms. Moreover, structural disarrays of thylakoids have also been reported in prolonged heat stress conditions, i.e. for 3 months. Injury to thylakoid structures is associated with a deterioration in chlorophyll contents which indicates the inhibition of PSII (Hu et al. 2020; Kadir et al. 2007). Hence, chlorophyll fluorescence may help to identify changes in photosynthetic apparatus as an indicator for heat stress tolerance in grape cultivars (Kadir et al. 2007).

Leaf transpiration increases under elevated temperature as observed by Greer (2019) that transpiration rates in grapevine increased up to five times for the corresponding increase in temperature from 15 to 40 °C. This increase in transpiration activity was from 0.5 mmol m^{-2} s^{-1} to about 2.5 mmol m^{-2} s^{-1}; however, further increases in temperature (45 °C) did not affect leaf transpiration. Similarly, for cv. Semillon, substantial increase in transpiration was observed with increase in leaf temperature above 35 °C; the increase is mainly to meet up the enhanced evaporative cooling demands (Keenan et al. 2010). In another related study, four time increases in transpiration of cv. Chardonnay were noticed as the temperature increased from 15 to 30 °C, while this rate was even higher for cv. Cabernet Sauvignon at 35–40 °C (Keller 2010). A linear trend for the transpiration rates was noticed with temperature increase from 20 to 40 °C. Moreover, genotypes have varying responses to temperature, e.g. relatively higher transpiration rates have been observed for cv. Semillon vines compared to many other cultivars (Rogiers et al. 2009); thus, its cooling capacity owning to better transpiration may help to retain the canopy temperature relatively lower than the atmospheric temperature. In addition to climatic variables, the quality and growth of grapevine vegetative and reproductive growth, ripening and yield may also be affected by vineyard management such as pruning type, crop load, training systems, grafting and timings of cultural practices as discussed by Winkler (1974). It is highly crucial to acquire the knowledge of the varietal specificities for high-quality grape production (Jones and Davis 2000).

Henceforth, optimizing vineyard management is required for enhancing vineyard productivity and profitability.

22.6 Adaptation Strategies for Viticulture in the Wake of Climate Change

The elaborated climate change impacts on viticulture make it imperative to plan and apply suitable adaptation measures. It included short-term adaptation measures and changes in viticulture management practices and techniques, such as irrigation scheduling, protection from sun burns, improving water use efficiency (WUF) and devising long-term adaptation strategies such as selection of suitable varieties and identifying new suitable viticulture regions for a sustainable crop production (Fraga 2019) in consultation with stakeholders is an upheaval task for modeller, policy makers and viticulturists.

In order to adapt viticulture, physiologists and breeder must focus on improving water use efficiency (WUE) to minimize the impact of elevated CO_2 and climate change by integrating the knowledge from genomics and phenomics to incorporate characteristics from promising QTLs. Moreover, improvements in photosynthetic efficiency and WUE by introducing C4-like characteristics in C3 plants coupled with modelling approaches need to be focused (Ahmed and Ahmad 2019). Climate change necessitates identifying new genotypes and incorporating resilience such as heat and drought tolerance from wild cultivars. Moreover, the existing viticulture may not remain suitable for premier-quality table and wine grape cultivation under future climate; hence, identifying new viticulture zones based on crop heat unit requirements is the need of time. Furthermore, improving vineyard management practices, e.g. pruning, thinning and canopy management for maintaining vine balance, is necessary to cope with these challenges.

22.7 Conclusion

Currently, global viticulture is facing sustainability challenge owing to climate change. Rising CO_2 coupled with high temperature and lower rainfall negatively affected grapevine production. Phenological advancements with poor inflorescence development, less fruit set and low yield have been observed in many viticulture regions. Although elevated CO_2 levels may have some positive impacts on photosynthetic activity, the overall impact in conjugation with increasing temperature and water stress would be negative. Moreover, the physiological activities of vines such as photosynthesis activity, stomatal conductivity and water use efficiency are also severely affected under heat and drought stress. Similarly, key quality attributes of wine and table grapes, e.g. berry sugar, acidity levels, polyphenols and anthocyanin, may not reach desirable levels for premier-quality grape production. The impact of climatic trends on viticulture would be more in the coming decades, e.g. major grapevine cultivars originating from cooler climates would not be able to withstand heat stress. Indigenous and wild grapevine germplasm from relatively warm and dry regions may serve as an alternative. Henceforth, it is crucial to identify the key components of grapevine regulatory networks controlling heat stress response and acquisition of tolerance against environmental stresses for sustainable viticulture.

References

Acevedo-Opazo C, Ortega-Farias S, Fuentes S (2010) Effects of grapevine (*Vitis vinifera* L.) water status on water consumption, vegetative growth and grape quality. An irrigation scheduling application to achieve regulated deficit irrigation. Agric Water Manag 97(7):956–964

Ahmed M, Ahmad S (2019) Carbon dioxide enrichment and crop productivity. In: Agronomic crops. Springer, Singapore, pp 31–46

Arrizabalaga-Arriazu M, Morales F, Irigoyen JJ, Hilbert G, Pascual I (2020) Growth performance and carbon partitioning of grapevine Tempranillo clones under simulated climate change scenarios: elevated CO_2 and temperature. J Plant Physiol 252:153226

Ben-Asher J, Tsuyuki I, Bravdo BA, Sagih M (2006) Irrigation of grapevines with saline water: I. Leaf area index, stomatal conductance, transpiration and photosynthesis. Agric Water Manag 83(1):13–21

Bensalem-Fnayou A, Bouamama B, Ghorbel A, Mliki A (2011) Investigations on the leaf anatomy and ultrastructure of grapevine (*Vitis vinifera* L.) under heat stress. Microsc Res Tech 74:756–762

Bernardo S, Dinis LT, Machado N, Moutinho-Pereira J (2018) Grapevine abiotic stress assessment and search for sustainable adaptation strategies in Mediterranean-like climates. A review. Agron Sustain 38(6):1–20

Bhat ZA, Padder SA, Ganaie AQ, Dar NA, Rehman HU, Wani MY (2017) Correlation of available nutrients with physicochemical properties and nutrient content of grape orchards of Kashmir. J Pharmacogn Phytochem 6(2):181–185

Bindi M, Fibbi L, Miglietta F (2001) Free air CO_2 enrichment (FACE) of grapevine (*Vitis vinifera* L.): II. Growth and quality of grape and wine in response to elevated CO_2 concentrations. Eur J Agron 14:145–155

Blancquaert EH, Oberholster A, Da-Silva JMR, Deloire AJ (2018) Effects of abiotic factors on phenolic compounds in the grape berry – a review. S Afr J Enol Vitic 40:1–14

Caffarra A, Eccel E (2011) Projecting the impacts of climate on the phenology of grapevine in a mountain area. Aust J Grape Wine Res 17:52–61

Cameron W, Petrie PR, Barlow EWR, Patrick CJ, Howell K, Fuentes S (2021) Is advancement of grapevine maturity explained by an increase in the rate of ripening or advancement of veraison? Aust J Grape Wine Res 27(3):334–347

Chaves MM, Zarrouk O, Francisco R, Costa JM, Santos T, Regalado AP (2010) Grapevine under deficit irrigation: hints from physiological and molecular data. Ann Bot 105:661–676

Christensen JH, Hewitson B, Busuioc A, Chen A, Gao X, Jones R, Kolli RK, Kwon WT, Laprise R, Magana Rueda V (2007) Regional climate projections. In: Solomon S, Qin D, Manning M, Chen Z, Marquis M, Averyt KB, Tignor M, Miller HL (eds) Climate change 2007: the physical science basis. Contribution of Working Group I to the Fourth Assessment Report of the Intergovernmental Panel on Climate Change. Cambridge University Press, Cambridge/New York

Costa JM, Ortuno MF, Lopes CM, Chaves MM (2012) Grapevine varieties exhibiting differences in stomatal response to water deficit. Funct Plant Biol 39:179–189

Costa R, Fraga H, Fonseca A, De Cortazar-Atauri IG, Val MC, Carlos C, Reis S, Santos JA (2019) Grapevine phenology of cv. Touriga Franca and Touriga Nacional in the Douro Wine Region: modelling and climate change projections. J Agron 9:210

Cramer GR, Van Sluyter SC, Hopper DW, Pascovici D, Keighley T, Haynes PA (2013) Proteomic analysis indicates massive changes in metabolism prior to the inhibition of growth and photosynthesis of grapevine (*Vitis vinifera* L.) in response to water deficit. BMC Plant Biol 13:49

Creasy GL, Creasy LL (2018) Grapes, vol 27. CABI

De Orduna RM (2010) Climate change associated effects on grape and wine quality and production. Food Res Int 43:1844–1855

Duchene E, Schneider C (2005) Grapevine and climatic changes: a glance at the situation in Alsace. Agron Sustain Dev 25:93–99

Duchene E, Huard F, Dumas V, Schneider C, Merdinoglu D (2010) The challenge of adapting grapevine varieties to climate change. Clim Res 41:193–204

Ebadi A, Coombe BG, May P (1995) Fruit-set on small Chardonnay and Shiraz vines grown under varying temperature regimes between budburst and flowering. Aust J Grape Wine Res 1:3–10

Edwards EJ, Unwin DJ, Sommer KJ, Downey MO, Mollah M (2016) The response of commercially managed, field grown, grapevines (*Vitis vinifera* L.) to a simulated future climate consisting of elevated CO2 in combination with elevated air temperature. Acta Hortic 1115: 103–110

Edwards EJ, Unwin D, Kilmister R, Treeb M (2017) Multi-seasonal effects of warming and elevated CO_2; on the physiology, growth and production of mature, field grown, shiraz grapevines. OENO One 51:127–132

Esteban MA, Villanueva MJ, Lissarrague JR (2002) Relationships between different berry components in tempranillo (*Vitis vinifera* L.) grapes from irrigated and non-irrigated vines during ripening. J Sci Food Agric 82:1136–1146

Ewart A, Kliewer WM (1977) Effects of controlled day and night temperatures and nitrogen on fruit-set, ovule fertility, and fruit composition of several wine grape cultivars. Am J Enol Vitic 28:88–95

FAOSTAT (2016) Food and agricultural commodities production. FAOSTAT

Ferrandino A, Lovisolo C (2014) Abiotic stress effects on grapevine (Vitis vinifera L.): focus on abscisic acid-mediated consequences on secondary metabolism and berry quality. Environ Exp Bot 103:138–147

Ferreira MI, Conceicao N, Malheiro AC, Silvestre JM, Silva RM (2015) Water stress indicators and stress functions to calculate soil water depletion in deficit irrigated grapevine and kiwi. In: VIII international symposium on irrigation of horticultural crops, vol 1150, pp 119–126

Ferris R, Ellis RH, Wheeler TR, Hadley P (1998) Effect of high temperature stress at anthesis on grain yield and biomass of field-grown crops of wheat. Ann Bot 82:631–639

Field SK, Smith JP, Holzapfel BP, Hardie WJ, Emery RJN (2009) Grapevine response to soil temperature: xylem cytokinins and carbohydrate reserve mobilization from budbreak to anthesis. Am J Enol Vitic 60:164–172

Fraga H (2019) Viticulture and winemaking under climate change. Agronomy 9(12):783

Fraga H, Santos JA (2017) Daily prediction of seasonal grapevine production in the Douro wine region based on favourable meteorological conditions. Aust J Grape Wine Res 23:296–304

Fraga H, Malheiro AC, Moutinho-Pereira J, Santos JA (2012) An overview of climate change impacts on European viticulture. Food Energy Secur 1(2):94–110

Fraga H, Malheiro AC, Moutinho-Pereira J, Santos JA (2013) An overview of climate change impacts on European viticulture. Food Energy Secur 1(2):94–110

Fraga H, Malheiro AC, Moutinho-Pereira J, Santos JA (2014) Climate factors driving wine production in the Portuguese Minho region. Agric Meteorol 185:26–36

Fraga H, Atauri IG, Santos JA (2018) Viticultural irrigation demands under climate change scenarios in Portugal. Agric Water Manag 196:66–74

Fraga H, Pinto JG, Santos JA (2019) Climate change projections for chilling and heat forcing conditions in European vineyards and olive orchards: a multi-model assessment. Clim Chang 152:179–193

Girona J, Marsal J, Mata M, Del Campo J, Basile B (2009) Phenological sensitivity of berry growth and composition of tempranillo grapevines (*Vitis vinifera* L.) to water stress. Aust J Grape Wine Res 15:268–277

Goncalves B, Falco V, Moutinho-Pereira J, Bacelar E, Peixoto F, Correia C (2009) Effects of elevated CO_2 on grapevine (Vitis vinifera L.): volatile composition, phenolic content, and in vitro antioxidant activity of red wine. J Agric Food Chem 57:265–273

Greenspan M (2005) Integrated irrigation of California wine grapes. Prac Winery Vineyard 27(3): 21–79

Greer DH (2019) Stomatal and non-stomatal limitations at different leaf temperatures to the photosynthetic process during the post-harvest period for *Vitis vinifera* cv. Chardonnay vines. N Z J Crop Hortic Sci 48:1–21

Greer DH, Weedon MM (2012) Modelling photosynthetic responses to temperature of grapevine (Vitis vinifera cv. Semillon) leaves on vines grown in a hot climate. Plant Cell Environ 35: 1050–1064

Greer DH, Weedon MM (2013) The impact of high temperatures on Vitis vinifera cv. Semillon grapevine performance and berry ripening. Front Plant Sci 491(4):1–9

Greer DH, Weston C (2010) Heat stress affects flowering, berry growth, sugar accumulation and photosynthesis of Vitis vinifera cv. Semillon grapevines grown in a controlled environment. Funct Plant Biol 37:206–214

Hedhly A, Hormaza JI, Herrero M (2005) The effect of temperature on pollen germination, pollen tube growth, and stigmatic receptivity in peach. Plant Biol 7(5):476–483

Hu S, Ding Y, Zhu C (2020) Sensitivity and responses of chloroplasts to heat stress in plants. Front Plant Sci 11:375

Intrigliolo DS, Castel JR (2010) Response of grapevine cv. 'Tempranillo' to timing and amount of irrigation: water relations, vine growth, yield and berry and wine composition. Irrig Sci 28(2): 113–125

IPCC (2014a) Climate change 2014: synthesis report. In: Core Writing Team, Pachauri RK, Meyer LA (eds) Contribution of Working Groups I, II and III to the Fifth Assessment Report of the Intergovernmental Panel on Climate Change. IPCC, Geneva, p 151

IPCC (2014b) Climate change 2014: mitigation of climate change. Contribution of Working Group III to the Fifth Assessment Report of the Intergovernmental Panel on Climate Change. Cambridge University Press, Cambridge/New York

Jarvis C, Barlow E, Darbyshire R, Eckard R, Goodwin I (2017) Relationship between viticultural climatic indices and grape maturity in Australia. Int J Biometeorol 61:1849–1862

Jones GV, Davis RE (2000) Climate influences on grapevine phenology, grape composition, and wine production and quality for Bordeaux, France. Am J Enol Vitic 51:249–261

Jones G, Snead N, Nelson P (2004) Geology and wine 8. Modeling viticultural landscapes: a GIS analysis of the terroir potential in the Umpqua Valley of Oregon. Geosci Can 31(4):167–178

Junquera P, Sanchez de Miguel P, Linares R, Baeza P (2006) Study of influence of irrigation rates and distribution in the time. In: Agronomic behaviour of vineyard to different water availability

Junquera P, Lissarrague JR, Jimenez L, Linares R, Baeza P (2012) Long-term effects of different irrigation strategies on yield components, vine vigour and grape composition in cv. Cabernet-sauvignon (*Vitis vinifera* L.). Irrig Sci 30(5):351–361

Kadir S, Von Weihe M, Khatib KA (2007) Photochemical efficiency and recovery of photosystem II in grapes after exposure to sudden and gradual heat stress. J Am Soc Hortic Sci 132:764–769

Keenan T, Sabate S, Gracia C (2010) Soil water stress and coupled photosynthesis-conductance models: bridging the gap between conflicting reports on the relative roles of stomatal, mesophyll conductance and biochemical limitations to photosynthesis. Agric For Meteorol 150:443–453

Keller M (2005) Cluster thinning effects on three deficit-irrigated *Vitis vinifera* cultivars. Am J Enol Vitic 56(2):91–103

Keller M (2010) The science of grapevines: anatomy and physiology. Elsevier, Inc, Amsterdam, p 400

Keller M, Tarara JM, Mills LJ (2010) Spring temperatures alter reproductive development in grapevines. Aust J Grape Wine Res 16:445–454

Kizildeniz T, Mekni I, Santesteban H, Pascual I, Morales F, Irigoyen JJ (2015) Effects of climate change including elevated CO_2 concentration, temperature and water deficit on growth, water status, and yield quality of grapevine (*Vitis vinifera* L.) cultivars. Agric Water Manag 159:155–164

Kliewer WM (1977) Effect of high temperatures during the bloom-set period on fruit-set, ovule fertility, and berry growth of several grape cultivars. Am J Enol Vitic 28:215–222

Koch B, Oehl F (2018) Climate change favors grapevine production in temperate zones. Agric Sci 9:247–263

Kose B (2014) Phenology and ripening of *Vitis vinifera* L. and *Vitis labrusca* L. varieties in the maritime climate of Samsun in Turkey's Black Sea Region. S Afr J Enol Vitic 35(1):90–102

Koufos GC, Mavromatis T, Koundouras S, Jones GV (2020) Adaptive capacity of winegrape varieties cultivated in Greece to climate change: current trends and future projections. Oeno One 54(4):1201–1219

Kuhn N, Guan L, Dai ZW, Wu BH, Lauvergeat V, Gomes E, Li SH, Godoy F, Arce-Johnson P, Delrot S (2013) Berry ripening: recently heard through the grapevine. J Exp Bot 65(16): 4543–4559

Kun Z, Bai-Hong C, Yan H, Rui Y, Yu-an W (2018) Effects of short-term heat stress on PSII and subsequent recovery for senescent leaves of Vitis vinifera L. cv. Red Globe. J Integr Agric 17: 2683–2693

Lamaoui M, Jemo M, Datla R, Bekkaoui F (2018) Heat and drought stresses in crops and approaches for their mitigation. Front Chem 6:26

Liu M, Fang Y (2011) Effects of heat stress on physiological indexes and ultrastructure of grapevines. Sci Agric Sin 53:1444–1458

Lovisolo C, Perrone C, Carra I, Ferrandino A, Flexas J, Medrano H (2010) Drought-induced changes in development and function of grapevine (Vitis spp.) organs and in their hydraulic and non-hydraulic interactions at the whole-plant level: a physiological and molecular update. Funct Plant Biol 37(2):98–116

Luo HB, Ma L, Xi HF, Duan W, Li SH, Loescher W, Wang JF, Wang LJ (2011) Photosynthetic responses to heat treatments at different temperatures and following recovery in grapevine (Vitis amurensis L.) leaves. PLoS One 6(8):23033

Mackenzie DE, Christy AG (2005) The role of soil chemistry in wine grape quality and sustainable soil management in vineyards. Water Sci Technol 51(1):27–37

Magalhaes N (2008) Tratado de viticultura: a videira, a vinha eo terroir. Chaves Ferreira, Lisboa

Magalhaes N (2015) Tratado de Viticultura: A Videira, a Vinha e o Terroir. Esfera Poética, Lisboa, p 605

Malheiro AC, Campos R, Fraga H, Eiras-Dias J, Silvestre J, Santos JA (2013) Winegrape phenology and temperature relationships in the Lisbon wine region, Portugal. OENO One 47(4): 287–299

Martinez-Luscher J, Morales F, Sanchez-Diaz M, Delrot S, Aguirreolea J, Gomes E (2015) Climate change conditions (elevated CO2 and temperature) and UV-B radiation affect grapevine (*Vitis vinifera* cv. Tempranillo) leaf carbon assimilation, altering fruit ripening rates. Plant Sci 236: 168–176

McCarthy M (2005) Water stress at flowering and effects on yield. In: Garis K, Dundon C, Johnstone R, Partridge S (eds) Transforming flowers to fruit. ASVO, Adelaide, pp 35–37

Meinshausen M, Smith SJ, Calvin K, Daniel JS, Kainuma ML, Lamarque JF, Matsumoto K, Montzka SA, Raper SC, Riahi K, Thomson AG (2011) The RCP greenhouse gas concentrations and their extensions from 1765 to 2300. Clim Chang 109(1):213–241

Mosedale JR, Wilson RJ, Maclean IMD (2015) Climate change and crop exposure to adverse weather: changes to frost risk and grapevine flowering conditions. PLoS One 10(10):e0141218

Moutinho-Pereira J, Correia C, Falco V (2006) Effects of elevated CO2 on grapevines grown under Mediterranean field conditions–impact on grape and wine composition. Aust J Grape Wine Res 6:2–12

Moutinho-Pereira J, Goncalves B, Bacelar E, Cunha JB, Coutinho J, Correia CM (2009) Effects of elevated CO_2 on grapevine (*Vitis vinifera* L.): physiological and yield attributes. Vitis 48(4): 159–165

Mullins MG, Bouquet A, Williams LE (1992) Biology of the grapevine. Cambridge University Press, Cambridge

Munitz S, Schwartz A, Netzer Y (2016) Evaluation of seasonal water use and crop coefficients for cabernet sauvignon' grapevines as the base for skilled regulated deficit irrigation. Acta Hortic 1115:33–40

Munitz S, Netzer Y, Schwartz A (2017) Sustained and regulated deficit irrigation of field-grown merlot grapevines. Aust J Grape Wine Res 23(1):87–94

Munitz S, Netzer Y, Shtein I, Schwartz A (2018) Water availability dynamics have long-term effects on mature stem structure in *Vitis vinifera*. Am J Bot 105(9):1443–1452

Naor A, Bravdo B, Hepner Y (1993) Effect of post-veraison irrigation level on sauvignon blanc yield, juice quality and water relations. S Afr J Enol Vitic 14(2):19–25

Neethling E, Barbeau G, Quenol H (2012) Change in climate and berry composition for grapevine varieties cultivated in the Loire Valley. Clim Res 53:89–101

Neethling E, Petitjean T, Quenol H, Barbeau G (2017) Assessing local climate vulnerability and winegrowers' adaptive processes in the context of climate change. Mitig Adapt Strateg Glob Chang 22:777–803

Nievola CC, Carvalho CP, Carvalho V, Rodrigues E (2017) Rapid responses of plants to temperature changes. Temperature 4:371–405

O'Neill SD (1983) Role of osmotic potential gradients during water stress and leaf senescence in Fragaria virginiana. Plant Physiol 72(4):931–937

OIV (2010) Criteria for the methods of quantification of potentially allergenic residues of fining agent proteins in wine. Resolution OIV/OENO, p 427

OIV (2013) Description of world vine varieties. L'Organisation Internationale de la Vigne et du Vin, Paris

OIV (2019) Statistical report on world viti-viniculture. International Organisation of Vine and Wine, Paris

Pagay V, Collins C (2017) Effects of timing and intensity of elevated temperatures on reproductive development of field-grown Shiraz grapevines. OENO One 51(4). https://doi.org/10.20870/oeno-one.2017.51.4.1066

Parker A, Garcia I, Chuine I, Barbeau G, Bois B, Boursiquot JM, Cahurel JY, Claverie M, Dufourcq T, Geny L (2013) Classification of varieties for their timing of flowering and veraison using a modelling approach: a case study for the grapevine species *Vitis vinifera* L. Agric For Meteorol 180:249–264

Pellegrino A, Lebon E, Simmoneau T, Wery J (2005) Towards a simple indicator of water stress in grapevine (*Vitis vinifera* L.) based on the differential sensitivities of vegetative growth components. Aust J Grape Wine Res 11(3):306–315

Poni S, Lakso N, Turner JR, Melious RE (1994) Interactions of crop level and late season water stress on growth and physiology of fieldgrown Concord grapevines. Am J Enol Vitic 45(2): 252–258

Poudel PR, Mochioka R, Beppu K, Kataoka I (2009) Influence of temperature on berry composition of interspecific hybrid wine grape 'Kadainou R-1' (Vitis ficifolia var. ganebu $\times$ V. vinifera 'Muscat of Alexandria'). Am J Enol Vitic 78(2):169–174

Prasad PVV, Craufurd PQ, Summerfield RJ (1999) Fruit number in relation to pollen production and viability in groundnut exposed to short episodes of heat stress. Ann Bot 84:381–386

Rajasekaran K, Mullins MG (1985) Somatic embryo formation by cultured ovules of Cabernet Sauvignon grape: effects of fertilization and of the male gameticide toluidine blue. Vitis 24:151–157

22 Climatic Challenge for Global Viticulture and Adaptation Strategies

Rogiers SY, Greer DH, Hutton RJ, Landsberg JJ (2009) Does night-time transpiration contribute to anisohydric behaviour in a *Vitis vinifera* cultivar. J Exp Bot 60:3751–3763

Rogiers SY, Holzapfel BP, Smith JP (2011) Sugar accumulation in roots of two grape varieties with contrasting response to water stress. Ann Appl Biol 159(3):399–413

Romeroz P, Gil-Munoz R, Del Amor FM, Valdes E, Fernandez JI, Martinez-Cutillas A (2013) Regulated deficit irrigation based upon optimum water status improves phenolic composition in monastrell grapes and wines. Agric Water Manag 121:85–101

Rossouw GC, Smith JP, Barril C, Deloire A, Holzapfel BP (2017) Implications of the presence of maturing fruit on carbohydrate and nitrogen distribution in grapevines under postveraison water constraints. J Am Soc Hortic Sci 142(2):71–84

Ruel JJ, Walker MA (2006) Resistance to Pierce's disease in Muscadinia rotundifolia and other native grape species. Am J Enol Vitic 57(2):158–165

Salazar-Parra C, Aguirreolea J, Sanchez-Diaz M, Irigoyen JJ, Morales F (2012) Climate change (elevated CO2, elevated temperature and moderate drought) triggers the antioxidant enzymes' response of grapevine cv. Tempranillo, avoiding oxidative damage. Physiol Plant 144:99–110

Salon JL, Chirivella C, Castel JR (2005) Response of cv Bobal to timing of deficit irrigation in Requena, Spain: water relations, yield and wine quality. Am J Enol Vitic 56:1–8

Santesteban LG, Miranda C, Royo JB (2011) Regulated deficit irrigation effects on growth, yield, grape quality and individual anthocyanin composition in *Vitis vinifera* L. cv. 'Tempranillo'. Agric Water Manag 98:1171–1179

Sharma A, Kumar V, Shahzad B, Ramakrishnan M, Sidhu GPS, Bali AS, Handa N, Kapoor D, Yadav P, Khanna K (2019) Photosynthetic response of plants under different abiotic stresses: a review. J Plant Growth Regul 39:509–531

Shellie KC (2006) Vine and berry response of merlot (Vitis vinifera L.) to differential water stress. Am J Enol Vitic 57:514–551

Snider JL, Oosterhuis DM, Loka DA, Kawakami EM (2011) High temperature limits in vivo pollen tube growth rates by altering diurnal carbohydrate balance in field-grown Gossypium hirsutum pistils. J Plant Physiol 168:1168–1175

Staudt G (1982) In vivo pollen germination and pollen tube growth in Vitis and dependence on temperature. Vitis 21:205–216

Tomasi D, Jones GV, Giust M, Lovat L, Gaiotti F (2011) Grapevine phenology and climate change: relationships and trends in the Veneto Region of Italy for 1964–2009. Am J Enol Vitic 62:329–339

Uriarte D, Intrigliolo DS, Mancha LA, Picon-Toro J, Valdes E, Prieto MH (2015) Interactive effects of irrigation and crop level on tempranillo vines in a semiarid climate. Am J Enol Vitic 66(2):101–111

Uriarte D, Mancha LA, Moreno D, Bejarano D, Valdes E, Talaverano I (2017) Effects of timing of water deficit induction on Dona Blanca white grapevine under semiarid growing conditions of South-Western Spain. In: Marsal J, Girona J (eds) ISHS Acta Hortic, pp 1150–1168

Van Leeuwen C, Destrac-Irvine A (2016) Modified grape composition under climate change conditions requires adaptations in the vineyard. OENO ONE 51:147–154

Van Leeuwen C, Destrac-Irvine A (2017) Modified grape composition under climate change conditions requires adaptations in the vineyard. OENO One 51:147–154

Van Leeuwen C, Seguin G (2006) The concept of terroir in viticulture. J Wine Res 17:1–10

Van Leeuwen C, Friant P, Chone X, Tregoat O, Koundouras S, Dubourdieu D (2004) Influence of climate, soil, and cultivar on terroir. Am J Enol Vitic 55(3):207–217

Van Leeuwen C, Destrac-Irvine A, Dubernet M, Duchene E, Gowdy M, Marguerit E, Pieri P, Parker A, De Resseguier L, Ollat N (2019) An update on the impact of climate change in viticulture and potential adaptations. J Agron 9(9):514

Vanden HJ, Centinari M (2021) Under-vine vegetation mitigates the impacts of excessive precipitation in vineyards. Front Plant Sci 1542:713135

Wang LJ, Fan L, Loescher W, Duan W, Liu GJ, Cheng JS, Luo HB, Li SH (2010) Salicylic acid alleviates decreases in photosynthesis under heat stress and accelerates recovery in grapevine leaves. BMC Plant Biol 10:34

Webb LB, Whetton PH, Barlow EWR (2007) Modelled impact of future climate change on the phenology of winegrapes in Australia. Aust J Grape Wine Res 13:165–175

Wen PF, Chen JY, Kong WF, Pan QH, Wan SB, Huang WD (2005) Salicylic acid induced the expression of phenylalanine ammonia-lyase gene in grape berry. Plant Sci 169:928–934

White MA, Diffenbaugh NS, Jones GV, Pal JS, Giorgi F (2006) Extreme heat reduces and shifts United States premium wine production in the 21st century. PNAS (USA) 103:11217–11222

Winkler AJ (1974) General viticulture. University of California Press

Wohlfahrt Y, Smith JP, Tittmann S, Honermeier B, Stoll M (2018) Primary productivity and physiological responses of *Vitis vinifera* L. cvs. under free air carbon dioxide enrichment (FACE). Eur J Agron 101:149–162

Wohlfahrt Y, Collins C, Stoll M (2019) Grapevine bud fertility under conditions of elevated carbon dioxide: this article is published in cooperation with the 21th GIESCO International Meeting, June 23–28 2019, Thessaloniki, Greece. Guests editors: Stefanos Koundouras and Laurent Torregrosa. Oeno One 53:2. https://doi.org/10.20870/oeno-one.2019.53.2.2428

Wohlfahrt Y, Patz CD, Schmidt D, Rauhut D, Honermeier B, Stoll M (2021) Responses on must and wine composition of *Vitis vinifera* L. cvs. riesling and cabernet sauvignon under a free air CO_2 enrichment (FACE). Foods 10:145

Xiao F, Yang ZQ, Lee KW (2017) Photosynthetic and physiological responses to high temperature in grapevine (Vitis vinifera L.) leaves during the seedling stage. J Hortic Sci Biotechnol 92:2–10

Yamane T, Jeong ST, Goto-Yamamoto N, Koshita Y, Kobayashi S (2006) Effects of temperature on anthocyanin biosynthesis in grape berry skins. Am J Enol Vitic 57:54–59

Yau IH, Davenport JR, Rupp RA (2013) Characterizing inland Pacific Northwest American viticultural areas with geospatial data. PLoS One 8(4):e61994

Zsofi ZS, Toth E, Rusjan D, Balo B (2011) Terroir aspects of grape quality in a cool climate wine region: relationship between water deficit, vegetative growth and berry sugar concentration. Sci Hortic 127(4):494–499

Zufferey V, Murisier F, Vivin P, Belcher S, Lorenzini F, Spring JL (2012) Carbohydrate reserves in grapevine (*Vitis vinifera* L. 'Chasselas') the influence of the leaf to fruit ratio. Vitis 51(3): 103–110